OCCUPATIONAL
THERAPY
With Aging Adults

OCCUPATIONAL THERAPY
with Aging Adults

Promoting Quality of Life through Collaborative Practice

Karen Frank Barney, PhD, OTR/L, FAOTA
Professor Emerita
Director, Reentry Program
Saint Louis University Prison Program
College of Arts & Sciences

Chair Emerita
Department of Occupational Science & Occupational Therapy
Edward & Margaret Doisy College of Health Sciences
Saint Louis University
St. Louis, Missouri

Margaret A. Perkinson, PhD, FGSA, FAGHE, FSfAA
Associate Research Scientist
Department of Sociology and Anthropology
University of Maryland Baltimore County
Baltimore, Maryland

Editor-in-Chief
Journal of Cross-Cultural Gerontology

Emeritus Faculty and Director of Gerontology Component
NAPA-OT Field School in Antigua, Guatemala

ELSEVIER

ELSEVIER

3251 Riverport Lane
St. Louis, Missouri 63043

International Standard Book Number: 978-0-323-06776-8

Content Strategy Director: Penny Rudolph
Content Development Manager: Jolynn Gower
Publishing Services Manager: Julie Eddy
Designer: Margaret Reid

Printed in the United States of America

Last digit is the print number: 9   8   7   6   5   4   3   2   1

In memory of two models of optimal aging who taught in our *Occupational Therapy with Aging Adults* course at Saint Louis University for a decade: Augusta R. Feehan, 106 years, Matriarch of Christ Church Cathedral, St. Louis, Missouri, and Gus G. Sotiropulos, 89 years, DDS, MS, Director, Orthodontia Clinic, Center for Advanced Dental Education. Always in good humor, Gus and Gussie regaled OT students with stories and wisdom about the aging process and the secrets of their full, occupationally engaged lives. They both sustained active work and social lives until shortly before their deaths.

To my husband, Steve, my soulmate and best friend—a feminist prior to the Women's Movement. In 1965, the year that the St. Louis Gateway Arch came together and Medicare was enacted, we married, grew older through the intervening years, and continue to experience the best there is to be along the way.

KFB

In loving memory to my first and foremost guides for growing older with grace and resilience, my parents, William (Bill) H. Perkinson, Jr., who made life joyous with his generous spirit and vibrant sense of humor, and Rose M. Tlapek Perkinson, who fostered me with her gentle wisdom and strength. I had the great fortune to be embraced by their unconditional love.

MAP

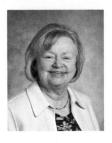

Karen Frank Barney is an occupational therapist with nearly 50 years of experience in geriatric practice and occupational therapy higher education. Dr. Barney received her Bachelor of Science in Occupational Therapy and Master of Science in Adult Education degrees from the University of Wisconsin–Madison, and her PhD from the Saint Louis University School of Public Health in Health Services Research. Dr. Barney has worked in a variety of medical and community settings in Wisconsin, Kentucky, and Missouri, including a decade in skilled nursing facilities, providing consultation and direct services. She served on an American Occupation Therapy Association (AOTA) Conference national planning committee on long-term care, and as newsletter editor for the AOTA Gerontology Special Interest Section (GSIS). Since 1980, her consulting and direct practice have been primarily in community settings. She taught in university settings for 33 years, serving as primary faculty for the aging-related courses in three university programs; served as faculty and resource consultant and director of the Occupational Therapy Geriatric Scholar Program for the Gateway Regional Geriatric Education Center (GEC), funded by the Health Resources Services Administration (HRSA), at Saint Louis University for 22 years; and continues to provide mentorship for occupational science students and master's degree projects and dissertations. Throughout her years of work within the GEC, she published numerous injury prevention manuals and related primary prevention tools used in the community. Dr. Barney served on the Editorial Board for the *American Journal of Occupational Therapy*, and as a reviewer for *Disability and Health Journal, Open Rehabilitation Medicine Journal, Archives of Physical Medicine & Rehabilitation*, and *Quality of Life Research*. She was enrolled in the Roster of Fellows by the AOTA in 1998, and is the recipient of awards for service to the profession, from Saint Louis University, and from the communities in which she has resided. She accepted a nomination to the American Occupational Therapy Foundation Leaders & Legacies Society in 2015. As Professor Emerita, she served as the interim director of the Saint Louis University Prison Program, within which she is leading the development of a model interprofessional re-entry program. Her research interests focus on interdisciplinary service models, older adult injury prevention, and health-related quality of life, including within jail and prison settings.

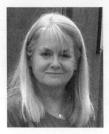

Margaret A. Perkinson is a medical anthropologist and social gerontologist with over 35 years of experience in research and applied anthropology with older adults. Dr. Perkinson's doctoral degree is in Human Development and Aging with a focus on Medical Anthropology from the University of California–San Francisco. She has conducted gerontological research in urban and rural settings across the United States and abroad. Dr. Perkinson's research interests include family caregiving of older adults, dementia care, diabetes management, residential options and service delivery for older adults, participatory action research, and global aging. She taught aging-related courses in two occupational therapy departments for a total of 10 years and worked for 8 years as a senior research scientist at the Polisher Research Institute of the Philadelphia Geriatric Center, a major interprofessional research center based in a long-term care facility. With Karen Barney and colleagues Gelya Frank and others, she helped to establish the National Association for the Practice of Anthropology (NAPA) Occupational Therapy (OT) Field School in Antigua, Guatemala, an international field school for occupational therapy and anthropology graduate students, and directed its gerontology component. More recently, she assisted as a consultant in the development of a continuum-of-care retirement community (CCRC) in Changzhou, China. She has published in numerous peer-reviewed journals, including *Human Organization, The Gerontologist, Journal of Gerontology: Social Sciences, Medical Anthropology, Mental Health and Aging, Contemporary Gerontology, Physical and Occupational Therapy in Geriatrics, Gerontology and Geriatrics Education, Practicing Anthropology, Journal of Geriatric Social Work,, Journal of Intergenerational Relationships, Journal of Women and Aging*, and *Generations: Journal of the American Society on Aging*. Dr. Perkinson co-edited a special issue of *Physical and Occupational Therapy in Geriatrics* that was later published as a book, *Teaching Students Geriatric Research*. She served as president of the Association for Anthropology and Gerontology (AAGE), executive board member and treasurer of the Association for Gerontology in Higher Education (AGHE), member of the executive board of the Behavioral and Social Sciences Section of the Gerontological Society of America (GSA), and member of the Committee for Human Rights for the American Anthropological Association (AAA). She has been editor-in-chief of the *Journal of Cross-Cultural Gerontology* since 2005 and has served on the editorial boards of *Anthropology and Aging Quarterly* (charter member), *Physical and Occupational Therapy in Geriatrics, Care Management Journals, Journal of Aging Studies*, and *Occupational Therapy Journal of Research*. She is an elected Fellow of three professional organizations: GSA, AGHE, and the Society for Applied Anthropology (SfAA).

Wajiha Z. Akhtar, PhD, MPH
Epidemiologist & CAREWare Administrator
District of Columbia Department of Health
Washington, DC

Steven M. Albert, PhD
Professor and Chair, Department of Behavioral and
    Community Health Sciences
Graduate School of Public Health
University of Pittsburgh
Pittsburgh, Pennsylvania

Elena M. Andresen, MA, PhD, FACE
Professor of Epidemiology and Interim Dean
Oregon Health & Science University
School of Public Health Initiative
Portland State University
Portland, Oregon

Judith C. Barker, PhD
Professor, Department of Anthropology, History, and Social
    Medicine
School of Medicine
University of California—San Francisco
San Francisco, California

Jane Bear-Lehman, PhD, OTR/L, FAOTA
Professor and Inaugural Chair, Department of Health
    Studies
College of Health Professions
Pace University
Pleasantville, New York
Adjunct Associate Professor
Psychosocial Research Unit on Health, Aging, and
    the Community
College of Dentistry
New York University
New York, New York

Althea Barry, BSc OT
Occupational Therapist
Former Program Developer, Grandmothers Against Poverty
    and AIDS (GAPA)
Part-Time Lecturer, University of Cape Town, Occupational
    Therapy
Current HIV Outreach Occupational Therapy Coordinator
NSW Department of Health
Sydney, Australia

Margaret Newsham Beckley, PhD, OTR/L, SCLV, CLVT, COMS
Blind Rehabilitation Outpatient Specialist
St. Louis Veterans Administration Medical Center
St. Louis, Missouri

Shirley Kharasch Behr, PhD, FAOTA
Founding Chair, Department of Occupational Science &
    Occupational Therapy
Doisy College of Health Sciences
Saint Louis University
St. Louis, Missouri

Shirley Blanchard, PhD, ABDA, OTR/L, FAOTA, FHDRTP
Associate Professor, Occupational Therapy
School of Pharmacy & Health Professions and School
    of Medicine
Creighton University
Omaha, Nebraska

Judith E. Bowen, MPA, FAOTA
Founding Chair, Department of Occupational Therapy
University of Texas—El Paso
Sedona, Arizona

Sherylyn H. Briller, PhD, FSfAA
Associate Professor of Anthropology
Faculty Associate in the Center on Aging and the Life
    Course (CALC)
Department of Anthropology
Purdue University
West Lafayette, Indiana

Kathleen Brodrick, MSc OT UCT
Specialisation in Gerontology
Founder, Grandmothers Against Poverty and AIDS (GAPA)
Khayelitsha, South Africa

David C. Burdick, PhD
Director, Stockton Center on Successful Aging
Professor of Psychology
Stockton University
Galloway, New Jersey

Michael Bradley Cannell, PhD, MPH
Assistant Professor, Department of Biostatistics and
    Epidemiology
University of North Texas Health Science Center
Fort Worth, Texas

David B. Carr, MD
Alan A. and Edith L. Wolff Professor of Geriatric Medicine
Professor, Medicine and Neurology
Clinical Director, Division of Geriatrics and Nutritional
    Science
Washington University School of Medicine
St. Louis, Missouri

Tracy Chippendale, PhD, OTR/L
Assistant Professor, Department of Occupational Therapy
Steinhardt School of Culture, Education, and Human
    Development
New York University
New York, New York

Abhilash K. Desai, MD
Board Certified Geriatric Psychiatrist
Medical Director, Idaho Memory & Aging Center,
    PLLC
Boise, Idaho

Kate de Medeiros, PhD
Robert H. and Nancy J. Blayney Professor Gerontology
Department of Sociology and Gerontology
College of Arts & Science
Miami University
Oxford, Ohio

**James W. Ellor, PhD, D Min, ACSW, LCSW, BCD, DCSW,
CGP, LCPC, CSW-G**
Professor, School of Social Work
Baylor University
Waco, Texas
Editor, Journal of Religion, Spirituality, and Aging, A
    Routledge Journal

Joseph Flaherty, MD, BCIM, BCIM-G
Professor & Associate Director, Geriatric Medicine
Division of Geriatric Medicine, Internal Medicine
Co-Medical Director, Home Care Program
Medical Director, Nursing Home and Hospice Agency
Saint Louis University School of Medicine
St. Louis, Missouri

Kimberly A. Furphy, DHSc, OTR, ATP
Associate Professor and Director, Occupational Therapy
    Program
Stockton University
Galloway, New Jersey

Laura N. Gitlin, PhD
Director & Professor, Center for Innovative Care in Aging
School of Nursing, Department of Community-Public Health
School of Medicine, Department of Psychiatry and Division
    of Geriatrics
Johns Hopkins University
Baltimore, Maryland

Chris Gonzalez-Snyder, MA, OTR/L
Director of Rehabilitation Services
SSM Rehabilitation Hospital—Bridgeton
Bridgeton, Missouri

George T. Grossberg, MD
Professor, Department of Neurology & Psychiatry
Department of Anatomy and Neurobiology
Department of Internal Medicine
Division of Geriatric Medicine
School of Medicine
Saint Louis University
St. Louis, Missouri

Areum Han, PhD, OTR/L
Assistant Professor, School of Occupational Therapy
Texas Woman's University
Denton, Texas

Clarice Harrison*
Case Study Consultant
Sheffield Hallam University
Sheffield, United Kingdom

Ann M. Hayes, PT, DPT, MHS, OCS
Associate Professor, Department of Physical Therapy and
    Athletic Training
Doisy College of Health Sciences
Saint Louis University
St. Louis, Missouri

Julia Henderson-Kalb, MS, OTR/L
Instructor, Department of Occupational Science and
    Occupational Therapy
Doisy College of Health Sciences
Faculty Practitioner, Saint Louis University Geriatric
    Primary Care Clinic and Amyotrophic Lateral
    Sclerosis Association Certified Treatment Center of
    Excellence
Saint Louis University
St. Louis, Missouri

Margaret M. Herning, PT, PhD
Professor Emerita
Department of Physical Therapy and Athletic
    Training
Doisy College of Health Sciences
Saint Louis University
St. Louis, Missouri

*Deceased

Clare Hocking, PhD, MHSC(OT), NZROT
Professor, Department of Occupational Science and
    Occupational Therapy
School of Clinical Sciences
Faculty of Health and Environmental Sciences
Executive Editor, *Journal of Occupational Science*
Auckland University of Technology
Auckland, New Zealand

Linda Hunt, PhD, FAOTA, OTR/L
Professor, School of Occupational Therapy
Director, Graduate Certificate in Gerontology for
    Healthcare Professionals
College of Health Professions
Pacific University
Hillsboro, Oregon

Susan Hyde, DDS, MPH, PhD
Associate Professor of Clinical Preventive and Restorative
    Dental Sciences
Chair, Division of Oral Epidemiology and Dental Public
    Health
Interprofessional Education Faculty Lead, Dentistry
Director for Dentistry, Multidisciplinary Fellowship in
    Geriatrics
University of California—San Francisco School of Dentistry
San Francisco, California

Shirley J. Jackson, PhD, OTR/L, FAOTA
Associate Dean, College of Nursing and Allied Health
    Sciences
Associate Professor, Department of Occupational Therapy
Howard University
Washington, DC

Cindy Kempf, MA, OTR/L
Director of Clinical Services RPI Therapy Services
Adjunct Faculty, Department of Occupational Science &
    Occupational Therapy
Doisy College of Health Sciences
Saint Louis University
St. Louis, Missouri

Heather Turek Koch, MS, OTR/L
Occupational Therapist
Rusk Rehabilitation Center
Columbia, Missouri

Mary Krieger, MLIS, RN
Assistant Director for Information Services
Medical Center Library
Saint Louis University
St. Louis, Missouri

Helen Lach, PhD, RN, GCNS-BC, FGSA
John A. Hartford Foundation Claire Fagin Fellow
Associate Professor, School of Nursing
Saint Louis University
St. Louis, Missouri

Soo Lee, MD
Assistant Professor, Autism Assessment, Research,
    Treatment, and Services [AARTS] Center
Department of Psychiatry
Rush University Medical Center
Chicago, Illinois

Hedva Barenholtz Levy, PharmD, BCPS, CGP
Director, HBL PharmaConsulting
St. Louis, Missouri

Debra Lindstrom, Ph, OTR/L
Professor, Department of Occupational Therapy
Western Michigan University
Kalamazoo, Michigan

Daphne Lo, MD
Clinical Fellow, Division of Geriatric Medicine
Department of Internal Medicine
University of California—San Francisco
San Francisco, California

Helene Lohman, OTD, OTR/L, FAOTA
Professor, Department of Occupational Therapy
Creighton University
Omaha, Nebraska

Lisa M. Luetkemeyer, JD
Attorney, Husch Blackwell, LLP
St. Louis, Missouri

Catherine L. Lysack, PhD, OT(C)
Deputy Director, Institute of Gerontology
Professor, Department of Health Care Sciences,
    Occupational Therapy and Gerontology
Eugene Applebaum College of Pharmacy and Health
    Sciences
Wayne State University
Detroit, Michigan

Joan M. McDowd, PhD
Professor, Department of Psychology
Director, SilverRoo Research Laboratory
Director, UMKC Consortium for Aging in Community
Director, Doctoral Program in Psychology, Experimental
    Health Psychology Option
University of Missouri, Kansas City
Kansas City, Missouri

Phyllis Meltzer, PhD, MSG
Founder, Life Course Publishing
Redondo Beach, California

Louise A. Meret-Hanke, PhD
Associate Professor, Health Management and Policy
College of Public Health and Social Justice
Saint Louis University
St. Louis, Missouri

John E. Morley, MD
Dammert Professor of Gerontology
Director, Division of Geriatric Medicine
Acting Director, Division of Endocrinology
School of Medicine
Saint Louis University
St. Louis, Missouri

Miriam S. Moss, MA (retired)
Behavioral Research Institute
Sociology and Anthropology Department
Arcadia University
Glenside, Pennsylvania

Keli Mu, PhD, OTR/L
Associate Professor and Chair, Department of Occupational
    Therapy
Creighton University
Omaha, Nebraska

Carol A. Needham, JD
Saint Louis University
School of Law
St. Louis, Missouri

Linda Orr, MPA, OTR/L
Program Coordinator, Occupational Therapy Assistant
    Program
Lewis & Clark Community College
Godfrey, Illinois

Kathy Parker, MS, OT
Director of Programs and Outreach
American Stroke Foundation
Mission, Kansas

Amish Patel, MD
Geriatric Medicine
UnityPoint Clinic—Senior Health at Methodist Atrium
Peoria, Illinois

Amy Paul-Ward, PhD, MSOT
Associate Professor
Department of Occupational Therapy
Florida International University
Miami, Florida

Catherine Verrier Piersol, MS, OTR/L
Clinical Director
Jefferson Elder Care
Jefferson Center for Applied Research on Aging and Health
Thomas Jefferson University
Philadelphia, Pennsylvania

Linda Pollard
Care Worker
Sheffield, United Kingdom

Nick Pollard, PhD
Senior Lecturer in Occupational Therapy
Faculty of Health and Wellbeing
Research Coordinator, Centre for Health and Social Care
    Research
Sheffield Hallam University
Sheffield, United Kingdom

Graham D. Rowles, PhD
Professor of Gerontology
Director, Graduate Center for Gerontology
Chair, Department of Gerontology
University of Kentucky
Lexington, Kentucky

Charlotte B. Royeen, PhD, OTR/L, FAOTA
Dean of College of Health Sciences
Professor of Occupational Therapy
Rush University
Chicago, Illinois

Dikaios Sakellariou, PhD, FHEA
Lecturer—Occupational Therapy
School of Health Care Sciences
Cardiff University
Cardiff, United Kingdom

Carole Schwartz, MS, OTR/L
Research Public Health Analyst
RTI International
Chicago, Illinois

Jaclyn K. Schwartz, PhD, OTR/L
Assistant Professor, Department of Occupational
    Therapy
Florida International University
Miami, Florida

Lauren R. Schwarz, PhD
Assistant Professor, Department of Neurology and
    Psychiatry
Saint Louis University
St. Louis, Missouri

Virginia C. Stoffel, PhD, OT, BCMH, FAOTA
President, American Occupational Therapy Association
    2013-2016
Associate Professor
Department of Occupational Science and Technology
College of Health Sciences
University of Wisconsin—Milwaukee
Milwaukee, Wisconsin

Donghua Tao, MA, MS, PhD
Reference Librarian
Associate Professor
Library—Medical Center
Saint Louis University
St. Louis, Missouri

Susan C. Tebb, PhD, MSW, RYT-500
Professor
School of Social Work
College for Public Health and Social Justice
Saint Louis University
St. Louis, Missouri

Nina Tumosa, PhD
Project Officer, Medical Training and Geriatrics Branch
Division of Medicine and Dentistry
Bureau of Health Workforce
Health Resources Services Administration
Rockville, Maryland

Laura VanPuymbrouck, OTR/L
Graduate Research Assistant, Department of Occupational
    Therapy
PhD Candidate, Disability Studies and Human
    Development
University of Illinois—Chicago
Chicago, Illinois

Mirtha M. Whaley, PhD, MPH, OTR/L
Assistant Professor and Director of Academic Affairs
Department of Occupational Therapy
Nova Southeastern University
Tampa, Florida

FOREWORD

This book is a call. At one level, it is a call to celebrate. It celebrates the global success of aging populations, which calls to mind the possibilities of aging adults' occupational potentials. At another level, this book is a call to challenge. In doing so, it beckons gerontological occupational therapy to be essentially collaborative in nature. And, at the same time, this book is a call to action. It calls forth, into full view, the appreciation of gerontological occupational therapy's highly specialized nature.

Writing this foreword from New Zealand, I offer another understanding of this book being a call. For Māori, the indigenous people of New Zealand, the *karanga*, or call, is a formal call of welcome as visitors are ceremonially welcomed onto the *marae*, or tribal meeting place. It is a welcoming into conversation. A call comes back in response. The *kaikaranga* (the women who call) are usually elder women. "The best callers have ethereal but carrying voices, in the words of an informant 'like a bird, high, light and airy'. Their calls are long and effortless" (Salmond, 2009, p. 137). In the same way, Karen Barney and Margaret Perkinson, the editors of this book, raise their voices in the call. They welcome you, the reader. They offer you safe passage as you are drawn into a conversation about advancing gerontological occupational therapy practice; a practice specialty whose time has come in the context of the global aging population.

This foreword, like all forewords, is an introduction to what awaits you in this book. To understand its origins and intent, I engaged in a conversation with Karen Barney and Margaret Perkinson. I know them as colleagues, and I visited them when I was last in St. Louis, Missouri. I have had chance meetings with them at gerontology, or occupational therapy, conferences in different places around the globe when we are all far from home. And I know I will meet up with them at conferences in the future and continue our conversations about what makes excellent practice with aging adults. I had known, for some time, this book was in the making. Yet, until our conversation about what inspired this project, I had not appreciated the depth of human spirit imbued in this book. It is deeply embedded in the editors' aspiration for aging adults being enabled to live occupationally rich lives, regardless of the changes that may come with advanced age. Their original ambition was to influence how gerontological occupational therapy might be best practiced as a highly specialized discipline. It raises thinking, and professional reasoning, well above any low ground in which pervasive, negative biases about the status of practice with aging adults might persist.

Karen Barney and Margaret Perkinson embarked on what I consider to be an inspirational journey in the making of this book. They took for granted that gerontological occupational therapy was never meant to be practiced in isolation. They believed practice would be at its best when practiced collaboratively. In accord, they set out to identify specialists in diverse disciplines across the gerontology spectrum, from community to medical settings. They engaged with gerontologists practicing, for example, law, epidemiology, anthropology, human development and aging, geography, library science, dentistry, psychology, geriatric medicine, geropsychiatry, nursing, physical therapy, endocrinology, sociology, pharmacy, neurology, theology, public health, social work, and occupational science. They introduced the science specialists to gerontological occupational therapists practicing in the field. Many chapters in this book emerged from new interdisciplinary professional collaborations. I couldn't help but notice that most authors are situated in North America, yet that is not where the book's relevance resides. Because it speaks to aging adults' changing life contexts and embodied capacities, it speaks to gerontological occupational therapy practice across continental boundaries. While the way of practice may need to be interpreted by gerontological occupational therapists globally, the human science underpinnings are transferable. Another thing that appeals to me, is how each chapter is unashamedly evidence-based in nature. Each offers the contemporary science on the topic and critically considers what sound gerontological occupational therapy, as a specialist practice, would look like.

This book is expansive yet deliberately focused. It breathes new life into gerontological occupational therapy for it to be all it can be. I expect, as you are already reading this foreword, you are already imbued with the spirit to be the best gerontological occupational therapist you can be. Aging adults, personally and collectively, will be the benefactors.

Valerie A. Wright-St Clair, PhD, MPH, DipProfEthics, DipBusStudies (Health Management), DipOccTherapy

Salmond, A. (2009). *Hui: A study of Maori ceremonial gatherings* (3rd ed). North Shore, Auckland: Penguin Group (NZ).

This textbook was developed to address requests by occupational therapy educators for a comprehensive resource for practice with older adults that could also serve as an update for those already in the field. Also, given the growing emphasis on interprofessional health care and community-based teams, this book introduces non-OT members of such teams to up-to-date gerontological developments in the field. Why the sense of urgency?

By the 2020s, demographic trends both in the United States and on the global level are likely to have a profound effect on economic growth, living and moral standards, and the shape of the world order. As the unprecedented growth in the number of elders and the unprecedented decline in the number of youth over the next several decades are experienced worldwide, the demand for services with older adults will surely increase. Incoming OT students (and those already in the field) have the opportunity and responsibility to equip themselves for this work by becoming familiar with the rich body of current gerontological evidence and by learning to use it to enrich their practice.

Current OT practice in developed countries typically works to address the needs of adults as a collective entity, but fails to recognize ongoing biopsychosocial developmental transitions as well as the unique characteristics and needs of later life. Physical rehabilitation textbooks typically provide comprehensive approaches for age-related conditions (e.g., arthritis, stroke) but do not address the complex systemic associated changes with aging that impact functional outcomes. Additionally, in the United States historically and currently, OT textbooks have focused specifically upon the role of occupational therapy in service provision with older adults, with limited commentary on global demographic issues, the role of other providers of services, and the systems within which services are provided. Coverage of diversity and differing cultural issues is limited to those that present primarily in North America, through occupational therapy perspectives. Most textbooks that are used in OT education regarding aging related issues are somewhat limited in scope, typically confined to either a medical model perspective or current related intervention strategies. To address these gaps, this textbook utilizes a global, holistic, evidence-based approach to target the needs and enhance the occupational performance potentials of persons 60 years and older. The overall emphasis is upon collaboration with the client (i.e., as an individual, group, agency, or community) to address the interaction of aging-related changes with physical and sociocultural environments and to optimize occupational performance, occupational engagement, and interpersonal relationships, thus enhancing overall well-being and quality of life.

The goal of this work is to inspire occupational therapists, occupational therapy assistants, and members of other disciplines with whom they collaborate to work holistically, cross-culturally, and collaboratively in the manner in which they serve aging adults. Furthermore, role competencies, including *intradisciplinary* (to maximize the understanding and utilization of service extenders in the profession) and *interprofessional* processes (as compared with less integrated interdisciplinary roles and functions) are explored and encouraged, to maximize the impact of services provided.

Collaboration is a highly intentional theme throughout the textbook: the title implies that interventions are planned and executed *with* (not for) the client, whether that client represents an individual older adult and his or her support system, an aging group, or a population. The title also implies collaboration both intraprofessionally (e.g., OT, OTA) and interprofessionally (e.g., different disciplines), wherever relevant. Within both types of collaboration the emphasis is on understanding, appreciating, and complementing each others' perspectives to optimize efforts as a service delivery team.

Additionally, in the spirit of *collaboration*, the editors themselves represent an interprofessional approach, reflecting the emerging collaborative work of occupational therapists, anthropologists, and others working in occupational therapy, occupational science, and other related areas. With their collective experience, including their own aging, they are well suited to conceptualize this textbook. Both editors have extensive backgrounds working with older adults, their families, and numerous types of agencies in aging service delivery systems in the U.S. within their respective disciplines.

The authors of nearly every chapter also reflect this collaborative, interprofessional approach to their respective subjects. A wide variety of professionals in the field of gerontology contributed chapters to this text, in order to accomplish a number of purposes. First, some provided an expanded view of the needs of older adults and a greater level of detail regarding the role of their respective disciplines in their work with older adults. Others contributed perspectives on interprofessional and intraprofessional opportunities to collaborate in service provision with older adults and their significant others. This approach was utilized in addressing case examples in a care plan/intervention format for each relevant topic. Additional contributors provided expertise to support evidence- and occupation-based practice.

Advances in the use of evidence guided by current theories and conceptual models, which include occupational science (OS) and OT theory, occupation-centered practice, and theories from other disciplines, are presented; each chapter is evidence-based. Readers will find strategies for identifying and applying evidence relevant to practice with older adults. This information is interfaced with content related to the occupational therapy processes that include screening, evaluation, intervention, and targeting of outcomes with older clients.

The impact of globalization increasingly affects many aspects of the lives of recipients of services, as well as the services providers, and requires consideration of needs, resources, and dynamics on multiple levels. To do so, the book's authors employed theoretical models from a variety of sources, proceeding from macro- to micro-level influences on practice that include (but are not limited to): the World Health Organization, international health systems, U.S. government and public health sources, and the disciplines of occupational science and occupational therapy, with the AOTA *Occupational Therapy Practice Framework* (OTPF) as the predominant model. Coverage of macro-level influences on aging and OT practice represents a unique contribution of this book. To augment our global perspective, examples of international medical and social models of service provision are included within varying cultural contexts, reflecting actual or potential occupational therapy practice.

The editors selected chapter topics with the intent of providing thorough, contemporary coverage across a full range of gerontological occupational therapy practice areas. This process resulted in 30 chapters, divided into six sections: Conceptual Foundations, Age-related Biological System Changes, Age-Related Psychosocial Changes, the Functional Environment of Aging Adults, Continuum of Care, and Trends and Innovations in Care with Aging Adults. In addition to coverage of traditional topics related to development and pathology in later life, this book addresses factors rarely included in aging and OT texts, such as ethical and legal approaches, epidemiology of global aging, nutrition and oral health concerns, pharmacological issues, low vision interventions, assistive technology supports for aging individuals, issues of occupational justice for older adults, and community-based models of practice.

Since occupational therapists customarily work collaboratively with other disciplines, almost all chapters are co-authored by one or more gerontological experts and one or more occupational therapists specializing in OT practice related to that chapter's topic. The professional backgrounds of our 74 chapter authors reflect the interdisciplinary perspective of the book: law, public health, epidemiology, library science, anthropology, physical therapy, medicine and geriatrics, sociology, dentistry, pharmacology, psychology, physiology, geriatric psychiatry, theology, social work, human development and aging, geography, health policy and administration, and nursing, in addition to occupational therapy and occupational science. While most of our authors are well-established senior scholars and practitioners, renowned for their mastery and depth of knowledge in their respective fields, we also included community activists and more junior, up-and-coming professionals for fresh perspectives on their given areas of expertise. Some teams of co-authors came to this project with long histories of collaboration. Other chapter co-authors were new to each other, and collaborating on the chapter afforded new insights into each other's disciplinary perspectives.

Most interprofessionally authored chapters share the same basic structure, with the intent of providing a two-pronged approach to each topic. Typically first, the gerontological expert presented an overview of relevant, cutting-edge research on the given chapter topic. The gerontological occupational therapist then discussed how that research evidence could be incorporated into OT practice. The reader should approach each chapter for an explication of the most recent and essential research-based knowledge and scholarly resources on a given topic and for clearly stated guidelines for using that knowledge to enrich his or her work. For the OT readers, each chapter should lead the way toward a practice that is evidence-based. For the non-OT gerontologists, each chapter provides a window into the often-misunderstood field of occupational therapy and guidance toward achieving informed collaborations in interprofessional gerontological work.

ACKNOWLEDGMENTS

We would be remiss if we did not acknowledge the following individuals . . .

Our publisher, Elsevier, and their publishing staff:

Kathy Falk, Executive Content Strategist, inspired Karen Barney to consider developing this textbook and guided the initial process; Jolynn Gower, Content Development Manager, worked patiently with us for several years as we progressed, then together with Penny Rudolph, Content Strategy Director, provided the exceptional guidance necessary to complete the production process. Megan Fennell and Alex Kluesner supported important infrastructure processes during the editing phase, and the Marketing staff worked closely with us to launch the publicity for our textbook. Without the expert collaborative spirit of this publishing team, we could not have produced this work.

Research Assistants: It was a privilege to work with the following Saint Louis University Occupational Science and Masters in Occupational Therapy students, whose effort greatly supported the development of numerous chapters: Samantha Chen, Andrea Nelson, Morgan Seier, and Fatihat Salako.

Valerie Wright-St Clair, PhD, OT, offered early in the development of this work to review the textbook upon completion. Seeking to include a global scholarly gerontological perspective on this work, we are incredibly indebted to her for her enthusiastic willingness to write the foreword. Her beautifully written piece heralds our call of welcome to the field of gerontological occupational therapy.

We extend our unending appreciation to each one of our 74 chapter contributors. We are proud and honored to include such esteemed colleagues in this work and to showcase their considerable expertise. The logistics of coordinating a publication of this scale would have been even more daunting without their prompt responses to requests and queries and their continued patience with the process.

We also would like to acknowledge the people who inspired us along the way:

Some of my most profound professional experiences have included the nurturing from others in my discipline. I believe that Kathy Saunders first hired me at Madison General Hospital in Madison, Wisconsin since our cross-cultural spirits resonated—mine is lifelong. My first extensive exposure to service provision with older adults was due to Sr. Pat, who left her hospital and consulting roles with a skilled nursing facility in Madison, asking me to take her place. I therefore moved from pediatrics to geriatric practice, when, in the late '60s, these were very unique roles for OTs. While in that role for a decade, I also consulted with other skilled nursing facilities, adult day centers, and continuum of care communities, during which University of Wisconsin-Madison faculty Betty Hasselkus and Jean Kiernat provided strong encouragement and guidance. Jean recruited me as OT staff for their pioneering community based services supporting independent living for older adults. Betty especially encouraged me to write, and through the years greatly impacted my view of scholarship and modeled meaningful occupation in academic roles. I'm eternally grateful for their encouragement and career-long friendships. My University of Wisconsin BSOT classmate, Toni Walski, former Occupational Therapy Assistant Program Director at Madison Area Technical College, had the foresight that OT higher education would be a good match for me. Teaching with Teri Black, Carol Holmes, Catherine Wilson, and Toni instilled within me a career-long allegiance to intraprofessional practice merits. Joy Anderson, Program Director at Eastern Kentucky University (EKU) Department of Occupational Therapy, provided me with my first opportunity to teach at the professional level fulltime, when our family relocated to Kentucky. At EKU, Penny Benzing, known at that time as a gerontic OT specialist, encouraged me to immerse myself in related local and national aging-related associations. I'm deeply grateful to Carolyn Baum for hiring me in the Program in Occupational Therapy at Washington University School of Medicine, due to our relocation to St. Louis, Missouri, my home town, when my parents' health was deteriorating. She enabled my appointment to the Gateway Geriatric Education Center core faculty group, headed by John Morley, Saint Louis University School of Medicine. Subsequently, I served with this interdisciplinary geriatric team for 22 years; this afforded me a wealth of opportunities to evolve our interprofessional geriatric relationships, including Joseph Flaherty, George Grossberg, Helen Lach, Louise Meret-Hanke, Sue Tebb, and Nina Tumosa, all of whom are contributing authors for this textbook. My gratitude extends also to James Kimmey, founder of the St. Louis University School of Public Health, Greg Evans, Ana Maria Murgueytio, and James Romeis, for facilitating my entry and progression through the Health Services Research doctoral program. I am also extraordinarily grateful to Shirley Behr, founding Chair of the Department of Occupational Science & Occupational Therapy at Saint Louis University, for enabling the last chapter of my fulltime academic career, and to Ruth Zemke and Gelya Frank, who have supported and expanded my Occupational Therapy and Occupational Science circles and international collaborations.

Upon making the decision to publish this textbook, I immediately sought collaboration with my dear colleague, compatriot, and friend, Peggy Perkinson, a Medical Anthropologist, with whom I taught at Saint Louis University. Her global interprofessional gerontological connections have hugely facilitated the transdisciplinary collaborations that have resulted in this textbook. I'm thus greatly indebted to her for this and her astute editing prowess contributions to our publication process.

Finally, my husband and soulmate, who has been my constant cornerstone and unconditional support through 50 years of aging and the entire publishing process, must be recognized. Without his wise counsel and monumental influence, I could not have undertaken my OT career as it has unfolded, including this work.

Karen Frank Barney

I appreciate this opportunity to acknowledge those who mentored and inspired me during the process of developing this book and the path that led to it. I have been blessed to have been at the right places at the right times in terms of gerontological "hot spots" throughout my career. Sincere thanks go to my early mentor Irwin Press, who first introduced me to the field of anthropology and so strongly supported my initial professional development; other early mentors Robert Habenstein and Donald Cowgill, who introduced me to what was then the relatively new field of gerontology as an area of intellectual challenge and personal fulfillment; Irving Rosow, David Chiriboga, Margaret Clark, Len Pearlin and many other teachers and mentors at University of California, San Francisco, who guided me through my doctoral work and inspired me with their brilliance and the intensity of their commitment to their work; M. Powell Lawton, Robert Rubinstein, Rachel Pruchno, Steve Albert, Mark Luborsky, Allen Glicksman, Patricia Parmelee, Miriam Moss, Kimberly Van Haitsma, and Athena McLean, my mentors, colleagues, and good friends at the Polisher Research Institute at the Philadelphia Geriatric Center, who showed me the heights that can be achieved when working in truly generative, motivated research teams; Carolyn Baum, the visionary who introduced me to the field of occupational therapy; Gelya Frank, my model for integrating anthropology, occupational science, and occupational therapy in international work; Linda Breytspraak, who encouraged my initial involvement in the professional associations of gerontology and my many subsequent mentors, colleagues, and friends in the Association for Gerontology in Higher Education (AGHE), Gerontological Society of America, (GSA), and the Association for Anthropology and Gerontology (AAGE). I am truly blessed to have worked with these esteemed leaders of the past and current development of the field of gerontology and to be able to count all as close personal friends. All have contributed to my knowledge and understanding of gerontology and occupational therapy and thus to the development of this book.

Special thanks go to my co-editor, mentor, colleague, and close friend, Karen Barney. We co-taught graduate-level gerontology and research courses in occupational therapy for many years and shared every detail of the development of this book on an almost daily basis. She instigated this book and, with her many years of experience in OT, provided its core expertise. I am very grateful to her for inviting me to collaborate on what has become a mission and labor of love.

Thanks also go to my friends and many relatives who cheered me on with boundless support. And final thanks to David Rockemann, my closest colleague, best friend, and spouse, who was my constant sounding board and unending support throughout, and whose incredible ability to keep things in perspective continues to keep me on track.

Margaret A. Perkinson

CONTENTS

CHAPTER 1

Gerontological Occupational Therapy: Conceptual Frameworks, Historical Contexts, and Practice Principles

Margaret A. Perkinson, PhD, FGSA, FAGHE, FSfAA, Karen Frank Barney, PhD, OTR/L, FAOTA

In spite of illness, in spite even of the archenemy sorrow, one can remain alive long past the usual date of disintegration if one is unafraid of change, insatiable in intellectual curiosity, interested in big things, and happy in small ways.

Edith Wharton

I grow more intense as I age.

Florida Scott-Maxwell

As we grow old . . . the beauty steals inward.

Ralph Waldo Emerson

CHAPTER OUTLINE

OBJECTIVES

- Review basic gerontological concepts and theories
- Discuss theoretical frameworks of gerontology within occupational science and occupational therapy theoretical perspectives
- Provide historical and global contexts that underscore the significance of the field of gerontology in general and gerontological occupational therapy in particular
- Provide an overview of the history of and the challenges and opportunities inherent in gerontological occupational therapy
- Discuss the contributions and application of gerontological concepts to occupational therapy interventions
- Provide conceptual guidelines for facilitating occupation-based interventions with older adults

These are exciting times to be a gerontologist, both for researchers and practitioners. Long-held negative notions of old age are giving way to more complex, nuanced understandings of late-life experiences and processes. These newly refined understandings, based on a growing body of gerontological research, should inform and guide those in positions to assist older adults in the search for an enriched later-life stage suffused, as the earlier quotes suggest, with an alive, intense state of inward beauty. Given the purview of occupational therapy, that is, "achieving health, well-being, and participation in life through engagement in occupation,"[7] as well as its holistic approach and emphasis on client-centered care and quality of life, occupational therapists are especially well suited to benefit from and contribute to contemporary gerontological theory and practice. This chapter introduces the basic concepts, theoretical and disciplinary orientations, and goals that underlie this book. It also provides historical and global contexts that explain why the current epoch may well be considered revolutionary in respect to old age, and why this aging-related revolution is especially relevant to the field of occupational therapy. After an overview of the history of and challenges inherent in gerontological occupational therapy (OT), we underscore the significance of current gerontological debates to the development and implementation of gerontological OT interventions.

Basic Concepts and Theories of Old Age

Evolution of Gerontological Concepts and Theory Regarding Late-Life Activity/Occupation

Early gerontologists framed aging largely in negative and universal terms. Old age was equated with physical decline, cognitive dysfunction, social disengagement, and marginalization. Disengagement theory predominated, claiming universal processes of decline and mutual withdrawal of the aged from society and society from the aged. This presumably played out when older adults voluntarily relinquished former roles and activities to embrace peace and quiet. At the same time, representatives of the immediate social group or larger society presumably perceived older members as unable to fulfill the requirements of former work and social roles and reallocated those roles (and the attached resources) to the up-and-coming younger generation. The period of late life was both problematized and medicalized as entailing inevitable, "incurable" biological and psychological declines that warranted little more than custodial care or occasional efforts at rehab for those who showed less decrement or possessed more resources.

Subsequent theorists disengaged from disengagement theory, replacing it with its polar opposite, activity theory. Life satisfaction ebbed and flowed, depending on the levels of activity in which an older adult engaged. Whereas disengagement theory posited a direct positive relationship between life satisfaction and decreased activity in later life, activity theory claimed a similar relationship between life satisfaction and increased activity in old age. The relationship between activity and aging has remained a central focus of gerontological theory, a focus that parallels the central domains of occupational science and occupational therapy, that is, fostering quality of life through participation in requisite, life-sustaining, and meaningful activities or occupations.

The new "positive gerontology" extends this line of thought, replacing earlier assumptions of inevitable decline with concepts such as successful aging, productive aging, and civic engagement as appropriate and attainable goals in later life.[37,51,59] (See Chapter 4 and Chapter 18 for more extensive discussions of the evolution of gerontological theory as it pertains to occupational therapy.) Although it contributed to the advancement of the field in terms of theory, scholarship, and policy, positive gerontology is not without its critics.[49,50,61]

Deeply rooted in individualistic, contemporary U.S. values of independence, autonomy, activity, and progress, the precepts of positive gerontology may not hold in alternate cultural contexts,[43,62,63,64] for example, in societies that value interdependence over self-sufficiency. In addition, by continuing to equate "success" in aging with the maintenance of good physical and mental health, substantial sectors of older adults with functional limitations (or lacking financial resources to access the means to optimal health) would be doomed, by definition, to the status of "failure."

Critical social gerontologists have contributed to the discussion by examining the influence of cultural, historical, and political factors on the construction, experience, and valuation of aging. Neither equating aging with deficits nor denying the reality of age-related losses, critical social gerontologists stress the potential to achieve personal mastery and a sense of meaning and continued growth—what some may call resilience—in the face of loss of whatever nature.

Current Concepts and Theory in Occupational Therapy Relevant to the Understanding and Facilitation of Late-Life Activity/Occupation

The Person-Environment-Occupational-Performance (PEOP) model[14] provides an ecological transactional systems framework central to the organization of this book (Figure 1-1). It represents the most recent refinement of a model that has been widely used in the fields of occupational science and occupational therapy and that underlies the predominant intervention guidebook, *Occupational Therapy Practice Framework: Domain and Process* (3rd ed.).[7]

In the PEOP model, well-being is a function of the interactions among personal factors, the physical and sociocultural environment, the demands and qualities inherent within a given occupation or activity, the nature and level of performance skills and patterns pertaining to that occupation or activity, and subsequent participation or engagement.[7,14] The updated version of the model underscores the client-centered dimension of the occupational therapy process. That process entails collaboration with the client to synthesize and interpret information elicited from the client's narrative story. This collaborative effort seeks to identify and verbalize client perceptions, choices, interests, needs, and goals. Therapist and client continue to work together, using the narrative input to formulate a plan to achieve client-defined goals, given the resources and barriers available to the client to address occupational performance needs.

The revised PEOP model reinforces relatively recent forays into community-based occupational therapy by offering a definition of "client" that includes persons, groups, and populations.

Conceptual Framework of the Book: Late-Life Experience from an Occupational Perspective

The definition of aging that guided the conception of this book represents a synthesis of current thought in gerontology

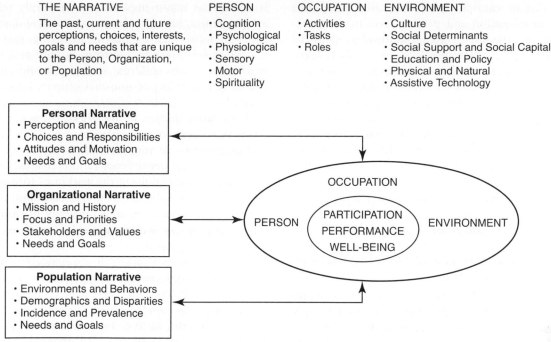

THE NARRATIVE
The past, current and future perceptions, choices, interests, goals and needs that are unique to the Person, Organization, or Population

PERSON
• Cognition
• Psychological
• Physiological
• Sensory
• Motor
• Spirituality

OCCUPATION
• Activities
• Tasks
• Roles

ENVIRONMENT
• Culture
• Social Determinants
• Social Support and Social Capital
• Education and Policy
• Physical and Natural
• Assistive Technology

FIGURE 1-1 Occupational performance (doing) enables participation (engagement) in everyday life that contributes to well-being (health and quality of life). (From Baum, C., Christiansen, C, & Bass, J. (2014). The person-environment-occupation-performance model. In C.H. Christiansen, C. Baum & J. Bass (Eds). *Occupational therapy: Performance, participation and well-being* (pp. 49-55). Thorofare, NJ: Slack, Inc.)

and occupational science/therapy. We regard aging as an ongoing biopsychosocial process that is interactive, situated, and negotiated within specific sociocultural, temporal, and physical contexts.[7,54] We view this definition from an occupational perspective, using the conceptual lens of the PEOP model.[14]

Aging is a complex, multidimensional, and dynamic process, requiring transdisciplinary approaches to both research and practice. This process occurs over a lifetime, within a changing constellation of personal factors (e.g., physical, cognitive, and psychological status and function; personal life experiences and their interpretations; immediate and long-term goals) and environmental factors (e.g., the built and natural environment and social, cultural, and historical contexts). As an aging individual encounters the challenges inherent in a given occupation or activity, these personal and environmental factors come into play to influence the nature of the performance of that occupation and ultimately the extent of participation or engagement in it. The significance and meaning ascribed to the occupation and to its performance and participation by the aging individual (and possibly by relevant reference group figures) are critical to the resulting sense of well-being or lack thereof. Significance and meaning can be self-generated or can derive from culturally prescribed and shared patterns of meanings and values. These patterns are actively interpreted, manipulated, and/or modified by the individual in light of past personal experiences, as well as current, ongoing, and anticipated interactions.

The Study of Aging in Historical Context

The Demographic Transition

It is no exaggeration to describe the current changes in global populations as a demographic revolution. Never in the history of humankind have so many people lived so long.[25] To put this into perspective, physical anthropologists suggest that, on average, Neanderthals could expect to live little more than 20 years; only a small percentage reached age 40.[25] Over subsequent millennia, average life expectancy barely budged. Around the turn of the twentieth century, however, conditions changed. Advances in public health in developed countries struck a blow to infectious diseases, greatly reducing infant and child mortality and allowing more people to live longer lives. In 1900, 4% of the U.S. population (approximately 3.1 million people) lived to age 65 or beyond. By 2040, those numbers are expected to increase to 21%, and a total of 79.7 million.[4] Since World War II, average life expectancy on the global level has increased from 45 years to 69.6 years. In addition, the percentage of the oldest old (those aged 80 and over) worldwide is rising rapidly and is projected to increase 233% between 2008 and 2040.[42] As a species, we have made greater gains in average life expectancy in the past 70 years than in the previous 132,000 years.

The relatively recent global decline in birth rates represents the second major factor fueling the demographic transition. In the mid-1950s the average number of children per woman worldwide equaled 5.0. That number has plummeted due to various social and historical factors (e.g., increased education and participation in the workforce for women, transition from agricultural to industrial economies making large families less economically feasible). The global average number of children per woman is now 2.7, with some countries experiencing birth rates below replacement levels. The decline in birth rates has a significant impact on the proportion of older adults both globally and in given societies. In the near future those aged 65 and over will outnumber children under age 5 for the first time in history,[42] and researchers expect the global difference in percentages between the two age groups to continue to grow (Figure 1-2). (See Chapter 3 for a more detailed discussion of global demographic changes and their implications.)

Resulting Social Changes and Their Implications for Later-Life Occupations

It is difficult to exaggerate the effect of the global demographic transition on both individual and societal levels. Life experiences and social institutions that many now take for granted, such as retirement and empty-nest households, are modern phenomena, previously encountered by the very few.[2,31] Major changes in the family, workforce, health and health-care systems, and lifestyles resulting from population aging have a direct effect on related occupations. These occupations are changing radically or are newly available for older adults. With new or altered occupations come new challenges to performance and participation for older adults, challenges that may be more easily met with the help of occupational therapists trained in gerontology.

Current demographic changes have had a direct effect on average family size and composition. Compared with families of past eras, contemporary families are more likely to include multiple generations, with fewer members in each succeeding generation. This transformation in family structure has major implications for family relationships and dynamics, for example, the nature of spousal relationships in longer-lasting post-childrearing marriages, the nature of relationships between parents and their older and fewer adult children and grandchildren, and the changing availability of informal support for care of older adults.[52]

The relative decline in the size of younger cohorts portends significant societal changes as well. As the numbers and proportions of young members in the workforce decline, the old-age dependency ratio increases; that is, there are fewer younger adults in the workforce to support growing numbers of older retirees. Out of desire or necessity, greater numbers of older adults may opt to either integrate partial employment with retirement or postpone retirement altogether.

With the growth of older cohorts, especially the oldest old, chronic conditions are supplanting acute episodes of disease as primary health concerns (see Chapter 3 for a more detailed discussion). The epidemiologic transition will, perforce, transform health-care systems, and a greater proportion of health-care providers will by necessity shift primary attention from diagnosis and cure to health promotion, rehabilitation, and maintenance of function supportive of personally meaningful well-being until the end of life. Chronic illnesses by definition admit no cure; thus therapeutic goals for older adults are more likely to be framed as facilitating continued participation in occupations of choice, rather than attaining a predisease state.

In the past, the life course entailed a widely shared and fairly predictable sequence of roles (i.e., student, spouse, parent, worker) that provided structure to both daily life and transitions to the next life stage. The typical woman was widowed before the last child left the household. The typical man died while still employed. Only the very few spent their later years retired from work or from childrearing.[19] Today's growing cohorts of older adults now face a stage of later life that is largely unchartered, lacking widely shared roles and cultural expectations,[26,58] other than to avoid burdening those around them or perhaps to remain "busy."[28] It is a new life era that is at once exhilarating and free, open to new possibilities, and yet daunting and uncertain, with no clear guideposts in sight. As noted, never before have so many lived so long. Many current attitudes toward aging and the aged emerged from an earlier time, a time with far fewer older people and greatly differing social patterns and institutions. These outdated attitudes may impede our ability to embrace both the challenges and the opportunities of population aging in the twenty-first century. Today's older adults are in a sense reinventing the experience of aging, negotiating new later-life models in active construction and pursuit of meaningful occupations. The times cry for a cadre of occupational therapists to specialize in gerontology, to use the wisdom and skills of the discipline to join in this effort to reinvent old age by identifying, supporting, and creating meaningful occupations in later life.

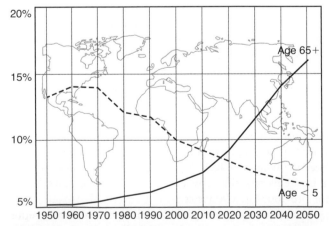

FIGURE 1-2   From Kinsella, Kevin and Wan He U.S. Census Bureau, International Population Reports, P95/09-1, An Aging World: 2008, U.S. Government Printing Office, Washington, DC, 2009.

Implications of Current Gerontological Debates for the Practice of Occupational Therapy

The conceptual distinctions discussed in the earlier section are not simply ephemeral abstractions. They directly influence what is considered to be a "good" old age. The subsequent logic of our practice models and theories may lead to very different definitions of optimal aging (which in turn help to define optimal therapeutic outcomes) and imply differing routes to attainment of optimal states. The theories and conceptual frameworks that individual therapists select (either consciously or not) and the discipline endorses are critically important because they help to define desired intervention goals—that is, what a therapist attempts to achieve in partnership with a client as determined by their shared definition of "good" old age, and the steps the therapist and client choose to take to achieve or at least approximate that optimal state.

The concept of "occupational possibilities" would seem especially relevant to understanding and supporting optimal late life as it is defined and experienced in contemporary times. Occupational possibilities are "the ways and types of doing that come to be viewed as ideal and possible within a specific sociohistorical context, and that come to be promoted and made available within environments."[60,61] Occupational possibilities thus represent shared, taken-for-granted notions of what people think they can and should do.[61] This is precisely what today's cohort of older adults is in the throes of negotiating—occupational possibilities appropriate for a stage of life that, for the masses, is new and relatively unchartered. Because they are yet to be fully and clearly articulated, the occupational possibilities of late life remain nebulous and thus somewhat elusive, to be determined on an individual or collective basis. Viewed within the PEOP model, the emergent nature of late-life occupational possibilities represents an aspect of the sociocultural environment that, depending on the resources of the individual or associated reference group, may offer an exhilarating opportunity for creative life design or a terrifying encounter with the existential void. Assisting older individuals or groups of older adults to realize appropriate occupational possibilities in later life is the privilege and challenge of contemporary occupational therapists in gerontology.

Positive gerontology may be seen as the discipline's attempt to document (or possibly guide) the ongoing negotiation of late-life occupational possibilities. As noted by Rudman,[61] however, contemporary discourses of positive aging may be seen as limited and "present a narrow range of ideal occupations focused on consumption, production, and self-maintenance." One might argue that we, as gerontologists and/or occupational therapists, have a responsibility to assume a client-centered approach in helping to identify and promote the legitimacy and health-promoting qualities of a wide range of age-appropriate occupational possibilities and work to minimize barriers and maximize resources to enable and empower older adults to attain them.

The Evolution of Gerontological Occupational Therapy

Historically, occupational therapy with aging adults has lacked the prominence of other OT specialties, such as pediatrics. We use the term *gerontological* here, rather than *geriatric*, as it expresses neutrality with regard to settings in which OTs practice collaboratively with older adults, and is thus more descriptive of practice that spans community-based and medical OT settings.

The accumulated body of OT research and practice with older adults represents a distinguished and highly relevant foundation to guide contemporary occupational therapists in the field. The potential of therapeutic activity to engage individuals in meaningful, health-promoting processes was first recognized in the late nineteenth and early twentieth centuries, resulting in the formalization of occupational therapy as a discipline in 1917 with the founding of the National Society for the Promotion of Occupational Therapy.[6,13,] During the first several decades following that formalization, emphases on medical care and rehabilitation with returning soldiers[16] and other mainstream-society populations were the prevailing forms of occupational therapy practice. Specialization in gerontological OT practice occurred relatively late in the history of the field. As a result of Naida Ackley's[3] and Lela Llorens's[47] lifespan-oriented Slagle Lectures, the profession took greater notice of geriatric population needs. The late 1960s therefore witnessed the emergence of both hospital- and community-based models of therapy with older adults.[40] During the early 1970s, organizers of the American Occupational Therapy Association (AOTA) Annual Conference included the Chronic Illness and Aging planning committee led by Betty Hasselkus and Jean Kiernat,[29,33] because chronic illnesses and related disabilities have historically served as a focus for OT interventions in adults. Additionally, these gerontological OT pioneers, as well as Joan Rogers,[55,56] Lela Llorens,[47,48] and others, claimed that the aging process itself presented special intervention opportunities for practitioners, as well as challenges, and developed innovative programs to address both aspects. Related programs first presented nationally at the AOTA conference included independent living supports that emphasized injury and fall prevention, home safety, maintenance of activities of daily living (ADLs) and instrumental activities of daily living (IADLs), meaningful occupational participation, and mental health interventions in long-term care settings.[34,39-41]

In recognition of the evolving demographics and the need for organizational support of these program developments, in 1987 AOTA published *The Role of Occupational Therapy with the Elderly (ROTE): Faculty Guide.* Written and edited by Linda Davis et al.,[27] ROTE urged OT educators to develop curricula that focused on the additional aging-related needs in providing interventions. Considering that pediatrics was already an established specialty practice in the profession, with the "graying of America," it seemed intuitive that the needs of persons at the other end of the age spectrum also should be targeted for attention. During the same period AOTA added a Geriatric Special Interest Section (GSIS), which has historically published a quarterly newsletter for members and attracts OT practitioners in geriatric programs to related conference presentations. Further recognition for occupational therapists who practice with older adults evolved within the past decade with the AOTA Board Certification in Gerontology credential development.[8]

During the 1990s, the first randomized control trial (RCT) within the profession was conducted by Florence Clark and her team of interdisciplinary scholars at the University of Southern California (USC). This study of community-dwelling older adults had a significant interdisciplinary professional influence when it was published in the *Journal of the American Medical Association.*[35] Their outcomes study, Occupational Therapy for Independent-Living Older Adults, served as the first of several successive RCTs by the USC group to demonstrate the effectiveness and efficacy of preventive health programs that utilize occupational therapy interventions.[36] The second Well Elderly study further demonstrated the significant value of the role of OT in health promotion with diverse community-based populations. These studies that validated the use of OT with aging adults have consistently focused on a variety of health-promoting OT interventions for various geriatric populations.[21,22,35,36,38] The work of these researchers, as well as that of other occupational therapists and interdisciplinary scholars, has advanced the development of geriatric practice in the profession and promoted extensive application of similar interventions.[30,45,46]

Creative intervention models that are based on an increasing awareness of aging-adult needs have stood the test of time. These models involve occupational therapists in a variety of roles within settings such as health promotion and injury prevention programs, continuum-of-care settings, geriatric education centers, and aging agencies. The geriatric OT intervention models historically spanned the spectrum of meaningful occupation; continuum-of-care offerings, including environmental and activity program planning and assessment; and related consultation. Some of these freestanding programs, such as Independent Living, Inc. in Madison, Wisconsin, and private practices continue today, 30 to 40+ years after their initial development, because they provide basic supports for aging-related changes and the associated needs of older adults.

Characteristics of Occupational Therapy Practice with Aging Adults

In state-of-the-art practice, evidence-based approaches are considered integral to the screening, assessment, and intervention processes with all ages. The *Occupational Therapy Practice Framework: Domain and Process*[7] (*OT Practice Framework*) mentioned earlier provides the current guidelines for the scope of occupational therapy practice. These guidelines encompass the entire operationalization of the

OT process, which includes evaluation, intervention, and outcomes. The following discussion considers how these guidelines can be utilized to address the specific needs, challenges, and resources of older adults. The remainder of the book elaborates on various aspects of this theme.

In addressing the processes set forth in the *OT Practice Framework,*[7] occupational therapists who work with older adults should select evaluation instruments that have demonstrated reliability and validity when applied to similar aging populations. Chapter 6 specifies the process indicated for evaluating geriatric clients.

When intervening with older adults, numerous reflective questions regarding the older client and/or the client's family or other support systems should be pondered. Whether 50, 70, or 90 years of age or older, the client is an individual with years of living and associated roles, identities, transitions, and related occupational performance in activities that may range in associated personal meaning from low to extremely high. These life experiences and personal dimensions should be considered whenever interacting with the individual. The PEOP model discussed earlier as underlying the *OT Practice Framework*[7] can be used to generate age-relevant questions to inform assessment and development of interventions for older clients. Figure 1-3 addresses the need to consider, foremost, the aging individual's well-being and quality of life.

As presented in Figure 1-3, well-being and quality of life are the interdependent outcomes of the person/client intrinsic elements, plus clients' extrinsic contexts/environments that afford their occupational options, which in turn result in clients' occupational performance patterns and participation. These symbiotic elements apply regardless of age-related changes, comorbidities, and overall level of function, whether as a senior athlete or an individual with highly reduced occupational potential at the end of life. These dimensions of well-being and quality of life complement the PEOP model while addressing aging-related needs.

In concert also with the *OT Practice Framework,*[7] the questions in the next section provide examples of topics to explore with the older client and/or family members regarding each component contributing to the individual's well-being and quality of life. Ideally, such questions elicit personal narratives that provide a picture of the client's life, as well as insight regarding the individual's current occupational needs and interests. During the initial interview, or later if deemed to be more appropriate, the therapist should empathetically and objectively inquire about each of the categories included in this model. Note also that when the client is a group, agency, or community, these same categories can be utilized, with adaptations to the nature of the questions, in order to reflect the collective dynamics and needs of the client.

Person-Related Questions

How are intrinsic factors uniquely expressed in this older individual, and how may function be different now

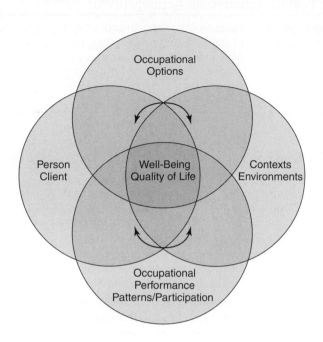

Person/Client: How are intrinsic factors uniquely expressed in this older individual/group; how may function be different now compared with the past?

Contexts/Environment: What are the contexts/environments in which occupational options are grounded?

Occupational Options: What are the activity participation possibilities? What does this older adult/group want/need to do; what are the current priorities and goals?

Occupational Performance/Participation: What comprises enactment of activities within the individual's/group's context?

Outcome Goal for OT Intervention: What will enable performance of and engagement in priority activities to support overall well-being and quality of life?

FIGURE 1-3 Aging components of well-being and quality of life. (Modified from Person-Environment-Occupation-Performance/Participation [PEOP] model [Christiansen et al., 2005] applied to geriatric OT practice [copyright SLACK, Inc.]; and Barney, K. F. [2012]. Geriatric occupational therapy: Achieving quality of daily living. In A. Sinclair, J. Morley, & B. Vellas [Eds.], *Pathy's principles and practice of geriatric medicine* [5th ed., p. 1718]. Chichester, West Sussex: John Wiley & Sons, Ltd.)

compared with the past? Person-related questions should inform the therapist regarding inherent factors about the individual client. These factors include gender, age, and racial or ethnic origins; all body structures and functions that are physiologic, including sexual, psychological, mental, sensory, and neuromusculoskeletal function; and spiritual attributes. For example, what are the individual's values, beliefs, and cultural background? Does the client express spirituality; if so, how? If the expression of the individual's identity and function is altered due to mild cognitive impairment (MCI), dementia, or other cognitive disability, the therapist should ascertain whether caregivers can provide insight into the older adult's intrinsic characteristics and performance.[32]

CASE EXAMPLE 1-1: 85-y/o Male, Diagnosis (Dx): Congestive Heart Failure (CHF)

Alex Milosovic spent nearly 50 years farming land that had been in his family for generations. After having completed an agricultural degree, he'd been so successful that he acquired much more acreage through the years, resulting in a large farm corporation that his sons now run. When referred to OT by his primary care physician for congestive heart failure (CHF) intervention to better manage his daily living, he will very much appreciate recognition of his Slavic identity and Orthodox faith. His commitment to continuing his church work is instrumental to his well-being, regardless of his cardiac status.

CASE EXAMPLE 1-2: 94-y/o Female, Dx: Post-Hip Fracture (fx)

Beatrice Henderson has been widowed for 30 years. She spent her adult life employed until the age of 68 as a secretary for several leaders of a national civil rights organization advocating on behalf of her racial group. Long-term goals in a successful therapeutic assessment and intervention process will supportively address her need to continue to advocate against the racial disparities that she has experienced throughout her life. Her condition is temporary, and should not preclude her resolve for continued participation in these advocacy activities.

CASE EXAMPLE 1-3:   72-y/o Female, Dx: Post-Cerebrovascular Accident (CVA)

Nancy Dalton immigrated to the United States from England after World War II with her American soldier husband. Since that time they raised two daughters, both of whom are married with children and live in other parts of the country. As a devout Roman Catholic, through the years Nancy has served in her parish by heading the wedding committee because of her ongoing commitment to supporting the lives of younger members. When referred to OT in a subacute care unit following a cerebrovascular accident (CVA), she expects that her long-term commitment to her church will be respected and related participation will be considered as a long-term goal in her intervention plan.

CASE EXAMPLE 1-4:   60-y/o Male, Dx: Mild Cognitive Impairment (MCI), with Probable Early-Onset Dementia

Formerly a well-loved physician, Kim Hu has been married for 40 years, with four grown children and six grandchildren. Cognitive deficits that presented a few months ago and his diagnoses resulted in his early retirement from practice. His neurologist referred Dr. Hu to OT for a baseline and ongoing assessment process in an effort to sustain his optimal participation. His spouse is totally committed to his well-being and will also benefit from services. Together, they seek support to sustain their lifestyle for as long as possible.

Context-/Environment-Related Questions

What are the contexts/environments in which occupational options are grounded? Having an understanding of the client's sociocultural context and both physical and social environments where the client functions will provide a current foundation for what is possible for participation. The client's context includes how society relates to the client's gender identity, age, race/ethnicity, and educational and socioeconomic status; cultural norms regarding occupational performance and participation; and access to and use of technology and virtual environments (if any). The occupational therapist should inquire as to whether any constraints to the client's participation are present in the environment (e.g., occupational justice issues such as ageism, racism, or sexism). Further, an understanding of the client's natural, built, and social environments facilitates the therapist's understanding of how best to evaluate and intervene with the individual. During the evaluation process, the occupational therapist should carefully note the client's preferences for participation in meaningful occupations. The clinical reasoning process should also consider that the context/environment may constrain participation. Thus the occupational therapist should collaborate with the client in considering alternative contexts and environments, to expand the individual occupational options. Consider the case examples provided earlier, and reflect upon the nature of questions that should be asked to understand the contextual/environmental factors that affect these clients' occupational performance and participation.

Occupational Options–Related Questions

What are the client's activity participation possibilities? Occupational options represent a composite of the client's fundamental attributes, functional capacity, and abilities, including skills and acquired knowledge, together with what the client's contexts and environments support. The range and limits of occupational options are based upon this interface. Essentially, if the client has capacity and capability, and the client's social, physical, and/or other contexts/environments are supportive, then the aim to participate in occupations may be realized. Otherwise, if there is not a "goodness of fit" between the desired occupation(s) and the client's capacities, and/or the client's contexts/environment, the client, the occupation(s), and/or the client's surroundings will need to be adapted in order for the client to participate in the desired occupation.

What does this client want and/or need to do, what has the client enjoyed in the past, and what are the client's current priorities? These types of questions should inform the therapist about the client's life experience, both past and present. What are the current most relevant identities the client prefers to be known for, both past and present? The therapist also should identify what the client does not want to do or is unable to do for whatever physical, cognitive, psychological, sociocultural, or logistical reasons. Where possible, in establishing therapeutic rapport, begin with determining the client's occupational participation motivation. Typically, beginning with these priorities will assist in developing rapport with the individual. Consideration of the activity demands of the client's expected or preferred occupations will include a need to acquire knowledge of the space, social environment, process elements, any required objects, and personal physical and/or mental function needs for client participation. Consider the case examples provided earlier, and reflect upon the nature of questions that should be asked to understand these clients' desired activities, related requisite abilities, and the contexts that affect occupational performance.

Occupational Performance/Participation–Related Questions

All activities present inherent occupational demands that require occupational performance attributes and/or skills in order to be performed. These implicit performance requirements include motor, process, and/or social interaction skills and abilities,[7] yet the requirements typically vary with each activity. When intervening with an older client, the occupational therapist should reflect upon the nature of the occupations that the individual prefers, needs, and/or is motivated to perform, and either observe (preferred method) or question the individual about the relevant requisite performance skills. The individual's context and intrinsic factors must also be considered in planning, to determine the extent to which participation in the occupation is realistic. Additionally, the individual's prior performance patterns (e.g., habits, routines, rituals, and roles [7]) should be taken into account when evaluating and planning to intervene with the individual, group, or population. Consider the case examples provided earlier, and reflect upon the nature of questions that should be asked to understand these clients' performance skill factors required to participate in their preferred occupations.

Following the initial observation, interaction, and reflection just described, the occupational therapist should develop a client-centered occupational profile that is sensitive to current and future aging-related needs. From that point, goals are established and related interventions are planned to address the client's health-supporting occupational engagement needs.

Outcomes-/Participation-Related Questions

Occupational therapy interventions with aging adults optimally represent collaboration between the client and therapist, and may also include family members or other support systems, resulting in mutually desired targeted outcomes. These outcomes should support the aging client's access to participation, role competence, overall health, well-being, and quality of life.[7] Measureable outcomes are preferred in order to document progress; however, qualitative feedback captures nuances and personalized elements of meaningful occupational engagement or barriers to meaningful engagement that measurement may not accomplish. Thus the occupational therapist should utilize a mixed-methods approach to gathering feedback data. The type of data to be collected is identified early in the intervention process in order to capture all relevant information. Data collected may relate to prevention aspects, occupational justice, and/or the client's occupational performance, adaptation, level of health and wellness, degree and nature of participation, quality of life and well-being, role competence, and self-advocacy.[7]

Understandings that are based on a client's responses to these questions can inform the development of individually tailored interventions that maximize the individual's potential to successfully perform occupations of his or her choice.[5,12,21,23,24,44,56]

Fundamental Intervention and Outcome Considerations with Older Clients

The following are fundamental intervention and outcome considerations with older clients:

- Understanding the older client's context and environment
- Clarifying the client's occupational performance and participation priorities, both short- and long-term

- Collaborating in setting functionally appropriate and meaningful intervention priorities
- Promoting safety, accessibility, and mobility with all relevant medical, social, or other precautions
- Facilitating optimal participation in the activities that are most important to the client, and assisting in establishing short-term adaptive approaches, where indicated
- Ensuring probable continued performance and participation in priority occupations and roles with family, friends, and social groups, to the extent feasible, including short- and long-term planning
- Identifying salient caregiver needs, where indicated, as well as resources to promote optimal client occupational performance

The overarching outcome goal for OT intervention is to enable the client's priorities for participation (e.g., occupational engagement in desired activities) in order to support overall well-being and quality of life. The model in Figure 1-4 expresses this application of the performance components in this process.

In this model, what comprises *elder well-being (EWB) and quality of life (QoL)* is dependent on and a function of the *personal (or population) attributes (PAs),* based upon the client's unique demographic factors, health status, functional potential, and motivation, plus *environmental factors (EFs)* that include all salient contextual aspects that support (or hinder) the *occupations/activities (OAs)* that the client needs and wants to pursue based upon the client's *performance skills and patterns (PSPs),* allowing *participation (P)* in society, to the satisfaction of the client in meeting the client's requisite needs and desires.

Challenges in Gerontological Practice and Research

Gaps in Occupational Therapy Curricula

As discussed earlier, throughout the early evolution of OT practice, despite its conceptual foundations of holism and association with health disciplines, the field has been largely aligned with medical disciplines and related reductionist treatment.[17,18,53] As a result, OT with adults has generally focused on conditions that are associated with

EWB + QoL = f (PA + EF + OA + PSP + P)	
EWB	Elder Well-Being
QoL	Quality of Life
PA	Person / Group / Population Attributes
EF	Environmental / Contextual Factors
OA	Occupations / Activities
PSP	Performance Skills & Patterns
P	Participation

FIGURE 1-4 Model: Components of aging, well-being, and quality of life.

medical systems of care, including hospitals, rehabilitation centers, home health care, and skilled nursing facilities.[11,12,27] In the United States the profession's accreditation standards emphasize application of therapeutic principles across the lifespan.[1] Students in entry-level OT programs historically have learned fundamental treatment approaches for medical conditions that occur throughout the adult age groups. Instruction without a particular focus on the aging-related physical, socioemotional, and developmental changes that occur as individuals transition through the life course has typified OT academic curricula. The ongoing proliferation of accreditation standards poses increasing challenges to entry-level professional programs to include comprehensive competency-based content and allows little room for the inclusion of aging-specific applications. Nevertheless, given the growing numbers of older adults, as discussed earlier, it is apparent that gerontologically informed content is needed to address the differentiated needs of older adults.

Image Issues

Over the course of time, OT employment opportunities in skilled care facilities, home health care, and continuing care retirement communities (CCRCs) have continued to steadily increase. Although therapists in these types of settings typically identify themselves as geriatric occupational therapists, ironically, informal communications with those who intervene with aging adults in acute care and rehabilitation settings indicate that these individuals do not identify themselves as geriatric occupational therapists, despite their large geriatric caseloads. Avoidance of self-identification with the status of geriatric/gerontological occupational therapist continues to be a problem for the field.

Reimbursement Structures, Standardization of Care, and Implications for Professional Development and Professional Identity

In the United States numerous health-care settings rely on reimbursement for services in a variety of forms, including fee-for-service structures based upon daily quotas or expectations for billable units of care. As a result, the need for a high level of quantifiable productivity drives much of the type of care that clients receive in these settings. Within this process therapists have little time to ponder fundamental geriatric concepts that may positively influence therapeutic outcomes. Consequently, interventions are typically provided across the adult age span in the same standardized manner. If this continues, rather than maturing in our development within the profession by creating increasingly better ways to meet the unique needs of older adults, OT personnel may remain static in how we practice with aging adult populations.

Benner[15] identified five levels of competency in clinical nursing practice. This model, tracing the stages of novice, advanced beginner, competent, proficient, and expert, may provide categories of professional development that are equally salient to OT practice with aging adults. The

constraints of the fee-for-service health-care environment described earlier, in which therapy is expected to follow routine, standardized procedures, may preclude mastery of basic skills, resulting in limited or delayed opportunities for the OT practitioner to progress past the novice and advanced beginner levels. Although the OT profession prides itself on providing holistic care, that orientation may be lost if too much emphasis in intervention is procedural. It is especially important to apply a holistic, client-centered approach when working with aging adults because of the uniqueness of each person. Aging and sociocultural factors may be dramatically different from one individual to another and require very different therapeutic approaches than simply applying procedural processes that work for younger age groups.[9-12] We run the risk of achieving less-than-optimal outcomes of care unless we are attentive to the unique intervention needs of aging adults. Tailoring interventions to each aging adult is not only the appropriate application of our craft, but also supports the full professional development of gerontological occupational therapists to the status of expert practitioners and influences their basic professional self-identity.

REVIEW QUESTIONS

1. Discuss how gerontological theory has changed over time. What are the implications of this change for occupational practice with older adults? Discuss the treatment plan you would develop if you were the therapist for Case Study 1-4, the 60 y/o male with mild cognitive impairment and probable early-onset dementia, using disengagement theory to guide your decisions regarding diagnosis and therapy. How would your work differ if you used the "positive gerontology" framework?
2. Discuss the contributions of "positive gerontology" to the way we think about later life. What are some of the arguments against this conceptual framework?
3. Discuss the PEOP model.
4. Discuss the social and cultural changes that have accompanied the demographic transition and the impact of these changes on the experience of later life.
5. Trace the emergence of geriatric/gerontologic practice as a specialty within the OT discipline.
6. Explain an optimal client/therapist intervention and outcome process with older adults, based upon guidelines presented in the chapter.
7. Identify at least one challenge in gerontological practice and in research, explaining potential ways to address each.

REFERENCES

1. Accreditation Council for Occupational Therapy Education (ACOTE ®). (2011). *Standards and interpretive guide (effective July 31, 2013), January 2012 Interpretive Guide Version.* Retrieved from https://sphhp.buffalo.edu/content/dam/sphhp/rehabilitation-science/acote-standards-2011.pdf.

2. Achenbaum, W. A. (1978). *Old age in the new land: The American experience since 1790.* Baltimore, MD: Johns Hopkins University Press.

3. Ackley, N. (1962). 1962 Eleanor Clarke Slagle Lecture. *The challenge of the sixties. American Journal of Occupational Therapy, 16,* 273–281.

4. Administration on Aging (AoA). (2012). *Profile of older adults.* Washington, DC: Administration on Aging.

5. Allison, H., & Strong, J. (1994). Verbal strategies used by occupational therapists in direct client encounters. *Occupational Therapy Journal of Research, 14,* 112–129.

6. American Occupational Therapy Association. (1940). *History. Occupational Therapy and Rehabilitation, 19,* 30.

7. American Occupational Therapy Association. (2014a). *Occupational therapy practice framework: Domain and process* (3rd ed.). Bethesda, MD: AOTA.

8. American Occupational Therapy Association. (2014b). *Board and specialty certifications.* Retrieved from http://www.aota.org/en/Education-Careers/Advance-Career/Board-Specialty-Certifications.aspx.

9. Barney, K. F. (1991a). From Ellis Island to assisted living: Considering the needs of older adults of diverse cultures. *American Journal of Occupational Therapy, 45*(7), 586–593.

10. Barney, K. F. (1991b). Occupational therapy strategies to promote health with an expanding population of well elderly. *Occupational Therapy Journal of Practice, 2*(3), 69–81.

11. Barney, K. F. (2006). Geriatric occupational therapy: Focus on participation in meaningful daily living. In M. S. Pathy, J. E. Morley, & A. Sinclair (Eds.), *Principles and practice of geriatric medicine* (4th ed., pp. 780–791). United Kingdom: John Wiley & Sons.

12. Barney, K. F. (2012). Geriatric occupational therapy: Achieving quality of daily living. In A. Sinclair, J. Morley, & B. Vellas (Eds.), *Pathy's principles and practice of geriatric medicine* (5th ed., pp. 1879–1888). Chichester, West Sussex: John Wiley & Sons, Ltd.

13. Barton, G. E. (1920). What occupational therapy may mean to nursing. *Trained Nurse and Hospital Review, 64,* 304–310.

14. Baum, C., Christiansen, C, & Bass, J. (2014). The person-environment-occupation-performance model. In C. H. Christiansen, C. Baum & J. Bass (Eds). *Occupational therapy: Performance, participation and well-being,* 4th ed., (pp. 49–55). Thorofare, NJ: Slack, Inc.

15. Benner, P. (1984). *From novice to expert: Excellence and power in clinical nursing practice.* Menlo Park, CA: Addison-Wesley Publishing Company.

16. Billings, F. (1919). Leaving too soon: The disabled soldier should remain in the hospital for full restoration, physical and mental. *Carry On, 1,* 8–10.

17. Bing, R. K. (1981). Occupational therapy revisited: A paraphrastic journey. *American Journal of Occupational Therapy, 35*(8), 499–518.

18. Christiansen, C. H., & Baum, C. M. (Eds.). (1997). *Occupational therapy: Enabling function and well-being* (2nd ed.). Thorofare, NJ: SLACK Incorporated.

19. Chudacoff, H. P., & Hareven, T. K. (1979). From the empty nest to family dissolution: Life course transitions into old age. *Journal of Family History, 4,* 69–83.

20. Clark, C. A., Corcoran, M., & Gitlin, L. N. (1995). An exploratory study of how occupational therapists develop therapeutic relationships with family caregivers. *American Journal of Occupational Therapy, 49,* 587–594.

21. Clark, F., Azen, S. P., Zemke, R., Jackson, J., Carlson, M., Mandel, D., & Lipson, L. (1997, October 22/29). Occupational therapy for independent-living older adults: A randomized controlled trial. *Journal of the American Medical Association, 278*(16), 1321–1326.

22. Clark, F., Jackson, J., Carlson, M., Chou, C., Cherry, B., Jordan-Marsh, M., & Azen, S. (2012). Effectiveness of a lifestyle intervention in promoting the well-being of independently living older people: Results of the Well Elderly 2 Randomized Controlled Trial. *Journal of Epidemiology in Community Health, 66*(9), 782–790.

23. Corcoran, M. A. (1993). Collaboration: An ethical approach to effective therapeutic relationships. *Topics in Geriatric Rehabilitation, 9,* 21–29.

24. Crepeau, E. B. (1991). Achieving intersubjective understanding: Examples from an occupational therapy treatment session. *American Journal of Occupational Therapy, 45,* 1016–1025.

25. Crews, D. E., & Gerber, L. M. (2003). Reconstructing life history of hominids and humans. *Collegium Antropologicum, 27*(1), 7–22.

26. Cutler, S., & Hendricks, J. (2001). Emerging social trends. In R. Binstock & L. K. George (Eds.), *Handbook of aging and the social sciences* (5th ed., pp. 462–480). San Diego: Academic Press.

27. Davis, L. J. (1987). *The role of occupational therapy with the elderly: Faculty guide.* Rockville, MD: The American Occupational Therapy Association.

28. Ekerdt, D. (1986). The busy ethic: Moral continuity between work and retirement. *The Gerontologist, 26,* 239–244.

29. Gainer, F. E. (2013 November 25). *Personal communication.*

30. Gitlin, L. N., Corcoran, M., Winter, L., Boyce, A., & Hauck, W. W. (2001). A randomized, controlled trial of a home environmental intervention: Effect on efficacy and upset in caregivers and on daily function of persons with dementia. *The Gerontologist, 41,* 4–14.

31. Hareven, T. (2001). Historical perspectives on aging and family relations. In R. Binstock & L. George (Eds.), *Handbook of Aging and the Social Sciences* (5th ed., pp. 141–159). San Diego, CA: Academic Press.

32. Hasselkus, B. R. (2007, January/February). Everyday occupation, well-being, and identity: The experience of caregivers in families with dementia. *American Journal of Occupational Therapy, 61*(1), 9–20.

33. Hasselkus, B. R. (2013). *Personal communication.*

34. Hasselkus, B. R., & Kiernat, J. M. (1989). Not by age alone: Gerontology as a specialty in occupational therapy. *American Journal of Occupational Therapy, 43*(2), 77–79.

35. Jackson, J., et al. (1998). Occupation in lifestyle redesign: The Well Elderly Study occupational therapy program. *American Journal of Occupational Therapy, 52*(5), 326–336

36. Jackson, J., Mandel, D., Blanchard, J., Carlson, M., Cherry, B., Azen, S., & Clark, F. (2009). Confronting challenges in intervention research with ethnically diverse older adults: The USC Well Elderly II trial. *Clinical Trials, 6*(1), 90–101.

37. Johnson, K., & Mutchler, J. (2014). The emergence of a positive gerontology: From disengagement to social involvement. *The Gerontologist, 54*(1), 93–100. doi: 10.1093/geront/gnt099.

38. Jordan-Marsh, M., Forman, T., White, B., Granger, G., Knight, B., & Clark, F. (2009). Confronting challenges in intervention research with ethnically diverse older adults: The USC well elderly II trial. *Clinical Trials, 6*(1), 90–101.

39. Kiernat, J. M. (1976). Geriatric day hospitals: A golden opportunity for therapists. *American Journal of Occupational Therapy, 30*(5), 285–289.

40. Kiernat, J. M. (1979a). Adaptive living and accident prevention for the aged. *Allied Health & Behavioral Sciences, 2*(1), 61–79.

41. Kiernat, J. M. (1979b). The use of life review activity with confused nursing home residents. *American Journal of Occupational Therapy, 33*(5), 306–310.

42. Kinsella, K., & He, W. (2009). U.S. Census Bureau, International Population Reports, P95/09-1, *An Aging World: 2008,* Washington, DC: U.S. Government Printing Office.

43. Lamb, S. (2014). Permanent personhood or meaningful decline? Toward a critical anthropology of successful aging. *Journal of Aging Studies, 29,* 41–52.

44. Law, M., Baptiste, S., & Mills, J. (1995). Client-centered practice: What does it mean and does it make a difference? *Canadian Journal of Occupational Therapy, 62,* 250–257.

45. Levine, R., & Gitlin, L. (1990). Home adaptations for persons with chronic disabilities: an educational model. *American Journal of Occupational Therapy, 44*(10), 923–929.

46. Levine, R., & Gitlin, L. (1993). A model to promote activity competence in elders. *American Journal of Occupational Therapy, 47*(2), 147–153.

47. Llorens, L. A. (1970). 1969 Eleanor Clarke Slagle Lecture. Facilitating growth and development: The promise of occupational therapy. *American Journal of Occupational Therapy, 24,* 93–101.

48. Llorens, L. A. (1984). Changing balance: Environment and individual. *American Journal of Occupational Therapy, 38*(1), 29–34.

49. Martinson, M., & Minkler, M. (2006). Civic engagement and older adults: A critical perspective. *The Gerontologist, 46*(3), 318–324. doi: 10.1093/geront/46.3.318.

50. Moody, H. (2005). From successful aging to conscious aging. In M. Wykle, P. Whitehouse, & D. Morris (Eds.), *Successful aging through the lifespan: Intergenerational issues in health* (pp. 55–68). New York, NY: Springer Publishing Company.

51. Morrow-Howell, N., Hinterlong, J., & Sheridan, M. (2001). *Productive aging: Concepts and challenges.* Baltimore, MD: Johns Hopkins Press.

52. National Institute on Aging. (2007). *Why population aging matters: A global perspective.* Publication No. 07-6134, Washington, DC: NIA.

53. Pattison, H. A. (1922). The trend of occupational therapy for the tuberculosis patient. *Archives of Occupational Therapy, 1,* 19–24.

54. Perkinson, M. A., & Solimeo, S. (2014). Aging in cultural context and as narrative process: Conceptual foundations of the Anthropology of Aging as reflected in the works of Margaret Clark and Sharon Kaufman. Remembering our roots [Special issue]. *The Gerontologist, 54*(1), 101–107. doi: 10.1093/geront/gnt128.

55. Rogers, J. C. (1981a). Gerontic occupational therapy. *American Journal of Occupational Therapy, 35*(10), 663–666.

56. Rogers, J. C. (1981b). Home care: A practical alternative to extended hospitalization. *American Journal of Occupational Therapy, 35*(10), 678.

57. Rosa, S. A., & Hasselkus, B. R. (2005, March/April). Finding common ground with patients: The centrality of compatibility. *American Journal of Occupational Therapy, 59*(2), 198–208.

58. Rosow, I. (1974). *Socialization to old age.* Berkeley, CA: University of California Press.

59. Rowe, J., & Kahn, R. (1997). Successful aging. *The Gerontologist, 37,* 433–440.

60. Rudman, D. L. (2005). Understanding political influences on occupational possibilities: An analysis of newspaper constructions of retirement. *Journal of Occupational Science, 12*(3),149–160.

61. Rudman, D. L. (2006). Positive aging and its implications for occupational possibilities in later life. *Canadian Journal of Occupational Therapy/Revue Canadienne D'Ergotherapie, 73*(3), 188–192.

62. Rudman, D. L., Cook, J. V., & Polatajko, H. (1997). Understanding the potential of occupation: A qualitative exploration of senior's perspectives on activity. *American Journal of Occupational Therapy, 51*(8), 640–650.

63. Rudman, D. L., & Dennhardt, S. (2008). Shaping knowledge regarding occupation: Examining the cultural underpinnings of the evolving concept of occupational identity. *Australian Occupational Therapy Journal, 55*(3), 153–162.

64. Torres, S. (1999). A culturally-relevant theoretical framework for the study of successful ageing. *Ageing and Society, 19*(1), 33–51.

65. United Nations Department of Economic and Social Affairs, Population Division. (2005). *World Population Prospects. The 2004 Revision.* New York: United Nations.

Ethical and Legal Aspects of Occupational Therapy Practice with Older Adults

Carol A. Needham, MA, JD; Lisa Luetkemeyer, JD, MHS, CCC-SLP; Helene Lohman, PhD, OTR/L, FAOTA; Keli Mu, PhD, OTR/L

CHAPTER OUTLINE

OBJECTIVES

- Explain ethical principles and how they relate to practice with older adults
- Discuss legal obligations of occupational therapy practice
- Describe client errors and appropriate responses to errors made
- Explain aspects of professional liability
- Discuss how to address fraud and abuse in occupational therapy practice

Professionals draw on a variety of sources to guide their behavior both in and out of the workplace. Past experiences, personal values, legal requirements, and professional codes of conduct are but some of the influences that direct a clinician's professional practice. When working with vulnerable populations, the implementation of a code of ethics becomes even more important to ensure the safety and well-being of clients and maintain the high standards of the profession. The Oxford English Dictionary defines ethics as "[t]he science of morals; the department of study concerned with the principles of human duty."[66]

Ethical Principles

To ensure that members of the occupational therapy (OT) profession maintain high standards of behavior and client care, professional organizations across the globe publish codes of ethics to guide their members in all aspects of practice. Generally, these codes require assurance of confidentiality, respect for client autonomy and informed consent, and nondiscriminatory practices.

In the United States, the American Occupational Therapy Association (AOTA) publishes the *Occupational Therapy Code of Ethics and Ethics Standards*.[18] Other professional associations, such as the College of Occupational Therapists in the United Kingdom[30] and the Australian Association of Occupational Therapists,[20] publish similar codes to which their practicing professionals are encouraged to adhere. These publications guide professionals to make ethical choices when interacting with clients, families, caregivers, and co-workers.

In 2015 the AOTA published its most recent *Occupational Therapy Code of Ethics and Ethics Standards* (Box 2-1).[18] It is "a public statement tailored to address the most prevalent ethical concerns of the occupational therapy profession. It outlines Standards of Conduct the public can expect from those in the profession." It serves as a force in "guiding ethical dimensions of professional behavior, responsibility, practice, and decision making."[18] The *Code of Ethics and Ethics Standards*

| BOX 2-1 | The American Occupational Therapy Association (AOTA) *Occupational Therapy Code of Ethics and Ethics Standards* |

Principle 1. Occupational therapy personnel shall demonstrate a concern for the well-being and safety of the recipients of their services.

Principle 2. Occupational therapy personnel shall refrain from actions that cause harm.

Principle 3. Occupational therapy personnel shall respect the right of the individual to self-determination, privacy, confidentiality, and consent.

Principle 4. Occupational therapy personnel shall promote fairness and objectivity in the provision of occupational therapy services.

Principle 5. Occupational therapy personnel shall provide comprehensive, accurate, and objective information when representing the profession.

Principle 6. Occupational therapy personnel shall treat clients, colleagues and other professionals with respect, fairness, discretion, and integrity.

(From American Occupational Therapy Association. [2015]. Occupational therapy code of ethics. Retrieved from http://www.aota.org/-/media/Corporate/Files/Practice/Ethics/Code-of-Ethics.pdf. Also see American Occupational Therapy Association. [2007]. Enforcement procedures for the occupational therapy code of ethics and ethics standards. Retrieved from http://www.aota.org/Consumers/Ethics/54232.aspx.)

consists of seven principles that are intimately in alignment with the general ethical principles and virtues: They address professional conduct in all areas of practice and with all stakeholders. Foundational to these principles are ethical reasoning and reflection. Thus based on these principles therapists apply mindful reflection to guide their actions.[18] These principles are:

- Beneficence
- Nonmaleficence
- Autonomy and confidentiality
- Social justice
- Procedural justice
- Veracity
- Fidelity

Beneficence

Beneficence is the bioethical principle underlying the duty to act in the best interests of the client. Beneficence implies action of "kindness, mercy, or charity"[18,22] toward others. According to the AOTA's *Code of Ethics and Ethics Standards*,[18] examples of application of beneficence include demonstrating concern for the well-being of those receiving OT services through referral to other health-care professionals when appropriate and providing current assessment and intervention.[18] A specific example of application of this principle to gerontological practice would be making an extra effort to locate reasonable community services for an older adult client with a low income.

Nonmaleficence

Nonmaleficence, in more familiar terms, means "do no harm." To act with nonmaleficence, the therapist must have a basic knowledge of client diagnosis, needs, and appropriate treatment protocols. In addition, the therapist must provide the appropriate standard of care and take precautions not to cause needless injury or harm. The AOTA standards include the policy that occupational therapists "avoid exploiting any relationship established as an occupational therapy clinician, educator, or researcher to further one's own physical, emotional, financial, political, or business interests at the expense of recipients of services, students, research participants,

employees, or colleagues."[18] The code lists many other examples to illustrate this principle. By adhering closely to these professional standards, practitioners reduce the chance of negatively affecting their clients. An example of a possible violation of this principle would be a therapist inexperienced with shoulder injuries providing intervention to an older adult client without seeking out information on correct intervention protocols, or finding an appropriate mentor.

Autonomy

Autonomy is the right of individuals to be self-determining and in control of their own destiny. Because the client is the best judge of personal values, wants, and needs, the client is also the most qualified person to make health-care decisions for him- or herself—the client knows his or her personal values, wants, desires, and needs better than anyone else. AOTA guidance states that practitioners should "establish a collaborative relationship with recipients of service and relevant stakeholders, to promote shared decision making" and should "fully disclose the benefits, risks, and potential outcomes of any intervention; the personnel who will be providing the intervention; and any reasonable alternatives to the proposed intervention."[18] After fully informing clients and their families of the risks and benefits of treatment, the principle of autonomy also requires therapists to respect the client's right to refuse services (informed consent and the client's right to refuse treatment are discussed later in this chapter).

Confidentiality

Confidentiality includes respecting the client's privacy with regard to his or her medical condition and treatment and also following state and federal privacy laws and regulations, such as the Health Insurance Portability and Accountability Act (HIPAA) of 1996.[35,45,46] Confidentiality also applies to students in educational programs, such as when doing research and with provision of client information.[18]

Justice

In health-care settings, providers should also strive for justice—both social and procedural. Social justice requires that health-care providers perform services equally and fairly across all client groups—stressing access to care regardless of cultural, ethnic, or physical differences. Advocating for our older adult clients illustrates this principle. Educating clients, staff, and referral sources (such as treating physicians) about the benefits of OT becomes an important aspect of client advocacy. Providing pro bono (free) services or services at a reduced cost is an example of application of this principle.

Although access to care and social justice are crucial aspects of practice, procedural justice dictates that professionals have an ethical duty to comply with the rules and policies of their employers, the laws of the state or country where they are employed, and professional standards of conduct outlined by the licensing or credentialing authority. Licensing is discussed later in this chapter. In gerontological practice, complying with Medicare regulations is an example of applying procedural justice.

Veracity

The ethical principle of veracity—truth and honesty—pervades all aspects of OT practice. From truthful education of clients, families, and staff to documentation of client care to billing codes and minutes, it is ethically and legally expected that health-care professionals provide honest and accurate information. Not only could incorrect information negatively affect client care in one isolated instance, it could undermine the reputation of OT in the public's eye because veracity is based on trust. Breakdown of the profession's reputation in the health-care field may also affect reimbursement policy in the future. Therefore therapists should take care to be honest, truthful, and law-abiding individuals in all situations. An example of violation of this principle in gerontological practice would be providing fraudulent Medicare documentation.

Fidelity

Fidelity involves treating service providers, clients, and others with respect. Working in a collegial manner with members of the interprofessional gerontological team exemplifies this principle. Trends in health care encourage interprofessional team collaboration.[34] Furthermore, fidelity involves adhering to the AOTA *Code of Ethics and Ethics Standards* and avoiding conflicts of interest with practice or research. An example of application of this principle in gerontological practice is to foster communication with the interprofessional team to maximize client care.

Legal Obligations

As professionals, therapists in gerontological practice, as well as all areas of practice, are expected to adhere to not only ethical standards but also legal standards as set forth by federal and state law. Many of these legal obligations codify the ethical standards. Legal duties discussed in this chapter are standards of care and duty of care, licensure, documentation, informed consent, and confidentiality.

Standard of Care and Duty of Care

Although there is not a medical definition for *standard of care*, the term is commonly used in medical situations.[74] Generally, standard of care refers to "a diagnostic and treatment process that a clinician should follow for a certain type of client, illness, or clinical circumstance"[56] or in legal terms "the degree of care that a reasonable person should exercise."[43] Thus standard of care is the acceptable and appropriate care that an occupational therapist provides for a client's condition.

Occupational therapists apply standard of care in practice by utilizing, as much as possible, evidenced-based practice with intervention approaches and by having practice guided by the AOTA's *Occupational Therapy Practice Framework*[17] and the standards of practice for occupational therapy.[14] In the United States, standard of care may be outlined by the state licensure board by which the professional is admitted to practice. For example, to maintain a license in Pennsylvania, occupational therapists must adhere to ethical principles and standards of professional conduct outlined in the state regulations in that state. These regulations require the therapist to maintain confidentiality of client information, respect the legal rights of the client, and perform only those functions for which the therapist is trained and competent. *Duty of care* is a term more commonly found in the United Kingdom and is clearly explained in the *Code of Ethics and Professional Conduct* published by the College of Occupational Therapists.[30] It states that "[a] duty of care arises when a referral is received by an occupational therapy service or practitioner. The duty of care would require [the therapist] to assess the suitability of the potential [client] for occupational therapy with reasonable care and skill, following usual and approved occupational therapy practice."[30] Furthermore, duty of care has been defined as "a moral or legal obligation to ensure the safety or well-being of others."[66] Thus duty of care involves an element of concern for safety. In this chapter the terms *standard of care* and *duty of care* are both utilized.

Licensure

In most states, occupational therapists are required to be licensed by a state board before practicing. State boards regulating occupational therapy are generally comprised of a combination of occupational therapists, occupational therapy assistants, and members of the general public. Some state boards may also incorporate licensed professionals from other health professions, such as licensed physicians. The board members meet on a regular basis to vote on admission of new professionals, whether they are new graduates fresh out of school or seasoned professionals who seek licensure in a new state. In addition, the board serves as the disciplinary authority, determining whether rule infractions have been committed and doling out the appropriate sanctions. Although most states have a state occupational therapy board, in some states licensure is managed under an advisory council, the state's medical board, or another state regulatory body or department.[51]

Requirement for licensure allows states to oversee the practice of health professionals to ensure the safety and well-being of state residents. Licensing of health-care professionals is regulated by state law and regulation, and accordingly licensure requirements vary from state to state.[15] State-specific requirements generally include graduation from an accredited OT program, passage of the National Board for Certification in Occupational Therapy NBCOT examination, completion of supervised fieldwork, and payment of fees.[15] As of 2013, forty-nine (49) states require licensure to practice as an occupational therapist, and only one, Hawaii, requires professional registration.[15] Although both licensure and registration are mechanisms of the state, licensure requirements are generally more stringent than registration.

The purpose of professional licensure is to regulate entry into the profession to ensure that licensees have obtained a minimum level of skill and training. In addition, the applicable state regulatory body determines the scope of practice for the profession; the level of supervision required for assistants, techs, aides, and students; the amount of annual continuing education required; and the level of discipline indicated for infractions.

Therapists need to understand how to comply with legal and ethical duties in the supervision of occupational therapy assistants and, as discussed, supervision guidelines can come from state licensure boards or other entities. In gerontological practice therapists will supervise more OT assistants than in other areas because skilled nursing facilities are OT assistants' primary area of practice.[13] As a general rule, assistants may not perform assessments or create or alter treatment plans. In addition, it is the therapist's responsibility to ensure that the assistant is properly trained to implement the delegated tasks and appropriately supervised. Supervising therapists should always review all notes from the OT assistant before signing them. Remember that if an error is made, the supervising therapist's license is on the line as well as the assistant's. Taking a few extra minutes to thoroughly review documentation is well worth the time and effort. By signing an assistant's notes, the therapist is asserting that the notes are truthful, accurate, and appropriate. Doing so without proper review can endanger both the client's health and the therapist's licensure.

Documentation

Documentation involves legal and ethical obligations and is a means of communicating information to other professionals on the care team. Although face-to-face communications play an integral role in relaying information to nursing staff and physicians, documentation in the patient chart provides a lasting record. Documentation allows medical and nursing staff who may not be present to speak with the therapist the opportunity to review patient performance and progress at any time. Thorough documentation provides vital information to the care team regarding pain management, patient functioning, and progress.[9]

In addition to providing a means of communication among members of the treatment team, patient documents also serve as a legal record of patient care. Should an investigation be conducted pursuant to a lawsuit or a complaint lodged with a payor such as Medicare or a private insurer, documentation may be accessed and examined. Providing potentially fraudulent documentation may trigger a focused Medicare review[27] and relates to the ethical standards of procedural justice and veracity.[18] Documentation needs to be truthful and compliant with regulations and workplace policies and procedures. Therefore all health-care providers should make an effort to ensure that documentation is clear, timely, and accurate.

Documentation standards are a product of statute, licensure regulations, facility standards, payor mandates, and professional association guidelines. The AOTA requirements, as outlined in Guidelines for Documentation of Occupational Therapy,[9] include documenting in a professional and legal fashion such that the contents are "organized, legible, concise, clear, accurate, complete, current, grammatically correct, and objective."[9] Medicare regulations provide specific information regarding guidelines that should be reflected in documentation to justify reimbursement, such as that intervention is of a reasonable time frame and amount and appropriate for the client's condition.[11,28] In most practice arenas with older adults, payors outline specific requirements for intervention and documentation. Therapy should reflect skilled service and, as such, requires a high level of interpretation and analysis of client performance and progress. This should be reflected in the notes. In current practice most documentation is entered into an electronic health record. Although in an electronic format, such documentation should comply with the same basic guidelines as those for written documentation (Box 2-2).

Careful and thoughtful documentation serves to protect the client, provider, and facility. The client benefits because documentation reflects provided intervention and client progress. Documentation should demonstrate consideration for client welfare through a client-centered focus. Documentation can provide justification for continuity of care. The providers benefit because documentation demonstrates evidence of an appropriate standard of care, includes the client's informed consent, and should demonstrate completion of a client-centered plan. If documentation is thorough and appropriate, it can help the professional refute charges of negligence in client care. The facility benefits because client documentation can provide a source of information for quality measurement and support for reimbursement.

Informed Consent

All health-care professionals have the ethical and legal obligation of obtaining informed consent from their clients whether in a medical or a community setting. As stated in Principle 3 of the AOTA *Code of Ethics and Ethics Standards*, "individuals have the right to make a determination regarding care decisions that directly affect their lives. In the event that a person lacks decision-making capacity, his or her autonomy

BOX 2-2   General Guidelines for Documentation

1. Because the patient chart is also a legal document, the therapist should carefully, accurately, and specifically record evaluations, assessments, and notes.
2. Avoid generalities with documentation. For example, if a client refuses to complete a task, the therapist should avoid simply documenting that "the client was noncompliant." Instead, note that the "client refused to complete dressing activity" or whatever task was asked of the client.
3. To maintain objectivity, document the client's own words, rather than general descriptions, if the client reports discomfort or any other concern. Instead of stating that the "client was tired," the therapist could document that the "client said she was sleepy because she did not take a nap."
4. The therapy record should contain documentation of the care provided, the client's response—including refusal to participate or noncompliance (see discussions of both later in this chapter)—and changes in medical condition.
5. Document any relevant discussions about the client made to family, caregivers, or staff as well as any teaching or education provided, whether over the phone or in person.
6. To justify reimbursement or continued authorization to treat, show clinical judgment and a plan in all documentation and avoid solely documenting observations.
7. Be objective and only include information relevant to the health and treatment of the client. Do not use ambiguous terminology (e.g., "client performed poorly"). Be specific.
8. Maintain professionalism in the chart. Do not document arguments or disagreements with other health professionals.
9. Never chart a verbal order unless one was received.
10. Only document care personally provided or observed physical findings.
11. Do not sign notes as a supervisor unless they have been reviewed for accuracy and appropriateness.
12. Do not backdate notes or alter a record. This may be considered fraudulent. If information from a prior session was accidentally omitted, document the information in a new note with the current date and write "late entry."
13. When documenting electronically, change the system password regularly and do not share it. Position the computer screen away from others and don't forget to log out.

(From HPSO Risk Advisor. [2007]. Document defensively: Here's how. *HPSO Risk Advisor.* Retrieved from http://www.hpso.com/pdfs/newsletters/2007/HPSO07_All.pdf; and Sames, K. M. [2005]. *Documenting occupational therapy practice.* Upper Saddle River, NJ: Pearson/Prentice Hall.)

should be respected through involvement of an authorized agent or surrogate decisionmaker."[12,18]

Informed consent shows respect for the client's autonomy by allowing the client to be the master of his or her own course of intervention and provides control in what the client may experience as an upsetting, out-of-control situation. Obtaining informed consent is one means to approach intervention as client-centered and in an ethical manner.

A major consideration when obtaining consent is the client's health literacy, which is the ability of the client to comprehend information provided about a specific medical procedure, condition, or intervention. In 2003 the National Assessment of Adult Literacy revealed that between 10% and 13% of all individuals between the ages of 16 and 64 have problems accessing, reading, understanding, and using health-care information.[61] In contrast, 29% of adults aged 65 and over demonstrate below-basic health literacy skills.[77] A 2007 study revealed that older adults with inadequate health literacy were more likely to die in the next 6 years than those with adequate health literacy.[21]

Factors that influence health literacy include socioeconomic status, education level, cognition, and overall health. To ensure that older adults are empowered to truly make informed decisions about their course of intervention and therapy goals, occupational therapists must either informally assess their client's health literacy level through a thorough client history, chart review, and interview or by consulting other professionals on the care team, such as the speech-language pathologist or social worker. Then, client education should be tailored to that specific client's needs.

Because many adults encountered in gerontological practice settings may exhibit some sort of cognitive impairment, therapists must also consider cognition as a complicating factor of informed consent. Knowing that a person has a diagnosis of Alzheimer's disease does not provide enough information to determine whether he or she has the cognitive capacity to provide consent. It is important to critically consider the person's stage of dementia[24] and the individual's "social and situational" context.[29] In Buckles et al.'s[24] study, researchers examined the subjects' understanding of informed consent across the range of dementia from very mild to moderate. They found that subjects in the very mild to mild categories understood informed consent with a minimal-risk protocol. However, for subjects with moderate dementia they suggested including a caregiver in the consent process.

Completing a simple interview may not provide enough information to determine whether a person with Alzheimer's disease has the cognitive capacity to provide informed consent. Cole[29] suggested that to make an opinion about the person's capabilities practitioners should consider doing a formal assessment of decision-making skills (e.g., the MacArthur Competence Assessment Tool for Clinical Research Version [MacCAT-CR] and consider the individual aspects of the person's situation.[19]

Recent research considered informed consent and mild cognitive impairment (MCI), a condition that can be a precursor to dementia. A study published in *Neurology* concluded that clients with MCI demonstrated significant impairments in medical decision-making capacity compared with healthy adults.[65] Those clients with MCI exhibited impaired cognitive and emotional capacity, which adversely affected their ability to make decisions about whether to accept or refuse a particular medical treatment or select among intervention options.

Therapists must be sensitive to the cognitive level of their clients and either alter their communication style to ensure client understanding of education (simple language, visual or written aids, repetition of information) or consult with the physician to determine whether the client is in need of assistance in the decision-making process.

For a client to truly provide informed consent, three requirements must be met:[22,40]

1. Adequate information
2. Client competency
3. Voluntary decision making

Client Must Be Adequately Informed

For the client to make an informed decision, he or she must be provided with all of the information necessary to make the decision. The therapist must disclose and explain all of the following aspects:[3]

- Diagnosis
- Nature, purpose, and probability of success of the proposed treatment
- Risks and benefits of the proposed treatment
- Any alternatives to the proposed treatment
- Risks and benefits of alternative proposals
- The risks and benefits of no treatment at all

In general, down-to-earth, everyday vocabulary should be used to describe the client's condition and plan of care. It may be best to avoid medical terminology and jargon with which the client may be unfamiliar. Information should be simplified as much as necessary and follow-up questions should be posed to the client to ensure comprehension. The client should be encouraged to ask questions or request clarification of anything that was difficult to understand. Asking the client to explain the information back to the therapist can be useful in making sure that the key points have been understood.

When providing client education, the therapist should allow adequate processing time as well as time for the client to formulate questions. With the client's permission, a family member or friend may be invited to take part in the session to provide support to the client. Most important, the therapist should strive to maintain an open and supportive relationship with the client. The more comfortable the client is, the more likely he or she will be to ask questions and voice concerns.

Client Must Be Competent

If a client cannot comprehend that to which he or she is consenting, then the consent is not truly informed. Competence

is a key aspect of making an informed decision. Unfortunately there are no established criteria to determine the level of competency necessary for informed consent. Essentially, the client must be capable of understanding the risks and benefits of the proposed intervention. If there are any concerns that a client may not be competent to make medical decisions, the facility's social worker and the client's treating physician should be notified. The physician may assess the client to determine whether he or she is competent to make medical decisions.[44] If the client is deemed incompetent by the physician, a surrogate decision maker must consent to treatment. Surrogate decision makers are client-designated next of kin or other appointed individuals who are expected to make the same treatment decisions as the client if he or she was capable.[72] The legal right to assign a surrogate decision maker is determined by the Patient Self-Determination Act. This act addresses the ability to make decisions about health care, to formulate advance directives, and to be informed of institutional policies regarding life-sustaining treatments.[42] The act "provides clear ethical and legal recognition of the authority of patients and surrogates in the healthcare setting by affirming the control which they have in making many decisions about their lives and what transpires in them."[76]

In the general population, circumstances under which a client may need a surrogate decision maker are most commonly the result of a sudden event resulting in brain damage such as a traumatic brain injury or cerebrovascular accident (CVA) or a progressive disease process affecting cognition. Generally clients are considered competent to make medical decisions unless they are legally determined unable to do so.[53] In those instances, a surrogate decision maker may be appointed to make those decisions if a health-care power of attorney has not already been selected by the client to make health decisions. If the client fails to select a health-care power of attorney, the physician generally makes the determination of competence at the bedside, and a surrogate decision maker is appointed. State law sets forth the persons authorized to make medical decisions on behalf of an incompetent individual absent a legal guardian or durable power of attorney. However, it is in the best interest of the client to have that decision made ahead of time and thus all clients—gerontological or not—should be encouraged to complete an advance directive and appoint a durable health-care power of attorney while still in good health.

In the gerontological population, competence becomes a more prevalent issue. Mental status is dependent on many variables, including medical diagnosis (e.g., traumatic brain injury, CVA, dementia). Disease states (e.g., urinary tract infection) and medications can alter a person's mental status (see Chapter 13). Please refer to Chapters 9, 14, 15, and 16 for additional information on aging and mental status changes. In addition, mental acuity may vary throughout the day. A client who is coherent in the morning may exhibit diminished decision-making ability as the day progresses either due to fatigue or sundowning. Sundowning refers to the increased confusion and agitation later in the day that is often found among people with cognitive impairments.

When facilitating comprehension, one should be aware of the normal changes involved in the aging process. The client's senses may be less acute. Therefore the therapist should make accommodations for known sensory deficits. If hearing is an issue, background noise should be kept to a minimum and the therapist should face the client when talking. If the client has vision problems, the therapist should use large print, ensure that the client is wearing glasses or contact lenses if needed, and provide adequate light in the environment.[47] (See Chapter 10 for additional information.)

Client Decision Must Be Voluntary

Consent to medical treatment must be voluntary. Each client has the right to participate in—or refuse—therapy without pressure from medical staff. Although health-care professionals may make multiple attempts to persuade the client to participate in intervention and may even provide multiple opportunities to participate in care, it is ultimately the client's decision whether or not to participate; clients have the right to refuse treatment.[33] This decision must be respected by the therapist. Under the federal Patient Self-Determination Act of 1990[56] (discussed earlier), every hospital, long-term care facility, hospice, and home health agency receiving Medicare and Medicaid funds must provide clients with a statement of their rights, including the right to refuse treatment.[42]

Autonomy

The voluntary consent requirement is merely an extension of the principle of autonomy discussed in Principle 3 of the *Occupational Therapy Code of Ethics*.[18] In health care a client's autonomy is affected by the setting. A client receiving home health services has more autonomy in the home than a client in a long-term care setting or hospital. In institutional settings, activities, meals, treatments, and even showers may be regimented and generally left to the staff to schedule, with little control left to the client. Clients are often left feeling like a cog in the wheel without any control over aspects of their daily lives. In these types of settings it is even more important to respect each client as an autonomous individual who deserves the dignity of self-determination. Because facility residents and clients may have minimal control over their environment, it is imperative to allow them as much control as possible over every aspect of care. Including clients in the planning process gives them more control and a more vested interest in their treatment. The current revision of the required screening tool for skilled nursing facilities that receive federal funding (Minimal Data Set [MDS] 3.0) includes client input through interviews.[26]

Confidentiality

Confidentiality is also included in Principle 3 of the AOTA *Code of Ethics and Ethics Standards*.[18] Because therapists often spend large quantities of contact time with clients, they have the unique opportunity among health professionals to learn more about the client on an intimate personal basis than many other practitioners on the care team. The large amount of contact time spent with each client on a recurring basis allows the therapist to monitor change over time and be among those serving as a first line of defense against status changes or medical complications. That said, there are limits on when and how much information may be shared with whom.

Health Insurance Portability and Accountability Act

Although occupational therapists have been required to honor client confidentiality through the AOTA *Code of Ethics and Ethics Standards*, state licensure requirements, and internal employer policies, the Health Insurance Portability and Accountability Act of 1996 (HIPAA)[46] federally mandated this obligation.[35] HIPAA was passed to help ensure the protection of private client information, called protected health information (PHI) in the act, in light of the increased use of emerging technologies such as the Internet and electronic databases and the security risks associated with their use. The Health Information Technology for Economic and Clinical Health Act (the HITECH Act),[45] part of the American Recovery and Reinvestment Act of 2009, widened the scope of privacy and security protections available under HIPAA. The HITECH Act also increased the legal liability of health-care professionals for noncompliance and increased enforcement.[31]

Under HIPAA, health-care providers are required to maintain the confidentiality of PHI, which includes a client's medical history or diagnosis, treatment records, and billing information. PHI is protected in all forms: writings, verbal communications, and electronic records.[35,68,71] Although providers are required to take measures to maintain client confidentiality, their actions are generally scalable to their size, resources, and sophistication. This notion of scalability carries with it a reasonableness approach but does not serve to completely insulate a provider from exposure to liability under HIPAA.

Most documentation is done electronically, and electronic records include those stored on computer disks, hard drives, networks, and the Internet.[36] To safeguard electronic information, clinicians should protect their passwords and restrict access to handheld electronic devices and laptop computers. Client information may be faxed between health-care providers so long as reasonable measures have been taken to assure protection of the information, such as confirming that the fax number is correct, putting a notice on the cover sheet to destroy the information if the fax is mistakenly misdirected, and calling to confirm receipt of the fax. If a disclosure that is not permitted by HIPAA without specific client authorization is desired, the client's written authorization is required before such disclosure takes place.

PHI must be protected for all clients, whether living or deceased, and may be disclosed only to that specific client, to other authorized individuals, or to authorized organizations; it may be used or disclosed without authorization for treatment, payment, or health-care operations.[35] In the event of an inappropriate disclosure of a client's PHI, HIPAA requires that an entity implement breach notification procedures to inform all affected individuals that their PHI may have been disclosed. The specific notification procedures required depend on how many clients are affected and whether the information is protected through encryption or some other means. If a clinician becomes aware of a breach of PHI, he or she should immediately notify a supervisor or the risk manager for the organization so that an investigation can be conducted and the appropriate actions may be taken.

Penalties for violating HIPAA (including the HITECH Act) include civil penalties of fines ranging from $100 to $50,000 with repeated violations for HIPAA beyond a one-time violation at $1,500,000 and potential criminal penalties.[46] Although penalties for HIPAA violations were rarely enforced in the past, the HITECH Act increased enforcement mechanisms, and thus health-care providers should anticipate more scrutiny in the future. In recent cases, criminal sanctions have included probation and prison time. In 2009 an Arkansas physician was sentenced to 1 year of probation and 50 hours of community service and was required to pay a $5000 fine for accessing a client's records without any legitimate purpose.[41] In 2010, a former surgeon at the UCLA School of Medicine was sentenced to 4 months in federal prison for illegally accessing medical records.[38] In 2011 several breaches involved accessing records of known people with penalties resulting in fines, probation, termination, and suspended privileges.[52]

Confidentiality in Practice

Although it is necessary to protect client privacy, there are many instances when the therapist needs to communicate with family members and other caregivers. Many clients need help and support from family and friends during recovery from hospitalization and acute illness. In taking on the role of caregiver, a spouse or adult child may require education regarding precautions, mobility or range of motion, transfer techniques, activities of daily living (ADLs), and adaptive equipment use. To provide information or education to family or friends, the therapist should first obtain permission from the client. Once consent is obtained, it should be documented immediately in the client's chart and necessary precautions should be taken to ensure that information is only released to those for whom the client consents.[39] If speaking to a caregiver or family member over the phone, necessary precautions may include requiring a password to verify that the family member is authorized to receive private information. In addition, the therapist should confirm that person's identity. Directly calling the family member provides assurance that the correct family member was contacted. Finally, all communications as well as precautions taken should be documented in the client's chart.

To ensure continuity of care and a complete assessment and appropriate intervention, client information may be disclosed to other members of the health-care team. However,

only the minimum amount of information necessary for adequate assessment and intervention should be relayed. Although the client's relevant medical history and preillness condition may be relevant to the other therapists treating the client, knowledge of the client's personal history, however interesting, is usually not necessary for the provision of services or daily care. Be cognizant of what information is important to relay for improvement of the client's health and only provide necessary information. That said, there are some necessary exceptions to confidentiality in the cases of potential physical harm and/or abuse.

Exceptions to Confidentiality Rules
Potential Harm by the Client
If a client appears to be a danger to self or others, the therapist has a duty to report these concerns to a supervisor, the treating physician, and possibly authorities. In addition, if a client threatens harm to another person, the therapist may be required to warn that person of the threat. In that event, the therapist should consult the risk manager of the facility for guidance on reporting requirements.

Potential Harm by Others
According to the National Center on Elder Abuse,[62] abuse of older adults is a hidden problem that can be difficult to monitor. Although it can be difficult to obtain specific statistics, the National Center reports an increasing trend. As health-care providers, occupational therapists are considered mandatory reporters of elder abuse in most states.[1] Generally, if a therapist has a reasonable belief that a vulnerable adult has been abused, neglected, or exploited, this concern should be reported. Examples include a lack of basic hygiene, a verbally demeaning caregiver, a lack of adequate clothing, or inadequately explained cuts or bruises.[2] When you have a sense that something about the client's situation is just not right, find out more. Unfortunately, the most likely abusers are those closest to the abused adult: adult children, spouses, and other caregivers. (Box 2-3).

If abuse is suspected the therapist should follow company policies regarding reporting concerns in addition to calling the state's elder abuse hotline. The state-specific numbers as well as general statistics and information on elder abuse identification and prevention may be accessed at the National Center's website at www.ncea.aoa.gov.[63]

When Errors Are Made

"To err is human."[50,67] As with any other health-care professionals, occupational therapists do make errors.[54] In a series of research studies centered on OT practice errors,[54,59,70] researchers found that occupational therapists make various errors ranging from minor errors (e.g., ripping fingernails or causing client fatigue) to severe ones (e.g., rupturing tendons or leaving a hot pack on too long, resulting in burns).[59] In a study on errors in gerontological practice,[54] researchers found errors related to internal factors or external factors as well as

---

BOX 2-3	Risk Factors and Signs of Older Adult Abuse

Risk Factors	Signs
Financial or other family problems	Depression/anxiety
Past history of abusive relationships	Passive and compliant
Social isolation and dependence	Fearful
Physical, functional, or cognitive deficits in caregivers	Socially withdrawn
Inadequate housing or unsafe conditions in the home	Change in financial behavior
	Unexplained or repeated injuries
	Delays in seeking medical attention for an injury
	Elusive explanations for medical conditions
	Inconsistent laboratory findings
	Signs of dehydration or malnutrition without a medical cause
	Evidence of poor care (e.g., poor hygiene)
	Muscle contractures due to restricted movement

(Data from Canadian Network for the Prevention of Elder Abuse. [n.d.]. Abuse of older adults: Signs and effects. Retrieved from http://www.winnipeg.ca/police/TakeAction/elderabusefacts/FactSheet_4.pdf; and World Health Organization. [2002]. Abuse of the elderly. Retrieved from http://www.who.int/violence_injury_prevention/violence/world_report/factsheets/en/elderabusefacts.pdf.)

---

technical and moral factors. Discussed internal factors were "poor judgment, inexperience, and lack of knowledge."[54] A typical example of an error from an internal factor was inattention resulting in an older adult falling. Discussed external factors were influences outside of the therapist's control, such as a wrongly written order regarding weight-bearing status for an older adult following hip surgery. Technical errors involved methods, skills, or approaches that led to physical harm, such as exceeding a client's limitations following a hip replacement. Moral errors related to behaviors that undermine the practitioner-client relationship or are ethically inconsistent, such as providing an unneeded service to obtain Medicare payment or being untruthful in documentation by exaggerating the level of function accomplished through therapy.[54,59] Unique to occupational therapists was the research finding of therapists being more likely to report moral errors and that therapists tended to judge moral errors as more concerning than technical ones.[54] Additionally, most practice errors occurred during the intervention phase of the OT process.[59]

These research studies on OT practice errors suggest that the causes of errors are from both individual and systemic factors. Examples of individual causes are lack of experience, lack of training, lack of assertive behavior, inadequate knowledge, and misjudgment. Unrealistic productivity pressure, unclear or illegible documentation, lack of timely and effective communication, inadequate orientation to specialized equipment, and inability to access clients' medical history are among the examples of reported systemic causes of errors. In the studies focused on gerontological practice,[54,59] system causes, such as influences from regulations related to prospective payment systems (PPSs) contributed to some practice errors. Among all the causes, the top causes of errors, according to a national survey study, are misjudgment, inadequate preparation, lack of experience, inadequate knowledge, and miscommunication. Regardless of how errors occurred, making errors affected therapists emotionally.[59]

The top causes of errors, misjudgment, lack of preparation and experience, and inadequate knowledge, are in stark contrast with the principle of beneficence of the AOTA *Code of Ethics and Ethics Standards*.[18] Beneficence requires OT personnel to "take steps (e.g., continuing education, research, supervision, training) to ensure proficiency, use careful judgment, and weigh potential for harm when generally recognized standards do not exist in emerging technology or areas of practice."[18]

Miscommunications among OT personnel and clients, client family members, and other health-care providers often lead to practice errors. Ensuring clear, sufficient, accurate, and concise communication (verbal and written) among all service providers and recipients is one key to preventing and reducing errors. Without doubt, errors are inevitable in OT practice even with the most experienced and diligent occupational therapists. The dilemma that occupational therapists face when errors happen is what to do and how to manage errors. Therapists learn from errors by gaining knowledge of safety strategies, changing practice procedures, and developing an understanding of how to morally manage errors.[70] The ultimate goal is to create a "culture of safety."[70] Acceptable ways to report and disclose errors and other methods to improve error reduction are discussed next.

Incident Reports

If a mistake by a therapist occurs and causes potential client harm, the error should be documented. Most facilities have established policies and procedures for reporting adverse events involving client care, often in the form of incident reports. These reports generally serve two purposes: (1) to protect the client by alerting management to possible safety hazards requiring investigation and correction and (2) to learn from the event and improve processes to avoid such errors in the future through quality improvement initiatives. Generally the occupational therapist should include the specific date and time of the occurrence, any witnesses who observed the event, and who was notified after the incident occurred.

An incident report should be filed any time a client is injured. If a therapist has observed an incident, he or she should document only what was observed firsthand. The event should be described in an objective and factual manner, using direct quotes if statements made by staff, the client, or others present are relevant. Documentation should be objective and as honest as possible. Although it may be tempting to the therapist to protect him- or herself or others from blame, falsification of the records potentially violates state and/or federal law and could cause additional harm to the client if information relevant to the client's care and course of treatment is left out. Finally, the therapist should include any assessment and care that was provided before, during, and after the incident. Ultimately, assuring client safety is paramount.

Disclosure of Errors

One of the most important aspects of intervention and care for a client is developing a trusting relationship. This begins from the first moment the client is seen. If a mistake is made, it is necessary to apologize to the client to maintain a trusting relationship. Everyone makes mistakes, and the therapist should feel no shame in admitting an error. When an apology is warranted, the therapist should verify the employer's policy on disclosure, file an incident report, and check with the organization's risk manager. A timely and appropriate apology can deepen the relationship with client and family, and safeguard the client.[48,49,82] Coalitions such as Sorry Works promote disclosure through apology and compensation to mitigate anger and reduce the likelihood of a lawsuit.[83]

Even with a movement toward full disclosure of errors, for past centuries and still today health-care providers are often trained to be perfectionists. In a perfectionism paradigm, making errors and disclosing errors to clients and families are unthinkable or irrational. Those against disclosure of errors believe such an act would diminish the trust of clients and the public in health-care providers, damage the fragile therapeutic relationship with clients, result in countless lawsuits, empower clients unnecessarily, destroy professional reputation, and result in loss of professional license. They argue that the nondisclosure is grounded firmly on the belief of therapeutic exception or therapeutic privilege. Therapeutic privilege refers to physicians withholding information that is felt to be contraindicated to share or could harm the client physically or psychologically.[23]

Proponents of disclosure of errors, however, argue that disclosure of errors is an ethical and obligated act (i.e., Principle 6, veracity, of the AOTA *Code of Ethics and Ethics Standards*). This principle includes honest, objective transmission of information and, as stated, therapists should "refrain from using or participating in the use of any form of communication that contains false, fraudulent, deceptive, misleading, or unfair statements or claims."[18] As recipients of health-care services, patients have the right to be informed

of accurate, comprehensive, and objective health-care information, including disclosure of errors. Furthermore, research findings specific to occupational therapists suggest that disclosure of errors more likely leads to "constructive coping mechanisms and changes in practice,"[59] as discussed in the next section.

Error Prevention and Reduction

As stated earlier, errors are inevitable even with the best-prepared and the most diligent OT practitioners. The encouraging news is that research literature on OT practice errors indicates that occupational therapists often use constructive strategies to prevent future errors and that OT practitioners become more vigilant in their practice after errors occur. Therapists reflected on and learned from errors, paid more attention to details, and altered their service approaches and methods.[54,59]

That said, there are strategies available to help prevent and reduce the likelihood of a practice error occurring. Specific error prevention and reduction strategies include the following measures:[58]
- Strengthen departmental orientations for newly hired occupational therapists.
- Implement performance-based competency checks to improve in-service and continuing education outcomes.
- Establish new policies and programs based on collected error data.
- Capitalize on the existing infrastructures of the facility.
- Establish or improve mentorship for new employees.
- Create non-punitive cultures and environments.

Strengthen Departmental Orientation

Strengthening on-site orientation for new therapists is an effective strategy for error prevention/reduction.[58] In addition to general orientation at the worksites, providing site-specific orientations to areas that are prone to error is important. These orientations must occur and be strengthened. Identification of these error-prone areas needs to be based on data generated from the input of administrators, safety personnel, therapists, and other stakeholders through a problem-solving process.

Implement Performance-Based Competency Checks

Outcomes-based in-service training and continuing education are effective ways to ensure professional competency of occupational therapists.[58] However, *knowledge* is not the synonym of *competency*. Merely attending an in-service training or continuing education program does not guarantee competency acquisition; therapists must advocate for performance-based competency checks to ensure and improve the outcomes of training. For example, new therapists could have a competency check on safe transfer procedures. Competency checks are especially essential for infrequently used skills such as implementing physical agent modalities, or newly acquired skills such as operating recently purchased equipment.

Establish New Policies and Programs

Establishing new safety policies and safety programs is another worksite approach to error reduction.[58] Examples of such initiatives or measures include the following:

- Policies to require confirmation of signed physician orders before initiating intervention
- Committees addressing patient safety concerns, such as patient skin integrity or falls

Capitalize on Existing Infrastructure

Existing infrastructures in treatment facilities may be used to prevent and reduce practice errors.[58] Such existing infrastructures include the following examples:

- Safety committees
- Quality assurance programs that collect patient error data and enable respective programs to design and/or strengthen orientations, in-service training, health care, and patient education

The Joint Commission (TJC) plays a significant role in error reduction and patient safety improvement. For instance, one current TJC standard mandates that two methods must be implemented to verify the identity of patients before initiating treatment.[75]

Establish a Mentorship Program for New Employees

Occupational therapists have voiced the importance of providing mentorship to new employees in research literature on practice errors in OT practice. Therapists asserted that mentors should be provided to all new graduates or to experienced occupational therapists who decide to enter a different practice area.[58]

Create a Non-punitive Culture

The value of creating a non-punitive culture and working environment cannot be overstated.[58] Creation of such a culture or environment is essential for practitioners to share their errors with others openly, which in turn will help everyone learn to prevent/reduce errors and improve patient safety. An anonymous and voluntary reporting system for OT professionals provides an open forum for practitioners to share errors, explore prevention/reduction strategies, and ensure lessons learned for all.

The notion of establishing a non-punitive culture and environment needs to be fostered early in professional education. OT professional programs should be educating students that practice errors are inevitable, and the most important thing is to learn from errors when they occur.

Consequences for Violating Professional Obligations

Occupational therapists work in a complex, ever-changing health care environment. Recent modifications in health care provision in response to the Affordable Care Act resulted in new systems for gerontological care being piloted and integrated into practice, such as accountable care organizations and bundling of care. Beyond the overall macro changes to the health care environment, therapists face day-to-day challenges in providing patient care. Sometimes it may seem difficult to get a handle on the complexity of issues that therapists face. Therefore it is important to refer to and apply a professional code of ethics as well as have system structures in place to help guide therapists' professional conduct in this era of increasingly complex practice. Beyond ethical standards, laws regulating health-care practice are created to protect the public's safety and to help influence actions. Laws are defined as "rule(s) of conduct or action(s) prescribed or formally recognized as binding or enforced by a controlling authority."[81] The next section includes a discussion of provisions in place to address violations of appropriate client care and practice.

Violation of Standard or Duty of Care

If a client feels that a therapist has violated the standard of care, there are many avenues through which to lodge a complaint. Some clients may verbalize their dissatisfaction by reporting concerns directly to the therapist. In this instance the therapist has the opportunity to rectify the situation before it escalates. Allowing the client or family time to voice concerns, receive validation, and suggest solutions to the problem should help the therapist resolve any issues the client may have and allow the therapist-client relationship to continue.

If the issues are not resolved to the client's satisfaction, further measures may be taken. First, the employer may be contacted and the therapist may be penalized in accordance with company policy. Another option available to clients is to file a complaint with a professional accrediting organization such as the AOTA. According to AOTA procedure, complaints against a member may be filed by anyone with knowledge of a suspected ethical violation by an association member. A signed, written complaint must be filed with the Ethics Commission (EC), and the EC shall make a preliminary assessment of the complaint and determine whether an investigation is warranted.[4,5] If the EC determines the event does rise to the level of an ethical violation, the EC may initiate a charge. If the member is found to have committed an ethical violation, the member may be sanctioned. Any sanctions may be appealed and presented to an appeal panel, whose decision is final.[18]

The NBCOT, the organization that certifies occupational therapists, may also investigate allegations of ethical misconduct. Disciplinary sanctions carried out by the NBCOT[60] include formal written reprimand, public censure, compulsory community service, probation with conditions, suspension of certification to practice for a specified term, ineligibility for certification, or revocation of certification.

Finally, clients may also file a complaint with the state[12] in which the therapist practices. If a therapist violates any licensure requirements or a client files a complaint, the licensure board, or other entity, in the applicable state will conduct an investigation.[10,16] If the licensee is found to be in violation, penalties may be assessed. Penalties for noncompliance vary according to state statute and regulation and degree of infraction. Sanctions may range from public reprimand, licensure suspension or revocation (e.g., Texas),[69] fines (e.g., $250 to $1000 in Georgia[32]), to (in extreme cases) imprisonment. Actions that violate state licensure laws may also violate federal laws; therefore, professionals may be exposed to additional liability for the same infraction.

Violating one's scope of practice and creating fraudulent documentation are two examples of issues that may be addressed by a licensure board. If a health professional acts outside the profession's scope of practice or provides fraudulent documentation, he or she may expose the client to risk of injury and expose her- or himself to civil and criminal sanctions, including licensure revocation, fines, and criminal charges.

Reimbursement Fraud and Abuse

When dealing with reimbursement issues, therapists should document intervention codes and minutes truthfully and accurately to avoid claims of fraudulent documentation. Health-care fraud occurs when a health-care professional knowingly, willfully, and intentionally makes a false statement or claim.[6,78,79] Making false statements or documentation to obtain program benefits, such as Medicare reimbursement when a provider would otherwise not be entitled to payment, is fraudulent. For example, submitting claims for services that were not provided or billing for more minutes than were provided to increase reimbursement level are fraudulent activities.

When determining whether fraud or abuse has occurred, the government may look to whether the services were reasonable and necessary, whether the charges were appropriate and accurate, and whether documentation supports the treatment provided.[55] Therefore, documentation serves as an important means for the therapist to substantiate the services provided.

False Claims and Penalties

Unfortunately fraud occurs in therapy practice and sometimes with rehabilitation corporations that employ therapists. In 2012 a therapist was convicted of submitting around $1.5 million in fraudulent claims to Medicaid and Medicare for therapy not provided. In 2004 the nation's largest provider of rehabilitation services agreed to pay $325 million to settle allegations that the company defrauded Medicare and other federal health-care programs.[37] The allegations included billing for physical therapy services provided by persons other than licensed physical therapists and billing for individual services when individual services were not rendered.[37]

The False Claims Act prohibits knowingly filing false or fraudulent claims against the U.S. government.[78] If an individual violates the False Claims Act by charging Medicare or Medicaid for services that were not rendered, anyone may bring a civil action on behalf of the government against that individual. Therefore a co-worker, a patient, or a patient's family member may report a violation. Under the act, fraud by a provider is considered a felony and is punishable by a fine of up to $25,000 and up to five years' imprisonment[80] and civil penalty fines up to $10,000 if the provider makes a false claim, bills for services not provided, misrepresents services provided, or falsely certifies that certain services were medically necessary. If an individual is proven to have submitted false claims, he or she may be fined from $5000 to $10,000 for each false claim[78] and the prosecutor has the discretion to triple the fine.[64] Additional sanctions include administrative actions such as licensure suspension or revocation. Therefore it is imperative to bill accurately and truthfully for services rendered because it could prove extremely costly financially and emotionally to submit false claims.

Whistleblower Protections

A private citizen who becomes aware of violations of the False Claims Act may bring a civil action against the individual or company in violation of the act on behalf of the government.[78] For example, in 2008 two employees, including an occupational therapist, of a corporation that provides gerontological services filed whistleblower lawsuits alleging that excessive therapy was being provided to increase reimbursement.[73] Any individual who brings such an action may share in the proceeds recovered as a result of the suit.[78] In addition, certain workplace protections are provided. An employee who lawfully reports violations, assists in such an investigation, or testifies regarding a violation may not be discharged, demoted, suspended, threatened, harassed, or discriminated against.[78] If an employer engages in any of the prohibited actions, the employee may be reinstated, receive two times the amount of lost wages, and receive compensation for any special damages sustained as a result of the discrimination, including litigation costs and reasonable attorneys' fees.[57,78]

Summary

Providing intervention in today's health-care world is becoming increasingly complex, and inevitably practice issues develop and mistakes occur. As a result, therapists need to be cognizant of ethical standards and legal protections to help guide practice. Applying the AOTA *Occupational Therapy Code of Ethics and Ethics Standards*[7,8,18] in daily practice is paramount for good care. Furthermore, understanding legal aspects of patient/client care helps to promote a better and safer client-care environment. Finally, therapists should seek out work in an environment that fosters good ethical care and one that provides a culture of safety and concern for clients.

Application Exercise

Read Case Study 2-1 and reflect upon the scenarios and answer the questions, applying the ethical/legal principles from this chapter.

CASE STUDY 2-1

Marylyn is a student doing her clinical rotation at a skilled nursing facility (SNF) with older adults covered under Medicare. Recently Marylyn experienced a couple of ethical/legal situations that made her pause to reflect on correct actions. The first situation involved Samantha, a newly employed occupational therapist in the department. Marylyn admired Samantha because she seemed to work hard and appeared to always have unusually high productivity. One day when Marylyn was in the OT clinic, she noted that Samantha was providing a group intervention with four residents. However, later in the main office she noted that Samantha documented the treatment of each of the residents as an individual treatment rather than as a group intervention.

The next situation occurred when Marylyn was working with Martha, an 84-year-old woman who was recovering from a total hip replacement. While assisting Martha with a transfer back to bed, Marylyn became distracted when her supervisor came into the room to ask a question. Within the couple seconds that Marylyn turned away from Martha to address her supervisor, Martha fell and sustained some minor injuries. Marylyn felt terrible and was quite tearful when she discussed the resident's fall with her supervisor.

Case Study Questions

What ethical principle(s) is Samantha possibly violating?
What should Marylyn do with her suspected finding about Samantha?
How should Marylyn handle the resident's fall?
What can Marylyn learn from both situations?

REFERENCES

1. American Bar Association. (2006). *Reporting requirements: Provisions and citations in adult protective services laws, by state.* Retrieved from http://www.abanet.org/aging/docs/MandatoryReportingProvisionsChart.pdf.
2. American Medical Association. (1993). Diagnostic and treatment guidelines on elder abuse and neglect. *Archives of Family Medicine, 2,* 371–388.
3. American Medical Association. (2013). *Informed consent.* Retrieved from http://www.ama-assn.org/ama/pub/physician-resources/legal-topics/patient-physician-relationship-topics/informed-consent.page.
4. American Occupational Therapy Association. (2000). *Ethics Commission advisory opinion on patient abandonment.* Retrieved from http://www.aota.org/ Practitioners/Ethics/Advisory/36510.aspx.
5. American Occupational Therapy Association. (2005). Occupational therapy code of ethics (2005). *American Journal of Occupational Therapy. 59,* 639–642.
6. American Occupational Therapy Association. (2005, August). *Fact sheet: Fraud and abuse basics.* Retrieved from http://www.aota.org/Practitioners/Reimb/ Resources/Fraud/ 37789.aspx.
7. American Occupational Therapy Association. (2006). Guidelines to the occupational therapy code of ethics. *American Journal of Occupational Therapy, 60,* 652–658.
8. American Occupational Therapy Association. (2007). Enforcement procedures for the occupational therapy code of ethics (edited 2007). *American Journal of Occupational Therapy, 61,* 679–685.
9. American Occupational Therapy Association. (2008). Guidelines for documentation of occupational therapy. *American Journal of Occupational Therapy, 62,* 684–690.
10. American Occupational Therapy Association. (2008, September). *Jurisdictions regulating occupational therapists.* Retrieved from American Occupational Therapy Association website: http://www.aota.org/Practitioners/Licensure/StateRegs/OTRegs/36459.aspx.
11. American Occupational Therapy Association. (2009, March). *Medicare rules for concurrent therapy.* Retrieved from http://www.aota.org/Practitioners/Reimb/Pay/Medicare/ FactSheets/37784.aspx.
12. American Occupational Therapy Association. (2010a). *Frequently asked questions about ethics.* Retrieved from http://www.aota.org/en/Practice/Ethics/FAQ.aspx.
13. American Occupational Therapy Association. (2010b). *Occupational therapy compensation and workforce study.* Retrieved from http://www.nxtbook.com/nxtbooks/aota/2010salarysurvey/index.php.
14. American Occupational Therapy Association. (2010c). *Standards of practice for occupational therapy.* Retrieved from http://www.aota.org/-/media/Corporate/Files/Practice/OTAs/ScopeandStandards/Standards%20of%20Practice%20for%20Occupational%20Therapy%20FINAL.ashx.
15. American Occupational Therapy Association. (2013a). *About state licensure.* Retrieved from http://aota.org/Students/Current/Licensure.aspx.
16. American Occupational Therapy Association. (2013b). *Colorado enacts licensure law for occupational therapy practitioners.* Retrieved from http://www.aota.org/News/Media/PR/2013-Press-Releases/CO-Licensure.aspx.
17. American Occupational Therapy Association. (2014). *Occupational therapy practice framework: Domain and process.* Bethesda, MD: American Occupational Therapy Association.
18. American Occupational Therapy Association. (2015). *Occupational therapy code of ethics.* Retrieved from http://www.aota.org/-/media/Corporate/Files/Practice/Ethics/Code-of-Ethics.pdf.
19. Appelbaum, P.S., & Grisso, T. (2001). *MacArthur Competence Assessment Tool for Clinical Research Version [MacCAT-CR].* Sarasota, FL, US: Professional Resource Press/Professional Resource Exchange.
20. Australian Association of Occupational Therapists. (2001). *Code of ethics.* Retrieved from http://otaus.com.au/sitebuilder/about/knowledge/asset/files/1/codeofethics.pdf.
21. Baker, D. W., Wolf, M. S., Feinglass, J., Thompson, J. A., Gazmararian, J. A., & Huang, J. (2007). Health literacy and mortality among elderly persons. *Archives of Internal Medicine, 167,* 1503–1509.
22. Beauchamp, T., & Childress, J. (2001). *Principles of biomedical ethics* (5th ed.). New York, NY: Oxford University Press.
23. Bostick, N. A., Sade, R., McMahon, J. W., & Benjamin, R. (2006). Report of the American Medical Association Council on Ethical and Judicial Affairs: Withholding information from patients: Rethinking the propriety of 'therapeutic privilege.' *The Journal of Clinical Ethics, 17,* 302–306.
24. Buckles, V. D., Powlishta, K. K., Palmer, J. L., Coats, M., Hosto, T., Buckley, A., & Morris, J. C. (2003). Understanding of informed consent by demented individuals. *Neurology, 61,* 1662–1666.

25. Canadian Network for the Prevention of Elder Abuse. [n.d.]. Abuse of older adults: Signs and effects. Retrieved from http://www.winnipeg.ca/police/TakeAction/elderabusefacts/FactSheet_4.pdf

26. Centers for Medicare and Medicaid Services. (2006). *Introduction to the MDS 3.0 evaluation study*. Retrieved from http://www.cms.gov/Medicare/Quality-Initiatives-Patient-Assessment-Instruments/NursingHomeQualityInits/downloads/MDS30Draft.pdf.

27. Centers for Medicare and Medicaid Services. (2009). Medicare program integrity manual. Chapter 6: Intermediary MR guidelines for specific services. Retrieved from http://www.cms.gov/Regulations-and-Guidance/Guidance/Manuals/downloads/pim83c06.pdf.

28. Centers for Medicare and Medicaid Services. (2010). *Medicare learning network: Medicare outpatient therapy billing*. Retrieved from http://www.cms.gov/Outreach-and-Education/Medicare-Learning-Network-MLN/MLNProducts/Downloads/Medicare_Outpatient_Therapy_Billing_ICN903663.pdf.

29. Cole, C. (n.d.). *Informed consent in people with Alzheimer's disease*. Retrieved from http://ana.nursingworld.org/MainMenuCategories/EthicsStandards/Resources/IssuesUpdate/UpdateArchive/IssuesUpdateSpringSummer2005/AlzheimersDisease.aspx.

30. College of Occupational Therapists. (2010). *Code of ethics and professional conduct*. Retrieved from http://www.cot.co.uk/sites/default/files/publications/public/Code-of-Ethics2010.pdf.

31. Coppersmith Gordon Schermer & Brockelman, P. L. C. (n.d.). *HITECH act expands HIPAA privacy and security rules*. Retrieved from http://www.azhha.org/member_and_media_resources/documents/HITECHAct.pdf.

32. Ga. Comp. R. & Regs. r. 43-28-16.

33. *Cruzan by Cruzan v. Director*, Missouri Dept. of Health, 110 S.Ct. 2841 (1990).

34. Cuff, P. A. (2013). *Interprofessional education for collaboration: Learning how to improve health from interprofessional models across the continuum of education to practice: Workshop summary*. Institute of Medicine. Retrieved from http://www.nap.edu/openbook.php?record_id=13486&page=R1.

35. Department of Health and Human Services. (2000). *Summary of the HIPPA privacy rule*. Retrieved from http://www.hhs.gov/ocr/privacy/hipaa/understanding/summary/privacysummary.pdf.

36. Department of Health and Human Services. (2007). *Security standards: Physical safeguards*. Retrieved from http://www.hhs.gov/ocr/privacy/hipaa/administrative/securityrule/physsafeguards.pdf.

37. Department of Justice. (2004). *Healthsouth to pay United States $325 million to resolve Medicare fraud allegations*. Retrieved from http://www.justice.gov/opa/pr/2004/December/04_civ_807.htm.

38. Dimick, D. (2010). Californian sentenced to prison for HIPAA violation. *Journal of AHIMA* [online journal]. Retrieved from http://journal.ahima.org/2010/04/29/californian-sentenced-to-prison-for-hipaa-violation/.

39. HPSO Risk Advisor. (2007). *Document defensively: Here's how*, 7, HPSO.

40. Faden, R., & Beauchamp, T. (1986). *A theory and history of informed consent*. New York, NY: Oxford University Press.

41. Federal Bureau of Investigation. (2009). *Doctor and two former hospital employees sentenced for HIPAA violations*. Retrieved from http://www.fbi.gov/littlerock/press-releases/2009/lr102609.htm.

42. Federal Patient Self Determination Act. (1990). Retrieved from http://euthanasia.procon.org/sourcefiles/patient_selfdetermination_act.pdf.

43. Garner, B. A. (Ed.). (2014). *Black's law dictionary* (10th ed.). St. Paul, MN: Thomson Reuters.

44. Guzman-Clark, J. R. S., Reinhardt, A. K., Wilkins-Schantz, S., & Castle, S. (2012). Decision-making capacity and conservatorship in older adults. *Annals of Long Term Care, 20*(9), 36–39.

45. Health Information Technology for Economic and Clinical Health Act (HITECH Act). (2009). Retrieved from http://www.hhs.gov/ocr/privacy/hipaa/understanding/coveredentities/hitechact.pdf.

46. HIPAA. (2005). *Everything you always wanted to know about HIPAA*. Retrieved from http://www.hopkinsmedicine.org/nursing/dry_run/benefits/hipaa_self_study_packet.pdf.

47. Hooper, C. R., & Bello-Haas, V. D. (2009). Sensory function. In B. R. Bonder & V. D. Bello-Haas (Eds.), *Functional performance in older adults* (3rd ed., pp. 101–128). Philadelphia, PA: F.A. Davis.

48. HPSO Risk Advisor. (2006). When and why you should apologize to patients. *HPSO Risk Advisor, 1*.

49. HPSO Risk Advisor. (2008). What to do when you make a clinical error. *HPSO Risk Advisor, 2, 1*.

50. Institute of Medicine. (1999). *To err is human: Building a safer health systems*. Washington DC: National Academy Press.

51. Jacobs, K., & McCormack, G. L. (2011). *The occupational therapy manager*. Bethesda, MD: AOTA Press.

52. NYU Langone Medical Center. (2011). *HIPAA security: Harsh fines, penalties are a wake-up call to us all*. Retrieved from http://compliance.med.nyu.edu/news/documenting-inpatient-admissions.

53. Leo, R. J. (1999). Competency and the capacity to make treatment decisions: A primer for primary care physicians. *Primary Care Companion Journal of Clinical Psychiatry, 1*(5), 131–141. Retrieved from http://www.ncbi.nlm.nih.gov/pmc/articles/PMC181079/.

54. Lohman, H., Mu, K., & Scheirton, L. (2003). Occupational therapists' perspectives on practice errors in geriatric practice settings. *Occupational Therapy in Geriatrics, 21*(4), 21–39.

55. Medicare Program Integrity Manual. (n.d.). Chapter 6: Intermediary MR Guidelines for Specific Services. Retrieved from http://www.cms.gov/Regulations-and-Guidance/Guidance/Manuals/downloads/pim83c06.pdf.

56. Medicinenet.com. (2013). *Definition of standard of care*. Retrieved from http://www.medterms.com/script/main/art.asp?articlekey=33263.

57. Morgan & Morgan Complex Litigation Group. (n.d.). *Whistle blower retaliation*. Retrieved from http://www.whistle-blower-attorneys.com/whistleblower-retaliation.html.

58. Mu, K., Lohman, H., Cochran, T., Scheirton, L., Coppard, B., & Kokesh, S. (2011). Improving client safety: Strategies to prevent and reduce practice errors in occupational therapy. *The American Journal of Occupational Therapy, 65*, e69–e76. doi:10.5014/ajot.2011.000562.

59. Mu, K., Lohman, H., & Scheirton, L. (2006). Occupational therapy practice errors in physical rehabilitation and geriatrics settings: A national survey study. *The American Journal of Occupational Therapy, 60*, 288–297.

60. National Board for Certification in Occupational Therapy. (2011). *Procedures for the enforcement of the NBCOT candidate/certificate code of conduct*. Retrieved from http://www.nbcot.org/pdf/Enforcement_Procedures.pdf.

61. National Center for Education Statistics. (2003). *The health literacy of America's adults: Results from the 2003 national assessment of adult literacy*. Washington, DC.

62. National Center on Elder Abuse. (n.d.). *Statistics/data*. Retrieved from http://www.ncea.aoa.gov/Library/Data/index.aspx.

63. National Center on Elder Abuse. (2009). *Homepage*. Retrieved from http://www.ncea.aoa.gov/NCEAroot/Main_Site/Index.aspx.

64. National Whistle Blowers Center. (2012). *False Claims Act/Qui Tam FAQ*. Retrieved from http://www.whistleblowers.org/index.php?Itemid=64&id=3.

65. Okonkwo, O., Griffith, H. R., Belue, K., Lanza, S., Zamrini, E. Y., Harrell, L. E., & Marson, D. C. (2007). Medical decision-making capacity in patients with mild cognitive impairment. *Neurology, 69*(15), 1528–1535.

66. Oxford English Dictionary. (2015). *Duty of care*. Retrieved from http://www.oxforddictionaries.com/us/definition/american_english/duty-of-care.

67. Pope, A. (n.d.). *An essay on criticism*. London: Printed for W.Lewis in Russel Street, Covent Garden; and Sold by W.Taylor at the Ship in Pater-Noster Row, T.Osborn near the Walks, and J. Graves in St. James Street. 1711. Retrieved 21 May 2015 via Google books.

68. Privacy Rights Clearing House. (2013). *HIPAA basics: Medical privacy in the electronic age*. Retrieved from https://www.privacyrights.org/fs/fs8a-hipaa.htm.

69. 40 Tex. Admin. Code § 374.1.

70. Scheirton, L. S., Mu, K., Lohman, H., & Cochran, T. M. (2007). Error and client safety: Ethical analysis of cases in occupational and physical therapy practice. *Medicine, Healthcare and Philosophy, 20*.

71. Searson, S., Hicks, Cole, J., Herzig, T., & Brooks, M. (2010). HIPAA for cancer educators: Are you correctly using PHI? *Journal of Cancer Education, 25*, 83–86.

72. Shalowitz, D. I., Garrett-Mayer, E., & Wendler, D. (2006). The accuracy of surrogate decision makers: A systematic review. *Archives of Internal Medicine, 166*, 493–497.

73. South, T. (2012). *Feds: Life care plan started at top*. Timesfreepress.com. Retrieved from http://www.timesfreepress.com/news/2012/dec/23/life-care-scheme-started-at-top-feds-say/.

74. Strauss, D. C., & Thomas, J. M. (2009). What does the medical profession mean by "standard of care"? *Journal of Clinical Oncology, 27*, e192–e193. Retrieved from http://jco.ascopubs.org/content/27/32/e192.

75. The Joint Commission. (2012). *National patient safety goals*, effective January 1, 2013. Retrieved from http://www.jointcommission.org/assets/1/18/NPSG_Chapter_Jan2013_HAP.pdf.

76. Ulrich, L. P. (1998). *The requirements of the patient self-determination*. Retrieved from http://academic.udayton.edu/lawrenceulrich/315psdame.htm.

77. U.S. Department of Education, Institute of Education Sciences, National Center for Education Statistics. (2003). *National assessment of adult literacy*. Retrieved from http://nces.ed.gov/naal/health_results.asp#AgeHealthLiteracy.

78. 31 U.S.C. §§ 3729-3733 (False Claims Act).

79. 31 U.S.C. §§ 3801-3802 (Program Fraud Civil Remedies Act).

80. 18 U.S.C. § 287.

81. Mish, F. C. (Ed.). (2003). *Merriam-Webster's Collegiate Dictionary* (11th ed.) Springfield, MA: Merriam-Webster, Inc., p. 704.

82. Winger, M. (2013). *HIPAA increases financial penalties for repeat violations to address increasing healthcare data breaches*. Retrieved from http://www.zephyrnetworks.com/hipaa-healthcare-data-breaches-financial-penalties/.

83. Wojcieszak, D., Banja, J., & Houk, C. (2006). The sorry works coalition: Making the case for full disclosure. *Joint Commission Journal on Quality and Patient Safety, 32*(6), 344–350.

84. World Health Organization. (2002). *Abuse of the elderly*. Retrieved from http://www.who.int/violence_injury_prevention/violence/world_report/factsheets/en/elderabusefacts.pdf.

CHAPTER 3

Looming Disease Burden Associated with the Aging Process: Implications for Occupational Therapy

Elena M. Andresen, PhD, Michael Bradley Cannell, PhD, Wajiha Z. Akhtar, PhD, Karen Frank Barney, PhD, OTR/L, FAOTA

CHAPTER OUTLINE

OBJECTIVES

- Introduce concepts that link public health and occupational therapy
- Discuss historic and current occupational therapy practice trends that emphasize these links
- Relate relevant theoretical models applied to public health and occupational therapy practice and research
- Describe the global aging and demographic population shifts currently under way
- Compare and contrast trends in health and aging between developed and developing nations
- Interpret predictions for the future of aging with special emphasis on the case of the United States
- Define major disease and health issues affecting aging and lifespan in the United States
- Define the context of aging, including the perspective of families and caregivers
- Articulate the significance and implications of the trends and predictions regarding aging populations in the United States and other countries for occupational therapy practice, research, and service

The population of our world is aging, a phenomenon that speaks of successes in improved health and longevity in both developed and developing nations. In considering the possibility that this trend could also seriously hamper our ability to provide health care and services to our populations, the phenomenon also might be termed a tsunami.

In this chapter, we describe the demographic shifts and their causes, and also the predictions about what the trends will produce during the twenty-first century. Furthermore, the case is made for an occupational therapy (OT) professional moral imperative to address the increased emerging needs of aging adult populations. Opportunities for intervention throughout the continuum of care will be emphasized, in order to support a steady state in the health of aging adults and overall quality of life for these older adults and their families or other support systems.

The experiences of aging, and the organization of health and social services for older adults, are quite different depending on the country or region of the globe. The probability of aging is very different in areas of Africa affected by the epidemic of human immunodeficiency virus (HIV) and acquired immunodeficiency syndrome (AIDS), natural disasters such as drought, and civil and military conflicts than in Western Europe or the United States, where both public health and health-care systems are complex and highly developed. However, there are broad differences in longevity and health within and among developed nations as well. Systems of health care and their financing may be highly centralized (e.g., Japan, Canada) or loosely defined "systems" and heterogeneously paid (e.g., the United States). Internal disparities between different groups also result from, and affect, how health care is delivered. This chapter provides an overview of the global experiences of aging; however, our focus case is the United States. This case allows us to more fully explore population perspectives of prevention relevant to the needs and problems related to older age and use extensive readily available data and statistics to demonstrate key issues.

As is discussed in more detail later in this chapter, the diseases of older age are primarily chronic diseases. Chronic diseases also make up the bulk of conditions that historically have involved gerontological occupational therapists in medical care settings, especially those working in home health, residential care, acute and subacute care, rehabilitation centers, skilled nursing facilities, and hospice programs. Prevention is a key concept for integrating gerontological OT with public health for chronic diseases. We introduce the public health model of prevention here so that OT roles that are described later in the chapter, such as promoting wellness and quality of life, can be set into a population perspective and in clinical and other forms of OT practice. Public health thinking about preventing and treating health conditions has moved to a socioecological framework in recent years.[16,17] This model of public health integrates aspects across the levels of individual, interpersonal, community, and society.

Although relatively new to public health disciplines, these concepts resonate with occupational science and OT science, because, for occupational therapists, intervention ideally occurs within the context of the client's environment. Prevention is considered at different levels in public health, and this perspective is especially useful in considering current health-care trends and the resulting expanded practice opportunities for occupational therapists working with aging populations.

Public health describes three different levels of prevention: primary, secondary, and tertiary.[9] When we seek to prevent disease at the primary level, for example, we reduce smoking or increase exercise to reduce the risk of heart disease. At the secondary level, early disease detection is important, so that we catch diseases at early stages when we can mitigate the effects. Mammography is a classic case of secondary prevention; early-stage breast cancers are easier to treat and women's outcomes are much better with early detection. Finally, when diseases and conditions are already advanced, we move to the tertiary level, where the goal is to mitigate complications and symptoms, and reduce mortality. For OT practice, these concepts are relevant before the more obvious stage of tertiary prevention. Tertiary prevention might mean mitigating the effects of stroke by improving a client's ability to perform self-care. However, each of the other prevention stages is also an OT opportunity. For someone with paralysis who uses a wheelchair, primary prevention may be directed at reducing the incidence of skin ulcers, contractures, diminished strength, and potential for diminished overall quality of life. Stroke survivors could be a target group for secondary prevention if a new technique for breast self-examination were promoted to improve women's abilities in early cancer detection, for example, and occupational therapists worked with clients to perform this examination manually, despite the clients' sensory and/or motor deficits or hemianopsia.

We reinforce the link between public health, chronic disease, and what occupational therapists treat and prevent in Table 3-1, which presents the 10 leading causes of mortality and the 10 leading conditions that result in disability. This focus on chronic diseases and older age is made especially relevant when examining the major causes of death in the United States. The mortality statistics in Table 3-1 combine data from all age groups in the United States, whereas the disability statistics focus on adults age 18 and older. The data in both lists make the point of the importance of chronic diseases. For mortality, eight of the 10 are chronic diseases, and flu, pneumonia, and septicemia are more likely to occur in people with existing chronic conditions. For disability, all are exclusively (or primarily) chronic diseases. Later in this chapter we also provide data from a comparison country, Turkey, with features of developing and developed nations.

TABLE 3-1 Leading Causes of Mortality and Disability in the United States

Leading Causes of Death (Deaths in 2013)*	Leading Causes of Disability (Estimated Population, 2005)+
Heart disease (611,105)	Arthritis or rheumatism (8,552,000)
Cancer (584,881)	Back or spine problems (7,589,000)
Chronic lower respiratory diseases (149,205)	Heart trouble (2,988,000)
Unintentional injuries (130,557)	Lung or respiratory problem (2,224,000)
Stroke (128,978)	Mental or emotional problem (2,203,000)
Alzheimer's disease (84,767)	Diabetes (2,012,000)
Diabetes (75,578)	Deafness or hearing problem (1,908,000)
Influenza and Pneumonia (56,979)	Stiffness or deformity of limbs/ extremities (1,627,000)
Kidney disease (47,112)	Blindness or vision problem (1,460,000)
Intentional self-harm-suicide (41,149)	Stroke (1,076,000)

*Source: National Center for Health Statistics (2013) *Deaths: Final data for 2013.* Retrieved from http://www.cdc.gov/nchs/fastats/leading-causes-of-death.htm (Accessed May 21, 2015.)
+Source: Centers for Disease Control and Prevention (2009). These are self-reported by persons in the Survey of Income and Program Participation (SIPP). Disability was defined as having difficulty with ADLs and IADLs.
Centers for Disease Control and Prevention (CDC) (2009). Prevalence and most common causes of disability among adults - United States, 2005. *Morbidity and Mortality Weekly Report, 58(16),* 421-426.

Population Demographic Shifts

Today, the older adult population (defined variously as age 60 or 65 years of age and over) is the largest it has ever been, and it is growing. As a starting place for the data on the global trend in aging, consider that the United Nations[33] reports that, globally, there were 205 million persons aged 60 and older in 1950. By 2013, the number had increased to 841 million. This trend is showing no signs of slowing, and the older population is expected to be the fastest-growing population worldwide for at least the next 50 years. Although aging is occurring in every region of the globe (Figure 3-1), it is not growing at the same rate or in the same time frame in all regions (Figures 3-2 and 3-3).

As is clearly demonstrated in Figure 3-2, the increase in the world population over age 65 is on a steep uphill slope, driven mostly by increases in this age group in the less developed nations. It is important to note that some are very rapidly developing nations such as China, India, and Brazil, to name a few. These three countries are still classified as less developed by the United Nations; however, their large populations and increasing average life expectancies still contribute to the rapidly growing older age group in the world. The more developed nations are also increasing in numbers of older adult individuals; however,

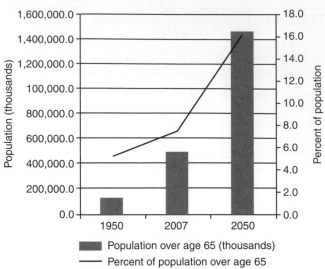

FIGURE 3-1 Population and percentage of population older than age 65: World, 1950, 2007, and projected for 2050. (Data from United Nations, Department of Economic and Social Affairs, Population Division. [2007]. *World population ageing 2007*. New York, NY: United Nations Publications.)

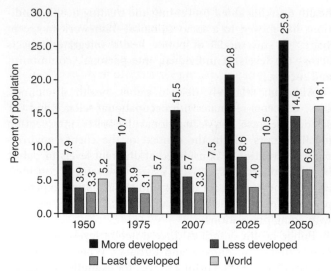

FIGURE 3-3 Percentage of population aged 65 or over by development area: 1950 to 2050. (Data from United Nations, Department of Economic and Social Affairs, Population Division. [2007]. *World population ageing 2007*. New York, NY: United Nations Publications.)

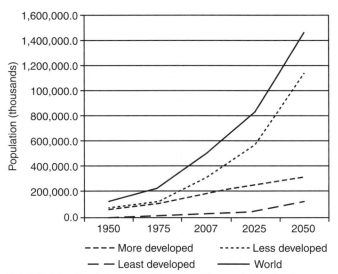

FIGURE 3-2 Population aged 65 or over (thousands) by development area: 1950 to 2050. (Data from United Nations, Department of Economic and Social Affairs, Population Division. [2007]. *World population ageing 2007*. New York, NY: United Nations Publications).

it is a much more gradual slope because much of the gain in longer life occurred decades ago. The same is true for the least developed nations, where life expectancy continues to be seriously compromised. Figure 3-3 shows the percentage of the population that is 65 and over in comparison with the estimated total number of people. This figure clearly shows that although the percentage of the population constituted by older adults is growing all over the world, the nations with the largest percentage of older adult population will remain in the more developed regions of the world for at least the next 50 years due to the much longer life expectancy of individuals in these regions.

All of the graphs and tables presented here demonstrate a concept that is central to this chapter. Population aging, simply

put, is the process by which older individuals become a proportionally larger share of the total population.[33] Generally speaking, the more developed a country is, the further along it is in the process of having an aging population.

Variation in the population-aging phenomenon is also shown in Table 3-2, which notes the percentage of the population age 65 or over for selected countries. There was significant variation in the age structures of these countries in the year 2000, with Japan having 17% of its population over the age of 65 and Nigeria having just 3%. The difference becomes even more striking when looking at the numbers projected for 2050. Japan will have an astonishing 36.4% of its population over age 65, whereas in Nigeria, the percentage will have only increased to 6.8%. The special case of Japan is raised again later in this chapter in the context of culture, aging, and caregiving.

Another way that we can visualize the phenomenon of population aging and differences among countries is through the use of a special type of chart known as a population

TABLE 3-2 Percent of Population Aged 65 or Over, Selected Countries: 1950, 2000, 2025, 2050

	1950	2000	2025	2050
United States	8.3%	12.3%	18.5%	21.1%
Bolivia	3.5%	4.0%	6.1%	11.6%
Egypt	3.0%	4.1%	7.6%	14.5%
India	3.3%	5.0%	8.3%	14.8%
Japan	4.9%	17.2%	28.9%	36.4%
Mexico	4.4%	4.7%	9.3%	18.6%
Nigeria	3.0%	3.0%	3.8%	6.8%
Poland	5.2%	12.1%	20.2%	27.9%
World	5.2%	6.9%	10.4%	15.6%

From Plassman BL, Langa KM, Fisher GG,, et al: Prevalence of dementia in the United States: The Aging, Demographics, and Memory Study, Neuroepidemiology 2007;29(1-2):125-132 pyramid. Population pyramids graphically show the age and sex structure of a country. Traditionally, there is a fairly even distribution of males and females protruding laterally from the center of the graph, as well as a large base of people in the younger age groups, tapering vertically to fewer people in the oldest age groups. This structure is what gives the population pyramid its name. As we have discussed, however, the population structure is changing, and the shapes of population pyramids are changing as well.

The more traditional-looking shape is said to be expansive: There are many more young people in the population than old, which is a pattern generally observed as a less developed nation is expanding. Figures 3-4 and 3-5 highlight the past, current, and projected future differences in the aging structures of the more developed and least developed parts of the world. In 1950 both the least developed and more developed parts of the world exhibited an expansive pyramid structure; however, the more developed regions were already beginning to change. By the year 2000, there was a very clear difference between the age structures in the two areas. Whereas the least developed nations continue to exhibit the expansive structure, the more developed nations are clearly constrictive—they begin to look like a "column" of age groups. Finally, according to the projections for the year 2050, the more developed regions will be stationary in structure, whereas the least developed nations will begin to transition from an expansive to a constrictive structure. However, the rate of aging in the less developed regions of the globe is expected to outpace that of more developed regions in the next 50 years.[33]

Driving Forces

The health and demographic forces that lead to these different population pyramids are fertility rates, mortality rates, and longevity of older adults. As a result of decreases in the first two and increases in the latter, we see an aging of the population, and an increase in chronic diseases. As shown in Figure 3-6, these trends are observable. Life expectancy at birth has been, on average, rising steadily since 1950. Additionally, the world fertility rate has been declining since 1950; however, its rate of decline has started to slow somewhat. Add these trends to reductions in late-life mortality, and it is no wonder that the world's population is aging.

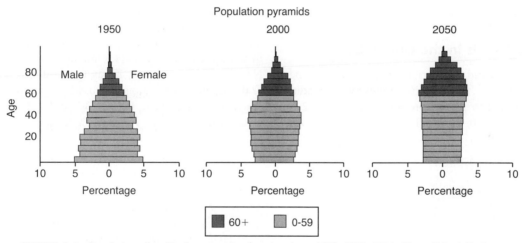

FIGURE 3-4   Population pyramids for more developed nations: 1950, 2000, 2050. (From United Nations, Department of Economic and Social Affairs, Population Division. (2007). World Population Ageing 2007. New York, NY: United Nations Publications.)

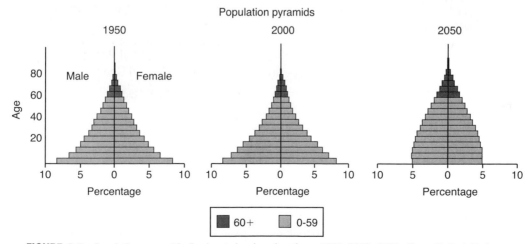

FIGURE 3-5   Population pyramids for least developed nations: 1950, 2000, 2050. (From United Nations, Department of Economic and Social Affairs, Population Division. (2007). World Population Ageing 2007. New York, NY: United Nations Publications.)

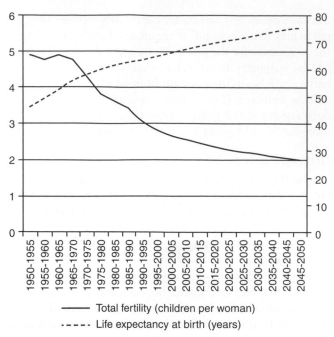

FIGURE 3-6 World fertility and life expectancy, 1950 to 2050. (Data from Population Division of the Department of Economic and Social Affairs of the United Nations Secretariat. *World population prospects: The 2008 revision.*)

Demographic Trends in the United States

Just as the rest of the world is experiencing population aging, so too is the United States. In the United States the older adult population is expected to grow from 43 million in 2012 to about 80 million in 2040, at which time older adults will

make up about 21% of the population.[1] The number of people aged 85 and over is expected to grow from approximately 6 million (1.9% of the population) to approximately 14 million (3.7% of the population).[1]

One interesting contributor to this demographic shift is the phenomenon we call the "baby boom" generation, resulting from a sharp increase in fertility after World War II. People born between 1946 and 1965 make up the baby boom generation. The oldest of the baby boomers turned 65 in 2011, and the youngest of them will be 65 by 2030. Not only is this a large cohort of individuals, it is also unique in the history of the United States (and other developed Western nations) in terms of increased levels of education, wealth, and diversity. Baby boomers are also unique in the fact that they have significantly fewer children than did previous generations. All of these factors have important implications for each level of prevention (discussed earlier), and clinical care. As described by the Institute on Aging, people in the United States aged 65 and older "will be markedly different from previous generations, with higher levels of education, lower levels of poverty, more racial and ethnic diversity, and fewer children."[19]

Population aging can also be considered at the subcountry level. Even in the United States, the proportion of older persons in the population varies considerably by state, with some states experiencing much greater growth in their older populations. In 2012 about half (51%) of persons aged 65+ lived in nine states: California (4.6 million), Florida (3.5 million), New York (2.8 million), Texas (2.8 million), Pennsylvania (2.0 million), and Illinois, Ohio, Michigan, and New Jersey (each over 1 million).[1] Figures 3-7 and 3-8 provide graphic information about the variations among states.

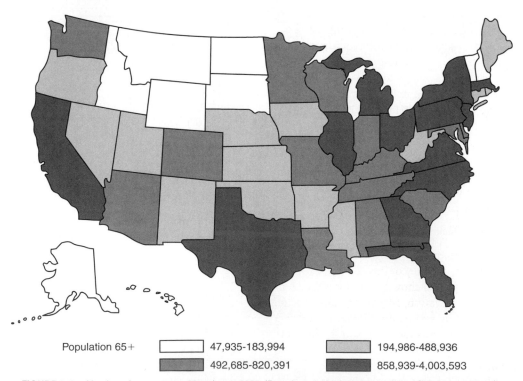

FIGURE 3-7 Number of persons age 65 and over, 2007. (Data from Administration on Aging. [2009, July 16]. U.S. population estimates for states by age: July 1, 2007. Retrieved from http://www.aoa.acl.gov/Aging_Statistics/Profile/2008/docs/2008profile.xls.)

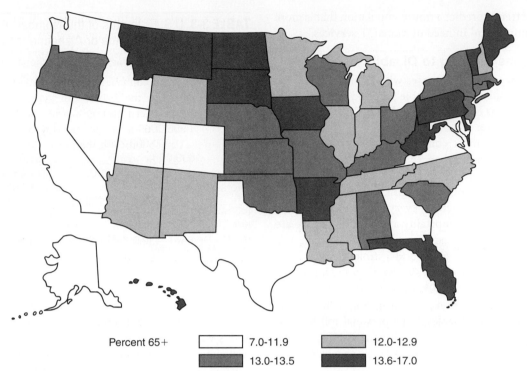

Percent 65+		
☐ 7.0-11.9	☐ 12.0-12.9	
☐ 13.0-13.5	☐ 13.6-17.0	

FIGURE 3-8   Percentage of population 65 and over, 2007. (Data from Administration on Aging. [2009]. U.S. population estimates for states by age: July 1, 2007. Retrieved from http://www.aoa.acl.gov/Aging_Statistics/Profile/2008/docs/2008profile.xls.)

Disability in the United States

Chronic physical, mental, and emotional conditions can limit the ability of adults to perform important basic activities of daily living (ADLs) and instrumental activities of daily living (IADLs), such as working and doing everyday household chores. With advancing age, an increasing percentage of adults experiences limitation of activity.[35] In the United States we have a wealth of data to help us describe the health of our population over time. There is actually good news from these data. The National Health Interview Survey (NHIS),[26] National Long Term Care Survey (NLTCS),[27] and Survey of Income and Program Participation (SIPP)[34] all indicate that since the 1980s there has been a decline in the relative percentage of individuals needing help with self-care (ADLs and IADLs).[15] Unfortunately, because of demographic shifts, the absolute numbers of older adults with limitations are still on the rise. The NLTCS also demonstrates that along with the decline in the percentage of those with limitations, there has been an increase in the severity of those limitations.[15] Census Bureau data (Survey of Income and Program Participation [SIPP]) from 2010 show that among the civilian noninstitutionalized population, 18.7% had some level of disability and 12.6% had a severe disability.[5] Figure 3-9 shows that, not surprisingly, the older a person is, the more likely he or she is to develop disability, severe disability, and the need for assistance.

Looking again at Figure 3-1, this dramatic increase in both crude numbers of individuals and percentage of the population age 65 and over is evident. Although the population of

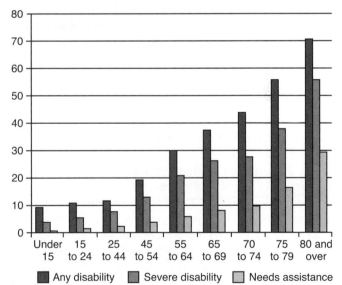

FIGURE 3-9   Disability prevalence and the need for assistance, by age, 2005. Note: The need for assistance with activities of daily living was not asked of children under 6 years. (Data from Brault, M. W. *Americans with disabilities: 2005. Current population reports, P70-117.* Washington, DC: U.S. Census Bureau, 2008.)

those 65 and over increased roughly fivefold in the 57 years between 1950 and 2007, it is projected to increase by almost thirtyfold in the next 43 years. Not only are the total numbers projected to rise, but there is also clearly a dramatic increase in the slope of the line showing the percentage of the population over age 65 compared with younger age groups. Taken together, these trends predict a future population that is more functionally limited and in need of more OT services.

Key Conditions Leading to Disability

We highlight three chronic diseases with high prevalence in gerontological populations (see Table 3-1) and with very different needs in terms of gerontological OT. These are stroke, arthritis, and dementia.

Stroke is the fifth most common cause of death in the United States, killing more than 128,978 people in 2013, the most current year for which complete data are available.[35] The American Heart Association estimates that someone in America has a stroke, on average, every 40 seconds.[3] Perhaps even more important than mortality as a result of stroke are the other costs to survivors, caregivers, and the nation as a whole. In addition to its financial costs, stroke clearly affects quality of life. Among those who survive a stroke, functional limitations affect as many as 20% of survivors at a level that requires institutional care after 3 months: 15% to 30% of survivors are permanently disabled.[3] The personal toll is highlighted by a study by Samsa and colleagues (1998),[31] who found that 45% of those at risk of stroke view survivorship as an outcome worse than death.

Demographic factors contribute to stroke risk. Age increases risk (8% of adults over 65 versus less than 1% of adults 18 to 44), as does being a member of an ethnic or racial minority. Native American, multiracial, and African American groups are at higher risk of stroke compared with white and Asian Americans.[14] Stroke rehabilitation needs are expansive and varied. Based on the population sample of adults in the Framingham Heart Study, among ischemic stroke survivors who were aged 65 and over, about 50% had some hemiparesis, 35% had depressive symptoms, 30% were unable to walk without some assistance, 26% were dependent in activities of daily living, 26% were institutionalized in a nursing home, and 19% experienced aphasia.[32]

Another common condition that contributes to functional impairment is arthritis.[35] Reports by the Centers for Disease Control and Prevention (CDC) based on results from the 2012 National Health Interview Survey (NHIS)[26] are that "21% of adults had ever been told by a doctor or other health care professional that they had some form of arthritis, rheumatoid arthritis, gout, lupus, or fibromyalgia, and 26% had chronic joint symptoms (e.g., pain or stiffness in or around a joint in the past 30 days that began more than 3 months ago)."[26]

As with stroke, incidence of arthritis increases with age, and 49% of adults of age 75 are diagnosed as having arthritis compared with 7% of adults 18 to 44 years of age. Arthritis also is more common among women (59% of cases), and among Native Americans, African Americans, and Caucasian Americans as compared with Asian Americans.[26] Risk factors for arthritis and arthritis-attributable activity limitation include obesity and physical inactivity. Obese individuals are almost twice as likely to report arthritis (29.3%) than are normal-weight individuals (17.4%).[13]

TABLE 3-3 U.S. Estimates of the Number of Individuals with Dementia or Alzheimer's Disease, 2002

Age (years)	All dementia Number (95% CI)	Alzheimer's disease Number (95% CI)
71-79	712,000 (375,000-1,050,000)	332,000 (181,000-483,000)
80-89	1,996,000 (1,590,000-2,401,000)	1,493,000 (1,111,000-1,875,000)
90+	699,000 (476,000-922,000)	2,381,000 (1,849,000-2,913,000)
Total	3,407,000 (2,793,000-4,021,000)	2,381,000 (1,849,000-2,913,000)

Note: CI=confidence interval
Data from Plassman, B. L., Langa, K. M., Fisher, G. G., Heeringa, S. G., Weir, D. R., Ofstedal, M. B., et al. (2007). Prevalence of dementia in the United States: The Aging, Demographics, and Memory Study. *Neuroepidemiology*, 29(1-2) 125-132.

Dementia diagnoses also increase markedly with age. Dementia is a category of diseases that shares some similar signs and symptoms. The most common type of dementia is Alzheimer's disease, which accounts for 60% to 80% of cases.[2] Current estimates indicate that someone in the United States develops Alzheimer's disease every 67 seconds, and this number is expected to increase to every 33 seconds by the middle of the twenty-first century.[2] Dementia is very much an experience of aging populations and contributes to an increasing strain on health-care dollars, supportive care, and families, in addition to the individual's own experiences.

The Aging, Demographics, and Memory Study (ADAMS) has added significantly to our understanding of dementia at the population level in the United States.[29] ADAMS is a population-based study of dementia that includes individuals from all regions of the United States and aims to determine the prevalence of dementia. Based on ADAMS data (Table 3-3), 13.9% of all Americans age 71 and older have some form of dementia. However, there is a steep increase in prevalence during the eighth and ninth decades of life, and among those 90 years old, 37.4% have some form of dementia.[29] The study found no significant difference in rate of dementia between men and women. However, because there are more women among the oldest old, there are more women living with dementia.[2,29] A few risk factors that have been consistently associated with dementia other than age are lack of physical activity, lower levels of education, and presence of the APOE ε4 genotype.[29]

The Future of Disability in the United States

The Institute of Medicine recently tackled issues and predictions about disability.[18] The estimates of this 2007 report are that between 40 and 50 million Americans today are living with some type of disability or activity limitation.[18] Combining an aging population and an increase of disability with age means that the United States will continue to face increases in the sheer numbers of people and older adults with disability.

Alarmingly, this report also suggests that people now in the middle years are less healthy than earlier cohorts were, for example, because of increasing obesity. If this trend continues, the previous trend of decreasing disability prevalence in older age will be reversed and baby boomers will contribute to an increasing number and percentage of adults with disability.

Obesity as a Contributing Factor

The prevalence of certain conditions that contribute to disability—notably, physical inactivity, diabetes, and obesity—increases with older age. However, surveys also show a worrisome increase in overweight or obesity among children, young adults, and middle-aged adults. Based on childhood obesity rates, the future of disability prevalence is bleak.[18] Obesity is one of the most important, widespread, and costly epidemics the United States currently faces, and will in all likelihood continue to face for the foreseeable future. According to the CDC,[6] the prevalence of obesity has been steadily increasing for the past 30 years; approximately 15% of adults in 1976 to 1980 were obese, and the number increased to 32.9% in the 2003 to 2004 survey.[13] During the same time period, the prevalence of overweight for children aged 2 to 5 years increased from 5% to 13.9%.[14]

There is research into, and predictions about, both the long- and short-term implications of the U.S. obesity epidemic. One consequence is that we are now seeing diseases in children that were once thought to only afflict adults. Stephen R. Daniels discusses the effect of obesity on children's cardiovascular systems, metabolic systems, pulmonary systems, gastrointestinal systems, musculoskeletal systems, and psyche, and the economy. One very telling example to illustrate this point is the increase of children, some as young as 8 years old, with type 2 diabetes, once referred to as adult-onset diabetes.[14]

Obesity and overweight increase risk for many other chronic diseases and disabilities, including heart disease, high blood pressure, stroke, cancers, gallbladder disease, obstructive sleep apnea syndrome, metabolic syndrome, and general functional limitations, and adversely affect quality of life.[30] Therefore obesity should be regarded as one of the most significant influences on the future health, disability status, and quality of life of older adults in the United States. Obesity trends in other developed nations suggest an increasing global concern as well.

CASE EXAMPLE 3-1   Morbidity and Mortality in Turkey

Modern Turkey is a nation of nearly 82 million people that provides a mixed example of health care and population structure in regard to aging (see the Central Intelligence Agency [CIA] *Factbook* for more country details[8]). The country moved rapidly into a secular parliamentary structure beginning in 1923, unifying primarily Muslim groups that were part of the Ottoman Empire. Infrastructure developments including health-care facilities and delivery of universal health care have continued to be challenging. Turkey is about the size of the U.S. state of Texas and includes remote rural areas with sparse populations. It is bordered by countries that have had sustained military or civil conflicts that affect the health and health care of the citizens of the bordering nations (examples include Bulgaria, Georgia, Iran, and Iraq). Turkey has negotiated to be a candidate for joining the European Union and continues to work on aspects of its development that provide for equality of opportunity in health and health care. The country currently has an age structure that is 7% older adult (aged 65 and older) and 26% younger than age 15; the United States, in comparison, is at 15% and 19%, respectively.[8] Life expectancy at birth is 73 years, as compared with 80 in the United States. Twenty-six percent of the population is engaged in agriculture, as compared with less than 1% in the United States, and 73% of the population currently is urban.

Unlike countries like the United States, ongoing systematic heath surveillance and mortality data are not readily available. In order to have a more accurate representation of mortality and causes of death, the Turkish government conducted in-person surveys of 12,000 randomly selected households and augmented this with a registry of deaths.[23] Although infectious diseases are still common, the people of Turkey, especially in urban areas, are more likely to develop chronic conditions similar to those seen in developed nations. The 2002 report demonstrated the strong contribution of chronic conditions to mortality and morbidity (using a statistic called disability-adjusted life years that combines across both). Among the top 20 conditions, most resonate with the causes listed earlier in Table 3-1, for example, heart disease, stroke, cancer, arthritis, and mental health conditions. However, also included were conditions like diarrheal diseases, tuberculosis, and lower respiratory infections. In summarizing the findings, the Turkish government described differences between Turkish citizens' health and that of residents of other nations. Rural Turkish people have a preponderance of chronic diseases contributing to mortality and morbidity (62.2%); however, this compares to 78.2% for developed nations. The comparison to developing nations is sobering: In this group of countries, only about 40% of mortality and morbidity is due to chronic conditions, and much of the remainder is due to communicable diseases and maternal child health conditions that are much less common in developed nations. Turkey is thus a nation with similarities to both developing and developed nations, and its health care development, including aspects of rehabilitation and occupational therapy, will continue to need to breach these differences.

Selected Global Issues

Considerations of Caregiving

As the previous sections demonstrate, the global population is aging. Even with considerable intervention to promote healthy aging, the increase in sheer numbers of persons who live into advanced age suggests there is now, and will continue to be, an effect on caregiving at both the societal and family levels. More and more of our older adults rely on informal caregivers to assist in many of their everyday activities. When considering the effects of global aging, OT providers need to include considerations of the effects of clients on their larger social and family support systems (see Case Examples 3-2and 3-3).

CASE EXAMPLE 3-2   Caregiving in the United States

Data from the United States provide information on informal caregiving arrangements. According to the National Alliance for Caregiving (NAC), informal U.S. caregivers contribute 257 billion unpaid dollars annually. In the NAC random-digit-dialed survey, caregivers were defined as individuals 18 years of age or older who provided assistance with one or more ADLs or IADLs to an adult 18 years of age or older.[25] The NAC estimated that there are 44.4 million caregivers in the United States (21% of the adult population). This number equates to 22.9 million households. Based on the NAC definition of caregiving, fully one quarter of the caregivers of adults aged 60 and older reported that they provided care for someone with cognitive impairment. Also important, the NAC demonstrated that caregivers who had higher levels of caregiving (measured in terms of time and activities) also had poorer outcomes, for example, physical, emotional, and financial strains.

The Behavioral Risk Factors Surveillance System (BRFSS)[7] is another source of data that provides periodic reports on U.S. caregiving. The BRFSS is an ongoing state-based telephone survey conducted by the CDC that collects information on "health-related risk behaviors, chronic health conditions, and use of preventive services."[7] In 2000, a single BRFSS question asked about caregiving of adults aged 60 and older.[22] The prevalence of caregiving varied considerably. Nationally, 15.6% of adults reported they were caregivers. However, the levels were highest in the southeastern states where chronic conditions also are high (for example, 21.2% in Missouri, and 20.4% in West Virginia), and caregiving rates were the lowest in the far West (for example, Alaska, 9.9%; Hawaii, 10.5%).

Following this brief national query into caregiving, a number of states added a module of questions on caregiving to the BRFSS during 2006 to 2009.[4,12,13,24,28] The BRFSS defined caregivers as any person 18 years of age or older who provides care or assistance to a family member or friend, of any age, because of illness or disability. BRFSS estimates of caregiving ranged from 11.0% to 15.5% depending on the state.[12,13,28] In these expanded inquiries, caregivers reported that their role increased their own health, social, and economic problems. When asked the greatest difficulties from caregiving, the majority of respondents reported that caregiving creates stress, leaves too little time for self or family, and creates a financial burden. In combination with NAC data, these results suggest that caregiving is a common role and that although this role provides invaluable assistance for the recipients, it comes at a personal and perhaps societal cost.

Global estimates of the frequency of caregiving are not available. It is likely that the prevalence, effects, and importance of caregiving are at least as varied globally as they are among U.S. states. Social and cultural norms and traditions, women's work and family roles, geographic dispersement of nuclear families—all of these play some role in determining the likelihood that a person who ages with the need for assistance will have informal (family or neighborhood) support versus formal assistance.

CASE EXAMPLE 3-3   Caregiving in Japan

As noted earlier, Japan experienced dramatic increases in its older adult population following World War II. In 1950 about 4.9% of the population were older adults. In 1995 it was 12.8%, and in 2025 the projection is that 25% of the population of Japan will be aged 65 or older.[38] This gives Japan the distinction of having the oldest population in the world.[33] Although this is a marker of a successful society, there are also accompanying problems. Persons with dementia, for example, are projected to number 2.62 million by 2015.[38]

Japanese culture sets care of the aged as a responsibility of the succeeding generation. These expectations are part of cultural standards related to the patrilineal extended family.[38] Traditionally, as a couple aged, their first son's wife was expected to fulfill all the hands-on caregiving responsibilities for her parents-in-law.[38] This tradition has been successful even considering social changes in Japanese families. In 1992, 33.4% of older adults who were seriously limited (labeled "bedridden") were not institutionalized and were cared for by spouses of their children.[38] There have been significant social changes in women's roles in Japan in recent decades. About 12 million women were estimated to work outside the home in 1975, and by 1993, the estimate was 20 million.[38] There was an accompanying decline in the number of households that included three generations (19.2% in 1970 versus 12.5% in 1995).[38] More recently, men have taken on more of the caregiving role, so that they now constitute 15% of caregivers to older adults in Japan.[21] The demographic result is that the number of senior citizens living alone has quadrupled in the last two decades (611,000 to 2,360,000), suggesting that the traditional role of daughters-in-law is no longer a universal social assumption.[21]

Implications for Occupational Therapy Service Delivery

This epidemiologic foundation provides an understanding of changing U.S. and global demographics and associated current and projected effects on the incidence of disease and disability over time. The discussion specifically provides the history and projections of aging-associated morbidity and mortality to provide a basis for reflection regarding what types of OT interventions are needed currently and will be needed in the future. Furthermore, the knowledge shared on age-related disease and disability risk factors serves to inform OT personnel in reinforcing the use of health-supporting and health-promoting interventions. This information requires us to examine our current interventions to determine whether they address the current and emerging needs of the aging individuals and communities being served. In addition, the disease and disability risk data provide a roadmap for the development of new therapeutic approaches. We are called to apply continuous surveillance of both historical and new disease and disability patterns as they emerge. As holistic, quality-of-life-supporting practitioners, OT personnel are equipped to integrate this information into the changing health-care systems environment in any era. In doing so, the profession can also serve on the forefront of meeting the changing needs of society.

As indicated earlier, occupational services have historically been predominantly provided within medical health-care delivery systems (refer also to Chapter 23 on health-care systems). Community-based services providing home health care and support systems for individuals with mental illness have been available since the 1920s in the United States; however, these have been limited in scope and capacity for reimbursement. In 1978 the World Health Organization convened an international conference on primary health care that resulted in a declaration that health is a fundamental right of people around the globe.[37] The influence of this declaration, the implications of the changing demographics and related disease burden reported earlier, and the evolving health-care systems globally indicate expanded opportunity for occupational therapy personnel (OTP)—both occupational therapists and OT

assistants. Because demographic trajectories suggest increased numbers of aging adults and associated chronic conditions in both developed and developing countries, OTP are called to address health-related aging issues in health-promoting modes across the continuum of care. Nearly 50 years ago Leavell and Clark proposed an epidemiologic model of preventive medicine that covered the entire continuum of medical care (1965) and is well suited to the thinking of today with regard to the emphasis on health-promoting services.[20] Figure 3-10, based on Leavell and Clark's model, depicts the role of occupational therapy in health promotion activities throughout the continuum of care. To align with the age-related forecasts regarding disease, disability, morbidity, and mortality, OT providers can revise their clinical reasoning processes and their orientation to the provision of services. These can be expanded to "professional reasoning" and a health-promoting orientation, both of which fit all types of settings, whether clinical or community based. Furthermore, around the world and in the United States, the health-care reform era holds all providers accountable for population health—that of the communities served. Thus this adaptation is required in order to better serve the needs of individuals, communities, and other populations with whom OTP interact. Developed countries outside of the United States with government-funded health-care systems already have incorporated many of these elements and roles. Important health-promoting lessons may be learned from them because their morbidity and mortality rates are currently better than those of the United States.[36]

Occupational Therapy in Community-Based Primary Prevention

Until recently in the United States, most OT providers had not participated in primary care types of services. For at least 20 years, a few entrepreneurial therapists have engaged in health-promoting and health-protecting interventions in their private practices, which have addressed the needs of individuals and communities across the lifespan. The field of occupational therapy has always been inherently holistic, and can therefore address the primary health-promoting needs of aging populations.

Gerontological occupational therapy service opportunities				
No disease or condition identified		Disease or condition diagnosed		
Health promotion interventions	Specific protection and prompt treatment	Early diagnosis and prompt treatment	Disability limitation	Rehabilitation
Primary prevention		Secondary prevention		Tertiary prevention
Public health practice		Primary medical care	Secondary medical care	Long-term care/ hospice
Community-oriented		Individual and community orientation		Dual emphasis

FIGURE 3-10 Health promotion throughout the continuum of care. (Modified from Leavell, H. R., & Clark, E. G. [1965]. *Preventive medicine for the doctor in his community: An epidemiologic approach* [3rd ed.]. New York, NY: Blakiston-McGraw Hill.)

An example of a long-term, well-established health-promoting service agency for aging adults is Independent Living, Inc. (ILI). ILI was established in 1967 by Jean Kiernat, Betty Hasselkus, faculty at the University of Wisconsin–Madison, and social workers in Dane County, Wisconsin. These OT visionaries understood the concepts of occupational performance and engagement, and the social support needs of aging adults. Thus they founded ILI to provide services so that older adults could remain living at home for as long as possible. Initial OT services included home safety assessments and interventions by OTPs, as well as social work support services. These later evolved so that an *OTR* and a certified occupational therapy assistant (COTA) supervised a carpenter who made grab bar installations and built chair and sofa extenders, before their commercial availability. Services were initially funded by grants or contracts, and additionally included consultations and interventions to adapt the living environments of aging residents of congregate living facilities. Adaptations included a range of modifications, including adding or adjusting lighting, highlighting stair edges and appliances to accommodate age-related vision changes, supplying adaptive equipment for bathrooms, and educating residents on safety precautions to prevent falls and other injuries. Serving all of Dane County, Wisconsin, ILI has expanded and has continued to provide health-promoting services for 40 years.

An innovative and life-enriching community-based program for aging adults, OASIS, in St. Louis, Missouri, was established by an adult educator, Marylen Mann, in consultation with Carolyn Baum, of Washington University in 1982. OASIS initially began in a May Department Store in St. Louis. Over the years it expanded to sites throughout the United States and includes classes, intergenerational activities, and other health-promoting activities for adults of age 50 and over.

The Well Elderly series of randomized control trials, conducted by Florence Clark and her University of Southern California OT faculty associates, has demonstrated the effectiveness and the efficacy of OT intervention with independently living aging adults. These trials have continued since findings were first published in 1997 and have provided much needed evidence to support the role of OT in health promotion and reduced morbidity among multicultural study participants.[10,11] Overall findings have consistently demonstrated the effect of OT health promotion interventions on health and age-related changes, which typically result in functional decline. Their studies for the past two decades have used state-of-the-art interdisciplinary research design, including biomarker and quality-of-life measurement. Consistent results include improvement in general health and vitality, function, and quality-of-life domains.[10,11]

The American Occupational Therapy Association CarFit program is another example of a primary health promotion effort tailored for OT personnel to engage with aging adults in promoting driver, passenger, and societal safety. The program provides information and materials on resources that can enhance aging drivers' occupational performance and safety, and potentially increase their community mobility, thus positively affecting IADL function. (See also chapters 20 and 21).

Occupational Therapy in Secondary Prevention Services

Occupational therapy has played a role in community programs providing secondary prevention services for the Arthritis Foundation throughout the United States for at least four decades. These have primarily consisted of classes to educate groups and individuals with arthritis diagnoses about how to manage their lives despite their disease process. Classes led by OTs teach and promote joint protection techniques, assist in organizing activities to promote energy conservation, promote arthritis-related exercise and swim programs, and coach regarding strategies to plan older adults' everyday lives to include meaningful occupational balance.

In addition, OT has been instrumental in developing programs for early intervention for aging adults with mild cognitive impairment that evolved into different forms of dementia, including Alzheimer's disease. Throughout the years of increasing organizational development, occupational therapists have paired with the national and local Alzheimer's Association offices to plan and conduct numerous programs. These programs target the unique and diverse needs of those with dementia and their families and caregivers to support overall function and quality of life for all who are involved.

Occupational therapists serve on planning committees and as providers for other organizations that serve the more specific needs of those with dementia and their family and other support networks. They assist in determining and tailoring environmental and other cognitive supports for this population, including their caregivers.

Occupational Therapy Health Promotion in Tertiary Care

Tertiary prevention in rehabilitation and long-term care and hospice care settings is individually oriented and tailored to the specific needs of the individual, family, and/or other supports. Historically, regarding implementation of services for this population, the profession has typically thought of this aspect of care as medical treatment. However, based upon Leavell and Clark's epidemiologic model of preventive medicine, tertiary care should also be considered for health promotion interventions. Throughout the intervening years since its development, as thinking about supports for quality of life and cost containment evolved, this model has stood the test of time and thus represents a "goodness of fit" with ethical, economic, and quality-of-life approaches to health care. Thus we are challenged to view all levels of care as opportunities for health promotion, and OT is especially well aligned to meet this challenge. Hence, whether services are provided for an aging individual who sustained a hip or Colles fracture, cerebrovascular accident, or spinal cord injury, or who is certified for hospice care, a health promotion approach is optimal. Through a holistic approach in collaboration with the client and significant others, occupational therapists strive for creative problem solving and meaningful goals for each individual served.

REVIEW QUESTIONS

1. The population pyramid for developed nations is distinguished by which of the following?
   a. An inverse triangle, with more older adults than children
   b. A "column" with similar numbers of people across the age groups
   c. A bottom-heavy triangle with more young people than older people
   d. More developed and less developed nations having similar-looking population pyramids
2. The dramatic historical shifts in the age of the world population are the result of which factor?
   a. The move from infectious diseases to chronic conditions
   b. Decreased fertility rates
   c. Increased life expectancy
   d. All of these
3. In developed nations like the United States and countries in Western Europe, the current emphases on independent living for older adults will result in
   a. most rehabilitation taking place in the community.
   b. a mix of rehabilitation settings (e.g., acute care, nursing homes, outpatient centers, and the community).
   c. an increase in comorbidities.
4. _____ is the leading cause of mortality in the United States.
   a. Stroke
   b. Cancer
   c. Heart disease
   d. Alzheimer's disease
5. Which of the following is an example of a primary prevention intervention?
   a. Promoting a new technique for breast self-examination to improve women's abilities in early cancer detection
   b. Recommending barrier-free home adaptations for a person in a wheelchair to prevent and educate for possible obstacles and accidents
   c. Improving self-care for a client after a cerebral hemorrhage
   d. Screening a client with the Modified Mini-Mental State Examination to detect a decline in cognitive function
6. What characteristic of the baby boom generation is **not** different from characteristics of previous generations?
   a. Lower levels of poverty
   b. Fewer children
   c. More racial diversity
   d. More children
7. Which of the following is a reason why obesity should be regarded as one of the most significant influences on the future health and disability status of individuals in the United States and other developed nations, and quality of life in these nations?
   a. Obesity is a contributing factor to an array of chronic diseases.
   b. Obesity is completely preventable.
   c. Over the last 40 years the prevalence of obesity has increased by 10%.
   d. Scientists agree that the increase in childhood obesity will result in an end to the steady increase in life expectancy seen in recent years.
8. Which of the following is **not** a reason why Turkey can be characterized as a developing and developed nation?
   a. Turkey is run by two forms of government: secular and nonsecular.
   b. Maternal and child health conditions are not comparable to those of developed nations.
   c. Communicable diseases are still common in Turkey.
   d. Prevalence of chronic diseases in Turkish people is similar to that of individuals in developed nations.
9. In the BRFSS study, levels of caregiving were highest in southeastern U.S. states. This finding parallels what other (linked) southeastern characteristic?
   a. These states are characterized by low poverty rates.
   b. The BRFSS asks more questions about caregiving in the southeastern states compared with the rest.
   c. Of the caregivers of adults aged 60 and older in the southeastern states, 70% reported that they provided care for someone with cognitive impairment.
   d. Chronic diseases are more common (prevalence and incidence) in these states.
10. T F Health promotion as an OT approach is most appropriately applied throughout the continuum of care of services for young age groups, when the potential for growth is greatest.
11. T F Occupational therapy health promotion strategies emphasize prevention of psychological and physical deterioration via occupations.
12. T F Gerontological occupational therapy services have historically been provided primarily within medical care systems.
13. List the three levels of OT services provided within the continuum of care, and provide an example of an OT intervention with aging adults for each level.
14. Hospice is a form of palliative care; list two ways that occupational therapists can work with individuals to affirm life within this type of care setting.

ESSAY QUESTIONS

Answer one of the following three questions:
1. The demographics within a country have major implications for family structure. Discuss the differences between families living in a country with a high birth rate and few older adults and those living in a country with a low birth rates and greater number of older adults. How might family caregiving differ as a result of these differences?
2. You are the occupational therapist for a homebound older woman with dementia. How would you include the woman's family members in your practice?
3. You are working with an older person who is trying to decide whether or not to retire. What factors would you encourage him or her to consider?

REFERENCES

1. Administration on Aging, U.S. Department of Health and Human Services. (2013). *A profile of older Americans: 2013.* Retrieved from http://www.aoa.gov/AoAroot/Aging_Statistics/Profile/index.aspx.

2. Alzheimer's Association. (2015-2009). *2015 Alzheimer's disease facts and figures.* Washington, DC: Alzheimer's Association.

3. American Heart Association Statistics Committee. (2009). *Heart disease and stroke statistics—2009 update.* Dallas, TX: American Heart Association.

4. Bouldin, E. D., Akhtar, W., Brumback, B. A., & Andresen, E. A. (2009). *Characteristics of caregivers and non-caregivers–Florida, 2008.* Retrieved from http://fodh.phhp.ufl.edu/publications/docs/Caregiving%20in%20Florida_05-09-09.pdf.

5. Brault, M. W. (2012). *Americans with disabilities: 2010, current population reports, P70-131.* Washington, DC: U.S. Census Bureau.

6. Centers for Disease Control and Prevention (CDC). (2006). *NHANES data on the prevalence of overweight and obesity among adults: United States, 2003-2004.* Retrieved from http://www.cdc.gov/nchs/products/pubs/pubd/hestats/overweight/overwght_adult_03.htm.

7. Centers for Disease Control and Prevention (CDC). (2015). *BRFSS—about the BRFSS.* Retrieved from http://www.cdc.gov/brfss/about/.

8. Central Intelligence Agency (CIA). (2015). *The world factbook: Turkey.* Retrieved from https://www.cia.gov/library/publications/the-world-factbook/geos/tu.html.

9. Chacko, L. R., & Chacko, S. A. (2010). Modern public health systems. In E. M. Andresen & E. L. Bouldin (Eds.), *Public health foundations: Concepts and practices* (pp. 27–28). San Francisco, CA: Jossey-Bass/Wiley.

10. Clark, F. (2012). *Well elderly 2, Los Angeles, California, 2004-2008.* ICPSR33641-v1. Ann Arbor, MI: Inter-university Consortium for Political and Social Research [distributor].

11. Clark, F., Azen, S., Zemke, R., Jackson, J., Carlson, M., Mandel, D., & Lipson, L. (1997). Occupational therapy for independent living older adults: A randomized controlled trial. *JAMA, 278*(16), 1321–1326.

12. Crawford, A. C., Bouldin, E. D., Brumback, B. A., & Andresen, E. A. (2008a). *Characteristics of caregivers and care recipients—Kansas, 2007.* Retrieved from http://fodh.phhp.ufl.edu/publications/docs/Kansas_Report_Final_12_5_08.pdf.

13. Crawford, A. C., Bouldin E. D., Brumback, B. A., & Andresen, E. A. (2008b). *Characteristics of caregivers and care recipients—Washington, 2007.* Retrieved from http://fodh.phhp.ufl.edu/publications/docs/Washington CG Report_10-13-08.pdf.

14. Daniels, S. R. (2006). The consequences of childhood overweight and obesity. *Future of Children, 16*(1), 47–67.

15. Freedman, V. A. (2006). Late-life disability trends: An overview of current evidence. In M. J. Field, A. M. Jette, & L. Martin (Eds.), *Workshop on disability in America, a new look, summary and background papers* (pp. 101–112). Washington, DC: The National Academies Press.

16. Gebbie, K., Rosenstock, L., & Hernandez, L. M. (Eds.). (2003). *Who will keep the public healthy? Educating public health professionals for the 21st century.* Washington DC: The National Academies Press.

17. Institute of Medicine. (2002). *The future of the public's health in the 21st century.* Washington DC: The National Academies Press.

18. Institute of Medicine. (2007). In M. J. Field & A. M. Jette (Eds.), *The future of disability in America.* Washington, DC: The National Academies Press.

19. Institute of Medicine. (2008). *Retooling for an aging America: Building the health care workforce.* Washington, DC: The National Academies Press.

20. Leavell, H. R., & Clark, E. G. (1965). *Preventive medicine for the doctor in his community: An epidemiological approach* (3rd ed.). New York, NY: Blakiston-McGraw Hill.

21. Long, S. O., & Harris, P. B. (2000). Gender and elder care: Social change and the role of the caregiver in Japan. *Social Science Japan Journal, 3*(1), 21–36.

22. McKune, S., Andresen, E. M., Zhang, J., & Neugaard, B. (2006). *Caregiving: A national profile and assessment of caregiver services and needs.* Retrieved from http://www.rosalynncarter.org/publications/.

23. Ministry of Health (Turkey) & Başkent University. (2002). *National burden of disease and cost-effectiveness project, inception report.* Ankara, Turkey: Ministry of Health (Turkey).

24. Minnesota Department of Human Services Aging and Adult Services. (2009). *2008 Minnesota behavioral risk factor surveillance survey caregiving module.* St. Paul, MN: Author.

25. National Alliance for Caregiving & American Association of Retired Persons (NAC & AARP). (2004). *Caregiving in the United States.* Washington, DC: Author.

26. National Center for Health Statistics. (2014). Summary health statistics for U.S. adults: National health interview survey, 2012. Retrieved May 21, 2015, from http://www.cdc.gov/nchs/products/series/series10.htm.

27. National Long Term Care Survey. (n.d.). *What is the NLTCS?* Retrieved May, 20, 2015, from http://www.nltcs.aas.duke.edu.

28. Neugaard, B., Andresen, E. M., DeFries, E. L., Talley, R. C., & Crews, J. E. (2007). Characteristics and health of caregivers and care recipients: North Carolina, 2005. *Morbidity and Mortality Weekly Reports, 56*(21), 529–532.

29. Plassman, B. L., Langa, K. M., Fisher, G. G., et al. (2007). Prevalence of dementia in the United States: The aging, demographics, and memory study. *Neuroepidemiology, 29*(1-2), 125–132.

30. Salihu, H. M., Bonnema, S. M., & Alio, A. P. (2009). Obesity: What is an elderly population growing into? *Maturitas, 63*(1), 7–12.

31. Samsa, G. P., Matchar, D. B., Goldstein, L., et al. (1998). Utilities for major stroke: Results from a survey of preferences among persons at increased risk for stroke. *American Heart Journal, 136*(4), 703–713.

32. Thom, T., Haase, N., Rosamond, W., et al. (2006). Heart disease and stroke statistics—2006 update: A report from the American Heart Association Statistics Committee and Stroke Statistics Subcommittee. *Circulation, 113*(6), 85–151.

33. United Nations, Department of Economic and Social Affairs, Population Division. (2013). *World population ageing 2013.* New York, NY: United Nations Publications.

34. U.S. Census Bureau. (2006). Introduction to SIPP. Retrieved from http://www.census.gov/sipp/intro.html.

35. U.S. Department of Health and Human Services, Center for Disease Control and Prevention, National Center for Health Statistics. (2014). *Health, United States, 2013, with Chartbook.* Hyattsville, MD: U.S. Government Printing Office.

36. Woolf, S. H. (2012). The price of false beliefs: Unrealistic expectations as a contributor to the health care crisis. *Annals of Family Medicine, 10*(6), 492.

37. World Health Organization. (1978). *International conference on primary health care.* Declaration of Alma-Ata. USSR: Alma-Ata.

38. Yamamoto, N., & Wallhagen, M. (1997). The continuation of family caregiving in Japan. *Journal of Health and Social Behavior, 38*(2), 164–176.

CHAPTER 4

Theoretical Models Relevant to Gerontological Occupational Therapy Practice

Clare Hocking PhD, OTR/L, Phyllis Meltzer, PhD

CHAPTER OUTLINE

OBJECTIVES

- Identify theories and models of aging; gain understanding of the validity of and exceptions to universal applications of each theory
- Envision possible applications of theories and models of aging to occupational therapists' gerontology-based practice
- Interpret perspectives/theories of aging from an occupational viewpoint
- Interpret information derived from aged persons themselves regarding their views on elements of successful aging
- Compare similarities between the development of the disciplines of gerontology and occupational therapy
- Discuss attempts to define and identify successful aging from a variety of viewpoints

Older age can be conceptualized from multiple perspectives: as a biological progression, a developmental process, a social phenomenon, and a lived experience. Although phenomenological understandings of living in advanced age are relatively new, efforts have been made to bring the various perspectives together into a holistic understanding of aging. Occupational therapists are attuned to those efforts. Biopsychosocial theory, for example, was promoted to occupational therapists in the mid-1970s as being well suited to working in community settings and supporting their role in "teaching skills for living."[50] Ideas concerning healthful aging have a much longer history. Taoist, Islamic, Greco-Roman, Hebrew, and Christian scriptures have provided observations about health and aging, and through the centuries the different schools of thought became intertwined. For example, nineteenth-century philosophers influenced the thinking of twentieth-century biologists.[1]

Occupational perspectives, such as those occupational therapists and occupational scientists might propose, are largely absent from the multidisciplinary discourse on aging. For example, in the authoritative textbook *Handbook of Theories of Aging*,[9] the only mention of occupations besides caregiving relates to hunting and foraging, which apparently influenced the evolutionary determination of the human lifespan.[39] In this chapter, the focus is squarely on occupational perspectives of aging. This chapter brings together theoretical understandings of being aged, being occupied, being in context, and, as is the case for some individuals, being affected by a health condition.

To set the scene we consider a range of theories of aging, dwelling on those that speak to older people's engagement in the everyday world of doing. Acknowledging older people as occupational beings, we provide an overview of the theories occupational therapists draw from to explain the dynamic relationship between people, their environment, and their occupations, and how the things people do in older age affect their health and well-being. To further explicate the context of older people's participation in occupations, a frequently cited model that explains environmental influences on older adults' occupational engagement is described. Finally, because older age may be accompanied by the onset of chronic health conditions, that theoretical basis is supplemented by the World Health Organization's *International Classification of Functioning, Disability and Health* (ICF), which explains the relationship between participation in the activities of everyday life and having a health condition.[71]

Being Aged: The Emergence of Theories of Aging

Theories of aging, which attempt to answer the questions of how and what changes are part of the aging process, have a very long history. Drawing on Hippocrates (460-377 BCE), Aristotle (384-322 BCE) is credited with being the first Western person to propose firm ideas about aging.[1] The idea that aging was not a disease but a normal stage of life during which disease may occur is also longstanding, having been proposed by Seneca (4 BCE–65 CE), who emphasized quality of life over a diseased but long life. Cicero also maintained that old age might have advantages if people maintain their strength and interest in life.[1]

Current understandings of aging have been shaped by gerontology, which emerged as a scientific field of inquiry in the United States with the publication of E. V. Cowdry's *Problems of Aging: Biological and Medical Aspects* in 1939. The book was a compendium of the work of experts from various medical and biological disciplines who reviewed "the current state of theories and knowledge on aging in their disciplines."[1] A great number of "competing theories about senescence, explicating continuities and changes from the cellular to the societal levels"[1] followed, spurred by the founding of two professional organizations in the 1940s—the American Geriatrics Society and the Gerontological Society of America—which encouraged researchers to create theories with cooperation from researchers in other disciplines.

Sixty years later, the biomedical perspective prevails. Governments and individuals are alert to the lifestyle factors that give rise to heart disease, diabetes, and cognitive impairments, and the need to actively manage those conditions to stave off disability and death. Explanatory models, such as psychoneuroimmunology, seek to explain individuals' susceptibility to chronic and infectious diseases in terms of the links between their beliefs, psychological and stress responses, and neurologic and endocrine functioning. These views overshadow life-course and biodemographic perspectives, which acknowledge the influence of cumulative inequalities related to gender, race, low socioeconomic status, and sexual orientation on the early onset and poor outcomes of chronic health conditions.[9] Public policy perspectives also reveal how old-age policies are shaped by social processes and in turn shape the experience of being aged.[9]

Psychological theories of aging are also pervasive. Perhaps the best known was developed by Erik Erikson in his middle age.[23] Erikson's theory of ego development encompassed the lifespan and proposed that each stage, from infancy to old age, represented a choice or crisis. Old age, he believed, led to integrity and wisdom. Integrity should be the "dominant syntonic disposition, in search of balance with an equally pervasive sense of despair," whereas wisdom is a "detached concern with life itself."[23] Joan Erikson, in her later years, stated in a documentary film that these elements of the theory were not necessarily right—in fact, they were "just plain wrong." She revised the theory of old age to include coping and facing death as important components.[21]

History of Gerontology Theories: Gerontology as a Discipline

The emergence of gerontology as a discipline parallels that of occupational therapy in time and focus. During and following World War II, psychologists and people in related disciplines became aware of the need for theories that could guide the creation of programs and practices to enhance the lives of the aging. The goal became the search to identify the determinants of "successful aging." Early pioneers include James Birren, one of the founders of gerontology during the 1940s, who established much of the framework of modern gerontology theory.[10] Havighurst[30] defined one of the key concepts, successful aging, as a feeling of happiness and satisfaction with one's current and past life, and Butler[13] considered life review and reminiscence as meaningful. Rowe and Kahn[58] affected the vocabulary of gerontology by identifying the differences between "usual" and "successful" aging. Recently, older adults themselves, in focus groups and research surveys, are creating their own definitions of successful aging: considering themselves successful despite chronic physical conditions and functional difficulties.[64] Successful aging theories currently include, among others, the concepts of productivity,[58] adaptation,[12] and resilience.[29] New theories continue to be formulated in collaboration with allied health professions and social scientists.

Being Aged: Gerontological and Psychological Models of Aging

We discuss a range of psychosocial models of aging in the following sections, as these more clearly incorporate occupational perspectives. We start with disengagement theory, which is the most controversial.

Disengagement Theory

Disengagement theory is important, as it was the first theory of aging proposed by gerontologists. Disengagement theory purported that it was natural and inevitable that older people would withdraw from society and increasingly focus on personal meanings. Although allowing that there would be variations in timing,[22] the theory postulated that this withdrawal was mutual—members of society would also disengage from older people as their abilities, knowledge, and skills deteriorated and they ceased to perform the social roles associated with work, family, and marriage.[18]

Fifty years later, however, disengagement theory seems too accepting of the biomedical perspective that the years beyond retirement are characterized by increasing decrepitude, senile degeneration of physical and cognitive capacities, and pathologic processes. It also seems to perpetuate the ageist attitudes prevalent in Western societies, which frame older people as having less to offer than younger people and force them to withdraw, whether they wish to or not.[25] It is also controversial because potentially mediating factors such as race, gender, and social status were not recognized.[1] Further, disengagement theory may be based on a misinterpretation—that the withdrawal from society it postulates is not preparation for death, but rather a preference for interacting with the people closest to them. That possibility, as framed by socioemotional selectivity theory, suggests that people who perceive their time to be limited are more focused on the present, prioritize happiness over new learning, and seek "emotionally rich interactions with significant others."[61] The theory is given weight by evidence demonstrating its applicability to younger adults with life-threatening illness, who similarly perceive their time to be limited. Disengagement theory has largely been abandoned.[25]

Successful Aging

The concept of "active aging," which is diametrically opposed to disengagement theory, has been theorized since the early 1950s. It has taken on many guises over the years. One of these guises, the theory of successful (as opposed to normal) aging, was initially presented as a fact.[31] Defined as a feeling of happiness and satisfaction with one's current and past life,[30] some researchers operationalized successful aging as "life satisfaction, morale, happiness, and mental health."[46] More recent iterations have defined successful aging as "the ability to maintain three key behaviors or characteristics: low risk of disease and disease-related disability, high mental and physical function, and active engagement with life."[60] The hierarchical nature of these components suggests that the absence of disease and disability, and concomitant risk factors, makes it easier to maintain physical and mental functions, which in turn indicates the potential for activity. The aging adult must actually do some of the activities, whether pertaining to social engagement with other people or productive behavior.

However, social science researchers have challenged the parameters Rowe and Kahn[58] proposed, arguing that successful aging encompasses larger arenas of behavior and conditions. Older adults themselves certainly have a broader perspective. For instance, Strawbridge and associates[64] found that 867 older adults participating in the Alameda County Study rated themselves as aging successfully despite chronic physical conditions and functional difficulties that meant that none of them met Rowe and Kahn's criteria. Similarly, older adults who discussed successful aging in focus groups in California placed little emphasis on genetics, longevity, function, independence, or the absence of disease/disability. Rather, in their opinion, successful aging centered on four interrelated components: attitude/adaptation, security/stability, health/wellness, and engagement/stimulation, It also required a positive attitude, realistic perspective, and the ability to adapt.[57] In studies that have recruited an older cohort, however, such as the Leiden longitudinal study of people aged 85+, participants identified the effects that "longevity, physical, cognitive, psychological and social health and functioning" have on successful aging, and also acknowledged that it is a process of adaptation involving "effective coping, living circumstances (finances, neighborhood) and also overall life satisfaction."[12] Ongoing exploration may validate older people's multidimensional definitions and contribute to theory building.

Correlation studies also bring new understandings of what is required for successful aging. For instance, in their study of successful aging among 1825 Korean older adults, Jang, Choi, and Kim[37] measured a range of factors, including the presence of chronic diseases, physical functioning, history of mental illness and social activity participation, and subjective well-being.

They concluded that higher level of education was the most important socioeconomic factor because it explained correlations between successful aging and household and personal income, which the authors concluded was the result, for the most part, of educational opportunities.

There is some agreement emerging from the research that control of the social environment and material well-being are requirements for successful aging. Equally, research has not supported other assumptions, such as that minority older adults (in the United States) are disadvantaged compared with the larger population and that the additive effects of marginalization are greater in old age than in middle age. Rowe and Kahn's 1987 definition of successful aging has also been critiqued for not addressing ethnic differences, differences in experiences of life events and coping mechanisms,[69] and differences in how older adults themselves perceive successful aging. "Finally, criticism has been leveled on the successful aging paradigm for vesting too much responsibility within the individual for achieving this normatively desirable state, thus risking further marginalization of high-risk segments of society, such as the poor and older women."[69]

Activity Theory

Havighurst and colleagues'[30] activity theory proposed that normal aging is typified by continuing engagement in meaningful occupations and relationships. The specific relationship predicted was between social activities and life satisfaction, whereby higher levels of satisfaction would be associated with a higher frequency of activity and with informal social activities rather than formal or solitary activities.[49] Activity theory was more formally developed by Lemon, Bengtson, and Peterson,[44] who specified the relationship between activity and well-being.

Activity theory is partially supported by evidence from research. There is substantial support for a positive relationship between the number and frequency of activities older people participate in and their survival, functional and cognitive status, physical health, psychological well-being, social status, maintenance of skills and knowledge, and satisfaction with life. Evidence from the Aging in Manitoba Study (AIM), which is the largest and longest-running study on aging in Canada, showed that levels of everyday activity reported six years after the initial survey were positively related to happiness, as well as better function and reduced mortality. However, participation in solitary occupations was also related to happiness. Participants who engaged in handwork hobbies, playing or listening to music, attending the theater, or reading and writing were happier six years later than those who did not.[49]

Other studies, however, have reported that some occupations that might be considered solitary, such as listening to the radio and watching television, are negatively associated with well-being. Also, because the studies do not establish causality, it is not clear whether good health enables higher levels of activity, being more active promotes good health, or both. There is also some evidence that older people's activity levels can be irrational and excessive.[33,53] In addition, the evidence does not clearly show whether different kinds of activities confer different kinds of benefits. For example, productive activities might confer a sense of competence and usefulness, but if they are not physically demanding, they might not provide the known benefits of exercising. Finally, the proposed association between life satisfaction and social rather than solitary occupations has not been widely researched and is not clearly supported.[49]

Continuity Theory

Atchley's[4,5] continuity theory elaborated on activity theory by introducing a life-course perspective. It proposes that older adults persist with the activities, behaviors, opinions, beliefs, preferences, and relationships that characterized them in earlier stages of their lives, and that doing so is an adaptive strategy for managing changes in their physical, social, and mental status and the life events associated with growing older. That is, with the support of their network of relationships and social roles, older adults make decisions that preserve occupations that are highly meaningful and other activities that characterize their daily routines to sustain their self-concept and lifestyle.[40,43] Continuity theory is descriptive, focusing on the relationship between the things people do and their psychological functioning, rather than the extent of their involvement in various occupations.[53] It rests on the assumption that people's personalities are stable, and that personality influences the roles individuals assume, their interest in those roles, and their life satisfaction.[22]

Although the theory is supported to some extent by research findings, it does not account for the diverse outlooks older people have on their everyday activities and the future, the active choice some make to relinquish activities that worry them, or the transfer of tasks to younger people.[16] It does not encompass documented reductions in the range of activities with declining health or changes in the kinds of occupations people participate in as they age,[49] such as the shift toward activities that require less physical effort, and from outdoors to indoor activities. It also fails to account for older adults who initiate new occupations, such as widows who take up new hobbies and exercise routines, and men who begin to shop, clean, and cook after losing a spouse.[53]

Productive Aging

In the 1980s, active aging was reinterpreted as "productive aging," and in the United States, in the economic retrenchments of the Reagan administration, it was recast as civic engagement—"volunteerism that places the responsibility for solving social problems on the shoulders of American volunteers while government retreats."[47] Productive aging refers to "all activities … that create goods or services of value,"[58] including paid, unpaid, self-defined, culturally defined, and other activities. The concept of productive aging is supported by reports regarding the activities of older adults, such as one from the MacArthur Study of Successful Aging, which asserted that most older people do some productive work and that "all in all, the amount of such work is substantial; and … much of it continues throughout life."[58]

The link between remaining productive and successful aging lies in its outcomes. For example, older Japanese women in the northern Okinawan village of Kijaha are the main contributors to the occupation of *basho-fu* weaving. The fiber they use requires intense labor to prepare it for the weaving loom. As the women age they contribute less-intense physical labor, but remain active in some aspects of the preparation processes.[69] In exchange for their continuing skilled contribution, they receive symbolic capital,[11] which refers to the amount of honor and prestige possessed by a person with regard to existing social structures. Symbolic capital relates to the opinions of others as well as the individual, and it is accrued "through self-maintenance of health, continued engagement with society (in various cultural manifestations), and pursuit of productive activity."[69] Through their participation in *basho-fu*, the women are honored as living cultural treasures.

Reflections on Active Aging

Since the 1960s, postmodern perspectives have influenced research and theory development in at least two ways. First, researchers give more credence to people's perception of their own lives. Reflecting that credibility, members of a reference group of older adults living in the United Kingdom were asked for their opinion of active aging; they reported that they prefer the notion of "comfortable, healthy aging."[16] Second, there is increasing tolerance for diversity. That mind shift plays out in the recognition that active aging may manifest differently in early and later old age. Accordingly, the concept of active aging has been criticized for representing youthful or middle-aged perspectives that have been supported by research that has canvassed the views of people in early old age.[16]

Picking up on such concerns, researchers now recognize that older adults' perspective of being active may be less about actively working to achieve goals and more related to taking pleasure in everyday occupations, relationships, and events.[16] Researchers have also argued for the need to investigate how the "oldest old" age successfully, based on measured differences between the younger and older cohorts. People in the younger group are more physically and mentally fit than those of previous generations, retain the ability to learn, have greater emotional intelligence and wisdom than any other age group, and maintain their ability to adjust to changed circumstances and health status. Among the oldest old, even the healthiest have been found to have severely impaired ability to learn and show declines in life satisfaction, affect, identity, and psychological and medical status. Although there is no agreed-on demarcation between the young old and those living in advanced old age, a population approach might place the transition at the chronologic age where 50% of a cohort have died. In developed nations, that would be 75 to 80 or 80 to 85 years of age, depending on how the cut-off was calculated.[7]

Related Theories

Alongside the theory development and research that continues to explore successful, productive, and active aging, psychologists have developed concepts to explain the personal characteristics and behaviors of people who age well. One concept that is related to, but not coincident with, the definitions of successful aging is resilience. Harris[29] asserted that resilience should be the goal of aging, and proposed that resilience exists in a theoretical framework. Others believe that the focus of research on successful aging will shift toward greater understanding of "interindividual variation across the life span and will center around why and how some individuals show more resilience and others more decline at the same chronologic age."[26] Ryff and Singer,[60] who have contributed to the research literature on resilience, found that "persistent psychological strengths are linked with better health ... even among those with low educational status." As connections between biological and psychological strengths become apparent, so the goal of aging successfully may not be limited to those with "good" physical health, but enjoyed by those who are able to understand and adapt to the changes that aging brings.

Another explanatory theory is the theory of goal-achievement strategies (selection, optimization, and compensation), which proposes that people select goals in relation to their resources (time, energy, knowledge, skills, personal capacities, health, social support, socioeconomic status); acquire, refine, and allocate internal and external resources to achieve their goals (optimization); and use compensatory strategies when confronted with losses or decline.[2] This "dynamic model of development as a continuous process of specialization and loss"[73] provides a theoretical basis for Baltes's[6] theory of successful aging. In the 20 years since it was proposed, this theory has been applied to people in adolescence through to old age. In relation to older people, it proposes that abandoning less meaningful activities, focusing on the things that are most important or salient in their everyday lives, and devising new ways of doing things when confronted by diminishing abilities can be adaptive strategies that optimize emotionally meaningful experiences.[36] That might include spending more time on some occupations and routines, and reducing the time and effort invested in less satisfying activities.[42] Selective optimization with compensation may explain why older adults indicate well-being and low rates of depression despite poor physical health and loss of some functions. Those areas where individuals have achieved a high level of competence may remain stable, whereas other areas, not as well developed, may decline. Emotional regulation and the ability to avoid conflict may also contribute to feelings of well-being.[73]

Longitudinal data from the Berlin Aging Study provide general support for selective optimization with compensation, with older people with higher cognitive, sensorimotor, and social functioning found to be better able to implement such strategies.[42] A recent study conducted in Croatia also showed that older people who report higher levels of subjective well-being are typically more persistent and single-minded, devoting themselves to the things they want to achieve (optimization) and finding alternate ways or trying harder (compensation) if their usual ways of doing things

prove ineffective. Those with lower reported well-being resort to selecting one or two goals to pursue, concentrating all their efforts on a few things, and switching goals when they cannot achieve things as they did previously.[2] Additional support for the notion of compensation comes from independently developed categories of person- and environment-related compensatory strategies.[67]

There is an apparent alignment between these findings and research reported by occupational scientists and therapists. In particular, the process of "trading off" independence in some spheres of daily life to preserve important aspects of their lifestyles[62] supports the concept of selection, and evidence that older adults devise practical strategies to support participation in everyday occupations supports the concept of compensation.[54,51] Successful aging through the application of selection, optimization, and compensation strategies also provided the theoretical basis for the University of Southern California's Well Elderly Study.[15]

Critical Perspectives

A major shortcoming of the earlier psychosocial theories was their focus on "normal" aging—that is, they explicitly neglected older adults with chronic illness.[22] Generational differences, such as having lived through the Great Depression of the 1930s, and gender differences are also not sufficiently addressed. For example, there is accumulating evidence that retired men and women value social leisure activities differently,[36] and that although men derive benefit from watching and attending cultural events such as sports games, women report better health, greater satisfaction with life, and less anxiety and depression when they actively participate in activities such as taking art classes, singing in a group, learning a musical instrument, and the like.[20] Based on their knowledge of the relationship between occupation and health, occupational therapists and occupational scientists would also expect that the "quality" of the activity ought to be acknowledged. Supporting that assertion, a recent study of more than 5000 older women and men in England found that although socially productive occupations (e.g., working, volunteering, and caregiving) are associated with higher levels of well-being and reduced incidence of depression, that is only the case if individuals feel appreciated for the things they do. Significantly, those caring for an immediate family member (e.g., partner, child, parent, or parent-in-law) are less likely to feel appreciated than those caring for a friend, neighbor, grandchild, or other relative.[48]

Questions have also been raised about the way active aging is conceptualized at an individual level, given the influence of structural issues affecting older adults. For instance, Atchley's continuity theory has been critiqued for presenting continuity over the lifespan as a norm, when it is likely more typical of men than women.[56] Disengagement theory, activity theory, and continuity theory also fail to take account of structural issues such as experiences of unemployment, racism, and older women's history of restricted vocational choices and lower pay rates, which impose financial and societal barriers to being active.[17] These factors are important given the known association between mental health problems among older people and lower educational levels, economic hardship, declining social support, and chronic physical health conditions, all of which are likely to prevent them from actively engaging in valued activities.[16] The active aging theories also presuppose that people live in a stable society where access to significant others is positive and possible, and that there are opportunities to meaningfully engage in chosen occupations.[22]

International Uptake of Active Aging

The concept of active aging has been taken up in different ways in different contexts. The contemporary iteration, positive aging, emphasizes the known association between activity levels and health by somewhat zealously promoting the need to "use it or lose it."[16] Occupational therapists are responding to the positive aging agenda. A Canadian Association of Occupational Therapists Position Paper[14] linked active living for older adults to healthy aging. Wilcock[68] urged occupational therapists to engage in political activism to counter Western stereotypes of older adults being sedentary, and productive aging has been taken up as a Centennial Vision of the American Occupational Therapy Association.[51]

The World Health Organization (WHO)[72] has also taken up the concept of active aging, which it describes as allowing "people to realize their potential for physical, social, and mental well-being throughout the life course and to participate in society according to their needs, desires and capacities". Being active is further described as "continuing participation in social, economic, cultural, spiritual and civic affairs" and recognizes that even after retirement and despite illness, frailty, disability, and receiving care, people can continue to contribute to "their families, peers, communities and nations."[72] Accordingly, the WHO considers that active aging policy and programs should promote mental health and social connection as being equally as important as physical health status. Finally, because "ageing takes place within the context of others—friends, work associates, neighbours and family members" and is shaped by the opportunities and risks that individuals have experienced, concepts of interdependence, mutual aid, and support are considered to be vital.

The Organisation for Economic Co-operation and Development (OECD) is also promoting the active aging message, proposing public policy initiatives to foster active aging as a means of "maintaining prosperity in an ageing society."[55] Interpreting productive aging in the sense of paid work, it suggests initiating workplace reforms to increase job opportunities for older workers, removing incentives for early retirement, and providing more flexibility in how people transition to retirement. However, various commentators have argued that viewing older people in terms of their "economic usefulness"[24] is inequitable, imposing unattainable expectations on older adults who have not maintained good health and placing an additional burden on women who also provide the bulk of caregiving services.[47] As Rudman[59] reminds us, in framing societal perceptions about what is ideal and possible, positive aging discourses "limit occupational possibilities and promote occupational injustices".

Models to Explain Being Occupied

Gerontologists have developed theories that explain the activities of older adults, and occupational therapy theorists have generated a number of theoretical explanations of engagement in occupation across the lifespan, thus complementing the theories of aging discussed earlier. All of the theories of occupation encompass the person who is occupied, whatever his or her capacities; the activity that engages his or her energy and attention; and the environment in which it takes place. In this chapter we provide an overview of three of the models that have an explicitly occupational focus: Kielhofner's[41] Model of Human Occupation (MOHO), the Canadian Model of Occupational Performance and Engagement (CMOP-E),[65] and Baum and Christiansen's[8] Person-Environment-Occupation-Performance (PEOP) model. Rather than attempt to describe each in detail, we have chosen to draw out their differences, and to consider their fit with the concept of active aging and the theory of goal-achievement strategies.

The MOHO primarily focuses on explaining the volitional processes, roles, and habits that guide and structure people's participation in occupation; the motor, process, communication, and interaction skills that underlie performance; and the subjective experience of engaging in occupation. People are described as anticipating, choosing, experiencing, and interpreting the things they do and, through participation in occupation over the lifespan, developing their identity and learning about their values, preferences, and capacities. In comparison to the person engaged in occupation, the environment and occupation itself are much less theorized. The environment is described as affecting "what people do and how they do it."[41] It is made up of objects, spaces, occupational forms, and social groups, all of which are influenced by culture, the economy, and the political context. The environment provides opportunities and resources, but it also demands and constrains occupational performance. Occupation is conceptualized at three levels: participation in work, play, and daily living activities; performance of an occupational form; and the observable actions that exhibit a person's skill levels. Occupational adaptation is achieved when people develop a positive sense of their identity and competence, as a consequence of participating in occupation.

The MOHO explicitly addresses occupational change and development over the lifespan, describing older adults as confronting biological changes, social conventions, and accumulated losses that place them at risk of a diminished sense of personal causation, and as having less interest in work and more interest in family. Standards may be redefined, and values satisfied, in alternate ways. Although retirement may be liberating and allow more time to spend with family, some older adults will experience diminished roles, meaning, and self-worth. If habits are disrupted by changed circumstances and capacities, and activity choices are constrained, loneliness, boredom, and depression may result.[41] The overall sense is that older adults prefer being active and contributing to the lives of others, but that the intensity of engagement in occupation naturally declines.

The CMOP-E is elaborated in the context of client-centered practice, organized within an enabling, occupation-focused problem-solving process. People are conceptualized as occupational beings who have an occupational repertoire and pattern that make them unique. Spirituality is at the heart of the model, influencing the development and application of individuals' cognitive, affective, and physical capacities. Three realms of occupation are identified—self-care, productivity, and leisure—and occupation is understood to be "the bridge that connects person and environment."[65] Individuals are described as living in environments made up of physical, institutional, cultural, and social components. Personal, occupational, and environmental layers of the model are presumed to be mutually influential, but the nature of those interactions is not explored.

Engagement in occupation is described as being influenced by each person's skills and talents,[65] and to develop and change over the lifespan. Although transitions in response to illness are identified, the effect of aging on occupation is not discussed in the body of the theory, although the embedded case studies include intervention in long-term care environments. Recent theoretical developments have shifted the emphasis from occupational performance to occupational engagement, signaling that people need not physically perform an occupation to actively engage in it. Concepts embedded in the model that align with theories of active aging include capacity and competence, development, roles, and satisfaction. Other key concepts are occupational deprivation, identity, mastery, meaning, and occupational potential. Consistent with theories of active aging, engagement in occupation is presumed to enhance health. Acknowledgment that participation is affected by individuals' capacities and can be active or passive, sporadic or constant, novel or well established allows that activity levels might or might not support healthy aging. Notably, concepts such as adaptation and compensation for decreasing competencies are not included.

The PEOP model proposed by Baum and Christiansen[8] also provides a generic explanation of people's participation in occupation, without specific reference to older adults' developmental path or specific needs. Five intrinsic person factors are identified—psychological, cognitive, neurobiological, physiologic, and spiritual—which refer to meanings that "contribute to a greater sense of personal understanding about self and one's place in the world."[8] Occupation, meaning the things people want and need to do in everyday life, is described as a hierarchy of behaviors and abilities. Key concepts are the abilities that support performance, observable actions, tasks, and roles, which confer privileges and responsibilities and typically involve the performance of a range of occupations. Consistent with the MOHO and the CMOP-E, the environment is less theorized than other components of the model. It is described as comprising cultural values, social and economic systems, the built environment, technology, and social supports. Again, aging is not specifically addressed, and although the model evidences similar concerns to the theories of aging, it does not explicitly advance a perspective about remaining active into older age, or mechanisms by which people adapt and respond to changing capacities and environments.

Being in Context: Lawton's Ecological Model

Supplementing the propositions occupational therapists have advanced to explain people's interactions with their environment, insights can be gleaned from other disciplines. Older adults' homes, especially homes they have occupied for a long time, are recognized as holding "strong emotional, symbolic, material, and social meanings,"[28] and being attached to their place of residence is thought to promote a sense of control and security, and to support self-esteem and identity. However, older adults' interactions with their home environments are not static. Over time, the character of the neighborhood or their access to it might change, for example, if they no longer drive. Equally, if their homes fall into disrepair or an area becomes increasingly inaccessible, older adults might decide to modify the architectural features of their homes, incorporate assistive devices, or relocate.[28] Despite that complexity and the fact that a number of professionals, including occupational therapists, are concerned with designing or modifying environments that will support older people's participation, the field continues to develop "a unified and robust theoretical direction" in conceptualizing older people's transactions with the environment.[27]

One enduring and frequently cited attempt to provide conceptual clarity is Lawton and Nahemow's 1973 ecological model.[66] In broad outline, the model proposes that the environment serves three functions: maintenance, stimulation, and support.[27] It also addresses older people's adaptive responses to the environment,[28] proposing that there is a relationship between their competencies, which refers to their biological health, cognitive and affective functioning, motor skills, quality of life, financial resources, and sense of efficacy, and the "press" of the environment, meaning its physical and social demands.

Lawton's model posits that when they have the competencies required to respond to the environmental demands they encounter (i.e., there is a good "fit"), older adults are adaptive and exhibit competent behavior and positive affect. Slightly lower environmental demands result in comfort and relaxation; slightly higher press brings challenge and demands the person's attention. Higher or lower levels of competence or press result in negative affect and maladaptive behavior. The central idea, the environmental docility hypothesis, suggests that as people's competence decreases, their behavior is increasingly determined by the environment.[3,35,67] That is, the magnitude of the problem caused by an environmental barrier depends on the person's competencies. Thus individuals with lower competence are less able to independently change their situation because most of their energy is expended on adapting to environmental demands. Consequently, the effect of negative changes in the environment may be magnified, but, equally, minor improvements may have a big effect on their ability to function.[35]

Lawton later proposed a second hypothesis, proactivity, which allows that older people actively manage their environments to achieve important life goals and maintain their independence.[67] He also suggested that when older people's level of competence corresponds to environmental demands, they can make use of a greater variety of resources in the environment to satisfy their needs. Thus moving to a more supportive environment might enable older adults to better use the resources available to them to support participation.[66]

Recent research has tested the model, and there is some empirical support for the idea that older adults' home environments help maintain their functional abilities and provide a sense of normalcy despite other losses[27] and that older people's competencies support adaptation.[45] Research focusing on depression, however, has not demonstrated the interrelationship between affective functioning and environmental press that Lawton's theory predicts.[3]

Research conducted by occupational therapists supports Lawton's docility theory, confirming the proposition that vulnerability to environmental barriers increases as competencies decline, especially among frailer older adults.[35] It also shows that vulnerable older adults act to influence the environment,[70] that interventions to decrease environmental press can reduce the magnitude of barriers older adults experience and improve their performance,[63] and that environmental factors affect disability rates.[35] The model has limitations, however, in not addressing individual differences that might influence older adults' adaptive responses, such as older adults' preferences, attitudes, knowledge, and needs, although it has generated environmental measures, such as the Housing Enabler.[27,28,35] In addition, it does not fully explain how the environment acts as a resource if older people are sufficiently competent to use it or how older people reduce environmental demands. However Cutchin's concept of place integration, which is based on the philosophy of pragmatism,[19,32] has been recognized as providing insights into the transactional process of aging in place.[38]

Recent theoretical advances arising from research also suggest that older people are more attuned to hazards in the environment that they have experienced firsthand or if they know someone who encountered a problem with a particular product or feature of the environment; that loss of valued relationships, activities, or possessions destabilizes self-worth and self-concept; and that environmental change can be positive if perceived to enhance control, improve person–environment fit, or bring hope for the future. Theory development might also usefully address the nature of the activities older people engage in, whether "obligatory or discretionary, planned or unplanned, and how environmental incentives and constraints lead to the adoption or rejection of particular activities."[28]

Models of Functioning

Having addressed historic and more recent theories of aging, models that explain people's engagement in occupation, and how the environment shapes participation, our remaining task is to bring living with a health condition into the picture. It is easy to assume that health conditions that affect people's capacity to regulate their emotions or metabolism, sense the world around them, and move, think, or express themselves cause disabilities. The World Health Organization's *International Classification of Functioning, Disability and Health* (ICF),[71] which was developed in consultation with people with disabilities, paints a more complex picture. The ICF has two key components. One is a detailed classification system that itemizes the structures and functions of human bodies that might be impaired by health conditions, aspects of activity and participation that impairments can affect, and features of the human and nonhuman environment that can be barriers to participation for people with impairments. The classification can be used as a framework to gather health statistics, so that people's health status can be compared across different countries. It also serves as a checklist to establish all of the ways an individual's participation is affected by his or her health condition, and at a societal level, to compare the participation rates of people with and without impairments in important occupations such as education, paid work, and political life. The other component is the Model of Functioning and Disability, which explains the interrelationships among health conditions, body structures and functions, participation in the activities of everyday life, and personal factors—including being aged and individuals' life history of occupational choices and constraints (Figure 4-1).

The important feature of the model in relation to this discussion is that all of the relationships it describes are bidirectional, and each factor can influence all of the other factors. That is, as we have long assumed, impairments due to a health

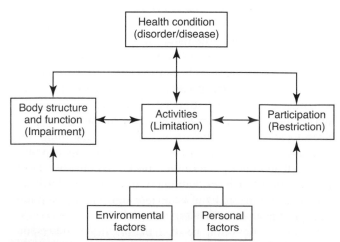

FIGURE 4-1 Interactions between the components of ICF. (From World Health Organization. [2001]. *International classification of functioning, disability and health.* Geneva: World Health Organization.)

condition can, but do not always, affect a person's ability to engage in activity and limit his or her participation, but the actual effect can be exacerbated or reduced by things in the environment or an individual's age, circumstances, personality, characteristic way of doing things, attitudes, and a multitude of other factors that make each person unique. Equally, however, the causal relationship might act in the opposite direction. Barriers to participation can exacerbate an existing health condition or cause another one, such as when restricted participation after a stroke leads to depression or, when participation is facilitated in some way, impairments are reduced or resolved through the health-giving properties of participating in occupation.

The other theories discussed in this chapter map onto the ICF fairly well, with each bringing its own focus and filling in the gaps left by the others. The theory of goal achievement,[2] for example, addresses the strategies older people use to support or enhance participation in meaningful occupations. The resources identified in the model include body structures and functions (such as personal capacities and energy), personal factors (knowledge, skills, time, and socioeconomic status), and aspects of the environment (material resources and social support). Health is also identified as a resource. The goals individuals select can be readily interpreted as relating to participation, and the proposal that older adults use compensatory strategies to reach their goals aligns with the ICF's emphasis on participation. The model complements the ICF in identifying personal factors that are relevant to continued participation and in naming the kinds of strategies older adults employ to promote participation—selecting goals, optimizing resources, and compensating for impairments due to health conditions or deficiencies in the environment. The goal-achievement model is inconsistent with the ICF, however, in identifying that older adults might select to abandon participation in less meaningful occupations.

Two of the models explaining human occupation (MOHO and CMOP-E) have encompassed the ICF concept of participation. They, and the PEOP model, are also broadly consistent with the ICF. That is, each encompasses the main elements of the ICF—occupation/participation, the environment, and aspects of the person including the structures and functions underpinning performance, each person's unique characteristics and life history, and the effects of a health condition—and each model recognizes the interrelatedness of those elements. Of the occupational therapy models, the CMOP-E's attention to the influence of the institutional environment best aligns with the ICF classification of services, systems, and policies that influence participation. There are, however, several points of difference. Where the ICF separates health conditions, body structures and functions, and personal factors, the occupational models integrate those concepts into understandings of the person. Each of the occupational models explains the nature of the relationship between people, the environment, and occupation, whether spiritual (CMOP-E and PEOP) or volitional and habitual (MOHO), whereas the ICF seeks only to explain participation in relation to health conditions. In addition, the occupational models attend to the quality of participation and people's subjective experience of and satisfaction with their participation, whereas the ICF is solely concerned with its extent, qualified by the level of difficulty in relation to the person's capacity and the assistance he or she receives. Interestingly, none of the occupational models addresses the influence of support, relationships, and others' attitudes in the detail given in the ICF.

Summary

As the discussion in this chapter shows, when the theoretical proposals advanced by gerontologists, psychologists, occupational therapists, and the World Health Organization are brought together, we generate a comprehensive understanding of older adults' participation in occupation. Older adults can be seen as actively responding to their circumstances by selecting occupations that are meaningful to them, optimizing their resources, and using compensatory strategies to adapt to shifts in the environment and their own abilities. It is also well recognized that the ability to adapt is constrained when there is a poor fit between a person's capacities and environmental demands. That might be due to a chronic health condition or financial, educational, and social disadvantages, but more research is needed to uncover the mechanisms by which those factors translate into barriers to participation. However, research recognizes that advanced old age, female gender, minority ethnic status, and the burden of caring for others create systematic disadvantages for some groups. A critical appraisal of contemporary theories of aging also reveals that although occupational therapists strive to enable older adults to participate, the concept of active aging has gathered a political overlay that slants the perspective of policymakers and members of society toward expecting older adults to remain active (to preserve their health) and productive (to avoid being a drain on the economy). Such perspectives will work against older adults whose life courses do not support successful aging.

REVIEW QUESTIONS

1. Discuss the merits (validity) of three theories of successful aging from data gathered from focus groups and theorists. Cite variables such as racial or socio-economic differences, expressions of productivity, etc.
2. Following Hurricane Katrina (or other major natural disaster), many people found themselves with no access to their usual occupations. What theories of successful aging can be applied in these cases? Provide examples.
3. How do current government policies affecting people who are aging define "success?"
4. Compare and contrast gerontology theories with occupational therapy/occupational science explanations on successful aging.
5. Discuss the effects of home environments or neighborhood on an individual's ability to age successfully and engage in meaningful occupations.

REFERENCES

1. Achenbaum, W. A. (2009). A metahistorical perspective on theories of aging. In V. L. Bengtson, M. Silverstein, N. M. Putney, & D. Gans (Eds.), *Handbook of theories of aging* (2nd ed., pp. 23–38). New York, NY: Springer.
2. Ambrosi-Randić, N., & Plavšić, M. (2011). Strategies for goal-achievement in older people with different levels of well-being. *Studia Psychologica, 53,* 91–106.
3. Aneshensel, C. S., Wight, R. G., Miller-Martinez, D., Botticello, A. L., Karlamangla, A. S., & Seeman, T. (2007). Urban neighborhoods and depressive symptoms among older adults. *The Journal of Gerontology, 62B,* S52–S59.
4. Atchley, R. C. (1971). Retirement and leisure participation: Continuity or crisis? *The Gerontologist, 11,* 13–17.
5. Atchley, R. C. (1989). A continuity theory of normal aging. *The Gerontologist, 29,* 189–190.
6. Baltes, P. B. (1997). On the incomplete architecture of human ontogeny: Selection, optimization, and compensation as foundation of developmental theory. *American Psychologist, 52,* 366–380.
7. Baltes, P. B., & Smith, J. (2003). New frontiers in the future of aging: From successful aging of the young old to the dilemmas of the fourth age. *Gerontology, 49,* 123–135.
8. Baum, C. M., & Christiansen, C. H. (2005). Person-environment-occupation-performance: An occupation-based framework for practice. In C. H. Christiansen, C. M. Baum & J. Bass-Haugen (Eds.), *Occupational therapy: Performance, participation, and well-being* (pp. 243–266). Thorofare, NJ: Slack.
9. Bengtson, V. L., Silverstein, M., Putney, N. M., & Gans, D. (Eds.). (2009). *Handbook of theories of aging* (2nd ed.). New York, NY: Springer.
10. Birren, J., & Schaie, K. W. (Eds.). (1990). *Handbook of the psychology of aging* (3rd ed.). New York, NY: Academic Press.
11. Bourdieu, P. (1984). *Distinction: A social critique of the judgement of taste.* (R. Nice, Trans.). Cambridge, MA: Harvard University Press. (Original work published 1979)
12. Bowling, A. (2007). Aspirations for older age in the 21st century: What is successful aging? *International Journal of Aging and Human Development, 64,* 263–297.
13. Butler, R. N. (1974). Successful aging and the role of life review. *Journal of the American Geriatrics Society, 22,* 529–535.
14. Canadian Association of Occupational Therapists. (2003). Position statement: Occupational therapy and active living for older adults. *Canadian Journal of Occupational Therapy, 70,* 183–184.
15. Carlson, M., Clark, F., & Young, B. (1998). Practical contributions of occupational science to the art of successful ageing: How to sculpt a meaningful life in older adulthood. *Journal of Occupational Science, 5,* 107–118.
16. Clarke, A., & Warren, L. (2007). Hopes, fears and expectations about the future: What do older people's stories tell us about active aging? *Aging and Society, 27,* 465–488.
17. Clarke, P., Marshall, V., House, J., & Lantz, P. (2011). The social structuring of mental health over the adult life course: Advancing theory in the sociology of aging. *Social Forces, 89,* 1287–1314.
18. Cumming, E., & Henry, W. E. (1961). *Growing old.* New York, NY: Basic Books.
19. Cutchin, M. P. (2003). The process of mediated aging-in-place: A theoretically and empirically based model. *Social Science and Medicine, 57,* 1077–1090.
20. Cuypers, K., Krokstad, S., Holmen, T. L., Knudtsen, M. S., Bygren, L. O., & Holmen, J. (2011). Patterns of receptive and creative cultural activities and their association with perceived health, anxiety, depression and satisfaction with life among adults: The HUNT study, Norway. *Journal of Epidemiological and Community Health, 1–6.* doi: 10.1136/jech.2010.113571.
21. Davidson, J. (Director). (1995). *On old age 1: A conversation with Joan Erikson* at 90 [Motion picture]. San Louis Obispo, CA: Davidson Films.
22. Ebersole, P. (2005). *Gerontological nursing and healthy aging.* Cambridge: Cambridge University Press.
23. Erikson, E. H., Erikson, J. M., & Kivnick, H. Q. (1986). *Vital involvement in old age.* New York, NY: W. W. Norton & Co.
24. Estes, C., Biggs, S., & Phillipson, C. (2003). *Social theory, social policy, and aging: A critical introduction.* London: Open University Press.
25. Fry, C. L. (2009). Out of the armchair and off the veranda: Anthropological theories and the experiences of aging. In V. L. Bengtson, M. Silverstein, N. M. Putney, & D. Gans (Eds.), *Handbook of theories of aging* (2nd ed., pp. 499–515). New York, NY: Springer.
26. Gans, D., Putney, N. M., Bengtson, V. L., & Silverstein, M. (2009). The future of theories of aging. In V. L. Bengtson, M. Silverstein, N. M. Putney, & D. Gans (Eds.), *Handbook of theories of aging* (2nd ed., pp. 723–738). New York, NY: Springer.
27. Gitlin, L. N. (2003). Conducting research on home environments: Lessons learned and new directions. *The Gerontologist, 43,* 628–637.
28. Golant, S. M. (2003). Conceptualizing time and behavior in environmental gerontology: A pair of old issues deserving new thought. *The Gerontologist, 43,* 638–648.
29. Harris, P. B. (2008). Another wrinkle in the debate about successful aging: The undervalued concept of resilience and the lived experience of dementia. *International Journal of Aging and Human Development, 67*(1), 43–61.
30. Havighurst, R. J. (1961). Successful aging. *The Gerontologist, 1,* 8–13.
31. Havighurst, R. J., & Albrecht, R. (1953). *Older people.* New York, NY: Longmans.
32. Heatwole Shank, K., & Cutchin, M. P. (2010). Transactional occupations of older women aging-in-place: Negotiating change and meaning. *Journal of Occupational Science, 17,* 4–13.
33. Hinterlong, J. E., & Williamson, A. (2006-7). The effects of civic engagement of current and future cohorts of older adults. *Generations, 30,* 10–17.
34. Hocking, C., Murphy, J., & Reed, K. (2011). Strategies older New Zealanders use to participate in day-to-day occupations. *British Journal of Occupational Therapy, 74*(11), 509–516.
35. Iwarsson, S. (2005). A long-term perspective on person-environment fit and ADL dependence among older Swedish adults. *The Gerontologist, 45,* 327–336.
36. Iwasaki, Y., & Smale, B. J. A. (1998). Longitudinal analyses of the relationships among life transitions, chronic health problems, leisure, and psychological well-being. *Leisure Sciences, 20,* 25–52.
37. Jang, S-N., Choi, Y-J., & Kim, D-H. (2009). Association of socioeconomic status with successful ageing: Differences in the components of successful aging. *Journal of Biosocial Science, 41,* 207–219.

38. Johansson, K., Josephsson, S., & Lilja, M. (2009). Creating possibilities for action in the presence of environmental barriers in the process of "ageing in place." *Ageing and Society, 29*, 49–70.

39. Kaplan, H., Gurven, M., & Winkling, J. (2009). An evolutionary theory of human life span: Embodied capital and the human adaptive complex. In V. L. Bengtson, M. Silverstein, N. M. Putney, & D. Gans (Eds.), *Handbook of theories of aging* (2nd ed., pp. 39–60). New York, NY: Springer.

40. Kelly, J. R. (1999). Leisure behaviors and styles: Social economic and cultural factors. In E. Jackson & T. Burton (Eds.), *Leisure studies: Prospects for the twenty-first century* (pp. 135–150). State College, PA: Venture Press.

41. Kielhofner, G. (2008). *Model of human occupation: Theory and application* (4th ed.). Baltimore, MD: Lippincott Williams & Wilkins.

42. Lang, F. R., Ricckmann, N., & Baltes, M. M. (2002). Adapting to aging losses: Do resources facilitate strategies of selection, compensation, and optimization in everyday functioning? *The Journals of Gerontology, 57B*, P501–P509.

43. Lawton, M. P. (1993). Meanings of activity. In J. R. Kelly (Ed.), *Activity and aging: Staying involved in later life* (pp. 25–41). Newbury Park, CA: Sage.

44. Lemon, B. W., Bengtson, V. L., & Peterson, J. A. (1972). An exploration of the activity theory of aging: Activity types and life satisfaction among in-movers to a retirement community. *Journal of Gerontology, 27*(4), 511–523.

45. Lichtenberg, P. A., MacNeill, S. E., & Mast, B. T. (2000). Environmental press and adaptation to disability in hospitalized live-alone older adults. *The Gerontologist, 40*, 549–556.

46. Maddox, G. L., & Campbell, R. T. (1985). Scope, concepts, and methods in the study of aging. In R. H. Binstock & L. K. George (Eds.), *Handbook of aging and the social sciences* (2nd ed., pp. 3–31). New York, NY: Van Nostrand-Reinhold.

47. Martinson, M. (2006–2007). Opportunities or obligations? Civic engagement and older adults. *Generations, 30*, 59–65.

48. McMunn, A., Nazroo, J., Wahrendorf, M., & Zaninotto, P. (2009). Participation in socially productive activities, reciprocity and well-being in later life: Baseline results in England. *Ageing and Society, 29*, 765–782.

49. Menec, V. H. (2003). The relation between everyday activities and successful aging: A 6-year longitudinal study. *The Journals of Gerontology, 54B*, S74–S82.

50. Mosey, A. C. (1974). An alternative: The biopsychosocial model. *American Journal of Occupational Therapy, 28*(3), 137–140.

51. Murphy, S. L. (2010). Centennial vision: Geriatric research. *American Journal of Occupational Therapy, 64*, 172–181.

52. Neugarten, B. L. (1964). *Personality in middle and late life*. New York, NY: Atherton Press.

53. Nimrod, G., & Kleiber, D. A. (2007). Reconsidering change and continuity in later life: Toward an innovation theory of successful aging. *International Journal of Aging and Human Development, 65*, 1–22.

54. Nygard, L. (2004). Responses of persons with dementia to challenges in daily activities: A synthesis of findings from empirical studies. *American Journal of Occupational Therapy, 58*, 435–445.

55. Organisation for Economic Co-operation and Development. (1998). *Policy brief: Maintaining prosperity in an ageing society*. Paris: OECD. Retrieved from http://www.oecd.org/dataoecd/21/10/2430300.pdf.

56. Quadagno, J. (2007). *Aging and the life course: An introduction to social gerontology* (4th ed.). Boston, MA: McGraw-Hill.

57. Reichstadt, J., Depp, C. A., Palinkas, L. A., Folsom, D. P., & Jeste, D. V. (2007). Building blocks of successful aging: A focus group study of older adults' perceived contributors to successful aging. *The American Journal of Geriatric Psychiatry, 15*(3), 194–201.

58. Rowe, J. W., & Kahn, R L. (1998). *Successful aging*. New York, NY: Pantheon Books.

59. Rudman, D. L. (2006). Reflections on … Positive aging and its implications for occupational possibilities in later life. *Canadian Journal of occupational Therapy, 73*, 188–192.

60. Ryff, C. D., & Singer, B. (2009). Understanding healthy aging: Key components and their integration. In V. L. Bengtson, M. Silverstein, N. M. Putney, & D. Gans (Eds.), *Handbook of theories of aging* (2nd ed., pp. 117–144). New York, NY: Springer.

61. Sneed, J. R., & Whitbourne, S. K. (2005). Models of the aging self. *Journal of Social Issues, 61*, 375–388.

62. Stanley, M. (2006). *Older people's understandings and perceptions of well-being: A grounded theory*. Adelaide, Australia: Unpublished doctoral dissertation, University of South Australia.

63. Stark, S., Landsbaum, A., Palmer, J. L., Somerville, E. K., & Morris, J. C. (2009). Client-centred home modifications improve daily activity performance of older adults. *Canadian Journal of Occupational Therapy, 76*, 235–245.

64. Strawbridge, W. J., Wallhagen, M. I., & Cohen, R. D. (2002). Successful aging and well-being: Self-rated compared with Rowe and Kahn. *The Gerontologist, 42*(6), 727–733.

65. Townsend, E. A., & Polatajko, H. J. (2007). *Enabling occupation II: Advancing an occupational therapy vision for health, well-being, and justice through occupation*. Ottawa, ON: CAOT Publications ACE.

66. Voelkl, J. E. (1993). Activity among older adults in institutional settings. In J. R. Kelly (Ed.), *Activity and aging* (pp. 231–245). Newbury Park, CA: Sage.

67. Wahl, H-W., Oswald, F., & Zimprich, D. (1999). Everyday competence in visually impaired older adults: A case for person-environment perspectives. *The Gerontologist, 39*, 140–149.

68. Wilcock, A. A. (2007). Active ageing: Dream or reality? *New Zealand Journal of Occupational Therapy, 54*, 15–20.

69. Willcox, D. C., Willcox, B. J., Sokolovsky, J., & Sakihara, S. (2007). The cultural context of "successful aging" among older women weavers in a northern Okinawan village: The role of productive activity. *Journal of Cross Cultural Gerontology, 22*, 137–165.

70. Wood, W., Womack, J., & Hooper, B. (2009). Dying of boredom: An exploratory case study of time use, apparent affect, and routine activity situations on two Alzheimer's special care units. *American Journal of Occupational Therapy, 63*, 337–350.

71. World Health Organization. (2001). *International classification of functioning, disability and health*. Geneva: World Health Organization.

72. World Health Organization. (2002). *Active ageing: A policy framework*. Geneva: Author. Retrieved from http://www.who.int/ageing/publications/active/en/index.html.

73. Zarit, S. H. (2009). A good old age: Theories of mental health and aging. In V. L. Bengtson, M. Silverstein, N. M. Putney, & D. Gans (Eds.), *Handbook of theories of aging* (2nd ed., pp. 675–691). New York, NY: Springer.

CHAPTER 5

Foundations of Evidence-Based Gerontological Occupational Therapy Practice

Mary Krieger, RN, MLIS, Donghua Tao, MLIS, MS, PhD, Charlotte B. Royeen, PhD, OTR/L, FAOTA

CHAPTER OUTLINE

OBJECTIVES

- Describe the evolution of and rationale for evidence-based practice within the occupational therapy profession and the relationship between evidence-based practice and ethical gerontological occupational therapy practice
- Describe the steps for implementing evidence-based practice and the online information tools and resources for acquiring research evidence
- Identify the research designs that are appropriate for answering different types of questions in occupational therapy practice and describe the techniques for evaluating these studies
- Describe practical strategies for implementing evidence-based practice in gerontological occupational therapy
- Describe future trends in applying and implementing evidence-based practice in occupational therapy

Rationale for Evidence-Based Practice

Research within the occupational therapy (OT) profession generates a body of knowledge upon which practice is built, tests the theoretical models and tools used in practice, and evaluates the process and outcomes of therapy.[51] Research demonstrates to clients, policymakers, referring physicians, and to the public at large that "the profession possesses the expertise and data-based evidence to accomplish what it purports to accomplish for its patients and students" (p. 347).[35] Furthermore, research demonstrates which OT services and interventions are efficacious in improving health, promoting wellness, and enhancing quality of life for clients, and it guides practitioners in providing the highest standard of care. Evidence-based practice (EBP) refers to a clinical decision-making process that integrates the best available research evidence with clinician expertise and patient background, values, and preferences to produce the best outcome for the patient.[82] According to Horowitz and Toto, using an evidence-based approach in gerontological OT is a "win-win situation for everyone. It demonstrates professionalism and ethical practice, supports effective interventions and improved client outcomes, and documents intervention rationale in case of reimbursement inquiries" (p. 30).[47] Most important, evidence-based practice is the right thing to do as professionals, and fosters the use of clinical reasoning with empirical data. In this manner, evidence-based practice is ethically based practice—something to which all therapists aspire for the good of society.

History and Scope of Evidence-Based Practice in Occupational Therapy

Although the concept of evidence-based practice originated in the field of medicine, this philosophy for clinical practice became firmly established within most of the health sciences disciplines by the middle to late 1990s, and evidence-based practice has expanded into other fields such as public health, psychology, education, and social work.[77] One of the earliest explicit references to evidence-based practice in the OT literature is a 1995 commentary calling upon OT professionals to publish research demonstrating the effectiveness of OT services—or else, this article notes, why would purchasers "buy it"?[20]

The concept of evidence-based practice, therefore, is relatively new. The actual work and implementation of evidence into practice are not. Based upon the work of A. Jean Ayres, evidence-based practice was the hallmark of the practice in sensory integration implemented by Virginia "Ginny" Scardina in her student training program of the 1970s. Some of the student occupational therapists who came out of this "movement" are well known today and still carry on in the tradition of evidence-based practice. They are (in alphabetical order): Joan Dostal, Linda Fazio, Jane Koomar, Shelly Lane, Charlotte Royeen, and Mary Schneider. Each day when a student arrived in the Cincinnati pediatric clinic where Virginia Scardina worked, there seemed to be a new way of doing things. Typically, it was because "Ginny" had just read research the night before that had implications for sensory integrative–based practice, and she implemented the research finding into practice the next day. That is what an evidence-based approach to health care is really all about. Thus some aspects of OT practice—as well as other practice areas—used evidence previously discovered long ago. This clinical model has greatly expanded so that today, there is a huge emphasis on getting everyone involved in evidence-based practice.

Although all OT practitioners may not realistically be expected to actively conduct research in addition to managing heavy caseloads, all therapists have a *duty* to be "consumers of research" and to implement current best evidence within their own practice.[27] There is often a perception that evidence-based practice is not feasible for frontline clinicians because of lack of time or lack of research appraisal skills. However, integrating evidence into OT practice is not a difficult task[47] and it benefits both the client and the therapist. Evidence-based practice can be viewed as a "toolbox of methods to aid clinical reasoning," which helps ensure that clients receive the best possible care. And, the use of independent, scientific evidence guards against personal bias in the selection of an intervention solely because a therapist may favor one particular type of intervention over another.[85] Many scholarly OT journals have published informative articles to help clinicians understand the principles of evidence-based practice and how to apply evidence in their clinical sites. Furthermore, professional associations, such as the American Occupational Therapy Association (AOTA), the British Association of Occupational Therapists (BAOT), and others, have developed guidelines that synthesize research findings that are critically important for clinicians. In these cases, experts have already synthesized the literature for the occupational therapist to read and use in practice. Thus no one can say their caseload prevents them from implementing evidence-based practice. The therapist only has to know where to find the syntheses of the needed information. In fact, it is well recognized that professional associations should and do assist their practitioners in sorting through evidence.

Evidence-based practice is an explicit standard of conduct in the ethical codes of the American Occupational Therapy Association,[46] the Canadian Association of Occupational Therapists,[12] and the College of Occupational Therapists in the United Kingdom,[15] and it is endorsed by the World Federation of Occupational Therapists.[57] Given that evidence-based practice is mandated in the codes of ethics for all of these professional organizations, it reinforces the fact that ethical practice is, in part, based upon evidence-based practice. Many practitioners labor under a false understanding of evidence-based practice, thinking that it is only based upon clinical trials research. The intent of initiatives regarding evidence-based practice was never to do away with clinical expertise and the knowledge gained via practice and other sources of client knowledge, but to supplement it with empirical data from systematic research to assist in clinical reasoning for improved client outcomes. In fact, Coppola and Elliot have presented a broader definition of "evidence" that includes three categories of evidence that are important to occupational therapists: evidence from research, evidence from the client in context, and evidence from reflective clinical experience. The integration and application of evidence from these three sources is considered to be one of the hallmarks of "best practice" in gerontological occupational therapy.[28]

Interprofessional Models of Evidence-Based Practice

Interprofessional collaboration and evidence-based practice are considered core competencies that all health professionals, regardless of discipline, should possess to provide optimum patient-centered care in the twenty-first century.[16] However, "work in evidence-based practice is often profession-specific, without exchange of theories, models, or tools in a unified approach focusing on a specific patient outcome" (p. 414).[69] The study designs that constitute "high-quality" evidence often vary among the professions. In medicine, quantitative methods such as meta-analyses and randomized trials are ranked at the top of the evidence hierarchy. In nursing, social work, and occupational therapy, qualitative research studies are also especially valued for their client-centered orientation, insight into patient experiences, and exploration of the issues that are important to clients.[41,77] These variations may reflect the sociologic level of development of the profession (is it a mature or emerging profession?) and the levels of research developing within the field. For example, it is a challenge to do proper clinical trials research if basic constructs and knowledge in the field are lacking (often called descriptive research). This, in part, is also why clinical trials in occupational therapy are challenging, because the profession has a limited quantity of descriptive studies.

Cognitive and social boundaries, such as different research cultures, knowledge domains, and values, may inhibit diffusion of evidence-based innovations across professions.[29] However, interprofessional organizations like the Cochrane Collaboration and the Joanna Briggs Institute are working to synthesize the high-quality research evidence from the professional literature of many different health-care professions to produce an evidence base that may be shared across the professions.

Since 1993, the Cochrane Collaboration has been a leading model of interprofessional collaboration in producing systematic reviews of the effectiveness of health interventions to support evidence-based practice. The Cochrane Collaboration is organized into review groups that focus on particular health areas, and participation by health professionals from all fields is encouraged within the groups. The Cochrane review groups investigate the efficacy of interventions for health problems such as dementia, stroke, musculoskeletal disorders, hypertension, and depression, which are relevant to gerontological occupational therapists and are areas in which occupational therapists possess considerable expertise.[62] There are significant benefits to individual therapists and to the OT profession as a whole from participating in the work of the Cochrane groups:

> Occupational therapy clinicians can use Cochrane systematic reviews to confirm, inform, and improve their practice and that of the teams in which they work. . . . For occupational therapists and occupational therapy students who are interested in better understanding research, the Cochrane site . . . incorporates resources to improve skills in appraising quality of clinical trials and enhancing understanding of systematic reviews. . . . For occupational therapy researchers, Cochrane systematic reviews identify gaps where further research is required. (p. 209)[62]

Participation of occupational therapists in the Cochrane Collaboration broadens the evidence base of the OT profession, validates the effectiveness of OT interventions in a highly visible and authoritative public forum, and strengthens the collaborative relationships with other professions working to improve outcomes for older adult clients. "In order for systematic reviews to be truly multidisciplinary, and of value to all, occupational therapy must be included as should other health professions" (p. 289).[65]

The Joanna Briggs Institute (JBI) is an international research and implementation collaboration incorporating the disciplines of nursing, medicine, occupational therapy, physiotherapy, nutrition and dietetics, podiatry, complementary therapies, aged care, and others whose mission is to improve health globally through evidence-based practice. JBI was established in 1996 and is currently based at the University of Adelaide in South Australia. JBI collaborating groups are composed of health-care professionals from over 40 countries who work to promote evidence-based health care through providing education and training, conducting systematic reviews, developing Best Practice Information Sheets, and integrating evidence into practice.[50] Like the Cochrane Collaboration, the JBI is a dynamic, working model of interprofessional collaboration in producing evidence to support health-care practice. Key members of the JBI team have also developed a conceptual model for the *process* of evidence-based practice that is built upon the earlier medical model of evidence-based practice proposed by Haynes and colleagues (Figure 5-1)[44] but is more inclusive in its definition of evidence. In the JBI model (Figure 5-2),[72] qualitative research, credible expert opinion, and authoritative textual sources such as books, journals, reports, and guidelines are considered valid sources from which evidence can be synthesized. The rationale for this more "pluralistic approach to what constitutes legitimate evidence" is that practicing clinicians must respond to patient/client needs "even if no evidence from research exists....The pragmatics of practice require clinicians to adopt a perspective that works and is the most appropriate in the circumstances" (p. 9).[72]

In 2007, health professionals from medicine, nursing, psychology, social work, and public health formed the Council on Evidence-Based Behavioral Practice (EBBP) with grant support from the National Institutes of Health. This interprofessional group is working to "improve research and practice training for psychosocial interventions, build the evidence

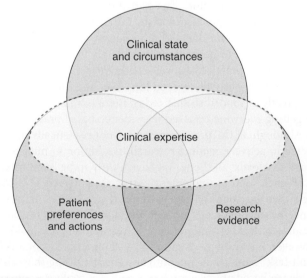

FIGURE 5-1 Haynes et al.'s evidence-based medicine model. (From Haynes, R. B., Devereaux, P. J., & Guyatt, G. H. [2002]. Clinical expertise in the era of evidence-based medicine and patient choice. *ACP Journal Club, 136,* A11-A14.)

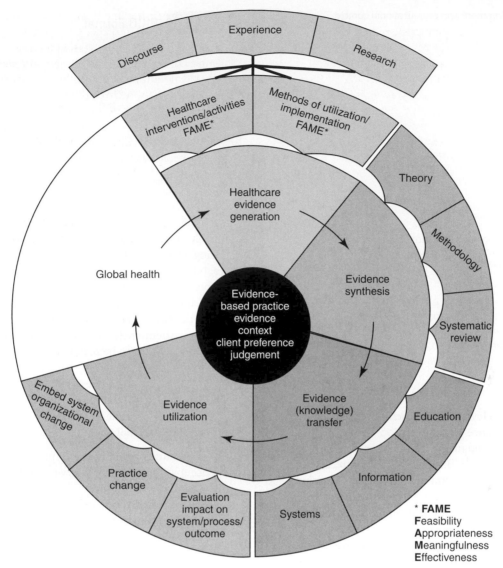

FIGURE 5-2   Model of evidence-based practice. (From Pearson, A., Wiechula, R., Court, A., & Lockwood, C. [2005]. The JBI model of evidence-based healthcare. *International Journal of Evidence-Based Healthcare, 3*, 207-215.)

base for behavioral treatments, and upgrade evidence-based behavioral practice." Behavioral practice seeks to influence behavioral and social factors such as smoking, obesity, poor nutrition, and physical inactivity that contribute to illness and poor health outcomes.[80] Members of the EBBP Council have developed a transdisciplinary conceptual model of evidence-based practice, that is, a model that works across disciplines (Figure 5-3),[77] which incorporates the important concepts that each profession has contributed to evidence-based practice and attempts to minimize the deficiencies in the individual profession's model.[77]

An important point to note here is that the *models* of evidence-based practice have evolved over time from the earliest model that described the process of EBBP from the perspective of a single profession (medicine) to models that are designed to be interprofessional in their scope and work across

the health-care disciplines. The OT profession can and should "use evidence from a variety of disciplines and professions to support and improve practice" (p. 290),[27] and it is likely that initiatives to produce and share evidence across professions will continue to grow. "The potential to affect improvements in the quality of care delivered through interdisciplinary teams informed by evidence is the opportunity of the decade" (p. 416).[69]

Implementation of Evidence-Based Gerontological Occupational Therapy Practice

Straus and colleagues have developed five steps for implementing evidence-based practice, which can be summarized with the "5A" memory aid: (1) **a**sking a clinical question, (2) **a**cquiring the evidence, (3) **a**ppraising the evidence critically

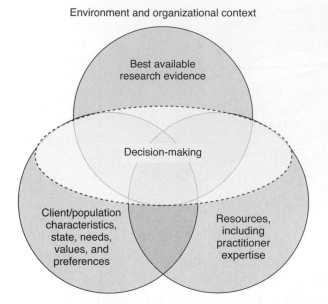

Environment and organizational context

FIGURE 5-3 Transdisciplinary model of evidence-based practice. (From Satterfield, J. M., Spring, B., Brownson, R. C., Mullen, E. J., Newhouse, R. P., Walker, B. B., & Whitlock, E. P. [2009]. Toward a transdisciplinary model of evidence-based practice. *The Milbank Quarterly, 87,* 368-390.)

for validity and relevance to the client or population, (4) applying the evidence in conjunction with patient preferences and clinician judgment, and (5) assessing the effectiveness of this process.[77,82] The first two steps are discussed in detail in the following section of this chapter, "Searching and Selecting the Literature." Steps 3 and 4 are described subsequently in the section "Critiquing and Conceptually Applying the Literature to Current Practice." The following clinical question is used as an example throughout these sections to illustrate each of the steps:

If utilized with older adults living in the community, does a preventive OT intervention targeting activity of daily living (ADL) skills improve daily functioning and maintain the ability of individuals to live independently at home?

Searching and Selecting the Literature

Asking a Clinical Question

The first step in evidence-based practice is to formulate a clear, precise question about a specific client's problem or a problem that is common in the population of older adults. In occupational therapy, the question frequently focuses on one of three tasks: (1) identifying an occupational performance issue, (2) selecting an assessment tool, or (3) planning an intervention.[85] Straus and colleagues[82] have defined four elements that comprise a well-constructed clinical question, expressed as the PICO format (Box 5-1).

The PICO format identifies the important elements in a clinical question, such as the client characteristics and intervention of interest, and it helps to focus the therapist's "scarce

| **BOX 5-1** | PICO Format |

P—Patient/population/problem of interest
I—Intervention (this can be a treatment, diagnostic test, assessment measure, or other activity planned for the patient or occurring with the patient)
C—Comparison intervention (if relevant to the clinical situation)
O—Outcome of interest to the patient and to the clinician

(From Straus, S. E., Richardson, W. S., Rosenberg, W., & Haynes, R. B. [2005]. *Evidence-based medicine: How to practice and teach EBM* [3rd ed.]. New York, NY: Elsevier Churchill Livingstone.)

learning time" on evidence that directly supports client care.[82] The PICO format should serve as a guide or template for choosing search terms that will be entered in online databases, but it is important to note that not all of the words or concepts in the PICO format have to be used in the search strategy. It is best to begin the search using search terms that describe the two most important PICO elements, which are usually the patient/client and the intervention. Then, if the set of results is too large to be scanned in a reasonable amount of time, the terms that express the outcome element can be added to the search. The question concerning the efficacy of home-based occupational therapy in helping clients to maintain independence might appear in this manner when rewritten in the PICO format:

P—older adults living in the community
I—occupational therapy intervention targeting ADL/ IADL skills
C—compared with no intervention
O—improve function; maintain independence and ability to live at home

Acquiring the Evidence to Inform Practice

The next step in evidence-based practice is to gather the information or evidence to address the problem or question. External sources of evidence to support clinical decision making can be high-quality research studies published in peer-reviewed journals, authoritative textbooks for background knowledge, professional association websites that publish clinical practice guidelines, and specialized online databases that synthesize and summarize research. For OT practice with older adults, individualized evidence gathered from the client and from family members within the context of their daily lives should be considered an equally important source of evidence upon which to base treatment decisions. The client is the authority on the occupations that are meaningful to him or her, the interventions that have been successful in the past, and the outcomes that are most important for his or her well-being and quality of life.[28,85]

Acquiring the external evidence to guide clinical decisions is a two-step process: (1) identifying the appropriate information resources for the question and (2) creating and executing an effective search strategy within those resources.

Information Resources for Occupational Therapy

As has been previously stated, a first step for any occupational therapist is to determine whether there are practice guidelines or other resources that may be available from professional occupational therapy associations to address the question at hand. It may or may not be necessary to go beyond what these organizations have available. If a particular question or issue is beyond the resources provided by the professional organizations, an online bibliographic database may be used to search for articles published in peer-reviewed journals to address the question. Some of these databases are freely available to the public, whereas others require a paid subscription for access. Consultation with a health sciences librarian is highly recommended because the librarian can provide a list of the resources available at a given site and can assist with creating effective search strategies. The investment of a few hours of time with a librarian at the beginning of the information retrieval process can save hours of time for the busy clinician in the long run. Many outcomes of interest to occupational therapists working with older adults, such as client safety, improved quality of life, health promotion, and client education, are shared by other health-care professionals. Research studies pertaining to these outcomes can be found in the literature of a variety of health sciences disciplines, including medicine, nursing, psychology, geriatrics, and rehabilitation. Therefore, a comprehensive literature search on any given topic most often requires the use of multiple online databases.

Bibliographic Citation Databases

Bibliographic citation databases contain the citations (author, title, and source information) and abstracts for a select group of journals, depending on the scope or coverage area of the database. Often these databases index the higher-quality, peer-reviewed journals in the designated subject areas, and they may or may not contain links to full-text articles. Bibliographic citation databases are one of the most important sources for finding research for evidence-based practice.[23] They provide access to the original research articles that are the foundation for professional guidelines and for specialized, evidence-based online tools that will be discussed in more detail later in this chapter.

There are several discipline-specific bibliographic databases that are particularly effective for retrieving high-quality literature related to the practice of gerontological occupational therapy. The benefit of using the discipline-specific databases is that they contain a thesaurus, or "master list," of subject terms, which helps the searcher find the most relevant information on a topic. The drawback is that each database must be searched separately with the terminology unique to that database to get the best results, which can be a more time-consuming task. The databases described here would be appropriate to use in searching for evidence about the efficacy of preventive OT interventions with older adults.

OT SEARCH

The **OT SEARCH** is an online index of the contents of the American Occupational Therapy Foundation (AOTF) Wilma L. West Library. It aggregates the journal and book literature of occupational therapy and supporting materials from the rehabilitation, education, and psychology disciplines into one convenient database, a type of "one-stop shopping" for information related to occupational therapy. The OT SEARCH thesaurus contains subject terms that precisely describe the physiologic assessments, therapeutic techniques, and theories used by occupational therapists. OT SEARCH is accessed by paid subscription only, but members of the American Occupational Therapy Association (AOTA) receive a substantial discount in price. More information about this database can be obtained at the AOTF website (http://www.aotf.org/).

MEDLINE/PubMed

MEDLINE/PubMed is the premier database for retrieving biomedical journal literature, and it covers virtually all health-care disciplines. It indexes approximately eight occupational therapy journals and 100 rehabilitation journals, along with the core peer-reviewed clinical and research journals in medicine, geriatrics, nursing, and related health sciences disciplines. MEDLINE has a comprehensive thesaurus of medical subject headings (known as MeSH), and the terms are arranged in a logical, hierarchical tree structure that allows the searcher to "explode" a subgroup of search terms to broaden a search. MEDLINE also has a "Restrict to MeSH Major Topic" feature that allows users to narrow a search to subject terms that are the main focus of the article. PubMed is the interface to the MEDLINE database that is freely available to the public and can be accessed worldwide.

The Cumulative Index to Nursing and Allied Health Literature

The Cumulative Index to Nursing and Allied Health Literature (CINAHL) database covers the literature of nursing, physical therapy, occupational therapy, nutrition and dietetics, and other health-related professions. CINAHL indexes approximately 13 occupational therapy–related journals not covered by MEDLINE and includes citations to books, book chapters, and dissertations. Access to CINAHL is by paid subscription only. There is some overlap of journal content coverage between MEDLINE and CINAHL, but both databases should be searched to achieve comprehensive retrieval of the OT literature related to a clinical question.

AgeLine

Another discipline-specific database relevant for occupational therapy, the AgeLine database, contains citations to journal articles, books, book chapters, and reports on all aspects of aging (50+ years), including economics, public policy, psychology, social work, and health. When using the AgeLine database, the searcher has less need to use limiters or keywords to restrict the retrieval to articles about older adults, which is required in the other databases. The highly focused subject areas and relatively small size of the AgeLine and OT SEARCH databases often make it easier to locate relevant articles that are buried in the larger databases such as MEDLINE. Access to the AgeLine database is by paid subscription only.

Scopus and Web of Science

There are two large, multidisciplinary bibliographic citation databases, Scopus and Web of Science, which cover the journal literature in a broad array of scientific, medical, and social sciences journals, including the humanities. These databases require a paid subscription and they can be used for subject searching and for cited-reference searching—that is, for retrieving articles that cite a particularly relevant reference article or to view the cited references of a relevant article. The benefit to using these broader databases is that one search will retrieve articles from many different subject disciplines, which is beneficial for occupational therapy because the knowledge base of the profession covers or relates to so many disciplines and fields of study, and because it saves time for the searcher. The disadvantage is that these databases lack some of the search tools—for example, the "explosion" of subject terms in the thesaurus and the ability to designate subject terms as a major focus of the article—that the MEDLINE and CINAHL databases provide.

When preparing a literature review or performing a comprehensive database search for evidence related to client care, it is best to use multiple databases that cover the literature related to the topic to reduce the chance of missing relevant article citations.

It should be noted that when searching in all of these databases—OT SEARCH, PubMed, CINAHL, AgeLine, Scopus, and Web of Science—the bibliographic records for journal articles, *not* the full text of the articles, will be retrieved. The clinician will be able to read abstracts for many of the articles, and some of these databases contain links to the full text of journal articles. Depending on the institution for which the occupational therapist works, there may be direct access to paid subscription journals from a tool within the databases. Therapists may consult the librarians at their individual institutions or clinic sites to find out what journal resources and subscription-based bibliographic citation databases will be available to them.

Specialized Evidence-Based Practice Resources

During the early years when evidence-based practice was being defined and hierarchies of evidence were being developed, the bibliographic databases like MEDLINE that indexed primary research studies were the major and sometimes sole source of acquiring evidence. In the last decade, however, specialized information systems and services have evolved to support the needs of busy clinicians for rapid, efficient, and authoritative access to high-quality evidence, including databases that contain summaries or syntheses by subject experts of individual or multiple well-conducted research studies.[43] One such synthesis of research is the systematic review, a summary and critique of a select group of high-quality

research studies on a given intervention. Occupational therapists, like all health-care professionals, face the challenge of keeping up to date with the volume of relevant research published in their field and related fields, and the systematic review can be a useful resource to inform practice.[3]

One specialized evidence-based practice resource, OTseeker, is a database that contains the citations to systematic reviews and randomized controlled trials relevant to the practice of occupational therapy. OTseeker should not be confused with the OT SEARCH database described earlier in the chapter. OTseeker is freely available to occupational therapists and to the public, and its content is limited to only systematic reviews and randomized controlled trials, a very select group of research studies that are considered to have the strongest evidence for practice. OT SEARCH is more inclusive in gathering together all types of literature, research and nonresearch, that are relevant for OT practice. The systematic reviews and randomized trials in OTseeker are located by rigorous searching of key databases, such as MEDLINE, CINAHL, and others, and by hand searching key journals relevant to occupational therapy. The randomized controlled trials in OTseeker are rated on their methodological quality using a scale that was developed for the Physiotherapy Evidence Database (PEDro). The rating scale helps users determine which studies have higher internal validity and are less subject to bias.[8] OT seeker is updated continuously as new studies are published, which is essential for maintaining the currency of the evidence. In a 2007 survey, users of OTseeker reported that it was a valuable resource for finding evidence related to practice, and it was ranked as the third most frequently used resource after the MEDLINE and CINAHL databases.[9]

The Cochrane Collaboration website, as discussed previously, is another important resource for finding systematic reviews of the effectiveness of health-care interventions related to gerontology and occupational therapy. The abstracts and summaries of the systematic reviews are freely available on the website http://www.cochrane.org/; access to the full text of the reviews is by paid subscription only.

Other Internet Resources

Although general Internet search engines, such as Google, have the ability to retrieve an immense body of electronically published information, they lack the selectivity in content and precision in searching that the bibliographic citation databases possess. However, Internet resources that can be valuable for evidence-based practice are the professional websites for the national and international occupational therapy associations, such as the World Federation of Occupational Therapists (WFOT) and the American, Australian, British, and Canadian occupational therapy associations. All of these associations have web pages devoted to evidence-based practice tools and resources. Some of the content may be restricted to members only, but there is a wealth of freely available content.

Another Internet resource that is extremely useful for finding evidence-based practice guidelines is the National

Guideline Clearinghouse (NGC). NGC is an initiative of the Agency for Healthcare Research and Quality (AHRQ) of the U.S. Department of Health and Human Services. Although it is based in the United States, this database provides access to clinical practice guidelines from many different countries and from many different health-related disciplines that seek to improve the quality and safety of health care.[1] Clinical practice guidelines from national and international professional societies, such as the American Geriatrics Society or the European Federation of Neurological Societies, are also published in journal articles, and these can be retrieved by performing a subject search in PubMed and applying the "Practice Guideline" limit.

Developing a Search Strategy for Bibliographic Databases

Once the appropriate databases have been identified, search terms can be selected to represent the concepts in the PICO statement, and a search strategy is constructed based on the syntax and query modes of the databases. Literature searching skills, like other clinical skills, improve with practice, experience, and familiarity with different techniques and different databases. There are a few key searching techniques common to most bibliographic databases and to general Internet search engines that can be used by searchers to effectively retrieve the evidence needed for practice. Before beginning the search process in any database, it is most helpful to review the Help documentation for that database to determine how the elements discussed in the following sections are handled.

Useful Techniques for Database Searching
Keyword versus Thesaurus (Controlled Vocabulary) Searching

In bibliographic databases, a keyword search, also called text word or natural language searching, retrieves a set of citations that match the character string that is entered, most commonly in the title, abstract, and subject heading fields of the bibliographic records. The use of keywords is effective when searching for very new concepts in the literature or unique terms within a discipline, but it has several drawbacks. Because keyword searching retrieves only the exact

character string that is entered, synonyms must be used when a comprehensive retrieval is desired. For example, when attempting to retrieve all of the articles that pertain to or describe the population of older adults, there are a large number of keywords (e.g., *older adults*, *elderly*, *aged*, *geriatric*) that must be used or potentially relevant articles may be missed.

In databases that contain a thesaurus or master index of subject headings, such as the Medical Subject Headings (MeSH) in MEDLINE/PubMed, index terms are chosen to represent major concepts in the literature covered by the database. Each bibliographic record in the database is assigned subject headings that describe the important concepts or content discussed in the corresponding articles. When the subject heading (versus a keyword) is used in a search, all of the records related to that subject heading are retrieved and a more comprehensive, precise retrieval of articles is achieved. The MEDLINE and CINAHL databases have subject headings such as "aged," "aged 80 and over," "frail elderly," "geriatric assessment," "health services for the elderly," and others, and both databases have age group limits that can be applied to effectively retrieve articles relevant to gerontology. When a subject heading is used, the database will generally display a field tag enclosed in brackets in the search history, for example, "Activities of Daily Living"[MeSH] in PubMed.

Finally, keywords and subject heading terms may be used in combination within a single search; it is not necessary to restrict a strategy to one method or the other. An example of this is shown later in the chapter (see Figure 5-4) where MeSH terms and keywords are both used in a PubMed search for articles about the efficacy of home-based occupational therapy in helping clients to maintain independence.

Boolean Operators and Nesting

After choosing the appropriate subject headings or keywords, these terms are connected by Boolean operators that designate the mathematical operations the computer will perform on the sets of citations. The Boolean operators most frequently used in database searching are AND, OR, and NOT. Combining search terms with the Boolean operator AND means that the resulting set of article citations will contain all of the search terms. Use of the AND operator makes the

	Patient/Population	AND	Intervention	AND	Intervention	AND	Outcome
	Aged[MeSH]		Occupational Therapy[MeSH]		Activities of Daily Living[MeSH]		home
OR			occupational therapist		activities of daily living		community
OR			occupational therap*				independen*

FIGURE 5-4 Concept diagram of PICO elements (shown above). The final search strategy entered into PubMed was: ("Aged"[MeSH]) AND ("Occupational Therapy"[Mesh] OR occupational therapist OR occupational therap*) AND ("Activities of Daily Living"[Mesh] OR "activities of daily living") AND (home OR community OR independen*)

resulting set smaller and more focused. Combining search terms with the Boolean operator OR means that the resulting set of articles will contain at least one of the search terms. The OR operator is frequently used to connect terms that are synonyms, and it will nearly always make the result set larger. The Boolean operator NOT can be used to exclude citations from the result set that contain a particular term. Figure 5-4 is a concept diagram of the search strategy in PICO format for preventive OT services in older adults showing the Boolean operators that will connect the concepts.

The technique of nesting helps to preserve the logic of a search query when multiple terms and Boolean operators are used. When a query contains terms that are joined by the same Boolean operator, for example, aged OR elderly OR geriatric, the order in which the terms are entered generally does not affect the result set. When a search query contains more than one type of Boolean operator, for example, rehabilitation AND aged OR geriatric, nesting is used to tell the database to process one query as a unit, then to process the results of that query with another query, and so forth. A set of parentheses ( ) is used in most databases for nesting. The query rehabilitation AND (aged OR geriatric) would retrieve a set of citations containing the term *rehabilitation* and would combine that set with a set of citations that contain either of the terms *aged* or *geriatric*.

Truncation or Stemming

Truncation or stemming is a technique used in keyword searching that allows for the retrieval of multiple forms of a word using a designated character, such as the "*," "?," or "$." Depending on the database, truncation may be used at the beginning or middle of a word, but is most commonly used at the end of a word to retrieve multiple endings. In PubMed, the truncated keyword disab* would retrieve citations containing the words *disable*, *disabled*, *disability*, and *disabilities*.

Phrase Searching

It is important to determine how each database processes keywords that are intended to represent a phrase, for example, *motor control*, *physical activity*, or *activities of daily living*. Some databases like PubMed will automatically insert the Boolean operator AND between each term that is entered in the query box. To search for keywords as an exact phrase, it is often necessary to enclose the phrase in double quotation marks, for example, "activities of daily living." When subject headings are selected from a database thesaurus, the use of quotation marks for phrase searching is not needed because the computer automatically inserts the punctuation and field tags.

Summary

The first two steps in the process of finding evidence about the efficacy of a preventive OT intervention in maintaining the independence of older adults living at home have been demonstrated. The MEDLINE, CINAHL, OT SEARCH, OT-seeker, AgeLine, Web of Science, and Scopus databases were identified as relevant information resources for questions regarding OT interventions with older adults. The question was articulated in the PICO format and a concept diagram of search terms and Boolean operators was prepared. The diagram is used as a model when entering the search strategy into the different databases to provide consistency and thoroughness for the retrieval in each system. The techniques of subject headings, keywords, Boolean operators, truncation, and phrase searching were used to prepare a search strategy for the PubMed database (see Figure 5-4) from which articles will be selected for appraisal and application of evidence.

Critiquing and Conceptually Applying the Literature to Current Practice

After acquiring the relevant research literature, the next step is to "identify the strengths and weaknesses of a research article in order to assess the usefulness and validity of research findings."[91] This process is called critical appraisal. This section will introduce general principles, criteria, and tools for evaluating research literature, as well as specific criteria for different types of study designs. Because the final goal of evaluating evidence is to choose appropriate therapeutic interventions for patients, factors for conceptually applying the valid literature to current practice are also discussed. Sample literature and study designs related to gerontological occupational therapy are used to explain the appraisal and application techniques.

Research Design and Levels of Evidence

The common types of study designs in the biomedical sciences include clinical trials (randomized or nonrandomized, controlled or uncontrolled, and blinded or unblinded), case-control studies, cohort studies, cross-sectional studies, case series, case-report studies, systematic reviews (including meta-analysis), narrative reviews, and qualitative studies. These designs can involve both humans and animals. As occupational therapy focuses on clinical patient care, the designs covered in this chapter are the designs that involve humans.[21]

Certain research designs are suitable for answering certain research questions. For example, experimental studies, such as randomized control trials (RCT), are typically good for answering questions about therapy, diagnosis, exposure to harm, and screening and prevention; case-control studies or cohort studies are typically good for finding causes, incidence, risk factors, or prognosis for a disease or condition; cross-sectional studies are good for reporting prevalence or frequency of factors, as well as determining the status of a disease or condition; case series or case reports represent a description of rare cases; qualitative studies explore patients' concerns, issues, feelings, and subjective understandings of their lives and experiences.[7,21,91]

Based on different classification schemes, one study design can fall into different categories. Depending on whether a study collects raw data, studies can be classified as primary research or secondary research. Primary research studies collect data from study subjects or an existing data source, then analyze the data. Secondary research studies summarize or

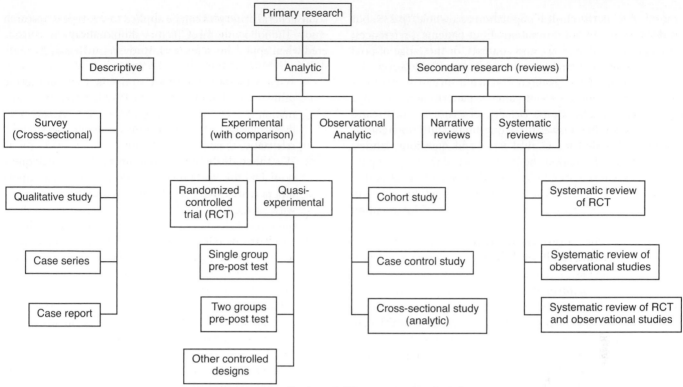

FIGURE 5-5   Classifications of different types of study designs.

synthesize the findings of existing research. Based on this scheme, systematic reviews and narrative reviews are secondary research, whereas the other study designs can be viewed as primary research. Primary research studies can be divided into descriptive studies, which simply describe a population,

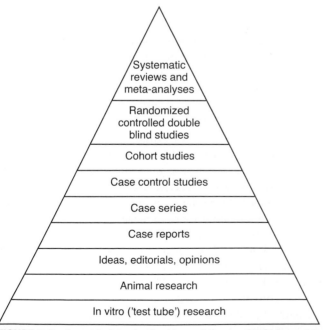

FIGURE 5-6   Pyramid of levels of evidence. (Source: SUNY Downstate Medical Center. Medical Research Library of Brooklyn. Evidence Based Medicine Course. A Guide to Research Methods: The Evidence Pyramid. (http://library.downstate.edu/EBM2/2100.htm)

or analytic studies, which quantify the relationship between factors.[14] Depending on whether the data of analysis in a study are numerical or words, pictures, or objects, the research design can be categorized as a quantitative study or a qualitative study; depending on whether some intervention was performed or the study subjects were merely observed, study designs are classified into experimental or observational studies.[21] Adapted from a diagram developed by the Centre of Evidence Based Medicine,[14] Figure 5-5 presents types of study designs incorporating different classification schemes.

According to the American Occupational Therapy Association (AOTA) Literature Review Project,[40,60] by referring only to the rigor of experimental design and to the degree to which results can be considered credible and generalizable, there are five levels of evidence: (1) systematic reviews, meta-analyses, and RCTs; (2) two-group pre- and posttest studies, cohort studies, and case-control studies; (3) one-group pre- and posttest studies; (4) case series; and (5) narrative reviews and case reports (Figure 5-6). Holm[46] used a similar scheme in her 2000 Eleanor Clarke Slagle lecture. In contrast to this hierarchical model of research designs, there is a growing trend toward use of a "mixed methods" approach, collecting both quantitative and qualitative data and thus combining the strengths of each to answer research questions.[19] Selection of research design should depend upon the particular research goals, questions, and aims of the study, rather than a preordained ranking of approaches.

This standard hierarchical structure of levels of evidence is useful for evaluating studies that examine "an intervention's causal effect in the clinical population as a whole,"(p.235) but it does not provide information about patients' preferences, perceptions, occupations, and contexts, or the range of possible intervention strategies and outcomes.[89] However, the philosophy of client-centered practice in occupational therapy requires evidence about patients' patterns and the range of possible interventions. Usually, descriptive studies and qualitative studies answer these questions. With different information needed for clinical tasks and questions, studies that provide information about patterns and the range of possible interventions should be viewed as equal to studies that investigate the causal effect of a single intervention, and all of them should be evaluated to provide the "best" intervention choice to the current patient.[89]

Another type of publication is related to the levels of evidence just described, especially to systematic reviews. This specific type of publication is called *evidence-based clinical practice guidelines*. Simply speaking, clinical practice guidelines provide recommendations on diagnosis, management, and treatment in a specific area of health care by using the information in systematic reviews of evidence and an assessment of the benefits and harms of alternative care options.[17] The difference between clinical practice guidelines and systematic reviews is that guidelines typically define appropriate actions or incorporate values after synthesizing systematic reviews and other sources of evidence so that guidelines provide recommendations, strategies, or information that assists health-care practitioners and patients in making health-care decisions in specific clinical circumstances.[76] As guidelines provide action-ready recommendations, the quality of guidelines is closely associated with benefiting or harming both patients and health-care practitioners, thus affecting health-care outcome. Knowing how to evaluate and appraise clinical practice guidelines is especially important. The criteria of appraising clinical practice guidelines are detailed in the following section.

Appraisal of Research Literature
General Appraisal Principles

Critical appraisal is a systematic process of examining research to assess its relevance to clinical problems, validity of methodology, and clinical significance.[11,49,91] The primary goal of critical appraisal is to determine the quality of research design and results in research evidence, and to judge whether the effectiveness of evidence is based on rigorous research design. The function of critical appraisal is to provide high-quality research evidence for occupational therapists so that they can choose appropriate interventions for patients by integrating the evidence with clinical expertise and patient values. Through critical appraisal, occupational therapists can determine quickly whether studies are reliable and identify whether studies are worth the time to take a closer look.

Different study designs are prone to various sources of system bias, which make the methodological criteria for critical appraisal vary according to the design.[91] However, some general principles can be applied to any type of research study. The following three factors should always be considered when appraising a research study, regardless of its study design:[11,37,91]

1. What is the purpose of the study? Is it relevant to the problems of the current practice? Will it meet the information needs for the current practice? Answers to these questions help determine whether the study is relevant to the clinical problem.
2. Was the study design appropriate for the research question? Did the study methods address the most important potential sources of bias? Was the study conducted with methods to minimize bias? The answers to these questions help determine the methodological validity. Valid study design and study methods determine whether the study results being considered are credible and generalizable.[40] There are two kinds of validity: internal validity and external validity. Internal validity indicates the degree to which one can be certain that findings are a result of treatment and not chance occurrences.[40] To achieve a study's internal validity, biases should be minimized to the greatest extent. External validity indicates the degree to which results can be generalized to the larger population.[40] The results of a study with high internal validity are often difficult to generalize to a wide range of patients in an occupational therapist's daily practice because the researchers attempted to control study subjects and study settings precisely.[49]
3. Do the data justify the conclusion? Was there any overemphasis, or were important differences missed? Were the study results clinically important to the problems of current practice? The answers to these questions help determine the clinical significance of studies.

In addition to these three general criteria that can be applied across all different types of evidence, there are lists of questions to evaluate each different type of evidence by research question[11,82,86] and by research design. Because various sources of bias are inherent in different study designs, the appraisal checklists for specific study designs are useful to assess the quality of different types of studies. The following sections provide a checklist of questions for appraising each type of study design, followed by a sample citation retrieved from the PubMed search on the effectiveness of a home-based OT intervention related to activities of daily living (ADLs) in maintaining the functional independence of older adults. These checklists guide occupational therapists in evaluating research studies, yet they are not inclusive lists. The studies to be evaluated may meet some of the major design requirements on the list, but not all. In such cases, a judgment call is needed to analyze the possible applicability of the evidence to the current practice with the existing biases.

Systematic Reviews

A systematic review is a summary of available evidence completed by systematically identifying, appraising, and synthesizing individual studies on a particular topic.[4,91] The individual studies identified in a systematic review can be experimental or observational studies, such as a systematic review of RCTs. Some systematic reviews statistically combine the results from individual studies to produce an overall conclusion. This type of systematic review is called meta-analysis.

Although systematic reviews and meta-analyses have been recognized as the most reliable evidence because rigorous methodology is used to identify and evaluate relevant studies,[56,84,87] a risk of bias still exists. Biases include the selection of studies, quality of primary studies, publication delays, failure to publish, published studies with positive findings, and others.[32,91] Because of these biases, systematic reviews can vary in quality. The following checklist can be referred to for assessing the quality of systematic reviews:[4,32,73]

1. Does the review clearly and explicitly address a focused question?
2. Is it clear how the primary studies were retrieved?
3. Are the inclusive criteria to select the studies clearly stated?
4. Is the quality of the included studies systematically assessed using explicit and predetermined criteria?
5. Have the reasons for any differences between the results of individual studies been explored?
6. Is it clearly stated exactly what data were extracted from individual studies?
7. Were the decisions about the inclusion of studies, quality assessment, and data extraction checked by more than one person?
8. Are the findings of the included studies appropriately synthesized?
9. Are the reviewers' conclusions supported by the evidence they cite?

A good example of a systematic review is the following resource:

Steultjens, E. M., Dekker, J., Bouter, L.M., Jellema, S., Bakker, E. B., & van den Ende, C.H. (2004). Occupational therapy for community dwelling elderly people: A systematic review. *Age and Aging, 33*(5), 453-460. (PubMed ID: 15315918)

Controlled Trials, Randomized and Nonrandomized

Experimental studies in medicine that involve humans are called clinical trials.[21] Depending on whether or not they have a control group, clinical trials are classified as controlled trials and uncontrolled trials. In controlled trials, depending on whether study subjects are randomly allocated to the study group or to the control group, controlled trials fall into two categories: randomized control trials and nonrandomized control trials.

Randomized control trials (RCTs) are good for answering research questions about the effectiveness of an intervention, which includes therapy, treatment, diagnosis, screening, and even managerial interventions.[32] The RCT has been viewed as the "gold standard"[74,90] because "it provides the strongest evidence for concluding causation; it provides that best

insurance that the result was due to the intervention."[21] A rigorously designed RCT study should report the following key design elements to minimize biases: same baseline characteristics of control and experimental groups and randomization (selection bias), equal treatment of both control and experimental groups (performance bias), treatment withdrawal and loss of follow-up (attrition bias), and "blind" outcome assessment (detection bias).[11,32,37,40] Statements about how these biases have been minimized in an RCT study can usually be found in the methodology section of the abstract and the article. A checklist for appraising the methodological quality of RCTs is as follows:[32,37,73]

1. Did the study ask a clearly focused question?
2. Was this an RCT and was it appropriately so?
3. How were the study participants recruited? Were they equal in age, sex mix, socioeconomic status, presence of coexisting illness, and so on?
4. Were participants appropriately allocated to intervention and control groups? Was the method of allocation described?
5. Were participants, staff, and study personnel "blind" to participants' study groups?
6. Were data collected in the same way? Were participants treated at the same time intervals, and did they receive the same amount of attention from researchers and health workers?
7. Were all of the participants who entered the trial accounted for at its conclusion? Was there loss of participants for follow-up? Were all the study participants' outcomes analyzed by the groups to which they were originally allocated (intention-to-treat analysis)?
8. Did the study have enough participants to minimize the play of chance? Was there a statistical power calculation?
9. What outcome was measured and how? Was the instrument tested for reliability and validity? Was follow-up long enough for the effect of the intervention to be reflected in the outcome variables?
10. How were the results presented and were they precise? Was a confidence interval or a P value reported?

A good example of an RCT is the following resource:

Gitlin, L. N., Hauck, W. W., Dennis, M. P., Winter, L., Hodgson, N., & Schinfeld, S. (2009). Long-term effect on mortality of a home intervention that reduces functional difficulties in older adults: Results from a randomized trial. *Journal of the American Geriatrics Society, 57*(3), 476-481. (PubMed ID: 19187417)

Cohort Study

A cohort study observes the effects of risk factors, incidence, and prognosis of diseases[21,32,91] by following two or more groups of patients over a certain period of time. It answers the question of "what will happen" and is prospective.[21] A cohort study can be a good alternative when an RCT cannot be undertaken due to reasons of cost, acceptance, ethical concerns, or other factors.

The major source of bias for a cohort study is selection bias, or bias in cohort recruitment, specifically, whether all subjects were recruited in a defined time period and whether the groups had the same characteristics. Another major source of bias is selective drop-out, i.e., when participants leave the study due to non-random factors. The following questions can be used to appraise the quality of a cohort study:[32,73,91]

1. How was the cohort recruited? Was the cohort representative of a defined population? Was everybody included who should have been included?
2. Have the instruments used for measurement or outcome variables been validated?
3. Have authors taken account of the confounding factors in the design and/or analysis?
4. Was the follow-up of subjects complete and long enough?

A good example of a cohort study is the following resource:

Petersson, I., Kottorp, A., Bergström, J., & Lilja, M. (2009). Longitudinal changes in everyday life after home modifications for people aging with disabilities. *Scandinavian Journal of Occupational Therapy, 16*(2), 78-87. (PubMed ID: 18821447)

Case-Control Study

Case-control studies start with the outcome of interest, for example, a disease, and then look backward in time to detect possible causes or risk factors for that disease.[21] A case-control study answers the question of "what happened" and is retrospective. The study group is comprised of individuals who have the disease, and the control group includes individuals who have not developed the disease. Ideally, there should not be any differences in other characteristics between the individuals in the study group (case) and the control group other than those with or without the disease. A case-control study is useful for the identification of the causes of disease and side effects of treatment. It can be conducted in a shorter time period than a cohort study and is relatively less expensive to undertake.[32]

In a case-control study, selection of appropriate control individuals and the possibility of recall bias (a patient interprets the possible causes of his or her disease by recalling events or experiences) are two major sources of bias. A checklist of appraisal questions for a case-control study is as follows:[73,91]

1. Were the cases clearly defined?
2. Were the cases representative of a defined population?
3. How were the controls selected, and were they drawn from the same population as the cases?
4. Did the authors identify confounding factors, such as genetic, environmental, and socioeconomic factors?
5. Were study measures identical for cases and controls?
6. Were study measures objective or subjective, and is recall bias likely if they were subjective?

A good example of a case-control study is the following resource:

Stott, D. J., Buttery, A. K., Bowman, A., Agnew, R., Burrow, K., Mitchell, S. L., et al. (2006). Comprehensive geriatric assessment and home-based rehabilitation for elderly people with a history of recurrent nonelective hospital admissions. *Age and Aging, 35*(5), 487-491. (PubMed ID: 16772361)

Cross-Sectional Study

A cross-sectional study collects data of both exposure and outcome at the same short period of time.[91] It answers the question of "what is happening."[21] A survey is usually a cross-sectional design. A cross-sectional study reports the status or stage of a disease, looks for reasons or explanations, and examines study participants' thoughts, opinions, and perceptions.

The following four questions should be asked when appraising a cross-sectional study:[91]

1. Was the study sample clearly defined?
2. Was a representative sample achieved? Was the response rate sufficiently high?
3. Were all relevant exposures, potential confounding factors, and outcomes measured accurately?
4. Were patients with a wide range of severity of disease assessed?

A good example of a cross-sectional study is the following resource:

Dahlin-Ivanoff, S., & Sonn, U. (2004). Use of assistive devices in daily activities among 85-year-olds living at home focusing especially on the visually impaired. *Disability and Rehabilitation, 26*(24), 1423-1430. (PubMed ID: 15764362)

Case Series or Case-Report Studies

Case series or case-report studies describe clinical conditions with no comparison group. Due to a lack of a comparison group, no conclusion should be drawn about an association between an intervention and an outcome. In addition, case series or case-report studies usually do not report how patients were selected. Authors usually report the favored intervention and patients with the best outcomes; negative results are usually not reported.[21] Due to these biases, case series and case reports are not ranked as high-level evidence. However, they can be useful for hypothesis generation and in designing studies to evaluate causes or to explain conditions. Therefore these descriptive studies should be viewed as "hypothesis-generating and not as conclusive."[21] The only question to ask when assessing case series and case-report studies is: "Is the article a description of a clinical case from its symptoms, diagnosis, treatment (intervention), prognosis, and outcomes as if it is telling a story?"

An example of a case-report study is the following resource:

Swagerty, D. L. Jr. (1995). The impact of age-related visual impairment on functional independence in the elderly. *Kansas Medicine, 96*(1), 24-26. (PubMed ID: 7666637)

Narrative Reviews

A narrative review study is a type of secondary research because it summarizes the literature on specific health-care topics. Different from systematic reviews, narrative reviews do not describe how the literature is retrieved and selected as relevant, nor is information about the validity of selected studies provided.[22] It often presents authors' opinions. Therefore, narrative reviews usually are viewed as informative documents and should not be relied upon to draw conclusions about the effectiveness of an intervention. As a review study, narrative reviews also have commonalities as systematic reviews. Some of the following questions for assessing systematic reviews are also applicable to assessing narrative reviews:[22,32,73]

1. Does the review clearly and explicitly address a focused question?
2. Are the findings of the included studies appropriately synthesized?
3. Are the reviewers' conclusions supported by the evidence they cite?

An example of a narrative review study is the following resource:

Stav, W. B. (2008). Occupational therapy and older drivers: Research, education, and practice. *Gerontology & Geriatrics Education*, *29*(4), 336-350. (PubMed ID: 19064470)

Qualitative Studies

Qualitative studies aim to acquire an in-depth understanding of human behaviors, and they explore experiences, beliefs, perceptions, and values.[49] Qualitative studies can answer questions of *why* and *how*,[49] for example, why services are not used and how successful service delivery can be ensured. Data in the qualitative studies are nonnumeric, such as words, pictures, or objects, and are collected through interviews, focus groups, observations, and other forms of data-collection methods. Research design and data collection in qualitative studies can be flexible as the study unfolds, which is completely different from quantitative studies, in which the study design is finalized before the data are collected. These inductive and subjective characteristics of qualitative studies historically raised questions about study validity from proponents of quantitative studies and caused struggles of gaining acceptance within the quantitative domain of evidence-based medicine.[78] Now, however a mixed-methods approach is viewed as an optimal approach for numerous research questions that are best addressed from developing multiple perspectives and a complete understanding about a research problem or question.[67,92,93,94] For a more extensive discussion of research methods, especially mixed methods, and OT, see the Depoy & Gitlin textbook.[23]

Although carrying special characteristics and limitations, qualitative research has been recognized to be congruent with the client-centered practice philosophy in occupational therapy. Client-centered occupational therapy is an "approach to service which embraces a philosophy of respect for, and partnership with, people receiving services"(p. 253).[55] According to this philosophy, a customized OT service plan should be designed to fit the individual client in terms of the client's beliefs, preferences, and expected outcomes. The patient's beliefs and experiences about diseases and the causes of illness should be considered in the process of occupational therapy. During the client evaluation and interventions design process, it is often useful to discuss with clients the outcomes that they perceive to be useful rather than what is defined by occupational therapists as useful. In this sense, qualitative studies are good at providing information about client values, which is an important component of evidence-based practice.

A list of key questions for appraising qualitative studies to determine the appropriateness of the study, given the purpose and context, is as follows:[32,41,56,59]

1. Was the purpose and/or research question stated clearly?
2. Was relevant background literature reviewed? Did previous work expose gaps in current knowledge?
3. What was the study design? Was the design appropriate to the study question?
4. Was a theoretical perspective identified?
5. What research method was used? Was it congruent with the research question?
6. Was the process of purposive selection described? Was sampling done until redundancy in data was reached?
7. Was adequate information about data-collection procedures provided, for example, gaining access to the site, field notes, and training of data gatherers?
8. Were data analyses inductive?
9. Was the process of data analysis described adequately?
10. Was the reasoning process for identifying categories or themes reported?
11. Was the researchers' level of participation clearly reported?
12. Was triangulation reported, such as using multiple data-collection methods or involving multiple researchers in one method?
13. Were the conclusions appropriate given the study findings?
14. Did the findings contribute to theory development and future occupational therapy practice/research?

A good example of a qualitative study is the following resource:

Häggblom-Kronlöf, G., Hultberg, J., Eriksson, B. G., & Sonn, U. (2007). Experiences of daily occupations at 99 years of age. *Scandinavian Journal of Occupational Therapy*, *14*(3), 192-200. (PubMed ID: 17763201)

Clinical Practice Guidelines

As defined by Institute of Medicine (IOM), clinical practice guidelines are "systematically developed statements to assist practitioner and patient decisions about appropriate health care for specific clinical circumstances."[30] More than 3700 clinical practice guidelines from 39 countries are collected in the Guidelines International Network (GIN) database, and nearly

2700 guidelines are disseminated through the National Guidelines Clearinghouse (NGC).[17] With such a large number of clinical practice guidelines available, it would be challenging to determine which guidelines are of high quality. The high quality of a guideline largely depends on the rigorous guideline development process. Both the IOM[17] and the Conference on Guideline Standardization (COGS)[79] provide standards for developing an unbiased, scientifically valid, and trustworthy clinical practice guideline. In line with the standards of the guideline development process, appraisal criteria have been developed to evaluate guidelines after completion. The Appraisal of Guidelines Research & Evaluation (AGREE) instrument has been widely used to evaluate guideline quality.[2,76] The NGC[66] also publishes its inclusion criteria to collect guidelines that meet certain quality standards. The following questions should be asked when evaluating the quality of a clinical practice guideline:[36]

1. Are the overall objectives, the clinical question(s) covered by the guideline, and the patients/clients to whom the guideline is meant to apply specifically described?
2. Does the guideline development group include individuals from all of the relevant professional groups?
3. Have the patients' views and preferences been sought?
4. Are the target users of the guideline clearly defined?
5. Was the guideline piloted among target users?
6. Were systematic methods used to search for evidence?
7. Are the criteria for selecting the evidence clearly described?
8. Are the methods used for formulating the recommendations clearly described?
9. Were the health benefits, side effects, and risks considered in formulating the recommendations?
10. Is there an explicit link between the recommendations and the supporting evidence?
11. Was the guideline externally reviewed by an expert panel before publication?
12. Is a procedure for updating the guideline provided?
13. Are the recommendations specific and unambiguous?
14. Are the different options for management of the condition clearly presented?
15. Are key recommendations easily identifiable?
16. Is the guideline supported with tools for application?

A good example of a clinical practice guideline is the following resource:

> Canadian Task Force on Preventive Health Care. (1994, revised 2012). *Recommendations on screening for type 2 diabetes in adults*. NGC:009362. Retrieved from http://guideline.gov/content.aspx?id=38473.

Appraisal Tools

For further exploration of general and design-specific critical appraisal criteria, various guidelines and assessment tools have been developed. Some examples are presented as follows:

- Agency for Healthcare Research and Quality. (2002). *Systems to rate the strength of scientific evidence.*

  Evidence Report/Technology Assessment No. 47, Publication No. 02-E019. Retrieved form http://www.ahrq.gov/clinic/epcsums/strengthsum.htm.
- Centre of Evidence Based Medicine. (2009). *Critical appraisal*. Retrieved from http://www.cebm.net/index.aspx?o=1157.
- Moher, D., Schulz, K. F., & Altman, D. (2001). The CONSORT statement: Revised recommendations for improving the quality of reports of parallel-group randomized trials. *JAMA, 285*(15), 1987-1991.
- Greenhalgh, T. (1997). How to read a paper: Assessing the methodological quality of published papers. *BMJ, 315*, 305-308.
- Guyatt, G., Rennie, D., Meade, M. O., & Cook, D. J. (2008). *Users' guides to the medical literature: A manual for evidence-based clinical practice* (2nd ed.). New York, NY: McGraw-Hill Medical.
- Public Health Resource Unit. (2008). *Critical Appraisal Skills Programme (CASP)*. Retrieved from http://www.phru.nhs.uk/Pages/PHD/resources.htm.
- Straus, S. E., Richardson, W. S., Glasziou, P., & Haynes, R. B. (2005). *Evidence-based medicine: How to practice and teach EBM* (3rd ed.) [CD-ROM accompanying the book]. New York, NY: Elsevier Churchill Livingstone.

Conceptually Applying Evidence

Through the critical appraisal process, research evidence that is relevant to the current practice question and has a valid research design and clinically important study findings is distilled from the retrieved literature. The next step is to consider whether or not the valid and potentially useful evidence can be applied to current practice.

Based on Straus et al. (p. 1),[82] evidence-based practice requires "the integration of the best research evidence with our clinical expertise and our patient's unique values and circumstances." In the OT profession, this traditional evidence-based practice definition may need to be expanded. Application and integration of evidence into an OT clinical or other intervention decision need to consider both *client context* (preferences and values, occupation, and environment) and *therapy context* (clinical expertise, practice setting, information resources, financial resources, and other resources available to the therapist).[6,7] Both clients and their families or caregivers should be included in the decision-making process. Due to this highly context-driven practice characteristic, three factors should be taken into account for the application of evidence into the current practice: appropriateness, acceptability, and feasibility.

Appropriateness of evidence refers to the applicability of study results to clients in the current practice. Attention needs to be paid to the variations among a study population and the patients in question. Clients' values and preferences, age, gender, socioeconomic status, ethnicity, occupation history, and severity of disease, and the environment in which these individuals live, are some of the factors that may affect the application of the study results to the current patients.[49,85,87] In addition, client-centered practice in occupational therapy is deeply concerned with the individuals' needs and goals for treatment or other intervention,[90] which are important to consider when an intervention or a clinical practice guideline, proven effective by research, is applied to the current practice. When the study population differs in significant ways from the patients or clients in question, applying the study treatment or intervention may result in very different outcomes. Questions like "Do the results apply to my clients?," "Do my clients differ in significant ways from those in the study?," and "Does the intervention fit in with my clients' values, preferences, and special needs?" should be asked to analyze the applicability of the evidence to the current practice.[7]

After considering patient/client context for identifying the appropriateness of the evidence, the context of therapy also needs to be analyzed. Acceptability and feasibility of the evidence for the current practice are determined by the answers to such questions as "Will occupational therapists and staff accept the evidence?," "Will patients/clients accept the intervention?," and "Is it feasible to implement the intervention considering the cost, equipment, and other resources in the current practice setting?"[7,86]

Many clinical questions in occupational therapy deal with general patterns and individual variation in occupation and occupational performance, methods for assessing occupation and occupational performance, and planning and implementing the most effective intervention that satisfies patients' general well-being.[61,90] Traditional evidence that is dominated by quantitative methods is not appropriate for answering all of these types of clinical or other types of practice-related questions. For example, an RCT masks individual variations among study subjects in its use of the group-comparison design, which loses the "art" of occupational therapy.[90] In RCTs, random allocation of individuals to intervention and control groups is conducted from the perspective of research design rather than considering individual choice and the environmental context. Therefore, the intervention in the RCT study may be potentially irrelevant to some, within their own environmental contexts. The "art" of occupational therapy requires consideration of client preferences, along with analysis of the occupations and environments relevant to each individual,[90] to design an individualized treatment or other intervention plan. To engage in "meaningful occupation,"[90] the therapist should consider both client-generated evidence as well as retrieved research evidence.

Therefore, occupational therapists recognize multiple types of evidence, which include not only research literature, but daily influences such as clinical expertise, consultation with experts and colleagues, and practice-based experience.[58,74] It has been suggested that the best available evidence should be applied from "a variety of designs based on the 'goodness of fit' to the research question (p.106)"[5] and be integrated with clients' choices and needs and practitioner expertise.

Evidence-based practice is a toolbox of methods to "integrate research study evidence into the clinical reasoning process" (p. 537).[85] It must serve the older client's needs. Sometimes no evidence can be found to answer specific clinical questions due to insufficient research or due to novel situations. In such cases, clinical expertise and practice experience play important roles. Often, available evidence may not provide the exact answers for the clinical questions or may provide conflicting results.[45,61] In such cases, critically appraising multiple types of evidence, applying the best available evidence to current patients/clients, advising them of the bias and limitations inherent in the evidence in a straightforward manner, and encouraging patients/clients to participate in the decision-making process are the strategies to achieve the optimal outcome.[7,86,88]

How to Implement Evidence-Based Practice: Challenges and Strategies

Although evidence-based practice has been viewed as essential for providing quality patient care, implementing it and changing prevailing daily practice is quite challenging, and both systemic and individual strategies are needed to overcome the barriers. This section discusses the challenges in and strategies for implementing evidence-based practice in gerontological occupational therapy at the individual level, organizational level, and disciplinary and professional level.

Challenges and Strategies at the Individual Level

The most frequent complaint from occupational therapists about applying evidence-based practice is that their time is fragmented with patient evaluation and individual/group treatment sessions[3] and they have no time to conduct a thorough search for current evidence. In addition, finding, evaluating, and applying evidence may take longer than expected. Most of the time, an occupational therapist who works on one case by going through this intellectual process still needs to manage other clinical cases.[10,74] Therefore, using time effectively is the goal of providing both high-quality and high-quantity patient/client care with the current best evidence.

To overcome the challenge of lack of time, and using the literature search strategies reviewed earlier in this chapter, the following strategies can be considered:

1. Retrieve the clinical practice guidelines of professional occupational therapy associations (e.g., AOTA) first, and supplement these by consulting guidelines provided by other organizations (e.g., American Cancer Society) and government agencies (e.g., American Healthcare Research and Quality [AHRQ]).
2. Consult secondary resources that collect reviews with critical assessments of the effectiveness of interventions, such as Cochrane Library, Database of Abstracts of Reviews of Effectiveness (DARE), American College of Physicians (ACP) Journal Club, PEDro, and OT-seeker; search PubMed Clinical Queries, which provides filters to retrieve studies on therapy, diagnosis,

and prognosis. This can save the time and effort involved in searching primary databases, such as PubMed, and sifting through thousands of papers with varying quality. As noted earlier, in PEDro and OTseeker, trials have been critically appraised and rated to assist occupational therapists in evaluating their validity and interpretability. With these ratings, occupational therapists will be able to easily determine the quality and usefulness of trials for informing clinical interventions.[70]

3. Set up search filters or alerts in My NCBI, a tool developed by the National Center for Biotechnology Information (NCBI), to simplify the search process and to read up-to-date publications.

4. Join a listserv provided by a professional association or an internal professional occupational therapy group.[87] A listserv is a virtual information exchange channel that an occupational therapist can use to ask clinical questions and acquire evidence that listserv members may have encountered before.

5. Attend a journal club.[53,87] A journal club provides opportunities to review articles on a topic of interest and discuss the findings from those articles among occupational therapists and other professionals.

6. Keep records of relevant articles (either the full text or citation records) on various clinical or other practice-setting related questions and organize them by clinical (or other contextual) questions. This strategy seems to take more time; however, in the long run, it will save time when searching for relevant articles from this well-organized and targeted evidence database. Additionally, the program ENDNOTE (http://endnote.com) is a helpful tool for maintaining a personal database of references.

Another potential barrier for implementing evidence-based practice is that occupational therapists may lack skills in acquiring, understanding, appraising, and using the evidence.[45,48,74]

Increasing numbers of research articles in the medical sciences are published each year. Each week, more than 12,000 new articles, including over 300 RCTs, are added to the MEDLINE database.[25] In addition, these research articles are published in a wide range of journals, not only in profession-specific journals, which makes it more difficult for occupational therapists to search for evidence, evaluate evidence, and select good-quality information.[4] Various research designs and complicated statistical methods also create difficulties in understanding terminology and study results for all fields.[56]

Evidence-based practice education should be additionally strengthened and required in occupational therapy degree programs. Contextualized research instruction[53] with the opportunity to participate in research projects helps students understand how to conduct a rigorous research study and why the criteria for appraising research evidence are set up in the way they are. The skills involved in conducting research and interpreting research should be taught together.[82]

This kind of training promotes a "research frame of mind" in students,[81] so that in future professional practice students can use their knowledge of research to evaluate research literature and to apply the findings within their own practice. The Accreditation Council for Occupational Therapy Education (ACOTE) and American Occupational Therapy Association (AOTA) have developed standards and made the commitment to evidence-based practice education and research.[46]

Attending continuing education workshops (e.g., continuing medical education [CME]) and conferences can help occupational therapists keep up to date. Interactive small-group meetings that feature discussions of evidence, local consensus, peer feedback on performance, and the development of personal and group learning plans[38] are good continuing education practices. To achieve these goals, organizations should develop mechanisms to establish such a learning culture and release time for occupational therapists to participate in continuing education activities to improve knowledge and skills in evidence-based practice.

Challenges and Strategies at the Organizational Level

There are often insufficient resources available in the practice settings for occupational therapists to use research evidence and implement interventions. This shortage of resources is especially significant in rural areas and in developing countries. The shortage includes lack of access to computers; lack of access to information resources, especially commercial information resources such as online databases and e-journals; and lack of librarians available to assist with acquiring and evaluating evidence.[61,71,74] HINARI (**www.who.int/hinari**) attempts to address this issue: HINARI is a program set up by the World Health Organization (WHO) to enable low- and middle- income countries to gain access to online biomedical and health literature at no or highly discounted cost from the many major publishers that participate in this program.

Organizational support for evidence-based practice by providing access to information resources and encouraging literature searching during daily practice can influence practitioners' behavior.[9,70] Studies have found that the frequency of use of evidence databases is associated with practitioners' perceptions of their employers' support for using evidence databases as a legitimate part of work practice.[9,33,34] To facilitate access to information resources and encourage the use of evidence in practice, organizations can provide funds to subscribe to academic and professional journals or negotiate with the professional associations to provide journal access to the organization's members,[31] provide release time for reading and evaluating research, offer funding for and allow work time to attend continuing education events and participate in research, invite researchers or experts to provide workshops, and offer other supportive avenues.[53]

Although education interventions for occupational therapists can improve their knowledge and skills in evidence-based practice, changes in behavior may not happen in day-to-day practice.[64] Substantial changes in practice behavior require more system support and organizational interventions. Studies have found that occupational therapists see use of research to validate their interventions as a secondary concern because their employers do not demand them to do so.[26,54] Attitudes of managers and administrative personnel play important roles in building an organizational culture that supports evidence-based practice. A few methods can be used to facilitate the changes in practice:[52,53,63]

1. Highlight evidence-based practice in business plans, annual reports, and performance appraisals.
2. Demonstrate a belief in the value of research so that evidence-based practice becomes visible in the organization.
3. Create an environment where change is viewed as desirable.
4. Use local opinion leaders' influence. It was found that therapists relied heavily on peers for learning and applying new knowledge, and "educationally influential" therapists may be an effective way to help move research into practice.[75]
5. Hire an expert facilitator to help people understand what they have to change (attitudes, habits, skills, ways of thinking and working, etc.) and how they can change it to achieve the desired outcome.
6. Support interprofessional collaborations in practice and research activities. See Chapter 27 for descriptive information on this topic.
7. Organize patient/client education programs to provide information about the possible changes in practice and obtain patient/client adherence.

An organization may adopt various strategies to enhance the acceptance of research-proven interventions in real practice. None of the approaches is superior for all changes in all situations, and a combination of strategies appropriate to the specific patient and practice setting is suggested.[38]

Challenges and Strategies at the Disciplinary and Professional Levels

A research–practice gap has been identified in the OT profession, which is represented by two aspects: (1) limited amount of gerontological OT research evidence,[10,42,61,74] and (2) discrepancies between real practice situations and research findings.[83] These gaps hinder the application of research findings to real patient/client practice and also create difficulties in the uptake of the research evidence into daily practice.

The limited availability of gerontological OT research can be due to the difficulties of conducting RCT studies, along with lack of time and funding to conduct research.[68] However, the tradition in the OT profession that emphasizes the practice experience may cause occupational therapists to view conducting research as something external to their daily practice.[27] When the evidence-based practice philosophy and method are given prominence, occupational therapists gradually pick up the trend that reading research and applying research results to their daily practice are the skills they need to possess. From the profession perspective, a professional culture of conducting practice-based research and publishing

research findings is beginning to be developed and formed as a routine in the OT profession.

To increase practice-based research studies, conducting research that addresses practical issues in real-world contexts should be encouraged in the profession. In addition, researcher-practitioner partnerships can be established, with researchers teamed up with practitioners at the research sites[87] or occupational therapists increasing their involvement with research.[58]

Occupational therapists may perceive that study findings will challenge routine practices considered to be effective, and professional competency.[26] This conflict of acknowledged value of evidence-based practice and behavior changes in real practice is thought provoking to the whole profession. How can the profession replace this conflict with harmony? As early as 1999 it was recommended that occupational therapists improve their skills in evaluating evidence and cultivate a professional culture that uses research evidence as part of practical competence and a client-based practice philosophy.[26] The field is making progress in this direction and for years has required mastery of research as a basic competency in OT degree programs. The upcoming cohorts of OT practitioners should be more adept in incorporating research evidence into their work.

Resources for Implementation of Evidence-Based Practice

The previous section described and discussed challenges and strategies for facilitating the implementation of evidence-based practice in gerontological occupational therapy. To achieve an effective implementation, the resources for changing practice with evidence-based research at different levels of health care are needed. These resources include innovation itself (i.e., research evidence); individual occupational therapists with the knowledge and skills of evidence-based practice; patients'/clients' attitude toward and compliance with the intervention; organizational context in culture, leadership, administration, facilitation, and feedback mechanisms; social context in terms of colleagues' opinions and multidisciplinary collaborations; and economic and political context in terms of financial support, policies, and regulations.[39,52]

These resources interrelate and interact with each other. Kitson[52] proposed a multidimensional framework to demonstrate the relationships among these resources. Instead of a hierarchy or linearity of cause and effect, a three-dimensional matrix was suggested and described with a function, which is that successful implementation is a function of the relation between the nature of the evidence, the context in which the proposed change is to be implemented, and the mechanisms by which the change is facilitated.[52] It would be unrealistic and impossible to implement evidence-based practice until all or most of the resources are available. A needs analysis of occupational therapists and environmental scanning should be conducted in the organization that plans to implement evidence-based practice, to learn which resources are lacking and what barriers exist for the occupational therapists in that organization. Based on these investigations, tailored strategies and interventions can be planned and performed to achieve optimal implementation outcome.

Future Applications and Trends in Evidence-Based Practice

The three-level challenges and strategies of implementing evidence-based practice in occupational therapy are not exclusive from each other. The implementation and application of evidence-based practice philosophy and method in occupational therapy will not be successful if only individual practitioners try hard to improve their literature search and evaluation skills and their organizations do not provide either management support or resource support. The same result would occur if no macro-level policy and regulations had been drafted that support evidence-based occupational therapy, although both individual practitioners and management believe in evidence-based practice and plan to implement it in their daily practice. The National Health Service (NHS) in England provides a dual framework that involves a shift from "individual approaches toward a whole system of service improvement across primary, secondary, and community care (p. 351)."[48] The framework includes three levels of effort from clear standards of service, to dependable local delivery, to monitored standards. An implementation of evidence-based practice in occupational therapy needs to "place the traditional, individual practitioner-focused strategies within an organizational framework of service improvement (p. 351)."[48] In this way, organizations and individuals share the risks, resources, and responsibilities needed to make sure patients receive safer and more effective interventions.

With economic globalization, more and more people travel all over the world for business, leisure, and their health needs to be cared for in the countries where they travel. In this trend, health-care resources need to be shared globally and health-care practice guidelines need to be standardized across the countries, for the benefit of local communities and travelers. Occupational therapists in the international community are aware of this change and are trying to catch up with the trend. In 2004 an international conference on evidence-based occupational therapy was held in Bethesda, Maryland.[18] The conference discussed the development and promotion of evidence-based occupational therapy from a more global perspective, which included international evidence-based practice education, exchange of information, and access to publications in the international community.

Past challenges to implementing evidence-based practice in occupational therapy, i.e., limited numbers of published OT research studies and research findings that are irrelevant to daily practice with older adults, are beginning to no longer hold. Producing more research that is relevant to practice[58,83] and increasing the published OT research in gerontology would correspond with the aging of the population and the demand for increased services for older adults.[13]

REVIEW QUESTIONS

1. What is the first source occupational therapists should check when looking for evidence to answer a clinical question?
   a. Guidelines or other resources from professional occupational therapy associations
   b. Cochrane Collaboration website
   c. Bibliographic databases such as MEDLINE/PubMed
   d. AHRQ website

2. Which of the following statements most accurately describes bibliographic citation databases?
   a. All citation databases provide access to full-text articles.
   b. Citation databases must be searched using controlled vocabulary.
   c. Citation databases contain the title, source information, and abstracts for journal articles.
   d. Most of the citation databases are available for free.

3. Which of the following is true with regard to PICO statements?
   a. All elements of the PICO statement should be used in a database search.
   b. PICO does not need to be used for occupational therapy questions.
   c. The outcome in a PICO statement is the most important term to use in a search.
   d. The PICO statement is a guide to help therapists identify important elements of a clinical question.

4. Which of the following databases are freely available to the public, and therapists will have access no matter where they are employed?
   a. OT SEARCH and AgeLine
   b. PubMed and OTseeker
   c. Scopus and CINAHL
   d. PubMed and Web of Science

5. Which of the following statements is true with regard to bibliographic database search techniques?
   a. All bibliographic databases have a thesaurus that contains subject headings.
   b. Bibliographic databases may be searched with a combination of keywords and subject headings.
   c. The same subject headings (thesaurus terms) can be used in multiple databases.
   d. Synonyms are not necessary when a keyword search is performed.

6. How are clinical practice guidelines different from systematic reviews and other types of evidence?
   a. Systematic methods are used to search for scientific studies.
   b. The criteria for selecting scientific studies are clearly described.
   c. Clinical practice guidelines provide action-ready recommendations by using the information from systematic reviews and other types of evidence.
   d. Focused questions are clearly and explicitly described.

7. Which statement correctly notes the differences between systematic reviews and narrative reviews?
   a. Systematic reviews are a type of secondary document.
   b. Systematic reviews clearly report how the primary studies were retrieved and selected.
   c. Systematic reviews clearly and explicitly address a focused question.
   d. Systematic reviews synthesize the findings of individual studies that are retrieved.

8. Challenges of implementing evidence-based practice include which of the following?
   a. Lack of time
   b. Lack of skills in finding scientific evidence
   c. Shortage of resources, such as computers, no access to bibliographic databases, etc.
   d. Limited available evidence on occupational therapy practice
   e. All of these

9. Critically evaluating the evidence is one step in the evidence-based practice process. Which of the following will determine whether the study results being considered are credible and generalizable?
   a. Valid study design and study methods
   b. Patient circumstances
   c. The database used to find the study
   d. None of these

REFERENCES

1. Agency for Healthcare Research and Quality, U.S. Department of Health and Human Services. (2009). *National guideline clearinghouse.* Retrieved from http://www.guideline.gov/.
2. The AGREE Collaboration. (2003). Development and validation of an international appraisal instrument for assessing the quality of clinical practice guidelines: The AGREE project. *Quality & Safety in Health Care, 12,* 18–23.
3. Bannigan, K. (1997). Clinical effectiveness: Systematic reviews and evidence-based practice in occupational therapy. *British Journal of Occupational Therapy, 60,* 479–483.
4. Bannigan, K., Droogan, J., & Entwistle, V. (1997). Systematic reviews: What do they involve? *Nursing Times, 93*(18), 54–44.
5. Bartlett, D. (2008). Introducing the evidence to practice commentary. *Physical & Occupational Therapy in Pediatrics, 28*(2), 105–108.
6. Bennett, S. (2005). Practicing and teaching evidence-based health care in other clinical specialties. 3. Occupational therapy [CD-ROM accompanying the book]. In D. L. Sackett, S. E. Strauss, W. S. Richardson, W. Rosenberg, & R. B. Haynes (Eds.), *Evidence-based medicine: How to practice and teach EBM* (3rd ed.). New York, NY: Elsevier Churchill Livingstone.
7. Bennett, S., & Bennett, J. W. (2000). The process of evidence-based practice in occupational therapy: Informing clinical decisions. *Australian Occupational Therapy Journal, 47,* 171–180.
8. Bennett, S., Hoffmann, T., McCluskey, A., McKenna, K., Strong, J., & Tooth, L. (2003). Introducing OTseeker (Occupational Therapy Systematic Evaluation of Evidence): A new evidence database for occupational therapists. *American Journal of Occupational Therapy, 57,* 635–638.
9. Bennett, S., McKenna, K., Hoffmann, T., Tooth, L., McCluskey, A., & Strong, J. (2007). The value of an evidence database for occupational therapists: An international online survey. *International Journal of Medical Informatics, 76,* 507–513.
10. Bennett, S., Tooth, L., McKenna, K., Rodger, S., Strong, J., Ziviani, J., et al. (2003). Perceptions of evidence-based practice: A survey of Australian occupational therapists. *Australian Occupational Therapy Journal, 50*(1), 13–22.
11. Burls, A. (2009). *What is critical appraisal?* Retrieved from http://www.medicine.ox.ac.uk/bandolier/painres/download/whatis/What_is_critical_appraisal.pdf.
12. Canadian Association of Occupational Therapists. (2007). *Code of ethics.* Retrieved from http://www.caot.ca/default.asp?pageid=35.
13. Case-Smith, J., & Powell, C. A. (2008). Concepts in clinical scholarship—research literature in occupational therapy, 2001–2005. *American Journal of Occupational Therapy, 62,* 480–486.
14. Centre of Evidence Based Medicine. (2009). *Study designs.* Retrieved from http://www.cebm.net/study-designs/.
15. College of Occupational Therapists. (2005). *Code of ethics and professional conduct.* Retrieved from http://www.cot.co.uk/Mainwebsite/Resources/Document/Code-of-Ethics.pdf.
16. Committee on the Health Professions Education Summit; Board on Health Care Services; Greiner, A. C., & Knebel, E. (Eds.), (2003). *Health professions education: A bridge to quality.* Washington, DC: National Academies Press.
17. Committee on Standards for Developing Trustworthy Clinical Practice Guidelines, Board on Health Care Services, Institute of Medicine of National Academies; Graham, R., Mancher, M., Wolman, D. M., Greenfield, S., & Steinbert, E. (Eds.), (2011). *Clinical practice guidelines we can trust.* Retrieved from http://www.iom.edu/Reports/2011/Clinical-Practice-Guidelines-We-Can-Trust.aspx.
18. Coster, W. (2005). International conference on evidence-based practice: A collaborative effort of the American Occupational Therapy Association, the American Occupational Therapy Foundation, and the Agency for Healthcare Research and Quality. *American Journal of Occupational Therapy, 59*(3), 356–358.
19. Creswell, J. W., Klassen, A. C., Plano Clark, V. L., & Smith, K. C. for the Office of Behavioral and Social Sciences Research. National Institutes of Health. (2011). *Best practices for mixed methods research in the health sciences.* Retrieved from. http://obssr.od.nih.gov/mixed_methods_research.
20. Culshaw, H. M. S. (1995). Evidence-based practice for sale? *British Journal of Occupational Therapy, 58,* 233.
21. Dawson, B., & Trapp, R. G. (2004). Study designs in medical research. In *Basic and clinical biostatistics* (4th ed., pp. 7–22). New York, NY: Lange Medical Books/McGraw-Hill, Medical Publishing Division.
22. Delfini Group. (2003). *Problems with narrative reviews (aka overviews).* Retrieved from http://www.delfini.org/Delfini_Primer_NarrativeReviewProbs.pdf.
23. DePoy, E. & Gitlin, L. (2015). *Introduction to research: Understanding and applying multiple strategies* (5th ed.). Philadelphia, PA: Elsevier Mosby.
24. Dieter, M. G., & Kielhofner, G. (2006). Searching the literature. In G. Kielhofner (Ed.), *Research in occupational therapy: Methods of inquiry for enhancing practice* (pp. 437–451). Philadelphia, PA: F. A. Davis.
25. Druss, B. G., & Marcus, S. C. (2005). Growth and decentralization of the medical literature: Implications for evidence-based medicine. *Journal of the Medical Library Association, 93,* 499–501.

26. Dubouloz, C.-J., Egan, M., Vallerand, J., & von Zweck, C. (1999). Occupational therapists' perceptions of evidence-based practice. *American Journal of Occupational Therapy, 53*(5), 445–453.

27. Eakin, P. (1997). The Casson Memorial Lecture 1997: Shifting the balance—evidence-based practice. *British Journal of Occupational Therapy, 60,* 290–294.

28. Elliott, S. J., & Coppola, S. (2008). Best practice in gerontology. In S. Coppola, S. J. Elliott, & P. E. Toto (Eds.), *Strategies to advance gerontology excellence: Promoting best practice in occupational therapy* (pp. 319–347). Bethesda, MD: American Occupational Therapy Association.

29. Ferlie, E., Fitzgerald, L., Wood, M., & Hawkins, C. (2005). The nonspread of innovations: The mediating role of professionals. *Academy of Management Journal, 48,* 117–134.

30. Field, M. J., & Lohr, K. N. (Eds.), (1990). *Clinical practice guidelines: Directions for a new program. Institute of Medicine.* Washington, DC: National Academies Press.

31. Finlayson, M. (2008). Increasing access to evidence. *Canadian Journal of Occupational Therapy, 75*(5), 259–260.

32. Gary, M. (2009). Appraising the quality of research. *Evidence-based healthcare and public health: How to make decisions about health services and public health* (pp. 125–180). New York, NY: Elsevier Limited.

33. Gosling, A. S., & Westbrook, J. I. (2004). Allied health professionals' use of online evidence: A survey of 790 staff working in the Australian public hospital system. *International Journal of Medical Informatics, 73*(4), 391–401.

34. Gosling, A. S., Westbrook, J. I., & Coiera, E. W. (2003). Variation in the use of online clinical evidence: A qualitative analysis. *International Journal of Medical Informatics, 69,* 1–16.

35. Grady, A. P. (1987). Research: Its role in enhancing the professional image. *American Journal of Occupational Therapy, 41,* 347–349.

36. Graham, I. D., & Harrison, M. B. (2005). Evaluation and adaptation of clinical practice guidelines. *Evidence Based Nursing, 8,* 68–72.

37. Greenhalgh, T. (1997). How to read a paper: Assessing the methodological quality of published papers. *BMJ, 315,* 305–308.

38. Grol, R., & Grimshaw, J. (2003). From best evidence to best practice: Effective implementation of change in patients' care. *The Lancet, 362,* 1225–1230.

39. Grol, R., & Winsing, M. (2004). What drives change? Barriers to and incentives for achieving evidence-based practice [Supplement]. *MLA, 180,* S53–S60.

40. Gutman, S. A. (2009). How to appraise research: Elements of sound applied design. *American Journal of Occupational Therapy, 63*(2), 123–125.

41. Hammell, K. W. (2002). Informing client-centred practice through qualitative inquiry: Evaluating the quality of qualitative research. *British Journal of Occupational Therapy, 65,* 175–184.

42. Hayes, R. L. (2000). Evidence-based occupational therapy needs strategically-targeted quality research now. *Australian Occupational Therapy Journal, 47,* 186–190.

43. Haynes, R. B. (2006). Of studies, syntheses, synopses, summaries and systems: The "5S" evolution of information services for evidence-based healthcare decisions. *Evidence-Based Medicine, 11,* 162–164.

44. Haynes, R. B., Devereaux, P. J., & Guyatt, G. H. (2002). Clinical expertise in the era of evidence-based medicine and patient choice. *ACP Journal Club, 136,* A11–A14.

45. Hilton, S., Bedford, H., Calnan, M., & Hunt, K. (2009). Competency, confidence and conflicting evidence: Key issues affecting health visitors' use of research evidence in practice. *BMC Nursing, 8,* 4–11.

46. Holm, M. B. (2000). Our mandate for the new millennium: Evidence-based practice—the 2000 Eleanor Clarke Slagle Lecture. *American Journal of Occupational Therapy, 54*(6), 575–585.

47. Horowitz, B., & Toto, P. (2005). Infusing evidence-based practice in gerontological occupational therapy. *Gerontology Special Interest Section Quarterly, 28,* 1–4.

48. Ilott, I. (2003). Challenging the rhetoric and reality: Only an individual and systemic approach will work for evidence-based occupational therapy. *American Journal of Occupational Therapy, 57*(3), 351–354.

49. Jerosch-Herold, C. (1998). Evidence-based practice: How to critically appraise a research paper. Part 1: Assessing the purpose and methods of a study. *British Journal of Hand Therapy, 3*(2), 18–20.

50. Joanna Briggs Institute. (2011). *About us.* Retrieved from http://www.joannabriggs.edu.au/About%20Us.

51. Kielhofner, G. (2006). The necessity of research in a profession. In G. Kielhofner (Ed.), *Research in occupational therapy: Methods of inquiry for enhancing practice* (pp. 1–9). Philadelphia, PA: F. A. Davis.

52. Kitson, A., Harvey, G., & McCormack, B. (1998). Enabling the implementation of evidence based practice: A conceptual framework. *Quality in Health Care, 7*(3), 149–158.

53. Koch, L. C., Cook, B. G., Tankersley, M., & Rumrill, P. (2006). Utilizing research in professional practice. *Work, 26*(3), 327–331.

54. Kornblau, B. (2004). Presidential address: A vision for our future. *American Journal of Occupational Therapy, 58,* 9–14.

55. Law, M., Baptiste, S., & Mills, J. (1995). Client-centred practice: What does it mean and does it make a difference? *Canadian Journal of Occupational Therapy, 62,* 250–257.

56. Law, M., & Baum, C. (1998). Evidence-based occupational therapy. *Canadian Journal of Occupational Therapy, 65,* 131–135.

57. Law, M., & Bennett, S. (2009). *Evidence-based occupational therapy.* Retrieved from http://www.otevidence.info/.

58. Lencucha, R., Kothari, A., & Rouse, M. J. (2007). Knowledge translation: A concept for occupational therapy? *American Journal of Occupational Therapy, 61*(5), 593–596.

59. Letts, L., Wilkins, S., Law, M., Steward, D., Bosch, J., & Westmorland, M. (2007). *Critical review form—qualitative studies* (version 2.0). Retrieved from http://www.srs-mcmaster.ca/Portals/20/pdf/ebp/qualreview_form1.doc.

60. Lieberman, D., & Scheer, J. (2002). AOTA's evidence-based Literature Review Project: An overview. *American Journal of Occupational Therapy, 56,* 344–349.

61. Lopez, A., Vanner, E. A., Cowan, A. M., Samuel, A. P., & Shepherd, D. L. (2008). Intervention planning facets—four facets of occupational therapy intervention planning: Economics, ethics, professional judgment, and evidence-based practice. *American Journal of Occupational Therapy, 62*(1), 87–96.

62. Martin, E., Baggaley, K., Buchbinder, R., Johnston, R., Tugwell, P., Maxwell, L., & Santesso, N. (2008). Occupational therapists should be more involved in the Cochrane Collaboration: The example of the Australian Cochrane Musculoskeletal Review Group. *Australian Occupational Therapy Journal, 55,* 207–211.

63. McCluskey, A. (2006). Managing change and barriers to evidence-based practice. In A. Kielhofner (Ed.), *Research in occupational therapy: Methods of inquiry for enhancing practice* (p. 685). Philadelphia, PA: F. A. Davis Company.

64. McCluskey, A., & Lovarini, M. (2005). Providing education on evidence-based practice improved knowledge but did not

change behavior: A before and after study. *BMC Medical Education, 5,* 40–51.

65. Miller, E., & Willis, M. (2000). The Cochrane Collaboration and occupational therapy: An emerging partnership. *British Journal of Occupational Therapy, 63,* 288–290.

66. National Guideline Clearinghouse. (2014). *Inclusion criteria.* Retrieved from http://guideline.gov/about/inclusion-criteria.aspx.

67. National Institutes of Health Office of Social and Behavioral Sciences Research. *Best Practices for Mixed Methods Research in the Health Sciences.* Retrieved from http://obssr.od.nih.gov/scientific_areas/methodology/mixed_methods_research/section2.aspx# When should mixed methods be used.

68. Nelson, D. J., & Mathiowetz, V. (2004). Randomized controlled trials to investigate occupational therapy research questions. *American Journal of Occupational Therapy, 58*(1), 24–34.

69. Newhouse, R. P. (2008). Evidence and the executive. Evidence-based behavioral practice: An exemplar of interprofessional collaboration. *Journal of Nursing Administration, 38,* 414–416.

70. OTseeker. (2009). OTseeker tutorial. Retrieved from http://www.otseeker.com/tutorial.htm.

71. Pain, K., Magill-Evans, J., Darrah, J., Hagler, P., & Warren, S. (2004). Effects of profession and facility type on research utilization by rehabilitation professionals. *Journal of Allied Health, 33*(1), 3–9.

72. Pearson, A., Wiechula, R., Court, A., & Lockwood, C. (2005). The JBI model of evidence-based healthcare. *International Journal of Evidence-Based Healthcare, 3,* 207–215.

73. Public Health Resource Unit. (2008). *Critical Appraisal Skills Programme* (CASP). Retrieved from http://www.phru.nhs.uk/Pages/PHD/resources.htm.

74. Rappolt, S. (2003). The role of professional expertise in evidence-based occupational therapy. *American Journal of Occupational Therapy, 57,* 589–593.

75. Rappolt, S., & Tassone, M. (2002). How rehabilitation therapists gather, evaluate, and implement new knowledge. *Journal of Continuing Education in the Health Professionals, 22,* 170–180.

76. Rosenfield, R., & Richard, N. (2009). Clinical practice guideline development manual: A quality-driven approach for translating evidence into action. *Otolaryngology–Head and Neck Surgery, 140,* S1–S43.

77. Satterfield, J. M., Spring, B., Brownson, R. C., Mullen, E. J., Newhouse, R. P., Walker, B. B., & Whitlock, E. P. (2009). Toward a transdisciplinary model of evidence-based practice. *The Milbank Quarterly, 87,* 368–390.

78. Savin-Baden, M., & Taylor, C. (2001). Conference report: Qualitative evidence-based practice. *American Journal of Occupational Therapy, 55*(2), 230–232.

79. Shiffman, R. N., Shekelle, P., Overhage, M., et al. (2003). Standardized reporting of clinical practice guidelines: A proposal from the conference on guideline standardization. *Annals of Internal Medicine, 139,* 493–498.

80. Spring, B. (2007). *EBBP: Evidence-based behavioral practice. Background.* Retrieved from http://www.ebbp.org/aboutus.html.

81. Stern, P. (2001). Occupational therapists and research: Lessons learned from a qualitative research course. *American Journal of Occupational Therapy, 55*(1), 102–105.

82. Straus, S. E., Richardson, W. S., Rosenberg, W., & Haynes, R. B. (2005). *Evidence-based medicine: How to practice and teach EBM* (3rd ed.). New York, NY: Elsevier Churchill Livingstone.

83. Sudsawad, P. (2005). A conceptual framework to increase usability of outcome research for evidence-based practice. *American Journal of Occupational Therapy, 59*(3), 351–355.

84. Taylor, M. C. (1997). What is evidence-based practice? *British Journal of Occupational Therapy, 60,* 47–474.

85. Tickle-Degnen, L. (1999). Evidence-based practice forum. Organizing, evaluating, and using evidence in occupational therapy practice. *American Journal of Occupational Therapy, 53,* 537–539.

86. Tickle-Degnen, L. (2000a). What is the best evidence to use in practice? *American Journal of Occupational Therapy, 54*(2), 218–221.

87. Tickle-Degnen, L. (2000b). Gathering current research evidence to enhance clinical reasoning. *American Journal of Occupational Therapy, 54*(1), 102–105.

88. Tickle-Degnen, L. (2000c). Monitoring and documenting evidence during assessment and intervention. *American Journal of Occupational Therapy, 54*(4), 434–436.

89. Tickle-Degnen, L., & Bedell, G. (2003). Heterarchy and hierarchy: A critical appraisal of the "levels of evidence" as a tool for clinical decision making. *American Journal of Occupational Therapy, 57,* 234–237.

90. Tse, S., Blackwood, K., & Penman, M. (2000). From rhetoric to reality: Use of randomized controlled trials in evidence-based occupational therapy. *Australian Occupational Therapy Journal, 47,* 181–185.

91. Young, J. M., & Solomon, M. J. (2009). How to critically appraise an article. *Nature Reviews Gastroenterology and Hepatology, 6,* 82–91. doi:10.1038/ncpgasthep1331

92. Creswell, J. W., & Plano Clark, V. L. (2011). *Designing and conducting mixed methods research.* (2nd ed.). Thousand Oaks, CA: Sage.

93. Morgan, D. L. (2007). Paradigms lost and pragmatism regained: Methodological implications of combining qualitative and quantitative methods. *Journal of Mixed Methods Research, 1*(1), 48–76.

94. Song, M., Sandelowski, M., & Happ, M. B. (2010). Current practices and emerging trends in conducting mixed methods intervention studies in the health sciences. In: A. Tashakkori & C. Teddlie (Eds.), *Handbook of mixed methods in social & behavioral research* (2nd ed., pp. 725–747). Thousand Oaks, CA: Sage.

CHAPTER 6

Approaches to Screening and Assessment in Gerontological Occupational Therapy

Jane Bear-Lehman, PhD, OTR/L, FAOTA, Tracy Chippendale, PhD, OTR/L, Steven M. Albert, PhD

CHAPTER OUTLINE

OBJECTIVES

- Describe selection of assessment tools that suit continuous quality improvement concepts within an evidence-based, client-centered care model
- Identify the methods, challenges, and uses of assessment in gerontological occupational therapy
- Describe considerations in assessment instrument selection for good practice, including utility of standardized and nonstandardized instruments, determination of reliability and validity, and suitability for client sample

The overriding aim of gerontological occupational therapy (OT) is to improve the ability of older adults to attain satisfactory and successful achievement of their occupations, including completion of daily life task performance, and fulfillment of roles and responsibilities in their home and community that may have become or have the potential to become difficult because of age-related changes, onset of disease, or the development of disability.[3,11] Human occupation and client-centered care are the two main concepts that direct the OT evaluation process. *Occupation* is an important component of the OT assessment of health and performance, and for the determination of an older adult's ability to interact effectively with his or her living environment to complete tasks and gain satisfaction through these transactions. Thus the OT evaluation is designed to measure how the client's strengths, skills, weaknesses, and limitations affect functioning in a specific personal environment. In a *client-centered evaluation,* the client is considered an essential part of the evaluation process in that the evaluation will determine what the occupational therapist will do in partnership with the client and what occupational goals are appropriate.

The specific OT evaluation is carefully selected to assess the client in the client's environment. In selecting the assessment tools for the evaluation, the occupational therapist determines the need for the assessment, the intended uses for the assessment, and the purpose of the assessment. An OT evaluation is initiated once a physician—or, in some states, a nurse practitioner—writes a referral directly to the OT or rehabilitation team (medical referrals are not required for some primary and secondary care OT services, e.g., community education programs and home safety assessments). Occupational therapists often work as integral members of an interdisciplinary team that may include the client, physicians, nurses, physical therapy practitioners, speech-language pathologists, psychologists, and social workers. Team consultation can help determine which team members can best meet the client's needs and help the client accomplish goals.

The selection and application of assessments for the OT evaluation are influenced by the occupational therapist's knowledge, skills, and clinical/professional reasoning, and are selected to be in accordance with both the needs of the client population and the requirements of the practice setting. But occupational therapists must also choose from among a great many assessments. These differ in quality, suitability for clients or assessment environments, and complexity, and in the kinds of information they produce. In this chapter, we review some of the factors occupational therapists must take into account when choosing or designing assessment tools.

Measurement and Assessment

Types of Measures

An initial important distinction is the source of assessment information. Does the assessment yield reports of performance from a client or the client's designated representative (when a client is unable to respond to questions), or does the assessment directly assess performance? Self-reports introduce a number of biases, even when these reports are elicited by occupational therapists or trained research assistants. A senior may deny or exaggerate deficits consciously, or not report accurately because of loss of insight related to cognitive deficit. Surrogates may not report accurately because of similar biases, or because they themselves are overwhelmed by caregiving challenges and cannot perceive older adult competencies accurately. Still, for some older adults self-reported function is perhaps more accurate than performance-based assessments. For these older adults, self-reports involve appraisals of habitual behaviors that cannot always be captured well in a single, short-term assessment of performance.

In considering performance-based assessments, it is important to distinguish between fully standardized tests (e.g., donning a pre-specified blouse or making change in a simulated shopping transaction) and assessments of ecologically valid tasks, such as a task habitually performed by an older adult in his or her home environment. The former offers the advantage of greater standardization and reliability (see discussion of reliability later in this chapter), and perhaps greater likelihood of access to population or clinical norms. But the latter is likely to offer greater validity—that is, a more accurate assessment of functional ability (see discussion of validity later in this chapter). Assessing daily activities actually performed by an older adult in his or her home environment is likely to give a truer picture of needs or competencies.

A second consideration is the degree of intrusiveness of assessments. Does the assessment require great investment of attention or effort by older adults? Or can it be performed simply in the normal course of an older adult's daily activity? The first offers the advantage of stress or challenge that may reveal deficits, but this sort of assessment also demands great motivation from clients. The second captures a baseline level of daily activity but may underestimate occupational competencies if older adults have unnecessarily restricted their activity.

Finally, a third consideration is the complexity of the assessment. Assessments range from simple checklists or score sheets (a simple global rating, for example, of bathing ability) to quite complex multidimensional assessments that require ratings of each ergonomic and cognitive element of a task.

The best assessment is the one that yields the most accurate information with the least intrusiveness and the most flexibility in administration. Of course, such an assessment is not always available. Hence the development of instruments and assessment technologies to overcome these trade-offs remains a major research concern for occupational therapy.

Levels of Data

A further consideration is what kinds of data an assessment produces. Are these data *nominal*, that is, simply categorical, denoting a type or kind of attribute, such as type of residence, without any true numerical significance? Or are the data *ordinal*, implying a rank ordering as, for example, in the following three grades of independence: "able to live independently," "able to live independently with supervision," and "not able to live independently"? Or, finally, are the data *interval*, with constant differences between values? For example, an interval measure would allow the investigator to say one older adult is able to live independently across 80% of his or her activities and another across only 40%, suggesting that the second senior is twice as impaired as the first. Each type of data allows different levels of sophistication in analysis.

Many OT functional assessments involve the summing of nominal or ordinal data to create an index of the client's functional ability.[15] For clinical purposes, this level of sophistication in data may seem reasonable and customary. However, many rehabilitation professionals now question the validity of assessments that simply total all of the nominal and ordinal data to determine a quantitative functional outcome score regardless of the type of metric that the question or observation is, or the level of achieved constructive validity of the tool and its components. Rehabilitation professionals are now calling for the application of Rasch modeling in the actual design of the functional tools. Rasch modeling relies on item response theory (IRT) to improve the level of the data so that valid comparisons can be made, and so that the interval or even *ratio* levels of data (measures that allow a true zero value) outcome values have a goodness of fit and are meaningful.[15,26]

Evaluating Assessment Tools

An assessment tool is obviously not useful if it gives a different result with repeated administration to the same client. In this case we say it is *unreliable*. An assessment is also not useful if what it measures does not provide information about what we are trying to measure. In this case we say the assessment is *invalid*. Tests may be good at identifying a case (for example, dementia or a balance disorder), in which case we say the assessment is *sensitive*. But the same test may also identify many noncases as cases, giving the test poor *specificity*. Finally, a test or assessment may be efficient in each of these domains but still fare badly in tracking change in a client over time. In this case we say the assessment is *nonresponsive*.

In choosing an OT assessment, it is important to consider each of these elements. Often, an assessment will be strong in one area but weaker in another, requiring the occupational therapist or researcher to decide which element is more important for the clinical task at hand.

Reliability

Reliability is the extent to which a measurement instrument yields consistent results when repeated multiple times. Think of getting on a scale several times in a row: Does the scale always read the same value? If so, that scale is reliable. Reliability is relatively easy to determine, and, in general, is assessed as a correlation between repeated administrations (test-retest reliability), multiple raters (interrater reliability), or related content or ability areas (internal reliability). Unreliable assessments introduce error that makes it difficult to see true relationships between the assessment and underlying clinical conditions.

Validity

Validity is the extent to which an assessment reflects the concept or quantity that it is intended to measure. The assessment should be considered a surrogate or proxy for the entity we really want to understand. If that surrogate or proxy is a good indicator of the underlying entity, then the assessment is valid. A measure can be reliable but not valid, but a valid assessment must always be reliable. Otherwise, error from the assessment itself (i.e., poor reliability) will make it difficult to gauge how well the assessment measures the clinical condition or concept in question.

Just as reliability takes many forms, so too does validity. Face (or content) validity suggests that a measure includes a reasonable set of indicators to assess the concept or clinical condition we seek to measure. Construct (or convergent) validity indicates that an assessment is highly correlated with other indicators of the underlying clinical condition. Divergent validity is indicated by a low or absent correlation between the assessment and indicators *not* hypothesized to be related to the underlying condition. Criterion validity assesses the extent to which a measure correlates with another indicator of some underlying true value. External validity, or generalizability, suggests that an assessment may be useful across different client or clinical settings.

As an example, think of the occupational therapist–elicited report of activities of daily living (ADLs), originally developed by Katz and colleagues.[19] The ADL assessment identifies the individual's ability to perform competencies considered essential for personal self-maintenance. Older adults self-report their degree of difficulty with bathing, dressing, personal grooming, transfer, continence, and use of the toilet. The underlying measurement quantity or concept is "personal self-maintenance competency," and the assessment is a count of the number of ADL tasks older adults report they have difficulty performing. The measure has face or content validity in that it elicits the degree of difficulty in performing a wide range of basic adult competencies. The tasks are not gender specific, optional, or subject to variation in lifestyle. The measure has construct validity in that people reporting ADL disability are likely to have motor, cognitive, or psychiatric conditions that compromise a person's ability to perform self-maintenance activities without difficulty; indeed, ADL disability is correlated with severity of these disease conditions. The measure has criterion validity to the extent that ADL disability increases the risk of mortality, hospitalization, and nursing home placement. Finally, the ADL measure has external validity in that the measure correlates with these indicators both in community and long-term care populations.[19]

The ADL measure yields ordinal data. That is, ADL tasks can be numerically ranked. The tasks differ in levels of complexity, and in motor and cognitive demand. As a result, ADL competencies appear to be gained and lost in a generally consistent (but not necessarily fixed) order. Early on, Katz et al.[19] suggested that the order in which ADL tasks are acquired in childhood development (first, feeding and transfer; later, toileting and dressing; last, bathing) is the reverse of the order in which they are lost in chronic disease (so that the first lost is bathing, the most complex of the tasks). He noted as well that the order in which they are regained in recovery from stroke or brain injury repeats the sequence for childhood development (so that the last competency reacquired is again bathing).

Katz's early research showed that the disability status of almost all older adults in a skilled care setting adhered to this rough hierarchy of preservation and loss of task ability. That is, people who were unable to do just one task from this set of tasks almost always had lost the ability to bathe. People who could perform only one task independently from the set of ADLs were likely to have retained the ability to feed themselves. The ability to group tasks according to complexity suggests a particular approach to scale development, with meaningful thresholds. It is no accident that variants of the ADL measure have become standard in gerontological assessment.

Sensitivity and Specificity

It is important to know the *sensitivity* and the *specificity* of an assessment for its capacity to detect the presence or the absence of a given characteristic among those who have a disease or condition. Sensitivity tells us how likely it is that the assessment will detect the presence of a characteristic among those who have the disease or condition, whereas specificity testing shows how likely it is that the assessment detects the absence of a characteristic in someone known not to have the disease or the condition. The assessment's predictive value scores provide the likely false-negative rate about the extent to which the assessment wrongly says someone does not have a deficit when he or she actually does. Sensitivity and false-negative rates are the key measures of the utility of an assessment. They tell us how good an assessment is in identifying cases for targeting interventions.

Assessments can also lead us to wrongly categorize a healthy person as either diseased or having a characteristic of a disease or a condition. This error is captured by the *specificity* of the assessment. Among those without the disease, what proportion is wrongly identified as a case? Specificity tells us whether a test goes too far and identifies people as having the disease when they really do not.

Very rarely is an assessment both highly sensitive and specific. Consider an assessment with a threshold score to define disability. If we lower this score, we will capture all cases, making the test maximally sensitive, but we will increase the likelihood of netting noncases and falsely labeling them as such (decreasing specificity). In practice, it is perhaps best to err on the side of increasing sensitivity so that cases will be identified and therapies offered. False-positives can be assessed with more sensitive tools and reclassified as noncases in follow-up assessments, if these are not too intrusive.

Responsiveness

If a client's status has changed, assessments should be able to detect this change in clients over repeated assessments. Responsiveness is a measure of how well an assessment captures change in clients. Thus, in a client with declining cognitive ability, a good assessment will register slower performance, or perhaps a greater number of errors, in a performance test of cooking or cleaning, relative to baseline values. The "minimal clinically significant difference" is the degree of change in an assessment associated with a change in performance or status perceived to be meaningful to a client or occupational therapist.

Selection of Assessment Instruments and Type of Practice Setting

Occupational therapists need to be aware of the specific, real-life factors discussed in the next sections when selecting and using assessments for the specific practice setting.

Length of Administration

The amount of time available and the goals of the practice setting need to be considered in the selection of the tool. Some assessments, such as the Cognitive Competency Test (CCT), which helps provide information about how individuals will perform their daily living tasks from a cognitive perspective, could require upwards of an hour to administer.[32]

Opportunities to conduct assessments may depend on how long clients are in a particular setting, which in turn depends on the setting of health-care delivery, residential arrangements associated with each type of facility, and Medicare guidelines. The occupational therapist who works with older adults who are hospitalized in an acute care facility, rehabilitation center, or intermediate care facility (ICF), or who delivers in-home health care or center-based outpatient rehabilitation, needs to be aware of diagnosis-based Medicare benefits and guidelines that specify the type of service delivery and the length of stay for in-client services or the duration of intervention for in-home or outpatient intervention. Rest home facilities, family care households, day-care facilities, and retirement communities are usually not covered by Medicare; thus the length of stay or the duration of intervention is determined by the individual, family, or facility. Similarly, hospice care for the terminally ill older adult client is covered by Medicare for the duration of the client's life and place of care; but in the home or facility, it is determined by the client and his or her family.

Cultural Congruence

The client's cultural background can directly influence health perceptions, health behaviors, and acceptance of therapeutic regimens.[7,24] Not just older adults from ethnic communities, but all persons, tend to demonstrate greater adherence to directives that are congruent with their own cultural health beliefs. Culturally influenced health perceptions and behaviors may be detected by the use of a client-centered OT evaluation that gleans an appreciation for the client's own relationship between culture and occupation by looking at the choices the client makes relative to activity level and engagement in particular occupations, and the value the client attaches to his or her occupations. The occupational therapist asks the client to identify his or her own occupational concerns and goals to design an intervention that recognizes how the client's cultural values influence his or her response to the compromised occupations and life satisfaction.[7,22]

Training of Occupational Therapists Recertification

Registered occupational therapists have at a minimum a bachelor's degree, whereas a minimum of a master's degree is required for occupational therapists graduating in or after 2007. Certified OT assistants (COTAs) have an associate's degree. Most states require registered occupational therapists and OT assistants to also hold a state license. Occupational therapists conduct the initial evaluations, design the interventions, and supervise the OT assistants who implement interventions and may contribute to the evaluation or reevaluation process.[3]

In addition, some assessments require the practicing occupational therapist to acquire advanced training or certification in the assessment. For example, occupational therapists require advanced training to use the Functional Independence Measure (FIM™), which is designed to document the severity of client disability and measure outcomes of medical rehabilitation in a uniform way. Occupational therapists also must satisfactorily complete certification requirements to evaluate ADL task performance using the Assessment of Motor and Process Skills (AMPS).[15,16]

Assistive Technologies

Because OT helps the older adult individual maintain daily life performance tasks (including basic and instrumental activities) and maintain familiar social roles and activities while encouraging new ones, the occupational therapist must often consider use of assistive technologies in assessments as a way to compensate for a change in functional capacity. The occupational therapist will conduct an assistive technology assessment with the client to determine whether the client has the capacity to use the technology effectively.

BOX 6-1 List of Instruments Reviewed

AAD: Assessment of Awareness of Disability[31]
AMPS: Assessment of Motor and Processing Skills[15]
Beck Depression Inventory[4]
Braden Risk Assessment[5]
CDC's home fall prevention checklist for older adults (http://www.cdc.gov/homeandrecreationalsafety/falls/adultfalls.html)
CCT: Cognitive Competency Test[32]
COPM: Canadian Occupational Performance Measure[23]
Dynavision Performance Battery[20]
FIM: Functional Independence Measure[16]
FPS: Faces Pain Scale (http://www.geriatricpain.org/Content/Assessment/Intact/Pages/FACESPainScale.aspx
FM: Functional Reach[13]

GDS: Geriatric Depression Scale[34]
GUG: Get Up and Go[25]
Hamilton Rating Scale for Depression[17]
I-HOPE: In-Home Occupational Performance Evaluation[29]
Katz ADL[19]
KTA: Kitchen Task Assessment[2]
MMSE: Mini-Mental Status Exam[12]
Mini-Cog[8]
Occupational Profile[1]
PAINAD: Pain Assessment in Advanced Dementia[33]
SLUMS: Saint Louis University Mental Status[30]
Timed Up and Go[28]
VAS/NRS: Visual analog scale/numeric rating scale[9]

Practical Considerations in Selecting Assessment Tools

In addition to type of practice setting, there are several specific practical considerations regarding assessment that should be considered when selecting assessment instruments (Box 6-1).

Assessments in the Public Domain

Some assessments are in the public domain, which means that they can be obtained at no cost to the user, such as the Katz ADL Index mentioned earlier. Some instruments may have originally been in the public domain but were later removed,* such as the Mini Mental Status Exam (MMSE) and the semistructured, client-centered Assessment of Awareness of Disability (AAD). The MMSE, a widely used instrument to detect dementia, can only be obtained through Psychological Assessment Resources (PAR); the AAD requires credentialing from the Karolinska Institute in Stockholm before use.[12,31] Occupational therapists may consider the Saint Louis University Mental Status scale (SLUMS), which is designed for early detection of mild dementia in its 11-item questionnaire; SLUMS demonstrates validity with the MMSE and is available in the public domain.[30] A scientific review of the utility and the validity of the tests and measures will provide the necessary determination for suitability and access.

Changes in Normative Values

As the population of older adults has grown in size and there is noteworthy increased longevity, it is important to consider whether the scores on standardized assessments suit those who are to be measured. Only recently, age-specific impairment scores for 5-year increments above the age of 70 years have been published for a number of measures, such as hand strength.[6]

Suitability for Setting

The format of the assessment may call upon the occupational therapist to direct observation of an individual or a group of individuals, or administer a performance-based measure, or elicit reports using a written or oral questionnaire. The suitability of a given assessment format depends on features of the client population, for example, whether clients can complete a paper-and-pencil or electronic questionnaire on their own.

Goodness of Fit

In reviewing the assessment, it is important to determine whether the construct in the assessment tool is standardized on a population similar to the one in the practice setting, and whether the items on the assessment are good representations of the underlying construct and sensitive enough to detect the level of function or change in function that is desired to be measured.[15] Moreover, it is critical that the assessment is well suited for the demographic characteristics, cultural group, and clinical or community-based needs of the population to be assessed.

Cost

Some instruments, particularly those with standardized protocols and normative data tables, may have a cost for the assessment manual, tools, and data-collection sheets, whereas others may require a specific training course or credentialing.

Human Resources

The occupational therapist needs to meet the training requirements for the selected assessments, and determine whether the format of the assessment is conducive for the practice setting. If the assessment is a self-report

---

* Official versions of instruments that have a change in the right to publish, licensing, or intellectual property agreements are removed from the public domain and must be obtained from the publisher that holds the copyright.

questionnaire, it may seem that many clients could complete the assessment on their own. However, if there are clients who require assistance in manual skills to complete the form, or who require cognitive cues to appreciate the question being asked, then additional staff time will be required to complete the assessment.

Computerized Assessments

In addition, the assessments that the occupational therapist administers may require specific computer technology or software during the test administration. For example, whereas the Assessment of Motor and Process Skills (AMPS; http://www.innovativeotsolutions.com/content/amps) requires the usual physical setup for the occupational therapist to observe the client completing carefully selected routine daily life tasks (such as making a sandwich or sweeping the floor), specific computer software is required to score test results. Alternatively, occupational therapists conducting off-the-road driving assessments require the use of simulators and computerized programs, such as DriveABLE (http://www.driveable.com) or Dynavision Performance Battery, during the assessment process.[20]

Client Considerations

Client-Centered Evaluation

Before choosing an assessment, there are a number of factors to consider. First, based on the client's diagnosis and medical history, it is imperative to take into consideration appropriate precautions. For example, in the case of someone with a recent orthopedic injury, the occupational therapist needs to consider weight-bearing status and range-of-motion restrictions before initiating further assessment. In the case of a client with a cardiopulmonary condition, the occupational therapist must determine any activity restrictions or surgical precautions. *Pain levels* should also be noted before administering any assessment. For performance-based assessments in particular, it is important to time the assessment with a client's pain medication. In addition to pain levels and precautions, the client's *cognitive status* should be considered, as this will affect the client's ability to follow directions, as well as the client's safety, during performance-based assessments. *Sensory impairments* including vision and hearing loss should also be considered. In some instances, hearing loss is misconstrued as cognitive impairment when a client provides inappropriate responses to questions because they were not heard clearly. Or, a client may struggle with a pen-and-paper assessment because of vision loss. For some performance-based assessments and home safety assessments, a client's *mobility status* and use of an assisted device should be noted. For example, a client going home in a wheelchair will require different home safety considerations than someone who uses a cane or rolling walker.

Sociodemographic factors need to be considered as well. *Language skills* are important for most assessments, but for accurate cognitive assessment in particular. Therefore assessments should be administered in the client's native language whenever possible. Some standardized assessment tools, such as the MMSE, have been translated into many languages.[12] *Education level* can also affect the results of cognitive assessments. In these cases, assessments identify low levels of education rather than true cognitive loss.

Finally, *practice setting* will influence assessment choice. An occupational therapist working in home care will encounter clients at a different functional level and in a very different context than an occupational therapist working in subacute or acute care. For example, an occupational therapist who works in a subacute care center may be concerned with kitchen safety and administer a standardized assessment, such as the Kitchen Task Assessment (KTA), to assist with discharge planning. In the acute care setting, this type of assessment may be inappropriate due to a client's limited strength, mobility, and activity tolerance at this stage of the client's recovery.[2]

Client-Centered Practice

Client-centered practice is a philosophy of practice that emphasizes client autonomy, client choice in decision making, respect for the individual, partnership with the client, and a need to ensure services are accessible and fit the client's context.[23] It includes a therapeutic relationship rooted in strong communication and trust. Therefore client centeredness affects the quality of interactions between clients and occupational therapists. This being the case, a client-centered approach affects not just the assessments chosen but the way in which they are administered. Occupational therapists who are client centered engage the client as an active participant in the therapy process. Specifically, they discuss with the client the assessment tools to be used, the purpose of the assessment, and the assessment findings.

In a client-centered evaluation, the occupational therapist helps the client prioritize activities and occupations that the client may want or need help with because of current or anticipated age-related functional decline. Clients are evaluated for the full spectrum of functional performance capacities; occupational therapists often use the Occupational Profile to begin assessment of cognitive and functional status to identify the limitations in occupation that can be improved from interventions and to determine strengths that can be used to compensate for weaknesses.[1] Often, age-related changes may produce functional limitations that can be remediated through intervention or compensatory strategies to improve achievement in the desired activity performance or occupation.

In addition to the occupational therapist's interaction with a client, some assessment tools themselves are client-centered with regard to the types of information they gather. Client-centered assessment tools involve exploring a client's values and preferences, beliefs, hopes, ways of dealing with adversity, and sense of what is important. A client-centered assessment takes into consideration information about the client's family and other contextual data.[14] It also allows for the recording of a client's goals and treatment/intervention preferences. Examples of client-centered assessment tools include the Assessment of Motor and Process Skills (AMPS) and the Canadian Occupational Performance Measure (COPM). The AMPS allows the client or a family member to select a specific ADL or an instrumental ADL (IADL) task to be used during the assessment. This translates into an assessment that is relevant to the client's life and cultural background. The COPM includes a client rating of importance for areas of occupation that are identified as problematic. This aspect of the assessment tool facilitates collaborative goal setting between the client and occupational therapist.

There are a number of documented benefits to a client-centered approach. These include improved care and quality of life, reduced depression and anxiety for the client, and a means to address ethnic and socioeconomic disparities. Moreover, this approach is ethically and morally superior to purely occupational therapist–driven approaches.[14]

Occupational Therapy Assessment and Continuous Quality Improvement

Continuous quality improvement (CQI) originated from the industrial sector, where the focus has been on improving the quality of goods by enhancing the manufacturing process. It has been adopted by the health-care industry and has gained increasing importance due in part to a scarcity of resources. This scarcity requires health-care organizations "to do more with less."[27] In the health-care setting, CQI is viewed as a philosophy of care. Health-care providers and administrators who embrace this philosophy strive to continually improve the quality of care provided to clients or "customers," a term that highlights the importance of client centeredness.[21] It is continual in that it is an ongoing process rather than one with a distinct beginning and end. Unlike most assessments or reassessments by health-care providers, CQI focuses not just on the end result or outcomes of care but on measuring and improving the processes that produce outcomes.[27] For example, if a long-term care facility wanted to decrease the incidence of dehydration, it might institute a program where staff members from different departments offer fluids throughout the day. The CQI committee would not only collect data on the number of cases of dehydration before and after the program was put in place, but it would also collect information about who offered fluids and how often, as well as how much each resident consumed throughout the day. This way the process and the final outcome of the program can be evaluated.

Although CQI initiatives are coordinated internally within the organization itself, outside agencies are also involved in improving and monitoring quality of care. These organizations are described later in this chapter.

Types of Quality Improvement Initiatives

A CQI project may be at the *individual* level, meaning the goal is to improve the care for one specific client. An example of this is decreasing the number of episodes of incontinence or decreasing pain levels for one client through collaboration between nursing, occupational therapy, and medical services. At the *group* level, the focus is on improving the quality of care for one hospital unit or for client groups with a particular vulnerability or risk. This type of CQI initiative may involve assessment tools that assign clients to risk groups. One example is the Braden Risk Assessment Tool, which puts people into risk categories for developing pressure ulcers.[5] Examples of CQI projects at the group level include reducing falls or decubitus ulcers by implementing a multicomponent, multidisciplinary program. At the *system* level, CQI initiatives strive to improve quality of care in the facility or across the organization. Examples include projects to decrease length of stay in subacute rehabilitation or reduce the number of repeat hospitalizations.

CQI Implementation

CQI takes a grassroots approach, where grassroots literally means involving "common or ordinary people," as opposed to the leadership in an organization. Every employee regardless of his or her position is empowered to identify problems and potential quality improvement projects. In other words, the ideas for improvement come from those who interact with clients on a daily basis rather than those in administrative positions. For example, a staff occupational therapist may note that clients are at risk for pressure ulcers and that a positioning program offered by an occupational therapist can resolve the problem. Or a member of the housekeeping staff notices unmet care needs, such as clients waiting for toileting assistance for extended periods of time during shift change. In some facilities, one or more employees may be hired to coordinate and oversee CQI projects. In many cases, multidisciplinary committees are organized to plan, carry out, and evaluate programs. Occupational therapists are important contributing members of these committees.

CQI Evaluation

Quality improvement projects can be evaluated in a number of ways. One is by reviewing the medical chart to collect information from initial assessments and reassessments, care plans, and daily notes, both pre- and post-program implementation. Electronic medical records in particular are useful to assess the process of care because these include time- and location-stamped notes. This helps to determine how often and where care was provided. Observation by noncare providers can be helpful to assess the quality of care provided, as opposed to documented care. Two independent observers are ideal to ensure the reliability of information collected.[27] Another way to evaluate the outcome of quality improvement projects is through client satisfaction surveys. Many organizations collect this kind of information when a client is discharged from a health-care facility or from home care services.

Quality Assessment from Outside Agencies

Assessment of quality of care can also be carried out by outside agencies. In other words, individuals who are not employed by the facility or health-care organization itself review quality standards. For example, the state sends a team of health-care professionals annually to evaluate the overall quality of care provided at each health-care institution. This includes both a thorough examination of medical records as well as on-site observations of care. Although the state requires any deficiencies in quality of care to be addressed, CQI is considered just one approach in addressing and preventing deficiencies, and therefore is not mandated.

The Joint Commission on Accreditation of Healthcare Organizations (JCAHO) is an independent, nonprofit organization that provides accreditation to facilities and organizations that achieve quality standards. Health-care organizations that contract their services are provided with education and advice to help achieve these standards. JCAHO provides accreditation of organizations and certification for specific programs across the health-care continuum, including hospitals, nursing homes, and home health agencies.[18]

Applying Assessment Tools

To see how occupational therapists make assessment tool decisions, consider Case Example 6-1.

CASE EXAMPLE 6-1   Mr. Gomez

Social Background

Mr. Gomez is a 92-year-old bilingual Spanish- and English-speaking widower who has been residing in an assisted living environment for the past 3 years. At the insistence of their daughter who lives 2 hours away, he and his wife moved into the assisted living center due to Mrs. Gomez's declining medical and functional status. Mrs. Gomez passed away 2 years ago, and Mr. Gomez continued to reside in the apartment they shared together in the center. He retired from being a jeweler when he was 85 to be home full time for his wife, whose health had begun to decline. Mr. Gomez speaks with his daughter daily and enjoys the ability to connect with his grandchildren on the Internet. His daughter visits two to three weekends each month and always wants to move Mr. Gomez to an assistive living center near her home, but Mr. Gomez enjoys being close to his friends in the center and those few friends who still reside in that town.

Mr. Gomez limits his driving to daytime and maintains a car in the assistive living center garage. The assisted living center provides housekeeping, two meals a day, and a network of friends. Mr. Gomez enjoys playing bridge, collecting coins, singing in the assisted living center's choir, and acting in the center's theater group. He and his group of friends enjoy music and museum outings that are sponsored by the center.

Medical History

Mr. Gomez was first admitted to the local acute care hospital following a fall incurred while stumbling over a sidewalk crack. He was treated for his hip fracture with open reduction internal fixation; a joint replacement was not needed. Three days after surgery, he was transferred to the subacute rehabilitation skilled nursing facility adjoining his place of residence.

His past medical history is significant for hearing loss in both ears, right more than left; heart attack 10 years ago; history of elevated blood pressure and cholesterol; and an old left shoulder rotator cuff football injury.

Assessment upon Admission to the Subacute Rehabilitation Facility

Mr. Gomez is very determined to return to his apartment in the assisted living center, reunite with his friends, and restore his usual and customary activities as soon as possible. Using the client-centered model, each proposed

assessment was discussed with Mr. Gomez with regard to the purpose and procedure. Findings will be shared with Mr. Gomez and discussed immediately.

The occupational therapist interviews the client to clarify the medical and social history from his perspective and to understand his living context. First, the occupational therapist needs to verify surgical or medical precautions related to his precipitating hip injury and his past cardiac-related diagnoses.

The occupational therapist should assess self-reported pain at the outset of the assessment. Because this bilingual client does not have a diagnosis indicating dementia, a visual analog scale (VAS) rating for pain (0-10, where 0 is no pain and 10 is the worst pain experienced) is selected (Figure 6-1). There are a number of reliable and valid pain scales to choose from had there been noted issues about language or severe cognitive impairment. In that case, other tools, such as the self-report Faces Pain Scale or the occupational therapist–administered Pain Assessment in Advanced

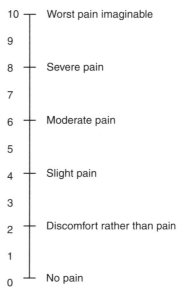

FIGURE 6-1   Visual analog scale for pain. (Adapted from O'Brien, P. D., Fitzpatrick, P., & Power, W. [2005]. Patient pain during stretching of small pupils in phacoemulsification performed using topical anesthesia. *Journal of Cataract & Refractive Surgery, 31*[9], 1760-1763.)

Continued

CASE EXAMPLE 6-1   Mr. Gomez—cont'd

0 NO HURT	1 HURTS LITTLE BIT	2 HURTS LITTLE MORE	3 HURTS EVEN MORE	4 HURTS WHOLE LOT	5 HURTS WORST

FIGURE 6-2 Faces Pain Scale. (Adapted from Hockenberry, M. [2014]. *Wong's nursing care of infants and children* [10th ed.]. St. Louis, MO: Elsevier.)

Dementia Scale (PAINAD), could be considered.[33] The Faces Pain Scale provides a visual facial expression associated with numeric values commonly used on the VAS that can help guide a client to anchor a pain level with a numeric level (numeric rating scale [NRS]) by the facial expression (Figure 6-2).[9] The PAINAD is specifically designed for the occupational therapist to assess pain in older adults who are unable to communicate their pain experiences or responses reliably due to cognitive impairments.

Even though Mr. Gomez's fall was caused by stumbling over a crack in the sidewalk, a hazardous environmental condition, the occupational therapist should be mindful to observe for safety and awareness during the functional assessments.

In order for Mr. Gomez to return to his own apartment at the center, it will be necessary for him to be independent in ADL tasks; he will need to ambulate with either a straight cane or a walker, not a wheelchair (Figure 6-3). Therefore, the assessment will address:

- physical measures of range of motion, strength, and sensation, recognizing that the left shoulder will be compromised from the old football injury
- bed mobility assessment for rolling, supine to sit, sit to supine
- transfer from the wheelchair to bed, toilet, and chair, with the goal to increase standing tolerance and balance to engage in ADL without need for a wheelchair

Due to the cardiac history, vital signs need to be monitored at rest and following activities. They must also ensure monitoring of vital signs during the early standing, mobility, and balance program.

The goal is to increase functional mobility over all surfaces (e.g., carpeted, uncarpeted, uneven surfaces), improve balance, and foster self-confidence and independence to safely complete ADL and IADL tasks using only a straight cane or walker. The larger personal goal is to return Mr. Gomez to his active lifestyle. Achievement of this goal can be measured by ADL and IADL measures and the Get Up and Go Test for fall risk assessment.[25]

The occupational therapist needs to note clinical signs that could be interrupting performance during the assessment process. For example, Mr. Gomez appears to have difficulty following verbal directions during the physical performance assessment and requires physical cues. The occupational therapist may question whether his need for physical cues indicates an undetected cognitive deficit or an unaddressed problem with hearing.

A cognitive screening is first performed to determine whether further assessment of cognition is indicated. The occupational therapist considers two reliable and valid cognitive screening tools: the Folstein MMSE and the Mini-Cog.[8] However, the occupational therapist uses the Mini-Cog because of its specificity and sensitivity and because it can be administered quickly (in about 5 minutes).

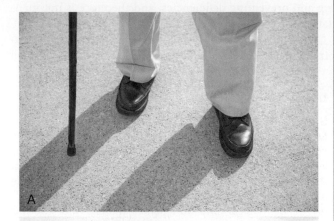

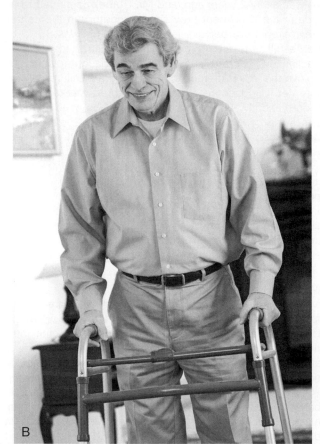

FIGURE 6-3 A, Using a straight cane. B, Using a walker. (Photos © istock.com.)

The Mini-Cog tool is readily accessible; it is in the public domain. The occupational therapist observes for how Mr. Gomez responds to verbal cues and questions during the course of the ongoing assessments to determine whether to make a recommendation for a hearing assessment.

CASE EXAMPLE 6-1 Mr. Gomez—cont'd

After the preliminary OT assessment, the occupational therapist schedules a bedside ADL to assess Mr. Gomez's self-care tasks when they are usually performed in the morning along with help from the nursing staff. The occupational therapist assesses level of assistance, independence, and safety in personal ADL performance of bathing, dressing, grooming, and toileting; and the occupational therapist completes the corresponding section of the FIM related to personal care. The FIM is a multidisciplinary tool that requires certification and training for use. The scores established for the FIM are useful to set weekly goals to monitor progress.

Assessment after 2 Weeks in the Subacute Rehabilitation Facility

Based on comments made by Mr. Gomez during OT treatment, the occupational therapist is concerned about his mental health. After a discussion with Mr. Gomez, the occupational therapist and client mutually agree that a screening for depressive symptoms is warranted. There are a number of assessments to identify depression, including the Hamilton Rating Scale,[17] Beck Depression Inventory,[4] and Geriatric Depression Scale (GDS).[34] The occupational therapist chooses the GDS because it was designed and developed specifically for use with older adults. It is also in the public domain. Mr. Gomez scores in the mildly depressed range on the GDS and likes the idea of a referral to psychiatry for further assessment.

The occupational therapist and client discuss fall risk and decide that further assessment is warranted. There are a number of assessment tools available, including the Functional Reach Test and the Timed Up and Go (TUG).[13] Although both are quick, easy to administer, and reliable, the occupational therapist uses the TUG because of its sensitivity with regard to detecting fall risk. Goals are set based on this evaluation to improve Mr. Gomez's balance so that he will be in a low-risk fall category.

The client no longer requires the wheelchair for indoor mobility within the subacute rehabilitation facility and relies only on a straight cane to complete mobility-related personal ADL tasks independently and safely. Furthermore, he ambulates within the facility for scheduled appointments and to visit his friends.

The client expresses concern with regard to his ability to return to the same apartment in the assisted living center and to complete instrumental tasks safely. Specifically, he mentions the ability to make his own lunch, which is not provided at the center. Although a number of tools can be used to assess meal preparation and other IADLs, such as the KTA, the occupational therapist chooses the client-centered AMPS because it incorporates not just the cognitive but also the physical demands of the task. Although the occupational therapist has not yet been trained in its use, the occupational therapist knows that the lead occupational therapist is AMPS-certified and has time this week to assist with the evaluation. The client chooses a kitchen task from the list of options, and the assessment is completed according to the standardized procedure.

Assessment at the Assisted Living Center

Once Mr. Gomez returns home to his apartment, the occupational therapist in the assisted living center completes a home safety assessment to ensure there are no environmental risk factors. The occupational therapist has the option of an environmental checklist such as the one developed by the Centers for Disease Control (CDC), "Check for Safety: A Home Fall Prevention Checklist for Older Adults." (http://www.cdc.gov/homeandrecreationalsafety/falls/adultfalls.html). This type of assessment requires the occupational therapist to conduct a survey of the physical home environment only.[10]

The occupational therapist adds the In-Home Occupational Performance Evaluation (I-HOPE), a more comprehensive client-centered option, to observe the client complete ADL and IADL tasks in the natural environment.

Mr. Gomez returns to his apartment in the assisted living center with a raised toilet seat and a bathtub seat. The assisted living center occupational therapist incorporated these into the I-HOPE[29] assessment. Based on the assessment, the occupational therapist also discusses with the client other options to decrease fall risk within his apartment.

The occupational therapist and Mr. Gomez go outdoors together to identify issues with safety, comfort, and level of independence in a community mobility challenge, walking to a local store to shop. This is a routine Mr. Gomez routinely completed before his hospitalization that he wishes to resume. The occupational therapist will note his ability to navigate curbs safely, any environmental obstacles in his regular route to the store (such as uneven sidewalks or lack of curb cuts), and his ability to cross the street safely with the traffic light. The OT will assess his activity tolerance and how many rest breaks are needed to make the return trip, as well as the availability of any benches for resting. Goals are set to increase safety awareness for outdoor environmental hazards and to increase independence with shopping. Goals are also set to increase standing and activity tolerance for the purpose of returning to the theater group.

A physical therapist continues to work with the resident on his gait, balance, and endurance, and collaborates with the occupational therapist to help the client meet his goals without duplicating services.

Shortly after Mr. Gomez's return home, the client's daughter approaches the residence staff with regard to her concerns about her father's driving. She is encouraged by the care coordinator to talk to the occupational therapist. The occupational therapist begins a conversation with Mr. Gomez and his daughter about driving fitness (see, e.g., http://www.aota.org/olderdriverweek). Based on this conversation, the occupational therapist plans to assess the client for any underlying deficits that could potentially affect driving health. These include visual acuity and visual scanning ability; visual field screening; visual perception; reaction time; cognitive skills, including attention, memory, insight, and judgment; and potential musculoskeletal changes, such as upper extremity, lower extremity, and neck range of motion (ROM). Depending on the results, the occupational therapist may suggest that the client be referred to a driving specialist for a more detailed assessment, including an on-road assessment. See Chapter 20 for more information regarding driving assessments.

Once these goals have been met and the client is satisfied with his performance on his ADLs, IADLs, and leisure activities, or he has reached his highest level of functioning, the client is discharged from the OT service.

Summary

In this chapter, we identify the methods, challenges, and uses of assessment in gerontological OT. We provide criteria to aid occupational therapists in the selection of assessments for their clients. A case example is presented with the intention to illuminate the decision-making process for the selection of assessments at three stages in the continuum of OT service provision. The chapter defines the standards and criteria for determining assessments that suit continuous quality improvement concepts within a client-centered care model. Suggestions are made to help the occupational therapist select assessments relative to availability of standardized and nonstandardized instruments, determination of reliability and validity, and suitability for client samples across care levels during the trajectory of daily living status.

REVIEW QUESTIONS

1. Before beginning an initial assessment, the occupational therapist should take which action?
   a. Review the chart to determine the client's medical history.
   b. Determine any precautions.
   c. Consult with the client's family.
   d. Both a and b are correct.
2. Before choosing an assessment tool, the occupational therapist checks to make sure that regardless of whether she or one of her co-workers administers the assessment, they will likely get the same results. This is an example of
   a. reliability.
   b. validity.
   c. sensitivity.
   d. specificity.
3. An occupational therapist searches for a tool to assess fall risk. The occupational therapist comes across a tool that is able to identify fallers 85% of the time, but incorrectly classifies people as fallers 50% of the time. This is an example of a tool with which characteristics?
   a. High sensitivity and low specificity
   b. Low sensitivity and high specificity
   c. High sensitivity and high specificity
   d. None of these
4. Mrs. Cho, an 86-year-old widow, is admitted for subacute rehabilitation for reconditioning following a prolonged hospital stay. The client indicates that independence in shopping is an important goal for her. Important client considerations with regard to the performance-based assessment of this IADL include which of the following?
   a. Pain level should be assessed.
   b. Determine any precautions first.
   c. Cognitive status should be considered.
   d. All of these are correct.
5. Which of the following is *false* with regard to CQI?
   a. CQI projects can be suggested by frontline workers such as occupational therapists.
   b. It is state mandated.
   c. Projects can be implemented for the benefit of one client.
   d. It can be evaluated in part using a chart review.
6. An occupational therapist considers which ADL assessment is most helpful for goal setting—that is, the tool that will be most useful in measuring small changes in functional status. This is an example of which of the following?
   a. Levels of data
   b. Validity
   c. Responsiveness
   d. None of these
7. Considerations when selecting an appropriate cognitive assessment include which of the following?
   a. The occupational therapist should consider the client's educational level.
   b. The amount of time available to complete the assessment should be factored in.
   c. Any advanced training needed to administer the assessment should be noted.
   d. All of these are correct.
8. An example of a self-report bias on a short-term assessment of performance is noted when a senior
   a. denies his functional deficits.
   b. exaggerates her functional deficits.
   c. or his surrogate does not report the deficits accurately.
   d. all of these.
9. Which of the following assessments would be most likely to give a truer picture of the needs or competencies of a senior?
   a. An actual ADL assessment performed by an older adult in his home
   b. A self-report ADL assessment completed by the older adult
   c. The score on the FIM while hospitalized in the acute care facility
   d. The Mini-Mental Status Exam (MMSE)
10. ADL is a critical dimension to be monitored among older adults because a change in ADL function and status
    a. indicates capacity to perform tasks based on complexity.
    b. often begins with a loss of the ability to self-feed.
    c. can be viewed with hierarchical indicators.
    d. can be measured sufficiently by self-report measures alone.

REFERENCES

1. American Occupational Therapy Association. (2014). Occupational therapy practice framework: Domain and process (3rd ed.). *American Journal of Occupational Therapy, 68*(Suppl. 1), S1–S48.

2. Baum, C., & Edwards, D. F. (1993). Cognitive performance in senile dementia of the Alzheimer's type: The Kitchen Task Assessment. *The American Journal of Occupational Therapy, 47,* 431–436.

3. Bear-Lehman, J., & Miller, P. (2006). *Occupational therapy. The Merck manual of geriatrics* (4th ed.). West Point, PA: Merck. http://www.merck.com/mrkshared/mmg/sec3/ch30/ch30a.jsp.

4. Beck, A. T., Steer, R. A., & Carbin, M. G. (1988). Psychometric properties of the Beck Depression Inventory: Twenty-five years of evaluation. *Clinical Psychology Review, 8,* 77–100.

5. Bergstrom, N. (1987). The Braden Scale for predicting pressure sore risk. *Nursing Research, 36*(4), 205–210.

6. Bohannon, R. W., Bear-Lehman, J., Desrosiers, J., & Massey-Westropp, N. (2007). Average grip strength: A meta-analysis of data obtained with a Jamar Dynamometer from individuals 75 years or more of age. *Journal of Geriatric Physical Therapy, 30,* 28–30.

7. Bonder, B. R., Martin, L., & Miracle, A. W. (2004). Culture emergent in occupation. *American Journal of Occupational Therapy, 58,* 159–168.

8. Borson, S., Scanlan, J. M., Chen, P., & Ganguli, M. (2003). The Mini-Cog as a screen for dementia: Validation in a population-based sample. *Journal of the American Geriatrics Society, 51*(10), 1451–1454.

9. Carlsson, A. M. (1983). Assessment of chronic pain. I. Aspects of the reliability and validity of the visual analogue scale. *Pain, 16,* 87–101.

10. Chippendale, T., & Bear-Lehman, J. (2010). Enabling "aging in place" for urban dwelling seniors: An adaptive or remedial approach. *Physical & Occupational Therapy in Geriatrics, 28*(1), 57–62.

11. Chippendale, T., & Bear-Lehman, J. (2011). The issue is—falls, older adults, and the impact of the neighborhood environment. *American Journal of Occupational Therapy, 65,* 1–6. doi: 10.5014/ajot.2011.000729.

12. Crum, R. M., Anthony, J. C., Bassett, S. S., & Folstein, M. F. (1993). Population-based norms for the Mini-Mental State Examination by age and educational level. *The Journal of the American Medical Association, 269*(18), 2386–2391.

13. Duncan, P. W., Weiner, D. K., Chandler, J., Studenski, S. (1990). *Functional Reach: A new clinical measure. J. Ger, 45,* M192–197.

14. Epstein, R. M., Fiscella, K., Lesser, C. S., & Strange, K. C. (2010). Why the nation needs a policy push on client-centered health care. *Health Affairs, 29,* 1489–1495.

15. Fisher, A. G. (1993). The assessment of IADL motor skills: An application of many faceted Rasch analysis. *American Journal of Occupational Therapy, 47,* 319–329.

16. Hamilton, B. B., Laughlin, J. A., Fiedler, R. C., & Granger, C. V. (1994). Interrater reliability of the 7-level Functional Independence Measure (FIM). *Scandinavian Journal of Rehabilitation Medicine, 26*(3), 115.

17. Hamilton, M. (1960). A rating scale for depression. *Journal of Neurology, Neurosurgery, and Psychiatry, 23*(1), 56.

18. Joint Commission on Accreditation of Healthcare Organizations. (May 12, 2015). Retrieved from http://www.jointcommission.org/default.

19. Katz, S., Ford, A. B., Moscowitz, A. W., Jackson, B. A., & Jaffee, M. W. (1963). Studies of illness in the aged: The index of ADL: A standardized measure of biological and psychosocial function. *The Journal of the American Medical Association, 185,* 914–919.

20. Klavora, P., Gaskovski, P., Heslegrave, R. J., Quinn, R. P., & Young, M. (1995). Rehabilitation of visual skills using the Dynavision: A single case experimental study. *Canadian Journal of Occupational Therapy, 62,* 37–43.

21. Kowal, C. E., Kagen-Fishkind, J. E., Sherlin, M. M., Newell, G., McCaffrey, E., & Gentes, J. M. (1997). An educational model to introduce staff nurses to continuous quality improvement/total quality management concepts. *Journal of Nursing Staff Development, 13,* 144–148.

22. Krefting, L. H., & Krefting, D. V. (1991). Cultural influences on performance. In C. Christiansen & C. Baum (Eds.), *Occupational therapy: Overcoming human performance deficits* (pp. 102–122). Thorofare, NJ: Slack.

23. Law, M., Baptiste, S., Carswell, A., McColl, M.A., Polatajko, H., & Pollock, N. (2005). *Canadian Occupational Performance Measure* (4th ed.). Toronto, ON: CAOT Publications ACE.

24. Lewis, C. B. (1996). *Aging: The health care challenge* (3rd ed.). Philadelphia, PA: F. A. Davis.

25. Mathias S, Nayak U. S. L., Isaacs B. (1986). Balance in elderly patients: the "get-up and go" test. *Arch Phys Med Rehabil, 67,* 387–389.

26. Rasch, G. (1960). *Probabilistic models for some intelligence and attainment tests.* Copenhagen: Danmarks Paedagogiske Institute.

27. Schnelle, J. F. (2007). Continuous quality improvement in nursing homes: Public relations or a reality? *Journal of the American Medical Directors Association, 8,* S2–S5.

28. Shumway-Cook, A., Brauer, S., & Woollacott, M. (2000). Predicting the probability for falls in community-dwelling older adults using the Timed Up & Go test. *Physical Therapy, 80,* 896–903.

29. Stark, S. L., Somerville, E. K., & Morris, J. C. (2010). In-Home Occupational Performance Evaluation (I-HOPE). *American Journal of Occupational Therapy, 64,* 580–589.

30. Tariq, S. H., Tumosa, N., Chibnall, J. T., Perry, M. H. III, & Morley, J. E. (2006). Comparison of the Saint Louis University Mental Status Examination and the Mini-Mental State Examination for detecting dementia and mild neurocognitive disorder—a pilot study. *American Journal of Geriatric Psychiatry, 14*(1), 900–910.

31. Tham, K., Bernspang, B., & Fisher, A. G. (1999). Development of the Assessment of Awareness of Disability. *Scandinavian Journal of Occupational Therapy, 6,* 184–190. doi: 10.1080/110381299443663.

32. Wang, P., & Ennis, K. (1986). *Clinical neuropsychology of intervention.* Boston, MA: Martinus Nijhoff.

33. Warden, V., Hurley, A. C., & Volicer, L. (2003). Development and psychometric evaluation of the Pain Assessment in Advanced Dementia (PAINAD) scale. *Journal of the American Medical Directors Association, 4,* 9–15.

34. Yesavage, J. A., Brink, T. L., Rose, T. L., Lum, O., Huang, V., Adey, M., & Leirer, V. O. (1983). Development and validation of a geriatric depression screening scale: A preliminary report. *Journal of Psychiatric Research, 17*(1), 37–49.

CHAPTER 7

Occupational Therapy Intervention Process with Aging Adults

Catherine L. Lysack, MSc, PhD

CHAPTER OUTLINE

OBJECTIVES

- Describe the major steps in the occupational therapy intervention process
- Understand why it is important to encourage client input and client choice in occupational therapy goal setting
- Explain how life roles and meaningful occupations change in later life
- Describe three actions occupational therapy practitioners can take during therapy with their older adult clients to enhance their clients' participation in meaningful occupations
- Give examples of how knowledge about the ethnicity and socioeconomic background of the client can enrich the practice of occupational therapists

Overview

The purpose of this chapter is to describe the occupational therapy (OT) intervention process. The chapter takes a functional approach, providing foundational concepts and models to guide OT interventions delivered by clinicians, and simple descriptions of the range of unique issues confronted by people as they age that can affect the services they receive from occupational therapy. OT interventions with older adults work best when much younger therapists understand the client and the client's real-life situations. Thus this chapter describes what the OT intervention process is and shows how critical it is to assess the person in context, which includes the personal backgrounds of older adult clients as well as their broader social, physical, and cultural environments.

The chapter is organized into five main sections: (1) Unique Issues Confronted by Adults in Later Life, (2) Conceptual Models That Inform the Intervention Process, (3) Steps in the Intervention Process, (4) Occupational Therapy Process with Individual Older Clients, and (5) Occupational Therapy Process with Groups. The first section describes several major events that can occur in later life (e.g., new health conditions, retirement from work, death of spouse, etc.) that challenge OT interventions. The second section describes two theoretical models, the International Classification of Functioning, Disability, and Health (ICF) model[42] and the Person-Environment-Occupation (PEO) model.[17] These models recognize the importance of client context and support the ideal of full participation in society for older adults, irrespective of health limitations, and therefore help to guide OT practice. The third section describes the basic steps involved in delivering all OT interventions. The fourth section describes how interventions are best delivered with individual older adult clients, and the fifth section discusses more novel situations when the OT intervention is delivered to groups of older adults and in areas of practice. The goal of this chapter is to provide knowledge that is useful to clinicians across a range of practice settings with older adults.

How Do Occupational Therapists Help Older Adult Clients?

Occupational therapy is a practical helping profession. When a client is referred to OT, the therapist begins by critically analyzing the presenting problem and the activities the person needs and wants to do. The successful therapist will find a way to maximize the abilities of the client, and modify and strengthen the environmental context so that necessary and desired activities can be achieved. Think for a moment about an older widow discharged from the hospital in a wheelchair after a debilitating stroke. She will be eager to return home, likely apprehensive about her ability to manage tasks, but also looking forward to "getting back to normal" and resuming what she likes to do, whatever that happens to be. What kind of intervention plan can the therapist develop that considers the client's abilities, optimizes the environment to support these activities, and also places the most meaningful life roles and passions this woman enjoys at the forefront of the intervention? The therapist will include activity of daily living (ADL) skills training in the intervention, perhaps teaching the client new ways of bathing and getting dressed, for example. The therapist might also undertake a home visit and make recommendations for simple modifications to the bathroom, kitchen, and laundry room to make self-care and other necessary household activities easier to perform. Will it be enough for this woman to be independent and safe at home alone? Rogers and Holm[30] write: "The occupational therapy process is the therapeutic problem-solving method used by occupational therapy (OT) practitioners to help clients improve their occupational performance" (p. 479). They stress that "a problem-solving stance" and "ability to critically analyze activities" are essential. In addition however, it is essential for all occupational therapists to consider that every older adult lives in a wider context that includes the physical environment (e.g., house, neighborhood), which may be more or less accessible, and a social environment (e.g., friends, family, co-workers, the public), which may hold more or less positive attitudes and be more or less supportive. The overarching goal of OT is to find ways to facilitate a client's return to the specific kind of daily life he or she would like to have. This means putting the meaningful occupations of clients at the center of our intervention efforts. It follows, then, that the goal-setting process must be a genuine collaborative partnership between the therapist and the client.[8] According to OT theory, if our interventions are designed correctly they will provide the "just right challenge" to clients because they optimize the best of what the client can do within the specific environment the client is in. Most important, OT interventions must be very attentive to identifying the most meaningful activities and occupations in clients' lives and working intentionally to integrate those meaningful activities and occupations into the intervention process. Think again about the widow discharged home after a stroke. Therapeutic activities during in-patient rehabilitation aimed at improving the functioning of her affected arm and hand could include repotting houseplants, for example, if gardening is a favorite activity. If swimming has been a fun recreational interest, then an aqua-fit class and return to the pool might also be recommended. If the therapeutic intervention focuses on what is most important to the client, then the intervention will be much more interesting, engaging, and motivating. When the client's wishes and choices are well integrated into the therapeutic process, there is a greater chance that the rehabilitation goals will be achieved.

Unique Issues Confronting Adults in Later Life

Aging and Disability

OT interventions for older adults have much in common with interventions designed for younger adults. Yet there are many experiences that are unique to later life or only occur if you have lived for many years and have given those events a chance to happen. All hold the potential to affect the OT intervention process, positively or negatively. The first issue is that older adults, on average, have poorer health and more chronic conditions than younger adults.[24] In part this is due to normal aging, which brings with it some declines in the senses, for example, vision and hearing, and also in the musculoskeletal system, for example, range of motion and strength (Chapters 8, 9, 10, and 12 are additional resources for these and related topics). This is not the same thing as pathological aging, that is, when a disease process is involved. Yet even normal aging means that older adults will take longer to perform daily tasks, and communication may be slower too. Imagine, then, a rehabilitation client referred to OT with a stroke or with Parkinson's disease or a hip fracture, for example. The intervention process could be quite straightforward and no different from the approach taken for the same client who is 20 years younger. However, in later life, the chance of comorbidities rises considerably, and this implies a more complicated assessment and intervention process. An older client may be diagnosed with a hip fracture, for example, but if the client also had a stroke 5 years earlier and did not recover completely and now the client is also dealing with diabetes and hypertension, then assessment and intervention will be more complicated and time consuming. It is also highly probable that older clients are taking medications for some or all of their health conditions. A national study shows that four out of five seniors are taking at least one prescribed medication, and a startling one in three take more than five medications.[29] It is in the clinical setting where the sickest seniors are found, and that is for whom occupational therapists most commonly design interventions. Healthy community-dwelling older adults may never find themselves receiving rehabilitation services of any kind. Thus therapists need to be attuned to the expected therapeutic effects of the medications on their clients but also how side effects of medications can adversely affect clients' function. (For more on this issue, see Chapter 13, which covers medication side effects in detail.)

Comorbidities, Medications, and Age-Related Fall Risk

Older clients with multiple comorbidities taking multiple medications are also at increased risk of other problems. Among the most serious are falls.[10] Because an injurious fall can precipitate admission to hospital and a downward spiral of functional decline, assessment of fall risk is a priority for therapists working with older adults in all acute care, rehabilitation, and long-term care settings, whether or not this is the primary reason for their referral to OT.[34] Fear of falling is also a serious concern.[15] Once an older person has fallen, the risk of having another fall increases significantly, and this can trigger a negative psychological response, fear. In turn, fear of falling leads to even greater activity restriction and deconditioning, which further diminishes balance and fitness, the very abilities needed to prevent a fall in the first place. The OT practitioner must be prepared for this. Therapists have many assessments available to them, and careful review of the best evidence-based screening tools and assessments available is always important (see Chapter 6). For the common situation of assessing fall risk, a brief screening tool like the Short Activities-Specific Balance Confidence (ABC-6) Scale[28] is frequently used to assess fall risk and then the data are used to help the therapist make very specific design changes to treatment plans.

Don't Forget Successful Aging!

Despite some expected age-related impairments, gerontology research reminds us that later life is not only a time of physical and cognitive decline. Later life can be a time of very good health and psychological resilience, creativity, and wisdom. Theorists have variously described this more positive view of aging as "successful" or "productive" aging (Additional resources on these topics are in Chapters 17 and 18). In one version of this general idea called *continuity theory*, Atchley[3] proposes that the people who age most successfully are those who carry forward the habits, preferences, lifestyles, and relationships from midlife into late life. A closely related theory is *selective optimization and compensation*, or SOC,[4] in which successful aging references the ability of older adults to learn, adjust, and adapt to the myriad of changes associated with age. According to SOC, older individuals have fewer resources and must select the goals or activities they wish to pursue and optimize their performance by devoting resources to those particular goals. These ideas are closely aligned with OT thinking. Therapists, especially in very busy clinical settings, must recognize how easy it is focus only on the older adult's impairments; they need to understand older client's strengths and abilities, too, and find ways to draw on the client's own reservoir of resources, supports, and optimism that he or she has developed by getting through difficult times in the past. Older adults, by virtue of their advanced years, bring an expertise about living life that young adults, including many occupational therapists, simply don't possess because they are too young! The 2010 Occupational Therapy Compensation and Workforce Study[1] reports that 56% of occupational therapists are under age 40 and one in five is under age 29. Do young therapists, many unmarried, know what it would be like for an older adult client to struggle in rehabilitation at the same time as the individual is dealing with the death of a spouse? Such major life events exert an enormous influence on the therapeutic environment.

Diversity: Seeing Life from the Client's Point of View

Age is not the only factor that separates occupational therapists from their older clients. Ethnicity and economic status do, too. For example, occupational therapists are overwhelmingly white; only 2.2% of practitioners are African American.[1] Most occupational therapists are also middle class and have benefited from substantial family support, both emotional and financial, throughout their lives. How well do young middle-class occupational therapists understand the lives of low-income older adults? Do they understand how much more difficult their lives are when they cannot afford to own or have access to a car, or even have sufficient funds to take the bus? Fortunately, occupational therapists in all settings have the opportunity, and the responsibility, to draw on the reservoir of life experience of the older client him- or herself. This will take effort when the life experiences of the older adult are difficult for the therapist to imagine. But it is an enormous opportunity to understand the client, which is a critical step in truly understanding how to address the client's needs. How does the client manage to do the things he or she needs to do in daily life? How can the therapist build on strategies that have served the client well in the past? Therapists need to listen to their clients, who bring a lifetime of experience of learning about and listening to their own bodies and dealing with life in general. Many have crafted workable solutions to survive and even thrive despite their difficulties, health and otherwise. Successful therapists will learn from their older clients and encourage them to put their personal knowledge and skills and strengths toward the rehabilitation issue at hand. That is the meaning of client-centered and occupation-based care, two concepts this chapter will discuss. Thus, to be effective, occupational therapists need to learn who the client is as an individual, and learn what goals are most meaningful to the client. Therapists just need to ask, listen, and respond.

Knowing how to specifically plan OT interventions with "older adults" is a challenge for younger occupational therapists for other reasons, too. First, the category refers to a very diverse group in terms of chronologic age. Typically, we understand "senior citizen" or "older adult" to mean persons age 65 years and older, mostly because, historically, 65 was the typical age of retirement from employment and the point where a person became eligible for government benefits such as Social Security and Medicare. People are living much longer than they used to, which means a much expanded period of older age (Note foundation information in Chapter 3). This makes it rather difficult to generalize from an "older adult" to the individual older client. The term *older adult* applies to persons in their 60s who are healthy and active *and* persons in their 90s or even older who might be quite unhealthy and inactive. And, of course, the opposite could be true. Age is generally an indicator of health and functioning but certainly not always. Further, the events we expect to happen in later life do not happen to everyone. Consider retirement, for example. A teacher or a government employee might retire at age 65 because he or she is working in a state with mandatory retirement or he or she is eligible for a full pension at this age, or both. However, a lawyer or a doctor might work for many years beyond 65 and never retire. On the other end of the spectrum are those who have had very prolonged periods of unemployment, and those who retire earlier than age 65 for health reasons. In other words, there can be a significant mismatch between chronologic age and the roles we assume older adults have. The therapist should not make assumptions. As stated earlier in this chapter, occupational therapists must ask questions and listen to their clients, to understand who they are and how to mobilize the personal resources of that person in the therapeutic effort to achieve the habilitation or rehabilitation goals.

From Young Old to Oldest Old

Given the diversity of older adults, specifically in regard to their health, the terms "young old" and "oldest old" have entered the lexicon.[25] These are functional terms or a shorthand way to describe the expectable functioning (or occupational performance) of an older adult. A "young-old" client is typically defined as 55 to 74 years. These clients are generally thought to be "well" individuals, mostly on the basis of age. On the other end of the function spectrum are the "oldest old," typically defined as 85+ years. Someone in this category is more likely to be struggling to maintain his or her health and independence. Consider for a moment how different OT after hip replacement would be for a "young-old" person who is a healthy 70-year-old living at home with her supportive spouse, versus an "oldest-old" 90-year-old who lives alone and has other serious health problems. Of course, age itself should not form the basis of the occupational intervention, nor should it be used to predict rehabilitation outcomes in individual clients. Occupational therapists need to be vigilant about this. There are many 90-year-olds who are living their lives very well without the involvement of any health-care professionals whatsoever. Because occupational therapists, like all health-care professionals, spend the vast majority of their time working with older clients who have the most serious illnesses and chronic health conditions, they may forget that most older adults never see an occupational therapist or undergo rehabilitation for any reason. The government report *Older Americans 2012: Key Indicators of Well-Being*[24] reports that only 4.2% of all adults over age 65 live in a long-term care facility such as an assisted living center or a nursing home; the remainder live at home independently in the community. Such data provide a necessary correction to stereotypes that too often portray older adults as frail and in need of professional care. It must be remembered that late life is also often a time of generativity and the passing along of one's skills and wisdom to the next generation. Attuned to this, OT practitioners should look for ways to encourage older adults to use their personal talents, in therapy and in their lives more broadly. In OT we know how important it is to our health and well-being to feel useful and productive. Later life is not always a time of decline; for many it can be a time of positive growth, discovery, and enjoyment.

Aging and Social Losses

By virtue of their advanced years, some older adults will confront declines in physical and cognitive functioning. These declines will often be viewed as "losses," and, as a result, they may feel that the social dimensions of their lives are narrowing. For example, a person who has lost confidence and stopped driving at night because of poor vision or a serious new health problem might not attend as many fun events with family and friends. When this happens, the individual will perceive losses not only in physical functioning, but in social functioning, too. This is just one example, but there are a variety of other "social losses" in later life. In Case Example 7-1, Erma is still feeling the loss of her husband. Her grief may be contributing to her loneliness and lack of interest in previously enjoyable activities. Older women will be a growing focus for occupational therapists as the demographics of the population change. It is well known that the population is aging, but old age is increasingly becoming a women's issue. Women tend to marry men who are older, and women live longer than men. This means that many women will live their later years as widows, like Erma. According to the U.S. Census, 80% of women will live more than a decade, on average, after the death of their spouse.[38] Widowhood is stressful. Research shows that women who are recent widows (widowed in the past year) have substantially higher rates of depressed mood, decreased social functioning, poorer mental health, and limited physical functioning for up to 3 years after the husband's death compared with women of the same age who are not recently widowed.[41] Because women at all ages are already at a two- to threefold risk of depression compared with men,[11] occupational therapists need to be especially alert to the signs of depression after bereavement.

CASE EXAMPLE 7-1   Erma

Erma Oldfield is 78 years old and lives alone in a two-bedroom bungalow with her two cats. She became a widow 3 years ago when her husband of 50 years passed away. Erma is healthy for her age. She takes no prescription medications and she rides her bicycle for an hour each day on a neighborhood trail. Erma is independent in all her housework and most of her outdoor yard work, although she relies on a handyman for heavier chores like cleaning her gutters each fall and washing her windows each spring. Erma still drives, although she has had three minor car accidents in the past year. No one was hurt in these collisions, but they were distressing to Erma and her grown daughter, Cindy. Erma has decided to ride with a friend to church and to her Wednesday night bridge club now, instead of driving herself. Although Erma describes herself as "doing better than many others my age," Cindy sees a different picture. Cindy believes her mother "hasn't been the same" since her father died. Cindy is also concerned to see her mother lose interest in baking, something she loved to do throughout her life. Erma has stopped hosting Sunday dinners, too. Several times when Cindy dropped by, she noticed how little food was in the fridge, and days can go by without Erma driving anywhere or talking to anyone. Erma has admitted to feeling "downhearted and blue," and Cindy thinks her mother may be depressed. Cindy wants her mother to be more forthcoming about her health issues so together they can find solutions.

Social Isolation, Grief, and Caregiver Burden

Caregiving for others, as Erma did for her husband in Case Example 7-1, is also a common feature of women's late-life experience. Caregiving, even when done willingly as a "labor of love" can still be exhausting and stressful. If not properly addressed, a sense of "caregiver burden" can emerge, and also a growing sense of loneliness and social isolation. This is not healthy. Social isolation can lead to depression. Unfortunately, too many mental health problems go unrecognized in later life (Chapter 16 covers age-related mental health conditions). Late-life depression is one of these. Depression in community-dwelling older adults is underrecognized and undertreated,[7,19] even by rehabilitation practitioners who work closely with older clients.[33]

With solid assessment data, clinicians can make better clinical decisions. In Case Example 7-1, there is some evidence that Erma may be depressed. Fortunately, through the use of valid and reliable screening and assessment tools, the therapist can identify and strengthen leisure interests and meaningful life roles, and also screen for things like depression(Chapter 6 covers screening approaches). Research shows that behavioral activation techniques are effective in reengaging older adults in activities that give them pleasure and meaning.[23] One place to start is using a brief screener like the 15-item Geriatric Depression Scale.[36] If depression is identified, the therapist can work to reincorporate "pleasant events" back into the person's daily routine. "Pleasant events therapy" is a nonpharmacologic intervention based on cognitive-behavioral principles. This approach invites the client to actively participate in actions to improve his or her mood. Research shows that occupational therapists can become knowledgeable about these simple interventions and deliver them effectively.[21] In many health-care settings, the physical diagnosis of the older client becomes the exclusive focus of the OT intervention. Therapists must remember that the social context of the client, which includes the client's personal history and current life circumstances, exerts an enormous influence too.

Late-Life Role Changes

The roles assumed by older adults are different from those of younger adults. For example, some older adults continue to be parents and grandparents, but they may not be relied upon to be "providers" on a daily basis. Thus, in midlife and through later life, after children leave home and establish lives of their own, parents must restructure their time and activities. When an occupational therapist has a new client who is an older adult, retired or working, it is essential to conduct a careful review of the client's work history, life roles, and leisure interests. The context of the client's home life is also important. The assessment data gathered will provide invaluable information to inform the occupational intervention. The Role Checklist,[26] for example, can be used to identify roles and the extent to which each is viewed as valuable. In Case Example 7-1, Erma assumes the role of mother, grandmother, friend, and churchgoer, among others. The Role Checklist will identify how personally meaningful each of these roles is and whether there are existing roles where Erma's participation can be strengthened or made more satisfying. Likewise, if Erma has lost a meaningful role, perhaps the therapist can assist Erma to identify a new role where Erma feels useful and productive. Leisure interests can be assessed too. Are there recreational, educational, artistic, sporting, and cultural activities that could occupy some of Erma's "free time" and be interesting to her? The Interest Checklist, originally developed by Matsutsuyu[22] and recently reevaluated,[16] is an 80-item list of leisure interests that takes about 15 minutes to administer. Therapists can use the Interest Checklist to evaluate how strong each interest is, and the degree to which participation in a pleasurable leisure interest may have fallen away in the face of some recent illness. Baum's Activity Card Sort (ACS) is another useful tool.[5] The Card Sort is a measure of occupation that enables OT practitioners to help clients describe their instrumental, leisure, and social activities. The ACS gives clinicians the occupational history and information they need to help clients rebuild their meaningful routines and healthy activities. It includes photographs of 20 instrumental activities, 35 low-physical-demand leisure activities, 17 high-physical-demand leisure activities, and 17 social activities. The ACS provides important data to inform the planning of occupation-based interventions in a way that is maximally customized to the individual client.

Residential Relocation in Later Life

Some older adults choose to make a downsizing community-based move when they determine that the physical demands of keeping up a large home and property have become too difficult.[9] Others undertake residential moves to be closer to family or to escape long, cold winters. However, research shows that older adults do not actually move very much, and when they do, the primary reason is because of an unexpected health "shock."[27,35] In Case Example 7-2, the care needs of Cookie may eventually outstrip Roland's ability to meet them. At that point, a move for Cookie may be unavoidable. Sudden relocations and unwelcome relocations are stressful. Not only is the individual (or couple, or family) dealing with the loved one's serious health problems, the individual must adjust to losing a much-loved familiar home at the same time as he or she is trying to reorient to new habits and routines in a new setting with new people.[13] Residential moves also require significant "downsizing" of possessions, which can be surprisingly difficult.[14] Another complication is learning how to manage downsizing decisions within the wider sphere of family life and cultural expectations.[20] The most challenging move situations of all, however, are the so-called "last moves," where older adults leave their longstanding homes where they have lived for many years independently into a more supported environment, such as an assisted living facility or nursing home, where they are dependent on others for care.

CASE EXAMPLE 7-2   Roland and Cookie

Roland Sawchuck has farmed for his entire life. He lives with his wife Constance ("Cookie") on a small farm in South Dakota. They travel to town every 3 days or so for groceries and farm supplies and sometimes stop at the local library for books. They lead a quiet life. They never had any children of their own but they were always friendly with the neighboring farm families. Over the decades, though, most of the children have moved to larger urban centers for higher education and better-paying jobs. One of two elementary schools in town is closing because of declining enrollment. Their church congregation is shrinking, too. Roland always said he would like to live on his farm forever. Perhaps he will, but he is facing the realization that if he does, he may have to live without Cookie. Cookie was diagnosed with

Alzheimer's disease last winter and her cognitive decline has been rapid. She is not safe at home alone. She wanders away from the house and yard, and there are days she is not sure who Roland is. There is a 20-bed nursing home in town, but Cookie loves the outdoors and the nursing home is old and has no garden, no walking paths, and no specialized dementia care unit. To receive advanced dementia care Cookie would have to move to a nursing home more than 4 hours away. Roland has decided he will just do the best he can. He refuses to "put Cookie in a home," especially not in one she will not like. Roland is worried, though. He is convinced that Cookie's doctor will decide that he cannot provide adequate care for Cookie, and Roland fears his wife of 60 years will be taken away.

Place Attachment and Residential Moves

Gerontology research has demonstrated the strength of "place attachment" in older people's lives.[31,32] (Chapter 19 covers the role of the environment in age-related well-being and quality of life.) A survey undertaken for the AARP by Bayer and Harper[6] found that 92% of community-dwelling adults aged 65 to 74 years wished to remain in their current homes as long as possible; the numbers rise to 95% for age 75+. Although respondents recognize that they may have assistance needs in the future, 82% wished to receive that assistance and care in their current home—that is, they preferred to "age in place." Therapists who work in the field of aging will be familiar with the phrase "aging in place."[39] Therapists may work with older clients and also families to modify and renovate spaces in the home so older adults can remain independent at home (See Chapter 26 for more detailed information). When a move is needed, however, occupational therapists must assist the older client and his or her family members by providing comprehensive assessment data about the client's function so that the best possible decisions can be made. What type of facility would be best? Will the client receive the needed care, and will the environment and other residents provide social and occupational enrichment? What steps can be taken to make the residential move easier for the relocating spouse and the spouse who is left behind? Thinking of Roland and Cookie from Case Example 7-2, what effects will Cookie's absence have on Roland? Will Cookie be able to adjust to a completely different living situation without Roland and without the familiar structure of her old habits and routines? Occupational therapists can play an integral role in finding clients optimal housing that fits their needs and managing the residential transition. Assessment is part of the equation, but so is up-to-date knowledge about the range of community services and assistance (paid and unpaid) available (Chapter 23 covers a wide range of OT services that relate to community services). Occupational therapists must also remember the value of theories and models that recognize the centrality of meaningful occupation and full participation in life as the foundation for overall health and well-being.

Conceptual Models That Inform the Intervention Process

The design of interventions and treatments for older adults is aided by theoretical frameworks or models that organize key concepts and knowledge. There are many models that guide practice in OT, as noted in Chapter 4. Therapists need to be familiar with them. The two models discussed next are important to OT because they include a strong emphasis on the environments in which clients work, play, and live. These models provide a "big-picture" view and remind the busy clinician that an older adult's personal situation and broader environment exert a significant influence on the older adult's occupational performance.

The International Classification of Functioning, Disability, and Health

The World Health Organization (WHO) provides a model called the International Classification of Functioning, Disability and Health (ICF).[42] The ICF model views a person's functioning as a dynamic interaction between health conditions and contextual factors. In this model, contextual factors are divided into personal and environmental factors. Personal factors are internal influences on functioning, such as age and gender, for example. Environmental factors are external influences on functioning that include features of the physical, social, and attitudinal world. Thus, in the ICF model, disability is viewed as an interaction between features of the person and features of the overall context in which the person lives. This is in contrast to a more traditional medical model that views disability as a feature of the person, directly caused by disease that requires medical care. The ICF model provides valuable guidance to OT practitioners because it underscores the role that personal and environmental factors play in shaping a client's participation in activities and life situations. The ICF model is also a universal model reminding us that everyone has a range of functional abilities, whether disabled or not. Further, the model can be seen to empower persons with functional needs because it underscores the right all

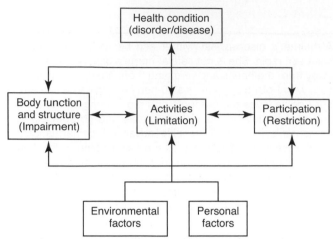

FIGURE 7-1   Interaction of concepts in the ICF model.

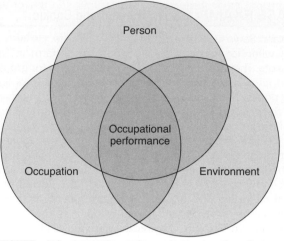

FIGURE 7-2   Interaction of concepts in the Person-Environment-Occupation model.

human beings have to participate in society. Under the ICF model, people are not defined as "dis-abled"; they are viewed instead as having a basic human right to participate in the activities and life situations they choose (Figure 7-1).

The Person-Environment-Occupation Model of Occupational Performance

Within the profession of OT, there are various models to guide clinical practice. One widely used model is the Person-Environment-Occupation (PEO) model, developed by Mary Law, Ph.D., OT, and which preceded the Person-Environment-Occupation-Participation model. The PEO has the concept of "occupation" at its core. Occupational performance is defined as a transactive relationship between people, their occupations and roles, and the environments in which they live, work, and play.[17] This model emphasizes the interdependence of persons and their environments, and the changing nature of occupational roles over time. The three components of the model are dynamic and constantly changing and sometimes overlapping, dependent on the roles an individual assumes. Under this model, the goal of OT is to find the "best fit" between the components. According to these theorists, optimal occupational performance occurs when an optimal balance is achieved between the person's occupational goals and the environment. The ICF and PEO models have pushed the profession to think about how people really live, and to not focus only on the remediation of their health problems, devoid of the context (Figure 7-2).

Steps in the Intervention Process

OT begins with a referral and ends when the client's therapeutic goals are achieved. The entire process can be as short as a few hours or as long as several weeks or even months. Irrespective of the time taken, however, the steps in the process are the same. After a referral is received, the process is one of information gathering, problem definition, goal setting, implementation, and finally evaluation:

1. Referral
2. Assessment
3. Problem identification
4. Goal setting
5. Implementation
6. Evaluation

The first step in the process is referral. This is the step where information is received by the therapist, who will then determine whether the client can benefit from OT services. Step 2 involves gathering information about the occupational performance of the client. This step is needed so the therapist can obtain a clearer view of the client's abilities and identify specific problems a client may be experiencing. The therapist may administer a short set of screening tools and assessments and even role and interest checklists to better understand the occupational and functional profile of the client—not only the narrow diagnostic reason for the medical referral. Therapists are also strongly urged to ask clients what they think their needs and strengths are. Step 3 is the problem identification and definition step. Based on data, which may come from observation, conversations with the client, and standardized and nonstandardized assessments, the therapist identifies the functional challenges the client faces. Guided by models like the ICF and PEO models, the therapist considers the social and physical context of the client, too, not only the client's functional limitations. The fourth step is goal setting. In this step the therapist works in partnership with the client to understand the client's views, and it is at this point in the process that the client's goals assume center stage. Working together, the therapist and client develop an individualized plan of action. This plan is the treatment plan or intervention. Step 5 is the actual intervention step. Intervention refers to the purposeful, directed actions taken by the therapist to put the plans into action. This is the "doing treatment" step. The therapist's actions are informed by the best evidence from the scientific literature (Refer to Chapter 5) combined with the therapist's clinical experience, clinical reasoning, and judgment, with a great deal of valuable input from the client him- or herself. The intervention can include physical rehabilitation, education, environmental modifications, the use of assistive devices (see Chapter 21), and additional services such as the use of personnel to help the client with mobility and transportation, money management, and the like. The final step in the OT process is evaluation. In this step, the original goals are revisited and the client's progress is measured against those goals. Typically, adjustments to the original intervention plan may be needed as the client's needs change. Evaluation and reevaluation continue as the client progresses and, it is hoped, achieves the therapeutic goals.

The OT intervention process may appear step-wise and linear, but it is not. The process is fluid and dynamic, responsive to the changing conditions of the client and the environment. The best interventions are interactive, creative, and flexible as the therapist engages *with* the client in a collaborative relationship where goals are set, possible client futures are imagined, and interventions are explored and undertaken together. An OT intervention process that is responsive to the client's own perceived needs and reflective of the client's real-life situation and future hopes provides a firm foundation for therapeutic success.

Occupational Therapy Process with Individual Older Clients

The ICF and PEO models remind occupational therapists to consider the personal background and contextual situation of older adults as they make their decisions. These models also underscore the importance of the client's preferences and choices. Fundamentally, occupational therapists believe that for treatment to be effective, the treatment must "match" the occupational needs of their clients. Thus we return to the two most fundamental concepts in OT interventions, occupation and client-centeredness.

Occupation-Based Interventions

Christiansen and Townsend[12] state that "to be occupied is to use and even seize control of time and space (or place)" (p. 2). These authors argue that the scholarly study of occupation may hold the key to understanding the art and science of daily life. Further, they argue that occupation is much more than activities or tasks. They say occupations are "invested with a sense of purpose, meaning, vocation, cultural significance, and (even) political power" (p. 2). These theorists urge their clinical colleagues to systematically evaluate how their clients "occupy" their time, through observation and formal assessments of time use and occupational activity. Individuals' use of time reveals a great deal about who people are and what they care about, which provides clues to how they might be best occupied in OT. The value and purpose of OT are to support the health and participation of clients by adapting the environment and engaging them in their desired occupations.[2,37] OT interventions are therefore based on thorough assessment, activity analysis, clinical reasoning, and attention to the centrality of meaningful occupations in clients' lives.

Client-Centered Interventions

Client-centeredness refers to placing the client's preferences and concerns at the center of the OT practitioner's therapeutic actions. To be a client-centered practitioner means the therapist respects the client's choices, supports and facilitates the client's occupational performance in accordance with the client's wishes, is flexible in designing and implementing interventions, and also recognizes the centrality of the person-environment-occupation relationship.[18] In short, to be client centered is to customize therapy for each individual client. Therapists must work even harder to be client centered when the cognitive status of the client makes it difficult to ascertain the client's goals and wishes. In cases of Alzheimer's disease and other types of cognitive impairment, it may be difficult for therapists to know if their interventions are meeting their clients' needs because they cannot rely on the client to tell them (note additional discussion of dementia and communication in Chapter 15). In these situations, therapists must work closely with family members who know the client and can share important insights about who that person is and what he or she values and enjoys. In more advanced stages of client cognitive impairment, the therapist is fortunate if family members are available to provide guidance about personal preferences and abilities and difficulties that are hidden from view as a result of the client's cognitive impairment. Although the occupational therapist in these situations will not receive direct input from the client, close consultation with the client's family and friends almost always provides information that the therapist can use to support the participation of even severely disabled older adults in activities that bring as much comfort and pleasure as possible.

Occupational Therapy Process with Groups

Emerging Areas of Practice

OT practice is expanding. *The 2010 Occupational Therapy Compensation and Workforce Study* completed by the American Occupational Therapy Association in 2010 states that 26.2% of the OT workforce is employed in hospitals, 21.6% in schools, and 19.3% in nursing facilities; the remainder work in outpatient clinics, home health, early intervention and community settings, and mental health.[1] When the survey asked about the primary age group treated, it is interesting to note that 35.9% indicated they provided direct client care to individuals age 65 years and older. This was up from 29.6% in the 2006 survey. This increased emphasis on older clients is likely driven by the aging of the population overall. OT students and practitioners should expect that professional training programs will place an even greater emphasis on gerontology and aging in their curriculums in the years ahead (Chapter 25 addresses this need).

Although a significant proportion of all interventions delivered to older adults will be in more "medical environments" such as hospitals, rehabilitation centers, and subacute rehabilitation facilities, the scope of practice in aging and the scope of settings in which therapists will find themselves are broadening. Growing numbers of OT graduates are working in roles and settings with a much greater emphasis on health and wellness, not just disease. This often means a transition out of the medical environment and into the community (Chapter 29 frames innovative community-based OT roles). The therapy provided is also much more likely to be educational rather than hands-on therapy. In this way, therapists are assuming the role of educator and advocate, and the interventions provided are new knowledge rather than hands-on therapy. Occupational therapists already provide some educational interventions to groups in traditional rehabilitation contexts. Think, for example, about a therapist leading an energy conservation group for women with rheumatoid arthritis. In this role, the therapist is a teacher, explaining the benefits of a resting splint to decrease pain and inflammation in the wrist, for example, or demonstrating ways of completing necessary household tasks that put less strain on the joints of the hand. Similarly, the occupational therapists on a predischarge home visit will explain the type of bathroom equipment that could be installed, such as grab bars and a bath seat, to prevent injuries or falls. Consider a client with a stroke or a hip fracture. Perhaps you don't even think of how you get in and out of the shower, but an older adult recovering from a hip fracture or a stroke certainly must. Every movement needs to be well considered when someone has a completely or partially paralyzed limb, impaired sensation, decreased balance, and/or reduced strength. In this situation, the interventions of the therapist include things like well-reasoned alternative methods of completing simple tasks such as a bathtub transfer, broken down into manageable safe steps. In all of these efforts the intervention provided looks very much like the OT intervention provided in the case of direct hands-on therapy; it is just that the intervention is primarily educational. All of the key steps in the intervention process (assessment, problem definition, implementation of the intervention, evaluation) are the same, although there may be multiple clients. In the case of the arthritis group, there are multiple clients with arthritis. In the case of the home visit, there is the client and also quite often a spouse, a grown daughter, and perhaps even a home health worker who will temporarily provide services to the older adult to ease the transition home.

There are other settings where occupational therapists are engaged in even more novel types of interventions. Consider an OT practitioner who has developed expertise in home modifications, for example. This individual could form his or her own business focused on home accessibility and provide paid services to those who need expert consultation. He or she could also be hired by a larger business such as an architectural firm or a building contractor. Who better to provide expert advice on renovations to support older individuals to age in place? Another example is driving. Occupational therapists can become driving rehabilitation specialists with advanced credentials related to driving simulator evaluations and on-road driving testing and training (Chapter 20 covers this specialty area). In a setting like this, the therapist may have an individual older adult client, but the therapist could also be hired to provide training and instruction to older adults in groups. There are occupational therapists who work for the American Automobile Association and provide driver training courses

for older adults to maintain strong driving skills, despite their increased age and possible physical limitations. The AARP provides a similar Driver Safety program. In these settings, the OT intervention process still includes assessment, goal setting, and then evaluation of the outcomes; the steps will just look different because they focus on the key skills that require remediation and improvement. The opportunities for therapists to twin their knowledge about the aging client with the myriad of ways older adults can "live better" in their environments are endless. Think again about the occupational therapist doing home accessibility assessments. Could she use her experience with health conditions to improve the design and operation of kitchen appliances? Why not? Imagine an occupational therapist working for a large consumer appliance company like Frigidaire or Whirlpool who could bring better-designed appliances to market, appliances that incorporate universal design principles so that an older adult with low vision or limited hand function, for example, could operate them without difficulty. Who better to redesign elements of our homes than therapists trained to identify the best fit of an older adult to his or her environment? Today, occupational therapists who work with older adults will find new settings and roles for their talents. New technology is transforming our lives in countless ways, and our homes too (Chapter 21 covers assistive devices). A voice-activated door has been possible for many years, but consider a voice-activated oven and television, or a smartphone that controls the locks on our doors and the window shades. Smart home technology holds promise for older adults and persons with disabilities. New graduates are likely to use new emerging technologies in their interventions in the future even more than they do today. Perhaps you will be the first occupational therapist working for Apple designing smartphone apps for persons with vision and hearing impairments. Chrysler and General Motors already hire occupational therapists to ensure optimal ergonomic work situations for auto plant workers, but there is a role for occupational therapists in the design of various new devices and adaptations to motor vehicles that can compensate for the limitations of older adult and disabled drivers. When technology is used to enhance occupational performance, in individuals or in groups, and in the community, home, and workplace, the occupational therapist is still doing OT. Provision of hands-on therapy, education, and creative design contributions can all enhance the occupational performance of the client. It is an exciting time to be a graduating occupational therapist, knowing that the demand for services for older adults is growing.

Summary

Occupational therapy is a practical helping profession. As Mary Reilly, a preeminent occupational therapist in the 1960s, once said, "Man, through the use of his hands, as they are energized by mind and will, can influence the state of his own health." The belief that by "doing" one can become healthy is an idea that has influenced the profession for many years. Theorists since Reilly have pushed the profession even further and urged, in addition, much deeper consideration of our clients' lives and the things, people, and places that "occupy" them. Wilcock[40] argues that "occupation is the natural biological mechanism for health" (p. 2), and therefore occupational therapists must focus on the occupational nature of all human beings, not only the needs of a small group with occupational dysfunction of a medically determined nature. If this is done, Wilcock believes, the profession will expand its outlook, and its practice, to include how humans "become well," and that will bring with it interventions to address the occupational health of populations at large. To achieve this, occupational therapists will need to be more than masters of helping people to "do" things, they will need to inspire clients to imagine what might be possible and then support them "to become what they have the potential to become" (p. 7). Recall the earlier sections of this chapter, the case studies of Erma Oldfield and Roland and Cookie Sawchuck. Fundamentally, in these cases, the occupational therapist must understand the person within the context of the individual's daily life and meaningful occupations. This means the occupational therapist's primary occupation, perhaps even *preoccupation,* becomes the goal-directed actions aimed at achieving the occupational results desired by the client. Therapy becomes a practical plan, in a myriad of smaller steps, to work toward the outcomes that are most relevant and meaningful to the client. Thus the OT intervention process begins with an invitation to explore occupational possibilities. And then begins the dynamic and exciting journey that is new and different with every client—a genuine, respectful, and creative engagement between the client and the therapist to realize the client's occupational possibilities.

REVIEW QUESTIONS

1. Reflect on the environmental factors that affect occupational performance. Give one example of how an unexpected and negative change in your environment would affect your student role. Give another example of how an unexpected negative change in an older client's environment could affect the client's life roles.
2. Think of an older adult in your life. If this person were struggling with a serious new illness or injury, how would you begin to motivate and inspire him or her to participate in meaningful occupations, despite any limitations? Give examples of the specific things you might say and do.
3. Identify similarities and differences in the OT assessment and intervention process for older adults compared with younger adults. Provide one example of how you would "do OT" differently for an older adult client.
4. Careful assessment of the life roles of an older adult (past and present) provides invaluable clues to who the person was and is, and what types of activities may be motivating for that individual both during therapy and afterward. Try to list "10 fun things" an older adult might enjoy doing, and imagine how to encourage the individual to work on his or her occupational performance as a stepping stone toward those goals.

5. Imagine an older client with a stroke or other significant disability. Think about the client's decreased physical functioning and how he or she will manage and accomplish all of the necessary tasks of daily life. Think about the recommendations you can make to help the client be safe and independent at home. Now, think of how your recommendations will work if the client has little or no money. Think again. How can you provide low-cost sustainable advice to assist your older adult clients, even those with very limited financial resources?
6. Imagine meeting a person who is absolutely different from you, in terms of age, ethnicity, life experiences, sexual orientation, income, religion, and politics. Knowing that your life and his or her life are very different, and that you think very differently on many topics, how do you succeed in the OT intervention process with such a client? Give specific examples of what the therapist should do and say during interactions with clients who are very different from the therapist.

REFERENCES

1. American Occupational Therapy Association (AOTA). (2010a). *2010 occupational therapy compensation and workforce study.* Bethesda, MD: Author.
2. American Occupational Therapy Association (AOTA). (2010b). Occupational therapy's perspective on the use of environments and contexts to support health and participation in occupations. *American Journal of Occupational Therapy, 64,* 357-369.
3. Atchley, R. (1993). Continuity theory and the evolution of activity in later adulthood. In J. Kelly (Ed.), *Activity and aging* (pp. 5-16). Newbury Park, CA: Sage.
4. Baltes, P. B., & Baltes, M. M. (1990). Psychological perspectives on successful aging: The model of selective optimization with compensation. In P. Baltes & M. Baltes M. (Eds.), *Successful aging: Perspectives from the behavioral sciences* (pp. 1-34). New York, NY: Cambridge University Press.
5. Baum, C., & Edwards, D. (2008). *Activity Card Sort* (2nd ed.). Bethesda, MD: AOTA.
6. Bayer, A. H., & Harper, L. (2000). *Fixing to stay: A national survey on housing and home modification issues.* Retrieved from http://cq5.share.aarp.org/research/surveys/stats/surveys/public/articles/areserach-import-738.html.
7. Brown, E., McAvay, G., Raue, P., Moses, S., & Bruce, M. (2003). Recognition of depression among elderly recipients of home care services. *Psychiatric Services, 54*(2), 208-213.
8. Cain, P. (2002). "Partnership is not enough": Professional-client relations re-visited. In K. Fulford, D. Dickerson, & T. Murray (Eds.), *Healthcare ethics and human values* (pp. 48-49). Oxford: Blackwell.
9. Calvo, E., Haverstick, K., & Zhivan, N. (2009). Determinants and consequences of moving decisions for older Americans: prepared for the 11th Annual Joint Conference of the Retirement Research Consortium, August 10–11, 2009, Washington. DC (Working Paper 2009-16). Boston: Center for Retirement Research.
10. Centers for Disease Control and Prevention (CDC). (2008). Self-reported falls and fall-related injuries among persons aged >65 years, United States, 2006. *Morbidity and Mortality Weekly Reports, 57,* 225-229.

11. Centers for Disease Control and Prevention. (2013). *An estimated 1 in 10 U.S. adults report depression.* Retrieved from http://www.cdc.gov/features/dsdepression/.

12. Christiansen, C., & Townsend, E. (Eds.), (2004). *Introduction to occupation: The art and science of living.* Upper Saddle River, NJ: Prentice-Hall.

13. Diaz Moore, K., & Ekerdt, D. (2011). Age and the cultivation of place. *Journal of Aging Studies, 25,* 189-192.

14. Ekerdt, D. J., Sergeant, J. F., Dingel, M., & Bowen, M. E. (2004). Household disbandment in later life. *Journal of Gerontology: Social Sciences, 59B,* S265-S273.

15. Friedman, S. M., Munoz, B., West, S. K., Rubin, G. S., & Fried, L. P. (2002). Falls and fear of falling: Which comes first? A longitudinal prediction model suggests strategies for primary and secondary prevention. *Journal of the American Geriatrics Society, 50,* 1329-1335.

16. Klyczek, J. P., Bauer-Yox, N., & Fiedler, R. C. (1997). The Interest Checklist: A factor analysis. *American Journal of Occupational Therapy, 51*(10), 815-823.

17. Law, M., Cooper, B., Strong, S., Stewart, D., Rigby, P., & Letts, L. (1996). The person-environment-occupation model: A transactive approach to occupational performance. *Canadian Journal of Occupational Therapy, 63,* 9-23.

18. Law, M., & Mills, J. (1998). Client-centered occupational therapy. In M. Law (Ed.), *Client-centered occupational therapy* (pp. 1-18). Thorofare, NJ: Slack.

19. Li, L., & Conwell, Y. (2007). Mental health care status of home care elders in Michigan. *The Gerontologist, 47*(4), 528-534.

20. Luborsky, M., Lysack, C., & Van Nuil, J. (2011). Refashioning one's place in time: Stories of household downsizing in later life. *Journal of Aging Studies, 25,* 243-252.

21. Lysack, C., Lichtenberg, P., & Schneider, B. (2011). Effect of a DVD intervention on therapists' mental health practices with older adults. *American Journal of Occupational Therapy, 65*(3), 297-305.

22. Matsutsuyu, J. S. (1969). The Interest Checklist. *American Journal of Occupational Therapy, 23,* 323-328.

23. Matuska, K., Giles-Heinz, A., Flinn, N., Neighbor, M., & Bass-Haugen, J. (2003). Brief report-outcomes of a pilot occupational therapy wellness program for older adults. *American Journal of Occupational Therapy, 57,* 220-224.

24. National Center for Health Statistics. (2012). *Older Americans 2012: Key indicators of well-being.* Retrieved from http://www.agingstats.gov/agingstatsdotnet/main_site/default.aspx.

25. Neugarten, B. L. (1974). Age groups in American society and the rise of the young-old. *Annals of the American Academy of Political and Social Science, 415,* 187-198.

26. Oakley, F., Kielhofner, G., Barris, R., & Reichler, R. K. (1986). The Role Checklist: Development and empirical assessment of reliability. *Occupational Therapy Journal of Research, 6,* 157-170.

27. Oswald, F., & Rowles, G. D. (2006). Beyond the relocation trauma in old age: New trends in today's elders' residential decisions. In H. W. Wahl, C. Tesch-Romer, & A. Hoff (Eds.), *New dynamics in old age: Environmental and societal perspectives* (pp. 127-152). Amityville, NY: Baywood.

28. Peretz, C., Herman, T., Hausdorff, J. M., & Giladi, N. (2006). Assessing fear of falling: Can a short version of the Activities-Specific Balance Confidence scale be useful? *Movement Disorders, 21,* 2101-2105.

29. Qato, D. M., Alexander, G. C., Conti, R. M., Johnson, M., Schumm, P., & Lindau, S. T. (2008). Use of prescription and over-the-counter medications and dietary supplements among older adults in the United States. *Journal of the American Medical Association, 300*(24), 2867-2878.

30. Rogers, J., & Holm, M. (2009). The occupational therapy process. In E. Crepeau, E. Cohn, & B. Schell (Eds.), *Willard and Spackman's occupational therapy* (pp. 478-518). Philadelphia, PA: Lippincott Williams & Wilkins.

31. Rowles, G. D. (1993). Evolving images of place in aging and "aging in place." *Generations, 17,* 65-70.

32. Rubinstein, R. L., & Parmelee, P. A. (1992). Attachment to place and the representation of the life course by the elderly. In I. Altman & S. M. Low (Eds.), *Place attachment* (pp. 139-163). New York, NY: Plenum.

33. Ruchinskas, R. (2002). Rehabilitation therapists' recognition of cognitive and mood disorders in geriatric patients. *Archives of Physical Medicine and Rehabilitation, 83,* 609-612.

34. Schepens, S., Sen, A., Painter, J. A., & Murphy, S. (2012). Relationship between fall-related efficacy and activity engagement in community-dwelling older adults: A meta-analytic review. *American Journal of Occupational Therapy, 66,* 137-148.

35. Sergeant, J. F., & Ekerdt, D. J. (2008). Motives for residential mobility in later life: Post-move perspectives of elders and family members. *International Journal of Aging and Human Development, 66,* 131-154.

36. Sheikh, J. I., & Yesavage, J. A. (1986). Geriatric Depression Scale (GDS). Recent evidence and development of a shorter version. In T. L. Brink (Ed.), *Clinical gerontology: A guide to assessment and intervention* (pp. 165-173). New York, NY: Haworth Press.

37. Stark, S. (2003). Home modifications that enable occupational performance. In L. Letts, P. Rigby, & D. Stewart (Eds.), *Using environments to enable occupational performance* (pp. 219-234). Thorofare, NJ: Slack.

38. United States Census. (2003). *America's families and living arrangements 2003.* Retrieved from http://www.census.gov/prod/2004pubs/p20-553.pdf.

39. Wahl, H., Iwarsson, S., & Oswald, F. (2012). Aging well and the environment: Toward an integrative model and research agenda for the future. *The Gerontologist, 52,* 306-316.

40. Wilcock, A. (1998). Doing, being, becoming. *Canadian Journal of Occupational Therapy, 65,* 248-257.

41. Wilcox, S., Evenson, K. R., & Aragaki, A. (2003). The effects of widowhood on physical and mental health, health behaviors, and health outcomes: The women's health initiative. *Health Psychology, 22,* 513-522.

42. World Health Organization (WHO). (2001). *International classification of functioning, disability and health.* Geneva: Author.

CHAPTER 8

Musculoskeletal System

*Ann M. Hayes, PT, DPT, MHS, OCS, Margaret M. Herning, PT, PhD,
Chris Gonzalez-Snyder, MA, OTR/L*

OUTLINE

OBJECTIVES

- Describe how the aging process changes each of the musculoskeletal structures as it relates to functional task performance.
- Describe common musculoskeletal disorders in the older adult, particularly osteoarthritis, rheumatoid arthritis, osteoporosis, fractures, back pain, lumbar spinal stenosis, and degenerative lumbar spondylolisthesis.
- List and explain the principles of joint protection and adjunct interventions involved in the management of rheumatoid arthritis.
- Identify the three stages of rheumatoid arthritis and treatment goals associated with each stage.
- Describe the treatment choices that occupational therapists have for clients with lumbar spinal stenosis and degenerative lumbar spondylolisthesis.
- Describe the effects of changes that occur in the mobility of older adults.
- Describe the management, considerations and precautions, and importance of exercise in occupation-based intervention.
- List and describe the factors causing falls in older adults and the effects of musculoskeletal changes.
- Describe occupation-based interventions in the management of musculoskeletal conditions.
- Discuss the psychological effects of mobility impairments in older adults.

Through every developmental stage in life's journey there are changes that occur and affect our abilities to perform functional activities. For older adults these changes often lead to a decline in their functional status and increased risk for injury. Musculoskeletal disorders are one of the most debilitating and costly disorders that affect older adults around the globe. It is for this reason that the United Nations and the World Health Organization (WHO) endorsed the *Bone and Joint Decade 2000–2010* to recognize the major burden that musculoskeletal conditions place on individuals, health systems, and the social care systems throughout the world.[132] Leveille[74] reports, "well over half the older adults in the United States report chronic joint symptoms." When working with older adults in therapy, it is likely that a musculoskeletal issue will need to be addressed as either a primary or secondary condition for treatment.

Variations in Structure and the Normal Aging Process

Bone

Bones, comprising the endoskeletons of vertebrates, are organs that move, protect, and support the body. More specifically, the functions of bones involve mechanical, synthetic, and metabolic purposes. For example, the mechanical functions involve protecting the brain and other internal organs, giving shape and support to the body, and working with the muscles and nerves to provide movement (Figure 8-1). The synthetic function involves production of blood in the bone marrow. There are various metabolic functions: mineral storage, growth factor storage, fat storage, acid–base balance (by absorbing or releasing alkaline salts), and detoxification (removing heavy metals from the blood). Bone also acts as an endocrine organ through the release of the hormone osteocalcin, which contributes to the regulation of glucose.[71]

In both sexes, aging bones lose calcium and become more brittle. This affects the strength of the bone. Bone density reaches its peak during the 20s and is higher in males. Healthy individuals, who have had a diet rich in calcium from childhood on and have been physically active, have the best prognosis for maintaining strong bones. Weight-bearing activities and muscle contraction stimulate bone density.[62, 65, 117]

Bones changes take place throughout life in a process called *remodeling.* In this process osteoclasts reabsorb bone and osteoblasts lay down new bone. Remodeling is influenced by how much mechanical stress was placed on the bone; the levels of calcium, phosphate, and vitamin D; and the levels of certain hormones, such as parathyroid hormone, calcitonin, cortisol, growth hormone, thyroid hormone, and sex hormones.[31] With age, some bones can change shape. For example, the femur may become wider in diameter, and the mandible and maxilla may shrink. Because of changes in cartilage, the length and breadth of the nose and ears may increase.

Trabeculae comprise the spongy cancellous bone. Trabecular patterns are important within the femoral neck and greater trochanter areas of the femur because they form a type of bone organization that helps the bone to absorb compressive, loading, and shear-bending forces directed through the femoral neck. Where the bundles cross there is an increase in bone strength, but where there is little or no crossing there is an inherent weakness in the bone and a susceptibility for a fracture.[52]

Muscles

Taber's Medical Dictionary defines muscle as "a type of tissue composed of contractile cells or fibers that effects movement of an organ or part of the body."[126] There are three different types of muscle in the body: smooth, skeletal (striated), and cardiac. Muscle functions vary depending on the type of muscle (see Figure 8-1). The musculoskeletal system is composed of "skeletal" or "striated" muscle. For the purposes of this chapter, the following discussion will refer to skeletal muscle.

Skeletal muscles are typically spindle shaped and consist of a central portion called the muscle belly. The ends of the muscle have attaching sites with tendons that connect to bone. "The more stationary attachment to bone is called the origin; the more movable attachment is the insertion."[76] Skeletal muscle produces strength and movement of the connecting bones.

Muscle strength, like bone strength, peaks in the 20s. Muscle fibers are composed of fast twitch, Type II (which generate energy mostly through anaerobic metabolism and produce rapid, quick, powerful contractions), and slow twitch, Type I (which generate energy through aerobic metabolism and produce slow, sustained contractions recruited in postural activities).

Older adults experience a greater loss in Type II fibers.[105,127] This may be associated with nonuse and also genetic influences. Important, also, is type of use. For example, older marathon runners may not show the typical age declines in strength in their lower extremities and lower abdominals but may show these in their upper trunk and upper extremities.

Sarcopenia is a term associated with declines in muscle mass, strength, and endurance and is linked with physical inactivity. Women experience greater loss than men. The decline in both sexes is greater after 70 years. Research now points to a combination of sarcopenia and obesity in older adults in which muscle mass has been converted to fat.[104] Creatinine clearance is also important. Creatinine is released during muscle contraction and is a natural waste product in the blood. Creatinine clearance is reduced in aging and may indicate a muscle protein breakdown.[25]

Besides muscle strength, declines in muscle power (ability to generate force at a fast speed) and muscle endurance (ability to sustain a muscle contraction) play a significant role in aging. An older adult may slip because of the inability to produce a quick muscle contraction to avoid losing balance, or an older adult may have trouble standing for prolonged periods of time due to fatigue in the lower extremity and trunk muscles.

Joints

A joint, or place of articulation, is the location in the body where two or more bones make contact. Joints are constructed to allow movement and provide mechanical support,

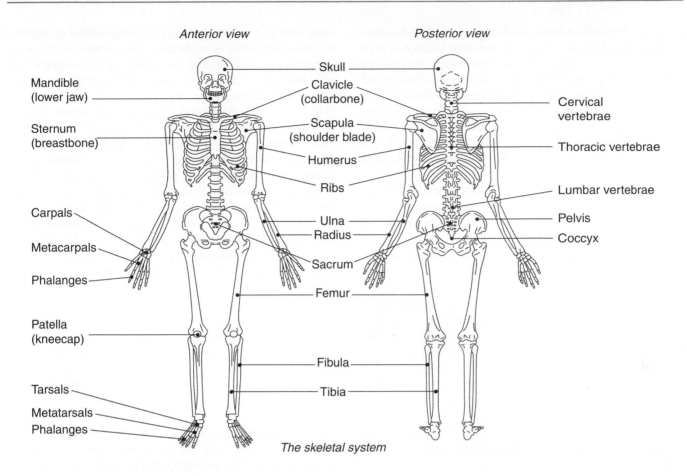

The skeletal system

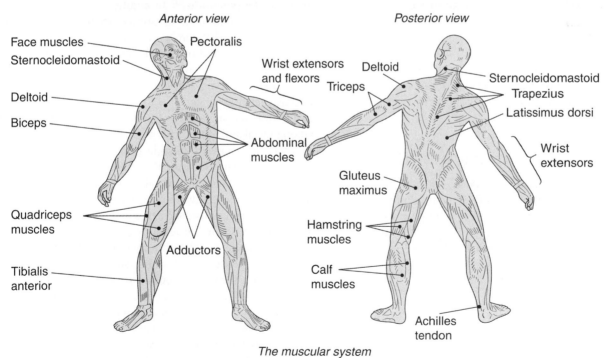

The muscular system

FIGURE 8-1 Muscles and the skeletal system. (From Hechtman, L. [2011]. *Clinical naturopathic medicine*. Edinburgh, UK: Churchill Livingstone.)

and they are classified based on their structure and function. For example, there are fibrous or immobile joints and there are cartilaginous joints. These are joints where the articular surfaces of the bones forming the joints are attached to each other by means of a white fibrocartilaginous discs and ligaments. These joints allow only a limited degree of movement. The most common type of joint in the body is the synovial joint. These joints allow for the greatest degree of mobility in the joint. See Box 8-1 for a list of characteristics of synovial joints.

Synovial joints can be further classified by the joint's function into different types based upon their movement. For example, there are gliding, hinge, ball-and-socket, pivot, and compound joints.

Degeneration in joints begins early in life, even in the teen years. Articular cartilage consists of collagen fibers and does not have a direct blood supply. It responds to mechanical stimulation (exposure to compressive and decompressive forces) by thickening. Too much or not enough stimulation can damage this. With age, articular cartilage can erode, lose tissue compliance, and become more brittle and less able to cope with stresses. Aging cartilage also contains less water, making it even more noncompliant. Formation of bone spurs (osteophytes) within the joints is common. Ligaments and tendons also become less extensible. The results are joint stiffening and limited range of motion. Finally, joint proprioception declines with age, especially at the knee and ankle.[29,94,105]

Common Musculoskeletal Disorders in Older Adults

Osteoarthritis

Osteoarthritis (OA) is a nonsystemic musculoskeletal condition that includes the progressive deterioration of articular cartilage and its underlying bone (commonly referred to as

---

| BOX 8-1 | Characteristics of Synovial Joints |

- The joint cavity is filled with synovial fluid.
- The synovial fluid provides nutrition and lubrication to the articular cartilage that covers the ends of the articulating bones.
- The joint is enclosed by a connective tissue that forms the articular capsule.
- The articular capsule is composed of two distinct layers and reduces friction at the joint.
- The internal layer consists of a thin synovial membrane, which secretes synovial fluid into the synovial cavity and lubricates the joint.
- The external layer is a fibrous layer composed of dense connective tissue that supports and/or controls specific motions in the joint (e.g., dislocation of the joint during normal movement).
- The joint capsule is supplied with blood vessels, sensory nerves, and pain and proprioception receptors.

(From Neumann, Donald A. [2002]. *Kinesiology of the musculoskeletal system: Foundations for physical rehabilitation.* St. Louis, MO: Mosby.)

---

subchondral sclerosis), as well as an overgrowth of periarticular bone that forms osteophytes at the margins of the joint. Before the age of 50, the prevalence of OA is higher in men than women, but after 50 years of age, women are more likely to be affected, especially in the hand, foot, and knee (Figure 8-2).[38] The disease exhibits progressive worsening with age, rising two- to tenfold in people from 30 to 65 years of age.[34] When it occurs in middle age with no known cause (i.e., degenerative joint disease [DJD]), it is classified as being idiopathic. Osteoarthritis can also be classified as secondary if it occurs in response to an injury, deformity, or a disease process. Traumatic osteoarthritis can occur due to a single macrotraumatic injury or it can be caused by cumulative microtrauma. The incidence and prevalence of OA in different regions of the body vary depending on how they are defined—either by clinical symptoms, radiologic findings, or a combination of the two—as well as factors such as gender, age, and genetics. According to a summary of "Stepping Away from OA," a multidisciplinary conference sponsored by the National Institute of Arthritis and Musculoskeletal and Skin Diseases in 1999, osteoarthritis can be prevented. In addition, this conference acknowledged that OA involves all joint tissues, and formally stated that OA is mechanically driven, biomechanically mediated, and dominated by attempted repair.[34]

Several risk factors have been identified for osteoarthritis, and the relative importance of these risk factors can vary depending on the joint that is involved, the stage of the disease, and whether the disease has been classified by radiographs or by symptoms.[137] In addition, risk factors are considered to be modifiable or nonmodifiable. Modifiable risk factors are those that can be changed; nonmodifiable factors are those that are out of an individual's control. In regard to nonmodifiable risk factors, besides age and gender, heredity appears to play a major role in the development of generalized osteoarthritis; a gene for the disease has been identified. In addition, the prevalence of OA and the joints it affects vary among racial and ethnic groups.

There are many modifiable risk factors that need to be considered when discussing the etiology of osteoarthritis. As early as 1997 Slemenda et al.[110] reported that decreased muscle strength, relative to body weight, could play a role in the development of osteoarthritis. In their study of individuals without a history of knee pain, isolated quad weakness was strongly associated with radiographic evidence of osteoarthritis of the knee. This study suggested that decreasing body fat and increasing muscle strength may assist in the prevention of OA; if nothing else, the intervention could be an effective tool for decreasing pain and improving function. Since Slemenda et al.'s initial work, multiple other studies have supported the idea of muscle weakness playing a role in the development and progression of OA. It should be noted, however, that at least one study has acknowledged that although strength increases seem to have a protective effect in healthy joints, increased strengthening may possibly encourage OA progression in malaligned joints secondary to the increased joint reaction forces sustained across the articulating surfaces.[106]

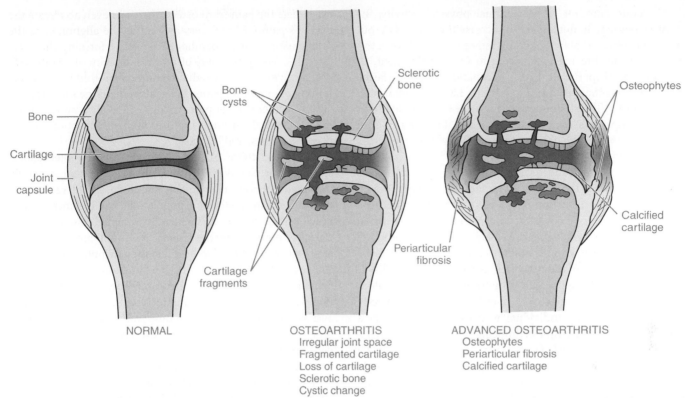

FIGURE 8-2 Schematic presentation of the pathologic changes in osteoarthritis. (From Ulbricht, C. [2010]. *Natural standard herbal pharmacotherapy.* St. Louis, MO: Mosby.)

Decreased joint proprioception has also been cited as a possible risk factor because it has been linked to joint instability and decreased shock absorption, both of which can lead to muscle weakness, and therefore possibly osteoarthritis.[107] However, in the case of proprioception, there is no consensus on whether decreased proprioception is the cause or the result of the osteoarthritis,[107] and some recent literature suggests that the link between OA and deficits in proprioception may not be as strong as previously thought.

There is increasing support in the literature suggesting that strengthening and aerobic exercise programs improve mobility, reduce pain, and increase muscle strength and joint proprioception in clients with osteoarthritis.[10,85,106,121] Because physical inactivity among geriatric individuals appears to play a role in the development of disease processes with long-term consequences that can contribute to the individual's loss of functional independence, encouraging activity and exercise makes sense.[95]

Obesity has also been shown to play a role in the development of OA, possibly due to the excessive loading on the joint surfaces of the lower extremities that increases the biomechanical stresses across the articulating surfaces. An association has been shown to exist between obesity and the progression of knee OA.[9,17,89] According to "The Arthritis, Diet, and Activity Promotion Trial" in 2004, older adults experienced decreased pain and improved function with weight loss and exercise.[83] Unfortunately, the evidence for obesity and the progression of hip OA is not as strong, but there is evidence that obesity increases the risk for the development

of bilateral hip OA.[51] In any case, according to recommendations published by the Osteoarthritis Research Society International (OARSI) in 2010, there was significant improvement in disability with weight loss.[136]

A history of joint trauma, such as a transarticular fracture or meniscal tear, and the presence of a bony deformity, such as developmental dysplasia of the hip, are also modifiable risk factors for the development of osteoarthritis.[11,32,122] In all of these situations, mechanical forces seem to be the underlying cause, but not necessarily because they directly damage the joint. Instead, it is hypothesized that these physical forces stimulate mechanical receptors in the chondrocytes that produce cytokines and enzymes that degrade the cartilage and surrounding joint tissues in an attempt to repair the damaged tissue.[84]

In addition to mechanical forces, congruency of the articulating surfaces seems to play a role in the development of osteoarthritis; the more incongruently the joints are aligned, the greater the chance that OA will develop. For example, developmental hip dysplasias are associated with the development of hip OA in young adults.[5,101] Recent studies have started looking at whether femoroacetabular impingement might be a risk factor for the development and progression of hip OA.[100] There is evidence to support that malalignment of the knee joint is a risk factor for progression of knee OA due to the fact that the malalignment changes the load distribution over the joint surfaces.[120] Leg-length inequalities are also associated with knee OA, but it is unclear as to whether they are a cause or consequence.

Moderate amounts of recreational physical activity, including jogging, do not appear to increase the risk of OA, but strenuous physical activity and/or intense competitive activity throughout life may contribute to OA development. In addition, participating in active occupations, such as farming, and those that require heavy lifting has been associated with hip OA.[60] The risk of developing knee OA in individuals whose occupations require squatting and kneeling is even higher in those individuals who are overweight, so it appears there is a summative effect with risk factors.[102]

Last, contrary to long-term beliefs, aging does not cause OA, but it is one of the strongest risk factors for the disease.[69] It has been obvious for a number of years that just because we age, it does not necessarily mean that we are going to develop OA; however, aging does play a role in the progression of the pathology and should be considered in relation to our past experiences and activities, as well as comorbidities. This statement is supported by multiple examples of older individuals who experience OA in only one joint of the body as well as the young individual who experiences OA at a joint secondary to multiple orthopedic injuries. In summary, then, if we take all risk factors into account, it should be stated that there is no single predisposing factor for OA; rather, it is a disease process to which there are a multitude of contributors.

OA is the result of tissue damage to a joint and the immune reaction that occurs as a result of that damage. Initially, swelling of the cartilage is seen as the chondrocytes attempt to repair the damage by increasing the production of proteoglycans. As the disease process continues, though, there is a decrease in the level of proteoglycans, a reduction in the thickness of the joint surface, and a loss of elasticity in the cartilage that contributes to its softening and ultimate deterioration.

Ask anyone who has OA and they will succinctly list the clinical signs and symptoms of OA: joint pain that worsens with activity and is relieved by "rest," joint stiffness (commonly referred to as "movie-goer's knee") and achiness, swollen and "tight" joints, malaligned and/or subluxed joints, and instability of the joint usually due to ligamentous laxity. In addition, clinical impairments include joint effusion that ultimately leads to joint enlargement, crepitus, decreased physiologic and accessory range of motion (ROM), muscle weakness, and posture abnormalities.

Chronic pain and functional dependency are not necessarily inevitable consequences of aging with joint disease. In developing intervention plans for osteoarthritis, the first level is to try to prevent OA from occurring; therefore, knowing the risk factors of OA, identifying them early in clients, and eliminating them as soon as possible are key aspects. Sometimes this is not possible, because some risk factors are modifiable, whereas others, such as age and gender, are not. After reviewing a client's major risk factors and eliminating or reducing them as much as possible, the next step of intervention is to reduce pain and improve function by individualizing the specific needs of the client based on his or her impairments. Regular, moderate-level exercise does not exacerbate the pain from osteoarthritis or even accelerate the disease's pathologic process as long as the alignment of the problematic joint is maintained while performing the exercises. Increasing the level of physical activity in clients with osteoarthritis helps to reduce pain and morbidity. In determining intervention plans, the goals remain the same for any level of client: control pain, increase flexibility, and improve muscle strength through the use of client education principles, modalities, and exercise.

Currently, there are no "gold standard" intervention strategies for clients with osteoarthritis; clinicians generally interpret the body of evidence found in the literature and generalize it to their client population. For instance, as was previously discussed, it is generally accepted that lower limb muscles, particularly the quadriceps, influence knee joint load, which is believed to be a major contributor to knee OA. Impairments in muscle function, including weakness and altered activation patterns, are commonly found in association with knee OA. Therefore, most clinicians will use exercise as a key component of conservative management programs for knee OA. Whether exercise influences disease development and progression requires further research, but currently, because exercise has been found to be effective in symptom reduction, most clinicians will support its use with clients with OA. Recently, evidence-based practice has received support by various groups that are heavily involved in the care of those with OA, for example, the Orthopedic section of the American Physical Therapy Association (APTA), the Osteoarthritis Research Society International (OARSI), the Ottawa Panel, and the American Academy of Orthopedic Surgeons (AAOS). Each of these groups has either developed clinical practice guidelines or made recommendations concerning the evaluation of and intervention with those who have hip and knee OA.[56,121,134,137] Although the techniques used to develop these guidelines and recommendations differ slightly depending on the group, the general principles in developing them are similar—a group of dedicated experts in the field reviewing research evidence that was available within a certain time period. All of the guidelines and criteria have been, and will continue to be, reviewed and updated as more evidence becomes available. In developing these guidelines, the panel of experts summarized the level of evidence that supports these interventions, the extent of consensus of agreement for each recommendation, and the strength of recommendation for each proposition. Allied health clinicians find these guidelines extremely useful in developing intervention plans for their clients with osteoarthritis.

Rheumatoid Arthritis

Rheumatoid arthritis (RA) is a systemic autoimmune disease process that exhibits both articular and periarticular impairments that include, but are not limited to, joint pain and stiffness. Although some of the impairments might be reversed over time, others cannot be, and these impairments ultimately interfere with the performance of functional activities (Figure 8-3). In comparing rheumatoid arthritis with osteoarthritis (OA), the main difference between the two is the

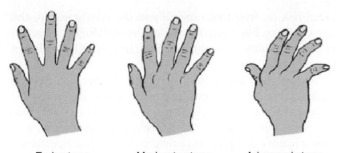

Early stage   Moderate stage   Advanced stage

FIGURE 8-3 Rheumatoid arthritis. (From Jonas, W. [2005]. *Mosby's dictionary of complementary and alternative medicine.* St. Louis, MO: Mosby.)

fact that RA is a systemic disease and OA is not. In other words, with RA, all systems of the body (e.g., visual, cardio-vascular, integumentary, renal, etc.) can be affected by the disease process, not just the musculoskeletal system.

Untill recently, a diagnosis of RA was confirmed when at least four of the seven criteria determined by the American College of Rheumatology (ACR) were fulfilled, and the first four criteria were present in the individual for at least 6 weeks.[3] However, in 2010, the ACR and the European League against Rheumatism (EULAR) collaboratively developed a new classification scheme focused upon early features of the disease process rather than later ones.[1] By redirecting the classification of RA, those involved in this process were hopeful that individuals would be classified earlier and effective disease-suppressing drug therapies initiated sooner, thereby encouraging more successful outcomes. The most recent set of criteria for classifying RA includes the presence of synovitis in at least one joint, the absence of a better diagnosis for the synovitis, and a total score of 6 or greater (out of a possible 10) in four areas: number and site of involved joints, serologic abnormality, elevated acute-phase response, and symptom duration. Because allied health practitioners are frequently the individuals initially recognizing the signs and symptoms of RA and referring clients to rheumatologists for further workup, diagnosis, and medical management, they should be aware of these new classification criteria. However, because the ACR does not want to exclude anyone with a later course of RA, health practitioners should continue to be aware of the older criteria as well, in order that any connective-tissue-type symptoms are not ignored. Even though the client may not have RA, there are many connective tissue disorders with similar symptoms that would still benefit from diagnosis and treatment.

The ACR has developed several classification systems that are helpful to clinicians in describing and defining the stages and functional levels of individuals with RA. The first classification system defines the course of the disease process. Type I RA is primarily self-limiting. Type II, which is mildly progressive, can typically be controlled with conservative treatment. Type III RA, which is severely progressive, typically cannot be controlled with conservative interventions, and therefore requires the most aggressive types of treatment. The Global Functional Status system describes a client's level

of function (Box 8-2).[57] This classification system is probably the most useful one for those involved in the rehabilitation and conservative care of clients with RA because it addresses which activities clients can do independently versus those in which they require assistance. By using this classification system, health-care professionals can understand exactly how a client is functioning because everyone is using the same language. Although it is understandable that clients will never be "cured" of their RA, it is possible that their health and functional status will improve, and the ACR Criteria for Evaluating Clinical Improvement in RA defines the specific criteria that must occur for this designation (Box 8-3). For instance, in order for improvement to have occurred in a

---

BOX 8-2   Global Functional Status

Class I: Independent in all self-care, vocational and avocational
Class II: Independent in self-care and vocational; limited in avocational
Class III: Independent in self-care; limited in vocational and avocational
Class IV: Limited in self-care, vocational and avocational
Usual self-care activities include dressing, feeding, bathing, grooming, and toileting. Avocational (recreational and/or leisure) and vocational (work, school, homemaking) activities are client-desired and age- and sex-specific activities.

(From Hochberg, M. C., Chang, R. W., Dwash, I., et al. [1992]. The American College of Rheumatology 1991 revised criteria for the classification of global functional status in rheumatoid arthritis. *Arthritis Rheumatology, 35*, 498-502.)

BOX 8-3   The 2011 ACR/EULAR Definitions of Remission in Rheumatoid Arthritis Clinical Trials

Boolean-based definition:
   At any time point, client must satisfy all of the following:
   Tender joint count ≤ 1*
   Swollen joint count ≤ 1*
   C-reactive protein ≤ 1 mg/dL
   Client global assessment ≤ 1 (on a 0–10 scale)**
Index-based definition:
   Simplified Disease Activity Index score of ≤ 3.3***

* For tender and swollen joint counts, use of a 28-joint count may miss actively involved joints, especially in the feet and ankles, and it is preferable to include feet and ankles also when evaluating remission.
** For the assessment of remission we suggest the following format and wording for the global assessment questions. Format: a horizontal 10-cm visual analog or Likert scale with the best anchor and lowest score on the left side and the worst anchor and highest score on the right side. Wording of question and anchors: For client global assessment, "Considering all of the ways your arthritis has affected you, how do you feel your arthritis is today?" (anchors: very well—very poor). For physician/assessor global assessment, "What is your assessment of the client's current disease activity?" (anchors: none—extremely active).
*** Defined as the simple sum of the tender joint count (using 28 joints), swollen joint count (using 28 joints), client global assessment (0–10 scale), physician global assessment (0–10 scale), and C-reactive protein level (mg/dL).
(From Rheumatology.org.)

client with RA, there must be > 20% improvement in the number of tender and swollen joints that the client has, along with > 20% improvement in three out of the remaining five criteria. Clients with RA can be considered to be in "remission," defined as an absence of disease activity, if at least five of six specific requirements are fulfilled for at least two consecutive months. Defined in this way, remission is a "state" and not just a change or transition between stages. Last, the ACR has defined factors resulting in a "poor" prognosis for a client with RA: earlier age at onset of disease, high titer of rheumatoid factor, an elevated erythrocyte sedimentation rate (ESR), swelling in more than 20 joints, and extraarticular manifestations. An awareness of these characteristics is important for therapists as they determine intervention plans for their clients.

Osteoporosis

Osteoporosis is a disease of bone in which the bone mineral density (BMD) is reduced, bone microarchitecture is disrupted, and the amount and variety of proteins in bone are altered. These consequences can result in fragile, porous bones, placing individuals with osteoporosis at a higher risk for bone fractures. Table 8-1 presents relative risk factors for hip fracture.

The rate of calcium loss accelerates during the first 5 years after menopause in women. By the age of 80 years women lose 30% compared with men losing 20%. The World Health Organization has classified bone density as normal, low, osteoporotic, and severe osteoporotic as measured using dual x-ray absorptiometry (DXA). Those in the last two categories

TABLE 8-1   Factors Found to Be Risk Factors for Hip Fracture in Several Studies, But about Which Some Uncertainty Still Exists

Risk Factor	Comparison
Relative Risk ≥ 2.0	
Health status	Poor/fair vs. good/excellent
Parkinson's disease	Present vs. absent
Race	White vs. Hispanic
Weight change	20% weight loss
Relative Risk 1.1–1.9	
Coffee	> 2 cups/day vs. no coffee
Calcium intake	< 400 mg/day vs. ≥ 1000 mg/day
Fractures since age 50 years	Fracture vs. no fractures
Height	Per 10-cm increase
Hip axis length	Per 1-SD* increase
Psychotropic drugs	Users vs. nonusers
Smoking	Smokers vs. nonsmokers
Thiazides	Nonusers vs. users
Vision	Acuity worse than 20/40
Physical inactivity	Not walking for exercise vs. walking for exercise

*SD = standard deviation.
(From Cummings, R. G., Nevitt, M. C., & Cummings, S. R. [1997]. Epidemiology of hip fractures. *Epidemiologic Reviews, 19*[2], 244-257.)

are at risk for fractures, especially in the vertebrae, hip, and wrist.[88] Bone fractures depend on bone strength (density) and bone quality (microarchitecture, bone vitality, ability of bone to repair itself).[91]

Osteoporosis affects both genders but the incidence is higher in women. An estimated 10 million in the United States have osteoporosis. Individuals at greater risk are those who are older, inactive, and of slight build, and those who have a history of a previous fracture. Individuals may have a history of adverse health practices (such as use of alcohol, cigarettes, and caffeine; diet low in calcium and vitamin D). Other risk factors can include prolonged use of medications (such as corticosteroids) and certain medical conditions such as renal disease.[88]

Preventive treatment includes calcium (1500 mg/day), vitamin D (800–1000 IU/day), exercise, and, in certain individuals, hormones. Vitamin D has taken on increased significance today as older adults have difficulty absorbing calcium and need vitamin D to induce the calcium-binding protein to move calcium across the cell membrane and encourage absorption of calcium in the small intestine. Weight-bearing and resistive exercises are important, but exercise should stress those skeletal sites most at risk for fractures.[88,118,119] Current research suggests that the best exercise for bone metabolism and decreasing the risk of falls involves impact forces.[64]

Medical treatment includes taking medications to inhibit the action of osteoclasts and their effect on bone resorption (bisphosphonates) or taking parathyroid hormone (to stimulate bone formation). As with prevention, daily intake of vitamin D and of calcium is important, as is exercise. Surgery options include vertebroplasty and kyphoplasty.[80] Both involve injecting surgical bone cement into recently fractured vertebra. The results of surgery show good pain reduction and return to function.

Fractures

A fracture is defined as a break in bone or cartilage and can occur anywhere in the body where these tissues reside.[114] One of the most common fractures that occur in the geriatric client is a hip fracture, which is defined as a break in the upper quarter of the femur; a fracture of the acetabulum or hip socket itself is not considered a hip fracture.

According to Maxey and Magnusson, of all the possible bony injuries, a hip fracture is the one that requires surgical intervention the most frequently.[79]

Epidemiology of Hip Fractures

In 1990, it was estimated that there were 1.66 million hip fractures worldwide; it is projected that this number will rise to 6.26 million by 2050.[22,135] This increase is believed to be due to the increased aging of the population, but also due to an increase in the incidence of osteoporosis, diminished overall muscle volume, and decreased neuromuscular responses to physical challenges.[98] In addition, with the rise of an aging population, there are a greater number of medical comorbidities that complicate the aging individual's health status, such as cardiopulmonary diagnoses and dementia.

TABLE 8-2 Established Risk Factors for Hip Fracture
in Women

Risk Factor	Comparison
Relative Risk ≥ 2.0	
Bone mineral density of the femur	Per 1-SD* decrease
Fall on hip	Fall on hip vs. fall on other part of body
Neuromuscular impairment	Unable to rise from chair without using arms vs. able to rise from chair
Race	White vs. Asian (in Asia)
Ultrasound attenuation	Per 1-SD decrease
Relative Risk 1.1–1.9	
Age	Per 5-year increase
Bone mineral density at nonfemoral sites	Per 1-SD decrease
Falls in past year	≥ 2 falls vs. 0 falls
Hormone replacement therapy	Nonusers vs. users
Neuromuscular impairment	
Grip strength	Per 5-kg decrease
Gait speed	Per 0.2-m/sec decrease
Weight	Per 10-kg decrease

*SD = standard deviation.
(From Cummings, R. G., Nevitt, M. C., & Cummings, S. R. [1997]. Epidemiology of hip fractures. *Epidemiologic Reviews, 19* [2], 244-257.)

TABLE 8-3 Risk Factors for Poor Outcomes
in Hip Fracture Patients

Preexisting Factors	Preoperative Factors	Postoperative Factors
Age	Type of fracture	Overall prognosis
Baseline functional status	Open or closed fracture	Risk for nonhealing surgical repair
Baseline mobility	Additional injuries	Risk of severe agitation or delirium
Baseline cognitive status	Rhabdomyolysis	Risk of postoperative fall and injury
Dementia	Time since fracture	Risk of worsening nutritional status
Nutritional status	Delay in surgery	Risk of inability to extubate
ASA score	Delirium	
Severity of osteoporosis	Degree of pain	
Lung disease		
Cardiac disease		
Renal disease		
Anticoagulation		
Terminal illness		

American Society of Anesthesiologists (ASA) Score.
(From Cummings, R. G., Nevitt, M. C., & Cummings, S. R. [1997]. Epidemiology of hip fractures. *Epidemiologic Reviews, 19* [2], 244-257.)

Because fracture care and intervention has evolved and improved in the past decades, opportunities for individuals to sustain second fractures are becoming more commonplace.

In general, women have a greater incidence of hip fracture than men, and the highest rates have been reported in predominately white populations in the Northern Hemisphere. There appear to be two main risk factors for hip fractures: decreased bone strength that can occur with pathologies such as osteoporosis and cancer and/or occurrence of fall-related trauma (Tables 8-2 and 8-3).[24]

Hip fractures are typically classified by orthopedic surgeons according to the area of the femur that is involved. In the case of an intracapsular hip fracture, the head and neck of the femur are involved. About one-half of all hip fractures involve the femoral neck and necessitate opening the femoral joint capsule during surgery, which increases the risk of infection. An increased rate of infection can complicate the postoperative course of events for individuals who may already be at risk due to their possibly frail health status. Not all fractures are intracapsular; intertrochanteric and subtrochanteric fractures are considered extracapsular and do not require that the capsule be opened during fixation. An intertrochanteric fracture occurs between the femoral neck and the lesser trochanter, and a subtrochanteric fracture occurs within an area approximately 2½ inches inferior to the lesser trochanter.

For rehabilitation professionals involved in the postoperative care of clients with hip fractures, hip fracture classification is usually dependent on the surgical approach used, the soft tissue involved, and the client's potential for rehabilitation.[8,79] In this classification system, hip fractures are categorized as being in one of the following five categories: nondisplaced/minimally displaced femoral neck fractures, displaced neck fractures, stable intertrochanteric fractures, unstable intertrochanteric fractures, and subtrochanteric fractures. Currently most types of hip fractures, but especially those that are displaced, are treated surgically with an open reduction internal fixation (ORIF). If a client with a hip fracture does not have a surgical repair, it is usually because of comorbidities that prevent it or due to the client being nonambulatory before injury.

However, Raaymakers[98] encouraged physicians to consider nonsurgical early mobilization for clients with impacted femoral neck fractures as long as they are healthy, which is considered to be any individual under the age of 70 with one or less comorbidity. Most intertrochanteric fractures are managed by the surgeon using either a compression hip screw or an intramedullary nail. Both will allow for impaction at the fracture site in order that the fracture will heal, so the decision to use one type of fixation over another is typically based on the surgeon's preference and his or her expertise with using the hardware. Subtrochanteric fractures are usually fixated with a long intramedullary nail and screw or the use of screws alone. Occasionally, a plate may be used rather than a nail.

Regardless of the age of the individual, one of the most important elements to consider in the case of a hip fracture is whether there has been compromise to the femoral head's blood supply. If the blood supply was disrupted, the cartilage and underlying bone in the area may have not received an adequate blood supply, and avascular necrosis, or tissue death due to lack of blood supply, may occur. Vascular necrosis can result in the loss of the spherical shape of the femoral head, leading to incongruency of the hip joint. Over time, this incongruency can result in arthritis of the hip joint, as evidenced by an antalgic gait and impaired hip joint ROM. Eventually, a total hip arthroplasty may be needed. Intracapsular fractures are more likely to lead to avascular necrosis of the femoral head because the femoral neck has a thin periosteum and minimal amount of cancellous bone. Subtrochanteric fractures tend to require some type of implant device, such as a long intramedullary nail, plate, rod, or screws. With a mechanical device in place, along with the high stresses endured by this part of the femur, there is an increased tendency for the implant to ultimately fail. Stability of the hip is proportional to the severity of the fracture, the quality of the bone, and the expertise of the surgeon, but the client's functional success is most dependent on his or her premorbid physical and mental abilities.

Back Pain

Although lower back pain (LBP) is a common complaint of the population in general, it is the most frequently reported musculoskeletal problem among older adults and their most frequently reported symptom.[54] Of all the visits that are made to a physician for LBP, 20% are made by individuals over 65 years of age. In a study by Weiner and colleagues in 2003, 42% of the community-dwelling older adults who participated in the study reported at least one incident of LBP in the previous year.[131] However, despite the fact that many older individuals suffer from it, little research has been done to try to delineate the patho-anatomic cause(s) of LBP in the adult population over 65 years of age.[14] The most common diagnosis made in the senior population is "degenerative spinal disease," which could encompass a number of specific pathologies (e.g., spinal stenosis, degenerative disc disease, spondylolisthesis, degenerative facet disease, etc.). Why is specific diagnosis so difficult? First of all, degenerative disc disease is commonly found at all spinal levels in older adults, regardless of the specificity of the imaging technique used, and there is poor predictive validity for pain in adults between 53 and 70 years of age.[59]

Second, both degenerative disc disease (DDD) and degenerative facet disease (DFD) (which are included in the degenerative spinal disease category) have been associated with LBP, but there is disagreement as to the relationship between these pathologies and spinal pain. Last, it is felt that psychological factors may play a role in pain pathogenesis, a thought that is supported by Hicks, who in a 2009 study found that the severity of disc and facet disease was indeed associated with chronic LBP, but not with the pain complaints self-reported by those with chronic LBP.[54]

The breakdown of client diagnoses for a typical internal medicine clinic that sees primarily adult clients consists of compression fractures (4%), spondylolisthesis (3%), malignancies (0.7%), ankylosing spondylitis (0.3%), and vertebral osteomyelitis (0.1%).[70] For clinics seeing predominately older adults, the percentages for compression fractures and malignancies are slightly higher. Therefore, when examining older adult clients with LBP, it is critical to consider concomitant contributions such as medical comorbidities, nutritional status, bone mineral density, and activity levels. It has become apparent in health care that the older adult client's well-being is influenced not only by the status of the body's individual systems (such as the cardiac, pulmonary, and renal systems), but also by the interactions between these systems. Because of the complexity of these interactions, it is beneficial for clinicians to follow recommendations for the diagnosis and treatment of lower back pain, such as those suggested by the American College of Physicians and the American Pain Society, not only for their geriatric clients, but for any of their clients with general lower back pain.[19]

Lumbar Spinal Stenosis

Degenerative spinal stenosis is an acquired condition with an insidious onset that is commonly diagnosed in the older adult population. Spinal stenosis is defined as osteoarthritis of the intervertebral discs and facet joints along with hypertrophy of the ligamentum flavum. Most commonly, it begins between the disc and the vertebral bodies, but it can also start at the level of the facet joint. It is a cycle of degeneration; as the degeneration worsens, there is osteophyte formation at the level of the facet joint and disc, and calcification/hypertrophy of the ligamentum flavum. Because these degenerative changes decrease the amount of room available for lumbar nerve roots in the central canal, lateral recess, and neural foramina, classic symptoms such as neurogenic claudication are experienced. It is believed that the pain that is experienced by the client occurs due to mechanical compression on the nerve roots and its resultant compromise to the neural blood supply.[50] It is interesting to note that the prevalence of degenerative disc disease increases with caudal progression from the T12/L1 level to the L4/L5 level, with a mild decrease of the disease process noted at the L5/S1 level. This makes sense when correlating these findings with the progressively higher compressive loads that the spine must endure at those levels. At the level of L5/S1, shearing forces are the predominant load sustained by the joint, and therefore the degenerative effect on that joint level is different from the effect at the more cranial lumbar joints.

The neurogenic claudication that occurs with spinal stenosis can occur unilaterally or bilaterally, but it is almost always asymmetric and brought on by functional activity or extension of the lumbar spine.

Degenerative Lumbar Spondylolisthesis

Lumbar spondylolisthesis is defined by *Stedman's Concise Medical Dictionary* as a forward movement of the body of a lumbar vertebrae on the vertebra, or sacrum, below it.[114]

In the case of adults older than 50 years of age, spondylolisthesis is primarily degenerative in nature, differing from the spondylitic spondylolisthesis seen in younger populations. In spondylitic spondylolisthesis, there is a pars interarticularis defect, most commonly seen as a fracture, but in degenerative spondylolisthesis, the pars is intact and the vertebrae as a whole slips forward secondary to osteoarthritis of the facet joints and insufficient ligamentous support. Degenerative spondylolisthesis occurs most frequently at the L4/L5 level (compared with the spondylitic type, which occurs most often at L5/S1) and results in similar symptoms as spinal stenosis, because both include compromise of the vertebral canal. Although x-rays can often determine the nature of the spondylolisthesis and the grade of the slippage, magnetic resonance imaging (MRI) or computed tomography (CT) with myelogram can help evaluate any associated compression of the neural elements, as well as screen for differential diagnoses of LBP, such as vertebral compression fractures.

Occupational Therapy Intervention for Musculoskeletal Conditions in the Older Adult

Occupational therapy (OT) intervention should be guided not only by the disease process but also by the problems and limitations identified during the evaluation, the client's perception of his or her limitations, and the individual's adjustment to those limitations. For therapists to analyze functional activity and interpret the musculoskeletal components of functional performance, an understanding of kinesiology and the physiologic components of the musculoskeletal system is essential. With this foundation to guide their clinical reasoning, occupational therapists can interpret assessment findings and develop an intervention plan with the client.

The goal of OT intervention is to increase a client's functional independence and well-being. Intervention should integrate information regarding the client's musculoskeletal status with information regarding the client's sensory function, cognitive abilities, and psychosocial status. To design an intervention plan with clients experiencing acute or chronic musculoskeletal conditions, an occupational therapist may need to integrate a biomechanical approach into an occupation-based intervention design.

Client and Caregiver Education

Intervention should always begin with client and caregiver education. Findings from the evaluation should be explained and meaningful intervention goals developed with input from the client. If there is a primary caregiver or family members involved in the client's care, education should also include these individuals. Education needs to focus on the disease and/or projected healing process that the client is going through, the purpose of specific intervention strategies and home programs, safety precautions, adaptations for the environment, activities of daily living (ADLs) and instrumental activities of daily living (IADLs), and follow-up recommendations. Musculoskeletal disorders are often chronic conditions that require not only physical but also psychological

adaptations. The education provided during therapeutic intervention is critical in preparing the client for discharge and resumption of life in the community. Therapists and assistants should provide clients and caregivers with the knowledge needed to empower them to make healthy choices that will promote healing, health, and well-being long after the therapy intervention is over.

Osteoarthritis

The American College of Rheumatology (ACR) provides recommendations for pharmacologic and nonpharmacologic therapies to treat persons with OA of the hand, hip, and knee.[56] OT intervention should follow these guidelines. For management of hand osteoarthritis (OA), practitioners should evaluate the individual's ability to perform functional activities, instruct in joint protection techniques, provide assistive devices as needed to help clients perform ADLs and IADLs, instruct in use of thermal modalities, and provide splints for patients/clients with trapeziometacarpal joint OA.

For management of OA of the knee and hip, ACR recommendations that would apply to occupational therapy interventions include encouraging clients' participation in cardiovascular and/or resistance exercise programs; encouraging their participation in aquatic exercise or tai chi programs (for OA of the knee) based on clients' individual abilities and preferences; encouraging clients to lose weight if overweight; and encouraging their participation in self-management programs.[56] Although not expanded on by the ACR, self-management programs for persons with OA of the knee or hip may involve training in joint protection with specific ADLs and IADLs, use of adaptive equipment, energy conservation techniques, and home safety with the use of walking aids as needed and prescribed by a physical therapist. The use of psychosocial interventions and thermal agents is also recommended, as indicated by their condition.

Traditional OT intervention for persons with osteoarthritis includes training in joint protection principles. Instructing clients in these concepts and teaching them how to integrate them into their daily routines and activity patterns can help them maintain current levels of function, and may also help prevent further deterioration of their joints. Understanding a joint's anatomy, mechanics, and supportive structures is the foundation to determining protective techniques for specific joints. In general, clients should be educated to: (1) maintain the range of motion of the joint; (2) increase the strength of the muscles around the joint; (3) reduce excessive loading on the involved joint(s); (4) respect and avoid pain in the joint(s) during activity performance; (5) avoid keeping the joint in one position for prolonged periods of time; and (6) balance activity and rest throughout the day.

Maintain Joint Range of Motion

Maintaining joint range of motion involves maintaining the length of the agonist and antagonist muscles around the joint and maintaining full mechanical motion of the articulating bony surfaces in the joint. Maintaining range of motion is important to provide a biomechanical advantage in the use of the joint and thus optimize functional abilities. This principle is also important to prevent development of joint contractures.

Muscle Strength

Joint stabilization is provided by forces internal to the musculoskeletal system, particularly the passive forces of connective tissues, ligaments, and joint capsules. Muscles around a joint can also provide a stabilizing and protective force when maintained at a constant length, such as during an isometric contraction. When external forces are placed upon the joint, the strength of the muscles around the joint is also an important proactive mechanism for a joint in motion. Weak muscles can increase the risk for damage to a joint because they tire easily and respond more slowly. This can place more stress on the other supporting joint structures and can lead to the deterioration of the overall joint structure. Weak muscles also make the joint structure more vulnerable to damage during sudden and unexpected movement (e.g., during a fall).

It is generally accepted that lower limb muscles (particularly the quadriceps) influence knee joint load, which is believed to be a major contributor to knee OA. Impairments in muscle function, including weakness and altered activation patterns, are commonly found in association with knee OA. Therefore clinicians will generally integrate the use of exercise into the conservative management of OA of the knee. For OA of any joint, clients should be instructed to continue performing daily activities and exercise within limitation of their pain to prevent muscle disuse atrophy and to strengthen the muscles.

Reduce Excessive Loading on the Involved Joints

Basic principles of kinesiology explain the effect that external forces, or loads, can have on the musculoskeletal system. The same structures that can stabilize and move the body can also have the potential to injure or deform the joints involved in the muscle and joint interaction. Forces (loads) can produce various effects on a joint depending on the direction of the force being applied to the joint. For example, the load may produce tension, compression, bending, shearing, torsion, or a combined load, which is caused by two forces being applied in opposite directions. Understanding these principles can help the clinician explain the damaging effects that load can have on arthritic joints.

For example, lower extremity weight-bearing activity produces compression of the articular cartilage and transmits load onto the underlying subchondral bone. Both the articular cartilage and the subchondral bone act as shock absorbers. However, in people with OA in the knee joints, the cartilage may be too thin to protect against repetitive impact loading. This can produce destructive effects on the joint cartilage. Malalignment of bones may place additional biomechanical stress on one side of an involved joint, thus producing pain and further joint damage.

Avoid Pain in Activity Performance

Clients should be educated on the importance of respecting their pain. If joint pain is experienced during engagement in activities, it should be recognized as a useful symptom that may indicate joint stress that exceeds the limits of comfort, thus indicating further deterioration in the involved joint.

Balance Activity and Rest throughout the Day

Even though the type of fatigue that accompanies the systemic disease of RA does not exist in OA, continued use of affected joints can increase pain, and muscle fatigue around weakened joints will result. Clients should be taught to self-monitor their activity levels by recognizing onset of pain and discomfort within their routine daily schedules. For individuals with OA, intermittent rest to the affected joints should be worked into their schedules throughout the day.

Avoid Staying in One Position for Long Periods

Joints with OA often become stiff following periods of inactivity. This stiffness is referred to as "articular gelling." Although the exact causes of articular gelling are not confirmed, it is suspected that this occurs due to diminished lubrication of the articular lining by surface-active phospholipids (SAPLs) which have been shown to be deficient in osteoarthritic joints.[55] This stiffness can generally be reduced in less than 30 minutes with active ROM (AROM) and/or nonstrenuous use of the joint.

Adaptations and Environmental Modifications

Recommendations regarding adaptations and environmental modifications can improve a client's level of independence and safety while performing everyday tasks. Assistive devices, such as reachers (Figure 8-4A), jar openers (Figure 8-4B), sock aides, long handled shoe horns, or elastic shoelaces (Figure 8-4C), may be recommended for these reasons, especially when the client's condition is chronic (such as OA) or progressive. For clients with OA, adaptations and modification to their environment can prevent undue stresses to involved joints. When possible, it is ideal to evaluate a client in their actual home, leisure, or work environment. Home health therapists have the ideal opportunity to make significant interventions in this area. Activities that may have been given up due to the pain caused by performance can be assessed and modifications made to return the client to an activity that previously brought pleasure or meaning to their life. Therapists working in clinics can also make valuable recommendations regarding environmental or activity modifications through actual performance of tasks in a simulated environment.

Joint Protection Education through Activity Performance

Recent studies support OT intervention using "activity strategy training" (AST), which is designed to teach adaptive strategies for symptom control and engagement in physical activity.[87] Murphy explains that AST involves an approach that addresses not only the physical aspects of physical activity (weakness, joint protection, body mechanics, etc.) but also addresses the environmental and behavioral barriers involved with activity performance. Murphy et al.[87] explain that "the behavioral strategies taught are based on content of coping skills training that specifically

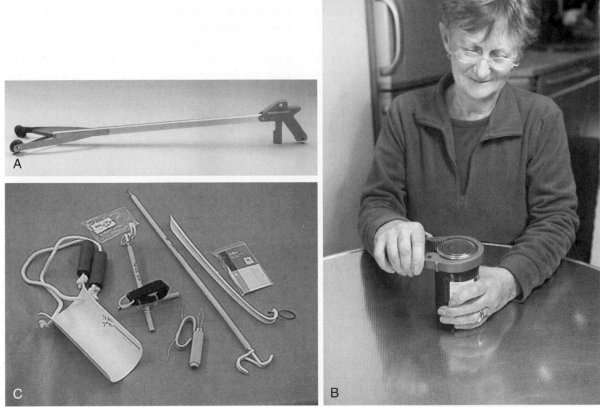

FIGURE 8-4   Assistive devices. A, Extended-handle reacher. B, Jar opener. C, Adaptive equipment used for dressing includes sock aid, adapted dressing stick, button aids, dressing stick, shoe horn, and elastic laces. (A from Early, M. B. [2013]. *Physical dysfunction practice skills for the occupational therapy assistant* [3rd ed.]. St. Louis, MO: Elsevier. B photo from istock.com. C from Sisto, S. A. [2009]. *Spinal cord injuries.* St. Louis, MO: Mosby.)

relates to activity performance (e.g., activity pacing, adding valued activities to daily routines)."

Murphy et al.[87] conducted a randomized controlled pilot trial, conducted at four sites (three senior housing facilities and one senior center) in southeastern Michigan. Fifty-four older adults with hip or knee osteoarthritis (mean age 75.3) participated. At each site, older adults were randomly assigned to one of two programs: exercise plus occupational therapy AST intervention (provided by an occupational therapist) or exercise plus health education (provided by a "health education interventionist"). This study concludes that although participants were involved in identical exercise programs, the participants who received AST tended to have larger increases in physical activity at posttest compared with participants who received health education.[87]

The importance of exercise for individuals with OA is being recognized by many in health care fields. Groups of clinical experts in the field of OA are establishing, and committed to updating, evidence-based clinical practice guidelines for the use of therapeutic exercise and manual therapy in the management of clients with OA.* In general, their recommendations include the use of therapeutic exercise (especially strengthening exercises), with or without manual therapy, for managing clients with OA, especially for pain management and improved functional status.

Rheumatoid Arthritis

Although the overall goal for every OT intervention is to improve or restore function and promote well-being, short-term goals for managing RA should include: (1) to decrease pain, (2) to prevent and/or control joint damage, and (3) to decrease the extraarticular manifestations of the disease. Medical management may involve pharmacologic therapy and/or surgical intervention, whereas OT personnel will focus upon lifestyle modification. These intervention approaches can be used in conjunction with each other or by themselves, and, of course, every client's plan of care will be different. When determining the intervention requirements on behalf of a client, decisions are based on the degree of joint synovitis, the amount of joint destruction and deformity, the client's pain tolerance, and their overall lifestyle. Goals for each client are dependent on the stage of disease that the individual is experiencing at the time.

Active Disease

If the individual is experiencing a flare-up of the disease process, he or she is considered to be in an "active" disease

---

*References 39,103,121,129,134, and 137.

stage; and the goals include reducing joint pain and conserving the client's energy, while trying to maintain the client's joint ROM. Modalities can be used to decrease pain as well as to reduce local intraarticular temperature and inflammation. Clients should be encouraged to "rest" their joints in a neutral position, and splints/orthoses (discussed in more detail later in this section) are appropriate for this goal. However, caution should be exercised because prolonged inactivity can lead to multiple undesirable outcomes, such as increased muscle weakness and loss of exercise tolerance. The client should be instructed in joint protection techniques and energy conservation principles (also to be further discussed in this section) because there is evidence that this type of intervention is effective.[46] Although some healthcare professionals feel that exercise is inappropriate at this stage, gentle active range of motion (AROM) or active assistive range of motion (AAROM) is beneficial for maintenance of joint motion and avoidance of soft tissue constriction; passive range of motion (PROM) should be avoided until inflammation subsides. Isometric exercises can be prescribed to prevent muscle atrophy, and the BRIME technique, as described by Gerber and Hicks in 1990, is a safe and effective means of doing this.[37] Although van den Ende and colleagues found that there were significant increases in strength with little to no changes in disease activity compared with controls, there is minimal evidence to support intensive exercise during this stage of disease activity.

Subacute Disease

As the acute flare-up resolves, the client moves into the subacute stage, in which preventing deconditioning and maximizing function become the primary objectives. However, the therapist must be constantly on guard to make sure that the intervention is not too aggressive; otherwise, the client might regress in his or her progress. Modalities are now used to heat tissues before performing PROM and stretching exercises. AROM is performed with an increase in frequency, and although isometrics are still appropriate to use at this time, repetitions and sets are increased. More aggressive strengthening exercises can be initiated through the use of resistance bands and progressive resistive training.[77] There is evidence to support the use of aerobic exercise in this stage,[125] and exercise modes such as the bicycle ergometer and swimming are encouraged to reduce stress on weight-bearing joints. Many clients enjoy water aerobics, dance therapy, and tai chi at this stage as well, which not only increases their aerobic conditioning, but also improves adherence to an exercise regime.[96,123]

Inactive Disease

Contrary to the opinions supporting intervention years ago, the American College of Rheumatology currently recommends strengthening exercises and aerobic conditioning for clients with inactive disease. In addition, the stage of disease inactivity is considered to be an optimal time for aggressively working toward improving muscle strength, joint mobility, flexibility, functional ability, and endurance. Joint protection

techniques and self-management education, which were integral parts of the treatment regime for those with active and subacute disease, are still critically important for the client's good health at this time.[45,46] In an article published in the journal *Physical Therapy*, the Ottawa Panel states that there is evidence for the use of therapeutic exercises, whole-body functional strengthening, low-intensity exercises, and general physical activity for clients with RA.[121] As for the amount and intensity of active exercise, multiple studies have supported the use of high-intensity, long-term exercise programs.[15] In 2003, Hakkinen and colleagues completed a study that confirmed that clients with both early and long-standing RA could safely improve their physical fitness levels by participating in a combined strength and endurance exercise program.[42] De Jong and colleagues found that long-term high-intensity exercise was more effective than usual care in improving functional ability in clients with RA, but that greater joint damage was sustained in both the experimental group as well as the control population who started with more structural damage and longer disease duration.[27] In a follow-up study in 2004, de Jong et al. concluded that a long-term high-intensity weight-bearing exercise program for clients with RA was effective in slowing down the loss of bone mineral density at the hip in clients with RA.[28] In 2005, Hakkinen et al. published a study that supported the theory that clients with RA who participated in a combined strength and endurance training program could increase their muscle mass, decrease their subcutaneous fat, and possibly decrease their cardiovascular risk.[43] Another study in 2005, by Munneke, found that high-intensity weight-bearing exercises appeared to accelerate the progression of damage in the large joints of the lower extremities in clients with RA if they had preexisting damage.[86] They concluded that clients with extensive large joint damage should refrain from activities that excessively load these joints. Therefore, based on these findings and results, the take-home message for clients with RA is that the benefits of both cardiovascular and neuromuscular exercise should not be ignored; however, caution is needed when prescribing exercises for clients with significant joint damage. In the case of these clients, exercises that unload the weight-bearing joints should be encouraged, and low-intensity aerobic exercises exchanged for high-intensity workouts.

For clients with rheumatoid arthritis, education regarding the disease process and symptoms is critical to help minimize or prevent potentially crippling joint deformities. A plethora of information regarding joint protection techniques can now be found on the Internet for clients' independent use, but these principles have been found to be more effective when demonstrated, assessed, and reinforced in actual performance of ADLs with therapists to provide education and feedback. For most individuals, ADLs and IADLs are routine activities that individuals perform in a specific manner throughout their entire lives; it takes a cognizant effort to perform such routine tasks in an atypical or new way. New habits of performance will need to be developed and reinforced in each client's daily life. A study conducted by Mathieux et al. evaluated the effects of an early OT program for clients with RA that included education regarding joint protection principles. The study involved a randomized, blind, controlled trial enrolling 60 clients with early RA. As with OA, findings support that OT intervention emphasizing joint protection education improved hand function in clients with early RA (Box 8-4).[78]

Respecting Pain

Joint pain during the inflammatory stage of RA is common and should be respected as the body's way to alert us to potential movements and/or stressors that may cause damage to the joint structure. Joint capsules are weakened and are more vulnerable to deformity during inflammatory phases. Trombly notes that the "pain-sensitive structures in the joint are the fibrous capsule, ligaments, fat pads, and periosteum. . . . [and that pain can] be elicited when attenuated ligaments and deranged joint spaces are aggravated through use that lengthens the ligaments further or resistive motion that compresses the joint spaces."[123] Clients should be educated to pay attention to their pain and either eliminate or modify activities that cause repeated and/or prolonged pain to joints during periods of inflammation.

Maintain Muscle Strength and Range of Motion

The muscles surrounding a joint provide stability and protection, and allow for movement. There needs to be balance between the agonist and antagonist muscles for proper joint mechanics. When there is an imbalance in strength between the agonist and antagonist, unstable joints are placed at greater risk for injury to the capsule, ligaments, and cartilage. In the presence of acute joint inflammation, when range can become limited, joint protection includes use of gentle, pain-free ROM exercise. Attempts to go beyond this range can raise intraarticular pressure and aggravate existing pain.[133]

Avoid Positions of Deformity and Forces in Their Directions

Clients should be taught to avoid external loads and internal forces that can facilitate deformity. For example, opening a door knob or jar lids in a manner that places an ulnar force on the digits can lead to ulnar drift of the metacarpophalangeal (MCP) joints. Teaching these basic principles to clients

---

BOX 8-4   Principles of Joint Protection

- Respect pain.
- Maintain muscle strength and range of motion.
- Use each joint in its most stable anatomic and functional plane.
- Avoid positions of deformity and forces in their direction.
- Use the largest, strongest joints available for the job.
- Ensure correct patterns of movement.
- Avoid staying in one position for long periods.
- Pace activities —energy conservation.
- Balance rest and activity.

(From Trombly, C. A., & Radomski, M. V. [2002]. *Occupational therapy for physical dysfunction*. Philadelphia, PA: Lippincott Williams & Wilkins, p. 1009.)

---

during actual activity performance can help the client gain confidence and independence in problem solving everyday tasks that may contribute to further deformity and/or pain.

Use the Largest, Strongest Joints Available for the Job

Using a larger joint to perform a task can prevent unnecessary force on smaller joints that are more vulnerable to damage. A commonly used example of this principle is carrying a purse with a strap over the shoulder instead of holding the weight of the purse over the smaller joints of the fingers. Therapists should observe clients perform various ADLs to analyze their task performance, to identify improper use of joints and opportunities for the client to integrate joint protection techniques into new methods of activity performance, and to help them develop new routines.

Ensure Correct Patterns of Movement

Maintaining proper alignment of joints during task performance, especially resistive activities, may help prevent pain, tenosynovitis, and possible deformity of joint capsules.

Avoid Staying in One Position for Long Periods

Prolonged static postures can lead to muscle fatigue, which can result in instability to the involved joint. This instability can lead to an imbalance of load and overstretching of the weaker muscles and surrounding ligaments.

Pace Activities—Energy Conservation

Often, principles that seem to be *obvious* or common sense are the ones most difficult for clients to integrate into their everyday lives. For example, people generally have routine activities that they perform in habitual ways day after day. For people who suffer from RA, the therapist should help them assess their lifestyles and analyze the pace at which they perform these tasks. Teaching them to incorporate energy conservation techniques may help them avoid fatigue and ultimately accomplish more priority activities throughout the day. Clients should avoid starting activities that cannot be interrupted or stopped.

Balance Rest and Activity

Balancing rest and activity is another principle that goes along with other energy conservation techniques. Because of the systemic nature of rheumatoid arthritis, people with this disease generally fatigue easily and need more rest than others. Educating clients to anticipate this fatigue and thus plan out their daily routines to balance activity with rest can help clients to feel they can prioritize tasks and accomplish more in their activity plans.

Modifications and Adaptations

Occupational therapists should make recommendations regarding environmental modifications and adaptive devices that may help prevent injury and fatigue and increase one's level of independence. As noted during the discussion of OA, this may occur in different ways—for example, changing the height of work surfaces, changing round door knobs to levers, or building up the size of handles to place less stress on small joints and weakened muscles.

Splinting and Orthoses for Joint Protection and Pain Reduction

Hand and wrist splints are often used, for varying reasons, with persons who have RA. Joint rest by means of immobilization has been found to reduce joint inflammation during the inflammatory process. Splints can be fabricated to provide support and reduce pain to unstable joints during functional performance. A metacarpal phalangeal (MCP) ulnar deviation orthosis can prevent misalignment of joints and overstretching of weakened joint capsules during occupational performance, and is often used to help to prevent ulnar deviation. To prevent hyperextension of the finger proximal interphalangeal (PIP) joints (swan-neck deformity), the use of a three-point, or "ring," splint may be used to allow for flexion of the PIP joints while preventing hyperextension. Dynamic splinting, using an orthosis with finger extension outriggers, is often used after finger MCP implant arthroplasty.

Osteoporosis and Fractures

Generally, osteoporosis does not lead to impaired functional performance unless fractures of a bone occur. For this reason, osteoporosis is generally not a primary condition resulting in OT intervention. It nonetheless is a very common comorbid condition that should be considered and integrated into treatment precautions and safety recommendations. It is a common condition seen by therapists working with adult and geriatric populations in areas of wellness and rehabilitation. As in other areas of musculoskeletal health, client education is critical to empower the affected individual to understand the effects of the condition on his or her body and how to make healthy choices that can reduce risks and often reverse the effects of the condition.

Vertebral Fractures

In general, therapeutic interventions for individuals who have sustained an osteoporotic fracture include reducing pain, healing in good alignment, reducing risk of further fractures, and maintaining/improving function.[82] Vertebral fractures are common in the older adult population. When working with individuals in the acute stage following vertebral fractures, therapeutic intervention should include education to teach individuals how to decompress their spines by lying on their backs on a firm mattress with their hips and knees flexed. Clients are taught to lie on the back and try to "lengthen" each leg.[82] Clients in the acute stage are also taught how to log roll, how to use adaptive devices with their ADLs, how to sit supporting their backs in straight-backed chairs, how to "hinge at the hips" when standing and reaching forward, and how turn by moving their feet and not twisting the trunk. In the acute stage, muscle strengthening may be limited to isometric contractions (such as lying supine and pressing the head and shoulders into the mattress).[82]

Individuals who progress to the post-acute stage of vertebral fractures may be referred to physical therapists who can perform a thorough examination, including measures of height and of thoracic and lumbar curves. Posture examinations include checking trunk and leg strength, protruding abdomen, and forward head. The space between the lower ribs and pelvic rim is measured because individuals lose vertebral height, which may progress to the lower ribs riding on top of the pelvic rim. By working as a team with physical therapists, information and techniques can be shared between the two disciplines that will enhance the client's recovery and functional gains.

Functional assessment and interventions should also address transfer training, limitations in range and strength, and cardiopulmonary response to activity. Often women with kyphotic spinal deformities from vertebral fractures will show a decrease in lung capacity and resultant difficulty in breathing.[99] Emphasis in the post-acute stage of vertebral fractures should include decreasing risk of further fractures and maintaining independence. Clients should be taught body mechanics for sitting, lying, standing, walking, bending, and lifting. Individuals should also be shown how to protect their spines when coughing or sneezing and substitute ways to carry out activities (such as washing hair by standing in shower and not bending at sink, dividing groceries into smaller bags for lifting, etc.).

Mobility for individuals who have had a vertebral fracture always centers on protecting the spine during any activity and consciously working on standing erect with a neutral spine posture (avoiding flexion of the upper spine).[94] Some individuals find that taping the upper back or wearing a modified back pack helps remind them to keep erect. Clients should be taught to avoid activities that place compressive loads on the back and how to strengthen their back muscles, especially the trunk and hip extensors.[109] Sinaki notes that bone health is dependent on weight-bearing activities.[111] Activities that provide impact and weigh bearing include brisk walking, going down stairs, and, with higher impact, jumping and hopping.

Hip Fractures

Other common fractures associated with the older adult population are hip fractures. The primary goal of rehabilitation for any of the categories of hip fractures is to return the individual to his or her previous functional level. The prognosis for attaining this goal can only be made with consideration of the type of surgical procedure performed on the client, the client's health status before the fracture, and any precautions given by the surgeon. Clinicians should be aware of the risk factors that can potentially lead to poor outcomes for clients who have sustained hip fractures[81] (see Table 8-3). According to a Cochrane Review in 2009, multidisciplinary rehabilitation is encouraged for individuals who have sustained a hip fracture; however, further research is needed in this area, because the results found in this review were not statistically significant.[48] There are few, if any, specific post–open reduction internal fixation (ORIF) clinical practice guidelines that clinicians can follow for working with these clients; however, a recent updated edition of a postsurgical rehabilitation text by Maxey and Magnusson is helpful for breaking down the process into three phases.[79] Phase I involves postsurgical intervention that is initiated in-hospital and should stress activities that encourage early mobilization of the client, prevent morbidities associated with bed rest, and prepare the client for discharge. The client's weight-bearing status and ROM limitations will depend on the client's fracture classification and the surgical technique used to reduce the fracture. This phase stresses exercises; functional self-care activities, including safe ambulation; and education in order that the client can be discharged from acute care. Occupational therapy in this phase will include functional transfers, generally regarding toileting and bed transfer training, and recommending and training in adaptive equipment such as a bedside commode or adaptive devices to perform ADLs. The physical therapist involved in the client's care will also address transfers in addition to gait training, AROM, and strengthening exercises to facilitate the healing process.

Intervention during Phase II is generally considered 2 to 4 weeks postsurgery. Clients who have progressed to Phase II should be free of any signs of infection and have decreasing pain levels. Their physical therapy exercise programs may be progressed to include PROM and more aggressive AROM to the hip joints, such as minisquats, along with continued gait/stair climbing as needed, and standing balance activities. During this phase the occupational therapist may be progressing the client to more challenging activities and educating in safety techniques for using the walker to perform ADLs. Functional transfer training should include car transfers to prepare the client for discharge and/or greater independence in the community. Progressive strengthening exercises with Theraband can be performed for the upper extremities because the client will be more dependent on upper extremity strength to perform transfers and for ambulation with a walker while the hip fracture is healing. Barring other comorbid conditions, by the end of this phase, the client should be independent in self-care ADLs, gait, and transfers; hip AROM should be 90 degrees; and the client should be ready for limited community ambulation.

The time frame for Phase III is generally 5 to 8 weeks after surgery, and intervention is generally reduced to only physical therapy on an outpatient basis. By the end of this phase, depending on prior level of functioning, clients should be able to self-manage their own exercise program, have increased strength in their lower extremities, be independent ambulators in the community, and have initiated a cardiovascular exercise program in addition to the post-rehabilitation plan of care.

Traditionally, clients with hip fractures have been cared for on the orthopedic floors of hospitals and rehabilitation centers. However, most of these clients have an overwhelming number of comorbidities that can result in death within 12 months postsurgery. Because of this, many units are combining the orthopedic management with input from a geriatrician, in the hopes that it would improve the care of older adult clients with hip fractures.

This approach was initially begun in the United Kingdom in the 1950s and continues to be more commonly utilized in Europe, but there is support in the literature for using the approach in all settings of geriatric rehabilitation.[18] A recent systematic review and meta-analysis by Bachmann et al. not only reinforced that inpatient rehabilitation programs specifically designed for clients with musculoskeletal conditions result in improved functional outcomes while decreasing nursing home admissions and mortality, but also found that these effects were sustained.[4] Unfortunately, as was noted in other articles describing orthopedic-geriatric models of care, there is currently no consensus on the characteristics that make these models successful.[7,44,128]

Back Pain

Clients suffering from acute muscular back pain are generally prescribed a period of activity modification along with medication by their physicians to relieve pain and diminish inflammation in the involved area. After this initial period of reduced or modified activity, in most cases, light activity can actually speed the healing process. A therapist should assess the client's movements, postures, and positions used to perform ADLs, and recommend techniques to lessen or control pain and to prevent reinjury. Lifestyle changes may also be encouraged, such as weight loss, if such factors are contributing to a risk for reinjury. A client with acute back pain is generally referred to a physical therapist and prescribed a program of muscle stretches and strengthening exercises to stabilize and prevent further injury or reinjury. An occupational therapist may be a member of a back or pain team and may focus intervention on client education and helping the client return to previously performed activities. Education should also include techniques for proper lifting and body mechanics. Because back pain is a common musculoskeletal problem, occupational therapists will frequently be working with clients who have back pain as a comorbid condition. The following sections address interventions for two common musculoskeletal conditions that commonly cause back pain.

Lumbar Spinal Stenosis

The pain caused by lumbar spinal stenosis, commonly experienced in the lower extremities, can be relieved by discontinuing the exacerbating activity or by flexing the lumbar spine through activities such as walking uphill, bike riding, or walking behind a grocery cart or walker. During spinal flexion, the diameter of the spinal canal is enlarged, and the ligamentum flavum is flattened, thereby lessening or eliminating the pressure on the nerve root and decreasing the pain caused by the neurogenic claudication. It is critical that the healthcare provider distinguish whether the pain is due to neurogenic versus vascular claudication because they are treated with different regimens. One way to make this determination is to assess the pulses in the lower extremities; clients with vascular claudication will exhibit diminished pulses. In addition, as previously stated, the pain symptoms in neurogenic claudication can be relieved/eliminated by flexing the spine, even while still continuing to ambulate, so this can be correlated with the vascular assessment. With vascular claudication, any type of ambulation will exacerbate the pain in the lower extremities (primarily the calves), and the only way to relieve the symptoms is to totally cease the walking activity. For clients with neurogenic claudication, extension of the spine will decrease the diameter of the spinal canal and cause the symptoms to worsen. Therefore any activity that encourages spinal extension (such as walking without an assistive device, walking on level surfaces, or reaching for objects directly overhead) will cause the pain to worsen. If allowed to flex the spine, the client can continue to walk without pain, or at least with a minimal increase in pain.

In addition to a vascular assessment, it is important that a thorough neurologic examination be performed on these individuals because compromised autonomic innervation of the lower extremities may inhibit appropriate vasodilation response to increased muscle use. Initially, a motor examination performed on a client with spinal stenosis is normal, but as the condition progresses, lower extremity weakness or bowel/bladder dysfunction may occur. A decrease in deep tendon reflexes might also be apparent, especially at the Achilles tendon. Common imaging studies that are routinely performed on these individuals include plain x-rays (including flexion/extension stress films), and additional workup may include MRI and CT with or without myelography and electromyogram (EMG) studies. EMG can be helpful in ruling out peripheral neuropathy from other sources, such as diabetes. Nerve root blocks and facet or sacroiliac joint (SIJ) injections may help to reduce pain and might also assist in establishing a diagnosis. If no neurologic deficits are identified during the examination, the common intervention usually includes nonsteroidal antiinflammatory drugs (NSAIDs), and physical therapy that would involve lumbar flexion, abdominal strengthening exercises, braces, and epidurals. Although lumbar flexion is encouraged to decrease symptoms, therapists work with each client independently to find the least amount of flexion that will alleviate the symptoms. With this approach, long-term effects of poor positioning/ posturing are minimized. If the client's functional status is limited by the condition, occupational therapy may be referred to assess functional performance and to make recommendations regarding environment and task modifications to increase independence in specific ADLs and IADLs. The same principles regarding lumbar flexion and use of abdominal muscles during transfers and activity performance should be incorporated into the intervention plan.

Surgery is generally reserved for those with severe functional limitations and persistent impairments. Spinal decompression is the most common surgical intervention. Typically, a decompression surgery removes all structures contributing to the neurologic compression, but the type of decompression surgery is based upon the anatomic site of stenosis and the presenting symptoms of the client.

Degenerative Lumbar Spondylolisthesis

Only 10% to 15% of clients seeking treatment will undergo surgery for degenerative lumbar spondylolisthesis.[61] Nonoperative interventions should be utilized first, even for clients with neurologic symptoms. If conservative measures

fail after a 3-month trial period, and the client continues to experience persistent LBP, progressive neurologic deficit, and/or bowel and bladder symptoms, surgical treatment is then warranted. Surgical options include decompression by itself or decompression combined with a fusion. Because there are few randomized clinical trials discussing degenerative spondylolisthesis, there is no optimal treatment protocol for working with this client population. The most common conservative interventions include a course of NSAIDs, an aerobic conditioning program (most successfully performed on a bicycle ergometer), a weight reduction program (if needed), and careful medical management of any associated osteoporosis. Physical therapy is commonly recommended to restore ROM and flexibility, decrease pain, increase muscle strength, restore neural mobility, and improve spinal stability.[61] Occupational therapists working in a multidisciplinary pain program may also be involved in the client's care, and treatment choices should be determined based upon the client's functional limitations and should include client education regarding environmental and activity modifications, and physical and cognitive interventions that work to improve ADLs. There are limited studies showing that bracing can be effective in improving functional activities and decreasing pain levels, as well as preventing further slippage of the superior vertebrae. Several studies on exercise have supported the use of flexion-type exercises and/or isometric extension strengthening without active trunk extension, as well as trunk stabilization exercises to decrease pain and increase function.[40,53,93,109,112]

Occupational Performance Deficits in Older Adults

Decline in Mobility with Aging

The combined effects of changes in the skeleton and muscles directly affect posture in the older adult. Unless the individual faithfully works on strengthening antigravity muscles, the typical posture becomes one of generalized flexion of the head, spine, hips, and knees.[75] These changes can make it harder for older adults to stand erect and maintain balance. The changes in muscles can be linked to a threshold concept to identify what strength is needed to do a particular functional task (such as rising from a chair, climbing stairs, getting up from the floor, carrying groceries) and to recognize that a small strength gain can produce a considerable functional improvement. Skeletal and muscle declines affect gait. Older adults walk slower to conserve energy and to feel secure, but walking at speeds less than 1.4 m/sec can be dangerous (the threshold time needed to cross a street before a stoplight changes). Older adults also take longer to modify their gait to avoid obstacles. They also need to focus their attention on the task of walking and have difficulty doing a simultaneous task (such as carrying on a conversation) while walking.[33]

Poor muscle endurance limits the distance an older person can travel. As a result, many find it difficult or impossible to walk the distance required from a parked car to a store.

Functional Performance Deficits

Christiansen and Baum[20] define the term *occupational performance* as "the unique term used by occupational therapy to express function as it reflects the individual's dynamic experience of engaging in daily occupations within the environment". The term *functional performance* "can be defined as the ability to conduct a specific task that could be related to daily living activities."[113] These terms are often used interchangeably, but Stamm et al.[113] note that measures of occupational performance and functional performance typically differ in an important aspect: measures of *occupational performance* refer to what an individual does in his or her actual environment whereas *functional performance* refers to an individual's ability to execute a task in a standardized environment. This difference is also addressed in the World Health Organization's International Classification of Functioning, Disability and Health (ICF) distinction of performance and capacity.[113]

Older persons experiencing musculoskeletal changes often experience a decline in their abilities to perform functional activities. These limitations are referred to as *functional performance deficits*. Such deficits may be experienced gradually with the normal progression of muscle deterioration or from a chronic condition such as osteoarthritis, but often the decline has a sudden onset with an acute injury or illness that results in accelerated loss of motion and/or muscle wasting that may occur with immobility and bed rest. Harper and Lyles[49] discuss the physiologic changes and complications associated with prolonged bed rest. They note that loss of muscular strength may be as high as 5% per day with immobility. Prolonged bed rest can also contribute to decreased muscle oxidative capacity, which can contribute to decreased aerobic capacity, bone loss, and joint contractures.[48]

Whether gradual or sudden, many older adults experience a transition from being independent to a lifestyle requiring varying levels of assistance to complete ADLs. Older adults may experience fluctuations in their abilities to perform such tasks, and thus there may be a blurring in the line between gradual decline in function and disability.

From a purely physical perspective on the musculoskeletal system, functional performance may be affected in older adults by decreased strength and flexibility or joint problems that limit range of motion and/or result in pain. A thorough understanding of a client's occupational performance must also analyze associated pathology that may be superimposed on the physical limitations and that can also present limitations in the client's ability to adapt to challenges of everyday life activities. To identify other risk factors for functional decline in the older adult, Stuck et al.[116] performed a systematic literature review of longitudinal studies published between 1985 and 1997. This study identified risk factors for functional decline using statistical analysis and revealed that musculoskeletal deficits may be associated with one or more of the following factors (listed in alphabetical order): cognitive impairment, depression, disease burden (comorbidity), increased and decreased body mass index, lower extremity functional limitation, low frequency of social contacts, low level of physical activity, no alcohol use compared with moderate use, poor self-perceived health, smoking, and vision impairment. Stuck et al.[116] note that some risk factors, such as nutrition and physical environment, have been neglected in past research.

Basic and Instrumental Activities of Daily Living

Occupational performance encompasses the domain of *activities of daily living* (ADLs). ADLs, a term now widely used in health care, have been recognized for their significance throughout the history of occupational therapy. The physical as well as psychological benefits of performing everyday life activities is rooted in the philosophy and foundation of the profession. According to the Occupational Therapy Practice Framework: Domain and Process,[47] ADLs refer to activities that are oriented toward taking care of oneself. Such activities may also be referred to as basic activities of daily living (BADLs) and personal activities of daily living (PADLs) (Box 8-5).

Instrumental activities of daily living (IADLs) are activities that are oriented toward interacting with the environment and that are often complex (Box 8-6).[47]

The importance of ADL measurement is recognized in a 1990 report by the U.S. Department of Health and Human Services. This report points out that the ability to perform ADLs has been found to be significant predictor for admission

---

BOX 8-5 Examples of Basic or Personal Activities of Daily Living

- Bathing, showering
- Bowel and bladder management
- Dressing/grooming
- Eating
- Feeding
- Personal hygiene
- Functional mobility
- Sexual activity
- Sleep/rest
- Toilet hygiene

BOX 8-6 Examples of Instrumental Activities of Daily Living

Care of others (including selecting and supervising caregivers)
Care of pets
Childrearing
Communication device use
Community mobility
Financial management
Health management and maintenance
Home establishment and management
Meal preparation and cleanup
Safety procedures and emergency responses
Shopping

to a nursing home, use of paid home care, use of hospital services, living arrangements, use of physician services, insurance coverage, and mortality.[35] In addition to these factors, determining functional status and limitations is now common practice for Centers for Medicare and Medicaid Services (CMS) reimbursement. Whether for therapeutic intervention, outcome research, or reimbursement with older adult populations, determining one's ability to perform ADLs has become standard practice.

Assessments of Activities of Daily Living

Functional assessment of a client's abilities to perform ADLs and IADLs involves a therapist's ability to simultaneously analyze the biomechanics of an activity while assessing and integrating the multiple dimensions of a client's performance skills. This information allows the therapist to appropriately prescribe a treatment intervention (exercise, activity, or task) to remediate and/or develop skills required for activity performance.

There are multiple instruments used to assist occupational therapists in this process. ADL assessments are used to quantify levels of independence versus burden of care and to identify occupational performance deficits. Letts and Bosch[73] performed a systematic review of 83 ADL instruments. A list of 15 instruments was identified to meet the following criteria: clinical usefulness, current use for clinical or research purposes, existence of reliability and validity testing, and availability of information about the instrument through peer-reviewed publications. Box 8-7 is a summary of their findings (with the exception of pediatric-specific instruments not applicable to this chapter).

ADL instruments may involve self-reporting, direct observation, and standardized assessments to evaluate functional abilities. Among the various methods, literature shows self-reporting to be the least accurate assessment of actual burden of care,[26] but self-reporting tools can provide value in recognizing the client's perception, insights into what motivates the client, and quality-of-life information.

One of the most commonly used tools is the Functional Independence Measure (FIM), which was developed in 1996 by the Uniform Data System of Medical Rehabilitation (UDS).[124] It is an 18-item ordinal rating scale that was developed in an effort to resolve the problem of lack of uniform measurement and data on disability and rehabilitation outcomes. The FIM has been adopted by the CMS as the official tool for determining functional status of clients for reimbursement in in-patient rehabilitation facilities (IRFs).

Stamm et al.[113] compared the content of occupation-based instruments used in adult rheumatology and musculoskeletal rehabilitation to the conceptual framework regarding function and disability of the International Classification of Impairment, Disability, and Handicap (ICIDH). In this study, the following seven instruments were identified as occupation-based assessments: the *Canadian Occupational Performance Measure,* the *Assessment of Motor and Process Skills,* the *Sequential Occupational Dexterity Assessment,* the *Jebson Taylor Hand Function Test,* the *Moberg Picking Up Test,* the *Button Test,* and the *Functional Dexterity Test.* Stamm et al. state that the main focus of these instruments is on the ICF components of activities and participation.[113]

Occupation-Based Intervention

Management of Musculoskeletal Conditions

For all musculoskeletal conditions, therapeutic management involves the reduction of symptoms to improve daily functioning and promote healing, modification to the environment to decrease barriers to function and increase safety, and client education for long-term management and prevention of further disability. As noted previously in the discussion of specific musculoskeletal conditions, reduction of symptoms may involve techniques to decrease pain and inflammation, increase ROM, or strengthen weak muscles.

Considerations and Precautions

Older adults often present with multiple comorbid conditions that need to be taken into account before prescribing therapeutic activity. These conditions may include but are not limited to cardiopulmonary precautions, hydration and nutrition status, vascular disorders, and blood sugar levels or other secondary complications of diabetes. Information obtained in a thorough medical history is important and must be integrated into the intervention process.

Importance of Exercise in Musculoskeletal Intervention

For a growing number of older adults, physical exercise has become a routine and meaningful occupation during their adult lives. Summarized by Finch, et al, the 2003 International Health, Racquet, and Sportsclub Association (IHRSA) Health Club Trend Report, Americans over the age of 55 yielded the largest increase in health club memberships, growing 23% from 5.6 million members in 2001 to 6.9 million in 2002.[36] For individuals who routinely incorporate exercise into their lifestyles, the use of physical exercise in occupational therapy can

---

BOX 8-7	Activity-Specific ADL Instruments

Canadian Occupational Performance Measure (COPM)*
Patient Specific Functional Scale (PSFS)*
Arndottir OT-ADL Neurobehavior Evaluation (A-ONE)
Arthritis Impact Measurement Scales (AIMS2)
Barthel Index (BI)
Functional Autonomy Measurement System (SMAF)**
Functional Independence Measure (FIM)
Health Assessment Questionnaire (HAQ)
Katz Index of Activities of Daily Living
Melville Nelson Self Care Assessment**
Physical Self-Maintenance Scale (PSMS)**

* Activity of daily living (ADL) instruments that address client-identified ADL activities.
** Instruments designed specifically for older adults.
(Modified from Letts, L., & Bosch, J. (2005). Measuring occupational performance in basic activities of daily living. *Measuring occupational performance: Supporting best practice in occupational therapy.* Thorofare, NJ: Slack.

be an appropriate goal for treatment. For adults who do not consider routine physical exercise to be a meaningful, ultimate goal of treatment, the use of exercise as a preparatory intervention and/or incorporated into the overall intervention plan can enhance a client's functional abilities. Physical exercise and activity are an important part of the older adult's musculoskeletal health and conditioning.

The importance of physical exercise for older adults has been substantiated in a growing number of studies over the past decade.[67] "Recent guidelines regarding physical activity from the Centers for Disease Control and Prevention and the American College of Sports Medicine recommend that every adult should accumulate at least 30 minutes of moderate-intensity physical activity on most days of the week."[67] The results of this study suggest that even very old, frail, and clinically complex patients may benefit from physical activity.

Clarke[21] states that one common component that needs to be a part of physical activity and exercise for the older adult is "an increase in the levels of mechanical load placed on the body as a whole and skeletal muscle in particular." Exercise and increased physical activity can prevent or reverse some of the deterioration commonly observed in aged skeletal muscle.[21] "Recent studies employing resistive exercise protocols, such as weight training of the lower limbs, have suggested that sarcopenia can be reversed in aged (>65 years old) individuals. These studies have indicated that resistive exercise increases contractile protein synthesis resulting in an increase in myofiber CSA and muscle strength in aged muscle unloading—induced myofiber atrophy can also be reversed by resistive exercise." [21]

In a systematic review of the literature, Latham et al.[68] assess the effects of progressive resistance training (PRT) exercises designed to increase strength in older adults and to identify adverse effects. This review included 121 trials with 6700 participants. The study found that when PRT was performed two to three times per week and at a high intensity, there was generally a small but significant improvement in physical abilities. The authors conclude that PRT is an effective intervention for improving physical functioning in older people, including the improvement of strength and the performance of some simple and complex activities.[68]

Prescribing Therapeutic Activities

OT intervention strives to engage clients in meaningful activities as a means and a goal for therapeutic intervention. For many older adults, repetitive or aerobic exercise may not be valued as meaningful occupation. For these individuals, such intervention strategies may prove to have poor client participation and carryover. For many older adult clients, asking them to perform a meaningful activity, or one with personal preference, can be more motivating than repetitive exercise and stretching. For such individuals, intervention programs for strengthening, balance, flexibility, and endurance may include a variety of moderate-intensity occupation-based activities that incorporate the targeted performance skills.

Substantial literature is also available that supports the efficacy of physical activities such as leisure walking, gardening,

and house-keeping (Figure 8-5).[67] Other examples of therapeutic activities that have been shown to provide musculoskeletal benefits include swimming, water aerobics, dancing, and tai chi (Figure 8-6). To maintain muscle fitness of smaller musculoskeletal structures that affect fine motor skills, occupation-based intervention may involve playing the piano, playing board games, or cooking. Just as there is no one exercise protocol for every client, activity interventions need to be adapted to the needs and abilities of each client and designed to meet the client's desired goals. Weigl et al.[130] note that the use of recreational activities in the rehabilitation of musculoskeletal conditions can have a positive effect on one's body perception, expand skills, improve general conditioning, and recruit social support, all of which may enhance participation and carryover.

To design an occupation-based intervention plan, the clinician needs to identify the specific musculoskeletal components that are limiting the client's performance in the specific functional activities that have been identified as goals for treatment. These impairments may involve (but are not limited to) the following areas:
- Muscle, soft tissue, or joints
- Limitations in flexibility resulting in decreased range of motion

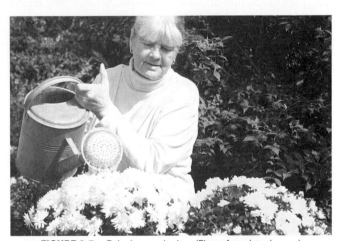

FIGURE 8-5   Enjoying gardening. (Photo from istock.com.)

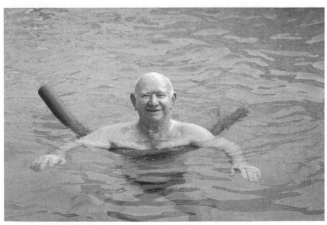

FIGURE 8-6   Water aerobics. (Photo from istock.com.)

- Decreased strength resulting in decreased range of motion
- Decreased motor endurance
- Impaired static and/or dynamic balance

The occupational therapist should interpret and prioritize the effects of these limitations through a functional perspective. After determining the basic and instrumental ADLs (BADLs and IADLs) that the client desires and/or needs to be able to perform, the therapist should design an intervention program that will aid in the remediation of the identified limitations. Often multiple areas of limitations, or component skills, can be addressed with one therapeutic activity. For example, a client with limited shoulder ROM also presents with decreased strength and endurance that affects the client's ability to perform upper-body dressing. Engaging the individual in a functional activity, such as placing the contents of a bag of groceries into an upper cabinet, incorporates active ROM at the shoulder joint to decrease joint tightness and increase ROM; if the client is lifting items (i.e., groceries) with the appropriate resistance determined by the therapist, motor strength can be increased. If the activity is graded appropriately with intermittent rest breaks, functional endurance can also be a target goal for this treatment intervention.

For musculoskeletal conditions, activity performance should be evaluated and treated with a biomechanical perspective. Functional limitations at joint-specific sites may be enhanced by joint mobilization to improving joint glide and/or stretch to imbalanced and tightened muscles; strengthening or immobilization of a joint may be needed to prevent damage at unstable joints. Activities that require muscle stretch (e.g., shuffle board) can be used to improve flexibility, which may in turn lessen the risk of muscular injury and ROM limitations and may also decrease joint and myofascial pain.[130]

If the client's cognitive skills allow, the therapist should educate the client about what skills are impaired and how this limits the client's ability to perform specific activities. With this approach, the therapist can work with the client to isolate specific skills for more focused intervention. Physical cues or assistance may be needed to stabilize joints during task performance. When functional activities are used to increase ROM, manual assistance may be needed for tight muscles to provide optimal stretch to muscle fibers. The therapist may need to apply manual stretch to the targeted muscles at end range and/or grade the activity so that task performance requires end-range stretch when appropriate.

If remediation is not realistic, modification of the environment or adaption of the activity must be pursued to help the client reach his or her highest level of independence. With chronic musculoskeletal conditions, modifying the environment or the way in which activities are performed can often help prevent pain and/or further deterioration to joints. With this said, providing clients with adaptive equipment early in their rehabilitation process should be critically analyzed so as to not inhibit a client's potential to regain maximal return of normal function.

For example, giving a client a reacher to assist in donning lower-body garments may quickly help the client regain independence in task performance, but it also eliminates the need for the client to use full hip and knee ROM, thus eliminating opportunities to improve these skills. The benefits, ranging from energy conservation to joint protection, should be weighed and integrated into the overall therapeutic intervention and discharge plans.

Prescribing therapeutic activities during the OT intervention process needs to take into account both personal and environmental barriers that may inhibit a client's performance of physical activities. Therapeutic approaches that offer only structured exercise have been shown to have small to moderate effects on arthritis pain/physical disability, and adherence to exercise typically wanes after the direct therapeutic intervention.[87] Occupational therapists should design their interventions to incorporate the previously noted techniques into everyday life tasks, which can be useful for sustaining ongoing physical activity performance and lifestyle changes.

Falls in Older Adults

A fall is considered an unintentional coming to rest on the ground, floor, or other lower level.[90] Falls increase with age, and a past history of falling is a red-flag warning. Every year more than one-third of individuals 65 years of age and older experience a fall. Among older adults, falls are the leading cause of death due to injury.[16]

Both extrinsic and intrinsic factors cause falls in older adults. Extrinsic factors reflect the environment, such as clutter in rooms, exposed cords, throw rugs that slip, poor lighting, spills, pets that are underfoot, broken steps, and steps without railings. Fall-prevention programs help older participants identify just what factors are present in their own homes and what resources are there to help them make their homes safer. This identification also includes activities to avoid, such as bathing without use of a handrail to hold onto or a shower seat, stepping up on a stool to reach an object, carrying objects with both arms while using the stairs, wearing shoes that are slippery, walking on slippery floors, and walking outside in icy conditions. The primary focus on extrinsic factors is to make individuals aware of the risks and modifications to the environment.

Intrinsic factors include poor vision; dizziness; decreases in cognition, muscle strength, sensation, balance, reaction time, and range; hypotension (orthostatic and postprandial); and loss of function due to the effects of multiple medications. The fear of falling can also increase the risk for falls.[66] A person may deny a fall or modify his or her activity to avoid anything that might lead to a fall.

Effects of Musculoskeletal Changes as They Contribute to Falls

Fall-related fractures are twice as high for women than for men.[115] In muscle strength, weak hip abductors and asymmetry in lateral stepping velocity cause a tendency to fall to the side, which presents a potential to fracture the neck of the femur.[23] Decreased strength in hip and knee extensors and decreased ankle strength can also contribute to falls.[6]

Balance testing can reveal individuals who are at risk for falls. Taking longer than 15 seconds to complete the Four Square Step Test (which involves stepping sideward, forward, and backward) or not being able to stand on one leg with eyes open for 5 seconds is considered a risk.[12,30] An individual who takes longer than 13.5 seconds to complete the Timed-Up-And-Go Test (which requires standing up from a chair, walking forward 10 feet at a comfortable pace, turning around, walking back to the chair, and sitting down) is at risk.[108]

Increased variability in walking patterns is associated with falls.[6] Other warning signs include walking very cautiously, keeping a wide stance, tilting the trunk to the side, grabbing for support, and inability to change speed and direction on demand.

A fall can cause a fracture depending on the direction of the fall, whether the person has protective muscle mass to absorb the fall, and the strength of the bone.[90] There are also instances of falls in extremely frail individuals when it is not known if the fracture preceded or followed the fall. The primary focus for intrinsic factors is to try to reverse those that are relevant.

Falls ultimately will restrict mobility as individuals seek to be safe in their environment and no longer challenge their potential. This then begins a downward spiral of hypokinetics. An activity program for those at risk for falls includes static-dynamic balance work, muscle strengthening, and gait training focusing on taking steps in different directions.[58]

Psychological Effects of Mobility Impairments in Older Adults

The physical and psychological effects of mobility impairments should not be separated when working with older adults. The loss of physical mobility, directly linked with independence in caring for oneself and performing lifelong tasks, can result in a lost sense of control and self-identity. The loss of independence can result in depression and sometimes despair. The American Association of Suicidology[92] reports that physical illness, uncontrollable pain, and the fear of a prolonged illness have all been identified as risk factors for suicide in the older adult population.

Antonopoulou and colleagues[2] found an association between musculoskeletal disorders and the quality of life and mental health of clients. This study found that depression is strongly correlated to most musculoskeletal disorders. Karp and Reynolds[64] discuss the relationship among depression, pain, and physical disability in older adults. They state that there is a high prevalence of older adults who suffer from chronic pain and depression, and they provide a potential explanation for this association. They explain that "similar brain regions [are] involved in both depression and pain (e.g., dorsolateral prefrontal cortex, anterior cingulated cortex, periaqueductal gray, insula cortex, and hypothalamus)." Understanding comorbid depression and pain is important in the care of older adults. Major depressive disorder (MDD) is not only common in older adults, but it "amplifies disability,

hastens cognitive and functional decline, increases risk of hospitalization, diminishes quality of life, and burdens caregivers."[63] Karp and Reynolds[63] conclude that depression and pain are mutually exacerbating and disabling; that they are risk factors for the onset of each other; and, when comorbid, that they can slow treatment outcomes for each other.

Poleshuck et al.[97] focus more specifically on the effects of psychosocial stress (e.g., unemployment and financial difficulties) and anxiety in clients with musculoskeletal conditions. In this study a cross-sectional sample of 500 primary care patients with musculoskeletal pain (250 with depression and 250 without depression) was conducted to "determine if psychosocial stress and anxiety were associated with depression severity in . . . patients with chronic musculoskeletal pain." The multilinear regression analysis in this study reveals that those clients with both musculoskeletal pain and depression report greater psychosocial stress and anxiety than those without depression. It also concludes that depressed clients also reported greater pain disability, more difficulties with financial security, and greater unemployment, suggesting an association between anxiety and psychosocial stressors and depression severity.

Reduced participation in treatment, which may be adversely affected by depression and other emotional stressors, has been associated with poorer functional outcomes.[72] Thus, for the rehabilitation therapist, it is clear that treating solely the physical aspects of musculoskeletal conditions would not be a comprehensive approach. Addressing and integrating a client's psychosocial stressors, anxiety, and depression may be necessary to fully engage the client in treatment participation and enhance carryover.

Interprofessional Interventions

"The evolution from the traditional mechanistic view of the human body to one encompassing a biopsychosocial approach has come about as a result of a greater understanding of the interrelationship between health, illness, and disease. . . . This inherent complexity of human health requires the involvement of individuals with disparate expertise collaborating in multidisciplinary teams to provide the best patient care." (p. 715)[13]

Current trends in health care emphasize the need for analysis of common practice to search for evidence that supports and justifies its effectiveness in client care. This includes not only specific treatment interventions, but the actual structures of our healthcare systems. Although more studies are needed in this area, there is a growing amount of literature that analyzes the benefits of multidisciplinary treatment interventions for musculoskeletal disorders.

Many avenues for research have yet to be undertaken in this area. The general philosophy that guides an interprofessional practice lies in the depth and quality of intervention that multiple disciplines contribute to a client when addressing the complexities of his or her problem(s) through different perspectives and with differing areas of expertise.

For example, Guzman and colleagues[41] provided a systematic literature review of 10 randomized, controlled trials to assess the effect of multidisciplinary biopsychosocial rehabilitation on clinically relevant outcomes in clients with chronic low back pain. The participants involved in the trials included a total of 1964 clients with disabling low back pain with a duration of more than 3 months. Guzman et al.[41] conclude that the reviewed trials provide strong evidence that intensive multidisciplinary biopsychosocial rehabilitation with functional restoration reduces pain and improves function in clients with chronic low back pain, and that less intensive interventions did not show improvements in clinically relevant outcomes.

Interprofessional collaboration and integration of interventions for clients with musculoskeletal conditions may vary from setting to setting. Typical members of a multidisciplinary care team for clients with musculoskeletal conditions generally include individuals from physical medicine, rheumatology, orthopedics, physical therapy, occupational therapy, social work, and clinical psychology. Weigl et al.[130] note that "there is evidence that multidisciplinary team care benefits patients with LBP, RA and fibromyalgia."

Summary

The musculoskeletal system involves the complex interactions of muscles, bones, and connective tissues. Throughout the lifespan it provides support and protection and allows for movement, and thus provides a means for us to engage in life. Each component of the musculoskeletal system varies in its structure and function, but there are similar patterns of change that occur as we age.

Understanding the physiologic and kinesiological aspects of the musculoskeletal system allows a therapist to evaluate and assess musculoskeletal conditions that limit clients in functional performance. An occupational therapist needs to understand the benefits of exercise and to integrate these principles into an occupation-based intervention plan with the goal of maximizing the client's functional status and well-being.

REVIEW QUESTIONS

1. Why is it important to reduce excessive loading on the involved joints of people with OA?
2. What are some treatments for people in an active phase of RA?
3. Describe the overall objective differences between the active, subacute, and inactive phases of RA.
4. Describe two therapeutic interventions to use with individuals in the acute phase of an osteoporotic vertebral fracture.
5. What is the typical posture of older adults who have experienced a decline in mobility? Name two functional tasks that may be impaired due to this decline.
6. What is the most commonly used tool in measuring a client's functional status, and why was it developed?
7. Name three specific musculoskeletal components/impairments that an occupational therapist must identify to design an occupation-based intervention plan.

True or False

8. Falls are the leading cause of injury deaths in older adults.
9. Chronic pain and functional dependency are inevitable consequences of aging with joint disease.

REFERENCES

1. Aletaha, D., Neogi, T., Silman, A., Funovits, J., Felson, D., Bingham, C., et al. (2010). 2010 Rheumatoid arthritis classification criteria: An American College of Rheumatology/European League Against Rheumatism collaborative initiative. *Arthritis & Rheumatism, 62*(9), 2569–2581.
2. Antonopoulou, M. D., Alegakis, A. K., Hadjipavlou, A. G., & Lionis, C. D. (2009). Studying the association between musculoskeletal disorders, quality of life and mental health. A primary care pilot study in rural Crete, Greece. *BioMed Central The Open Access Publisher, 10,* 143. doi: 10.1186/1471-2474-10-143.
3. Arnett F., Edworthy, S., Bloch, D., McShane, D., Fries, J., Cooper, N., Healey, L., Kaplan, S., Liang, M., Luthra, H., et al. (1988). The American Rheumatism Association 1987 revised criteria for the classification of rheumatoid arthritis. *Arthritis Rheum, 31*(3), 315–324.
4. Bachmann, S., Finger, C., Huss, A., Egger, M., Stuck, K., & Clough-Gorr, K. (2010). Inpatient rehabilitation specifically designed for geriatric patients: Systematic review and meta-analysis of randomised controlled trials. *British Medical Journal, 340,* c1718. doi: 10.1136/bmj.c1718.
5. Baker-LePain, J., & Lane, N. (2010). Relationship between joint shape and the development of osteoarthritis. *Current Opinion in Rheumatology, 22*(5), 538–543. doi: 10.1097/BOR.0b013e32833d20ae.
6. Barak, Y., Wagenaar, R. C., & Holt, K. G. (2006). Gait characteristics of elderly people with a history of falls: A dynamic approach. *Physical Therapy, 86*(11), 1501–1510.
7. Barone, A., Giusti, A., Pizzonia, M., Razzano, M., Palummeri, E., & Giulio, P. (2006). A comprehensive geriatric intervention reduces short- and long-term mortality in older people with hip fracture. *Journal of the American Geriatrics Society, 54*(4), 711–712.
8. Beaupre, L. A., Jones, C. A., Saunders, L. D., Johnston, D. W., Buckingham, J., & Majumdar, S. R. (2005). Best practices for elderly hip fracture patients. *Journal of General Internal Medicine, 20,* 1019–1025.
9. Belo, J., Berger, M., Reijman, B., Koes, B., & Bierma-Zeinstra, S. (2007). Prognostic factors of progression of osteoarthritis of the knee: A systematic review of observational studies. *Arthritis & Rheumatism, 57*(1), 13–26. doi: 10.1002/art.22475.
10. Bennell, K., Hunt, M., Wrigley, T., Lim, B., & Hinman, R. (2008). Role of muscle in the genesis and management of knee osteoarthritis. *Rheumatic Disease Clinics, 34*(3), 731–754. doi: http://dx.doi.org/10.1016/j.rdc.2008.05.005.
11. Blagojevic, M., Jinks, C., Jeffery, A., & Jordan, K. (2010). Risk factors for onset of osteoarthritis of the knee in older adults: A systematic review and meta-analysis. *Osteoarthritis and Cartilage, 18*(1), 24–33. doi: http://dx.doi.org/10.1016/j.joca.2009.08.010.
12. Bohannon, R. W., Larkin, P. A., Cook, A. C., Gear, J., & Singer, J. (1984). Decrease in timed balance test scores with aging. *Physical Therapy, 64*(7), 1067–1070.

13. Boon, H., Mior, S., Barnsley, J., Ashbury, F., & Haig, R. (2009). The difference between integration and collaboration in patient care: Results from key informant interviews working in multi-professional health care teams. *Journal of Manipulative and Physiological Therapeutics, 32*(9), 715–722.

14. Bressler, H., Keyes, W., Rochon, P., & Badley, E. (1999). The prevalence of low back pain in the elderly: A systematic review of the literature. *Spine, 24*(17), 1813–1819.

15. Cairns, A., & McVeigh, J. (2009). A systematic review of the effects of dynamic exercise in rheumatoid arthritis. *Rheumatology International, 30*(2), 147–158.

16. Centers of Disease Control and Prevention. (2014). *Health, United States.* Retrieved 9-7-15. http://www.cdc.gov/nchs/hus/injury.htm.

17. Chapple, C., Nicholson, H., Baxter, D., & Abbott, J. (2011). Patient characteristics that predict progression of knee osteoarthritis: A systematic review of prognostic studies. *Arthritis Care & Research, 63*(8), 1115–1125.

18. Chong, C., Savige, J., & Lim, W. (2010). Medical problems in hip fracture patients. *Archives of Orthopaedic and Trauma Surgery, 130*(11), 1355–1361.

19. Chou, R, Qaseem, A., Snow, V., Casey, D., Cross, J., Shekelle, P., & Owens, D. (2007). Diagnosis and treatment of low back pain: A joint clinical practice guideline from the American College of Physicians and the American Pain Society. *Annals of Internal Medicine, 147*(7), 478–491.

20. Christiansen, C., & Baum, C. M. (1997). *Occupational therapy: Enabling function and well-being.* Thorofare, NJ: SLACK.

21. Clarke, M. (2004). The effects of exercise on skeletal muscle in the aged. *Journal of Musculoskeletal Neuron Interact, 4*(2), 175–178.

22. Cooper, C., Campion, G., & Melton, L. J. (1992). Hip fractures in the elderly: A world-wide projection. *Osteoporosis International, 2*(6), 285–289.

23. Cummings, S. R., & Nevitt, M. C. (1994). Non-skeletal determinants of fractures: The potential importance of the mechanics of falls. *Osteoporosis International, 4*(Suppl. 1), S67–S70.

24. Cummings, R. G., Nevitt, M. C., & Cummings, S. R. (1997). Epidemiology of hip fractures. *Epidemiologic Reviews, 19*(2), 244–257.

25. Dagenais, S., Garbedian, S., & Wai, E. K. (2009). Systematic review of the prevalence of radiographic primary hip osteoarthritis. *Clinical orthopaedics and related research, 467*(3), 623–637.

26. Daltroy, L., Larson, M., Eaton, H., Phillips, C., & Liang, M. (1999). Discrepancies between self-reported and observed physical function in the elderly: The influence of response shift and other factors. *Social Science & Medicine, 48*(11), 1549–1561.

27. De Jong, Z., Munneke, M., Zwinderman, A. H., Kroon, H. M., Jansen, A., Ronday, K., & Hazes, J. (2003). Is a long-term high-intensity exercise program effective and safe in patients with rheumatoid arthritis: Results of a randomized controlled trial. *Arthritis & Rheumatism, 48*(9), 2415–2424.

28. De Jong, Z., Munneke, M., Zwinderman, A. H., Kroon, H. M., Jansen, A., Ronday, K., et al. (2004). Long term high intensity exercise and damage of small joints in rheumatoid arthritis. *Annals of Rheumatic Diseases, 63*, 1399–1405. doi:10.1136/ard.2003.015826.

29. Dieppe, P., & Tobias, J. (1998). Bone and joint aging. In R. Tallis, H. Fillit, & J. Brocklehurst, (Eds.), *Brocklehurst's textbook of geriatric medicine and gerontology* (pp. 1131–1135). Edinburgh: Churchill Livingstone.

30. Dite, W., & Temple, V. (2002). A clinical test of stepping and change of direction to identify multiple falling older adults. *Archives of Physical Medicine and Rehabilitation, 83*(11), 1566–1571.

31. Downey, P. A., & Siegel, M. I. (2006). Bone biology and the clinical implication for osteoporosis. *Physical Therapy, 86*(1), 77–91.

32. Englund, M., Guermazi, A., Gale, D., Hunter, D., Aliabadi, P., Clancy, M., & Felson, D. (2008). Incidental meniscal findings on knee MRI in middle-aged and elderly persons. *New England Journal of Medicine, 359*, 1108–1115.

33. Faulkner, K., Redfern, M., Cauley, J., Landsittel, D., Studenski, S., Rosano, C., Simonsick, E., Harris, T., Shorr, R., Avonayon, H., & Newman, A. (2007). Multitasking: Association between poorer performance and a history of recurrent falls. *Journal of the American Geriatrics Society, 55*(4), 570–576.

34. Felson, D., Lawrence, R., Dieppe, P., Hirsch, R., Helmick, C., Jordan, J., et al. (2000). Osteoarthritis: New insights. Part 1: The disease and Its risk factors. *Annals of Internal Medicine, 133,* 635–646. doi:10.7326/0003-4819-133-8-200010170-00016.

35. Fiedler, R. C., Granger, C. V., & Ottenbacher, K. J. (1996). The Uniform Data System for Medical Rehabilitation: Report of First Admissions for 19941. American journal of physical medicine & rehabilitation, 75(2), 125–129.

36. Finch, C., Donaldson, A., Mahoney, M., & Otago, L. (2009). Who chooses to use multi-purpose recreation facilities for their physical activity setting? *Sport Health, 27*(2), 16–18.

37. Gerber, L., & Hicks, J. (1990). Exercise in the rheumatic diseases. In *Therapeutic exercise* (5th ed.). Baltimore: Williams and Wilkins.

38. Goodman, C. C. (2009). Introduction to pathology of the musculoskeletal system. In Goodman, C. C., & Fuller, K. S. (Eds.), *Pathology implications for the physical therapist.* (4th ed., pp. 1-11). St. Louis, MO: W B Saunders.

39. Grainger, R., & Cicuttini, F. M. (2004). Medical management of osteoarthritis of the knee and hip joints. *Medical Journal of Australia, 180*(5), 232–236.

40. Gramse, R. R., Sinaki, M., & Ilstrup, D. M. (1980). Lumbar spondylolisthesis: A rational approach to conservative treatment. *Mayo Clinic Proceedings, 5*(11), 681–686.

41. Guzman, J., Esmail, R., Karjalainen, K., Malmivaara, A., Irvin, E., & Bombardier, C. (2001). Multidisciplinary rehabilitation for chronic low back pain: Systematic review. *British Medical Journal, 1*(322), 1511–1516.

42. Hakkinen, K., Alen, M., Kraemer, W., Gorostiaga, E., Izquierdo, M., Rusko, H., et al. (2003). Neuromuscular adaptations during concurrent strength and endurance training versus strength training. *European Journal of Applied Physiology, 89*(1), 42–52.

43. Hakkinen, A., Pakarinen, A., Hannonen, P., Kautiainen, H., Nyman, K., Kraemer, W., & Hakkinen, K. (2005). Effects of prolonged combined strength and endurance training on physical fitness, body composition and serum hormones in women with rheumatoid arthritis and in healthy controls. *Clinical and Experimental Rheumatology, 23*, 505–512.

44. Halm, E. A., Wang, J. J., Boockvar, K., Penrod, J., Silberzweig, S. B., Magaziner, J., & Siu, A. L. (2003). Effects of blood transfusion on clinical and functional outcomes in patients with hip fracture. *Transfusion, 43*(10), 1358–13365.

45. Hammond, A. (2008). Rehabilitation in musculoskeletal diseases. *Best Practice & Research Clinical Rheumatology, 22*(3), 435–449. doi: 10.1016/j.berh.2008.02.003.

46. Hammond, A., & Freeman, F. (2004). One-year outcomes of a randomized controlled trial of an educational-behavioural joint protection programme for people with rheumatoid arthritis. *Rheumatology*, 40(9), 1044–1051.

47. Hand, C., Law, M., & McColl, M. (2011). Occupational therapy interventions for chronic diseases: A scoping review. *American Journal of Occupational Therapy*, 65, 428–436. doi:10.5014/ajot.2011.002071.

48. Handoll, H. H. G., Cameron, I. D., Mak, J. C. S., & Finnegan, T. P. (2009). Multidisciplinary rehabilitation for older people with hip fractures [Review]. *The Cochrane Collaboration*, 4, 1–76.

49. Harper, C. M., & Lyles, Y. M. (1988). Physiology and complications of bed rest. *JAGS*, 36(11), 1047–1054.

50. Hart, E., Joyner, M., Wallin, B., & Charkoudian, N. (2012). Sex, ageing and resting blood pressure: Gaining insights from the integrated balance of neural and haemodynamic factors. *The Journal of Physiology*, 590(9), 2069–2079.

51. Heliövaara, M., Makela, M., Impivaara, O., Knekt, P., Aromaa, A., & Sievers, K. (1993). Association of overweight, trauma and workload with coxarthrosis: A health survey of 7,217 persons. *Acta Orthopaedica*, 64(5), 513–518.

52. Hertling, D., & Kessler, R. M. (2006). Assessment of musculoskeletal disorders and concepts of management. In D. Hertling & R. Kessler (Eds.), *Management of common musculoskeletal disorders: Physical therapy principles*. (4th ed., pp. 61–106).

53. Hicks, G. E., Fritz, M., Delitto, A., & McGill, S. M. (2005). Preliminary development of a clinical prediction rule for determining which patients with low back pain will respond to a stabilization exercise program. *Archives of Physical Medicine and Rehabilitation*, 86(9), 1753–1762.

54. Hicks, G. E., Morone, N., & Weiner, D. K. (2009). Degenerative lumbar disc and facet disease in older adults: Prevalence and clinical correlates. *Spine*, 34(12), 1301–1306. doi:10.1097/BRS.0b013e3181a18263.

55. Hills, R. A., & Thomas, K. (1998). Joint stiffness and articular gelling: Inhibition of the fusion of articular surfaces by surfactant. *British Journal of Rheumatology*, 37, 532–538.

56. Hochberg, M., Altman, R., Toupin April, K., Benkhalti, M., Guyatt, G., McGowan, J., et al. (2012). American College of Rheumatology 2012 recommendations for the use of nonpharmacologic and pharmacologic therapies in osteoarthritis of the hand, hip, and knee. *Arthritis Care & Research*, 64(4), 465–474. doi 10.1002/acr.21596.

57. Hochberg, M. C., Chang, R. W., Dwosh, I., Lindsey, S., Pincus, T., & Wolfe, F. (1992). The American College of Rheumatology 1991 revised criteria for the classification of global functional status in rheumatoid arthritis. *Arthritis & Rheumatism*, 35(5), 498–502.

58. Iwamoto, J., Suzuki, H., Tanaka, K., Kumakubo, T., Hirabayashi, H., Miyazaki, Y., & Matsumoto, H. (2009). Preventative effect of exercise against falls in the elderly: A randomized controlled trial. *Osteoporosis International*, 20(7), 1233–1240.

59. Jarvik, J. J., Hollingworth, W., Heagerty, P., Haynor, D. R., & Deyo, R. A. (2001). The longitudinal assessment of imaging and disability of the back (LAIDBack) study: Baseline data. *Spine*, 26(10), 1158–1166.

60. Jensen, A. N., Markwig, H., & Markwig, T. (2008). An algorithm for lifting points in a tropical variety. *Collectanea mathematica*, 59(2), 129–165.

61. Kalichman, L., Li, L., Kim, D., Guermazi, A., Berkin, V., O'Donnell, C. J., & Hunter, D. J. (2008). Facet joint osteoarthritis and low back pain in the community-based population. *Spine*, 33(23), 2560–2565.

62. Karinkanta, S., Heinonen, A., Sievänen, H., Uusi-Rasi, K., Fogelholm, M., & Kannus, P. (2009). Maintenance of exercise-induced benefits in physical functioning and bone among elderly women. *Osteoporosis International*, 20(4), 665–674.

63. Karp, J. F., & Reynolds C. F., III. (2009). Depression, pain, and aging. *Focus*, 7(1), 17–27.

64. Kort, W. M., Barry, D. W., & Schwartz, R. S. (2009). Muscle forces or gravity: What predominates mechanical loading on bone? *Medicine & Science in Sports & Exercise*, 41(11), 2050–2055.

65. Kukuljan, S., Nowson, C. A., & Bass, J. L. (2009). Effect of a multi-component exercise program and calcium-vitamin-D3-fortified milk on bone mineral density in older men: A randomized controlled trial. *Osteoporosis International*, 20, 1241–1251.

66. Lach, H. W. (2002). Fear of falling: An emerging public health problem. *Generations*, 3(Winter), 33–37.

67. Landi, F., Onder, G., Carpenter, I., Cesari, M., Soldato, M., & Bernabei, R. (2007). Physical activity prevented functional decline among frail community-living elderly subjects in an international observational study. *Journal of Clinical Epidemiology*, 60(5), 518–524.

68. Latham, N. K., & Liu, C. J. (2009). Progressive resistance strength training for improving physical function in older adults [Review]. *Cochran Review*, 3, 1–277.

69. Lawrence, T. M., Wenn, R., Boulton, C. T., & Moran, C. G. (2010). Age-specific incidence of first and second fractures of the hip. *The Journal of Bone and Joint Surgery*, 92(2), 258–261.

70. Lazaro, L., IV, & Quinet, R. J. (1994). Low back pain: How to make the diagnosis in the older patient. *Geriatrics*, 49(9), 48–53.

71. Lee, N. K., Sowa, H., Hinoi, E., Ferron, M., Ahn, J. D., Confavreux, C., & Jung, D. Y. (2007). Endocrine regulation of energy metabolism by the skeleton. *Cell*, 130(3), 456–469.

72. Lenza, M., Belloti, J. C., Gomes dos Santos, J. B., Matsumoto, M. H., & Faloppa, F. (2009). Surgical interventions for treating acute fractures or non-union of the middle third of the clavicle. Cochrane Database of Systematic Reviews, Issue 4. Art. No.: CD007428. doi: 10.1002/14651858.CD007429.pub2.

73. Letts, L., & Bosch, J. (2005). In M. Law, C.M. Baum, & W. Dunn (Eds.) *Measuring occupational performance in basic activities of daily living. Measuring occupational performance: Supporting best practice in occupational therapy*. (2nd ed., pp. 179-226). Thorofare, NJ: Slack Incorporated.

74. Leveille, S. G. (2004). Musculoskeletal aging. *Current Opinion in Rheumatology*, 16(2), 114–118.

75. Lewis, C. B., & Bottomley, J. M. (1990). Musculoskeletal changes with age: Clinical implications. In *Aging: Health care challenge* (2nd ed., pp. 135–160). Philadelphia, PA: FA Davis.

76. Lieber, R., & Bodine Fowler, S. (1993). Skeletal muscle mechanics: Implications for rehabilitation. *Physical Therapy*, 73(12), 844–856.

77. Marcora, S. M., Lemmey, A. B., & Maddison, P. J. (2005). Can progressive resistance training reverse cachexia in patients with rheumatoid arthritis? Results of a pilot study. *The Journal of rheumatology*, 32(6), 1031–1039.

78. Mathieux, R., Marotte, H., Battistini, L., Sarrazin, A., Berthier, M., & Miossec, P. (2009). Early occupational therapy programme increases hand grip strength at 3 months: Results from a randomised, blind, controlled study in early rheumatoid arthritis. *Annals of the Rheumatic Diseases*, 68(3), 400–403. doi: 10.1136/ard.2008.094532.

79. Maxey, L., & Magnusson, J. (2013). *Rehabilitation for the post-surgical orthopedic patient* (3rd ed.). St. Louis, MO: Mosby Elsevier.

80. McGirt, M. J., Parker, S. L., Wolinsky, J. P., Witham, T. F., Bydoon, A., & Gokaslan, Z. L. (2009). Vertebroplasty and kyphoplasty for the treatment of vertebral compression fractures: An evidenced-based review of the literature. *The Spine Journal, 9,* 501–508. http://www.ncbi.nlm.nih.gov/pubmed/19251485.

81. McNicoll, L., & Fitzgibbons, P. G. (2009). Optimal hip fracture management in high-risk frail older adults. *Geriatrics for the Practicing Physician, 92*(7), 250–252.

82. Meeks, S. M. (2005). The role of the physical therapist in the recognition, assessment, and exercise intervention in persons with, or at risk for, osteoporosis. *Topics in Geriatric Rehabilitation, 21*(1), 42–56.

83. Messier, S. P., Loeser, R. F., Miller, G. D., Morgan, T. M., Rejeski, W. J., Sevick, M. A., & Williamson, J. D. (2004). Exercise and dietary weight loss in overweight and obese older adults with knee osteoarthritis: The Arthritis, Diet, and Activity Promotion Trial. *Arthritis & Rheumatism, 50*(5), 1501–1510.

84. Middleton, R. P., Waldron, M. K., & Nielsen, N. (2011). U.S. Patent Application 13/996, *225.*

85. Mikesky, A. E., Mazzuca, S. A., Brandt, K. D., Perkins, S. M., Damush, T., & Lane, K. A. (2006). Effects of strength training on the incidence and progression of knee osteoarthritis. *Arthritis Care & Research, 55*(5), 690–699.

86. Munneke, M., de Jong, Z., Zwinderman, A. H., Ronday, H. K., van Schaardenburg, D., Dijkmans, B. A., & Hazes, J. M. (2005). Effect of a high-intensity weight-bearing exercise program on radiologic damage progression of the large joints in subgroups of patients with rheumatoid arthritis. *Arthritis Care & Research, 53*(3), 410–417.

87. Murphy, S. L., Strasburg, D. M., Lyden, A. K., Smith, D. M., Koliba, J. F., Dadabhoy, D. P., & Wallis, S. M. (2008). Effects of activity strategy training on pain and physical activity in older adults with knee or hip osteoarthritis: A pilot study. *Arthritis & Rheumatism, 59*(10), 1480–1487.

88. National Osteoporosis Foundation. (2008). *Boning up on osteoporosis: A guide to prevention and treatment.* Washington, DC: Author.

89. Neogi, T., & Zhang, Y. (2011). Osteoarthritis prevention. *Current opinion in rheumatology, 23*(2), 185.

90. Nevitt, M. C., Cummings, S. R., & Kidd, S. (1989). Risk factors for recurrent nonsyncopal falls: A prospective study. *JAMA, 261*(18), 2663–2668.

91. NIH consensus development panel on osteoporosis prevention, diagnosis, and therapy. (2001). Osteoporosis prevention, diagnosis, and therapy. *JAMA, 285,* 785–795.

92. Oordt, M. S., Jobes, D. A., Fonseca, V. P., & Schmidt, S. M. (2009), Training mental health professionals to assess and manage suicidal behavior: Can provider confidence and practice behaviors be altered? *Suicide and Life-Threatening Behavior, 39,* 21–32. doi: 10.1521/suli.2009.39.1.213.

93. O'Sullivan, P. B., Manip Phyty, G. D., Twomey, L. T., & Allison, G. T. (1997). Evaluation of specific stabilizing exercise in the treatment of chronic low back pain with radiologic diagnosis of spondylolysis or spondylolisthesis. *Spine, 22*(24), 2959–2967.

94. Pai, Y., Rymer, W. Z., Chang, R. W., & Sharma, L. (1997). Effect of age and osteoarthritis on knee proprioception [Abstract]. *Arthritis & Rheumatism, 40*(12), 2260–2265. doi: 10.1002/art.1780401223.

95. Peri, K., Kerse, N., Robinson, E., Parsons, M., Parsons, J., & Latham, N. (2007). Does functionally based activity make a difference to health status and mobility? A randomised controlled trial in residential care facilities (The Promoting Independent Living Study; PILS). *Age and Ageing, 37*(1), 57–63. doi: 10.1093/ageing/afm135.

96. Perlman, S. G., Connell, K. J., Clark, A., Robinson, M. S., Conlon, P., Gecht, M. P., & Sinacore, J. M. (1990). Dance-based aerobic exercise for rheumatoid arthritis. *Arthritis Care & Research, 3*(1), 29–35.

97. Poleshuck, E. L., Bair, M. J., Kroenke, K., Damush, T. M., Tu, W., Wu, J., & Giles, D. E. (2009). Psychosocial stress and anxiety in musculoskeletal pain patients with and without depression. *General Hospital Psychiatry, 31*(2), 116–122.

98. Raaymakers, E. L. (2006). Fractures of the femoral neck. *Acta Chirurgiae Orthopaedicae et Traumatologiae Cechoslovaca, 73*(1), 45–59.

99. Rao, R. D., & Singrakhia, M. D. (2003). Current concepts review; painful osteoporotic vertebral fracture: Pathogenesis, evaluation, and roles of vertebroplasty and kyphoplasty in its management. *Journal of Bone and Joint Surgery, 85-A,* 2010–2022.

100. Reid, G. D., Reid, C. G., Widmer, N., & Munk, P. L. (2010). Femoroacetabular impingement syndrome: An underrecognized cause of hip pain and premature osteoarthritis? *The Journal of Rheumatology, 37*(7), 1395–1404.

101. Reijman, M., Hazes, J. M. W., Pols, H. A. P., Koes, B. W., & Bierma-Zeinstra, S. M. A. (2005). Acetabular dysplasia predicts incident osteoarthritis of the hip: The Rotterdam study. *Arthritis & Rheumatism, 52*(3), 787–793.

102. Reijman, M., Pols, H., Bergink, A., Hazes, J., Belo, J., Lievense, A., & Bierma-Zeinstra, S. (2007). Body mass index associated with onset and progression of osteoarthritis of the knee but not of the hip: The Rotterdam study. *Annals of Rheumatoid Disability, 66,* 158–162. doi:10.1136/ard.2006.053538.

103. Roddy, E., Zhang, W., & Doherty, M. (2005). Aerobic walking or strengthening exercise for osteoarthritis of the knee? A systematic review. *Annals of the Rheumatic Diseases, 64*(4), 544–548.

104. Roubenoff, R. (2000). Sarcopenic obesity: Does muscle loss cause fat gain? *Annals of the New York Academy of Science, 904,* 553–557.

105. Rudy, T. E., Weiner, D. K., Lieber, S. J., Sladoda, J., & Boston, J. R. (2007). The impact of chronic low back pain on older adults: A comparative study of patients and controls. *Pain, 131*(3), 293–301.

106. Sharma, L., Dunlop, D., Andriacchi, T., Hayes, K., Song, J., Cahue, S., & Hurwitz, D. (2003, September). The adduction moment and knee osteoarthritis (OA), a longitudinal study. In *Arthritis and Rheumatism, 48*(9), S452–S452.

107. Sharma, L., Pai, Y. C., Holtkamp, K., & Rymer, W. Z. (1997). Is knee joint proprioception worse in the arthritic knee versus the unaffected knee in unilateral knee osteoarthritis? *Arthritis & Rheumatism, 40*(8), 1518–1525.

108. Shumway-Cook, A., Brauer, S., & Woollacott, M. (2000). Predicting the probability for falls in community-dwelling older adults using the Timed Up & Go Test. *Physical Therapy, 80*(9), 896–903.

109. Sinaki, M. (2002). Stronger back muscles reduce the incidence of vertebral fractures: A prospective 10 year follow-up of postmenopausal women. *Bone, 30*(6), 836–841.

110. Sinaki, M. (2003). Critical appraisal of physical rehabilitation measures after osteoporotic vertebral fracture. *Osteoporosis International, 14*(9), 773–779.

111. Sinaki, M. (2007). The role of physical activity in bone health: A new hypothesis to reduce risk of vertebral fracture. *Physical Medicine and Rehabilitation Clinics of North America, 18*(3), 593–608.

112. Sinaki, M., Brey, R. H., Hughes, C. A., Larson, D. R., & Kaufman, K. R. (2005). Significant reduction in risk of falls

and back pain in osteoporotic-kyphotic women through a Spinal Proprioceptive Extension Exercise Dynamic (SPEED) program. *Mayo Clinic Proceedings, 80*(7), 849–855.

113. Slemenda, C., Brandt, K. D., Heilman, D. K., Mazzuca, S., Braunstein, E. M., Katz, G. P., & Wolinsky, F. D. (1997). Quadriceps weakness and osteoarthritis of the knee. *Annals of Internal Medicine, 127*(2), 97–104.

114. Stamm, T. A., Cieza, A., Machold, K. P., Smolen, J. S., & Stucki, G. (2004). Content comparison of occupation-based instruments in adult rheumatology and musculoskeletal rehabilitation based on the International Classification of Functioning, Disability and Health. *Arthritis & Rheumatism, 51*(6), 917–924.

115. Stedman, T. L. (2005). *Stedman's medical dictionary* (28th ed.). Philadelphia, PA: Lippincott Williams & Wilkins.

116. Stevens, J. A. (2005). Gender differences for non-fatal unintentional fall related injuries among older adults. *Injury Prevention, 11*(2), 115–119.

117. Stuck, A. E., Walthert, J. M., Nikolaus, T., Büla, C. J., Hohmann, C., & Beck, J. C. (1999). Risk factors for functional status decline in community-living elderly people: a systematic literature review. Social science & medicine, 48(4), 445–469.

118. Suominen, H. (1993). Bone mineral density and long term exercise. *Sports Medicine, 16*(5), 316–330.

119. Swezey, R. L. (1996). Exercise for osteoporosis: Is walking enough? [Abstract]. *Spine, 21*, 2809–2813.

120. Swezey, R. L. (1997). Preventing osteoporotic fractures: The role of exercise, posture, and safety. *Journal of Musculoskeletal Medicine, 14*(4), 9–28.

121. Tanamas, S., Hanna, F. S., Cicuttini, F. M., Wluka, A. E., Berry, P., & Urquhart, D. M. (2009). Does knee malalignment increase the risk of development and progression of knee osteoarthritis? A systematic review. *Arthritis Care & Research, 61*(4), 459–467.

122. The Ottawa Panel. (2005). Ottawa Panel evidence-based clinical practice guidelines for therapeutic exercises and manual therapy in the management of osteoarthritis. *Physical Therapy, 85*(9), 907–971, 934–972.

123. Trombly, C. A., & Radomski, M. V. (2002). *Occupational therapy for physical dysfunction*. Philadelphia, PA: Lippincott Williams & Wilkins.

124. Uhlig, T., Fongen, C., Steen, E., Christie, A., & Odegard, S. (2010). Exploring tai chi in rheumatoid arthritis: A quantitative and qualitative study. *BMC Musculoskeletal Disorders, 11*(43). doi:10.1186/1471-2474-11-43.

125. U.S. Department of Health and Human Services, Wiener, J., & Handley, R. (1990). *Measuring the activities of daily living*. http://aspe.hhs.gov/daltcp/reports/meacmpes.pdf.

126. Van den Ende, C. H., Vlieland, T. V., Munneke, M., & Hazes, J. M. (1998). Dynamic exercise therapy in rheumatoid arthritis: a systematic review. *Rheumatology, 37*(6), 677–687.

127. Venes, D. (2013). *Taber's cyclopedic medical dictionary*. FA Davis.

128. Verdijk, L. B., Koopman, R., Schaart, G., Meijer, K., Savelberg, H. M., & Van Loon, L. C. (2006). Satellite cell content is specifically reduced in type II skeletal muscle fibers in the elderly. *AJP: Endocrinology and Metabolism, 292*(1), E151–E157.

129. Vidan, M., Serra, J. A., Moreno, C., Riquelme, G., & Ortiz, J. (2005). Efficacy of a comprehensive geriatric intervention in older patients hospitalized for hip fracture: A randomized, controlled trial. *JAGS, 53*, 1476–1482.

130. Vignon, É., Valat, J. P., Rossignol, M., Avouac, B., Rozenberg, S., Thoumie, P., & Hilliquin, P. (2006). Osteoarthritis of the knee and hip and activity: A systematic international review and synthesis (OASIS). *Joint Bone Spine, 73*(4), 442–455.

131. Weigl, M., Cieza, A., Cantista, P., & Stucki, G. (2007). Physical disability due to musculoskeletal conditions. *Best Practice & Research Clinical Rheumatology, 21*(1), 167–190.

132. Williams, M. A. (1998). Human development and aging. In *American College of Sports Medicine's (ACSM) resource manual* (pp. 501–506). Philadelphia, PA: Lippincott Williams & Wilkins.

133. Woolf, A. D., & Pfleger, B. (2003). *Burden of major musculoskeletal conditions* (9th ed., Vol. 81, pp. 646–656). Washington, DC: National Institutes of Health, U.S. National Library of Medicine.

134. Yood, R. A., & American College of Rheumatology Subcommittee on Rheumatoid Arthritis Guidelines. (2002). *Guidelines for the management of rheumatoid arthritis: 2002 update*.

135. Zhang, Y., & Jordan, J. M. (2010). Epidemiology of osteoarthritis. *Clinics in Geriatric Medicine, 26*, 355–369.

136. Zhang, W., Moskowitz, R. W., Nuki, G., Abramson, S., Altman, R. D., Arden, N., & Tugwell, P. (2008). OARSI recommendations for the management of hip and knee osteoarthritis, part II: OARSI evidence-based, expert consensus guidelines. *Osteoarthritis and Cartilage, 16*, 137–162.

137. Zhang, W., Nuki, G., Moskowitz, R. W., Abramson, S., Altman, R. D., Arden, N. K., & Tugwell, P. (2010). OARSI recommendations for the management of hip and knee osteoarthritis: part III: Changes in evidence following systematic cumulative update of research published through January 2009. *Osteoarthritis and Cartilage, 18*(4), 476–499.

CHAPTER 9

Physiological and Neurological System Changes with Aging and Related Occupational Therapy Interventions

John E. Morley, MD, Amish Patel, MD, Laura H. VanPuymbrouck, ABD, OTR/L, Carole Schwartz, MS, OTR/L, Karen Frank Barney, PhD, OTR/L, FAOTA

OUTLINE

OBJECTIVES

- Describe how the aging process changes physiologic and neurologic functions relative to occupational performance.
- Describe common physiologic and neurologic disorders in older adults, particularly cardiac, respiratory, genitourinary, gastrointestinal, integumentary, and neurologic; their sequelae; and implications for occupational therapy practice.
- Discuss energy conservation, work simplification, and conditioning strategies that occupational therapists typically use with aging adults to support occupational performance.
- Describe occupational-based interventions in the management of falls in the presence of physiologic and neurologic conditions.
- Discuss the psychological effects of physiologic and neurologic disorders in older adults.

Current medical advances have allowed people to experience longer and healthier lives. Although not all adults will challenge the formerly pervasive negative images of aging by running marathons, continuing to work throughout their 80s, and living physically active lives, each recent generation as a whole has shown an increase in making health-conscious lifestyle choices. Greater opportunities for older adults to participate in sustaining lifelong healthy lifestyles has changed the expectations for pushing back mortality and decreasing the extent of morbidity.[42] Advanced medical treatments are allowing once-fatal diseases to be eliminated or managed, resulting in longer lifespans. Each older adult is an individual whose prior lifestyle experiences and genetic makeup influence the changes that occur with advanced age. These fundamental physiologic and neurologic changes during life maturation are discussed in this chapter, including the variance in these changes during the aging process, because each adult ages differently. The focus of this discussion is on changes that may affect occupational performance, thus influencing overall health and well-being. For more detailed aging-related physiologic and neurologic information, readers are encouraged to consult current related scientific evidence, such as *The Merck Manual of Health & Aging* and other sources listed as references.[8] Refer to Table 9-1 for a list of commonly used abbreviations for conditions, and aging-related physiologic or neurologic changes and interventions. Occupational therapy (OT) plays an important role in mitigating the effects of aging changes during this later phase of life by optimizing client participation in meaningful occupation.

Occupation is known as "everything people do to occupy themselves, including looking after themselves . . . enjoying life . . . and contributing to the social and economic fabric of their communities."[30] The focus of intervention, therefore, is on maximizing clients' independence in performing meaningful activities of daily living, work and productive activities, and play and leisure activities.

The population of Americans of ages greater than 65 increased 11-fold from 1900 to 1994, according to the U.S. Census Bureau.[45] Older American adults numbered 1 in 8 in 1994 and will grow to the ratio of 1 in 5 by 2030. To improve our care for older adults, we need to understand the science behind what happens to the function of each bodily organ as individuals become older. Health-care professionals also need to learn from older adults, who are the experts on their

TABLE 9-1 Terms Associated with Aging-Related Physiological or Neurological Changes and Interventions

Term	Definition	Term	Definition
AAA	Abdominal aortic aneurysm	HR	Heart rate
AAROM	Active assistive range of motion	HTN	Hypertension (high blood pressure)
ADL	Activities of daily living	IADL	Instrumental activities of daily living
A.Fib.	Atrial fibrillation (cardiac arrhythmia)	ICP	Intracranial pressure
AICD	Automatic implantable cardio-defibrillator (pacemaker)	ICU	Intensive care unit
		IDDM	Insulin-dependent diabetes mellitus
ALS	Amyotrophic lateral sclerosis	I&O	Intake and output
AMA	Against medical advice	IVC	Inferior vena cava
Amyloid	Abnormal protein usually produced in bone marrow and can be deposited in any tissue or organ	L	Left
		LE	Lower extremity
		LBP	Low back pain
A/P	Anterior-posterior	LLQ	Left lower quadrant
AROM	Active range of motion	LOC	Loss of consciousness
AVR	Aortic valve replacement	LOS	Length of stay
BM	Bowel movement	LUQ	Left upper quadrant
BP	Blood pressure	MCA	Middle cerebral artery
B	Bilateral (both sides)	MET	Metabolic equivalent
BPH	Benign prostatic hypertrophy	MI	Myocardial infarction
CA	Cancer	MRI	Magnetic resonance imaging
CABG	Coronary artery bypass graft	MS	Multiple sclerosis
CAD	Coronary artery disease	MVP	Mitral valve prolapse
CHF	Congestive heart failure	MVR	Mitral valve replacement
CN	Cranial nerves (there are twelve)	NIDDM	Noninsulin-dependent diabetes mellitus
COPD	Chronic obstructive pulmonary disease		
COTA	Certified occupational therapy assistant	NKA	No known allergies
CPAP	Continuous positive airway pressure	NOS	Not otherwise specified
CPR	Cardiopulmonary resuscitation	NPO	Nothing by mouth
CRF or CKD	Chronic renal failure or chronic kidney disease	NREM	Nonrapid eye movement
		N & V	Nausea and vomiting
CS	Carotid stenosis	NWB	Non-weight, bearing
CSF	Cerebrospinal fluid	O_2	Oxygen
CT scan	Computed axial tomography (type of x-ray that shows 2-dimensional images of the parts of the body)	OA	Osteoarthritis
		OB/GYN	Obstetric and gynecology
		OOB	Out of bed
		OR	Operating room
CVA	Cerebrovascular accident (stroke)	ORIF	Open reduction internal fixation (typically used in orthopedic patients; may consist of screws and nails to correct a bone fracture)
CXR	Chest x-ray		
DNR	Do not resuscitate		
DM	Diabetes mellitus		
DME	Durable medical equipment		
DOB	Date of birth	OT	Occupational therapy
DOE	Dyspnea on exertion	PA	Physician's assistant
Dx	Diagnosis	PAM	Physical agent modality
ED	Emergency department	PE	Pulmonary embolism (blood clot in the lung)
EEG	Electroencephalogram		
EKG	Electrocardiogram	PEG	Percutaneous endoscopic gastrostomy (typically put in patients if adequate nutritional intake not being obtained due to malnourishment or dysphagia)
ENT	Ear, nose, and throat		
ESRD	End stage renal disease		
FTT	Failure to thrive		
f/u	Follow-up		
Fx	Fracture	PET	Positron emission tomography (used for cancer screenings and follow-up)
GAD	Generalized anxiety disorder		
GCS	Glasgow coma scale	PFM	Pelvic floor muscle rehabilitation
GERD	Gastroesophageal reflux	PID	Pelvic inflammatory disease
GYN	Gynecology	PMH	Past medical history
HA	Headache	PRBC	Packed red blood cells (used for a blood transfusion)
HD	Hemodialysis		
HEENT	Head, eyes, ear, nose, throat	PRN	As often as necessary
h/o	History of	PROM	Passive range of motion
		PT	Physical therapy

TABLE 9-1 Terms Associated with Aging-Related Physiological or Neurological Changes and Interventions—cont'd

Term	Definition	Term	Definition
PTCA	Percutaneous transvenous coronary angioplasty (balloon angioplasty)	SOAP	Subjective, objective, assessment, plan
PUD	Peptic ulcer disease	SOB	Shortness of breath
PVD	Peripheral vascular disease	s/p	Status post (following a procedure)
R	Right	ST	Speech therapy
RA	Rheumatoid arthritis	STD	Sexually transmitted disease
RBC	Red blood cells	sx	Symptoms
RCA	Right coronary artery	SW	Social worker
REM	Rapid eye movement	TAH	Total abdominal hysterectomy
RLQ	Right lower quadrant	TB	Tuberculosis
RN	Registered nurse	TBI	Traumatic brain injury
ROM	Range of motion	THA	Total hip arthroplasty
RPE	Rate of perceived exertions	THR	Total hip replacement
RT	Respiratory therapy	TIA	Transient ischemic attack
RUQ	Right upper quadrant	TKR	Total knee replacement
SCI	Spinal cord injury	TMJ	Temporomandibular joint
SDH	Subdural hematoma	TURP	Transurethral resection of the prostate
SLP	Speech-language pathology or pathologist	UI	Urinary incontinence
		UTI	Urinary tract infection
		WBC	White blood cells

lives; address their needs; recognize their strengths; and assist them in supporting their functional status.

Cardiovascular Function

Cardiac output typically decreases by 1% each year after age 50. Results of the aging process include the following changes in the cardiovascular system:
- Cardiac muscles are more resistant to endogenous and exogenous hormones, resulting in myocardial stiffness.
- Increased hypertension increases the risk of cerebrovascular accident (CVA), coronary artery disease (CAD), and congestive heart failure (CHF).
- In atherosclerosis, a thickening of the intima occurs, along with more deposition of calcium and phosphate, an increase in collagen in the media, and accumulation of cholesterol (Figure 9-1).

- Due to these conditions, together with decreased arterial flexibility, afterload (the aortic pressure the left ventricular muscle must overcome to eject blood) results.
- If a great amount of amyloid in the cardiac muscle is present, the combination of factors can lead to CHF.[25]

All of these changes in the cardiovascular system present an increased risk of mortality and morbidity, and frequently lead to the incidence of CAD, CHF, CVAs, and carotid stenosis.

Occupational Therapy Interventions Related to Cardiovascular & Cardiopulmonary Disease

The differing aging-related cardiovascular disease sequelae include the psychological, physical, and functional effects of the diagnosis on older adults' everyday living. Traditional OT cardiac interventions include conditioning programs and lifestyle management, such as energy conservation/work simplification. However, according to Bosworth et al., "Clinicians

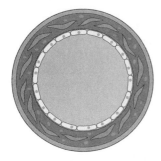
Normal arterial lumen

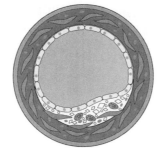
Atherosclerotic plaque deposit

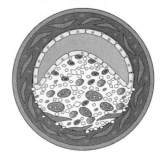
Advanced arterial atherosclerotic disease

FIGURE 9-1 Vascular arterial changes associated with aging. (From Frazier, M. S., & Drzymkowski, J. W. [2013]. *Essentials of human diseases and conditions* [5th ed.]. St. Louis, MO: Elsevier.)

must understand the full range of concerns affecting the [quality of life] QOL of their older patients with [congestive heart failure] CHF. The findings suggest that psychosocial aspects and patient uncertainty about their prognosis are important components of QOL among CHF patients."(p.83)[9] Careful attention to contextual factors such as cultural values and beliefs, spirituality, temporal issues, family and other relationships, and feelings regarding work or avocational-related losses should be a component of the occupational therapist's collaborative treatment plan with the patient, in addition to traditional treatment approaches. There are a number of interventions that occupational therapists may use during treatment sessions to instruct the older adult who has cardiovascular disease and other conditions, as described next.

Energy Conservation

Energy conservation involves the deliberate, planned management of one's energy through balancing rest and activity during times of high fatigue so that valued activities and goals can be maintained.[6, 37] Basic energy conservation strategies incorporate scheduled rest, principles of ergonomics, and home and activity modifications. Educating clients to adjust priorities by choosing how to spend energy, simplify activities so they require less energy, plan a balance of work and rest times, and change the time of day to do an activity are all part of the energy conservation approach used in occupational therapy.[37] This approach requires close collaboration between the client and the therapist or OT assistant and detailed activity analysis (Figures 9-2A and B).

Work Simplification

Evidence-based practice has demonstrated that when affected clients combine work simplification with energy conservation approaches, there is greater benefit to the client.[3] Work simplification objectives aim to minimize waste of labor, increase the effectiveness of each activity, eliminate duplication, and prevent fatigue. Examples of work simplification strategies that can be incorporated into intervention approaches with clients with cardiovascular or cardiopulmonary disease include the following:

- Replace heavy items with light ones.
- Eliminate unnecessary motions.
- Use adaptive equipment to assist in activities.
- Store supplies at the location where the task is performed.
- Arrange the environment to minimize fatigue or extraneous motions (e.g., replace standing with sitting while performing tasks).
- Carefully plan necessary and desired weekly tasks to ensure that difficult tasks are not all done on the same day or successive days.

Physical Conditioning

Conditioning programs focus on increasing strength and endurance; many facilities have cardiac conditioning rehabilitation programs for patients with any diagnosis of cardiopulmonary disease. Based on the evaluation of a client's various risk factors, the therapist custom designs the appropriate

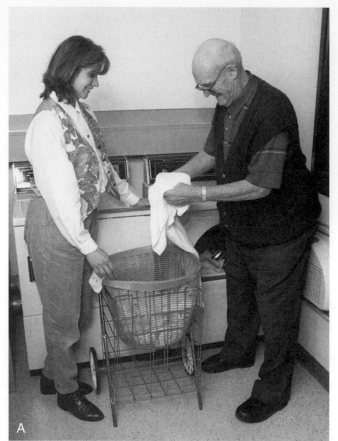

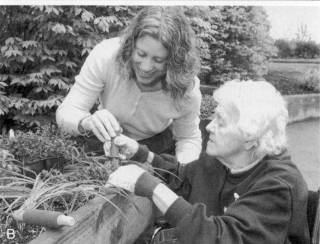

FIGURE 9-2   An Occupational therapist observes elders practicing energy conservation (A), while doing laundry and (B), while gardening. ([A] From Padilla, R., et al. [2012]. *Occupational therapy with elders*. St. Louis, MO: Mosby. [B] From Byers-Connon, S., et al. [2004]. *Occupational therapy with elders*. St. Louis, MO: Mosby.)

program of exercise intensity. Home programs developed by the therapist may focus on teaching clients to assess their physical response to exercise using the Borg Rate of Perceived Exertions Scale (RPE),[1, 44] as well as heart-rate monitoring. As the client increases his or her strength and endurance, the individual's ability to perform functional tasks at higher values of metabolic equivalency (MET) is expected to increase. This increased functional capacity in addition to lifestyle modifications will provide increased physical participation potential for a client with a cardiovascular or cardiopulmonary condition.

In summary, the occupational therapy personnel collaborate with the client and arrives at mutually agreed-upon goals to improve her or his performance of activities of daily living (ADL) and instrumental activities of daily living (IADL). Interventions used for clients with cardiovascular or cardiopulmonary conditions include work simplification, energy conservation methods, stress management, and increased awareness of cardiopulmonary distress symptoms, based upon the individual's medical status. If client, spouse/partner, or caregiver psychological needs are identified during therapy, these should also be addressed by the occupational therapist, who may also refer to other providers for professional assistance.

Respiratory System

Aging changes the respiratory and related systems, resulting typically in a moderate decline in pulmonary function. Typical changes affect the thorax, muscles of respiration, lung tissue, large and small airways, alveoli, pulmonary blood flow, and immune response. Vital capacity may decrease by 26 mL per year for men and 22 mL per year for women, after the age of 20. Total lung capacity typically stays the same, and vital capacity typically decreases because residual capacity increases. Further results of the aging process include the following changes in the respiratory system (Figure 9-3):

- Changes in the thorax that affect respiratory status include increased anteroposterior diameter, ossification of cartilage, and decreased vertebral disk space. Thus the chest wall is less mobile and compliant, resulting in less ability to move air rapidly. These changes result in a reduction of the maximal available force for both inspiration and expiration.
- Reduction of type IIA fibers in respiratory muscles (accessory, anterior abdominal, diaphragm, and intercostals) results in diminished strength and endurance and a stiffer chest wall. These changes result in the individual's greater use of all respiratory muscles, especially the diaphragm, because breathing is more difficult. Greater reliance on the diaphragm fosters heightened sensitivity to changes in body position or comfort following a large meal.
- Elastic recoil that opposes the elastic forces in the chest wall decreases with age, facilitating more compliant respiration against the stiff chest wall.

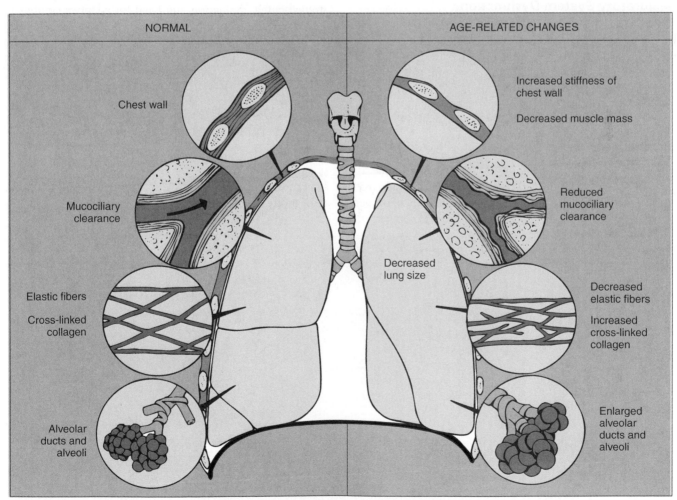

FIGURE 9-3 Respiratory System Changes Associated with Aging. (From Urden, L. D., Stacy, K. M., & Lough, M. E. [2015]. *Priorities in critical care nursing* [7th ed.]. St. Louis, MO: Elsevier.

- Although bronchial structures are generally unchanged, mucous production that protects lungs from infection is reduced with aging.
- Changes in alveolar structures appear microscopically similar to the changes that occur in emphysema, and are known as "senile lung." However, an individual may lose a maximum of 20% of the alveolar surface area without resulting effects on respiratory function.[32]
- Risk for aspiration increases with age, resulting from the changes described in previous list items.
- Infections may increase in older adults due to decreases in immune system function, and poor oral hygiene may also contribute to a decrease in the flow of saliva, which contributes to production of gram-negative bacilli. These conditions foster susceptibility to pneumonia, aspiration pneumonia, COPD, and lung cancer, especially in individuals who smoke tobacco.
- Causes that may additionally limit lung function include asthma, emphysema, chronic bronchitis, bronchiectasis, immobility due to bed rest, obesity, smoking, and surgical procedures that include anesthesia and/or postoperative complications.

Occupational Therapy Interventions Related to Respiratory System Dysfunction

The role of occupational therapy in working with aging adults with pulmonary conditions will vary with the treatment setting, depending on individualized protocols. The following steps describe the basic process for intervention:

1. First, the occupational therapist should review the chart to determine which pulmonary diseases the client has been diagnosed with; oxygen requirement if needed; radiology issues, if any; and medications.
2. Next, interview the client for preferences and difficulties in activities performed at home and outside the home.
3. Vital signs are very important to monitor, especially oxygen saturation and respiratory rate. The delivery of oxygen is of concern, because this relates to the severity of the client's pulmonary disease. Determination of the client's severity depends on the presence of a ventilator, tracheostomy collar, and nasal cannula—in that order. Blood pressure and heart rate are also important to monitor if the client is under any stress.
4. Upper extremities should be evaluated for limitations in strength, sensation, and range of motion (ROM).
5. Clients should be observed in their typical activities, including walking, carrying capacity, ADL, and writing. The client's symptoms are the most important indicator of pulmonary distress; therefore, always observe for shortness of breath (SOB), use of chest accessory muscles, cyanosis, respiratory rate, and depth of breathing before, during, and after therapy.

Within the following discussion, the intervention focus is on pulmonary rehabilitation programs, which are similar to those in other settings. In pulmonary rehabilitation the role of the occupational therapist is to assess and treat activity limitations associated with symptoms of COPD, including dyspnea and/or other pulmonary conditions. Goals are established to maximize the aging client's ability to participate in ADL and IADL, leisure activities, and vocational pursuits.[38] Additional treatment areas focus on upper extremity strengthening, evaluation and need for adaptive equipment or modifications of activities, and education in stress management and relaxation techniques. Work simplification and energy conservation, as described in the cardiopulmonary section, are also common components of a comprehensive treatment approach for clients with COPD.

Clients with pulmonary diseases often require supplemental oxygen during activity, and in more extreme conditions, there is a constant need for supplementation and close vigilance on the part of the therapist (Figure 9-4). The occupational therapist should be aware of this need and monitor O_2 saturation levels via a pulse oximeter (Figure 9-5). It is critical to be aware of the effect functional tasks have on the client's

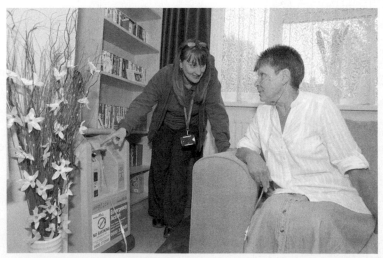

FIGURE 9-4   A patient with chronic obstructive pulmonary disease at home with oxygen. (From Broad, M. A., et al. [Eds.]. [2012]. *Cardiorespiratory assessment of the adult patient: A clinician's guide.* London: Churchill Livingstone.)

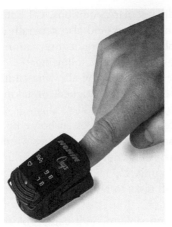

FIGURE 9-5 Pulse oximeter monitoring O_2 saturation levels. (From Garg, A. K. [2010]. *Implant dentistry*. St. Louis, MO: Mosby.)

oxygen saturation; typically if the levels fall below 90%, the activity is considered to be too strenuous for the client to perform. Educating the client and practicing controlled breathing techniques within the context of physical activity exertion is a recommended approach to OT intervention with clients who have COPD.[38] Controlled breathing techniques recognized as especially beneficial are diaphragmatic and pursed-lip breathing (Figure 9-6 AB, Boxes 9-1 and 9-2).

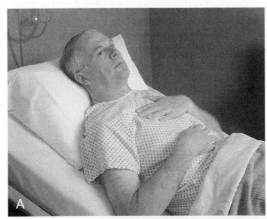

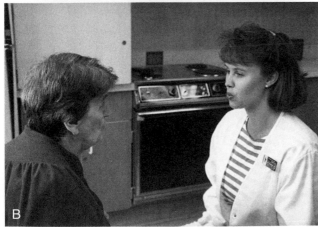

FIGURE 9-6   A. Client practicing diaphragmatic breathing; **B.** OT teaching pursed lip breathing. (From deWitt, S., et al. [2013]. *Fundamental concepts and skills for nursing* [4th ed.]. St. Louis, MO: Saunders.)

| **BOX 9-1** | **Steps in Teaching Diaphragmatic Breathing** |

Assist the client in identifying a comfortable, quiet place to sit or lie down, and instruct as follows:
1. Observe your breathing:
   - First, take a normal breath.
   - Next, try taking a slow, deep breath. The air coming in through your nose should move downward into your lower belly. Let your abdomen expand fully.
   - Now breathe out through your mouth (or your nose, if that feels more natural).
   - Take normal and deep breaths several times. Pay attention to how you feel when you inhale and exhale normally and when you breathe deeply. (Note that shallow breathing often feels tense and constricted, whereas deep breathing produces relaxation).
2. Practice diaphragmatic breathing for several minutes:
   - Put one hand on your abdomen, just below your belly button. Feel your hand rise about an inch each time you inhale and fall about an inch each time you exhale.
   - Your chest will rise slightly, too, together with your abdomen. Remember to relax your belly so that each inhalation expands it fully.
3. Breath focus practice: Once you've tried the previous steps, you can regularly practice *breath focus*.
   - Sit comfortably with your eyes closed and breathe while thinking of something you enjoy and a word or phrase that will help you relax.
   - Imagine that the air you breathe in brings peace and calm into your body. As you inhale, try saying to yourself: "Breathing in peace and calm."
   - When you breathe out, imagine that the air leaving your body carries tension and anxiety away with it. As you exhale, say: "Breathing out tension and anxiety."
   - Try 10 minutes of breath focus at first, and gradually add time until your breathing focus sessions are 15 to 20 minutes long.

Adapted from Take a deep breath. (2009, May). Retrieved from http://www.health.harvard.edu/staying-healthy/take-a-deep-breath.)

These techniques improve ventilation by releasing air that is trapped in the lungs, keeping the airways open longer, decreasing breathing demands, slowing the rate of breathing, relieving SOB, and fostering client relaxation.[15]

A third technique is lower rib breathing. This is achieved by having the client apply her or his own hands on either side of the lower section of the rib cage; with each expiration this force provides some tactile resistance that allows the ribs to expand during inspiration. Finally, relaxation techniques, such as progressive muscle relaxation, can be performed via a series of isometric contractions that are held for 7 to 10 seconds, followed by relaxation for 20 to 40 seconds.

Upper extremity muscle wasting also may accompany pulmonary diseases, resulting from disuse and the effects of prolonged steroid utilization.[44] A meta-analysis of randomized

Encourage the client to use this technique during parts of any strenuous activity (e.g., bending, lifting, stair climbing, walking more briskly, etc.), and instruct as follows:

- First, find a comfortable sitting position and relax your neck and shoulder muscles.
- Breathing normally, inhale slowly through your nose for two counts, keeping your mouth closed. It may help to count to yourself: inhale, one, two.
- Pucker (purse) your lips as if you were going to whistle or gently blow at a candle flame.
- Breathe out slowly and gently (exhale) through your pursed lips while counting to four. It may help to count to yourself: exhale, one, two, three, four.
- Practice this technique four to five times a day at first so you can get the correct breathing pattern; with regular practice, this breathing technique will seem natural to you.

(Adapted from Asthma. [2015, June]. Retrieved from http://www.lung.org/associations/states/minnesota/events-programs/mn-copd-coalition/patient-toolkit/coughingand-breathing.pdf and What to expect during pulmonary rehabilitation. [2015, June]. Retrieved http://www.nhlbi.nih.gov/health/health-topics/topics/pulreh/during).

control trials on unsupported upper extremity exercise (UUEE) and its effect on dyspnea concluded that "UUEE can relieve dyspnea and arm fatigue in clients with COPD during ADLs."[41] Also, a study by Costi et al. found that "unsupported upper extremity exercise training improved functional exercise capacity of patients with COPD."[13] Traditional means for OT to incorporate upper extremity exercise is through use of free weights, Therabands, or other forms of progressive resistive exercises. This approach would require careful attention to blood pressure, hypertension, pulmonary distress, and oxygen saturation levels; however, if within the physician-prescribed parameters, upper extremity exercise is recommended and beneficial.

Energy conservation and work simplification strategies, as discussed in the cardiovascular section, are critical components of interventions with clients with COPD. Part of this approach would include evaluation of work sites, including the client's home, to determine the need for adaptive equipment or environmental modifications. Finally, clients with COPD may benefit from stress management in conjunction with breathing technique instruction. Evidence for support for stress management for this population is found in an article by Cafarella et al., who noted, "In COPD, anxiety has been linked to greater disability, an increased frequency of hospital admissions for acute exacerbations and dyspnea."[12] A meta-analysis of trials with relaxation therapy in patients with COPD found statistically significant beneficial effects on both dyspnea and psychological well-being.[18] Cafarella et al. stated, "relaxation therapy encompasses breathing exercises, progressive muscle relaxation, biofeedback and meditation."[10] Using these techniques can help the client relax and better manage the physical and physiologic changes that can occur during a stressful situation.

As for cardiovascular conditions, OT interventions with respiratory conditions should also generally aim for including work simplification, energy conservation, and body mechanics strategies, such as the following:

1. Balance rest and work by allowing time to complete a task before becoming fatigued, or taking frequent rest periods during activities.
2. Ensure adequate ventilation at home by turning on the exhaust fan when cooking, having windows open, and using portable fans during the summer in homes without air conditioning.
3. Prioritize all tasks to reduce demands on the respiratory muscles.
4. Whenever possible, do not carry objects; instead slide them across the table or counter, use a multi-pocket apron, work in a sitting position, and have a cart on wheels to carry multiple items.
5. Shop by phone or online and use the related delivery services.
6. Avoid reaching and overhead movements by prearranging items that are frequently needed.
7. Use equipment with long handles for dustpans, sponges, squeegees, or any home care product.
8. Reduce steam during showering by turning on an exhaust fan, opening the bathroom window, opening the bathroom door (if possible), taking short showers, and running cold water before the hot water is turned on.
9. Use a bath seat during showers to conserve energy and a shower caddy within easy reach for shampoo, soap, and accessories (Figure 9-7).
10. Avoid spray cleaners, which may irritate bronchial airways.

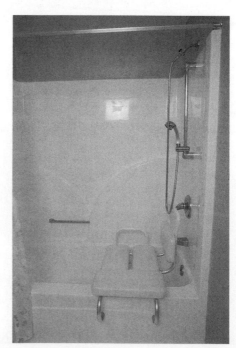

FIGURE 9-7 Shower bench, handheld shower head, and grab bar assist the weak patient. (From Monahan, F., et al. [2007]. *Phipps' medical-surgical nursing: Health and illness perspectives* [8th ed.]. St. Louis, MO: Mosby.)

11. To support lung function, exhale when bending or flexing at the trunk.
12. Select clothes to be worn the next day the night before, or gather all clothes for that day in one trip.
13. Wear loose clothes that allow the chest and abdomen to expand, and dress legs and feet first, because this requires the most energy.
14. Use long-handled dressing equipment, such as a dressing stick, long-handle shoe horn, and/or long-handle reacher, to conserve energy and prevent exhaustion during an activity/ADL (Figures 9-8).
15. Keep one's hairstyle simple to reduce energy expenditure.

All of these recommendations clarify a number of ways that aging clients can be taught to simplify their lifestyle when they have respiratory diseases.

Genitourinary System

The following list describes normal aging-related changes in genitourinary system structures and functions:

- Kidneys decrease in volume, size, and adaptability.
- Nephrons and tubules decrease in number, size, and function, and the concentrating and diluting functions of the kidneys are reduced. These changes may promote renal failure, especially in older adults with hypertension, diabetes mellitus, and dehydration.
- The bladder muscle weakens, with a decline in the ability to postpone voiding. Individuals younger than 65 have a bladder capacity of 500 ml to 600 ml; those older than 65 have a bladder capacity of 250 ml to 600 ml. Younger people have a sensation to void when the bladder is more

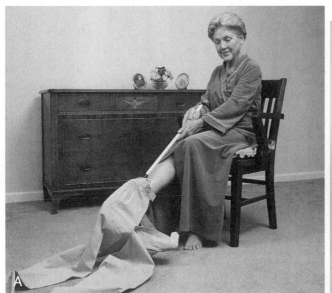
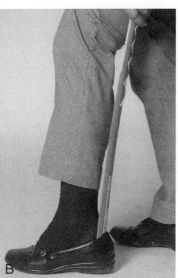
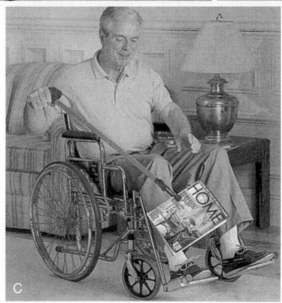

FIGURE 9-8 Collapsible dressing stick (A), long shoe horn (B), and long-handled reacher (C). ([A] Courtesy North Coast Medical Inc., [B] From Daley, T., et al. The role of occupational therapy in the care of the older adult. *Clinics in Geriatric Medicine*, 22(2), 281-290. [C] From Monahan, F., et al. [2007]. *Phipps' medical-surgical nursing: Health and illness perspectives* [8th ed.]. St. Louis, MO: Mosby.)

than half full, but older adults may have a reduction in sensation, resulting in sensing the bladder much later when the bladder is nearly full, or not at all, which can cause overflow incontinence.

- Glomeruli decrease in number; humans typically have 1 million glomeruli before age 40 and 700,000 at age 65.
- Creatinine clearance decreases with age, but creatinine levels change minimally because of the reduction in overall body muscle mass.
- Prostate hyperplasia increases with age and leads to urinary retention. Men aged 80 and over have a more than 90% chance of developing benign prostatic hyperplasia. This is due to the increased concentration of dihydrotestosterone in prostatic cells. Also, prostate cancer risk increases as males age.
- Maximum urethral closure pressure declines in both men and women with age.
- With age, the external and internal genitalia atrophy in males and females:
  - Females experience diminished secretions, thinning vaginal tissue, delayed arousal, and shorter orgasm; some experience decreased libido, which can be treated.
  - Males experience increased time in achieving erection, difficulty maintaining erection, and delayed ejaculation.[32]

During initial evaluations with older adult clients, occupational therapists and assistants should routinely include sexuality/sexual function and participation within an ADL/IADL assessment. Inclusion of this topic will allow for timely discussion, should the aging adult have questions or concerns. As with any other adult age group, occupational therapists can discreetly adapt client sexual participation approaches according to individual physical abilities and preferences.

The myth that incontinence is a part of normal aging can prevent older adults from seeking treatment for this treatable condition.[24] Occupational therapists who have specialized or advanced training in evaluating and providing interventions for urinary incontinence and pelvic floor disorders are valuable in addressing these treatable diagnoses. The occupational therapist provides a functional assessment and interviews the client or caregiver about the habits, routines, and behaviors of the client to analyze what factors may contribute to the etiology of the incontinence. The context in which the incontinence occurs is examined, as well as activity demands, to facilitate thorough inclusion of essential factors for a client-centered approach and a comprehensive evaluation. Occupational therapists with advanced training may decide a pelvic floor muscle (PFM) assessment is necessary to determine the cause of the incontinence.

Assessment of the strength, tone, isolation, and coordination of the pelvic floor muscles may be conducted. If indicated, the occupational therapist instructs the client in strength, endurance, and PFM coordination and relaxation as well as inhibition of problematic motor responses. Another technique that may be included is electromyography (EMG), or biofeedback, in addition to a home exercise program, if the individual is seen as an outpatient. For successful continence, the client can be instructed to concentrate on increasing times between toileting, thus using behavioral skills to avoid rushing to the toilet. Bladder training has been documented to reduce incontinence by at least 50%. These techniques may include increasing bladder storage capacity and changing behaviors or habits to extend the client's ability to resist voiding immediately, spreading the demand over a longer period. Other individuals may need to be trained to void more often, due to a larger-than-normal bladder, through the use of timed toileting techniques (self-cuing methods to ensure the toilet is used at specific intervals during waking hours).[19,24,40,46] Case Example 9-1 demonstrates an OT approach to urinary incontinence/overactive bladder.

Gastrointestinal System

Aging-related changes in the gastrointestinal system may be normal or pathologic, and are typically challenging to differentiate.[32] Furthermore, the changes that do occur typically do not affect gastrointestinal function in significant ways. The following are typical aging-related changes:

- Oral cavity: Changes in the oral cavity, including the teeth, soft tissues, salivary glands, mandible and joints, and taste buds, can affect appearance, nutrition, and resulting overall quality of life.[32]

CASE EXAMPLE 9-1: Urinary Incontinence/Overactive Bladder

Irene is a 72-year-old woman who was referred to occupational therapy for bladder urgency, urinary frequency, and urinary incontinence (UI). In the months before her referral her problem had gradually worsened, and her fear of having an incontinent episode in public had caused her to become homebound. Irene also had constipation, which affected her quality of life and contributed to her UI. The occupational therapist educated Irene on the role of diet and suggested that she reduce her caffeine intake and increase her dietary fiber. PFM reeducation was provided. As Irene gained better control of her pelvic floor muscles, she was taught how to inhibit bladder urges, particularly when she was out in the community when shopping, socializing with friends, attending church, or participating in other activities. She was also taught how to relax her pelvic floor muscles during a bowel movement. Over the course of therapy, Irene's bowel patterns became more regular and she was able to control her bladder urges, significantly reducing her urinary frequency and incontinence. As Irene's bladder control improved, she had the confidence to resume shopping on a more regular basis, attend church services, and engage in community activities. Also important to her overall health status and well-being, she was able to resume her twice-weekly exercise group.[19]

- Esophagus: The esophagus demonstrates decreased peristalsis (e.g., muscle contractions post-swallowing), with less sphincter function, which leads to increased transit time and potential for reflux. These changes may result in dysphagia and/or achalasia.
- Stomach: Delayed emptying of fluids and reduced production of hydrochloric acid increase the incidence of atrophic gastritis and hypergastrinemia, which can lead to premalignant lesions.
- Small intestine: Changes in the small intestine include increased absorption of vitamin A; reduced absorption of vitamin D, calcium, and zinc; and decline in lactase activity. Drug metabolism decreases with age because of the decrease in smooth endoplasmic reticulum.
- Large intestine: Changes in the large intestine include slower transit rate, decreased anal sphincter tone and strength, and less rectal compliance. These factors may lead to chronic constipation, the potential etiology for diverticulosis. Fecal incontinence may also occur and is one of the most psychologically traumatic experiences in older adults. Colon cancer risk also increases with aging.
- Pancreas, liver, gallbladder: Changes in these organs include reduced rate of blood flow and secretions, and enlargement of the bile duct, with an increase in cholelithiasis (30% of individuals older than 70).

Occupational therapists may use a similar approach for individuals with symptoms of bowel incontinence as for clients with urinary incontinence (see earlier example), always individualizing the approach to meet the individual client's needs.

Endocrine System

The basic function of the endocrine system, comprised of glands and organs, is to produce and secrete hormones.[9,29] Aging-related changes include the following:
- Pituitary gland: Changes in the pituitary gland affect several hormones:
  - Growth hormone: After age 30, a decline of approximately 15% per decade results in decreased lean body mass, resulting in increased fat mass, decreased bone density, and a general decrease in muscle mass.
  - Thyroid-stimulating hormone (TSH): Decline in production occurs with age.
  - Gonadotrophic hormones: Changes in gonadotrophic hormones affect the mammary glands, adrenal cortex, ovaries, and testes. Glandular tissue in female breasts is replaced by fibrous connective tissue; males may develop gynecomastia due to decreased testosterone production.
  - Estrogen: Decreased production with menopause precipitates bone mineral density changes, (e.g., osteopenia and osteoporosis) in women, and increases risk of fractures, especially in women.
- Thyroid gland: Limited changes occur with age, resulting in adequate function; parathyroid glands diminish in efficiency.

- Adrenal glands: Fundamental functions are generally intact.
- Pancreas: Changes include dilated pancreatic duct, slowing of enzyme and bicarbonate secretion, and decrease in insulin production. As adipose (fat) cells increase, insulin receptors decrease in quantity. These circumstances lead to type II diabetes mellitus (adult-onset hyperglycemia) in 15% to 25% of the older population in the United States.[9,29]

When working with clients with diabetes, occupational therapy personnel should be aware of the symptoms of hypoglycemia (low blood sugar level) and hyperglycemia (high blood sugar level).

Hypoglycemia can present with confusion, headache, lassitude, drowsiness, shallow respirations, tremulousness, anger, and nausea. To raise the blood sugar level, as soon as possible the individual should be given orange juice, candy, soda, a teaspoon of honey, or one amp of D50 or glucagon, if seen in a hospital setting. *Hyperglycemia* can present with fast and deep breathing, heartburn, excessive urination, nausea, headaches, blurred vision, constipation, and abdominal pain, and coma in diabetic ketoacidosis. If OT personnel observe symptoms of either hypoglycemia or hyperglycemia during a therapy session, these should be reported, so that appropriate action can be taken.

While working with persons who are diabetic, avoid any likelihood of injuries, because individuals with this diagnosis are more prone to infection and ulcers. For those who receive insulin injections at sites where they are receiving occupational therapy, the insulin may metabolize faster and the client can develop hyperglycemia. Clients with diabetes can also develop hypoglycemia after a therapy session if all the glucose is utilized during the session. Occupational therapists and assistants should review each client's chart for recent accuchecks and times of medication administration (Box 9-3).

Finally, as previously indicated, OT personnel can educate on energy conservation, work simplification, and time management, based upon the individual's priority activities. Note the OT Interventions: Overall Aging-Sensitive Approaches section for fundamental intervention approaches.

Integumentary System

Generally, more than any other organ system, the skin reflects the aging process. Changes in the hair, skin, and nails are typically apparent in aging adults.[9,32] Both intrinsic and extrinsic factors influence rates and degree of changes that occur on an individual basis. Intrinsic factors reflect genetic influences on aging, whereas extrinsic factors reflect environmental influences and lifestyle habits. *Photoaging*, for example, is a term referring to the cumulative changes related to the degree of environmental exposure and type of skin pigment.[32] The following list is a summary of aging-related skin changes that may influence occupational performance and overall well-being.
- Epidermis:
  - Thins in protected areas and thickens in unprotected (sun-exposed) areas; the turnover rate of epidermal cells declines 30% to 50% by age 80.

| BOX 9-3 | Intervention Tips for Clients with Diabetes Mellitus |

1. Encourage the client to monitor his or her blood sugar before and after exercise or any strenuous activity. If there are any symptoms of hyperglycemia or hypoglycemia, the client should check his or her blood sugar or obtain medical assistance.
2. Assist in insulin regulation and glucose control by increasing the client's strength, endurance, range of motion, and activity tolerance.
3. Provide aerobic exercise programming and graded upper extremity occupation-based activities that are meaningful to the client.
4. A client with a below-the-knee amputation as a result of diabetes should be reassured that she or he will receive a posterior knee conformer as soon as possible to minimize potential joint contractures.
5. Teach clients the importance of personal monitoring of the following:
   a. Check for sensory problems (e.g., changes in/decreased sensation), especially in the lower extremities.
   b. Inspect feet daily with a mirror; any cuts, abrasions, or openings should be reported for immediate medical attention. Until the client sees a healthcare provider, the client should apply triple antibiotic ointment and dry dressings.
   c. Wash feet daily in warm water, do not walk barefooted, use socks with no holes, and change socks daily.
   d. Keep toenails trimmed straight across; do not cut calluses or corns.
6. Clients may benefit from specially made shoes to prevent diabetic ulcers. Clients should wear wide-fitted shoes, and break in new shoes slowly.
7. Clients should be taught diabetic-related safety factors regarding the use of a stove and the importance of maintaining the water temperature not higher than 110 degrees, to prevent burns.
8. Any diet-related instructions provided to client

- Injured skin takes longer to repair, and sensitivity is decreased; in immobile individuals, an increased risk of decubitus ulcers occurs with aging.
- Dermis: The dermis contains blood vessels, nerves, glands, and hair follicles, with collagen comprising 79%. This layer thins with age, fostering fine and coarse wrinkles, and skin laxity, and making sedentary individuals more susceptible to decubitus ulcers.
- Glands: Sebaceous and sweat glands decrease production.
- Hair: Typically associated with the aging process are changes in color, growth, and distribution, especially changes to gray or white.
- Nails: With aging, nails become brittle, dull, dense, and thick, due to diminished blood supply to the nailbeds.

The incidence of skin disorders with aging is estimated to range between 40% and 70% of individuals, and may be either hereditary or related to other factors. Some disorders (e.g., diabetes, gout, liver disease, malignancies) foster skin disorders, as do some neurologic, metabolic, and vascular disorders. Environmental factors such as housing, neighborhood, and work setting may also contribute to the development of skin disorders. Pruritus, generalized itching, is very common in aging adults, and may be caused by internal, external, or psychological factors.[32]

Occupational therapists and assistants working with aging adults can encourage their clients to take measures to alleviate skin-related problems. Strategies to improve skin dryness and itching include reducing frequency of bathing, using nonirritating lotions and emollients, applying lubricants to moisten lips, and taking protective measures when environmental exposure is likely.

Musculoskeletal System

Note that Chapter 8, Musculoskeletal System, provides a comprehensive discussion of aging-related changes in the musculoskeletal system and related OT interventions. This chapter provides a supplemental discussion of topics that are pertinent to understanding physiologic aspects of aging in a comprehensive way.

Traditionally, occupational therapy will begin interventions for clients with orthopedic issues with a comprehensive OT evaluation. This would include an occupational profile and assessment of ROM, strength, hand and wrist function, skin changes, and the effects of any of these factors on performance of ADL/IADL. In addition, special considerations should be taken during the initial session with the client. These might include discussion and documentation of morning stiffness, if present, and its effects; percentages of "good days to bad days"; fatigue; and pain, both with and without activity with and without medication management. Initial documentation of the client's reports in each of these areas can be useful in determining the effectiveness of intervention strategies and improvement or decline in quality of life. Other areas that should be discussed or visually evaluated by the therapist or assistant with the client include:

- Body and extremity positioning at night and during leisure/work activities
- Use and height of seats in typically used spaces at home and work (if this applies)
- Amount of stair climbing required to access typically used environments (e.g., home and work; if this applies)
- Typical use and heights of work surfaces
- Need for and access to public versus private transportation
- Quality of mattress and pillow
- Current adaptive equipment and how it is currently being utilized

Immediate intervention strategies will be different within each realm of occupation for the client, depending on the stage or process that the client is currently experiencing. If the client is in an inflammatory stage of arthritis, for example, he or she will present with swollen and painful periarticular or extraarticular joints, making the need to reduce edema a priority (Figure 9-9).

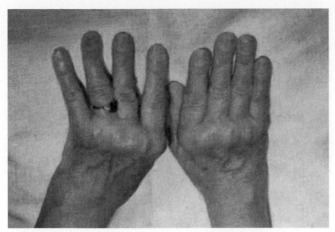

FIGURE 9-9   Rheumatoid arthritis of hands. (From Christensen, B. L., et al. [2010]. *Adult health nursing* [6th ed.]. St. Louis, MO: Mosby.)

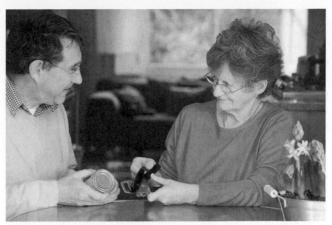

FIGURE 9-10   The OT practitioner shows a woman, who has arthritis, how to protect her joints while opening a can. Photo © istock.com

Reduction of stressors and proper positioning during ADL/IADL participation through incorporating adaptive strategies can help to reduce pain and potential deformity development. Typically, orthotic management is a useful intervention at this stage. Orthoses for osteoarthritis (OA) and rheumatoid arthritis (RA) are frequently used to decrease pain, minimize deformities, decrease inflammation, decrease stress to the joints, provide support for increased function, and assist with joint stability.[8]

Use of orthotics for reducing inflammation and protecting unstable joints during occupational performance is one method for eliminating joint stress; however, joint protection strategies should also be introduced and incorporated into the intervention process. "Joint protection and energy conservation tie in with basic science by understanding the process that occurs at the joint cartilage when joints are under prolonged stress."[8] Both for clients with OA and those with RA the stressors of performing everyday tasks in the usual way may aggravate the processes and hasten the destruction of joints. Evaluating the approach the client uses to open containers, carry items, and perform basic ADLs can facilitate collaboration in adapting these daily tasks to protect the joints, eliminate pain, and increase independence (Figure 9-10).

Therapeutic exercise programs for aging adults with OA and RA must always consider the amount of joint stability, muscle atrophy, and inflammation, if present.[7] Exercise recommendations and use of physical agent modalities (PAMs) in the treatment of arthritic conditions are common in OT practice. Because many clients with RA and OA report that beginning their day with a warm shower or bath results in temporary neuromuscular effects that decrease pain and muscle tension,[20] the occupational therapist or assistant may recommend bathing before engaging in exercise. Traditionally, exercise includes gentle active ROM (AROM), gentle progressive resistive exercises, and no- or low-impact aerobic activities. Careful attention to all symptoms and disease processes and individualization of program development are suggested for effective incorporation of exercise programs into the intervention of clients with arthritic conditions. Additionally, occupational therapists and assistants should ensure that their recommendations for exercise are balanced with the desired meaningful occupations that the individual pursues on a regular basis, to support optimal client quality of life.

Arthritis is a chronic condition that can benefit from the self-management strategies suggested earlier in this chapter. Lorig and Holman[33] designed the Arthritis Self-Management Program (ASMP), which incorporates components of the Chronic Care Model (CCM). The ASMP approach, to increase participants' perceptions of arthritis self-efficacy, is defined as perceived ability to control or manage various aspects of arthritis and was implemented in the United Kingdom in a randomized control study of the ASMP.[4] The program includes 6 weekly educational sessions of 2 hours each, led by mentor leaders, most of whom have arthritis. The topics for each session include the following:[4]

- General information about arthritis, and differentiated types
- Overview of self-management principles
- Rationale and implementation guidelines for exercise
- Cognitive symptom management, including relaxation and coping strategies
- Nutrition and health
- Strategies for communication with family and health-care providers
- Resources for various approaches and utilization

The results of this randomized control study demonstrated that at 4 and 12 month follow-ups, the ASMP was effective in terms of improving perceptions of control (i.e., arthritis self-efficacy), use of self-management techniques (e.g., cognitive symptom management, communication with physicians, and exercise), and health status (e.g., decreased fatigue, anxiousness, and depressed mood; and increased positive mood).[4] Therefore, successful OT intervention with clients who have been diagnosed with an arthritic condition should include exposure to traditional OT approaches and incorporation of a self-management program for long-term benefits and increased participation in occupation.

Neurologic System

This section provides an overview of aging-related changes in the brain and other neurologic system changes, to supplement the information provided in Chapter 10 on low vision, Chapter 14 on cognitive executive function, Chapter 15 on cognitive impairment and dementia, and Chapter 16 on mental health and psychiatry. Additionally, readers are encouraged to supplement their understanding with textbooks that focus on the anatomy and physiology of the nervous system, as well as general rehabilitation approaches utilized in OT services. To summarize, whenever one is working with an older adult with diagnosed or undiagnosed neurologic challenges, standard OT evaluation and intervention approaches should always holistically consider aging-related factors that contribute to the client's status, well-being, and overall quality of life. Structural changes in the nervous system result in declines in reaction time, lower nerve conduction velocity, and longer muscle action potentials. Additionally, the automatic functions of the central nervous system (CNS) are less efficient and the ability to maintain homeostasis is reduced; therefore, recovery from stress is affected, with extremes of cold, heat, and exercise especially presenting challenges[39] (Boxes 9-4 and 9-5).

For optimal outcomes, occupational therapy personnel should consider these age-related neurologic changes as they observe, evaluate, and intervene with each older client, taking immediate action if they represent high risk to the client. For some conditions, collaboration with or referral to other disciplines may ensure the best results and support for the OT client.

Occupational Therapy Interventions: Overall Aging-Sensitive Approaches

Occupational therapists are trained in providing treatment to persons who have incurred injury or disease affecting the neurologic system. Older adults are disproportionately represented in the population for impairments related to the diagnoses of Parkinson's disease, stroke, and dementia (including Alzheimer's disease). Older adults may also be seen for neurologic impairments caused by spinal cord or traumatic brain injury resulting from motor vehicle accidents and falls. The

treatment provided is customized to the needs of the individual, and consideration of comorbidities is essential, age notwithstanding. When clients have multiple conditions or impairments, the focus of treatment is on the multiple systems affected by the conditions or injuries as related to maximizing client independence and function.[44]

A thorough evaluation should be conducted to determine the older client's status. The individual's somatosensory, perception, and visuoperceptual performance and perception of position in space are assessed, and related interventions are included during OT intervention. When measuring older adults' visuoperceptual performance (e.g., using the Occupational Therapy Cognitive Assessment[26]) post-stroke, the clinician must be aware of any variance in performance that may be correlated to age.[36] Each assessment may vary according to subtests used, and thus it is important for the clinician to be mindful of aging-related factors when administering and interpreting results. The client's years of education can correlate with many subtests. Thus age and education should be considered as factors that may affect performance on tests, such as the Test of Visual-Perceptual Skills (TVPS),[34] during cognitive assessment.

Issues Regarding Self-Management of Chronic Illness

Physiologic changes that are more frequently observed in older adults may cause impairments in occupational performance that result in a physician's referral for a client to see an occupational therapist in a number of types of settings. An increase in symptoms may cause the client to be admitted to an acute care facility, or the combination of these symptoms in conjunction with another disease process may require the client to have extended inpatient, outpatient, or home-based therapy. These changes and chronic components of the disease process demand that the therapist incorporate self-management strategies into the treatment to allow for optimal quality of life for the client. Self-management of chronic illness implies that the patient/client is monitoring and managing symptoms, adhering to treatment regimens, keeping a healthy lifestyle, and managing the effects of the illness on daily functioning, emotions, and social relationships.[31,33,35,45]

The traditional approach of health-care providers treating clients with chronic illness, although well intentioned, fails to afford optimal clinical care or meet clients' needs to be effective self-managers of their illness.[14,32] For example, the traditional approach for working with a client with hypertension (HTN) is comprised of prescription and explanation of secondary prevention medication, explanation of stroke and risk factors, and possibly a discussion of lifestyle modification.[23] Gillham and Endacott[21] suggest that addressing lifestyle change has not been routinely and consistently implemented by health-care providers, with discussion of lifestyle recorded in only 37% of consultations, and with questionable effectiveness in improving self-reported lifestyle-related risk factors. The health-care provider working with clients with chronic conditions such as those described in this chapter must act as a teacher and collaborator in defining how to work with the

---

> **BOX 9-4**   Key Aging-Related Neurologic Changes
>
> - Neurons and glial cells: Structural changes and gradual decline in numbers
> - Synapses: Increased size, decrease in overall number
> - Nerve cells: Decreased lipids, increased accumulation of lipofuscin granules, differing signaling pathways
> - Muscles: Decline in muscle strength (due to decreased muscle mass), movement speed, and endurance; muscular vascular changes
>
> (From Millsap, P. [2007]. Neurological system. In A. Linton & H. Lach [Eds.], *Matteson & McConnell's gerontological nursing: Concepts and practice* [pp. 406-412]. St. Louis, MO: Saunders Elsevier.)

BOX 9-5   Aging-Related Changes That Affect Occupational Performance

- Reaction time: Slower cognitively and physically; however, same performance on psychomotor testing as younger adults
- Proprioception: Potential postural instability and falls; changes in joint-position sense during movement, but not at rest
- Balance: Postural control is affected by changes in sensory, motor, and CNS function, and often affected by a decrease in sensory cues and righting-reflex ability.
- Dizziness: Occurs when multiple sensory inputs are insufficient, uncoordinated, and not integrated well and is the most frequent complaint of adults 75 years and older. Spinning sensations (vertigo), light-headedness (presyncope), persistent unsteadiness (disequilibrium), and nonspecific dizziness are common forms.
- Syncope: This transient loss of consciousness and postural tone accompanies chronic conditions with associated medication use.
- Orthostatic hypotension: Changes in position from supine to standing position can precipitate a 20-mm Hg drop in systolic blood pressure or a 10-mm Hg drop in diastolic blood pressure. This condition may cause syncopal episodes and is typically caused by blood pooling in the lower extremities.
- Motor activity: Posture, movement, and reflexes are altered with aging.
  - Gait changes in men reflect a wide base and shorter steps, and a narrower base for women, sometimes described as "waddling."

- Benign essential tremor of the upper extremities, neck, and voice are common among older adults and are not related to Parkinson's disease.
- Thermoregulation: Older adults experience decreased homeostatic regulation.
  - Hypothermia: Early signs include apathy, confusion, cool skin, fatigue, and shivering.
  - Hyperthermia: Annually, approximately 3500 U.S. adults over age 60 die of heatstroke. Heat exhaustion symptoms include diarrhea, dizziness, dyspnea, feeling warm, headache, nausea, and vomiting; heatstroke symptoms include delirium, psychosis, loss of consciousness, and hot and dry skin.
- Sleep disturbance: More than 50% of adults over age 65 experience changes in their patterns of sleep; insomnia is the most frequent aging-related sleep complaint. Typical aging-related changes in the sleep cycle include lighter, more easily interrupted sleep, with more time spent in the lightest sleep stage (e.g., non-rapid-eye-movement [NREM] sleep) and less time in deeper/deepest sleep, which is the most restorative type of sleep. Rapid-eye-movement (REM) sleep time occurs earlier in the older person's sleep cycle as compared with younger adults. Comorbidities may affect sleep patterns, as may medications, smoking, and/or napping during the day or evening.

(From Millsap, P. [2007]. Neurological system. In A. Linton & H. Lach [Eds.] *Matteson & McConnell's gerontological nursing: Concepts and practice* [pp. 406-412]. St. Louis, MO: Saunders Elsevier.)

---

client to control the condition while optimizing the potential for participation in activities and occupations that are relevant and meaningful. The crux of appropriate care for chronic disease is a partnership between clients and health professionals in management over a period of time.[27]

In this partnership, health-care providers, such as occupational therapists, use self-management as a means to introduce and educate clients on managing health-behavior change.[16] The Chronic Care Model (CCM)[4] and the Expanded Chronic Care Model (ECCM)[4] are models that can guide this management. The CCM utilizes a "synthesis of evidence-based system changes intended as a guide to quality improvement and disease management activities."[4] The Expanded Chronic Care Model "broadens the CCM by directing additional efforts to reducing the burden of chronic disease, not just by reducing the impact on those who have a disease but also by supporting people and communities to be healthy."[5] Each of these models is grounded in behavior change theory and emphasizes the importance of including self-management education into a behavior change approach. According to the CCM, self-management interventions "emphasize the patient's crucial role in maintaining health and function and the importance of setting goals, establishing action plans, identifying barriers, and solving problems to

overcome barriers."[4] Lorig and Holman[33] created the Chronic Disease Self-Management Program (CDSMP) that outlines tasks and skills necessary to best manage chronic conditions. According to Trombly and Radomski,[41] "In basic and instrumental activities of daily living, the therapist helps the patient attain safety, maximum independence in priority activities, acceptance and optimal use of equipment, and energy-conservation participation." The collaborative self-management process described in the CDSMP can successfully address each of these issues.

A critical component of self-management is the use of a client-driven action plan. *Living a Healthy Life with Chronic Conditions*, a component of the CDSMP, uses an action plan that calls for a specific action or set of actions an individual can realistically expect to accomplish.[35] Action planning is seen to be a key variable in the volitional phase that influences the intention–behavior relationship.[11] Taking action involves getting people actively involved in behavior change.[33] The action plan involves a period of 1 or 2 weeks, and the targeted behavior must be very specific. For example, "This week I will walk around the block once before lunch on Monday, Tuesday, and Thursday." Next, it should be realistic or "doable." This means that the person should be able to achieve the behavior in that 1- to 2-week time frame. Finally, it should be something that the person is fairly confident he or she can accomplish.[33] Therapists might incorporate both self-management education and action planning into a therapy program.

Additional Intervention Strategies

Each section of this chapter highlights the increasing challenges that individuals must address for healthy aging. Despite older adults' declines in a variety of capacity areas, OT interventions can provide methods for clients to continue functioning in all meaningful life roles. However subtle, cumulative decline can increase the risk for devastating interruption of the ability to participate in meaningful occupations. For example, approximately 30% of people over 65 years of age living in the community fall each year.[22] This concern is highlighted here, and more information may be found in Chapter 24 on acute care. Falls in nursing care facilities and hospitals are common events that cause considerable morbidity and mortality for older people.[13] New recommendations for fall prevention by the American Geriatrics Society (AGS) and the British Geriatrics Society (BGS) were released in 2010. These recommendations include "assessment of ADL skills (including use of adaptive equipment and mobility aids); assessment of the individual's perceived functional ability and fear related to falling; and environmental assessment, including home safety; using exercise to improve strength, balance, and gait; managing medications, managing postural hypotension, and recommendations for appropriate footwear and existing foot problems."[21]

The *Occupational Therapy Practice Framework*[1] provides a guide for how these recommendations fit within the scope of OT practice. According to Jensen and Padilla, "Occupational therapy practitioners have a special opportunity for prevention and intervention because they are educated in the assessment and treatment of many of the factors associated with falls."[25] The March/April 2012 issue of the *American Journal of Occupational Therapy* was dedicated to occupational therapy's role in prevention of falls in the older population. A systematic review by Gillespie et al.[20] reported on two specific areas of intervention that were effective in decreasing the risk for falls. First of these was "exercise-based interventions that included two or more motor performance skills (e.g., balance, strengthening, endurance)," as well as "participation in group exercise, *Tai Chi*, and individually tailored home exercise programs" (Figure 9-11).[20]

Occupational therapists traditionally incorporate endurance, upper extremity strengthening, and balance exercises within treatment, and home exercise programs. The second recommendation by Gillespie et al. was for "home safety assessment and modification interventions"; they also noted that "these approaches were more effective when delivered by an occupational therapist."[20]

Occupational therapists are trained to evaluate functional capacity using a multifaceted approach that assesses all client and environmental factors that affect occupational performance. Thorough assessment and home modification, including adaptive equipment recommendation and training, assist older clients in reducing their risk of falling. "Common recommendations for home modification are to remove mats and throw rugs, to change footwear and to use nonslip bathmats."[17] Optimally, whenever possible, a thorough environmental assessment should be conducted, to include all usual and customary places where the client participates (e.g., home, neighborhood, etc.).

Prescription and training in the use of adaptive equipment are methods occupational therapy personnel use to enhance

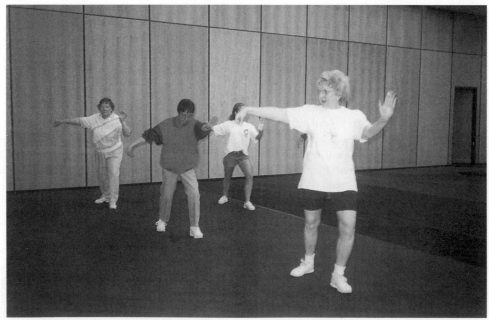

FIGURE 9-11 Older adults participating in a tai chi class. (From Deutsch, J., & Anderson, E. [2008]. *Complementary therapies for physical therapy: A clinical decision-making approach.* St. Louis, MO: Saunders.)

and maintain the occupational performance of older adults.[28] Typical adaptive equipment that occupational therapy practitioners recommend include bedside commodes, raised toilet seats, bath or shower benches and grab bars, and nonskid mats.[44] Additional equipment may be warranted, depending on the individual's specific conditions and preferences. Sufficient client and caregiver/support system training is necessary for successful use of this equipment. As with any prescribed tool, the therapist or assistant must ensure that clients and caregivers, if indicated, understand the purpose of the equipment and are safely independent in its use within the setting(s) in which the equipment will be utilized.

Occupational therapy practitioners should be mindful of fall potential when working with any individual; however, in older clients the results of a fall may affect health more significantly. According to the National Council on Aging, falls are the leading cause of both fatal and nonfatal injuries for people aged 65+.[40] Treatment/intervention focus areas can include:

- Fall-prevention assessment risk
- Interventions to reduce risk factors
- Evaluation of home and environment
- Recommendations for adaption or modification of the environment
- Education and training in adaptive equipment

The National Council on Aging[38] is a useful resource for occupational therapy personnel and for clients and family members. An example of one resource is "6 Steps to Protect your Older Loved One from a Fall." This consumer-friendly resource outlines simple, commonsense strategies that an occupational therapy personnel can review with a client and use as an adjunct within treatment. The guest editors of the special edition of the *American Journal of Occupational Therapy* dedicated to fall prevention, mentioned earlier, states: "In the context of fall prevention, the importance of developing, using, and evaluating diverse approaches to intervention (e.g., remediation, maintenance, compensation, disability preventions) described in the Occupational Therapy Practice Framework: Domain and Process cannot be overstated."[1] An OT intervention with any older client should consider the client's functional capacities and environments for assessment of fall risk and prevention.

Summary

The human body is comprised of a complex integration of multiple systems that work together for humans to survive and hopefully thrive. As a natural consequence of aging, the function of each organ declines as we become older. There are many interventions, however, that an occupational therapist and/or assistant can utilize to support the aging client's decline in function. These interventions support and/or improve performance in activities of daily living with exercise and other forms of training to increase activity tolerance. Strategies in energy conservation and work simplification are provided to support the aging adult's participation in her or his preferred activities. Furthermore, coping strategies, such as stress management and relaxation techniques, and home

safety assessments are incorporated, as indicated. Whenever appropriate, family members are educated about the interventions so that they can also improve and support the client's status, with an overall aim of supporting the individual's well-being and quality of life.

REVIEW QUESTIONS

1. Describe how the aging process changes physiologic and neurologic functions and may consequently affect occupational performance and resulting participation in ADL and IADL.

2. Discuss how energy conservation, work simplification, and conditioning strategies are utilized by occupational therapists and assistants to support occupational performance with older adults experiencing aging-related physiologic and/or neurologic conditions.

3. Describe occupational-based interventions to prevent falls with aging adults with physiologic and neurologic conditions.

4. Discuss how OT may appropriately intervene to mitigate common psychological effects of physiologic and neurologic disorders in older adults.

REFERENCES

1. American Occupational Therapy Association. (2014). Occupational therapy practice framework: Domain and process. (3rd ed.). *American Journal of Occupational Therapy*, 68(Suppl. 1), S1–S48.
2. Balady, G., Ades, P., Comoss, P., Limacher, M., Pina, I., Southard, D., et al. (2000). Core components of cardiac rehabilitation/secondary prevention programs: A statement for healthcare professionals from the American Heart Association and the American Association of Cardiovascular and Pulmonary Rehabilitation. *Circulation*, 102, 1069–1073.
3. Barlow, J., Turner, A., & Wright, C. (2000). A randomized controlled study of the Arthritis Self-Management Programme in the UK. *Health Education Research*, 15(6), 665–680.
4. Barr, V., Robinson, S., Marin-Link, B., Underhill, L., Dotts, A., Ravensdale, D., et al. (2003). The expanded Chronic Care Model: An integration of concepts and strategies from population health promotion and the Chronic Care Model. *Hospital Quarterly*, 7(1), 73–82.
5. Barsevick, A., Dudley, W., Beck, S., Sweeney, C., Whitmer, K., & Nail, L. (2004). A randomized clinical trial of energy conservation for patients with cancer-related fatigue. *Cancer*, 100, 1302–1310.
6. Beardmore, T. D. (2008). Rehabilitation of patients with rheumatic diseases. In J. H. Klippel (Ed.), *Primer on the rheumatic diseases* (13th ed. pp. 599–609). New York, NY: Springer.
7. Beasley, J. (2012). Osteoarthritis and rheumatoid arthritis: Conservative therapeutic management. *Journal of Hand Therapy*, 25(2), 163–172.
8. Beers, M. H., Jones, T. V., Berkwits, M., Kaplan J. L., & Porter, R. (2004). *The Merck manual of health & aging*. Whitehouse Station, NJ: Merck Research Laboratories.
9. Bosworth, H. B., Steinhauser, K. E., Orr, M., Lindquist, J. H., Grambow, S. C., & Oddone, E. Z. (2004). Congestive heart

failure patients' perceptions of quality of life: The integration of physical and psychosocial factors. *Aging and Mental Health*, *8*(1), 83–91.

10. Cafarella, P., Effing, T., Usmani, Z., & Frith, P. (2012). Treatments for anxiety and depression in patients with chronic obstructive pulmonary disease: A literature review. *Respirology*, *17*(4), 627–638.

11. Cleveland Clinic Foundation. Resources for Health Professionals. http://my.clevelandclinic.org/health/diseases_conditions/. Retrieved 06.25.15.

12. Conner, M. B., Sandberg, T., & Norman, P. (2010). Using action planning to promote exercise behavior. *Annals of Behavioral Medicine*, *40*, 65–76.

13. Costi, S., Crisafulli, E., Antoni, F., Beneventi, C., Fabbri, L., & Clini, E. (2009). Effects of unsupported upper extremity exercise training in patients with COPD: A randomized clinical trial. *Chest*, *136*(2), 387–395.

14. Crespo, R. & Shrewsberry, M. (2007). Factors associated with integrating self-management support into primary care. *The Diabetes Educator*, *33*(6), 126S–131S.

15. Cumming, R., Thomas, M., Szonyl, G., Frampton, G., Salkeld, G., & Clemson, L. (2001). Adherence to occupational therapist recommendations for home modifications for falls prevention. *American Journal of Occupational Therapy*, *55*(6), 641–648.

16. Devine, E. C., & Pearcy, J. (1996). Meta-analysis of the effects of pyschoeducational care in adults with chronic obstructive pulmonary disease. *Patient Educational Counseling*, *29*, 167–178.

17. Fantl, J. A., Wyman, J. F., McClish, D. K., Harkins, S. W., Elswick, R. K., Taylor, J. R., et al. (1991). Efficacy of bladder training in older women with urinary incontinence. *JAMA*, *265*, 609–613.

18. Fedorcsyk, J. M. (2011). The use of physical agents in hand rehabilitation. In T. M. Skirven, A. L. Osterman, J. M. Fedorcsyk, & P. C. Amadio (Eds.), *Rehabilitation of the hand and upper extremity* (6th ed. pp. 1495–1512). Philadelphia, PA: Elsevier.

19. Geusgens, C. M., Hagedoren, E., Jolles, J., & Wim, J. (2010). Environmental effects in the performance of daily tasks in healthy adults. *American Journal of Occupational Therapy [serial online]*, *64*(6), 935–940.

20. Gillespie, L. D., Robertson, M. C., Gillespie, W. J., Sherrington, C., Gates, S., Clemson, L. M., et al. (2012). Interventions for preventing falls in older people living in the community. *Cochrane Database of Systematic Reviews*, *12*(9), CD007146.

21. Gillham, S., & Endacott, R. (2010). Impact of enhanced secondary prevention on health behaviour in patients following minor stroke and transient ischaemic attack: A randomized controlled trial. *Clinical Rehabilitation*, *24*(9), 822–830.

22. Goldstein, M., Hawthorne, M. E., Engeberg, S., McDowell, B. J., & Burgio, K. L. (1992). Urinary incontinence. Why people do not seek help. *Journal of Gerontological Nursing*, *18*(4), 15–20. (PMID: 1569296).

23. Higginbotham, M., Morris, K., Williams, R., Coleman, R., & Cobb, F. (1986). Physiologic basis for the age-related decline in aerobic work capacity. *The American Journal of Cardiology*, *57*(15), 1374–1379.

24. Holman, H., & Lorig, K. (2004, May-June). Patient self-management: A key to effectiveness and efficiency in care of chronic disease. *Public Health Reports*, *119*, 239–243.

25. Jensen, L., & Padilla, R. (2011). Review of the evidence for the effect of interventions to prevent falls in persons with Alzheimer's disease and related dementias. *American Journal of Occupational Therapy*, *65*, 532–540.

26. Katz, N., Itzkovich, M., Averbuch, S., & Elazar, B. (1989). Loewenstein Occupational Therapy Cognitive Assessment (LOTCA) battery for brain-injured patients: reliability and validity. *American Journal of Occupational Therapy*, *43*(3), 184–192.

27. Kenny, R. A., Rubenstein, L. Z., Tinetti, M. E., Brewer, K., Cameron, K. A., Capezuti, L., & Peterson, E. W. (2011). Summary of the updated American Geriatrics Society/British Geriatrics Society clinical practice guideline for prevention of falls in older persons. *Journal of the American Geriatrics Society*, *59*(1), 148–157.

28. Law, M., Polatajko, H., Baptiste, W., & Townsend, E. (1997). Core concepts of occupational therapy. In E. Towsend (Ed.), *Enabling occupation: An occupational therapy perspective* (pp. 29–56). Ottawa, ON: Canadian Association of Occupational Therapists.

29. Linton, A. D. (2007). Respiratory system. In A. Linton & H. Lach (Eds.), *Matteson & McConnell's gerontological nursing: Concepts and practice* (pp. 353–356). St. Louis, MO: Saunders Elsevier.

30. Linton, A. D., Hooter, L. J., & Elmers, C. R. (2007). Endocrine system. In A. Linton & H. Lach (Eds.), *Matteson & McConnell's gerontological nursing: Concepts and practice* (pp. 525–542). St. Louis, MO: Saunders Elsevier.

31. Lorig, K., & Holman, H. R. (1993). Arthritis self-management studies: A twelve-year review. *Health Education Quarterly*, *20*(1), 17–28.

32. Lorig, K., & Holman, H. (2003). Self-management education: History, definition, outcomes, and mechanisms. *Annals of Behavioral Medicine*, *26*(1), 1–7.

33. Lorig, K., Holman, H. R., Sobel, D., Laurent, D., González, V., & Minor, M. (2000). *Living a healthy life with chronic conditions* (2nd ed.). Palo Alto, CA: Bull Publishing.

34. Martin, N. A. (2006). Test of visual perceptual skills. (TVPS-3). Flórida: PAR.

35. Matuska, K., Mathiowetz, V., & Finlayson, M. (2007). Use and perceived effectiveness of energy conservation strategies for managing multiple sclerosis fatigue. *American Journal of Occupational Therapy*, *61*, 62–69.

36. Migliore, A. (2004). Case report—improving dyspnea management in three adults with chronic obstructive pulmonary disease. *American Journal of Occupational Therapy*, *58*, 639–646.

37. Millsap, P. (2007). Neurological system. In A. Linton & H. Lach (Eds.), *Matteson & McConnell's gerontological nursing: Concepts and practice* (pp. 406–412). St. Louis, MO: Saunders Elsevier.

38. National Council on Aging. (2012). *Six steps to protect your older loved one from a fall*. http://www.NCOA.org.

39. Neumann, B., Tries, J., & Plummer, M. (2009). The role of OT in the treatment of incontinence and pelvic floor disorders. *OT Practice*, *14*(5), 10–13.

40. Peterson, E., Finlayson, M., Elliot, S., Painter, J., & Clemson, L. (2012). Unprecedented opportunities in fall prevention for occupational therapy practitioners. *American Journal of Occupational Therapy*, *66*(2), 127–130.

41. Radomski, M. V., & Trombly Latham, C. (2002). Assessment. In M. V. Radomski & C. Trombly Latham (Eds.), *Occupational therapy for physical dysfunction* (p. 177). Philadelphia, PA: Lippincott Williams & Wilkins.

42. Schreurs, K., Colland, V., Kuijer, R., de Ridder, D., & van Elderen, T. (2003). Development, content, and process evaluation of a short self-management intervention in patients with chronic diseases requiring self-care behaviours. *Patient Educational Counseling*, *51*(2), 133–141.

43. Shamliyan, T., Kane, R., Wyman, J., & Wilt, T. (2008). Systematic review: Randomized, controlled trials of nonsurgical treatments for urinary incontinence in women. *Annals of Internal Medicine [serial online], 148*(6), 459–473.

44. Tinetti, M. E., Inouye, S. K., Gill, T. M., & Doucette, J. T. (1995). Shared risk factors for falls, incontinence, and functional dependence: Unifying the approach to geriatric syndromes. *JAMA, 273*(17), 1348–1353. doi:10.1001/jama.1995.03520410042024.

45. U.S. Census Bureau. (1995). *Sixty-five plus in the United States, statistical brief.* http://www.census.gov/population/socdemo/statbriefs/agebrief.html. Retrieved March 14, 2015.

46. Wagner, E., Austin, B., Davis, C., Hindmarsh, M., Schaefer, J., & Bonomi, A. (2001). Improving chronic illness care: Translating evidence into action. *Health Affairs, 20*(6), 64–78.

CHAPTER 10

Occupational Therapy Interventions for Older Adults with Low Vision*

Margaret Newsham Beckley, PhD, OTR/L, BCPR, BCG, SCLV, FAOTA

CHAPTER OUTLINE

OBJECTIVES

- Define low vision.
- Identify diseases and conditions associated with low vision in older adults.
- Distinguish low vision from the typical vision changes associated with aging.
- Understand the function and components of vision.
- Identify components of low-vision evaluation.
- Understand how lighting, magnification, contrast, and working distance affect function.
- Identify strategies to improve the use of remaining vision for everyday tasks and occupations.
- Be familiar with referral sources to support older adults with low vision.
- Describe opportunities available for professional development for low-vision practice.

Low vision has been found to have an adverse effect on people's ability to participate in their everyday occupations.[4,19,32] An older adult with low vision may have difficulty with reading; writing; activities of daily living (ADLs); instrumental activities of daily living (IADLs); functional and community mobility; social, leisure, and spectator activities; or vocational tasks. As a result, there is a loss of independence, safety, and life roles and an increased potential for isolation and depression.

In 2000, the number of older adults (over 65 years of age) in the United States was 35 million, an increase of 3.7 million (11%) since 1990.[1] Of these older adults, approximately 1.3 million (4%) had a low-vision impairment.[24] The incidence of low-vision disorders among older adults is on the rise, and they make up two thirds of those diagnosed with a visual impairment.[27]

In 2008, the National Center for Health Statistics noted that 6.5 million older adults reported experiencing significant vision loss.[33] By 2030, experts in the field predict the rates of severe vision loss will double as the U.S. aging population increases.[34] These numbers do not include older adults in institutionalized living environments, such as skilled nursing facilities. Due to the large number of older adults currently with low vision and projections for an increase in that number, it is important for occupational therapy (OT) professionals to screen their clients for low-vision conditions and refer to an ophthalmologist or optometrist with a specialty in low vision for a full low-vision evaluation as needed.

---

*Dedicated to the Occupational Therapy Class of 2012, Barry University, Miami Shores, Florida

Functional Performance and Low Vision

Combined with the other physical changes associated with aging, the development of a low-vision impairment further challenges the functional performance and safety of those 65 years and older.[5] Furthermore, the psychological effects from the physical changes accompanying aging are compounded for those with a low-vision impairment.[38]

Low vision can be described as impaired visual perception due to visual acuity that is less than 70/200 or limited visual fields of 20 degrees or less, both of which result in limitations in a person's ability to participate in daily activities and occupations. It occurs as the result of a chronic visual disorder that cannot be corrected medically, surgically, or with conventional eyeglasses.[23] Low vision is different from typical vision changes associated with aging and, most often, results in a disability. According to a 2004 study by the National Eye Institute,[27] the four most common eye diseases leading to low-vision impairments are glaucoma, age-related macular degeneration, diabetic retinopathy, and cataracts.

Low vision may affect a person's safety and quality of life. For those with low-vision impairment, there is an increased risk of falls and fractures; these types of injuries can result in admission to a hospital or nursing home, and, for an older adult, can put the individual at risk of disability or premature death.[8] Another safety issue for someone with low vision is difficulty identifying medications. Misidentification of medications can lead to drug-related errors that affect the health of aging adults; these types of errors have become the fifth-leading cause of death among older adults. Forty percent of persons older than age 65 years of age take five or more prescription drugs each week, and 12% take more than 10,[13] increasing the chance even more for misidentifying medications. Depression is another concern for older people with low vision. Older people with vision impairments have a 57.2% risk of mild or moderate depression, compared with 43.5% of those without vision loss.[2]

Low Vision versus Age-Related Changes in Vision

Due to typical vision changes associated with aging, low-vision disorders may be dismissed as normal changes. Low-vision disorders are not the same as the normal vision changes that occur with aging. The typical age-related vision changes result from alterations in the cornea, pupil, lens, aqueous and vitreous humor, and macular pigment over time (Figure 10-1).[35]

As a result, visual acuity gradually decreases, making it difficult to read fine print. Contrast sensitivity, the eye's ability to detect subtle changes in light and dark objects, decreases and may result in reduced reading speed or facial discrimination when looking at photographs. There is an increased discomfort experienced with glare and an increased glare recovery time (the speed with which the visual system regains function following exposure to bright light). In addition, color discrimination decreases with age, causing some colors to appear more muted, particularly those along the blue–yellow axis.[35]

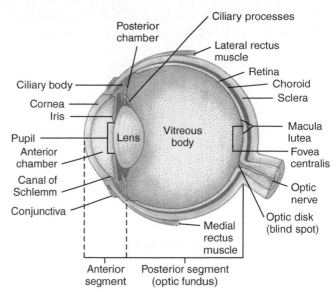

FIGURE 10-1 Anatomy of the eye. (From Ignatavicius, D. D., Workman, M. L., & Mishler, M. A. [1999]. *Medical-surgical nursing across the health care continuum* [3rd ed.]. Philadelphia, PA: WB Saunders.)

Low-contrast, low-lighting levels, and the presence of glare have been shown to reduce older adults' acuity levels as a result of age-related changes.[15] These typical changes associated with aging can be further compounded by a low-vision impairment that develops in later life, leading to greater functional impairment.

Older adults who develop low vision and mistakenly think it is a normal part of aging may not seek support services or be aware that services are available. In addition, older adults with low vision, more often than not, have a myriad of symptoms, conditions, and impairments. Interdisciplinary services that address the many areas affected by low vision have been found to improve the quality of life of older adults.[16,21] Whether service is direct intervention, team treatment, or a referral to another service provider, the various needs of an older adult client with low vision have a greater chance of being met through an interdisciplinary approach. The 5-year National Plan for Eye and Vision Research[27] identified interdisciplinary collaboration in low-vision treatment as a program goal. Related to this, *Healthy People 2020* also specifies objectives to increase the use of the various rehabilitation services by people with low vision and to increase the use of assorted visual and adaptive devices.[39] To this end, occupational therapists and OT assistants need to work in collaboration with other health and social service providers to ensure older adults with low vision receive necessary services and intervention.

An examination by an optometrist or ophthalmologist who specializes in low-vision therapy is usually the first step in the process. In addition to OT professionals, a certified low-vision therapist (CLVT) or a certified vision rehabilitation therapist (CVRT), formerly known as a rehabilitation teacher, can assist with many of the challenges one may face with ADLs and IADLs. Physical therapists can provide intervention with ambulation, transfers, safety, and balance. A certified orientation and mobility specialist (COMS) can also assist with managing safe mobility in the home, in addition to providing instruction for traveling safely and efficiently in the community. Additional services from members of the team can be provided by skilled nursing, a diabetic educator, a social worker or psychologist, and a family practice physician or geriatrician. The members of the low-vision rehabilitation team may vary depending on the service environment and funding sources. Occupational therapists and OT assistants need to be aware of the different service environments, delivery models, funding sources, and community resources associated with low-vision rehabilitation to provide effective client-centered care.

Function and Conditions of the Eye

Vision loss is an individualized condition. Two clients with the same diagnosis, the same age, and the same gender may have very different impairments. Vision is multidimensional. When working with older adults with an acquired vision loss, OT practitioners need to be aware of the five components that make up vision: visual acuity, visual field, contrast sensitivity, light modulation, and visual perception and interpretation (Table 10-1).[26]

TABLE 10-1   Visual Function Components and Definitions

Vision Function Components	Definitions
Visual acuity	Level of detail with which a person can see objects
Visual field	Total area one sees in a single view without turning the head or eyes
Central visual field	Area immediately surrounding the spot upon which the person is focusing
Peripheral visual field	Area beyond and surrounding the central field
Contrast sensitivity	Capacity to distinguish between similar shades of light and dark and to distinguish similar colors
Light modulation	Capacity to regulate light, control glare, and adapt to changing light conditions: light to dark or dark to light
Visual perception and interpretation	Correctly processing and interpreting the information the brain receives from the eyes via the optic nerve

(From Mogk, L. G. [2011]. Eye conditions that cause low vision in adults. In M. Warren & E. A. Barstow [Eds.], *Occupational therapy interventions for adults with low vision*, [pp. 27–46]. Bethesda, MD: AOTA Press.)

Physiology of Vision

When we see words, objects, faces, or landscapes, their reflections are carried by light through the eye to the retina. Light enters the eye through the cornea, then passes through the aqueous humor, pupil, and lens (see Figure 10-1). It continues to travel posteriorly through the vitreous humor to the first layer of the retina. The layers of the retina, from anterior to posterior are:

- internal limiting membrane
- axons
- ganglion cells
- inner plexiform layer
- inner nuclear layer
- outer plexiform layer
- outer nuclear layer (rod and cone cell bodies)
- external limiting membrane
- photoreceptors
- pigmented epithelium

Light is attracted to the internal limiting membrane and travels through the membrane to the axons, ganglion cells, inner plexiform layer, and then the inner nuclear layer. At the outer plexiform layer, light is converted into chemical energy. This energy then stimulates the rods and cones to become hyperpolarized, creating an electrical impulse. The electrical impulse is carried posteriorly through the external limiting membrane to photoreceptors and the pigmented epithelium. At this point, the collection of nerve fibers from the retina, known as the optic nerve, carries electrical impulse information from the retina, exiting the eye, to the optic tract (after chiasm), and then proceeds eventually to the visual cortex of the brain in the occipital lobe (Figure 10-2).

Pressure within the globe of eye needs to be maintained for accurate transmission of light, chemical energy, and electrical energy. The average range of intraocular pressure (IOP) is 10 to 22 mm Hg. Abnormally low IOP is when the pressure measures below 10 mm Hg. Abnormally high IOP is a measure of 30 mm Hg or higher, and very high IOP is considered to be 40 to 60 mm Hg. Abnormally high IOP results in glaucoma.

Pathology of Low-Vision Impairment

Low-vision impairments occur when there is a chronic deteriorating condition or an acute trauma that causes damage to the structures of the eye or the pathway from the retina to the visual cortex. A gradual loss of vision can occur with chronic conditions such as diabetic retinopathy or macular degeneration; an acute loss of vision can occur as the result of a sudden traumatic event, such as a stroke near the optic chiasm or visual cortex. Adjustment to acquired vision loss has been found to be more difficult than adjustment to congenital vision loss for older adults, and adjustment to an acute loss of vision is more challenging than adjustment to a gradual loss of vision.[4]

Conditions Causing Low-Vision Impairments

The four most common conditions causing low vision impairments in older adults are macular degeneration, diabetic

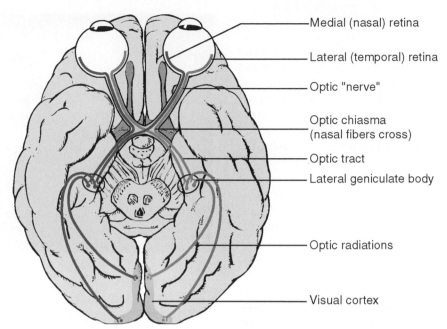

Medial (nasal) retina

Lateral (temporal) retina

Optic "nerve"

Optic chiasma
(nasal fibers cross)

Optic tract

Lateral geniculate body

Optic radiations

Visual cortex

FIGURE 10-2   Optic pathway. (From Liebgott, B. [2011]. *The anatomical basis of dentistry* [3rd ed.]. St. Louis, MO: Mosby.)

retinopathy, glaucoma, and cataracts.[27] Because older adults are more prone to a cerebrovascular accident (CVA), or stroke, than younger populations, acquired field loss due to stroke is another visual impairment that can affect this population.

Macular Degeneration

The most common eye condition that leads to low vision for older adults is macular degeneration (Figure 10-3), and it is found more frequently in Caucasian populations. Age-related macular degeneration (ARMD) occurs as a result of degeneration of the macula, the area of the retina that is responsible for central vision and much of color vision.[30]

When degeneration alone occurs, this is considered to be dry ARMD. For some people with ARMD, abnormal new blood vessels can form under the macula and leak,[10] which is referred to as wet ARMD. Macular degeneration usually progresses for several years, resulting in central scotomas. A person with ARMD will have reduced contrast sensitivity and color vision, with a preference for bright task lighting and a high sensitivity to ambient lighting.[10] Because the macula is responsible for central vision, ARMD impairs the ability to focus, affecting vision needed for activities such as reading, fine motor tasks, seeing faces in social situations, viewing pictures, and completing hobbies and leisure activities.

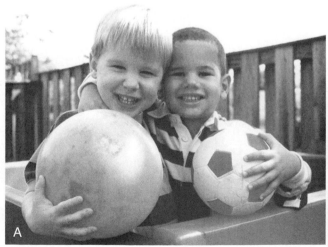
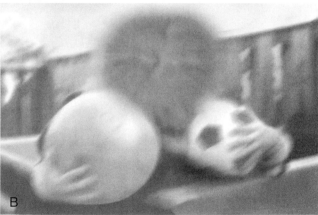

Normal Vision   Age-related Macular Degeneration

FIGURE 10-3   A, Normal vision. B, Simulated loss of vision with age-related macular degeneration. (From National Eye Institute, National Institutes of Health. [2010]. NEI photos, images, and videos. Retrieved from http://www.nei.nih.gov/photo/.)

Diabetic Retinopathy

Another leading cause of low vision in older adults is diabetic retinopathy (Figure 10-4). Diabetic retinopathy is found more frequently among African American, Hispanic, and Native American populations. Diabetic retinopathy is associated with diabetes and occurs when small blood vessels in the retina stop functioning properly.[30] Laser treatment or surgery may be used to stop the small-vessel leakage and stabilize the condition.[10] Vision may fluctuate based on dysregulated sugar levels, and the field of view that is affected depends on the areas of the retina that are damaged.[10] Someone with diabetic retinopathy has reduced contrast sensitivity and color vision, a preference for moderate task lighting, and a moderate sensitivity to ambient lighting.[10] In early stages of the disease, the small blood vessels in the retina may leak fluid into the retina, with the risk of impairing the entire retina, including the macula, and the vitreous humor, leading to distorted vision.[30] The degree of visual impairment can range from mild to total blindness. Depending on the location and amount of damage to the retina, someone with diabetic retinopathy can have difficulty with near, midrange, or distant activities.

Glaucoma

Glaucoma is another common cause of low vision in older adults and is found to run in families (Figure 10-5). The risk of developing glaucoma is five times greater in African Americans compared with Caucasians, and the rate for a visual impairment that results in blindness is six times greater for African Americans than it is for Caucasians.[30] Glaucoma is caused by an increase in intraocular pressure due to fluid buildup in the eye, resulting in compression of and damage to the optic nerve. Glaucoma can be treated successfully, if found early enough, through the use of eye drops that decrease intraocular pressure.[26] Someone with glaucoma will have reduced

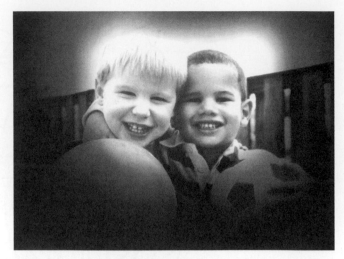

Glaucoma

FIGURE 10-5 Simulated vision with glaucoma. (From National Eye Institute, National Institutes of Health. [2010]. NEI photos, images, and videos. Retrieved from http://www.nei.nih.gov/photo/. Accessed 10.19.15)

contrast sensitivity and color vision, a preference for moderate task lighting, and a moderate sensitivity to ambient lighting.[10] The distinctive pattern of vision loss with glaucoma begins with initial loss in the midperipheral field, progressing toward the center and periphery.[26] Someone with glaucoma will have difficulty with mobility activities due to the midperipheral and peripheral field damage and, later, with near activities if the disease progresses to impairment of central vision.

Cataracts

The fourth common cause of low vision in older adults is cataracts (Figure 10-6). Cataracts cause clouding over the lens of the eye, decreasing the amount of light passing through the lens and limiting vision.[30] The most common form of cataracts affects distant vision, then near vision,

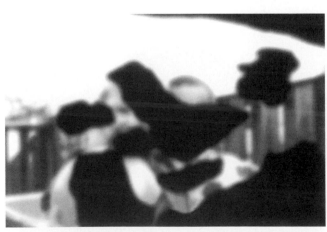

Diabetic Retinopathy

FIGURE 10-4 Simulated vision with diabetic retinopathy. (From National Eye Institute, National Institutes of Health. [2010]. NEI photos, images, and videos. Retrieved from http://www.nei.nih.gov/photo/. Accessed 10.19.15)

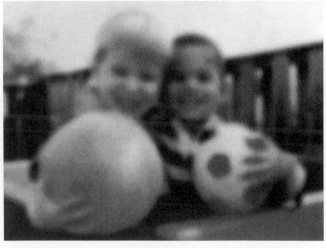

Cataract

FIGURE 10-6 Simulated vision with cataracts. (From National Eye Institute, National Institutes of Health. [2010]. NEI photos, images, and videos. Retrieved from http://www.nei.nih.gov/photo/. Accessed 10.19.15)

eventually causing blurriness and muted colors throughout the entire visual field.[26] Cataracts develop as a result of aging. Surgical removal of the lens is a viable option for most older adults, and vision becomes clear again with a replacement lens. For someone with an advanced cataract, visual acuity and details for distant, intermediate, and eventually near activities will be impaired.

Stroke

Visual field cuts that may result from stroke are not one of the common low-vision conditions; however, due to the effects on older adults who experience a field cut as the result of a stroke, it is frequently included in discussions of low-vision impairments in older adults. Visual field cuts that result from a stroke may involve one side of the visual field, known as homonymous hemianopsia, or a quadrant of the visual field, sometimes referred to as quadrantanopsia. The location of the damage along the optic pathway (Figure 10-7) determines the type of visual field deficit that may occur. If a lesion occurs along the optic tract or along the entire width of the optic radiations to the visual cortex, a contralateral hemianopsia will occur (Figure 10-8). For lesions at the

optic chiasm, preventing temporal field information from crossing to the contralateral optic tract, a bitemporal hemianopsia will occur (Figure 10-9). When the lesion occurs along the upper radiations of the optic tract that lead to the visual cortex, it will cause a lower quadrant contralateral field loss (Figure 10-10). In the first several months following a stroke, vision may improve. After this point, vision can be considered stable[10] and will not deteriorate any further due to the stroke. Field losses from stroke frequently cause difficulties with reading, finding items in a kitchen drawer, or bumping into objects in the environment as a result of not seeing the entire near, intermediate, or distant visual field.

Occupational Therapy Assessment and Intervention

Due to the large number of older adults currently with low vision and projections for an increase in that number through 2030,[34] it is important for OT professionals to screen their clients for low-vision conditions and refer to an ophthalmologist or optometrist with a specialty in low vision for a full low-vision evaluation as needed.

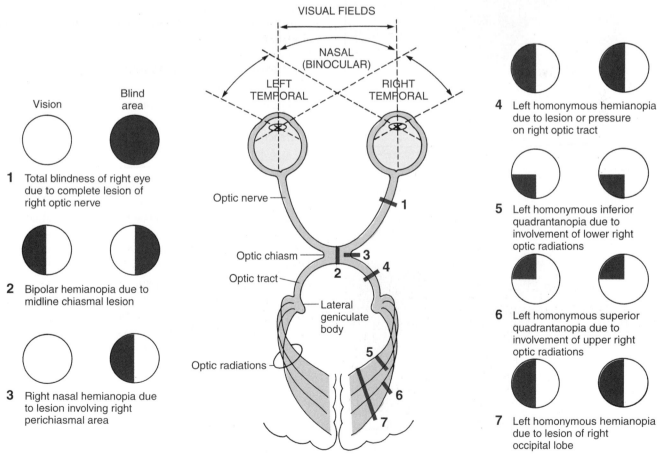

FIGURE 10-7 Homonymous hemianopsia. A right-sided brain stroke may cause lesions that disturb visual fibers and result in blindness in the left visual field. The optic pathway from the other side remains intact. (From Black, J. M, & Hawks, J. H. [2008]. *Medical-surgical nursing: Clinical management for positive outcomes* [8th ed.]. Philadelphia, PA: Saunders.)

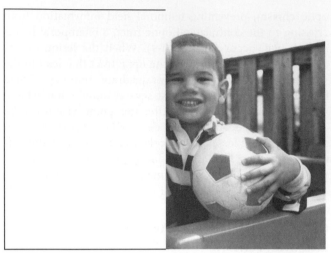

FIGURE 10-8   (From National Eye Institute, National Institutes of Health. [2010]. *NEI photos, images, and videos.* Retrieved from http://www.nei.nih. gov/photo/. Accessed 10.19.15)

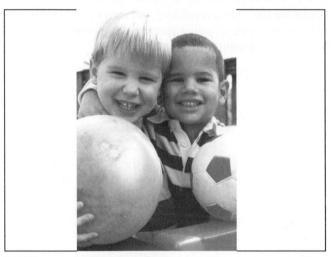

FIGURE 10-9   Simulated bitemporal hemianopsia following stroke. (From National Eye Institute, National Institutes of Health. [2010]. *NEI photos, images, and videos.* Retrieved from http://www.nei.nih.gov/photo/. Accessed 10.19.15)

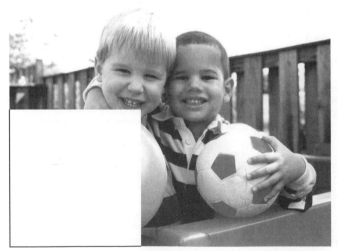

FIGURE 10-10   (From National Eye Institute, National Institutes of Health. [2010]. *NEI photos, images, and videos.* Retrieved from http://www.nei.nih. gov/photo/. Accessed 10.19.15)

When a client is referred for low-vision rehabilitation, it is necessary to review the report from the optometrist or ophthalmologist as part of the initial evaluation process. The content of a typical eye report includes ocular history, visual acuity with and without glasses, eye muscle function, intraocular pressure reading, contrast sensitivity, color vision, visual field test, pupillary response, photophobia, prescription, and prognosis. The eye report information is helpful in the assessment process in many ways. For instance, the visual acuity information can indicate the amount of magnification needed with optical devices, determine the degree of residual vision, and provide documentation to qualify a client for services.[6]

Although helpful when building the occupational profile, the occupational therapist needs to realize that the eye examination is completed in a controlled environment, without the lighting changes or distractions that are present in natural and everyday environments. In addition, the information from the eye report will not indicate how well a client with low vision can perform functional tasks. To determine the client's occupational performance skills and barriers to participation, the occupational therapist needs to assess the client in different environments and under various conditions. The results of the OT evaluation will help to identify intervention strategies, adaptive equipment and low-vision devices, and other professional low-vision services and community resources needed to improve a person's ability to complete daily activities and occupations.

Occupational Therapy Assessment

An important aspect of the low-vision evaluation is for it to be a positive experience for clients so that they are exposed to a success-oriented atmosphere related to their potential. This experience can relieve clients of some of the limitations and fears associated with vision loss and motivate them to accomplish their goals.

The OT low-vision assessment includes four components:[3] (1) the occupational profile, (2) evaluation of visual factors, (3) evaluation of environmental factors, and (4) evaluation of occupational performance.

Occupational Profile

The occupational profile, the "summary of the client's occupational history and experiences, patterns of daily living, interests, values, and needs,"[3] can be constructed from interviews, questionnaires, and previous medical, vision, and social histories. The occupational profile will help guide the development of intervention strategies and goals based on the client's priorities and interests. It may also reveal the need for referral to other professionals.

Gathering information for the occupational profile can be completed with a number of tools, including—but not limited to—the Occupational Therapy Practice Framework, 3rd edition; the Geriatric Depression Scale, short version;[37] or any other formal or informal data-collection tools that will provide a thorough appraisal of the client's occupational performance history. The questions in Box 10-1, for example, are

Reading and near-vision activities:

- What size print can you now read?
- Do you want to continue reading newspapers?
- Can you read your bills?
- Do you want to read the TV guide?
- Do you "spot" read more than you read novels or other books?
- Have you had low-vision devices, such as magnifiers, in the past? If so, do you still use them? If not, why not?

Everyday activities:

- Can you see to use a checkbook?
- Can you read your watch?
- Can you do regular household tasks, such as cleaning and laundry?
- Can you care for your personal grooming needs, such as shaving or applying makeup?
- Can you see to use the computer?
- Are you able to continue your hobbies?
- Can you watch television?
- Can you travel independently and safely?
- What, if any, difficulties are you having when traveling in your community?
- Are you still driving? If so, do you still feel safe driving?
- Does bright sunlight bother you?
- Has your vision problem affected your employment or educational studies?
- If you're a diabetic, can you see to fill your insulin syringes?
- Can you differentiate between your medications?

(From American Foundation for the Blind: VisionAware, www.VisionAware.org Accessed 10.19.15)

BOX 10-2   Occupational Therapy Evaluation of the Client's Visual Factors

- Assessing visual acuity at a distance
- Reading acuity for near vision
- Peripheral field testing
- Contrast sensitivity
- Scotoma assessment
- Reading assessment for reading speed

(From Scheiman, M., Scheiman, M., & Whittaker, S. [2007]. *Low vision rehabilitation: A practical guide for occupational therapists.* Thorofare, NJ: SLACK.)

from the VisionAware questionnaire and may provide useful vision-related data for the occupational profile.

Questions from the Low Vision Quiz from the National Eye Institute[28] are intended to gather information on a person's performance in typical daily activities with or without the use of prescription glasses, inquiring whether one has difficulty with the following activities:

- Recognizing faces of family and friends
- Doing things that require the person to see well up close, like reading, cooking, sewing, or fixing things around the house
- Being able to pick out and match the color of clothes
- Doing things at work or home in which lights seem dimmer than they used to appear
- Being able to read street and bus signs or the names of stores

Evaluation of Visual Factors

The second component of the low-vision assessment is evaluation of visual factors. This part of the assessment may vary, depending on the amount of information received from a client's optometrist or ophthalmologist. If the information from the eye doctor's clinical low-vision assessment is limited,

evaluation of visual factors can be completed by the occupational therapist as part of the functional low-vision assessment (Box 10-2).

Assessment of Visual Acuity at a Distance

Testing visual acuity at a distance can be completed with the Feinbloom Distance Test Chart, which is easily portable, or the ETDRS Chart (Figure 10-11), which is not as portable and can be illuminated.

Assessment of Reading Acuity for Near Vision

Reading acuity for near vision testing can be completed using the Minnesota Low Vision Reading Test, also known as the MN Read Card (Box 10-3). The MN Read Card has black print on a white background, and printed sentences change in incremental sizes. It is important to have proper task lighting on the MN Read Card and to position it so the client is reading at a 90-degree angle.

Peripheral Field Testing

Functional peripheral field testing can be completed with converging and/or dynamic activities to determine whether the client can detect an object or movement near and around him or her, and at what point. One method for testing for functional peripheral field loss is to have the client focus on a target or object straight ahead, while seated or standing, with the client's back to the occupational therapist. The client keeps his or her eyes and head facing forward. The occupational therapist stands next to the client's shoulder and proceeds to walk forward, parallel to the client's line of sight. The client indicates the point at which any part of the occupational therapist is visible. The process is repeated on the client's other side as well.[11] The distances from where the occupational therapist started and the points at which the occupational therapist came into the client's field of view constitute the measure of the client's restricted functional peripheral field for each side. There are other commonly used peripheral field testing procedures.[25,36] The selection of the testing procedure may be determined by the client's potential and goals. Peripheral vision testing is important because it is part of a client's early warning system, informing the client that something in the environment is moving, changing, or coming into the client's pathway. Being able to detect these changes is necessary for many functional activities, whether

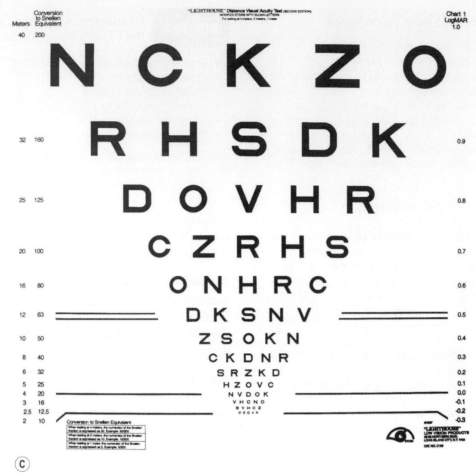

FIGURE 10-11   ETDRS Chart. (From Liu, G., et al. [2010]. *Neuro-ophthalmology diagnosis and management* [2nd ed.]. St. Louis, MO: Saunders.)

BOX 10-3	Helpful Websites

MN Read Card (Minnesota Low Vision Reading Test): http://gandalf.psych.umn.edu/groups/gellab/MNREAD/mnread.pdf

Low-vision products: http://www.shoplowvision.com/media/upload/docs/SLV-Products-for-Eye-Care-Professionals-2008.pdf

To find a certified driving rehabilitation specialist: http://www.driver-ed.org/i4a/pages/index.cfm?pageid=1

Eccentric viewing training: http://www.mdsupport.org/library/eccentric.html

Gardening tips: http://www.carryongardening.org.uk/gardening-for-blind-and-partially-sighted-people.aspx

---

the client is sitting at a table, using a wheelchair, walking, or driving.

Contrast Sensitivity

Contrast sensitivity is the ability to detect grayness and background[26] or distinguish between similar shades of light and dark.[30] There are a variety of testing charts for contrast sensitivity. Some are used for distance testing, such as the low-contrast ETDRS chart (see Figure 10-11) or the Mars Letter Contrast Sensitivity Test,[36] and others are used for near contrast sensitivity testing, such as Lea Numbers Low-Contrast Flip Chart or the Eschenbach Continuous Text Low Contrast Chart.[36] Whether testing for distance or near contrast sensitivity, the client reads or names the objects on the chart as the contrast of the objects is progressively reduced. The client will continue down the chart until he or she is unable to distinguish the letters, numbers, words, or figures from the background of the chart. Reduced contrast sensitivity may cause difficulties with reading, recognizing faces, or seeing a pedestrian in the crosswalk when driving on a rainy day.

Associated with contrast sensitivity is the need for adequate lighting. The low-vision assessment needs to include evaluation of a person's ability to discern the absence or presence of light, sensitivity to the degree of brightness of light, and the need to decrease or increase illumination.[18] Considerations in the area of lighting as it relates to assessment include the types of light, the position of the light, the client's ability to adapt to light and dark, and the effects of glare.[44] The occupational therapist should observe the client under various lighting conditions and determine the client's preferences for lighting during visual factor assessments. It is necessary to assess the client's lighting needs during various functional tasks. Therefore, assessment should include how well the client performs functional activities indoors and outside; determining how well the client manages the transition of moving into and out of bright lighting; and identifying the client's preference for light-absorbing lenses, shields, contrast lenses, dark lenses, and visors or hats.[18] In addition, a person with a greater need for light should be assessed in various situations, such as in a dimly lit room, at dusk, on a cloudy day, and with the provision of additional light,[18] and should be allowed time for his or her eyes to adapt when moving from a bright environment to a darker environment or vice versa.[7]

Although assessment of lighting can be completed informally by changing lighting conditions and glare-reducing devices as needed, there are specific lighting assessments available to the occupational therapist. Some of the specific assessment tools related to lighting include the Cone Adaptation Test, developed by Lea Hyvärinen; the Farnsworth D-15 Color Panel Test, developed by D. Farnsworth; and Foot-candle Reading Monitors,[7] which measure the amount of light coming from a surface. These types of assessment tools produce valuable information, although, in and of themselves, they do not give an indication of a client's overall functional performance. It is important to remember that two clients with similar low-vision diagnoses may have different functional performance levels. As such, the occupational therapist needs to consider all aspects of lighting in the assessment process to develop accurate and thorough baseline information on which to build the intervention plan.

Scotoma Assessment

A scotoma is a dense and localized visual field defect that creates a blind spot in the client's vision.[9] Scotoma testing completed by an optometrist or ophthalmologist gives very precise information about the size and location of a scotoma. When a person has a scotoma near or in the central visual field, reading and fine motor activities are difficult to complete. If information on the presence of a scotoma from a client's eye report is not available, the functional assessments discussed in the following sections can be used to determine whether a client has difficulty seeing in a particular area of the visual field.

Amsler Grid

The Amsler grid (Figure 10-12) is a tool used to measure the central 10 degrees of vision. Often this is the part of the visual field that we rely on to do close or meticulous work, such as placing tiny screws in a jewelry box. The Amsler grid is a one-dimensional square, 10 cm by 10 cm, made up of many smaller boxes. Most frequently, it is a white background with black lines making up the boxes and square; however, the contrast of the grid can be increased by using a black background and white lines. It is used to identify the presence of scotomas in a person's visual field, indicating changes in the macula. The test is completed with one eye at a time and with glasses if the client normally wears them. The grid is held 28 to 30 cm away, and the client is asked to look at the dot in

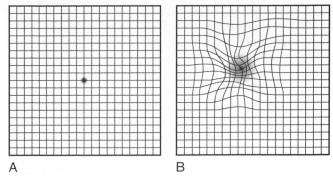

FIGURE 10-12 Amsler grid for monitoring age-related macular degeneration (AMD). *A,* How it would appear normally. *B,* How it might appear to someone with AMD. (From Ashar, B., et al. [2012]. *The Johns Hopkins Internal Medicine Board review: Certification and recertification* [4th ed.]. Philadelphia, PA: Saunders.)

the center of the grid. If the client does not see the dot in the center of the grid, it could be indicative of a scotoma. Then, the client is asked to look at all four corners of the square and to report if the corners are present or not. If the client does not see a corner, it could be indicative of the presence of a scotoma. And, last, the client is asked to report if the squares are all the same size and if any of the lines look wavy. If the squares do not all look equal or if some of the lines look wavy, it may indicate changes in the macula. The Amsler grid is not sensitive for clients with long-standing visual loss, which may be due the client unconsciously filling in the grid so it appears completely normal.[14]

Tangent Screen Test

Another test that can indicate scotomas in a client's visual field is the Tangent Screen Test.[36] This test is similar to the Amsler grid in that it measures the central part of the visual field. It is different from the Amsler grid in that it measures a larger field of view: 20 to 30 degrees. This is the part of the field of view used while reading. The Tangent Screen Test is completed with a large black felt screen mounted on the wall. Testing on the Tangent Screen is completed with one eye at a time and with glasses, if the client wears them. The client is seated facing the screen at a distance of 1 m. The client is told to focus on the white X in the middle while the occupational therapist moves a target in and out of the client's field of view to random locations. If a target is placed within the meridians on the Tangent Screen that correlate up to 30 degrees of central vision and the client does not report seeing it, it could be an indication of a scotoma. This type of testing is a good method to use when a client has had difficulty reading. If the client indicates having a blind spot to the right of the fixation mark, it may indicate a scotoma that is preventing the client from reading through a line of text.[14]

Clock Face Test

A third method to test for the possible presence of a scotoma is the Clock Face Test.[36] This method of testing is completed with one eye at a time and with glasses, if the client wears them. The client is seated facing the clock at eye level at a distance of approximately 2 ft. Using a clock face drawn on a white paper and a center focal point (Figure 10-13), the client is told to focus on the center. If the client cannot see the center, there is probably a scotoma directly in the client's central vision. If, while looking at the center focal point, the client reports being able to see the focal point but unable to see one of the numbers on the face of the clock, the location of the number that is not visible to the client could be indicative of the location of a scotoma. If, for example, the client reports not being able to see the number three, ask the client if focusing on the number nine causes the middle focal point to disappear. If so, there is a good chance the client has a scotoma in the right middle quadrant of the visual field. In addition, it may also indicate that the client could be a candidate for eccentric viewing as a compensatory strategy. Eccentric viewing is discussed later in the chapter as an intervention technique.

Reading Assessment for Reading Speed

The final visual factor testing is a reading assessment for reading speed. The Pepper Visual Skills for Reading Test (Pepper VSRT) is an evaluation available for use by occupational therapists to obtain a measure of reading speed and errors made while reading a series of unrelated letters and words. This evaluation tests vision with regard to word recognition ability, saccade control, return-sweep eye movement control, and scotoma placement while reading.[43] The Pepper VSRT scoring instructions suggest guidelines that will help the occupational therapist determine whether the client's reading performance would be described as "inaccurately and slowly, accurately but slowly, or with both speed and accuracy."[36] Another evaluation that can be used for reading assessment and reading speed is the Minnesota Low Vision Reading Test (MN Read Test) discussed earlier. Assessment of reading skills is important for

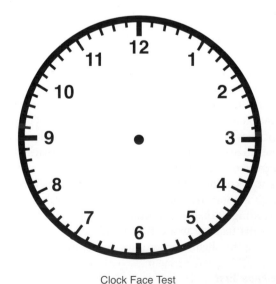

Clock Face Test

FIGURE 10-13   Clock Face Test. (From Scheiman, M., Scheiman, M., & Whittaker, S. [2007]. *Low vision rehabilitation: A practical guide for occupational therapists.* Thorofare, NJ: SLACK.)

reasons other than reading abilities and comprehension. The act of reading may also be an indicator of how a client with low vision performs with other near activities, such as bilateral fine motor tasks, writing, or needle-point.

Evaluation of Environmental Factors

The third component of an OT low-vision assessment is evaluation of environmental factors.[36] Consideration of environmental factors is important because it can make the difference in the client with low vision being able to complete a task successfully in one environment, yet failing to complete the same task when performed in another environment with different features. A difference in successful task completion can depend on the time of day and the amount of available light in a particular environment. It may be, for example, that a client is able to read at the kitchen table that sits next to an east-facing window in the early morning with only the use of a magnifier. However, by late morning, the kitchen may be flooded with light, causing too much glare for the client to see the words on the page.

In assessing the environment, the occupational therapist should evaluate: (1) available sources of light and glare; (2) possible positions for task lights, reading stands, and tables; (3) organization systems; (4) access to low-vision devices; (5) ergonomics of task performance; and (6) emergency response procedures.[36] Identifying environmental features that impair a client's performance may provide direction to a relatively simple solution that can mitigate or eliminate the problem. Consideration of all environments a client uses is important. Environments may vary greatly for some clients and may include, but are not limited to, various rooms of the home, various outdoor venues in different types of weather conditions, the grocery store, the senior center, shopping malls, museums, churches, medical office buildings, and restaurants. Asking a client to go through the schedule of a typical weekday and weekend day with you is one way to determine the different types of environments that may need to be considered in your evaluation.

Evaluation of Occupational Performance

The fourth component of the OT low-vision assessment is evaluation of the client's occupational performance.[36] Occupational performance is the ability to carry out activities of daily life, which includes areas of occupation. Areas of occupation include basic and personal ADLs, IADLs, education, rest, work, play, leisure, and social participation.[3] In the evaluation of a client's occupational performance, performance skills and patterns used in performance are identified, along with the other features that influence performance, such as client factors, activity demands, and context(s).[3] Therefore, in evaluation of the occupational performance of the client with low vision, multiple methods of assessment in relevant environments are necessary. Considering the assessment information that has already been discussed, the occupational therapist will know which assessments should be completed with the client to determine how low vision affects the client's performance.

Some assessments that may be chosen by the occupational therapist are those that are used with various populations and include tasks and activities that are found to be challenges for clients with low vision. Other assessments are designed more specifically for problems encountered by clients with low vision. In any case, it is important to consider the client factors, activity demands, and context(s) during the assessment of the client's performance in the various areas of occupation. As discussed previously, two clients with the same low-vision condition may have very different experiences and challenges. And, the same client with low vision may be able to perform an activity well, but when the context of the activity changes, the ability to succeed may change as well.

Assessments frequently used in the evaluation of the occupational performance of a client with low vision include the survey and observation of typical activities. Some of those assessments may include, but are not limited to, the Canadian Occupational Performance Measure (COPM), the Barthel Index, and the Performance Assessment of Self-care Skills (PASS)[17,20,22]. Activities that are particularly challenging and require routine assessment for clients with low vision include reading labels on medicine bottles and food containers, reading the newspaper and mail, pouring liquid, and using the microwave.[36] Depending on the facility, organization, or environment where an occupational therapist practices, other observational assessments may include basic and personal ADLs, IADLs, education, work, play, leisure, and social participation.

A standardized assessment of ADLs and IADLs developed specifically for occupational therapists' evaluation of the client with low vision is the Self-Report Assessment of Functional and Visual Performance (SRAFVP).[41] This assessment is made up of a 38-item self-report questionnaire and a seven-item observational assessment. The self-report questionnaire is the client's assessment of his or her performance of vision-dependent tasks, and the observation activities are an opportunity for the occupational therapist to confirm the client's reported visual abilities.[12]

As part of a comprehensive occupational performance evaluation, it is also important to consider the output of effort and energy on the part of the low-vision client.[36] Many times, older adults with low vision are considered independent with ADLs; however, this independence requires a significant amount of mental and physical effort on their part. This independence is achieved with an uncertain level of safety and little margin for error. As a result, the client is performing ADLs with maximal effort and has little to no reserve for other activities.[42]

During the evaluation process, the occupational therapist is developing and reviewing data that will be used to develop the client's goals and intervention plan. As part of the process, the occupational therapist must also assess the client's rehabilitation potential. For the client with low vision, the process of determining rehabilitation potential needs to consider the visual, movement, environmental, and cognitive components of tasks.[36] The goals and intervention plan need to be meaningful, achievable, and developed with the client to promote the client's ability to complete necessary and desired activities.

Intervention

The process of intervention is comprised of three components —intervention plan, intervention process, and intervention review—and leads to the client's outcome, which is engagement in occupation to support participation.[3] The intervention plan will guide actions taken and is developed in collaboration with the client. It is based on selected theories, frames of reference, and evidence, and it confirms the targeted outcomes for the client. Intervention implementation includes the ongoing actions taken to influence and support improved client performance. Interventions are directed at identified client outcomes, and the client's response is monitored and documented. The intervention review is a review of the implementation plan and process, and its progress toward targeted client outcomes.[3] The occupational therapist and OT assistant do not follow the components of the intervention process as linear steps; rather, OT practitioners continually reassess the intervention process based on how the client is responding, the influence of the environment, and the availability of resources, and adjustments are made as needed. The intervention process for the client with low vision allows the client to attain the desired outcome while the OT practitioner guides and adjusts the intervention process along the way.

The approach to intervention for the client with low vision will vary from one practice environment to another; however, there are components that should be included in any comprehensive OT plan. In addition, it is important to refer to other low-vision rehabilitation professionals to support the client's overall function, safety, and health as needed.

One approach to intervention is a seven-step sequential treatment plan developed by Scheiman, Scheiman, and Whitaker.[36] This approach includes the following course of intervention strategies:

1. Education (including the nature of the eye disease, the outlook for the future, and expectations of vision rehabilitation)
2. Therapeutic activities (including eccentric viewing, scanning, and reading skills)
3. Environmental modifications (including lighting contrast and glare)
4. Nonoptical assistive devices (including visual, tactile, and auditory)
5. Optical magnification
6. Computer technology in low-vision rehabilitation
7. Resources and handouts

This approach is comprehensive in nature and provides specific areas to include in an OT low-vision intervention plan. This is not to say it is the only approach; there are many others to consider.[40] Whatever approach the OT practitioner chooses to use with low-vision clients, it should be one that provides clients with strategies, resources, support, and confidence to successfully overcome the challenges of living with a low-vision impairment.

There are many aspects to occupational low vision intervention—too many to be covered in this chapter alone.

A general overview of the areas the OT practitioner needs to address will be presented, which includes many of the strategies described earlier:[36] client and family education, the use of optical and nonoptical devices, and the application of low-vision rehabilitation strategies. This overview provides fundamental information for general-practice OT professionals and students. For more extensive learning on the practice of OT in low-vision rehabilitation, further professional development is encouraged.

Client and Family Education

Initial OT sessions for the client with low vision may require a fair degree of client and family education. Clients with low vision have many questions and concerns about their eye condition; the prognosis with regard to whether they will be able to drive, read, care for children, socialize with family and friends, travel, work, or continue in particular roles and leisure activities; and whether they will go blind. It is helpful for the OT practitioner to be prepared for these types of questions ahead of time, giving the client general information about the disease process, and what the client may be able to accomplish through low-vision rehabilitation services, and referring more specific diagnostic and prognostic questions to the client's physician. The OT practitioner can prepare handouts on various topics to distribute to clients with low vision as needed. Helpful topics for handouts may include (1) OT services in low-vision rehabilitation; (2) tips for talking to the doctor; (3) information on conditions, such as low vision, glaucoma, macular degeneration, diabetic retinopathy, and cataracts; (4) national resources and support organizations (Box 10-4); (5) local community resources and organizations; and (6) tips for making print more readable (Box 10-5). Because OT sessions are limited in time, some of these resources may help the client with low vision and family members to pursue local opportunities on their own time. However, it is still the role of the OT practitioner to educate the client and family on how low vision affects occupational performance and how OT services may be able to reduce barriers to the client's engagement in occupation and support the client's participation.

Use of Optical and Nonoptical Devices

Clients with low vision frequently require devices to support the use of their remaining vision. Devices are usually categorized as either optical or nonoptical. Optical devices are magnifiers used to enlarge printed materials, medication labels, photographs, street signs, or any other items a client has difficulty seeing (Box 10-6). Nonoptical devices are small adaptive equipment items or materials that do not incorporate the use of a lens, and function to improve a client's ability to access visual information in the environment. Optical and nonoptical devices are usually not covered by insurance carriers; however, most states have funds available through Title VII of the Rehabilitation Act of 1973 to support the independence of older adults with visual impairments. Oftentimes, these funds are discretionary and can be used, in part, to pay for low-vision devices.[30] The OT practitioner would benefit from exploring the many devices and adaptive equipment items available to clients with low vision. Hands-on training opportunities are recommended to enable the OT practitioner to gain appropriate knowledge and skills before working with unfamiliar devices and adaptive equipment items.

Application of Low-Vision Rehabilitation Strategies

There are many strategies available to the OT practitioner to overcome barriers that result from low-vision conditions. Some of those strategies are identified here as they pertain to specific visual deficits (Table 10-2). A discussion of the use of those strategies will follow.

Lighting Strategies

To address lighting issues, the OT practitioner needs to consider the environment and the task at hand. There are circumstances in which a client would benefit from more light, which may be remedied with a task lamp, or would benefit from reduced light, which may be accomplished with a dimmer switch. At times, clients may be in need of a *portable* light source. A small high-powered liquid crystal display (LCD) flashlight improves readability of a menu in a dark restaurant or helps with mobility when directed to the floor or sidewalk in low-light or dark environments.

For indoor environments, lighting may include overhead fluorescent sources or incandescent, halogen, and/or combination bulbs typically found in lamps or ceiling fixtures in the home. In addition, natural light from the sun may enter through windows. Natural light can be an asset in the home or office when it is controlled with sheer panels, shades, or blinds on the windows. In the outdoors, natural light is more helpful in early or late parts of the day. Frequently, the use of a visor, sunglasses, or colored sun lenses will improve a client's vision. The OT practitioner needs to determine the best type of lighting and the best position for the light source to allow the client with low vision to be successful with everyday tasks (Figure 10-14).

When there is too much light in an environment, the client with low vision will experience glare. Glare can occur for several reasons, including reflected sunlight in an outdoor environment or reflected light indoors from surfaces such as floors, counters, and walls. It important for the OT practitioner to be aware of sources of glare for clients with low vision because glare can be discomforting at best, and disabling at its worst (Figure 10-15).

Contrast Strategies

To increase contrast, the OT practitioner needs to adapt a client's environment by using high-contrast colors and introduce nonoptical devices that will improve contrast with particular tasks (Figure 10-16). For instance, a simple use of colored electrician's tape along a door jamb, the edge of a step, a counter top, or along the edge of the bathtub can provide clients with low vision enough visual information to judge the depth, distance, or presence of an object. Other examples to improve contrast with reading and writing activities include the use of gel sheets, bold underlining for reading and writing, a writing

| BOX 10-4 | National Organizations for Low Vision |

Academy for Certification of Vision Rehabilitation & Education Professionals
3333 N. Campbell Ave., Suite 2
Tucson, AZ 85719
(520)887-6816
www.acvrep.org

American Academy of Ophthalmology
Street address:
655 Beach St.
San Francisco, CA 94109
Mailing address:
PO Box 7424
San Francisco, CA 94120-7424
(415)561-8500
www.aao.org

American Foundation for the Blind
AFB Senior Site
11 Penn Plaza, Suite 300
New York, NY 10001
1-800-232-5463
(212)502-7600
www.afb.org/seniorsite

American Council of the Blind
1155 15th St., NW, Suite 1004
Washington, DC 20005
1-800-424-8666
(202)467-5081
www.acb.org

American Occupational Therapy Association
4720 Montgomery Lane
PO Box 31220
Bethesda, MD 20824-1220
(301)652-2682
www.aota.org

American Optometric Association
243 N. Lindbergh Blvd.
St. Louis, MO 63141
1-800-365-2219
(314)991-4100
www.aoa.org

American Printing House for the Blind
1839 Frankfort Ave.
PO Box 6085
Louisville, KY 40206-0085
1-800-223-1839
(502)895-2405
www.aph.org

Association for Education and Rehabilitation of the Blind and Visually Impaired
1703 N. Beauregard St., Suite 440
Alexandria, VA 22311
1-877-492-2708
(703)671-4500
www.aerbvi.org

AWARE
PO Box 996

Mohegan Lake, NY 10547
(914)528-5120
info@visionaware.org
www.VisionAWARE.org

Blinded Veterans Association
477 H St., NW
Washington, DC 20001
1-800-669-7079
(202)371-8880
www.bva.org

Council of Citizens with Low Vision International
1859 N. Washington Ave., Suite 2000
Clearwater, FL 33755-1862
1-800-733-2258
(727)443-0350
www.cclvi.org

Independent Living Services for Older Individuals Who Are Blind
U.S. Department of Education, OSERS
400 Maryland Ave., SW
Washington, DC 20202-2800
1-800-872-5327
www.ed.gov/programs/rsailob/index.html

Lighthouse International
111 E. 59th St.
New York, NY 10022
1-800-829-0500
(212)821-9200
(212)821-9713 (TDD)
www.lighthouse.org

Low Vision Gateway
www.lowvision.org

National Association for Visually Handicapped
22 W. 21st St., 6th Floor
New York, NY 10010
(212)889-3141
(212)255-2804
www.navh.org

National Federation of the Blind
200 East Wells St. at Jernigan Place
Baltimore, MD 21230
(410)659-9314
www.nfb.org

National Library Service for the Blind and Physically Handicapped
Library of Congress
Washington, DC 20542
1-800-424-8567
(202)707-5100
(202)707-0744 (TDD)
www.loc.gov/nls

Resources for Rehabilitation
22 Bonad Rd.
Winchester, MA 01890
781-368-9094
www.rfr.org

BOX 10-5   Tips for Making Print More Readable

Low vision often makes reading a difficult task in the following situations:

- When a reduced amount of light can enter the eye
- When the image on the retina is blurred
- When the central portion of the retina (the macula) needed for reading is defective

The contrast of the print on its background is affected by reduced light and blurring. The damage to the central retina interferes with the ability to see small print, and to make necessary eye movements involved in reading.

The following guidelines make print more legible for individuals with vision problems and for the general public as well; therefore, they are important for universal design.

Print Size

Large-print type should be used, preferably 18 point, but at a minimum 16 point. Scalable fonts on the computer make this easy to do.

Font Type and Style

The goal in font selection is to use easily recognizable characters, either standard Roman or sans serif fonts. A good choice is Arial.

- Avoid decorative fonts.
- Use bold type because the thickness of the letters makes the print more legible.
- Avoid using italics or all capital letters. Both these forms of print make it more difficult to differentiate among letters.

Use of Color

The use of different colors of lettering for headings and emphasis is difficult to read for many people with low vision. When used, dark blues and greens are most effective.

Contrast

Contrast is one of the most critical factors in enhancing visual functioning, for printed materials as well as in environmental design. Text should be printed with the best possible contrast. For many older people, light lettering—either white or light yellow—on a dark background, usually black, is easier to read than black lettering on a white or light-yellow background.

Paper Quality

Avoid using glossy-finish paper such as that typically used in magazines and some journals. Glossy pages create excess glare, which makes it more difficult for people with low vision to read.

Leading (Space between Lines of Text)

The recommended spacing between lines of text is 1.5 lines, rather than single spacing. Many people who are visually impaired have difficulty finding the beginning of the next line when single spacing is used.

Tracking (Space between Letters)

Text with letters very close together makes reading difficult for many people who are visually impaired, particularly for those who have central visual field defects, such as older persons with macular degeneration. Spacing between letters should be wide—for example, a mono-spaced font such as Courier, which allocates an equal amount of space for each letter, is very readable.

Margins

Many low-vision devices, such as stand magnifiers and closed-circuit televisions (CCTVs), are easiest to use on a flat surface. An extra-wide binding margin makes it easier to hold the material flat. A minimum of 1 inch should be used; 1½ inches is preferable.

(From American Foundation for the Blind: VisionAware, www.VisionAware.org Accessed 10.19.15).

BOX 10-6   Four Fundamental Facts about Optical Devices

1. An optical device is not a cure and does not restore lost vision. It simply allows the user to have better function with the vision that he or she has remaining.
2. An optical device does not give clear vision to someone with a visual impairment. It can make an object appear larger and therefore be more readily identifiable, but it cannot make an object clearer when disease or trauma has caused the eye to lose its capacity for clear vision.
3. The low-vision physician prescribes optical devices in a specific manner for a given person for specific tasks.

To allow the client to self-prescribe or choose by trial and error and to think that this achieves the best result is a disservice.

4. To help a client use the prescribed device correctly, the practitioner must know precisely how the device works and how it should work for that person. Therefore, clear communication is necessary between the prescribing low-vision physician and the practitioner to ensure that therapy is effective. This will avoid the frustration and potential failure associated with using a device incorrectly.

(From Nowakowski, R. W. [2011]. Basic optics and optical devices. In M. Warren & E. A. Barstow [Eds.], *Occupational therapy interventions for adults with low vision* [pp. 75–103]. Bethesda, MD: AOTA Press.)

TABLE 10-2 Types of Visual Loss and Related Strategies to Improve Function

Type of Visual Loss	Strategies to Improve Function
Peripheral field loss	• Increasing lighting • Teaching scanning in vertical and horizontal planes • Increasing contrast • Teaching functional mobility skills to improve safety with mobility (For more complicated mobility tasks, such as multi-lane street crossings, refer the client to a certified orientation and mobility specialist [COMS].)
Central field loss	• Increasing lighting • Teaching eccentric viewing skills • Increasing contrast • Instructing client in the use of magnifiers for smaller printed items and dials
Decreased acuity (that cannot be corrected with eyeglasses)	• Increasing lighting • Increasing contrast • Instructing client in the use of magnifiers • Enlarging dials on appliances and numbers on phone

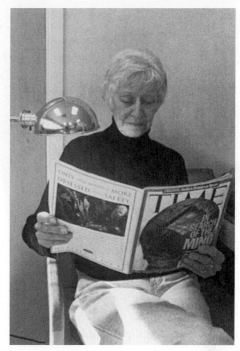

FIGURE 10-14 Use of a gooseneck lamp to increase effective task lighting without increasing lightbulb wattage. (From Guccione, A. A. et al. [2012]. *Geriatric physical therapy* [3rd ed.]. St Louis, MO: Elsevier.)

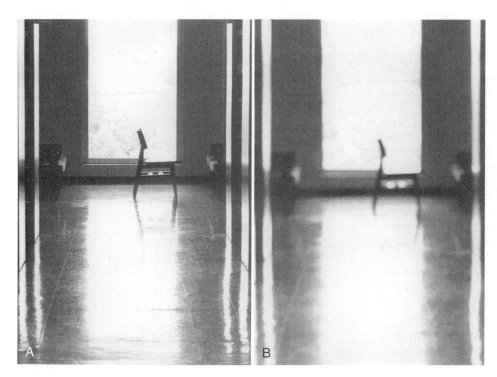

FIGURE 10-15 Glare perceived by a person with normal vision (A) and an older person whose eyes have undergone age-related changes (B). (From Linton, A. [2012]. *Introduction to medical-surgical nursing* [6th ed.]. St Louis, MO: Saunders.)

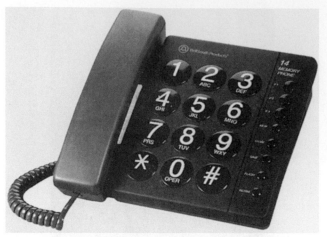

FIGURE 10-16 Black telephone with white lettering on the dial to enhance visual contrast. Large-button phone numbers also enhance visual acuity. (From Guccione, A. A. et al. [2012]. *Geriatric physical therapy* [3rd ed.]. St Louis, MO: Elsevier.)

guide, and a dark, thick felt pen (e.g., Sanford 20/20 Easy to Read Pen).

Scanning Strategies

Scanning is an effective technique to use with clients with visual field loss who have difficulty finding a landmark, the door to a business, or the edge of a page. When a client is outdoors, horizontal and vertical scanning techniques are effective in helping a client orient to the environment and locate an address, business, or door knob. The client is instructed to systematically view the environment, starting at the top and

scanning right to left, then left to right, until the object of interest comes into the visual field. The same technique can be used by scanning vertically, moving from top to bottom and bottom to top, working across the designated environment until clients find what they are looking for. In applying scanning techniques to near tasks, a client with a left-field deficit and the goal of reading effectively can benefit from the placement of a high-contrast border along the left margin of the reading material. The client would be instructed to scan to the left until the border comes into the line of sight. After reading the line of print, the client would be reminded to look for the border on the left to continue the reading process. Scanning techniques can be applied to many situations, allowing a client to orient and locate distant targets while aligning the visual field appropriately for both near and intermediate tasks.

Functional Mobility Strategies

Supporting the client with low vision in functional mobility skills is, in part, the responsibility of the OT practitioner. The client may need instruction for proper transfers in the bathroom, bedroom, living room, office, and car, to name a few. The client needs to be encouraged to keep pathways and furniture clear of clutter to avoid a fall or injury. Appropriate lighting and contrast in any given environment will aid clients with low vision in judging depth and distance during functional mobility tasks. The OT practitioner may also choose to instruct the client and caregiver in the use of sighted guide techniques (Box 10-7). These techniques will increase the client's safety in crowded or unfamiliar environments and areas that have poor lighting and uneven walking surfaces.

BOX 10-7 Sighted Guide Technique

Sighted guide is a technique originally developed for people who are blind, but it can also be helpful for people with low vision who are unsure of their bearings in an unfamiliar environment. **Remember: First always ask if any help is needed**, as not everyone needs sighted guide assistance.

The basis of the sighted guide technique is that the person who is blind or has low vision holds the guide's arm lightly above the elbow and allows the guide to walk one-half step ahead. This allows him or her to feel and follow the guide's direction.

1. To begin sighted guide, touch the arm of the person being guided with the elbow you prefer to use. He or she can then take your arm above the elbow. If someone needs extra support for walking, bend your supporting arm, parallel to the ground, so he or she can apply weight to your arm.

2. Give guiding signals just when a change in motion is needed. For example, pause briefly at the very edge of a curb. Signaling early can create confusion. Remember that verbal clues are also helpful, for example, "We are approaching a curb."

3. When going through a narrow door or passage, press your guiding arm backward toward the small of your back so the person being guided can move in single file behind you.

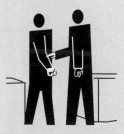

4. When approaching stairs, come to a stop at the edge of the first step and say whether the stairs go up or down and where the railing is located. The person being guided will follow one stair step behind, holding your arm with one hand and the handrail with the other. Pause after completing the stairs.

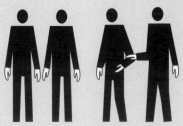

Continued

BOX 10-7   Sighted Guide Technique—cont'd

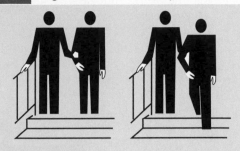

5. When approaching a curb, pause briefly at the very edge of the curb and say whether the curb goes up or down.

6. When coming to a door, stop first, then say whether the door opens toward or away from you, and whether it opens to the right or left. The person being guided can then move to the appropriate side. Open the door and proceed.

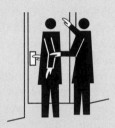

7. When approaching escalators and revolving doors, use techniques similar to those for stairs, curbs, and doors. If the person you are guiding is uncomfortable, use stairs or regular doors. Buildings with escalators or revolving doors are required to have stairs or regular doors.

8. When approaching a chair, place the hand of the person being guided on the back or side of the chair, if possible, so he or she knows where the chair is and which way it is facing. The individual can then decide where to sit.

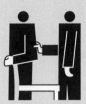

9. When helping a visually impaired person into a car, place one of this or her hands on the door handle and have the individual locate the edge of the car roof with his or her other hand. Then the person can seat himself or herself.

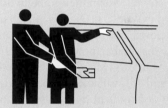

10. Increase or decrease the amount of assistance you give based on how comfortable the person being guided is with a sighted guide and whether he or she is carrying or using a white cane.

(Adapted with permission from *Sighted Guide Technique*, by SightConnection, 9709 Third Ave. NE #100, Seattle, WA 98115-2027.)

Functional mobility also includes the topic of transportation. When clients with low vision who have been driving for most of their adult lives are faced with the prospect of not being able to drive, it can be a difficult adjustment. Fortunately, a person with low vision can drive safely under the right circumstances.[31] There is not one isolated visual skill that can be associated with determining whether a person with low vision is fit to drive. It is best to refer clients with low vision who want to continue to drive to an occupational therapist who is also a certified driving rehabilitation specialist (CDRS) (see Box 10-3). These specialists are equipped with the knowledge and resources to intervene with clients with low vision who are interested in driving. For those clients who will not be driving, the OT practitioner can assist them in finding and using alternative transportation resources. Being familiar with public, private, and community transportation services in the local area will allow the OT practitioner to help clients with low vision make this transition with greater ease.

Eccentric Viewing Strategies

For clients with central field loss due to conditions such as macular degeneration, eccentric viewing is a strategy used to help them "look around" the blind spot in their field of view. With eccentric viewing, the client looks slightly away from their intended target, to bring it into view of the peripheral visual field. Once the client has determined the location of the scotoma or blind spot in the central visual field (as described earlier with the Clock Face Test method), training in looking around the scotoma is necessary to help develop eccentric viewing skills. The clock face, along with other visual tools, can also be used to further develop a client's eccentric viewing skills.

When using the clock face for eccentric viewing activities, the client with a scotoma in the center of the visual field is instructed to direct the scotoma to the right (toward the number three) to locate the center focal point. Then the client returns the scotoma to the center and is instructed to direct the scotoma upward (toward the number 12) to again locate the center focal point. This method of eccentric viewing training continues until the client is able to look around the scotoma with ease. Once a client has mastered the clock face, the client can progress to read lines of individual letters, then individual words, then lines of text, and finally to view pictures. Although some clients may have developed an eccentric viewing method subconsciously, for others it takes quite a bit of practice. Both the client and OT practitioner need to be patient with the process (see Box 10-3).

Magnification Strategies

Many times, clients with low vision benefit from magnification; however, it is not an intervention strategy that solves all low-vision problems.[29] When used properly, it can improve a client's functional visual abilities. There are several strategies for achieving magnification, including (1) use of a magnifier, (2) relative size magnification, (3) relative distance magnification, (4) angular magnification, and (5) projection magnification.[36]

Magnifiers are optical devices that use lenses to enlarge text and other materials. Magnifiers come in different powers and are measured in diopters (D). It is important to note that the stronger the power of a magnifier, the smaller the field of view; therefore, the higher-powered magnifiers will have smaller viewing windows. Magnifiers can be illuminated or nonilluminated and are available in different designs, such as stand magnifiers or handheld magnifiers (Figure 10-17). All of these features should be considered to meet the needs of individual clients.

Relative-size magnification is the process of increasing the size of an object to make it more visible. Simply put, relative-size magnification is an enlargement process.[36] This can easily be achieved when creating client handouts by using font features on the computer (see Box 10-5). Another method to achieve magnification is by decreasing the distance between the client and the object. This is known as relative-distance

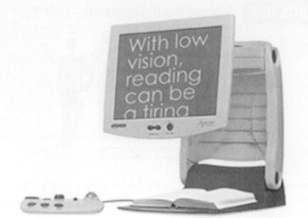

FIGURE 10-18 Computer with software for producing enlarged text. (From Guccione, A. A. et al. [2012]. *Geriatric physical therapy* [3rd ed.]. St Louis, MO: Elsevier.)

magnification. The closer the client is to an object, the larger the image becomes that is projected onto the retina.[36]

Angular magnification is achieved through the use of an optical device: the telescope. The use of a telescope allows an enlarged image of an object at a distance to be projected onto the retina.[36] This is very valuable for clients with low vision who need to read street signs, locate addresses, or identify a person from a distance. Another type of magnification is projection magnification. This type of magnification enlarges an image of an object by projecting it onto a screen.[36] This method is used in overhead projectors, closed circuit televisions (CCTVs), and portable electronic magnifiers (Figure 10-18).

The magnification devices and systems identified here are only a few of those that are available. It would be helpful for the OT practitioner to not only find hands-on training opportunities, but to also learn about the costs, and possible funding sources in the local community. Some of the devices and systems may be cost-prohibitive. However, many of the clients who require the more expensive items may be able to qualify for funding from a local agency. In addition, as with any type of adaptive equipment, if a client doesn't know how to use the magnifying devices and systems properly, they will not be used. It is important for OT practitioners to do all they can to make the most out of client education opportunities when it comes to the use of magnifiers. Clients have a great deal to gain if they're able to use the magnifiers efficiently and effectively.

Professional Issues in Low Vision

Professional Development

As the field of low-vision OT grows and expands, more skills are necessary to meet the needs of the low-vision OT client. As a result, occupational therapists and OT assistants would benefit from pursuing professional development opportunities in the area of low vision.

Professional development opportunities for low-vision practitioners include professional certification programs,

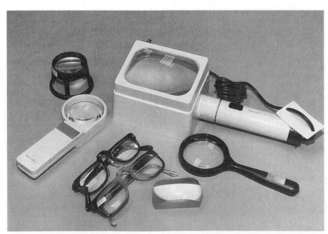

FIGURE 10-17 Some common optical aids used by individuals with low vision. (From Padilla, R. L. et al. [2012]. *Occupational therapy with elders* [3rd ed.]. St Louis, MO: Elsevier.)

graduate education with a focus in low-vision rehabilitation, face-to-face seminars, and online continuing education opportunities. The American Occupational Therapy Association's (AOTA) Board and Specialty Certification program provides an avenue for recognition in low-vision practice. Through a prospective and self-directed portfolio process, a specialty certification in low vision is available for occupational therapists (SCLV) and OT assistants (SCALV). Obtaining professional credentials indicative of advanced knowledge, skills, and experience in low vision provides OT practitioners the opportunity to have their expertise recognized by consumers, third-party payers, and professional peers.

Reimbursement

The Centers for Medicare and Medicaid Services (CMS) consider consumers with a low-vision diagnosis to have reduced physical functioning, and therefore such clients are covered for OT and physical therapy services related to mobility, ADLs, and other medically necessary goals. In 2002 the CMS authorized payment for physician-prescribed low-vision rehabilitation services provided by an occupational therapist (Table 10-3) or a physical

TABLE 10-3 Occupational Therapy Procedures for Low-Vision Rehabilitation

CPT Code	Description
97003	Occupational therapy evaluation
97530	Therapeutic activities (eccentric viewing training)
97532	Development of cognitive skills (compensatory skills)
97533	Sensory integrative techniques for enhanced sensory processing
97535	Self-care/home management training activities of daily living, meal preparation, safety, use of adaptive equipment
97537	Community/work integration (shopping, transportation, money management)

therapist. Current Procedural Terminology (CPT) codes are established by the American Medical Association for procedural billing purposes. For consumers with a low-vision diagnosis, optometrists (ODs) are considered physicians, and have the authority to prescribe low-vision rehab services.

CASE EXAMPLE 10-1   Mr. Smith

Mr. Smith is a pleasant 57-year-old married male with peripheral field loss in both eyes due to untreated glaucoma. He describes his field of view "as if I'm looking down a long cylinder and everything outside the cylinder is lost." He has two grown sons who are married. He retired early from his position as a university professor secondary to the limitations of the peripheral field loss in both eyes.

Mr. Smith is concerned about his visual limitations and has expressed worry about his ability to continue functioning on a level he is accustomed to around the house. In particular, Mr. Smith wants to maintain his role as caretaker of the yard—a role that allows him the enjoyment of being outdoors,

using his hands, and keeping his yard to support an attractive outdoor environment. He was referred to home health OT by his gerontologist to evaluate his ability to safely continue yard work. Mr. Smith's most recent evaluation by his ophthalmologist shows a loss of vision in the upper and lower quadrants of his visual field, along with the nasal and temporal fields.

Functional Visual Acuity Results
Mr. Smith was evaluated in the late afternoon, on a sunny day, both outdoors and inside his garage. The results of what he reported to see at various distances in each environment are as follows:

Outdoor and Indoor Environment:
Late-Afternoon Sunlight, Unless Specified
#1: some shadows

What Mr. Smith Reported to See
At 22 ft: can see tree trunk and three or four leaf bags

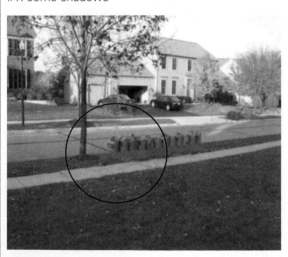

Continued

CASE EXAMPLE 10-1 Mr. Smith—cont'd

#2: some shading from neighbors' house

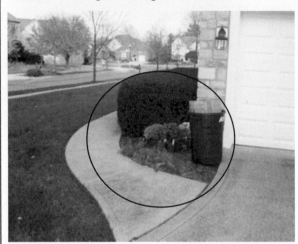

#3: some cloud coverage

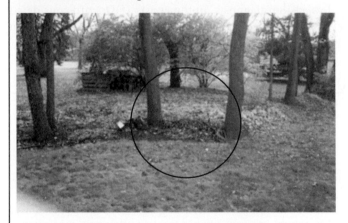

#4: some cloud coverage

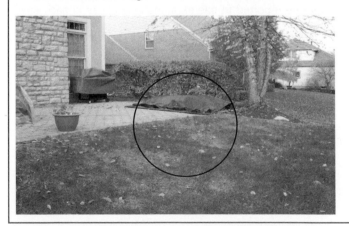

At 8 ft: can see part of 3.5-ft bush, most of sidewalk, flowers, and trash can; familiar with setup due to history in home

At 18 ft: can see brown objects—knows they are logs from earlier time; sees tree trunk on left

At 16 ft: can see blue tarp covering logs, grass and patio in forefront, and part of bush behind tarp

CASE EXAMPLE 10-1   Mr. Smith—cont'd

#5: in shadow of neighbors' house

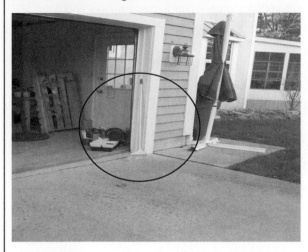

At 12 ft: can see broom, white frame of garage, gray siding, objects to lower left—not sure; part of piping to right

#6: less lighting in garage

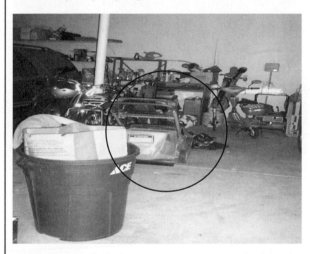

At 9 ft: sees the lawn mower and other things, familiar with setup and knows other yard tools to right of mower and slightly further into garage—does not distinguish them; sees green of yard waste receptacle in left-lower-corner view

#7: least amount of lighting, working further back into garage

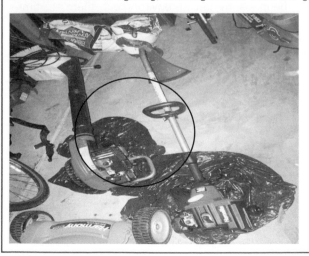

At 5 ft: can see portion of motor and black plastic casing of blower and black handle and rod of trimmer

Continued

CASE EXAMPLE 10-1 Mr. Smith—cont'd

#8: increased lighting toward outside view

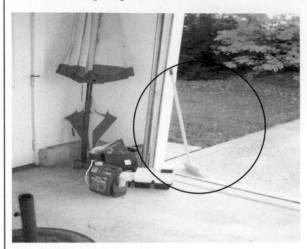

At 10 ft: can see grass in background, sidewalk to right, broom leaning on white frame; remarks about increased brightness when looking toward outside from garage

Functional Visual Fields

Mr. Smith's visual fields were evaluated outside, in an area somewhat shaded by the neighbors' house, and inside the garage, where there was less lighting available. Beginning inside the garage, viewing a near field of 5 feet with Mr. Smith looking straight at objects and not moving his eyes or head, he reported seeing portions of the leaf blower and the trimmer. An intermediate field for Mr. Smith was from 12 feet, and he could identify most of what was in his view, such as the broom, the white frame of the house, and gray siding, and he mentioned the objects to the right- and left-lower corners, although he did not identify them, and other objects in his field of view. The distance of 22 feet was used for Mr. Smith's far field of view. He stood in the shadow of the neighbors' house and looked out into shadows and sun. He was able to identify several bags of leaves, the grass, the tree trunk, and the sidewalk. Beyond the leaves, he did not identify much of anything and simply referred to that area as a general background.

Having the ability to move his head and eyes, Mr. Smith reported he could see most everything when scanning his environments from side to side and from up to down, if he knew to look for something; however, he is not sure he would always know to look for an object or person. He scanned in all areas of his visual field, not preferring any one area over another.

Mr. Smith has poor side-field awareness. When facing forward and looking ahead, Mr. Smith is unable to detect someone passing on his right or left side until the person is approximately 3 feet ahead of him. This type of impairment will impede Mr. Smith's functioning and safety if compensatory strategies, such as active scanning of his environment, are not incorporated into his functional routine.

Functional Visual Performance

Mr. Smith's usable vision in both eyes is 20/20 for distance and, with the use of glasses, for reading. The activities he needs to perform for maintaining the yard include raking, blowing, sweeping, trimming, bagging leaves and debris, moving logs, and planting flowers. At this time, Mr. Smith is not responsible for cutting the grass. Mr. Smith is able to complete the sweeping, raking, blowing, and trimming motions with similar positioning, posture, and scanning of his environment. He looks from right to left and back right, then up to down to up, but not in a methodical manner, for these tasks. For bagging leaves and debris, moving logs, or planting flowers, Mr. Smith's posture changes because he needs to lower himself down to the ground at times. He does this simply by bending down, using inefficient scanning methods to view the surface he is moving to (i.e., the ground), and then resting on a knee and foot, two knees (tall kneeling position), or two knees, while resting back on his heels. Mr. Smith tends to take a little longer to complete tasks because he often requires more time for locating the objects he needs for his yard tasks. When Mr. Smith is looking for a particular tool or is checking the progress of his work, he regularly scans his environment in all directions. When Mr. Smith is not anticipating an object, tool, or person to be in his immediate environment, there are times he may miss regularly scanning for them.

Intervention

Mr. Smith's motivation to maintain his caretaker role and yard routine is beneficial to the intervention process. In addition to OT, he would benefit from seeing a certified orientation and mobility specialist (COMS) to allow for him to safely and efficiently traverse the different surfaces and terrains in his yard.

OT intervention strategies to consider with Mr. Smith include:

1. Organize garage, work area, tools, and supplies for efficiency and to improve Mr. Smith's ability to locate needed items and/or avoid tripping over unexpected objects.
2. Provide adequate light in garage work and storage areas to improve Mr. Smith's ability to locate his tools and improve his safety.
3. Label items with high-contrast tape and markers to allow Mr. Smith to identify items more efficiently.

Case Example 10-1   Mr. Smith—cont'd

4. Incorporate efficient and effective scanning techniques to view yard, garage, and other work areas and support his ability to assess his work and progress, and locate items, tools, and landmarks (e.g., tree, driveway, garage door).
5. Consider distance from landmarks, tools, or other items to improve visual function during work tasks.
6. Incorporate use of dark visor or sunglasses to reduce glare as needed.
7. Investigate use of optical or electronic devices that may help to increase Mr. Smith's field of view in the yard, in the garage, or when reading labels.
8. Instruct in safety techniques and energy conservation techniques.
9. Develop schedule to work during the period of ideal daylight.
10. Refer to the local vision center for a thorough low-vision evaluation by an optometrist or ophthalmologist specializing in low vision. As a client at the vision center, Mr. Smith will also have access to support groups, social groups, additional resource information, social work services, and orientation and mobility services.

Summary

The OT practitioner who works to improve the occupational performance of older adults with low vision is providing them the opportunity to return to the roles and activities that give their lives meaning. It is an area of OT practice that is growing and should continue to grow for the next several decades, based on the projected increases in the older adult population.

REVIEW QUESTIONS

True or False

1. Typical vision changes associated with aging include macular degeneration, glaucoma, diabetic retinopathy, and cataracts.
2. Low-vision disorders are associated with visual-field deficits as opposed to impaired visual acuity.
3. A low-vision disorder can increase the risk of falls and fractures in older adults.
4. Clouding of the vitreous gel will affect the path of light from the cornea to the retina.
5. Vision loss is an individualized condition.
6. A low-vision examination by an optometrist or ophthalmologist will identify the rehabilitation potential of an older adult with low vision.
7. As part of an OT assessment of an older adult with low vision, the therapist needs to evaluate the client's visual factors.
8. The Feinbloom Chart and the low-contrast ETDRS Chart are used for testing visual acuity.
9. The Amsler grid is a tool used to measure the central 10 degrees of vision.
10. The approach to intervention for an older adult with low vision includes referring to other low-vision rehabilitation professionals as a means to additionally support the older adult's overall function, safety, and health.

REFERENCES

1. Administration on Aging. (2002). *Aging demographics.* Washington, DC: Dept. of Health and Human Services.
2. American Foundation for the Blind, Aging and Vision Loss Fact Sheet. http://www.afb.org/section.aspx?SectionID=68&TopicID=320&DocumentID=3374. Accessed 10.19.15.
3. American Occupational Therapy Association. (2014). Occupational therapy practice framework: Domain and process, 3rd ed. *American Journal of Occupational Therapy, 68*(Suppl. I), S1–S48. http://dx.doi.org/10.5014/ajot.2014.682006.
4. Beckley, M. N., Dickey, D., Manning, J., McCann, M., & Sewell, L. (2005). *Older adults with low vision: Exploring factors affecting occupation. Poster presentation.* Long Beach, CA: American Occupational Therapy Association Annual Conference and Exposition.
5. Beckley, M. N., Teaford, M. H., Kegelmeyer, D., Balaswamy, S., Flom, R., & Raasch, T. (2007). Interdisciplinary allied health education in treating older adults with low vision. *Journal of Allied Health, 36*(3), e192–e202.
6. Brilliant, R. L. (Ed.). (1999). *Essentials of low vision practice.* Boston, MA: Butterworth Heinemann.
7. Carter, K. (1983). Assessment of lighting. In R. T. Rose (Ed.), *Understanding low vision* (pp. 403–414). New York, NY: AFB Press.
8. Centers for Disease Control and Prevention (CDC), National Center for Health Statistics. (2001, March). *Trends in vision and hearing among older Americans.* http://www.cdc.gov/nchs/data/ahcd/agingtrends/02vision.pdf. Accessed 10.19.15.
9. Flom, R. (2004a). Visual functions as components of functional vision. In A. H. Lueck (Ed.), *Functional vision: A practitioner's guide to evaluation and intervention* (pp. 25–59). New York, NY: AFB Press.
10. Flom, R. (2004b). Visual consequences of most common eye conditions associated with visual impairment. In A. H. Lueck (Ed.), *Functional vision: A practitioner's guide to evaluation and intervention* (Appendix: 76–81). New York, NY: AFB Press.
11. Geruschat, D. R., & Smith, A. J. (2010). Improving the use of low vision for orientation and mobility. In W. R. Wiener, R. L. Welsh, & B. B. Blasch (Eds.), *Foundations of orientation & mobility* (Vol. III, 3rd ed., pp. 54–90). New York, NY: AFB Press.
12. Gilbert, M. P., & Baker, S. S. (2011). Evaluation and intervention for basic and instrumental activities of daily living. In M. Warren & E. A. Barstow (Eds.), *Occupational therapy interventions for adults with low vision* (pp. 227–267). Bethesda, MD: AOTA Press.
13. Gleckman, H. (2003). *Seniors' big drug problem.* Business Week. http://www.businessweek.com. Accessed 10.19.15.
14. Greer, R. (2004). Evaluation methods and functional implications: Children and adults with visual impairments. In A. H. Lueck (Ed.), *Functional vision: A practitioner's guide to evaluation and intervention* (pp. 177–275). New York, NY: AFB Press.

15. Haegerstrom-Portnoy, G., Schneck, M. E, & Brabyn, J. A. (1999). Seeing into old age: Vision function beyond acuity. *Optometry and Vision Science, 76*, 141–158.

16. Hinds, A., Sinclair, A., Park, J., Suttie, A., Paterson, H., & Macdonald, M. (2003). Impact of an interdisciplinary low vision service on the quality of life of low vision patients. *British Journal of Ophthalmology, 87*, 1391–1396.

17. Holm, M. B., & Rogers, J. C. (2008). The Performance Assessment of Self-Care Skills (PASS) In: In B. J. Hemphill-Pearson (Ed.), *Assessments in occupational therapy mental health.* (2nd ed. pp. 73–82), Thorofare, NJ: SLACK.

18. Koenig, A. J., Holbrook, M. C., Corn, A. L., DePriest, L. B., Erin, J. N., & Presley, I. (2000). Specialized assessments for students with visual impairments. In A. J. Koenig & M. C. Holbrook (Eds.) *Foundations of education* (Vol. II, 2nd ed., pp. 103–172). New York, NY: AFB Press.

19. Lamoureux, E. L, Hassell, J. B. & Keefe, J. E. (2004). The impact of diabetic retinopathy on participation in daily living. *Archives of Ophthalmology, 122*(1), 84–88.

20. Law, M., Baptiste S., McColl, M., Opzoomer, A., Polatajko, H., & Pollock, N. (1990). The Canadian occupational performance measure: An outcome measure for occupational therapy. *Canadian Journal of Occupational Therapy, 57*(2), 82–87.

21. Lovie-Kitchin, J. E., Devereaux, J., Wells, S., & Scupher, K. A. (2001). Multi-disciplinary low vision care. *Clinical & Experimental Optometry, 84*(3), 165–170.

22. Mahoney F. I., & Barthel D. (1965). Functional evaluation: The Barthel Index *Maryland State Med Journal, 14*:56–61.

23. Massof, R. (1995). *Issues in low vision rehabilitation: Service delivery, policy, and funding.* New York, NY: AFB Press.

24. Massof, R. (2002). A model of the prevalence and incidence among adults in the U.S. *Optometry & Vision Science, 79*(1), 31–38.

25. Meyers, J. R., & Wilcox, D. T. (2011). Low vision evaluation. In M. Warren & E. A. Barstow (Eds.), *Occupational therapy interventions for adults with low vision* (pp. 47–73). Bethesda, MD: AOTA Press.

26. Mogk, L. G. (2011). Eye conditions that cause low vision in adults. In M. Warren & E. A. Barstow (Eds.), *Occupational therapy interventions for adults with low vision* (pp. 27–46). Bethesda, MD: AOTA Press.

27. National Eye Institute. (2004). *National plan for eye and vision research.* Washington, DC: U.S. National Institutes of Health.

28. National Eye Institute. (2010). *Low vision quiz.* Bethesda, MD: National Institutes of Health. Retrieved from http://www.nei.nih.gov/health/lowvision/lowvision_quiz.

29. Nowakowski, R. W. (2011). Basic optics and optical devices. In M. Warren & E. A. Barstow (Eds.), *Occupational therapy interventions for adults with low vision* (pp. 75–103). Bethesda, MD: AOTA Press.

30. Orr, A. L. (1998). *Issues in aging and vision: A curriculum for university programs and in-service training.* New York, NY: AFB Press.

31. Peli, E. & Peli, D. (2002). *Driving with confidence: A practical guide to driving with low vision.* Singapore: World Scientific Publishing.

32. Perlmutter, M. S., Bhorade, A., Gordon, M., Hollingsworth, H. H., & Baum, M. C. (2010). Cognitive, visual, auditory, and emotional factors that affect participation in older adults. *American Journal of Occupational Therapy, 64*, 570–579.

33. Pleis, J. R., & Lucas, J. W. (2009). Provisional report: Summary health statistics for U.S. adults: National Health Interview Survey, 2008. *National Center* for Health Statistics. *Vital Health Statistics, 10*(242), 1–157.

34. Prevent Blindness America. (2002). *Vision problems in the U.S.: Prevalence of adult visual impairment and age-related eye disease in America.* Retrieved from http://www.preventblindness.org.

35. Rubin, G. S. (2000). Perceptual correlates of optical disorders of middle and later life. In B. Silverstone, M. A. Lang, B. P. Rosenthal, & E. E. Faye (Eds.), *The lighthouse handbook on vision impairment and vision rehabilitation* (Vol. 1, pp. 249–262). New York, NY: Oxford University Press.

36. Scheiman, M., Scheiman, M., & Whittaker, S. (2007). *Low vision rehabilitation: A practical guide for occupational therapists.* Thorofare, NJ: SLACK.

37. Sheikh, J. I., & Yesavage, J. A. (1986). Geriatric Depression Scale (GDS): Recent evidence and development of a shorter version. *Clinical Gerontology, 5*, 165–173.

38. Teitelman, J., & Copollilo, A. (2005). Psychosocial issues in older adults' adjustment to vision loss: Findings from qualitative interviews and focus groups. *American Journal of Occupational Therapy, 59*, 409–417.

39. U.S. Department of Health and Human Services. (2010). *Healthy people 2020.* Washington, DC: Author.

40. Warren, M. (2011). An overview of low vision rehabilitation and the role of occupational therapy. In M. Warren & E. A. Barstow (Eds.), *Occupational therapy interventions for adults with low vision* (pp. 1–26). Bethesda, MD: AOTA Press.

41. Warren, M., Bachelder, J., Velozo, C., & Hicks, E. (2008). *The self-report assessment of functional visual performance.* Birmingham, AL: Occupational Therapy Departments at University of Alabama at Birmingham and University of Florida at Gainesville.

42. Warren, M. L., & Lampert, J. (1999). Assessing daily living needs. In D. C. Fletcher (Ed.), *Low vision rehabilitation: Caring for the whole person. American Academy of Ophthalmology Series, Monograph 12.* San Francisco, CA: American Academy of Ophthalmology.

43. Watson, G., Baldasare, J., & Whittaker, S. (1990). The validity and clinical uses of the Pepper Visual Skills for Reading Test. *Journal of Visual Impairment and Blindness, 84*, 119–123.

44. Zimmerman, G. J., Zebehazy, K. T., & Moon, M. L. (2010). Optics and low vision devices. In A. L. Corn & Erin, J. N. (Eds.), *Foundations of low vision: Clinical and functional perspectives* (2nd ed. pp. 192–237). New York, NY: AFB Press.

CHAPTER 11

Nutrition, Occupational Performance, and the Phenomenology of Food in Later Life

Daphne Lo, MD, Abhilash K. Desai, MD, Julia Henderson-Kalb, MS, OTR/L, Miriam S. Moss, MA

CHAPTER OUTLINE

OBJECTIVES

- Understand how undernutrition can lead to poor overall health outcomes in older adults
- List three common nutritional deficiencies in older adults
- Understand the role nutrition plays in chronic disease
- Recognize that foods can often interact with commonly used drugs
- Describe appropriate occupational therapy interventions to assist older adults who have feeding problems, including interventions targeting food preparation
- List and explain the use of adaptive devices that can assist frail older adults with self-feeding
- Discuss factors that might impede eating and swallowing and related intervention approaches
- Summarize feeding techniques that caregivers should know to optimally assist an older adult with feeding problems
- Understand the relevance of social, cultural, and personal meanings of food and eating in the everyday lives of older adults
- Discuss gender differences in the meaning of food and eating in later life
- Comprehend various meanings of food among residents in long-term care settings

In the elderly, food is one of the major sources of possible pleasure; and it is a challenge for the health care providers to facilitate this enjoyment with their patients/clients for as long as possible. (p. 96)[10]

Activities surrounding food consumption represent health behaviors and occupations central to the lives and well-being of older adults. With aging, metabolism and physical activity slow down, sense of taste fades, and older adults may lose the opportunity to eat socially. Frailty can cause older adults to lose the capacity to shop, cook, prepare meals, eat, and clean up. These losses have significant biomedical and psychosocial implications, and older adults can easily develop malnourishment due to inadequate caloric and nutritional intake. Malnourishment in older adults can lead to decreased function, decreased quality of life, and increased mortality. This chapter will highlight important biomedical and occupational aspects of nutrition in older adults, as well as the cultural, social, and personal meaning of food and eating in older adults.

Nutritional Requirements in Older Adults

Slower metabolisms and less active lifestyles in older adults mean they do not require the standard 2000-calorie diet recommended for younger, more active adults. For those who are malnourished and/or experiencing situations requiring higher caloric intake (e.g., those recovering from surgery), it is important to consult a physician and a nutritionist to alter their daily caloric requirements. A daily diet for a healthy older adult should include 50% to 60% of total calories in carbohydrates, 15% to 20% of total calories in protein, and 30% of total calories in fat.[4]

In addition to calories, it is important for older adults to eat enough fiber and drink enough fluid to prevent constipation and dehydration because each can cause delirium, which can severely affect an older adult's health and function.[4] Fiber may be in the form of fruits and vegetables or dietary fiber supplements. Daily fiber requirements will vary between individuals and should be titrated to prevent and/or treat constipation without inducing diarrhea. Fluid requirements may fluctuate according to ambient temperature, but older adults should consume at least six to seven 8-oz glasses of fluids a day. Fluids can be any fluid the older adult wishes to drink, within reason. Many older adults will need reminders and encouragement to drink fluids because the body's ability to sense volume depletion and initiate thirst declines with age[20]. If an older adult's diet is lacking in fluid and fiber intake, it is important to ask about any concerns or problems with continence. Urinary incontinence and nocturia are often barriers to proper intake of fluids. Behavioral modifications such as scheduled toileting may help alleviate some concerns about urinary incontinence and help with improving fluid intake. Constipation can be a cause of perceived bowel incontinence due to leakage around an impaction.

The Undernourished Older Adult

Many older adults experience unintended weight loss, which negatively affects their function and well-being. As many as half of the older adults residing in nursing homes and 20% of community-dwelling older adults have below-average caloric consumption and body weight.[29,44] There are times when weight loss is associated with physical, emotional, or social factors that interfere with appetite and eating, and other times when weight loss is associated with end of life (see "Nutrition in End-of-Life Care" later in this chapter). Appetite naturally decreases with age, but pathologic weight loss is most commonly due to depression and medication side effects.[58] When caring for an older adult with unintended weight loss, one must correct controllable factors contributing to weight loss before attempting weight gain. When appropriate, nutritional supplements described later in the chapter may be used to promote weight gain in older adults.

Consequences of Undernourishment

Significant unintended weight loss across all ages is a matter of concern. In older adults, weight loss is associated with decreased bone mineral density and decreased muscle mass, both of which contribute to frailty and increased risk for loss of function and mortality.[29,44,58] In older adults who are already osteopenic or osteoporotic, further lowering bone mineral density can have disastrous consequences on function and well-being. Sarcopenia, the loss of muscle mass, is common even among healthy older adults, but can be accelerated or increased in those with poor nutrition.[11,58,85] Less muscle leads to muscle weakness, poor activity tolerance, and increased fall risk, all of which contribute to decreased function.[30,58]

Older adults residing in nursing homes who lose weight have a 30% risk of mortality in the next 6 months.[29,58] The risk of mortality can be reduced with weight stabilization or weight gain, creating a market for the nutritional supplements described later in the chapter.

Common Reversible Medical Causes of Malnutrition
Depression
Pathologic weight loss in older adults is often associated with depression. Treating depression can improve motivation for intake and socialization, thereby increasing intake. Mirtazapine is an antidepressant with potential side effects of promoting appetite, increasing weight, and improving sleep. This makes mirtazapine an often-prescribed drug for older adults with unwanted weight loss and comorbid depression. Unfortunately, studies have not consistently found significant weight gain in older adults using mirtazapine. Studies involving mirtazapine in older adults often enroll older adults who have comorbid depression, making it difficult to determine whether weight gain was due to the side effect of mirtazapine or improvement of depression.[29] Mirtazapine can cause drowsiness, which in turn can lead to falls. Because depression is a common cause of unintended weight loss, treatment of depression by any antidepressant tolerated by the older adult may reverse unintended weight loss.

Nutritional Supplements

Nutritional supplements given between meals (more than 60 minutes before the next meal) can help increase the energy consumption of older adults and promote weight gain.[85] Nutritional supplements, mostly in the form of shakes, come in a variety of brands and flavors. Aspects such as taste, consistency, and temperature can be important factors in an older adult's willingness to take a nutritional supplement and must be considered before providing a nutritional supplement.

Poor Dentition and Oral Health

Tooth decay and gum disease are prevalent in older adults and common reversible causes of malnutrition. Oral health problems from missing teeth, ill-fitting dentures, or infection can cause difficulty eating. Many medications commonly used by older adults cause dry mouth, leading to difficulty chewing and swallowing. Access to dental care often becomes more difficult for older adults. Furthermore, loss of self-esteem is associated with loss of teeth, leading to decreased socialization and depression, which in turn also increase risk of malnutrition. Older adults living in long-term care facilities and those with dementia are at increased risk for malnutrition related to poor dentition. (For more information, see Chapter 12 Oral Health for Aging Adults.)

Refeeding Syndrome

Special consideration is given here to older adults who may be recovering from severe malnourishment. Although it is important for these older adults to gain weight, reintroduction of calories must be done slowly and carefully to prevent refeeding syndrome.[11,76] First recorded in recovering Holocaust victims, refeeding syndrome is a condition seen with rapid reintroduction of calories in malnourished clients. It is characterized by a precipitous drop in intracellular (potassium, magnesium, and phosphorous) and extracellular (sodium) cations after refeeding of a malnourished person. The loss of cations may lead to fatal cardiac arrhythmias, edema, renal injury, and pulmonary injury.[11,76] Clients who are at risk of refeeding syndrome should be carefully monitored by a nutritionist and physician.

Common Nutritional Problems in Older Adults

Older adults are prone to certain nutritional problems due to poor food intake, which can result from various physiologic, psychological, and social changes in late life. The loss of social interaction during meals due to children moving out and/or loss of a spouse can decrease food intake. Comorbidities such as depression or pain may inhibit intake.[51] With age, absorption of nutrients is naturally decreased and abdominal surgeries may additionally impair nutrient absorption in the gut. Spinal cord compression due to osteoporosis can lead to decreased abdominal space and subsequent decrease in food intake. Common vitamin and nutritional deficiencies and related interventions in older adults are outlined in the following sections and in Table 11-1.

Vitamin D Deficiency

Vitamin D appears to play a large role in the health and well-being of older adults. Vitamin D is essential to bone health, and vitamin D deficiency is associated with increased fall risk, increased hip fracture risk, functional deterioration, muscle pain, and increased mortality. Aging naturally decreases the amount of vitamin D absorbed through the skin and in the gut. Due to a large public health initiative to encourage sunscreen use and ever-increasing numbers of older adults residing in institutionalized settings (i.e., long-term care facilities) where sun exposure is limited, nearly all older adult residents of long-term care facilities—and a large section of the general population—suffer from vitamin D deficiency.[59] It is important to measure vitamin D levels in older adults and provide supplements if serum levels are low to prevent osteoporosis and loss of function.

Iron-Deficiency Anemia

Anemia, a laboratory finding with multiple etiologies, is a state in which the number of red blood cells, or hemoglobin, is diminished. It can cause fatigue, activity intolerance, and decreased function.[51] Iron deficiency is a less likely cause in older adults compared with other causes such as chronic disease and vitamin B_{12} and/or folate deficiency. This is due to older adults' decreased need for iron. Usually, iron deficiency in older adults is due to chronic blood loss. Poor nutrition or medication interactions can also be a cause of iron-deficiency anemia in older adults.[47,51] In institutionalized older adults, the prevalence of iron-deficiency anemia is higher than that in the general population.[51] Thus when evaluating a client with increased fatigue or functional decline, it is important to consider anemia and causes of anemia because nutritional deficiencies can often be easily rectified.

Vitamin B_{12}/Folate (Vitamin B_9) Deficiency

Another cause of anemia is vitamin B_{12} and/or folate (vitamin B_9) deficiency. Vitamin B_{12} and folate deficiencies are common in older adults with "tea and toast" diets. Aging-related atrophic gastritis is the most common cause of vitamin B_{12} deficiency in older adults. Vitamin B_{12} deficiency is of particular concern in those with a history of gastrectomy or terminal ileectomy because both procedures severely impair the body's ability to absorb vitamin B_{12} from the gut. Vitamin B_{12} deficiency is associated with a syndrome involving poor cognition, loss of balance, and megaloblastic anemia. Folate deficiency is also associated with a decline in cognition.[59] When B_{12}/folate deficiency is suspected, it is important to check blood counts and vitamin levels. Diet changes and supplements may be needed to correct deficiencies.

Nutrition in Special Client Populations

Certain client populations may require specific diets to maintain health and prevent complications or loss of function from comorbidities. Certain dietary modifications have been shown to improve functional and cognitive health in older adults. Some common dietary modifications and their risks

TABLE 11-1 Common Nutritional Deficiencies, Consequences, and Interventions

Nutrient	Consequences	Intervention
Vitamin D	Increased fall risk Increased hip fracture risk Increased risk of mortality Increased risk of osteoporosis Functional deterioration	Screening for vitamin D deficiency Replacement if necessary Prophylactic vitamin D supplements for older adults in institutionalized settings
Iron	Anemia—fatigue, exercise intolerance	Screening for anemia Screening for possible causes of bleeding Replacement if necessary
Vitamin B$_{12}$	Poor cognition Loss of balance Megaloblastic anemia Increased risk of vascular disease Increased risk of depression Possible increased risk of age-related macular degeneration	Screening for vitamin B$_{12}$ deficiency, especially in those with history of abdominal surgery Replacement if necessary Prophylactic supplements for older adults with history of gastrectomy or terminal ileectomy
Vitamin B$_6$	Increased risk of vascular disease Increased risk of cognitive decline Anemia Increased risk of depression Possible increased risk of age-related macular degeneration	Usually borderline deficiency in older adults Improve diet Replacement with supplements if necessary
Folate	Poor cognition Megaloblastic anemia Increased risk of vascular disease Increased risk of depression Possible increased risk of age-related macular degeneration	Screening for folate deficiency Replacement if necessary
Calcium	Osteoporosis	Prophylactic vitamin D and calcium intake in the form of foods or supplements

(From Kaiser, M., Bandinelli, S.,& Lunenfeld, B. [2010]. Frailty and the role of nutrition in older people. *Acta Biomedica, 81*[Suppl. 1], 37-45; and Rohde, L. E., Silva de Assis, M. C., & Rabelo, E. R. [2007]. Dietary vitamin K intake and anticoagulation in elderly patients. *Current Opinion in Clinical Nutrition and Metabolic Care, 10,* 1-5.)

and benefits are described in this section. Keep in mind that most restrictive diets do not take into account older adults' personal food preferences or cultural and ethnic diets,[1] so changes such as no sweets for diabetics or salt restriction in those with heart failure can result in poor palatability of food and decreased intake leading to undernutrition in many older adults.

Diabetes

Blood glucose control is important to the health and function of older adults. Both hyperglycemia and hypoglycemia are associated with cognitive abnormalities. Hypoglycemia is known to cause falls, seizures, and delirium, three conditions that can severely affect an older adult's function and cognition. Hyperglycemia is also another common cause of reversible memory dysfunction.[59] Thus, it is important for older adults to maintain blood sugar control. Some older adults may require help from home health aides or family and friends to keep track of complicated drug and insulin regimens.

Dietary factors other than blood glucose control are also important. Diabetes increases the risk of other diseases that can threaten an older adult's health. The risk of atherosclerosis is increased with diabetes, which can result in stroke, myocardial infarction, and increased risk of vascular dementia. Multiple "silent strokes" or "ministrokes" over time can lead to vascular dementia, and major strokes can cause significant functional decline. Myocardial infarctions can lead to heart failure and possible death. Certain dietary considerations can help prevent or slow the progression of atherosclerosis (see the next section, "Cardiovascular Disease").

Those taking care of older adults with diabetes must also pay attention to signs of depression. Clients with diabetes are more prone to depression, which can cause fatigue, problems with concentration, poor nutritional intake, poor medication adherence, physical pain, and functional decline.[59]

Cardiovascular Disease

Two dietary modifications have been shown to improve cardiovascular disease risk. First is the Dietary Approaches to Stop Hypertension (DASH) diet, a primarily plant-based diet rich in fruits and vegetables and low-fat dairy with low levels of saturated fat, total fat, and cholesterol. Adhering to a DASH diet has been shown to decrease cardiovascular disease risk factors and was recently shown to decrease the 10-year coronary heart disease risk by almost 20%.[16]

The Mediterranean diet has also been found to improve cardiovascular health and reduce risk of cognitive decline. It contains high amounts of fruits, vegetables, and legumes; moderate amounts of whole grains; and small amounts of red meat. In addition, fish, nuts, and olive oil in the Mediterranean diet provide healthy fats.

Recently, specific nutrients such as flavanols and omega-3 fatty acids have been suggested to play a positive role in cardiovascular health. Unfortunately, studies are limited, and study design and control can vary substantially when testing these compounds that can exist as different isomers and in different amounts in various foods.

Flavanols, found in foods such as chocolate, grapes, and tea, have been shown in some studies to lower mortality from cardiovascular disease, although the evidence is not numerous or convincing enough to issue new guidelines in flavanol intake.[40] Despite the interest in omega-3 fatty acids, found in fish such as salmon, there is no conclusive evidence to show that supplementation with omega-3 fatty acids decreases mortality from cardiovascular disease in the long term.[27]

Congestive Heart Failure

Much attention is paid to maintaining fluid balance and limiting salt intake, but little research has been done to validate the effectiveness of salt and fluid restriction on preventing peripheral edema and shortness of breath, which are some of the major symptoms of congestive heart failure.[49] In clients whose symptoms are well controlled, a sodium-restricted diet of less than 3 g/day is recommended, and fluids do not need to be restricted. In clients with volume overload as evidenced by symptom exacerbation, it is recommended to limit sodium intake to less than 2 g/day with fluid restriction dependent on the severity of volume overload.[49]

Osteoporosis

Because protein forms about one sixth of bone volume in the form of collagen, it is important to improve protein intake as well as calcium and vitamin D supplements in clients with osteoporosis. Studies have shown increased animal protein intake to be associated with an increase in bone mineral density, and increased animal protein intake may increase calcium absorption from the gut.[22]

Those with osteoporosis are also encouraged to maintain adequate intake of calcium and vitamin D, either naturally or through supplements. For people aged 60 years and over, it is recommended to take in 300 mg of vitamin D per day and 1200 mg of calcium per day.[79] Recent research has studied the effect of calcium and vitamin D supplements on cardiovascular risk and mortality. Results are still inconclusive because many studies are not directly measuring cardiovascular disease as an end point and do not look at calcium or vitamin D supplements exclusively or in combination in a randomized controlled trial. Additionally, very few studies have examined natural dietary increase in calcium or vitamin D and their effect on cardiovascular disease risk.[79] It is important for all older adults, especially those with osteoporosis, to receive adequate vitamin D and calcium intake without taking in too much.

Nutrition in Dementia

Special attention is paid here to nutrition in older adults living with dementia. Although many older adults with dementia have the Alzheimer's type of dementia or mixed dementia (Alzheimer's plus vascular dementia), it is important to remember the other subtypes of dementia, such as Parkinson's disease dementia, frontotemporal dementia, Lewy body dementia, and alcohol-related dementia. Some types of dementia are potentially reversible (e.g., dementia due to nutritional deficiencies), and some (e.g., vascular dementia) are more preventable than others (e.g., Parkinson's disease dementia). Although the pathogenesis of dementia is a long process spanning two or more decades before the onset of symptoms, certain dietary modifications may decrease the risk of common dementia syndromes.

Reversible Dementia

Certain vitamin deficiencies and metabolic abnormalities are known to cause memory loss and dementia (see "Common Nutritional Problems in Older Adults" earlier in the chapter). Thiamine (B_1) and vitamin B_{12} deficiency can lead to dementia and may be reversed with early diagnosis and vitamin supplementation. Additionally, folate and B_{12} deficiency increase homocysteine levels, which may directly cause neuronal degeneration and/or increase the risk of cardiovascular disease and lead to a type of irreversible dementia.[5] Vitamin D deficiency has also been linked to poor memory (see discussion of vitamin D in "Common Nutritional Problems in Older Adults" earlier in the chapter).[5,17,59] As stated previously, hyperglycemia and hypoglycemia can also cause cognitive dysfunction, which may exacerbate any preexisting memory problems an older adult may have (see earlier discussion of diabetes in "Nutrition in Special Client Populations" section). Other potentially reversible dementias include alcohol-related dementia, medication-induced dementia, depression-related dementia, and dementia due to hydrocephalus.

Nutrition and Prevention of Dementia

Cardiovascular disease, such as atherosclerosis, may have a role to play in vascular dementia. Dietary modifications such as adhering to the Mediterranean diet or the DASH diet, switching to a plant-based diet, and controlling serum cholesterol levels during middle age may play an important role in preventing the onset of vascular dementia and Alzheimer's disease in later life.[30]

Unfortunately, few other dietary changes have been definitively proven to lower the risk of developing or altering the course of dementia, especially Alzheimer's dementia. Controlling serum cholesterol appears to have some effect on brain function. High levels of triglycerides may impair cognitive functioning by inhibiting the effects of leptin, a memory-enhancing hormone.[59] The role of cholesterol is complicated because cholesterol appears to have both a protective and detrimental effect on a client's risk of developing dementia. High levels of cholesterol during middle age are associated with an increased risk of dementia later in life, whereas high cholesterol in later life is associated with lower risk of dementia.[5]

One method of preventing brain aging and dementia is by restricting calories, a method shown to inhibit the body's natural aging process. Caloric restriction induces the production of neuroprotective molecules that help neurons resist damage. Unfortunately, dementia is a complex and lengthy disease, and any caloric restriction, unless enacted early in life, may be a case of too little, too late.[5]

There has been limited evidence to show that consumption of omega-3 fatty acids or free-radical antioxidants such as vitamin E may decrease the risk of dementia by decreasing the risk of strokes (see earlier discussion of cardiovascular disease in the "Nutrition in Special Client Populations" section).[5,17] Ultimately, clients are advised to eat healthily and lead healthy lifestyles to prevent or delay the onset of dementia.

Nutrition in Older Adults Diagnosed with Dementia

There is little evidence to support the use of diet to cure or stop the progression of dementia. To date, there are no guidelines for optimal diets in older adults with any type of dementia.[5] Recent studies have been conducted on "memory shakes," such as Souvenaid and Benevia, which claim to enhance memory. There is little evidence to support the benefit of these shakes, although one study showed some improvement in verbal memory in clients with early Alzheimer's dementia after finishing a trial of Souvenaid.[59] A small study found an improvement in verbal fluency with a trial of Benevia.[59]

Nutrition in Long-Term Care Communities

Growing numbers of older adults live in health-care communities such as assisted living facilities and nursing homes. Theoretically, living in a controlled environment can improve older adults' nutrition because they receive more nutritious diets that adhere to dietary restrictions based on health concerns, and residents may be prompted to eat by health-care staff. However, moving into a long-term care facility may put an older adult at risk for depression, further increasing the risk of undernutrition from poor intake. Personal food preferences and ethnic dietary norms frequently are ignored in long-term care settings, and choice of entrée or other dishes may be limited, resulting in dining experiences that may be less than optimal for residents.

Many disease-specific diet restrictions such as a no-concentrated-sweets diet for diabetics or a sodium-restricted diet in heart-failure clients have not been well studied or shown to be effective in older adult residents of long-term care communities. Thus, the American Dietetic Association (ADA) recommends foregoing restrictive diets to improve the food experience and palatability for older adults residing in health-care communities.[1]

Nutrition in End-of-Life Care

Food and nutrition are necessary to survival. Throughout this chapter, the importance of nutrition to health and well-being has been stressed. Severe neurologic injury can greatly prohibit a person from recognizing a need for nutrition and physically prohibit an individual from eating and/or swallowing. For many older adults, end-stage illnesses (e.g., terminal-stage dementia) may increase risk of aspiration. Feeding tubes do not alleviate and may even increase the risk of aspiration.[19] At these stages, nutrition can be less important to quality of life, bringing up many emotional and ethical issues for loved ones and health-care providers.

Should the decision be made to implement long-term enteral nutrition (also known as tube feeding), a percutaneous endoscopic gastrostomy (PEG) tube may be inserted into the stomach. A PEG tube is the most invasive means of giving long-term nutrition. A less invasive method is to insert a nasogastric (NG) tube through the nose extending into the stomach. Neither method comes without risk of aspiration. Many older adults, especially those with dementia, do not find tubes comfortable and may pull and dislodge them, increasing the risk of infection and possibly decreasing quality of life.[69] There is no definitive evidence to show that PEG or NG tubes improve mortality, decrease aspiration risk, or improve quality of life in older adults with terminal dementia,[31,69] which would be helpful information when writing health directives (see Chapter 2, Ethical and Legal Aspects of Occupational Therapy with Older Adults).

Food and Drug Interactions

The risk of adverse events from drugs must be balanced in older adults, who often require multiple medications for their comorbidities to improve their function. This section focuses on the important role food plays in drug metabolism and explains two common food-drug interactions.

The Role of Food in Drug Metabolism

Food and nutrition play vital roles in drug metabolism. Depending on the drug, food can alter the absorption of drugs from the gut. Certain drugs—such as the antibiotics cefuroxime and erythromycin, and lovastatin—can and should be taken with food to allow for better absorption.[34] Other drugs—such as the antibiotics ampicillin, ciprofloxacin, and doxycycline, and the blood pressure drug captopril—should be taken on an empty stomach for better absorption.[34] Table 11-2 lists common drug-food interactions. Unfortunately, having some drugs that require an empty stomach and others that require a full stomach can create a confusing and complicated drug regimen that may require the help of an older adult's pharmacist, family members, and home health aides.

Food can also affect the bioavailability of drugs by altering the function of liver enzymes responsible for breaking down drugs. One very common interaction between food and liver enzymes is described in the next section. Last, an older adult's nutritional status may affect the bioavailability of drugs: Poor

TABLE 11-2 Common Drug-Food Reactions

Drug	Clinical Use	Effect with Food
Acetaminophen	Analgesia	Slower absorption and later onset of analgesia
Captopril	Hypertension Heart failure	Decreased absorption with food
Ciprofloxacin	Antibiotic, often used for urinary tract infections	Substantially decreased absorption when taken with cations (calcium, zinc, iron, magnesium)
Digoxin	Heart failure	Decreased absorption with high-fiber food
Levodopa/carbidopa	Parkinson's disease	Decreased absorption, especially with high-protein meals
Metformin	Type 2 diabetes management	Decreased absorption, especially with high-fiber food
Warfarin	Anticoagulation	Decreased absorption Vitamin K effects
Aspirin	Anticoagulation Heart disease prevention	Increased absorption
Hydrochlorothiazide	Hypertension	Increased absorption with food
Simvastatin	Cholesterol management	Increased absorption with food
Tricyclic antidepressants (nortriptyline, amitriptyline, imipramine)	Depression, not recommended in older adults Neurologic pain	High-tyramine-containing foods such as cheese, alcohol, and liver can cause hypertensive crisis

(From Bressler, R. [2006, November]. Grapefruit juice and prescription drug interactions: Exploring mechanisms of this interaction and potential toxicity for certain drugs. *Geriatrics, 61*, 12-18.)

nutritional status will lower the amount of protein in the blood, potentially decreasing the body's ability to transport certain drugs throughout the body.[34]

Common Drug-Food Interactions

Vitamin K is necessary for the production of coagulation factors in the blood. Warfarin inhibits this vitamin K–mediated process of coagulation factor production. It is used to prevent blood clots from forming in clients known to have increased risk of forming life-threatening blood clots such as deep vein thromboses and pulmonary emboli. Theoretically, increased vitamin K intake can overcome the inhibitory actions of warfarin and increase production of coagulation factors. Although it is widely accepted that vitamin K intake affects warfarin therapy, the amount of daily vitamin K that is allowable and safe is not well studied. However, studies have shown that a stable intake of vitamin K may be necessary for proper anticoagulation, and fluctuations in daily vitamin K intake may affect anticoagulation.[64]

Another important food and drug interaction is the effect grapefruit juice can have on drug bioavailability. Grapefruit juice contains furanocoumarins, which directly inhibit the cytochrome P450 (CYP) family of enzymes. One member of this CYP family is CYP3A4, which is responsible for breaking down many drugs, such as antihypertensives, statins, antidepressants, and some potentially dangerous heart medications such as digoxin, in the liver. Grapefruit juice inhibits the action of CYP3A4, leading to both increased and decreased bioavailability of certain drugs depending on whether first-pass metabolism through the liver produces active or inactive metabolites. These effects can linger after the grapefruit juice

has been cleared out of the body. Various studies have shown that this effect is dose dependent, with most studies showing effects lasting for at least 24 hours and some residual activity occurring for up to 3 days.[12] Although the effect of grapefruit juice intake on serum drug levels is well documented, there is no conclusive evidence to state that this increases the risk and incidence of adverse events. Because of this theoretically increased risk of adverse drug events, it is recommended that clients taking medications targeted by CYP3A4 avoid grapefruit products.[12,34]

The Role of Supplements in the Nutrition of Older Adults

With increasing health consciousness and the focus on longevity, as many as 40% of older adults are taking supplements in the form of herbs, vitamins, and other over-the-counter (OTC) additives.[52] Although there is some evidence to suggest possible benefits of OTC supplements, there is also evidence to suggest that certain supplements do not have any added benefit to older adults' health and may sometimes cause harm. This section highlights misconceptions and concerns regarding dietary supplements, and provides guidelines for older adults wishing to take dietary supplements.

Herbal Supplements

Herbal supplements such as gingko biloba, ginseng, St. John's wort, and glucosamine often have origins in traditional medicine. Although traditional medicine specialists claim herbal supplements are safe and effective, consumers must keep in mind that the dosage and additives contained in one pill are unlikely to be the same formulation or dosage as what one might get from a traditional medicine specialist. Moreover, certain herbs are known to produce adverse effects in combination with other prescribed medications. Gingko biloba, often touted as a memory aid, can result in bleeding reactions when combined with warfarin or aspirin and can potentiate the effects of trazodone.[21] St. John's wort, often used for mood regulation, can decrease the effectiveness of amitriptyline and simvastatin.[21]

Herbal products are considered dietary supplements and are not strictly regulated by the Food and Drug Administration (FDA). There are no rigid guidelines for the dosage or formulation of each herbal product, making it difficult to control, monitor, and enforce quality and safety in these products. Certain compositions of herbal remedies may include potentially harmful chemicals that can directly harm an older adult or cause adverse drug reactions when combined with other OTC or prescription drugs. Variation in dosages and composition between products creates great difficulties for researchers seeking to study the benefits of an herbal remedy, contributing to the dearth of reliable information regarding OTC herbal remedies.[21] Should an older adult be interested in supplementing his or her diet with herbal remedies, consultation with a pharmacist or physician is highly recommended. Older adults should always inform their physicians of all OTC products they consume.

The Daily Multivitamin

With direct-to-consumer marketing toting benefits to bone health and the immune system, many older adults are now taking daily multivitamins in an effort to promote health and longevity despite no formal recommendation for older adults to take vitamin and mineral supplements. In a healthy older adult, the only vitamins and minerals needed in higher quantities are vitamin D, vitamin B_{12}, and calcium, and these requirements are generally not met by diet alone.[52] Most older adult individuals, especially those in long-term care facilities, are recommended to have vitamin D and calcium supplements. As stated in previous sections, other supplements are required only in times of vitamin or mineral deficiency when older adults may experience a loss of function and higher mortality. There is limited evidence to suggest that above-recommended daily intakes benefit overall health.[52] On the contrary, overfortification with certain vitamins such as vitamin A and vitamin D may actually cause harm (see the earlier discussion of osteoporosis in the "Nutrition in Special Client Populations" section). In older adults who are prone to kidney stones, overfortification of the diet with calcium may increase the risk of kidney stone formation.[52]

The use of daily multivitamin and mineral supplements may have the most benefit in older adults who are deficient in a vitamin or mineral due to poor nutrition or poor absorption.

In those who are susceptible to vitamin or mineral deficiencies, such as older adults with previous gastrectomies, and are prone to vitamin B_{12} deficiency or older adults living in nursing facilities with limited sunlight exposure, vitamin supplements may help prevent problems related to vitamin deficiencies. In healthy older adults, diet alone is likely to meet their vitamin and mineral requirements, although care should be taken to ensure older adults have adequate calcium and vitamin D intake.[13] If an older adult is concerned about micronutrient intake, consultation with a physician is recommended before beginning a supplement.

Occupational Therapy Evaluations for Feeding Disorders

To determine the issues that might be causing feeding difficulties for the older adult, it is important to complete a thorough feeding assessment. There are multiple feeding assessments that an occupational therapist can complete. Glantz and Richman[36] have created several assessments that work well. Whatever evaluation is completed, it is usually best to observe an entire meal in the setting in which the individual regularly dines. This allows for a more realistic evaluation of the entire feeding situation, including sitting position, environmental influences (e.g., lighting or noise), and dinnerware or adaptive equipment used.

Occupational Therapy Interventions for Feeding Disorders and the Older Adult

Treatment options for feeding issues with older adults are vast and are often similar to those for the non-older-adult population. As with all treatment in occupational therapy, the type of intervention used will depend on the person's diagnosis and functional level. The following sections list several options for intervention, and possible diagnoses that relate to particular interventions.

Grocery Shopping

Grocery shopping is often an overlooked but absolutely necessary part of food preparation and feeding. The older adult's ability to participate in this instrumental activity of daily living (IADL) may be impacted by income level and/or distance to grocery stores. Additionally, if an older adult has low vision, mobility issues, or low activity tolerance, grocery shopping might be a difficult activity. The scope of this discussion will focus on the act of shopping and not the physical act of getting to the grocery store, but note that many options do exist for transportation. Once at a grocery store, there are options for the older adult to make the shopping experience easier. Simply having a grocery cart to steady oneself can often be the only assistance an older adult needs.

However, if an individual is unable to walk distances within the grocery store due to decreased activity tolerance, loss of balance, or weakness, most stores provide motorized scooters with baskets to allow for greater mobility. Upon exiting the store, the older adult can ask for assistance from an employee to load heavy bags of groceries into a car.

If an older adult has difficulty getting around the grocery store or is unable to use transportation for one reason or another, there are still options for grocery shopping, depending on where the person lives. Some stores provide services for home delivery or in-store/curbside pick-up. These services allow a person to call in or go online and place a grocery order, and the grocery store will bag all of the items. Then the food is either delivered to the home or a person can go to the store and collect the order.[46] Most of the time there are fees associated with these services, but they can be invaluable for a person who needs them to live independently.

There are also food delivery services that are available to deliver groceries and already-prepared heat-and-serve meals. With these companies, a person can receive a catalog of available food options and order them online or over the phone. Then the food is delivered to the home. Such items can be heated and served or stored in a freezer for future use. Researching the options for the area in which a person lives can be a helpful reference for any older adult.

Food Preparation

For many older people, women especially, food preparation (cooking) can foster feelings of nostalgia. Giard[35] noted that "doing-cooking is the medium for a basic, humble, and persistent practice that is repeated in time and space, rooted in the fabric of relationships to others and to one's self, marked by the 'family saga' and the history of each, bound to childhood memory just like rhythms and seasons" (p. 157). Because of this, it is necessary to consider food preparation as an important occupation that must occur before feeding itself.

First consider the environment in which food is prepared: the kitchen space itself. Many adaptations can be made to the physical environment to make food preparation easier for the older adult.

Adaptations for an Older Adult in a Wheelchair

It is typically necessary to make special adaptations to the kitchen when an individual is in a wheelchair. The minimum turning radius for a wheelchair is 5 feet by 5 feet, so that amount of space is necessary to make a kitchen accessible for a wheelchair. If the space is not accessible via the wheelchair, most of the prep work can be done at a table outside of the kitchen. From a wheelchair level, it is easiest to complete kitchen tasks with lowered cabinets and knee space beneath counters and the sink (Figure 11-1).[43]

If lowering the cabinets is cost-prohibitive, removing the cabinet doors below the sink and a few cupboards can allow for an individual in a wheelchair to be in closer proximity to the countertops. If this is the chosen option, it is recommended that the hot water pipes either be removed or insulated with foam rubber or other protective material to prevent scalding. The garbage disposal might also need to be insulated.[43]

Adaptive equipment can also be used to make food preparation easier from a wheelchair level. To see what is being prepared on the stovetop burners, an oven-stove mirror may be installed. It is easiest for an individual who is in a wheelchair to use a stovetop with knobs on the front of the stove versus rear-mounted knobs (Figure 11-2). However, if rear-mounted knobs are the only option, a long stove knob turner may be used to reach the knobs.[68] (See also Chapter 21 for more information on adaptive technology.)

Adaptations for an Older Adult with Low Vision

For older adults who have difficulty with low vision, food preparation can be a difficult and dangerous task. Adapting the environment may be imperative for these individuals.

Lighting in the kitchen can be helpful or harmful for an older adult with low-vision deficits. Lighting levels for an older adult should be at least two or three times brighter than those comfortable for younger people. Fluorescent or halogen lights are often a better alternative to incandescent light bulbs. Painting the kitchen a light color also increases the amount of light interreflected in the room.[26]

There are also options to reduce the glare that some lighting creates. Using shades or sheers to filter natural light from windows can help reduce glare. It has been found that opaque or translucent light shades or covers reduce glare, so avoiding

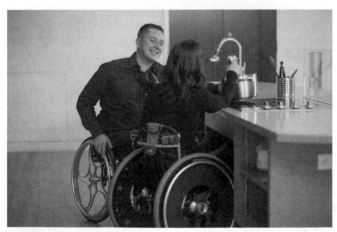

FIGURE 11-1   Space under the sink for a wheelchair. Photo © istock.com.

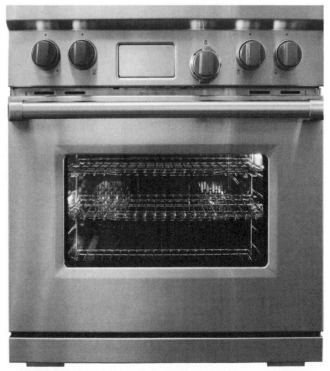

FIGURE 11-2   Stove with knobs on the front. Photo © istock.com.

clear-glass light fixtures is recommended. Shiny surfaces, such as linoleum tile or Formica countertops, can also cause glare. Matte-finish surfaces reduce glare, as does changing the position of the light source relative to the normal line of sight.[26] Wearing sunglasses or hats can reduce glare without changing the environment.

Using contrasting colors in food preparation can be helpful. A dark cutting board for light-colored foods and a light or white cutting board for dark-colored foods can allow an individual to more easily see the food being cut.[43] Other types of adaptive equipment are also available, such as a large-digit timer that can be easier to see for people with visual impairments. Also, liquid filling indicators are small gadgets that can be placed on any container and will make a buzzing sound when liquid has reached about 1 inch from the top of the container, to avoid overflow or spilling.

Adaptations for Energy Conservation

Preparing a meal takes energy. If the older adult has decreased endurance, meal preparation can be challenging. Multiple adaptations can be made to decrease the amount of energy it takes to prepare a meal. A general rule of thumb is to place the most-used kitchen items between eye and knee level to decrease the amount of stooping and reaching that an individual will need to do. A rolling cart can be used to move heavy items from one area of the kitchen to another; and sitting versus standing to prepare food will also conserve energy. Microwaves and toaster ovens are often easier to manage than standard ovens that are part of a stove, especially if located at counter height. Crockpots and food processers can also make cooking more manageable for an individual with limited activity tolerance. Instructing older adults on energy conservation techniques is also important so that meal preparation can be completed with little to no fatigue (Box 11-1).

Adaptive Equipment for Food Preparation

Many other pieces of adaptive equipment can be used for general food preparation. A nonslip material called Dycem, for example, can be used for a multitude of purposes, including but not limited to holding items in place while cutting and preparing food and providing additional grip when opening jars. A paring board may have several adaptations, including corner guards to support items being cut, prongs to hold items in place, and/or nonskid bases to prevent the paring board from sliding (Figure 11-3).[68]

BOX 11-1   Meal Preparation Techniques to Minimize Fatigue

- Plan ahead. Have all ingredients and utensils out before beginning a cooking task.
- Pace yourself. Rest while food is baking or items are boiling.
- Have a place to sit in the cooking area in case a rest break is needed.
- Sit while dicing, mixing, etc.
- Kitchen gadgets often save energy. Use a food chopper to dice food rather than manually completing the task. Use a blender or a food processor to blend food.
- If a kitchen is overly warm, prepare the majority of the food just outside of the kitchen. Excessive heat can decrease activity tolerance.
- Use a handled trivet on wheels to move a filled pot or pan along a countertop without having to carry it. Use a rolling utility cart to move heavy items from countertop to table.
- Allow dishes to air dry.
- Cook multiple meals at one time and freeze them in single-portion servings for future use.

Specialty Cookbooks and Websites*
- *Achilles, Elaine. **The Dysphagia Cookbook: Great Tasting and Nutritious Recipes For People With Swallowing Difficulties**. Nashville, TN: Cumberland House, 2004.*
- *Blakeslee, Mary E. **The Wheelchair Gourmet: A Cookbook For The Disabled**. New York, NY: Beaufort Books, Inc., 1981.*

- Davies, Ken. **Wheelchair Diet Plan.** Preston, UK: Help4U Publishing, 2001.
- **The Disabled Gourmet.** Orange Coast College Campus Colleagues Club. Costa Mesa, CA. Cookbooks by Morris Press, 1998.
- Evans, Henry and Jane Evans. **The Pureed Gourmet.** Scott Publishing, 2004.
- Greer, Rita. **Soft Options: For Adults Who Have Difficulty Chewing.** Great Britain: Souvenir Press, 1998.
- Klinger, Judith Lannefeld. **Mealtime Manual: For People With Disabilities And The Aging.** Thorofare, NJ: SLACK Incorporated, 1997.
- Relevant Websites:
  - Easy to Swallow http://www.easytoswallow.co.uk/
  - Mealtime Partner: Powered Dining Device www.mealtimepartners.com (enables people who cannot eat independently to feed themselves.)
  - Plum Organics http://www.plumorganics.com/ (gourmet line of frozen pureed food for those with swallowing problems.)
  - The Paraplegic Chef http://www.theparaplegicchef.com/
  - Erin's Cookin' http://erinscookin.com/ (quadriplegic cook, a percentage of the proceeds of her e-book goes to the Reeve Foundation.)

*Retrieved July 1, 2015, from the website: Cookbooks and Cooking for People with Disabilities
Christopher and Dana Reeve Foundation Paralysis Resource Center http://www.christopherreeve.org/atf/cf/%7B173bca02-3665-49ab-9378-be009c58a5d3%7D/COOK-BOOKS%20AND%20COOKING%20FOR%20PWD%203-11.PDF. See the website for additional cookbooks. Also, there are a multitude of "quick and easy" recipe books in bookstores today, and recipes for crock-pot cookery and one-pot meals. Multiple websites have guides for a week of cooking (or several days), with accompanying shopping lists.

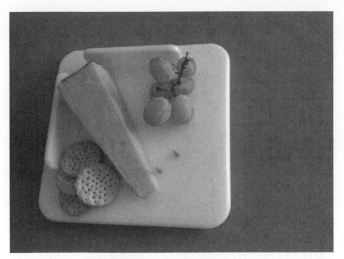

FIGURE 11-3   Nonslip cutting board.

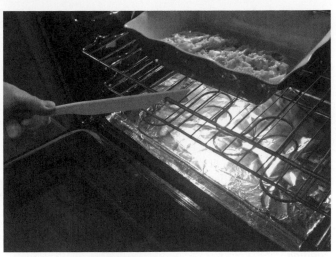

FIGURE 11-4   Push-pull helper.

For older adults with decreased strength, a bowl and beverage holder/tipper can hold large bowls or 1- to 2-gallon jugs and make tipping them over and pouring out their contents easier. For decreased grip strength, jar openers with long, nonslip handles can be useful to open jars, and long-handled levers on faucets can make it easier to turn on water.[68]

For the older adult who is having difficulty reaching items in a cabinet, reachers with circular rubber tips can be used to retrieve items. A push-pull helper may be used to retrieve or push in oven racks or hot dishes (Figure 11-4).[68]

Therapy staff can review adaptive equipment catalogs and select the appropriate pieces on an individual need or benefit basis. It is important to note that not every older adult will want or need a certain adaptation. Sometimes when an older adult is not familiar with a piece of adaptive equipment, it can be more confusing than beneficial. Introduce each item to the individual, and have him or her try using the equipment under the supervision of a therapist before using it independently. This approach can ensure appropriate use and adherence, as well as cost effectiveness.

Other Food Preparation Options

If preparing a meal becomes too difficult, there are other options for an older adult to obtain meals ensuring good nutrition. Meals on Wheels is a U.S. based national organization that provides fully cooked, ready-to-eat meals for older adults who are, for one reason or another, in need of them.[56] The cost of these programs varies, but the expense is usually very minimal. There are nearly 5000 of these nutrition centers throughout the country. Some programs serve meals at a specific location, whereas others deliver meals directly to a person's home. These programs usually deliver a meal at lunchtime, providing the older adult with at least one nutritional, hot meal each day.[56] Frequently, older adults report that the meals are of large enough portions that they can make two meals out of each one, providing food for lunch and dinner. If an older adult lives in a community that does not have a Meals on Wheels program, there is likely some similar service through a local church, temple, or senior center.

Case Example 11-1 describes an older adult struggling with food preparation.

CASE EXAMPLE 11-1   Older Adult Struggling with Food Preparation

Melba is an 85-year-old female who lives alone in a senior apartment complex across the street from her church. Approximately 2 years ago she was in a car accident that killed her husband and left her with several broken vertebrae in her cervical and thoracic spine. She had a history of osteoarthritis (OA) before the accident, and over the past 2 years has begun to demonstrate moderate to severe weakness in her neck and shoulders. She wears a neck brace most of the time to compensate.

After leaving her home of over 50 years and moving into the apartment, Melba was very determined to remain independent and maintain her ability to cook, a task that was always a central part of her life. But recently, she has begun

to struggle with some of the more involved aspects of cooking. This is only known because her daughter, who lives nearby, has observed her struggles and reported them to her physician, who wrote an order for an occupational therapy home health evaluation.

Through verbal report from her daughter and grudging agreement from Melba, it is reported that she has, on more than one occasion, dropped a plate or bowl when retrieving it from the cabinets. During the home health evaluation, it is noted that she has difficulties getting her pots and pans out from underneath the stove, where they are stored. She also becomes slightly short of breath with approximately 5 minutes of kitchen activity. Melba

Continued

CASE EXAMPLE 11-1 Older Adult Struggling with Food Preparation—cont'd

uses no assistive device for mobility, but she is observed holding onto the kitchen countertop, the kitchen table, or the refrigerator handle with one hand when carrying a pot in the other hand. When asked how she feels during the activity, Melba reports "I feel just fine—no complaints!"

Melba has a difficult time admitting that she is having any problems in the kitchen. She makes the comment, "I really miss my husband. Being in the kitchen is something that I can still do that I love. It reminds me of him a little bit."

Case Study Questions

1. What other questions might you ask Melba? What else would you like to observe during the evaluation?
2. List five environmental modifications and/or types of adaptive equipment that might be appropriate in this situation.
3. Would you recommend that Melba needs an assistive device for walking? If so, why and what type? If not, why not?
4. Are there any outside programs to which Melba could be referred?
5. List two short-term goals and one long-term goal for Melba.

Feeding

Once food is prepared, it is necessary to look at any issues the older adult might have with self-feeding. There are multiple reasons why a person may struggle with self-feeding. The issue may be neuromuscular, such as decreased grip strength following a stroke, or tremors in Parkinson's disease; or it could be cognitive, such as a person diagnosed with Alzheimer's disease who cannot cognitively initiate or continuously carry out the feeding process.[54] Regardless of the reason, it is important to help the older adult maintain self-feeding independence for as long as possible, and in such a way that is dignified for that particular individual. The following paragraphs discuss and Table 11-3 summarizes multiple adaptations that can be made so that a person can complete this task.

Utensils

For impaired grip, plastic utensils with built-up handles can be useful (Figure 11-5). Lightweight cylindrical foam padding can be purchased by the yard and can be cut to fit any utensil or food preparation item as well as pens, pencils, or anything that the older adult might be having trouble gripping. For those who are unable to grasp at all, a universal cuff (Figure 11-6) or a utensil holder (with or without wrist support) will allow the individual to self-feed without gripping a utensil. For people who have limited upper extremity movement or control, curved (angled) utensils (Figure 11-7) and extension utensils allow for food to be brought to the mouth with less upper extremity range of motion required. A person who experiences tremors might benefit from a weighted utensil or simply wrapping a wrist weight around the wrist at mealtimes. Research has demonstrated that weighted wrist cuffs, ranging from 1/5 to 4 pounds, decrease intention tremors. The amount of weight that is beneficial, however, is variable and specific to each individual person.[55] For those people who want to cut their own food for self-feeding or meal preparation but have limited wrist movement or grip strength, a rocker knife might be helpful.

Plates and Bowls

Frequently, older adults have difficulty seeing food on their plates due to multiple visual impairments. Using a plate that is the opposite color of the food being served can be helpful in visualizing food on a plate. For example, a dark-colored plate for lighter items, such as pasta or rice, can allow the person to see the food more clearly due to the contrasting colors.

There are multiple diagnoses that can cause a person to have difficulty scooping food onto a utensil or cause problems in pushing food off the plate in an effort to put the food on the spoon or fork. High-sided dishes or a compartment plate can make scooping food onto a spoon or fork much easier (Figure 11-8). Scoop dishes have a high side and a low side, allowing a person to use the side for easier scooping while still being able to move the feeding arm in at a lower, normal angle (Figure 11-9). If a person does not want to commit to a new plate, a clip-on food guard is a possibility. These clip on to any standard plate and can be used like a scoop dish. When using a scoop dish or a clip-on food guard, it is important to remember to angle the plate so that the high side is opposite of the individual's feeding extremity. For example, if a person wants to feed himself with his right hand, the high side of the plate should be placed on the person's left. This allows the right hand to push the food across the body in a natural motion and use the high side of the plate as a scoop at the end of the motion.

An easy-cut plate that has stainless steel pins to stabilize food can make it possible to cut food with one hand. Suction cups or nonskid material on the bottom of dinnerware can prevent plates or bowls from moving while the person is trying to eat.

Beverage Containers

Sometimes drinking liquids can be difficult for the older adult, causing frustration and possibly leading to decreased fluid intake. Inadequate fluid intake can often lead to dehydration.[9] For those individuals who simply have a problem with successfully bringing a cup to the mouth, there are many types of adaptive equipment that can help.

For individuals who have decreased grip strength, easy-grip cups with either one or two handles or a bilateral glass holder that can slip onto a glass of any size are excellent adaptations to maintain independence with self-drinking. If tremors are an issue, a weighted cup with a lid or once again simply using wrist weights (as stated in the utensils discussion of this chapter) would be an appropriate intervention.

TABLE 11-3 Impairments and Adaptations for Self-Feeding

Impairment	Adaptation	Comments
Impaired grip	Plastic built-up utensils Easy-grip cups with either one or two handles	Lightweight cylindrical foam padding can be purchased by the yard and can be cut to fit any utensil or food preparation item as well as pens, pencils, or anything that the older adult might be having trouble gripping.
	Bilateral glass holder	Glass holders can slip onto glasses of any size and are an excellent way to maintain independence with self-drinking.
Absent grip	Universal cuff Utensil holder (with or without support)	These devices will allow the individual to self-feed without gripping a utensil.
Limited upper extremity movement or control	Curved (angled) utensils Extension utensils	These utensils allow for food to be brought to the mouth with less upper extremity range of motion required.
Tremors	Weighted utensil Wrist weight	Research has demonstrated that weighted wrist cuffs, ranging from 1/5 to 4 pounds, decrease intention tremors.
	Weighted cup with a lid	The amount of weight that is beneficial is variable and specific to each individual person.[56]
Limited wrist movement or grip strength	Rocker knife	The utensil allows individuals to cut their own food and can assist in meal preparation activities.
Visual impairment	Dishes in a contrasting color to the food	Using a plate that is the opposite color of the food being served can help the individual to visualize the food on the plate. A dark-colored plate for lighter items, such as pasta or rice, can allow the person to see the food more clearly.
Difficulty scooping food	High-sided dishes Compartment plates Clip-on food guards	Scoop dishes have a high side and a low side, allowing a person to use the side for easier scooping while still being able to move the feeding arm in at a lower, more natural angle. Clip-on guards are good for older adults who prefer to use existing dishware. They clip on to any standard plate and can be used like a scoop dish. When using a scoop dish or a clip-on food guard, it is important to remember to angle the plate so that the high side is opposite of the individual's feeding extremity. For example, if a person wants to feed himself with his right hand, the high side of the plate should be placed on the person's left. This allows the right hand to push the food across the body in a natural motion and use the high side of the plate as a scoop at the end of the motion.
Only has use of one hand	Easy-cut plate Suction cups or nonskid mats	An easy-cut plate that has stainless steel pins to stabilize food can make it possible to cut food with one hand. Suction cups or nonskid material on the bottom of dinnerware can prevent plates or bowls from moving while the person is trying to eat.
Difficulty in tipping the head	Nosey cups Straws	Nosey Cups have a cutout in the cup that allows the individual to drink without extending the neck.
Needs to maintain neutral head alignment	Cup with a built-in straw	If the individual has difficulty using straws because the straws are difficult to control in the cup, a cup with a built-in straw or a straw holder might be the answer. Some straws have one-way valves that stay filled with fluid, eliminating the possibility of sucking in too much air when drinking.
Taking too large of a sip	Regulating drinking cups (with or without straws)	Regulating drinking cups allow for a certain measured amount of fluid to be released from the cup with any given sip. Sometimes these are controlled by a caregiver pressing and releasing a regulator trigger; other times the cup simply will only release a specific measured amount, such as 5 or 10 cc of fluid.

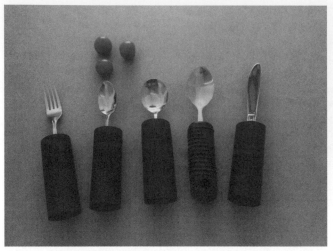

FIGURE 11-5   Eating utensils with built-up handles.

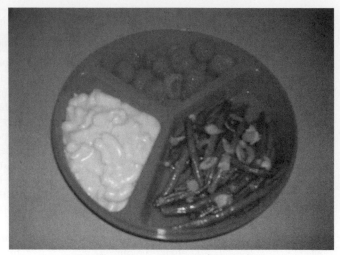

FIGURE 11-8   Compartment plate with lid.

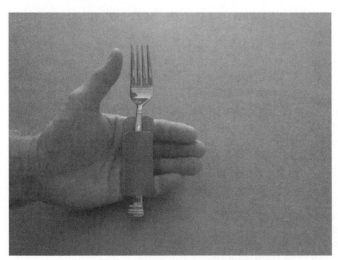

FIGURE 11-6   Universal cuff.

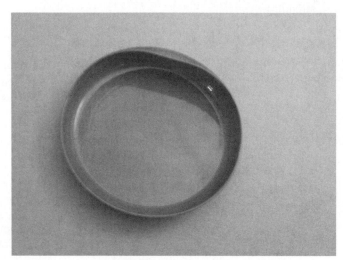

FIGURE 11-9   Scoop dish.

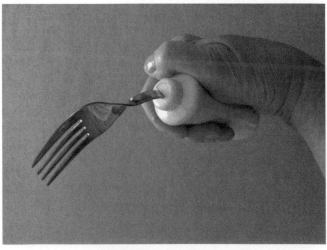

FIGURE 11-7   Bendable fork.

If the older adult has difficulty tipping the head back to drink, or if he or she simply needs to maintain a neutral head alignment, Nosey cups have a cutout in the cup that allows the individual to drink without extending the neck (Figure 11-10). A straw might also be used in this instance. If the individual has difficulty using straws because the straws are difficult to control in the cup, a cup with a built-in straw or a straw holder might be the answer. There are also straws that have one-way valves that stay filled with fluid, eliminating the possibility of sucking in too much air when drinking.

Many older adults have problems with taking too large of a drink at any one time, which can result in coughing or aspiration. Regulating drinking cups, either with or without straws, only allow for a certain measured amount of fluid to be released from the cup with any given drink. Sometimes these are controlled by a caregiver pressing and

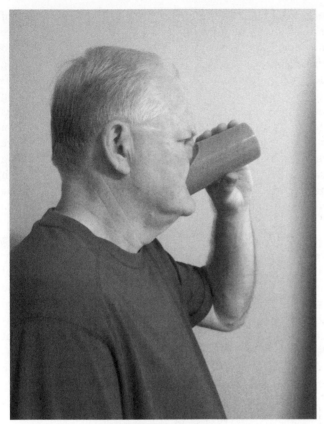

FIGURE 11-10   Nosey Cup.

releasing a regulator trigger. Other times the cup simply will only release a specific measured amount, such as 5 or 10 cc of fluid.

Positioning Options

The position in which a person is seated, either in a chair or a wheelchair, is an integral part of successful independent feeding. While eating, the ideal sitting posture is for the hips, knees, and feet to be at 90 degrees, with weight evenly distributed to both sides of the body.[81] The head should be upright and tilted slightly forward. It should be possible for the individual to move closer to the table so that his or her mouth can be 10 to 15 inches from the plate.[50]

Frequently, when an older adult with small stature is positioned correctly, he or she is in a shorter wheelchair (hemi-height). These wheelchairs normally have a seat-to-floor height of 17 to 18 inches, as opposed to a standard wheelchair, whose seat-to-floor height is 19 to 21 inches. The height of a standard dining table is 28 to 30 inches. Therefore, when a person requires a hemi-sized wheelchair, standard tables are too tall. Using an adjustable-height bed/chair table or a desk might be more useful.

It is important for a person to sit at a 90-degree angle when eating to facilitate proper digestion. Multiple positioning devices can be used for this:

- Although use of restraints is generally not encouraged, lap belts can be used to position the pelvis as close to midline as possible.[75]

- A solid seat or back insert can help maintain good posture and reduce the possibility of skin breakdown.[37]
- Lateral supports can prevent the older adult from leaning to either side.
- Several seat cushions may be used, including a pommel (abductor) cushion to prevent hip adduction and a wedge cushion to discourage forward leaning.
- There are also multiple head supports to maintain the head in a neutral alignment.[68]

When choosing a positioning device for an older adult, whether it is to increase independence in feeding or for any other reason, it is important to remember to select devices that will fit the unique needs of that individual.[37]

Eating and Swallowing

"Feeding, eating, and swallowing are interdependent activities, (p. 686)"[2] and therefore it is necessary for an occupational therapist to have the skills necessary to assess and intervene in all of these areas. Feeding, which is defined as "the process of setting up, arranging, and bringing food [or fluid] from the plate or cup to the mouth" (p. 686), has already been discussed. However, occupational therapists are also able to address eating and swallowing.

Eating, which is defined as "the ability to keep and manipulate food or fluid in the mouth and swallow it" (p. 686), and swallowing, defined as the "complicated act in which food, fluid, medication, or saliva is moved from the mouth through the pharynx and esophagus into the stomach" (p. 686), are both areas that are well within the occupational therapist's scope of practice.

As there are multiple issues that can cause feeding difficulties, there are also multiple issues that can affect eating and swallowing. Box 11-2 lists common eating and swallowing

---

BOX 11-2   Common Eating and Swallowing Issues

- Aspiration: The entry of secretions, fluids, food, or any foreign substance below the vocal cords and into the lungs; may result in aspiration pneumonia.
- Dysphagia: Difficulty with any stage of swallowing (oral, pharyngeal, esophageal); dysfunction in any stage or process of eating; includes any difficulty in the passage of food, liquid, or medicine during any stage of swallowing that impairs the client's ability to swallow independently or safely.
- Pocketing: Retention of food between the teeth and cheek.
- Reflux: Reflux of food, medication, liquids, and gastric juice from the stomach into the esophagus; also called gastroesophageal reflux disease. (GERD).
- Silent aspiration: Aspiration that occurs without coughing or overt choking; indication of motor and/or sensory deficits (if present) that inhibit protective responses.

challenges that an occupational therapist might encounter, and Box 11-3 discusses different techniques that might be used to treat these issues.

Routine

Warde and Hetherington noted, "For some people, what and where they eat is a very conscious expression of their personal identities and style of life" (p. 769).[80] Often when a person has been sick, becomes disabled, or has moved to a new location, routines are interrupted. This is true for mealtime routines. If it is possible to allow an individual to follow his or her normal mealtime routine, that person might consume more and perform the feeding task better. For example, if an older adult woman has moved to a skilled nursing facility and seems distracted during meals, an attempt could be made to allow the woman to a eat in her room or a quiet office. It might very well be that she is used to eating in a quiet location, and the noise of a dining room is too distracting.[39]

Caregiver Education

Many older adults depend on a caregiver to assist them in at least some aspect of the feeding process. Whether it is help with purchasing groceries, cutting up food, or bringing a utensil to the mouth, caregivers play an integral role in ensuring that older adults receive the proper amount of nutrition, calories, and fluids.[15] The amount and quality of care that an older individual receives might influence the intake of food and thus the individual's weight.[8] To maximize carryover from OT treatment to daily feeding activities, occupational therapists should educate the caregivers on any adaptive equipment or alternative feeding techniques that are being used with the older adult. It has been noted that ongoing caregiver education, rather than a 1- or 2-day education just before discharge, is more beneficial to everyone involved in the process. Ongoing caregiver education allows for improved follow-through and better relations between caregivers and therapists due to the collaborative effort required by all parties.[25]

A caregiver should be educated on any special techniques (e.g., energy conservation techniques used during cooking or a chin-tuck strategy during meals) or any adaptive equipment (e.g., a Nosey Cup or a divided plate) that are being used on a regular basis. They should also be made aware of any safety issues that the occupational therapist has noted. Besides some of the other areas discussed in this chapter, general feeding techniques might also be taught. Box 11-4 gives examples of feeding techniques on which an occupational therapist might want to instruct a caregiver.

Case Example 11-2 describes the feeding problems of a resident in a skilled nursing facility.

BOX 11-3   Common Swallowing Intervention Techniques

- Chin tuck: A strategy in which the head is flexed (chin tucked downward toward the chest) during the swallow, allowing the anterior structures of the pharynx posteriorly, resulting in a smaller entrance to the larynx; this strategy reduces the chance of food or liquid to fall into the airway.
- Clearing techniques: Strategies used to clear the mouth or pharynx of food or liquid residue.
- Diet liberalization: The relaxation of standards of accepted diets as ways to treat illness or decrease symptoms related to dysphagia.
- Double/multiple swallows: A swallow strategy whereby two or more attempts are used to swallow the food, medication, or liquid.
- Food consistencies: There are four levels of semisolid/solid foods proposed in the National Dysphagia Diet (NDD):
  - Regular: Normal food consistency
  - NDD Level 3 (i.e., Advanced): Soft foods that require more chewing ability
  - NDD Level 2 (i.e., Mechanical Altered): Cohesive, moist, semisolid foods, requiring some chewing
  - NDD Level 1 (i.e., Pureed): Homogenous, very cohesive, pudding-like, requiring very little chewing ability

- Liquid consistencies: There are four levels of liquid viscosity (i.e., thickness or resistance to flow):
  - Thin: Normal fluid viscosity
  - Nectar-like: Fluid viscosity that is slightly thicker than water
  - Honey-like: Fluid viscosity that is approximately that of honey
  - Spoon-thick: aka "pudding-like"; fluid viscosity that is approximately that of pudding
- Mendelsohn maneuver: A swallowing technique to facilitate prolonged laryngeal elevation during the swallow; results in keeping the upper esophageal sphincter open longer to allow passage of the bolus.
- Therapeutic feedings: Controlled delivery of food, medication, or liquid used to facilitate therapeutic outcomes to improve feeding, eating, and swallowing ability; not used as a primary source of nutrition or hydration.
- Thickening agent: Substance used to increase the viscosity of liquids.
- VitalStim: A method cleared by the Food and Drug Administration (FDA) to promote swallowing through the application of neuromuscular electrical stimulation to the swallowing muscles to strengthen and reeducate muscles and to facilitate motor control/function of the swallowing mechanism.

(From Cox, M., Holm, S., Kurfuerst, S., Lynch, A., Schuberth, L. M., et al. [2006]. Specialized knowledge and skills in feeding, eating, and swallowing for occupational therapy practice. *The American Journal of Occupational Therapy, 61*, 686-700.)

BOX 11-4 Caregiver Instructions for Feeding Techniques

- Keep distractions to a minimum; turn off the television and radio. If someone is easily distracted, eating alone might be better than eating with a group.
- Make sure that the individual is positioned properly; the ideal sitting posture is for the hips, knees, and feet to be at 90 degrees, with weight evenly distributed to both sides of the body.
- Try to prevent soiling of clothing; use a bib, an apron, towel, or one to two full-size napkins to cover clothing if an individual is at risk for spilling food. Have a box of moist, disposable washcloths nearby to clean off the hands and face. Remember that although many individuals can benefit from a clothing protector (i.e., bib or apron), some people might object to using one.

- Work with the individual to decide what is best for him or her.
- Give verbal cues as needed; using one-step commands, instruct the individual in each area that is needed. Speak in a calm, soothing voice and use words that are appropriate for adults. Remember that cues may need to be repeated.
- Give physical cues as needed; use hand-over-hand assistance to allow the individual to go through the motion of eating. Use verbal cues at the same time as the physical cues to reinforce the steps in feeding. Do not provide more assistance than is needed.
- Give praise freely and recognize even the smallest steps toward independent eating.

(Adapted from Litchford, M. (2005) Feeding instructions for caregivers. *Adult day care resource manual for the USDA Child and Adult Care Food Program*. National Food Service Management Institute. University, MS: University of Mississippi. Retrieved from http://www.nfsmi.org/documentlibraryfiles/PDF/20071128104309.pdf)

CASE EXAMPLE 11-2 Resident in a Skilled Nursing Facility

Jim is an 89-year-old male who entered a skilled nursing facility (SNF) approximately 15 months ago after falling at home and sustaining a right hip fracture. He underwent an open reduction–internal fixation (ORIF) procedure and came to the SNF for skilled therapy. Although he improved physically and was able to walk with a walker throughout the facility, his family decided that his diagnosis of mild Parkinson's disease along with his recent falls at home made for an unsafe living environment. They had a long talk with Jim, and it was decided that it was in his best interest to remain at the SNF for long-term care.

Since that time, Jim has become depressed. Although he understands that he needs to remain at the facility, he misses his home. He developed the flu last winter, and it caused his Parkinson's to become more progressed. He has begun to experience moderate intention tremors and has also begun to demonstrate mild dementia.

To ensure that the residents are not gaining or losing weight in an abnormal fashion, the facility performs monthly weight measures on all residents. When they weighed him, it was noted that Jim had an 8-pound weight loss in the last month. He completed a barium swallow diagnostic procedure, which came back negative for any swallowing issues. He has been referred to skilled occupational therapy (OT) for evaluation and treatment as indicated for feeding difficulties

As the occupational therapist, you arrive for lunch in the assistive-feeding dining room where Jim has recently

been placed. He is sitting slightly slumped forward in a wheelchair and there is a nursing assistant at the table with him, along with two other residents. The other two residents, both males, are falling asleep at the table. The nursing assistant is busy trying to wake them up and open up all of the containers on all of the trays. You observe Jim attempting to drink from a full juice glass. His tremors are such that the drink spills some onto his lap and Jim curses under his breath. He is able to eat a fish stick using his fingers but struggles in using utensils to eat his green beans and gelatin. Within approximately 10 minutes of beginning to eat, Jim throws down his fork in frustration and stares at the wall. Shortly thereafter, the nursing assistant begins to put food on a spoon and feed it to Jim, who grudgingly eats it.

Case Study Questions
1. What do you believe is the most important issue to address with Jim, and why?
2. List five separate adaptations that you could try with Jim to make his self-feeding more independent.
3. How might you address his sitting position during meals?
4. Do the caregivers at this facility need to be educated on feeding issues? If so, how would you educate them? If not, why not?
5. Write two short-term goals and one long-term goal for Jim.

Occupational Therapy: A Holistic Approach

It is important to remember that every older adult is an individual with a unique life story, not simply a client whom we are treating for a feeding issue. As Hasselkus so eloquently mentioned in the 2006 Eleanor Clarke Slagle Lecture:

And what does this all mean for the older woman who becomes disabled? As OTs, we might be advising her to no

longer do much cooking, to take shortcuts, to use more prepared foods, to let some other member of the family do most of the work now, to give up some of the usual family traditions, etc. Do we appreciate the emotional depths of these changes we are recommending? What can we do, with our expertise in homemaking skills, to better help such a client weather this huge wrench in her life patterns and identity within a family? (p. 634)[39]

As occupational therapists, we must do what is best for each individual older adult in each individual situation. If a certain approach does not work for someone, it is our job to try something else, and to focus on what is most appropriate within the context of that person's life. We must continuously strive to create a client-centered environment in which the older adult is able to function as independently as possible for as long as possible. The concluding section of this chapter offers a phenomenological perspective, to sensitize readers to the "emotional depths" to which Hasselkus refers.

A Phenomenological Approach to Food, Nutrition, and Frail Older Adults

As part of meaningful lived experience and a form of health behavior, eating is central to the lives and well-being of older persons. A phenomenological approach, focusing on the subjective experience of eating and nutrition, offers a unique opportunity to understand the world of frail older persons because food is a social and cultural object toward which people act, and a person's past and present attitudes, behaviors, and social position play a role in the meanings attributed to food.

As discussed earlier in this chapter, as an older adult becomes more frail, she or he may lose some capacities to shop, cook, prepare meals, eat, and clean up, and the opportunity to eat with family or other close persons. These losses have usually been assessed as limitations in performance of activities of daily living (ADL) and IADL and viewed through a biomedical lens as limiting nutritional intake and thus negatively affecting physical health. However, the influence of food and nutrition on an older adult's sense of personhood is equally significant. The following section examines the cultural, social, and personal meaning of food and eating in the everyday lives and activities of older adults.

Eating, as an activity or occupation, is central to an older person's identity and sense of competence and has particular meaning and value, as set forth by American Occupational Therapy Association.[3] Eating is clearly a meaningful, "goal-directed pursuit" (p. 628); it "reflect[s] cultural values, provide[s] a] structure for living" (pp. 628-629); and it enables "human needs to be met for self care, enjoyment and participation in society" (p. 629). Eating is certainly an activity "that people engage in throughout their daily lives to fulfill their time and give life meaning," (p. 629) and thus warrants the attention and care of occupational therapists.

Food is a biological given that is infused with cultural meanings. People speak of food in a social language with rich symbolic significance.[24] As part of the lived experience of older people, eating can offer us a way of understanding their world[53] and can be seen as associated with a sense of personal identity. An older person has a culturally constituted self, and food and person are mutually constituted.

Although occupational therapists and others have conducted significant research on the cultural and social meanings of meal preparation, eating, and food for older adults,*

relatively little research is available on the personal interpretation and understanding of the eating experience of frail older people. The following discussion primarily grows out of a multiyear study, the Culture of Food in Long-Term Care, funded by the National Institute on Aging (NIA 23775), that explored the cultural and personal meanings, processes, and transitions concerning eating and food for frail older people in settings ranging from an independent lifestyle in the community to life in assisted living facilities and nursing homes.[†] This discussion also is based on secondary data from the European Food in Later Life research project.[‡, 19,28] These research studies provide an additional, phenomenological lens through which OT professionals can view and understand food and eating in their efforts to be sensitive while improving the health, quality of life, and well-being of older persons.

Frail Persons Living in the Community

Understanding frail community-dwelling older adults' perceptions of food and meals provides a context to increase understanding of their lives and a baseline for understanding the meanings of food for persons residing in long-term care facilities. The following salient themes that emerged from interviews with community residents were based on the perspectives of three different groups: women, men, and persons who received home-delivered meals through Meals on Wheels.

Older Community-Dwelling Women

We start with women in outlining the meanings of food for frail old persons. This cohort of older adults consists mostly of individuals born in the 1920s and 1930s, at a time when household tasks associated with food and eating were primarily the province of women—their mothers. Preparing food for one's family, whether out of affection or out of obligation, is a significant part of the lived experience of most older women. Food traditionally tends to be important for gender identity,[33] with the cultural construction of the female role rooted in the cooking and giving of food.[61] Women's roles in planning, obtaining, and preparing meals have played a part in the continuing social construction of the family.[6,23]

*References 38, 42, 63, 71, 73, 83, and 84.
†Three long-experienced interviewers (with roots in gerontology, social work, and human development and gerontology) carried out qualitative ethnographic interviews focused on the meanings of "food," "eating," "meals," and similar constructs across late-life transitions. Study participants were frail men and women aged 75 years and over: persons living in the community (55), residents of assisted living facilities (39), and residents in nursing homes (43). Additionally, in six long-term care facilities, perspectives on food and meals were sought through interviews with long-term care staff (53), as well as researcher observations of mealtimes (40).
‡The European Food in Later Life Study focused on the activities and attitudes regarding food of community-dwelling older persons. It was based on a large sample of persons aged 65 through 90 years from eight European countries who were interviewed about food in their everyday lives.

Mealtime is a cultural habit or routine that has been part of these women's lives for decades, and men have tended to rely on women for their meals.

Our analysis focused on 18 frail widows living alone in an urban environment and their involvement in activities around food. In regard to food gathering, all of these women had help in shopping, largely because of mobility limitations or health conditions. Most depended on others for help in transportation or carrying heavy items. Each widow tried to maintain continuity with how she had shopped in the past. Food shopping, whether personally undertaken or guided by lists compiled by the widow, offered personal choice. For example, one woman said, "I don't eat anything I don't like. I'm privileged to do that because I shop for myself."

Meal preparation was often seen as a personal challenge: to lift heavy pans; to stand on one's feet or sit in one's wheelchair while preparing food. All widows said that they make themselves a plate from the stove rather than serving family style, and most prepared enough for more than one meal. Many had adapted by creating a purposely cluttered environment. As a wheelchair-bound widow said, "Well sometimes I can't reach too good. That's why you see everything sitting out and not put away because I can't get up there.... I keep things where I can reach them." What she liked most about her meals was "I can cook 'em and fix 'em the way I want them. That's what I like."

Cooking can enhance a sense of self. A widow whose mother taught her how to make soup said, "I cook it in a nice beautiful pot...vegetable and chicken soup. If I don't have that in the freezer, I feel like I'm undressed." Most women spoke of reducing their cooking for others at family occasions, and more than one said that they had "paid their dues," and it was time for others to do for them; this can be termed *delayed reciprocity.*

In response to our question, "When you think about food and eating, what comes to your mind?," more than half of the women spoke of their pleasure in eating. Choice was a big part of the enjoyment they found in their food. Less than half of the widows responded with thoughts of their health (e.g., their weight, cholesterol, or dental problems—the latter is a topic that has been rarely examined for its meaning to older persons). However, when asked if they think there is a connection between their health and what they eat, most of the women definitely agreed, and many stated that they should avoid, limit, or increase intake of certain foods. Eating was often thought of as a way of maintaining their personal survival. Typical of the statements of this group of women, one said, "My health keeps me from eating what I want to eat."

Women tended to view food preparation and meals as routine, and to find satisfaction in novelty—both in the food that they ate and their opportunity to socialize with others. A married woman described her pleasure in sharing a traditional Saturday activity with her husband: "We make all our own bread and marmalade...it's a little treat from having cereal during the week."[19] Women often stressed that they enjoyed breaking the routine and having special treats—finding a sense of novelty in their lives around food.

We asked women who lived alone about the **social context of eating**: whether they liked eating alone or preferred to eat with other people. Although over half of the widows said that they prefer to eat with others, most went on to explain that they had made good adjustments to eating alone most of the time. A widow of 38 years said, "I enjoy company; I like people. But I can eat alone too....I can still enjoy my food even when I'm by myself."

In the United Kingdom, widows referred to by Davidson, Arber, and Marshall[19] as "newly alone" tended to feel the loss of their routine of sharing regular meals with their husbands. Many sought to have social companionship that included meals with friends and neighbors, bringing to the fore the centrality for women of the theme of regarding food relationally. In the U.S. study, women often saw the food they prepared for others as a gift. An African American widow who loved to cook and share meals with her husband said, "Cookin' to satisfy him....When you live by yourself, that joy is taken away."

Overall, the widows indicated their acceptance of their frailty and their living and often eating alone, and they held on to their past in maintaining a sense of self-efficacy throughout the process of being maximally independent in procuring food, preparing it, and eating it.

Older Community-Dwelling Men

Next we turn to the rarely examined world of frail older men who live in the community. The few researchers who have explored the worlds of older men[§] have suggested that they strive to maintain a sense of masculinity, continuity, and self. Older men try to feel in control of their lives, emphasizing agency and purposive action. They may be challenged to maintain these attributes in the face of their own decline in health, strength, and control, and because they may have taken on increased responsibility for household tasks (e.g., cooking, shopping, and cleaning up) that are generally identified as women's work.

A web of meanings and themes underlie men's attitudes and behaviors in relation to food and eating. Four interrelated themes emerged from our interviews with 15 men; six were currently married and lived with their spouses, and all but one of the unmarried—who were mostly widowed—lived alone.

Eating to live was stressed when men spoke of eating as necessary to stay alive. When asked, "What are the best things about food and eating?," one 86-year-old widower said, "Well, you need it to survive, so I survive," and another widower said "...normally it's just something that I have to do to stay alive." Married men, however, often found pleasure in their meals; a 91-year-old, for example, said he ate out of sheer enjoyment. When the interviewer said, "Some people have suggested taking a pill instead of regular food," he replied, "Well, I get a joy out of a meal. It's a pleasure. It's taste, refreshing. It's something to take the monotony out of life." Davidson et al.[19] also found this pattern, differentiating men who lived alone from those who were married.

---

§References 14, 18, 57, 60, 66, and 78.

Importance of the physical body is seen as preserving health and self. Men often spoke of feeding the body as if it were a machine, and food as a fuel to maintain strength and functioning. In response to our question, "When you think of food and eating, what comes to your mind?," a man said, "Whether it's healthful, if it's good for my body. The food should provide my body with the proper nourishment." Men tended to see food not as way to improve their health, but to maintain their current level of functioning. Several men spoke of filling up: "You just fill up and you're happy. That's the best time of life."

Getting "filled up" is an example of how people often speak of food in a language rich in symbolic significance: In addition to the mechanical imagery, being filled up can be seen as a metaphor with meanings that are physical, cultural, and psychosocial. Thus, the body can be seen as material and as socially constructed.

Being a man is a theme that generally emerged when men spoke about their experience with food and meals in relation to their need to be strong, manly, able to perform and to do, to be in control—for example, "I'm no cook. I couldn't repeat how my wife made roast beef. I'm not a very good housekeeper."[77] Men tended to denigrate their skills in these feminine tasks.[78] Men tended to have a work orientation toward preparing meals. They spoke of the speed and effectiveness of their task performance. One widower said, "I never make a meal that takes more than 5 minutes." Another said, "This [microwave] is pleasure. Five, 6 minutes and I have a meal." A number of men spoke of women (neighbors, paid household help, daughters) who prepared or brought them meals, and each of these men indicated that he was in charge of the way women provided assistance. Men thus maintained a sense of independence and of control over their meals.

Eating and meals are typically **social events**, which is the fourth theme. In older adults' past decades of eating, throughout childhood and marriage, food and meals represent caring family concern and are typically social events. The salience of past memories and habits persists throughout a lifetime. A housebound widower who ate alone, had little appetite, and depended on daily supplements of Ensure recalled, "My mother could make herring and make it delicious." He also said, "My wife would soak hams and cook them with cabbage. Christ, I can almost taste it!"

Overall, continuity or changes in family ties and in community living arrangements tended to shape how the social context of meals was individually interpreted and experienced by older people. There were major differences in the social dimensions of eating between men living alone and married men.[18] Married men often expressed that they derived pleasure from eating, unlike men who lived alone, who often said they ate to live.[19] We asked a man who had been married over 50 years, "What are some of the nice things about eating together?" His wife, who often answered for her husband, pointed to the table where they eat: "I sit here and he sits there. I look at him. He looks at me. He's healthy; it's good for me. It's good to eat together." Married men emphasized the social satisfactions of shared meals and mutual

caring that couplehood represented. A never-married man said, "The worst thing you can do in life is to live alone and eat alone…but I manage to put up with it." Living and eating alone seemed to evoke the vulnerability of the isolated self. Men, and also women, who had always lived alone and continued to live alone tended to emphasize a flexible routine, with a sense of independence and self-reliance, leading them to indicate that they were satisfied with their food skills.

Meals on Wheels

When older persons have difficulty in shopping and preparing food and have a lack of money,[70] they often get assistance in meeting their nutritional needs from Meals on Wheels (MOW),[56] a program provided in the United States by federally funded Area Agencies on Aging or other community resources. Generally, one meal is provided daily at minimal or no charge, and recipients have little if any choice in selecting the meals that are delivered. MOW is often perceived as a way of enabling an older person to remain in his or her own home, with a sense of independence and autonomy.[45]

Sixteen recipients of MOW were interviewed; all but two were women. All had multiple health conditions that severely compromised their functional capacity; all but three lived alone. All recipients obtained additional food to supplement MOW—usually with the help of family, neighbors, or home care workers.

Three themes emerged from interviews with MOW recipients: autonomy in the face of dependency; importance of personal choice, within the context of limited possibilities; and a sense of acceptance and settling for the MOW as provided.

Autonomy persists in the context of dependency. We asked a 90-year-old woman, "When you think of food and eating, what comes to your mind?" She said, "I say work… to get it together and make it tasty.…I cooked myself until last year." She presented herself as a person who was and continued to be independent, although she now used MOW. A 76-year-old man who had no teeth and took medicines that sharply curtailed his appetite told us: "I force myself to eat.… I feel good because I can eat if I want."

Recipients of MOW often spoke of **choosing** what they will eat, sometimes adding spices or adding something to the meal that the recipients had cooked themselves. When asked about MOW, an 89-year-old woman said, "I really don't enjoy it, but I eat it.…When fish is delivered I don't even open it up; I throw it away." When asked about her favorite meal, she said, "I think lunch is my favorite meal because I eat what I want. You know that's my own. Like I have [buy] salmon, tuna fish…it's stuff I like."

Each day each person did choose when he or she would eat, what he or she would eat from the food at hand, where in the home he or she would eat it, and how he or she would clean up after the meal. The ability to make choices, even in grossly restricted circumstances, may enable older persons with limitations to regard themselves as autonomous and independent.[7,67] Thus for many MOW recipients, attitudes toward food and eating represented the continuity of a sense of agency and autonomy that appeared to be a metaphor for their attitudes toward life.

Nearly all of the MOW recipients indicated that they have just enough money to get along or that they can't make ends meet. Most told of a significant period in their lives when they were poor or had few financial resources. There was a strong theme of **acceptance**: "I'm not fussy about what I eat. It's food. It's there. You eat what's there." A 92-year-old woman said, "I have to put up with whatever it is….I have to eat whatever they send.…I've resigned myself to eat whatever they send." And a 75-year-old diabetic woman with a pacemaker and serious food allergies noted, "You eat because you're hungry. I don't see nothing enjoyable with it."

Acceptance and adaptation are central strategies for responding to age-related losses. Some older persons may have seen their decline as a diminished sense of everyday competence that could not be overcome and must be accepted, whereas others rejected acceptance and maintained an expectation that they would overcome their frailty.[74]

Acceptance and settling was not a theme for the six persons who indicated that they had briefly received MOWs in the past. These were mostly men, who generally reported that their money situation was "comfortable." They described MOW as "mediocre" and "inferior" food. They indicated that they exercised considerable choice and autonomy as they purchased frozen food and meals in markets where choice and quality were seen as better than in the MOW meals.

Meanings of and attitudes toward MOW constitute a prototype of other formal food services that are received by frail old persons (e.g., meals provided in long-term care; see following discussion)—denoting dependency, lack of autonomy, and lack of choice, although simultaneously allowing for some degree of independence, autonomy, and choice.

Food Insecurity

Food security can be defined as access at all times to enough food for an active, healthy life for all household members.[62] Conversely, food insecurity exists when the availability of and the ability to acquire nutritionally adequate and safe foods is uncertain or limited. Food insecurity is variably measured by the self-reports of older adults, particularly in response to the Food Security Supplement to the Current U.S. Population survey.[62] It is estimated that in the United States food insecurity occurs in over 8% of households with older persons.[48] Overall, food insecurity is associated with low income, limited mobility, poor health, high medical costs, and lack of availability of family support.[82]

Some research has reported that persons who receive home-delivered meals show improvement in dietary intake compared with a matched comparison group.[32] However, there is emerging evidence that older adults who receive home-delivered meals are particularly vulnerable to food insecurity.[48]

In the food study of frail community-dwelling older adults described earlier, fully half of those receiving MOW meals had evidence of food insecurity, whereas only 15% of the frail older adults not receiving MOW meals had evidence of food insecurity. In the light of research that has demonstrated that MOW meals reduce the food insecurity of older adults who regularly eat them,[32] it may be that the level of food insecurity of MOW recipients in our study might have been even higher were they to receive no home-delivered meals.

We now move to long-term care settings to describe how food patterns and themes of frail older adults in the community persist and are modified in an institutional context.

Meanings of Food and Meals in Long-Term Care

As we have described in the previous discussion of the meanings of food in the lives of older persons living in the community, there are many aspects of eating and of meals that give meaning to food: the ingredients in the food and the meal that follow cultural rules and habits about combinations and preparations of foods; the customs of what, where, with whom, and when we eat; and the symbolism of food in different contexts. When a person moves into a long-term care facility, much of the continuity of past eating habits and meals is potentially threatened—times for meals, with whom one shares a table at mealtime, what choices one has for each meal, and how the food is perceived to be similar to one's meals in the past. Additionally, the person's role in the food-to-meal process[28]—whether in selecting, planning, preparing, serving, and/or eating—is likely to shift abruptly.

The primary long-term care facilities in the United States are assisted living facilities (ALFs) and nursing homes (NHs). Although, as we will briefly indicate in the following discussion, they differ in structure and in the services they provide, the residents of both settings live in an institutional structure where all meals are provided, generally in a congregate setting. The content of the meals, the timing of the three daily meals, and the location of the dining room are determined by the administration of the facility.

In general, the cognitive functioning and the ability to undertake activities of daily living of NH residents are considerably lower than those of residents of ALFs. Most NH residents use ambulatory aids (walkers and wheelchairs). There are more medical and skilled nursing resources in NHs, more hands-on provision of daily ADL assistance, and more availability of specialized foods and assistance in the process of eating. The socioeconomic status of residents in ALFs tends to be considerably higher, reflecting the fact that most ALF residents or their families must pay for the cost of their care, whereas about two thirds of NH residents depend on coverage from Medicaid. The majority of residents in NHs in the U.S. Food Study were working class, and their educational backgrounds were considerably lower than those of ALF residents.

Central concerns and goals of long-term care facilities, however, tend to be similar: to provide good quality of care and quality of life for the residents, and to facilitate opportunities for personal control and choice in residents' daily lives.

Overall, we suggest that the similarities between ALFs and NHs tend to be more salient than the differences between them. For the purposes of this discussion, we generally will not distinguish between them.

Living in a long-term care facility is often seen and felt as a place where one *has* to be, not where one *wants* to be. A person generally has become a resident of long-term care when the person has difficulty managing to live in the community. Most residents are aware of their declining ability for self-care and increasing need for daily supports. Underlying their frailty is generally a significant degree of resilience.

General Themes

In the provision of meals for long-term care (LTC) residents, the meaning of food and mealtime goes well beyond consideration of the quality and quantity of food provided to a discovery and inclusion of resident-constructed understandings of their daily meals and the institutional context in which they eat their meals. Overall, meals tend to be seen as providing the central structure of each day. Meals can be seen as activities bounded by time periods with less structure and less expectation for resident participation. A retired teacher living in an NH was asked, "Tell me about your day yesterday. What were the main things that you did?" He responded, "Well, I got up and I had breakfast. And from then on, I was just, uh, you know, dangling in the wind, so to speak."

Four broad, strongly interrelated themes emerged from our research in long-term care: eating is a metaphor for living; the meaning of food is associated with a sense of personhood; the centrality of a social component in eating; and the interface between autonomy and dependency in meals and eating. Each of these themes was significant in the experience of frail older adults living in the community, and their salience persisted for long-term care residents.

Eating Is a Metaphor for Living

Residents, their family members, and the facility staff who provided care tended to equate eating with continuity of life, and not eating as portending death. When a resident continued to eat meals, family members generally expected that he or she would continue to live. A sister of one resident noted, "I was shocked by his death…. He did not need the nursing care, where you are actually like a vegetable…where they feed you, diaper you, put you in bed. He went to eat by himself: he ate breakfast, he ate lunch, he ate dinner." Again, eating was a major sign of living.

Attitudes toward food and meals are tied in with a wish to live and to survive. It was not unusual to hear residents talk about eating to live, rather than eating for pleasure. An older adult man was asked, "What do you think of the food here [in the NH]?" He responded, "I've almost forgotten what eating for one's pleasure means."

Meaning of Food Is Intertwined with a Sense of Personhood

Many of the women spoke about their personal competence and independence when we asked them about meals and food. When asked about cooking, an NH resident said, "I loved to cook, make cakes, pies. I used to make rolls, biscuits, cakes. I could cook anything. My daughter, when she first got married, she'd come to my house with her pots and pans and the meat, 'Mom, how you fix this?'" Women spoke with feeling of foods in their past, and saw the meals in the institution as not the same as past meals. In the LTC life space, women tended to relinquish the part of their identity that involved the role of food preparer and food giver, and as LTC residents they became food receivers.

Some family members attempted to protect their NH residents' vulnerable self in regard to food. A daughter, for example, complained about her mother being given ground-up food: "It was lunchtime, and I know what kind of person she is. She's a health nut. And the stuff that she was eating.…And I called the doctor and said 'You can't do this to her. You can't feed her mush.'" She saw her mother's attitudes toward food as a vital part of her sense of personhood.

Centrality of Social Dimension of Meals

When we asked ALF residents, "Whom do you sit with at mealtimes?," most residents were not able to give the names of their tablemates, but they generally identified tablemates in terms of gender, age, health status, and length of sitting together.

We observed limited social interaction at mealtimes between tablemates. Further, there was not much socialization between staff and residents at mealtime. Researchers have found that when staff members encourage residents' independence at mealtime, this tends to be associated with a decrease in social interaction between staff and residents.[72]

A very social widow had a unique positive attitude toward socializing at mealtime, as captured in the following dialog:

> Interviewer: What do you miss most about eating and meals when you lived in the community, when you were with your husband or by yourself?
> Respondent: I don't know. I just have happy feelings about when it gets to be quarter of twelve you know that you're going to go down and see your friends and sit and stuff like that so, I don't really have a lot of missings.

When she was asked about the highlight of her days, she said, "Meals would be a highlight because in addition to meals, you're meeting your friends that you haven't seen for like 6 or 7 hours and maybe they have something new to tell you or something like that."

Rather than this extremely positive picture of socialization at mealtimes, the modal descriptions of the social context at meals tended to reflect neutral or negative attitudes toward tablemates. One ALF resident said, "I think we're talked out. When you sit with the same people day in and day out, I'm sincere; I'm not being malicious. There's nothing to talk about; I'm done. So I leave the table, I finish my meal, and I asked to be excused, and they say okay."

Here are a few examples of the litany of criticisms of the behavior of tablemates:

The man is, he's a mess, in other words he yells out and he bangs on the table with a glass and a bunch of crap like that you know.

One lady, she slobbers all the time in her food. And the drips, you know, the saliva and all, just goes down and falls all over her. . . . It's constant, you know.

[In response to the interviewer's statement: "Some nursing homes say the people here just don't eat, they dine."] I was in the dining room and this guy reached over and took food off my plate, and ate it. How you going to call yourself dining?

To avoid this kind of problem, he ate most of his meals in his room.

Interface between Autonomy and Dependency

The change in living arrangements after moving to a LTC facility leads to modifications of the perceptions, attitudes, and behaviors of the new resident. The resident faces a new set of expectations in the institution, and he or she must respond to the new environment. Underlying much of the personal experience of residing in an LTC facility is the interface of residents' wish for autonomy and personal control of their daily lives and their need for support and assistance from staff members. Together, autonomy and dependency can enable them to maximize their quality of life.

Both **adjustment**, accepting the rules and expectations of the nursing home, and **adaptation**, a creative change in residents' behavior or attitude, are used by residents to enable them to take on the role of resident in the new living arrangement.

Adjustment

Residents tended to explicitly or implicitly recognize that they had very limited control over meals and food (what they eat, when, where, and with whom). A 93-year-old ALF resident said, "I guess you're not in control. You know you're not in control. And, uh [pause], that's the worst part of it I think." A 76-year-old man said, "A lot of times when you get your soup, it's cold...," and the conversation continued as follows:

Interviewer: So what do you do with the cold soup?
Respondent: Well, it goes back to the kitchen. You just don't eat it that day.

Another man said, "You either take what they give you, or you go without," and a woman said, "Oh, this morning my breakfast was so cold. I ate it." Another ALF woman said, "You can only select what they give you."

We asked a woman in the NH, "When you have a meal, what do you like the most about the meal?" She responded, "Just food; it's just food. As an Italian, it's not my food, but I'll eat it. . . . This—I'm adjusted to here. . . . This is eating. This is surviving. . . . If you don't get used to it, it's your fault. You're the one who's going to suffer."

The following dialogue took place with a female NH resident:

Interviewer: So, overall, how is the food here?
Respondent: Well, I'm really not adjusted to it, I'd say.
Interviewer: What's so hard about it?
Respondent: In the community I was living by myself. I got three meals, but it was what I wanted and how I wanted it. But here, it's different. It's not how you want

it or how you do it. It's how *they* do it. And so you have to eat the food. They can't have your likes every day.

Overall, these residents tended to reduce their expectations about food and mealtimes.

Adaptation

Special meals and occasions are often described as enjoyable. Going out for meals was frequently mentioned as a highlight of a day, and a way of being free from the limitations and constraints in the ALF.

We asked an ALF resident, "Tell me about your day yesterday; what were the main things that you did?" She responded, "I went for lunch with two high school friends. . . . I enjoy getting out any time I can and yet I'm not unhappy here. But I'm confined; I have a sense of lockdown [laughs] or something."

The idea of novelty, or a special treat, could be quite positive, particularly when it was associated with one's simple personal taste and memories of past foods—for example:

Interviewer: What do you like to eat out?
Respondent: I try to order something that I don't particularly get here.
Interviewer: Like what?
Respondent: Fried eggs.
Interviewer: Fried eggs. Oh, they don't make fried eggs [here]?
Respondent: No...everything's scrambled.

An 83-year-old widow did factory work at night for many years. When she moved to an ALF, she arranged to continue her sleeping and eating routine:

Interviewer: Do you consider this place to be your home now?
Respondent: Yes.
Interviewer: Okay. What makes it a home?
Respondent: Well I have my own laws, I can get up when I feel like, I can go to bed when I feel like, I go downstairs to meals, I can stay down there if I want to or come back up here and watch television. Now usually I'll have my breakfast at noontime when they have their main meal . . . and then at 5:00 I have dinner [when others have a light meal].

One NH resident provides an example of how resilience-emphasizing autonomy in the context of dependency could be played out within the confines of an NH. This NH resident was unique in that he chose to eat most all of his meals in his room. He also managed to find an interesting way to overcome some of the institutional constraints around food:

Interviewer: What foods do you miss [at breakfast]?
Respondent: They serve the same thing every day, watered-down powdered eggs, like they had in the army. . . . One day in Council meeting I said, "I just want some Raisin Bran," and they said, "Yeah, but we don't serve that no more." They serve me cornflakes every day.

To get what he wanted, he paid aides to buy him eggs and a box of Raisin Bran. He boiled the eggs in a teapot and kept the cereal in the closet. The aides kept it a secret.

Gender Differences

Here we briefly note some of the distinctions between men and women in their reactions to eating in ALFs and NHs.

Women

Some women asserted their positive attitude toward a break with continuity. An ALF resident said, "I deserve the privilege of letting somebody else fix the food and I'll eat it." And another said, "I don't miss cooking but I miss what I chose. The way I chose it. The way I cooked it."

For other women, there was a deep sense of relinquishment and regret. A 93-year-old widow said, "Now, I can't get up and walk, so there's nothing I can do to participate in the making of the meal, either serving or setting the table or anything like that."

Relinquishment involves a sense of personal vulnerability and dependency in the NH. Adaptation to institutional living involves "realization of losses."[64] In some ways, perhaps, relinquishment is a way of expressing personal efficacy, the ability to "adjust." Perhaps part of adjustment and adaptation involves relinquishment.

Men

Some men tended to spontaneously describe the LTC facility as a benign and caring place. In a way, they attributed to the NH or ALF feminine characteristics of caregiving. This may help us understand why the men seemed to be willing to complain about meals in the interviews, but they rarely said that they had complained to staff. Not infrequently they condoned or explained away their concern over meals and policies. Socially constructed ideas about masculinity may prevent an assertive response. The ability to "take it" may be adaptive for men. Additionally, it is difficult to speak truths to those in power.

This theme emerged from the voices of men who were LTC residents. For example, one resident said, "Oh —well, it's such a difficult job trying to please as many people as they do." Another conversation was as follows:

Interviewer: Do you have any choice about the people you sit with [at meals]?
Respondent: Not really.
Interviewer: So if you didn't like somebody, could you complain to somebody?
Respondent: Oh, I could move. But there's no need for it. For a half hour, forty-five minutes, I could put up with anything.

Here, "I can take it" was his metaphor for handling life's stresses, for asserting his autonomy within the context of dependency.

Food at the End of Life

Not eating rang an alarm bell for staff. An ALF administrator was asked, "Do you make use of hospice here?" The

administrator responded, "It's nice if we know they need hospice. We have a lady on hospice now....If they're not eating well, they're not thriving, then we'll bring hospice in."

Staff as well as residents viewed eating as a weapon against death, as in the following conversation with a nursing assistant in an NH:

Interviewer: Is there any other resident who might be closer to dying than the others...not doing very well?
Respondent: You know, Mr. D, he hasn't been looking too good lately. He's been looking real weak. He started stop eatin' a lot too. But when we see that, we make them like "feeders," so we can help them eat so they stay strong.

We asked a certified nursing assistant (CNA), "Are there any signs when a person dies that you have to deal with?" The CNA responded, "Signs? A resident may be eating one day and looking healthy, and the next day she might be tube fed, losing weight, or looking really sick."

Talking of a resident who recently died, a care aide indicated the importance of emotional labor,[41] suggesting there is more to giving food than placing it next to a resident:

She used to always [say] "Oh, I'm ready. Just take me now. I'm tired of living." I used to sit in there and try to talk to her. Me and her would talk all the time. . . . And I asked her why she was saying that. . . . You can't just give up. I would always go in there and make sure she got juice and stuff and drink it. . . . You need to sit there, not just give food to her and leave. . . . I would still go in there and try to give her a little water even if it's just to wet her mouth.

Providing food was a way of giving special attention to a resident, a way of operationalizing emotional labor. It was an opportunity for family and staff to give residents what they liked. When a resident no longer ate, family and LTC staff lost an important way of feeling helpful and close to the resident.

Summary

Clearly, food has the power to comfort or to control; to give pleasure or frustration; and to show love, concern, and care, or to demonstrate indifference, neglect, and personal suffering. When we eat "we are also consuming meanings and symbols" (p. 51).[6]

Useful Websites and Links
Ameds: Catalog of Home Medical Supplies & Equipment. http://www.ameds.com/daily-living-aids.
Caregiver Products. http://www.CaregiverProducts.com.
Sammons Preston/Patterson Medical. http://www.patterson-medical.com/.

REVIEW QUESTIONS

1. List three poor outcomes of undernutrition in older adults.
2. Discuss three common nutritional deficiencies in elders.
3. List three chronic diseases that may employ dietary restrictions as part of managing the chronic disease.
4. Discuss gender differences in the meanings of food and eating in later life.

REFERENCES

1. American Dietetic Association. (2010). Position of the American Dietetic Association: Individualized nutrition approaches for older adults in health care communities. *Journal of the American Dietetic Association, 110,* 1549–1553.

2. American Occupational Therapy Association. (2006). Specialized knowledge and skills in feeding, eating, and swallowing for occupational therapy practice. *The American Journal of Occupational Therapy, 61,* 686–700.

3. American Occupational Therapy Association. (2008). Occupational therapy practice framework: Domain and process (2nd ed.). *American Journal of Occupational Therapy, 62,* 625–683.

4. Baker, H. (2007). Nutrition in the elderly: Diet pitfalls and nutrition advice. *Geriatrics, 62*(10), 24–26.

5. Balenahalli, N., Rao, T. S., Prakasam, A., Sambamurti, K., et al. (2010). Neuronutrition and Alzheimer's disease. *Journal of Alzheimer's Disease, 19*(4), 1123–1139.

6. Beardsworth, A., & Keil, T. (1997). *Sociology on the menu: An introduction to the study of food and society.* New York, NY: Routledge.

7. Becker, G. (1994). The oldest old: Autonomy in the face of frailty. *Journal of Aging Studies, 8,* 59–76.

8. Berkhout, A. M. M., Cools, H. J. M., & VanHouwelingen, H. C. (1998). The relationship between difficulties in feeding oneself and loss of weight in nursing-home patients with dementia. *Age and Ageing, 27,* 637–641.

9. Bernstein, M., & Luggen, A. S. (2009). *Nutrition for the older adult.* Sudbury, MA: Jones and Bartlett Publishers.

10. Berry, E. M., & Marcus, E. M. (2000). Disorders of eating in the elderly. *Journal of Adult Development, 7,* 87–99.

11. Boateng, A. A., Sriram, K., Meguid, M. M., & Crook, M. (2010). Refeeding syndrome: Treatment considerations based on collective analysis of literature case reports. *Nutrition, 26,* 156–167.

12. Bressler, R. (November 2006). Grapefruit juice and prescription drug interactions: Exploring mechanisms of this interaction and potential toxicity for certain drugs. *Geriatrics, 61,* 12–18.

13. Buhr, G., & Bales, C. W. (2010). Nutritional supplements for older adults: Review and recommendations—part II. *Journal of Nutrition for the Elderly, 29*(1), 42–71.

14. Calasanti, T. (2005). Ageism, gravity and gender. *Generations, 29,* 8–12.

15. Chang, C. C., & Roberts, B. L. (2008). Feeding difficulty in older adults with dementia. *Journal of Clinical Nursing, 17,* 2266–2274.

16. Chen, S. T., Maruthur, N. M., & Appel, L. J. (2010). The effect of dietary patterns on estimated coronary heart disease risk: Results from the Dietary Approaches to Stop Hypertension (DASH) trial. *Circulation: Cardiovascular Quality and Outcomes, 3,* 484–489.

17. Cole, G. M., Ma, Q. L., & Frautschy, S. A. (2010). Dietary fatty acids and the aging brain. *Nutrition Reviews, 68,* S102–S111.

18. Davidson, K. (2004). Why can't a man be more like a woman?: Marital status and social networking of older men. *Journal of Men's Studies, 13,* 1–14.

19. Davidson, K., Arber, S., & Marshall, H. (2009) Gender and food in later life: Shifting roles and relationships. In M. Raats, L. de Groot, & W. van Staveren (Eds.), *Food for the aging population* (pp. 110–127). New York, NY: CRC Press.

20. Desai, A.K., Rush, J., Naveen, L., & Thaipisuttikul, P. (2011) Nutrition and nutritional supplements to promote brain health. In Hartman-Stein, P.E. & La Rue, A (Eds), *Enhancing Cognitive fitness in adults: A guide to the use and development of community-based programs* (pp. 249–269). New York, NY: Springer.

21. De Smet, P., & Wood, A. (2002). Herbal remedies. *New England Journal of Medicine, 347*(25), 2040–2056.

22. De Souza Genaro, P., & Martini, L. A. (2010). Effect of protein intake on bone and muscle mass in the elderly. *Nutrition Reviews, 68,* 616–623.

23. DeVault, M. (1991) *Feeding the family: The social organization of caring as gendered work.* Chicago, IL: University of Chicago Press.

24. Douglas, M. (1972) Deciphering a meal. *Daedalus, 101,* 61–82.

25. Elliott, S. J. (1997). Occupational therapy intervention for residents in a skilled nursing facility: A focus on atypical patients. *Occupational Therapy in Health Care, 10,* 53–74.

26. Figueiro, M. G. (2001). *Lighting the way: A key to independence.* http://www.lrc.rpi.edu/programs/lightHealth/AARP/pdf/AARPbook3.pdf.

27. Filion, K. B., El Khoury, F., Bielinkski, M., Schiller, I., et al. (2010). Omega-3 fatty acids in high-risk cardiovascular patients: A meta-analysis of randomized controlled trials. *BMC Cardiovascular Disorders, 10,* 24. Retrieved on October 13, 2015. http://www.biomedcentral.com/1471-2261/10/24.

28. Fjellstrom, C. (2009). The social significance of older people's meals. In M. Raats, L. de Groot, & W. van Staveren (Eds.), *Food for the aging population* (pp. 95–109). New York, NY: CRC Press.

29. Fox, C. B., Treadway, A. K., Blaszczyk, A. T., et al. (2009). Megestrol acetate and mirtazapine for the treatment of unplanned weight loss in the elderly. *Pharmacotherapy, 29*(4), 383–397.

30. Fratiglioni, L., Mangialasche, F., & Qiu, C. (2010). Brain aging: Lessons from community studies. *Nutrition Reviews, 68*(Suppl. 2), S119–S127.

31. Freeman, C., Ricevuto, A., & DeLegge, M. (2010). Enteral nutrition in patients with dementia and stroke. *Current Opinion in Gastroenterology, 16,* 156–159.

32. Frongillo, E. A., & Wolfe, W. S. (2010). Impact of participation in home-delivered-meals on nutrient intake, dietary patterns, and food insecurity of older persons in New York state. *Journal of Nutrition for the Elderly, 29,* 293–310.

33. Furst, E. L. (1997). Cooking and femininity. *Women's Studies International Forum, 20,* 441–449.

34. Genser, D. (2008). Food and drug interaction: Consequences for the nutrition/health status. *Annals of Nutrition and Metabolism, 52*(Suppl. 1), 29–32.

35. Giard, L. (1998). The nourishing arts. In M. de Certeau, L. Giard, & P. Mayol (Eds.), *The practice of everyday life* (Vol. 2, pp. 151–169). (T. J. Tomasik, Trans.). Minneapolis, MN: University of Minnesota Press.

36. Glantz, C., & Richman, R. (1986). *The dining experience.* Chicago, IL: Glantz/Richman Rehabilitation Associates.

37. Goodman, C. (2012). Wheel chair seating and positioning: Considerations for elders. In R.L. Padilla, S. Byers-Connon, & H. Lohman. *Occupational therapy with elders: Strategies for the COTA* (pp. 191–193). Maryland Heights, MO: Elsevier/Mosby.

38. Gustafsson, K., Andersson, I., Andersson, J., Fjellstrom, C., & Sidenvall, B. (2003). Older women's perceptions of independence versus dependence in food-related work. *Public Health Nursing, 20*(3), 237–247.

39. Hasselkus, B. R. (2006) The world of everyday occupation: Real people, real lives. *The American Journal of Occupational Therapy, 60,* 627–640.

40. Heiss, C., Keen, C. L., & Kelm, M. (2010). Flavanols and cardio-vascular disease prevention. *European Heart Journal*, *31*, 2583–2592.

41. Hochschild, A. R. (2003). *The commercialization of intimate life.* Berkeley, CA: University of California Press.

42. Hocking, C., Wright-St. Clair, V., & Bunrayong, W. (2002). The meaning of cooking and recipe work for older Thai and New Zealand women. *Journal of Occupational Science*, *9*(3), 117–127.

43. Infinitec.org. (n.d.) *Adaptive cooking.* Retrieved on October 13, 2015. www.infinitec.org/live/index.html.

44. Kaiser, M., Bandinelli, S., & Lunenfeld, B. (2010). Frailty and the role of nutrition in older people. *Acta Biomedica*, *81*(Suppl. 1), 37–45.

45. Keller, H. H. (2004) Identification of nutrition problems in older patients. *Geriatrics and Aging*, *7*, 62–65.

46. Kempiak, M. & Fox, M.A. (2002). Online grocery shopping: Consumer motives, concerns, and business models. *First Monday*, *7*(9), Retrieved July 1, 2015, http://firstmonday.org/ojs/index.php/fm/article/view/987/908.

47. Kheir, F., & Haddad, R. (2010). Anemia in the elderly. *Disease Monthly*, *56*, 456–467.

48. Lee, J. S., Fischer, J. G., & Johnson, M. A. (2010). Food insecurity, food and nutrition programs, and aging. *Journal of Nutrition for the Elderly*, *29*, 116–149.

49. Lenihan, D. J., & Uretsky, B. F. (2000). Nonpharmacologic treatment of heart failure in the elderly. *Clinical Geriatric Medicine*, *16*(3), 477–488.

50. Litchford, M. (2005). *Feeding instructions for caregivers. Adult day care resource manual for the USDA Child and Adult Care Food Program* (pp. 30–36). National Food Service Management Institute. University, MS: University of Mississippi. Retrieved June 30, 2015. http://www.nfsmi.org/documentlibraryfiles/PDF/20071128104309.pdf.

51. Lopez-Contreras, M. J., Zamora-Portero, S., Lopez, M. A., Marin, J. F., et al. (2010). Dietary intake and iron status of institutionalized elderly people: Relationship with different factors. *Journal of Nutrition, Health, and Aging*, *14*(10), 1–6.

52. Mackowiak, E. D., Bersntein, Y., & Paul, S. H. (2010). The adult vitamin and mineral supplement maze. *The Consultant Pharmacist*, *25*(4), 234–240.

53. Manton, C. (1999). *Fed up: Women and food in America.* Westport, CT: Burgin & Garvey.

54. Marcus, E. L., & Berry, E. M. (1998). Refusal to eat in the elderly. *Nutrition Reviews*, *56*, 163–171.

55. McGruder, J., Cors, D., Tiernan, A., & Tomlin, G. (2003). Weighted wrist cuffs for tremor reduction during eating in adults with static brain lesions. *The American Journal of Occupational Therapy*, *57*, 507–516.

56. Meals on Wheels of America.. (n.d.). Retrieved October 13, 2015 http://www.mealsonwheelsamerica.org.

57. Moore, A. J., & Stratton, D. C. (2002). *Resilient widowers: Older men speak for themselves.* New York, NY: Springer.

58. Morley, J. E. (2007). Weight loss in older persons: New therapeutic approaches. *Current Pharmaceutical Design*, *13*, 3637–3647.

59. Morley, J. E. (2010). Nutrition and the brain. *Clinical Geriatric Medicine*, *26*, 89–98.

60. Moss, S. Z., Moss, M. S., Kilbride, J. E., & Rubinstein, R. L. (2007). Frail men's perspectives on food and eating. *Journal of Aging Studies*, *21*, 314–324.

61. Murcott, A. (1995). Talking of good food: An empirical study of women's conceptualizations. *Food and Foodways*, *40*, 305–318.

62. Nord, M. (2003). Measuring food security of elderly persons. *Family, Economics and Nutrition Review*, *15*, 33–46.

63. O'Sullivan, G., Hocking, C., & Wright-St. Clair, V. (2008). History in the making: Older Canadian women's food-related practices. *Food and Foodways*, *16*(1), 63–87. doi:10.1080/07409710701885150.

64. Parnell, R. B. (2005). Perceived loneliness, helplessness and boredom of elderly residents in Eden nursing homes. [University of Hong Kong dissertation]. *Dissertation Abstracts International*, *66–07*, Section B, 3637.

65. Rohde, L. E., Silva de Assis, M. C., & Rabelo, E. R. (2007). Dietary vitamin K intake and anticoagulation in elderly patients. *Current Opinion in Clinical Nutrition and Metabolism Care*, *10*, 1–5.

66. Rubinstein, R. L. (1986). *Singular paths: Old men living alone.* New York, NY: Columbia University Press.

67. Rubinstein, R. L., Kilbride, J. C., & Nagy, S. (1992). *Elders living alone: Frailty and perception of choice.* New York, NY: Aldine.

68. *Sammons Preston/Patterson Medical.* Retrieved October 13, 2015 http://www.pattersonmedical.com/.

69. Sampson, E. L., Candy, B., & Jones, L. (2009). Enteral tube feeding for older people with advanced dementia [Review]. *Cochrane Database of Systematic Reviews*, *15*(2), CD007209. doi: 10.1002/14651858.CD007209.pub2.

70. Sharkey, J. R. (2002). The interrelationship of nutritional risk factors, indicators of nutritional risk, and severity of disability among home delivered meal participants. *The Gerontologist*, *42*, 373–380.

71. Shordike, A., & Pierce, D. (2005). Cooking up Christmas in Kentucky: Occupation and tradition in the stream of time. *Journal of Occupational Science*, *12*(3), 140–148. doi:10.1080/14427591.2005.9686557.

72. Stabell, A., Eide, H., Solheim, G. A., Solberg, K. N. & Rustøen, T. (2004), Nursing home residents' dependence and independence. *Journal of Clinical Nursing*, *13*, 677–686. doi: 10.1111/j.1365-2702.2004.00942.x.

73. Sydner, Y. M., Sidenvall, B., Fjellström, C., Raats, M., & Lumbers, M. (2007). Food habits and foodwork: The life course perspective of senior Europeans. *Food Culture and Society*, *10*(3), 367–387. doi:10.2752/155280107X239845.

74. Torres, S., & Hammarstrom, G. (2006). Speaking of "limitations" while trying to disregard them: A qualitative study of how diminished everyday competence and aging can be regarded. *Journal of Aging Studies*, *20*, 291–302.

75. Trefler, E., & Taylor, S. J. (1991). Prescription and positioning: evaluating the physically disabled individual for wheelchair seating. *The Journal of the International Society for Prosthetics and Orthotics*, *15*, 217–224.

76. Tresley, J., & Sheean, P. M. (2008). Refeeding syndrome: Recognition is the key to prevention and management. *Journal of the American Dietetic Association*, *108*(12), 2105–2108.

77. Van den Hoonaard, D. K. (2005). *When I cook it's nothing elaborate: Masculinity and older widowers' descriptions of housework.* Sheffield, UK: Presentation at the International Society for Critical Health Psychology.

78. Van den Hoonaard, D. K. (2007). Introduction: Aging and masculinity: A topic whose time has come. *Journal of Aging Studies*, *21*, 277–280.

79. Wang, L., Manson, J. E., Song, Y., & Sesso, H. D. (2010). Systemic review: Vitamin D and calcium supplementation in prevention of cardiovascular events. *Annals of Internal Medicine*, *152*, 315–323.

80. Warde, A., & Hetherington, K. (1994). English households and routine food practices: A research note. *Sociological Review, 42,* 758–778.

81. West, J. F. & Redstone, F. (2004). Feeding the adult with neurogenic disorders. *Topics in Geriatric Rehabilitation, 20*(2), 131–134.

82. Wolfe, W. S., Olson, C. M., Kendall, A., & Frongillo, E. A. (1996). Understanding food insecurity in the elderly: A conceptual framework. *Journal of Nutrition Education, 28,* 92–100.

83. Wright-St. Clair, V., & Hocking, C. (2005). Older New Zealand women doing the work of Christmas: A recipe for identity formation. *Sociological Review, 53*(2), 332–350. doi:10.1111/j.1467-954X.2005.00517.x.

84. Wright-St. Clair, V., Pierce, D., Bunrayong, W., et al. (2013). Cross-cultural understandings of festival food-related activities for older women in Chiang Mai, Thailand, eastern Kentucky, USA and Auckland, New Zealand. *Journal of Cross-Cultural Gerontology, 28*(2), 103–119.

85. Yeh, S. S., Lovin, S., & Schuster, M. W. (2007). Pharmacological treatment of geriatric cachexia: Evidence and safety in perspective. *Journal of the American Medical Directors Association, 8,* 363–377.

Oral Health for Aging Adults

Shirley Blanchard, PhD, ABDA, OTR/L, FAOTA, FHDRTP, Judith C. Barker, PhD, Susan Hyde, DDS, MPH, PhD

CHAPTER OUTLINE

OBJECTIVES

- Discuss the relationship between general health, oral health, and quality of life in older adults
- Relate the interprofessional roles of dentistry, occupational therapy, and nursing for older adults' access to oral care.
- Describe age-related changes in oral physiology
- Identify oral diseases that are prevalent among older adults and write a descriptive referral
- Explain how the *Occupational Therapy Practice Framework[3]* guides interventions for oral care
- Discuss the significance of the long-term care environment for oral health
- Identify risk factors and preventive measures for aspiration pneumonia
- Provide recommendations for oral hygiene and denture care for those who need assistance or are unable to care for themselves
- Recommend assistive technology for oral care for older adults with disabilities
- Identify strategies for addressing the challenges of providing oral care for clients with care-resistant behavior

For older adults, oral health both reflects and contributes to general health and quality of life (Figure 12-1). Eighty-five percent of older adults have at least one major chronic disease, and 50% have two or more chronic diseases.[9] Many studies have established associations between periodontal (gum) disease and chronic diseases such as cardiovascular disease, stroke, diabetes, and respiratory diseases. Systematic reviews have found that treating periodontal disease and improving oral hygiene has enhanced metabolic control for people with type 2 diabetes, prevented respiratory infections and death from pneumonia in clients in long-term care, and reduced cardiovascular disease.[15,55,67,68] Medications used to control chronic diseases often have oral side effects, including xerostomia (dry mouth), taste alteration, diminished bone health, and tissue overgrowth, swelling, inflammation, and ulceration.

Good oral health is required for three essential physiologic functions: mastication, speech, and protection. Tooth loss, precipitated by dental caries (tooth decay), periodontal disease, or injury, impairs both mastication and speech, and may also lower self-esteem, restrict social contact, and inhibit intimacy.[80] Diminished salivary flow, compromised by medications, irradiation, or disease, impedes both immunologic and mechanical protection. Oral and pharyngeal cancers result in significant disfigurement and have poor 5-year survival rates.[7] Oral pathogens can become blood-borne or aspirated, resulting in serious systemic disease. Poor oral health increases the risk of upper respiratory infection, aspiration pneumonia, febrile episodes, rheumatic fever, bacterial endocarditis, glomerulonephritis, diabetes, cardiovascular disease, and cerebral and myocardial infarction.[65,80] Pain from untreated oral diseases can hamper normal activities of daily living (ADLs) and disturb sleep.

CASE EXAMPLE 12-1   Mrs. Davidson

Mrs. Davidson is 88 years old and was admitted to a nursing care facility 2 months ago. Her medical history includes osteoarthritis, well-controlled hypertension, hyperlipidemia, and vascular dementia with subsequent memory loss. She has some teeth but has not had a dental check-up in many years. A dental screening revealed poor oral hygiene, inflamed and bleeding gums, only a few front teeth (no molars), and an area of irritation on the roof of her mouth.

Mrs. Davidson finished high school and worked intermittently as a cashier at a department store. She married and raised one son. She talks about missing her husband, son, and other friends who have passed away. She has few financial resources other than Medicare and Medicaid. Although she would have preferred to remain in her own home, she realized that she was unable to complete self-care and access the community. Admission to a long-term care facility provided an opportunity for assistance in managing basic activities of daily living.

At the nursing home's monthly client care plan meeting, Mrs. Davidson's health status and needs are reviewed by an interprofessional team of care providers. Mrs. Davidson, along with her remaining family member, her daughter-in-law, agreed to the following goals:
a. improve her ability to care for her own oral hygiene;
b. reduce her resistant behavior when staff try to provide assistance with daily oral hygiene;
c. improve her nutritional intake; and
d. request a referral to a dentist regarding the missing teeth, possible difficulty chewing, and sores found in Mrs. Davidson's mouth.

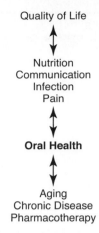

Quality of Life

↕

Nutrition
Communication
Infection
Pain

↕

Oral Health

↕

Aging
Chronic Disease
Pharmacotherapy

FIGURE 12-1   Oral health and aging.

Mrs. Davidson's scenario is an example of the oral health disparities often experienced by older adults; with dependence in ADLs and cognitive impairment as two important factors that contribute to these disparities.[29] Oral health disparities are defined as "diminished health status of population subgroups defined by age, socioeconomic status, geography, disability status, and behavioral lifestyles."[47]

Oral health disparities also include ethnic older adults who do not have access to adequate oral care.[26] Thirty-eight percent of community-dwelling older adults perceive their oral health to be fair or poor, African Americans report worse oral health and quality of life than whites, and edentulous adults (those without teeth) express worse quality of life than dentate individuals (those with teeth).[18,27,53,69] Oral health thus has a substantial effect on general health, nutrition, communication, and quality of life.

Fifty-four percent of community-dwelling adults aged 65 years or older typically have had a dental visit during the past year, and although this represents a steady increase in dental utilization by older adults during the past 40 years, access among minority older adults has not increased proportionally.[18,35] A major barrier to access to care is lack of dental insurance, which is typically not a retirement benefit. Neither Medicare nor the majority of state Medicaid programs cover preventive and/or restorative dental treatment for older adults; private insurance is often either unavailable or provides very limited coverage. As a result, older adults pay an increased portion of their dental expenses out-of-pocket, which may affect their treatment choices or ability to receive care.[26]

Long-standing federal legislation, the Omnibus Budget Reconciliation Act of 1987, requires skilled nursing facilities to provide for both routine and emergency dental services to meet the needs of each resident, and many states require additional measures to ensure the oral health of nursing home residents.[77] Despite these laws, poor oral health, inadequate mouth care, and limited access to dental care abound in long-term care settings.[70,84] Currently, there are no federal laws governing oral health in alternative long-term care facilities, such as group homes or assisted living centers, and state laws

provide only general guidelines for personal care assistance.[70] A survey of alternative long-term care facilities in Michigan found that fewer than 20% of the facilities had a written plan for oral health, provided a dental examination at admission, or had an agreement with a dentist to provide care.[70]

Although Medicare and most state Medicaid programs do not reimburse for preventive or restorative dental treatments for older adults, chronic diseases that result in diminished function that interferes with self-care (such as feeding, oral care, chewing, or swallowing) may demonstrate a medical necessity for skilled intervention in a nursing home, home health, or outpatient setting. Occupational therapists may initiate referrals to dentists based on results of an oral assessment, covered later in this chapter.

The health care reform proposed by the 2010 Federal Patient Protection and Affordable Care Act aims to provide health insurance coverage to those who are currently uninsured, slow the rising of health-care costs, reorganize the health delivery system, and improve the quality of care provided to all.[52] The broad goal is to create a more integrated and interprofessional public-health-oriented care-delivery system. Regrettably, dentistry and the importance of oral health were not included in this model of client-centered medical homes.[52] Viewing the causal dynamics of the oral health of older adults from a larger systems perspective illustrates the interplay of general health, nutrition, social engagement, quality of life, and policy on the development of effective oral health promotion and interventions.[46] Occupational therapists are important members of the interprofessional health-care team, and are more likely than dentists to interact with frail and institutionalized older adults. A working knowledge of the oral health issues associated with aging will greatly benefit interprofessional communication and referral for care.

Age-Related Changes in Oral Health

Normal aging occurs for oral physiology as it does for the other body systems. Teeth will wear, gingiva (gums) will recede, oral tissue will atrophy, chewing efficiency will diminish, and although the sense of taste may change slowly, a decreased sense of smell results in a loss of flavor perception and food enjoyment.[66] Normal aging does not involve tooth loss, dental caries (tooth decay), periodontal disease, xerostomia, infection, or pain, although these conditions are prevalent in older adults.

Despite improvements in many of the measures for the oral health of community-dwelling older adults during the past 40 years, disparities persist among racial and ethnic minorities and those with lower incomes and less education.[18] Nineteen percent of adults aged 65 years or older have no remaining teeth, and current smokers are more likely to have lost all their teeth (50%) (Table 12-1).[18,19] In general, seniors over age 65 years have an average of 19 remaining teeth, which is fewer than what is needed for an adequate functional dentition.[18,26] Older African Americans, however, have even fewer teeth, 15 on average.[18] Tooth decay and

TABLE 12-1 Oral Health and Access to Care for Community-Dwelling Older Adults

Oral Health Measure	65+-year-olds	65- to 74-year-olds	75+-year-olds
Tooth loss[1,6]			
Missing all teeth	18.6%	13.0%	25.8%
Mean remaining teeth	18.9	19.3	18.4
Untreated dental caries[1,6]	18.9%		
Coronal		18.5%	19.4%
Root		12.4%	16.6%
Periodontal disease[2]			
Moderate or severe	64.0%		
Xerostomia[3]	10% to 40%		
Candidiasis infection[4]			
Wears dentures	Up to 65%		
Orofacial pain[5]	17.4%		
TMJ (jaw joint)	7.7%		
Facial	6.9%		
Oral sores	6.4%		
Toothache	12.0%		
Burning mouth	1.7%		
Self-rated oral health[1]			
Good–excellent	61.6%	61.6%	61.7%
Fair–poor	38.4%	38.4%	38.3%
Dental visit past year[1]	54.5%	56.9%	51.6%

[1]Dye, B. A., Tan, S., Smith, V., Lewis, B. G., Barker, L. K., Thornton-Evans, G., . . . Li, C. H. (2007). Trends in oral health status: United States, 1988-1994 and 1999-2004. National Center for Health Statistics. *Vital Health Statistics, 11*(248), 1-92.
[2]Eke, P. I., Dye, B. A., Wei, L., Thornton-Evans, G. O., & Genco, R. J. (2012). Prevalence of periodontitis in adults in the United States: 2009 and 2010. *Journal of Dental Research, 91*(10), 914-920.
[3]Dental, Oral and Craniofacial Data Resource Center. (2002). *Oral health U.S., 2002.* Bethesda, MD: NIDCR/NIH.
[4]Akpan, A., & Morgan, R. (2002). Oral candidiasis. *Postgraduate Medical Journal, 78*, 455-459.
[5]Riley, J. L., Gilbert, G. H., & Heft, M. W. (1998). Orofacial pain symptom prevalence: Selective sex differences in the elderly? *Pain, 76*, 97-104.
[6]Dye, B. A., Thornton-Evans, G., Li, X., & Iafolla, T. J. (2015). Dental caries and tooth loss in adults in the United States, 2011-2012. *NCHS Data Brief*, No. 197. Hyattsville, MD: National Center for Health Statistics.

periodontal disease continue to be the leading causes of tooth loss.[20] Dental caries is as common a condition in older adults as it is in children, and is more likely to remain untreated.[25] Nineteen percent of adults aged 65 years or older in the general population have untreated dental caries, whereas 27% of older Mexican Americans have untreated caries.[19] Destructive periodontal disease affects 17% of adults aged 65 years or older, with higher prevalence and disease severity found among minorities, smokers, and those with lower incomes and less education.[18] Periodontal disease can contribute to local and systemic infection and inflammation, bad breath, and tooth loss.

Currently, there are no nationally representative data on xerostomia, but prevalence estimates range from 10% to 40% of older adults.[14] Xerostomia, or dry mouth, affects the ability to chew, taste, swallow, speak, and sleep. It can lead to increased plaque accumulation, dental caries, tooth loss, infections, inflammation, and uncomfortable dentures.[14] Xerostomia can result from decreased salivary flow, changed salivary composition, systemic disease, or as a side effect of medications. There are more than 500 medications for which xerostomia is a potential side effect, including tricyclic antidepressants, antihistamines, antihypertensives, and diuretics, all drug classes commonly used by older adults.[22]

Oral candidiasis (yeast infection) is the most common fungal infection in humans, and is underdiagnosed among older adults—up to 65% of those who wear dentures experience candidiasis.[1] Risk factors include decreased saliva, increasing age, antibiotic and steroid medications, dentures, high-carbohydrate diet, deficient vitamin B_{12} and iron, smoking, diabetes, and immunosuppressive disorders. Candidiasis can present as acute white plaques that when wiped away expose a painful, red, ulcerated surface; as chronic white or red tissue; or at the corners of the mouth as painful, fissured, and encrusted cracks. Untreated candidiasis can result in altered taste, burning mouth symptoms, and difficulty swallowing, and can disseminate throughout the body in immunocompromised clients, resulting in a mortality rate of 71% to 79%.[1]

Pain is often regarded as a normal part of aging, by both clients and their care providers. As a result, pain is underreported, underdiagnosed, and poorly managed in older adults.[28] Seventeen percent of older adults experience orofacial pain (often related to diabetes), including jaw joint pain, facial pain, oral sores, burning mouth, toothache pain, and reduced oral motility.[45,59,63] Chronic pain is associated with increased frailty, social withdrawal, decreased performance in basic and/or instrumental activities of daily living (IADLs), and diminished quality of life (Figure 12-1).[2,62]

How can a nondentist, specifically an occupational therapist, recognize these conditions and know when to make a dental referral? The Academic Geriatric Resource Center of the University of California, San Francisco, has developed an online learning module for nondental health professionals to conduct an oral health assessment to screen for disease, dysfunction, and discomfort (see Box 12-1 for helpful online resources).[78] The module outlines a systematic approach, beginning with an extraoral examination, followed by an intraoral examination, and concluding with an evaluation of the teeth and/or dentures. Both a Geriatric Oral Health Assessment screening tool and a demonstration video reinforce the learning material, and the module includes photos of the common oral conditions in older adults discussed earlier.

The Geriatric Oral Health Assessment screening tool was developed to aid in the evaluation and decision-making processes. The oral cavity can be prone to transient trauma, inflammation, and ulceration. These conditions often resolve themselves in 10 to 14 days. Therefore, if a soft tissue lesion is observed during the intraoral examination, it can be reevaluated in 2 weeks to determine whether it has healed. A lesion that is still present 2 weeks later requires a referral. When reporting your findings, note the lesion's general location, size, shape, and color; any pain or discomfort; whether there is blood or exudates; and whether the client knows how long it has been present. When writing a referral to a dentist, providing a description that includes these points greatly aids the dentist in focusing on the cause of concern.

Example of a referral note to a dentist on behalf of Mrs. Davidson: "Mrs. Davidson has only a few remaining teeth, her oral hygiene is poor, her gums bleed, and it has been many years since her last dental visit. Please evaluate the lesions on her upper left jaw, on the roof of the mouth, near the front teeth. There are two lesions, both of which are approximately 3 mm by irregular in shape, white, and not painful; no blood or pus is associated with the lesions; they cannot be removed by wiping with gauze; and the client was unaware of their presence."

Traditionally, in long-term care facilities, occupational therapists, speech pathologists, or nurses may assist the resident in the performance of oral hygiene, and as such are ideally suited to perform periodic oral health assessments.

Occupational Therapy Practice Framework for Oral Health

Occupational therapy practice is guided by the *Occupational Therapy Practice Framework* (OTPF).[3] The OTPF is based on the International Classification of Functioning, Disability, and Health (ICF).[83] The ICF and the OTPF consider the effects of the health condition and disability on the whole person. For example, the health condition of osteoarthritis may cause neuromuscular and sensory changes in body

---

BOX 12-1   Helpful Online Resources

Smiles for Life: A National Oral Health Curriculum (http://www.smilesforlifeoralhealth.com)
Smiles for Life provides the nation's only comprehensive online oral health curriculum. Developed by the Society of Teachers of Family Medicine Group on Oral Health and now in its third edition, this curriculum is designed to enhance the role of primary care clinicians in the promotion of oral health for all age groups through the development and dissemination of high-quality educational resources. The following curriculum modules are especially relevant for the occupational therapy practitioner:

    Module 1: The Relationship of Oral Health to Systemic
      Health
    https://www.perio.org/consumer/other-diseases
    Module 8: Geriatric Oral Health
    http://www.geriatricoralhealth.org/topics/default.aspx

Oral Care in Continuing Care Settings: Collaborating to Improve Policies and Practice (http://www.ahprc. dal.ca/projects/oral-care/default.asp)
This website focuses on oral health care for frail and dependent older adults, with particular emphasis on daily mouth care. Resources include information sheets, learning modules, video technique demonstrations, and research summaries.

Tooth Wisdom (http://www.toothwisdom.org/)
Oral Health America's online portal provides education for older adults and their care advisors, connects vulnerable populations to oral health care resources in their own local communities, provides evidence-based resources for health professionals, and advocates for policy that provides for the oral health of older Americans.

University of California, San Francisco (UCSF), Academic Geriatric Resource Center (http://www. gerigero-onlinecourse.ucsf.edu/)
The UCSF Academic Geriatric Resource Center has created an online curriculum in geriatrics and gerontology. The oral and dental health curriculum encompasses modules 4.2.5 to 4.2.15. Topics include oral health assessment, with a screening tool and video demonstration; common oral conditions in older adults; and guidelines for writing a dental referral.

The State of Aging and Health in America (http://www.cdc.gov/aging/data/stateofaging.htm)
The *State of Aging and Health in America* is a report series that began as a joint effort of the Centers for Disease Control and Prevention's (CDC's) Healthy Aging Program and the Merck Company Foundation, and evolved into an interactive data website where professionals can get current data at the national, state, and selected local levels for 15 key indicators of older adult health, including complete tooth loss (edentulism).

structures that cause physical limitations in participation (performing oral hygiene). Access to the environment (such as the bathroom) secondary to using an assistive device or dependent mobility may also impede participation. This inaccessibility may result in a change in context. For example, Mrs. Davidson's health condition of vascular dementia impedes her memory. She is unable to participate in oral hygiene secondary to her inability to problem solve and initiate the task. Reduced sensation related to osteoarthritis interferes with her ability to perceive objects in her hand and perform grip and pinch. Although the bathroom is the typical location to brush one's teeth, because of a limitation in access to the environment, she may need to brush her teeth in the kitchen or dining room, or sit rather than stand at the sink. Context must also be considered; it may be more confusing for Mrs. Davidson to perform oral care in a different room in the middle of the day than following her typical early-morning routine. Figure 12-2 summarizes the ICF model (how the health condition affects participation).

Figure 12-3 represents the Nagi Model, which offers another way to view the effects of chronic and acute disease on function and the client's resulting disability and impaired activity participation.[4] This disablement model is used in the *Physical Therapy Guide to Practice*. Again, Mrs. Davidson's medical condition is osteoarthritis, her impairment

limitations are strength and range of motion (ROM; difficulty reaching, placing, or manipulating oral care devices). The resulting activity limitations or barriers to function would manifest as reduced plate-to-mouth pattern and altered role for performing oral hygiene. An interprofessional collaboration between an occupational therapist, physical therapist, and dental hygienist may be warranted to reduce additional barriers to performance.

Occupational therapists use the occupational profile to ascertain the client's previous level of performance and what is meaningful to the client. The OTPF consists of occupations, performance skills, and client factors. ADLs are important occupations that include an older adult's ability to perform oral hygiene. Various performance skills are needed for oral care, including a stable head position in midline, upper extremity strength, gross and fine motor coordination, praxis (motor planning), visual perceptual skills, sensation, and cognition. Older adults may be limited in one or more of the aforementioned areas secondary to frailty, illness, injury, or disease sequelae. Table 12-2 depicts the interaction of Mrs. Davidson's occupational profile and factors that affect her engagement in the occupation of oral hygiene.

According to Katz et al.'s classic study "Studies of Illness in the Aged,"[35] older adults regain recovery in ADLs in a hierarchical or developmental fashion following an episode of illness. Katz and his colleagues suggest that basic ADLs are regained in the following order: grooming (oral hygiene), feeding (eating and swallowing), continence, transferring, toileting, dressing (upper and lower extremity), and bathing. Intervention typically begins with oral hygiene and progresses to more challenging ADLs, such as dressing; bathing requires the highest level of performance skill.[35]

Long-Term Care Settings

Occupational therapy practitioners provide a broad range of interventions in the long-term care setting. When providing interventions for older adults, who are often frail, it is important to consider barriers to performance. In addition to possible

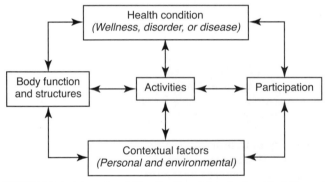

FIGURE 12-2 International Classification of Functioning, Disability, and Health (ICF).

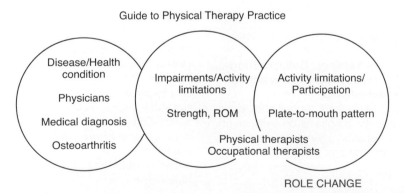

FIGURE 12-3 Interaction of disablement model and health professionals' Nagi Model. (Adapted from American Physical Therapy Association [APTA]. [2003]. *Guide to practice*. Alexandria, VA: American Physical Therapy Association.)

TABLE 12-2 Occupational Therapy Practice Framework Matrix

Occupational Therapy Practice Framework	Occupations (pp. S19-S21)	Client Factor (pp. S22-S24)	Performance Skill (pp. S25-S26)	Performance Patterns (p. S27)	Context and Environment (p. S28)	Types of Occupational Therapy Interventions (pp. S29-S31)	Activity and Occupational Demand (pp. S32-S33)	Outcomes (pp. S34-S35)
Domain p. S4	ADL IADL Rest and sleep Education Work Play Leisure Social participation	Values, beliefs, and spirituality Body functions Mental Sensory Neuromusculoskeletal (muscles, nerves, or other system)	Motor skills Process skills Social interaction skills	Person Habits Routines Rituals Roles Group or Population Routines Rituals Roles	Cultural Personal Temporal Virtual Environment Physical Social	Occupation and activities Preparatory methods (splints, assistive technology, wheeled mobility) Preparatory tasks Education and training Advocacy Group intervention	Relevance Object use/properties Space demands Social demands Sequencing/timing Required actions Required body functions Required body structures	Improvement Enhance Prevention Health and wellness Quality of life Participation Role Well-being Occupational justice
Client Profile 88-year-old female with osteoarthritis and impaired memory	ADL Oral hygiene IADL Health maintenance Decrease health risk behavior	Body functions ↓Memory (setup) Perception ↓Tactile sensation ↑Pain Neuromusculoskeletal ↓Joint mobility ↓Muscle power	Motor skills Grips and manipulates Process skills Locates and organizes items for oral care Sequences task Social skills Requests assistance appropriately	Habits Performs oral care daily Routine Follows morning sequence of oral care	Physical environment Accesses bathroom to perform oral care Social Expected to perform oral care by caregiver	Assistive technology Large-handle toothbrush Toothpaste dispenser	Object use Selects the appropriate utensils or devices for performing oral care	Improvement Perform oral care with setup ↓Joint pain with assistive technology ↑Self-efficacy Prevention Oral inflammation and gingivitis Bilateral upper extremity disuse atrophy

(Adapted from American Occupational Therapy Association. [2014]. Occupational therapy practice framework: Domain and process [3rd ed.]. *American Journal of Occupational Therapy, 68* [Suppl.1], S1-S48. Retrieved from http://dx.doi.org/10.5014/ajot.2014.682006.)

alterations in cognitive function, frailty among older adults is characterized by weight loss, fatigue, slowness, low activity level, and weakness. Collectively, impaired performance skills and frailty may result in the need for a higher level of care, and lack of performance.[6]

The Federal Nursing Home Reform Act, or OBRA (the 1987 Omnibus Budget Reconciliation Act), created a national minimum set of standards of care and rights for persons living in certified nursing facilities.[77] The Centers for Medicare and Medicaid (CMS) Minimum Data Set for nursing home resident assessment and care screening full assessment form (MDS) requires a reassessment of function every 30 days. Section G of the MDS includes performance of personal hygiene, which includes brushing teeth. The MDS uses a numerical rating scale from 0, which is independent, to 4, which is total assistance.[10] Occupational therapists who consistently participate in the monthly recertification process have the advantage of identifying residents who exhibit a change in function and who may benefit from skilled intervention.

Without intervention, older adults may experience altered roles and routines associated with good oral care and hygiene. For example, if there is loss of memory and the older adult is accustomed to brushing his or her teeth at a set time of day and no one is aware of this routine, this seemingly simple ADL task is lost in translation. In Mrs. Davidson's case, this may also be related to her resistance to having others assist her with oral hygiene. By completing a thorough client and family interview or occupational profile and focusing on context and environment, routines can be restored that help motivate Mrs. Davidson to perform oral care or to expect and accept caregiver assistance in reestablishing a consistent routine for this basic ADL.

Age is also associated with a reduced sense of taste and smell.[71] For older adults like Mrs. Davidson, who have concomitant conditions, it is important to assess client factors that may contribute to loss of oral function. Lack of oral sensation and taste are examples of deficits in oral structures that may increase the necessity and preference for soft, sticky, and sweet foods, which results in dental caries. Combined with a decrease in healthy oral habits and difficulty in brushing and flossing, this leads to increased risks for periodontal disease and systemic inflammation.

Client factors include body functions, such as oral motor muscle power, tone, sensation, and lingual control and coordination. Body structures, such as the cranial nerves, support the integration of facial and oral mechanisms required for oral motor performance. Cranial nerves and oral structures must be evaluated along with the aforementioned performance skills. Evaluation of the sensory and motor component of the cranial nerves may reveal loss of oral sensation, motor weakness, or a risk for dysphagia. Table 12-3 presents the overlap in sensory and motor functions of the cranial nerves. Wolf, Glass, and Carr[82] offer a diagram of the overlap between the sensory and motor functions of cranial nerves that contribute to oral motor performance (Figure 12-4). Any loss of oral sensory or motor function may contribute to dysfunction in any of the four stages of swallowing and result in an unsafe self-performance of oral care.

TABLE 12-3 Sensory and Motor Function of the Cranial Nerves

Cranial Nerve	Purpose
Trigeminal V	Sensation: forehead, face, and jaw; biting, chewing, proprioception
Facial VII	Facial expression, elevate larynx, salivation
Glossopharyngeal IX	Taste (posterior one third of tongue), salivation
Vagus X	Initiates swallow, peristalsis in the esophagus, phonation, taste
Accessory XI	Swallowing, elevate larynx and pharynx (flexion of head, lateral rotation—sternocleidomastoid)
Hypoglossal XII	Movement of tongue (position the tongue)
IX and X	Share gag reflex and phonation (speech production)

(Adapted from Bailey, P. [2004, April]. *Neurological representation of swallowing.* Retrieved from http://www.gbmc.org/documents%5CServices%5CDance%5Capril2004.pdf.)

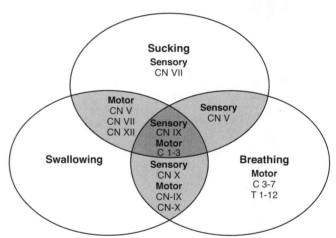

FIGURE 12-4 Overlapping function of the cranial nerves involved in sucking.

For example, upper motor neuron dysfunction may result in hypertonicity, a retracted tongue, and a positive bite reflex, whereas lower motor neuron dysfunction may result in oral and lingual hypotonicity, an imbalance of forces on the teeth, causing an open bite, altered facial expression, or problems with chewing, swallowing, drooling, and speaking.[49] Table 12-4 summarizes the four stages of swallowing and their relation to oral structures and oral hygiene.[33]

Aspiration pneumonia is the second most common nosocomial infection, accounting for 13% to 48% of infections in nursing homes, and is the major reason for hospital admission, with a 20% to 50% mortality rate.[68,72] Although aspiration occurs in both healthy and frail individuals, it does not lead to pneumonia in the presence of an intact coughing

TABLE 12-4 Stages of Swallowing and Client Factors

Stage of Swallowing	Client Factor	Barrier to Oral Hygiene
Stage I: Preparatory Stage	Impaired head and neck control Upper extremity muscle weakness, loss of sensation and gross and fine motor skills	Inability to perform plate-to-mouth pattern Unable to hold and/or detect toothbrush in hand Drooling and pocketing in the oral cavity Reduced oral aperture
Stage II: Oral Phase	Inner and outer oral motor weakness, impaired oral sensation, lingual incoordination Lip closure Lack of control of saliva (thin liquids and toothpaste) Reduced oral and lingual proprioception	Delayed swallow (oral pharyngeal weakness and pocketing) May aspirate on toothpaste, thin liquids, and mouthwash May be unable to detect toothbrush or food in the mouth Consider temperature and texture of mouthwash and fluoride treatment
Stage III: Pharyngeal Phase	Contraction of pharynx and elevation of larynx, upper esophageal sphincter (UES) relaxes	Loss of motility and bolus control, toothpaste stuck in lower throat
Stage IV: Esophageal Phase	Cricopharyngeus contracts to prevent reflux	Must remain in upright position following oral hygiene to prevent reflux or aspiration

(Adapted from Jenks, K. L., & Smith, G. [2013]. Eating and swallowing. In H. Pendleton & W. Schultz-Krohn [Eds.], *Pedretti's occupational therapy: Practice skills for physical dysfunction* [6th ed., pp. 617-621]. St. Louis, MO: Mosby.)

reflex, good lung function, and a healthy immune system.[68,72] Risk factors for aspiration pneumonia include compromised general health (particularly chronic obstructive pulmonary disease [COPD] and diabetes), multiple medications, smoking, assistance required for feeding or oral care, tube feeding, missing teeth, dental caries, periodontal disease, poor oral hygiene, and denture use.[38,72,73] The greatest risk factor for aspiration pneumonia is requiring feeding assistance.

Impaired head and body righting and positioning may result from decreased motor control, hypertonicity, hypotonicity, weakness, proprioception, and awareness of space or other perceptual dysfunction.[32] External supports, such as tumble forms or wheelchair seat inserts, may be used to improve base of support, posture, and midline head positioning (Figure 12-5).[52,76]

Studies have shown that receiving occupational, speech, and/or physical therapy to improve swallowing, positioning the client upright to maximize stability and support, feeding at a slower pace to allow longer chewing cycles before swallowing, and feeding smaller quantities per bite significantly reduced the incidence of aspiration pneumonia.[61,68,74] A systematic review of randomized clinical trials found that approximately one in 10 cases of death from pneumonia in long-term care residents may be prevented by improving daily oral hygiene.[68] Additional prevention measures include referral to a dentist to receive treatment for dental caries and periodontal disease, use of various strategies to reduce xerostomia, limitation of tube feeding, increasing time spent out of bed, and smoking cessation.[38,73]

Oral motor performance in older adults and persons with disabilities who reside in nursing care facilities may also be

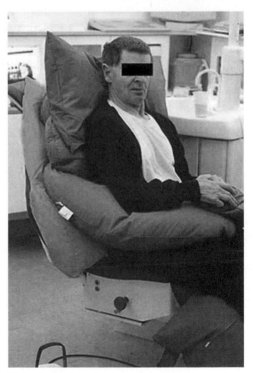

FIGURE 12-5   Positioning with external support for oral care (Picture adapted from Nunn, J., & Gorman, T. [2010]. Special care dentistry and the dental team. *Vital, 7,* 22-25.)

limited secondary to impaired oral aperture (how far one can open the mouth). Limited oral aperture may be observed in clients who have a diagnosis of scleroderma, scar tissue associated with facial burns, Parkinson's disease, and temporomandibular joint dysfunction. Preparatory methods, such as soft tissue mobilization, myofascial release (occipital release), electrical stimulation, or ultrasound, may be used to improve soft tissue extensibility. Mouth opening may be measured using assistive technology such as Therabite.[16,51,75] Naylor[50] reported that performing 18 weekly oral exercises using a stack of tongue blades may increase mouth opening for oral hygiene. When reduced oral aperture is chronic or not reversible, thickened liquids or a pureed diet may be recommended. A child-size toothbrush may be needed to clean the teeth and oral cavity.[50]

Successful follow-through with the care plan will depend on the level of interprofessional assistance provided and the environment. The Ecology of Human Performance model of occupation suggests that the social and physical environment also influences behavior and occupational performance. The long-term care setting may have a positive or negative effect on self-care participation.[17] For example, having an accessible sink and a toothbrush is positive; inadequate assistance based on process skills or impaired memory would be negative. The first therapeutic intervention proposed in this model is to establish and restore occupational performance. The occupational therapist will identify barriers to performance, then design interventions that improve performance. Mrs. Davidson, for example, would benefit from contextual supports, such as physical adaptations or environmental prompts.

Frail older adults often present with existing oral disease upon admission into long-term care due to their reduced ability to perform oral hygiene.[65] Despite families and caregivers preferring that dental services be delivered within the facility, fewer than 20% of residents receive dental treatment, and daily mouth care is often inadequate.[79,84] Barriers to receiving care within the facility include institutional-, client-, and provider-level impediments, such as complexity of the long-term care environment, lack of a dental operatory and equipment, challenging medical and behavior management, necessity of gaining informed consent, limited treatment options, time needed to provide service, unavailability of specialists, discomfort with providing treatment outside of a dental office setting, and low financial return.[42,84]

Certified nursing assistants (CNAs) provide daily hygiene, including oral care. Jablonski, Munro, Grap, and Elswick[29] report that CNAs have the least education about diseases associated with inadequate oral care but make up 65% of the staff in long-term care facilities. Pyle et al.[60] examined CNAs' knowledge of oral health, oral care-giving expectations, and oral care for 89 dependent residents. Results suggest that CNAs who had a history of tooth extraction were more likely to indicate that brushing teeth was important than those who had not experienced a tooth extraction.[60] Kaz and Schuhman[36] hypothesized that oral care provided by CNAs in nursing homes would improve with education provided through a mobile dental clinic. Results showed that CNA delivery of oral hygiene to residents was inadequate and did not meet state reviewer and federal facility expectations and guidelines.[36]

Wardt, Anderson and Sorensen[81] found that CNAs believed that oral care was more easily provided to residents

who had dentures and that oral care in general was repulsive but would improve quality of life. Other research found that CNAs did not dislike performing oral hygiene but were unsure how to perform this self-care task, especially when the resident was resistant to care or combative. CNAs shared that oral care was omitted most often when assigned duties could not be completed.[12] CNA knowledge and ability may improve with education by occupational therapists at the time of routine service delivery. Oral care performed in context and with demonstration by the occupational therapist may improve CNA self-efficacy.[12,81] Additional research is needed to support this premise.

Occupational Therapy Assessments of Oral Health

Several occupational therapy (OT) assessments aid in determining taste perception and oral motor performance, as described in the following discussion.

Mrs. Davidson rates her health as good and has few complaints except that she doesn't much care for the food: "it tastes like cardboard." Initially, the occupational therapist may complete a sensory assessment of basic taste perceptions by applying a stimulus to the corresponding areas of the tongue: sweet (front and tip), salty (anterior and lateral), bitter (posterior), and sour (lateral and middle). If Mrs. Davidson is unable to identify basic taste perceptions, the practitioner will also assess basic olfactory sensation because smell (processed in the temporal lobe) is a component of taste. Similarly, the sense of smell may be assessed by having the client identify five common scents (such as coffee, garlic, cinnamon, vanilla, and lemon). Scents are presented one at a time with one nostril compressed.[39,56,57,71] With age, the number of taste buds and the sense of taste are diminished. Extreme heat and cold sensations, oral infections, dry mouth, smoking, spicy and sour foods, and medications (such as beta blockers and angiotensin-converting enzyme [ACE] inhibitors) alter taste. A referral to a dentist and pharmacist would be beneficial to determine which factors may be contributing to her food tasting like cardboard. She needs some assistance with self-feeding and has poor dentition. Thus, a thorough oral assessment, including motor and sensory function of cranial nerves, is indicated.

The extraoral motor assessment (Table 12-5) suggested by Logerman[41] evaluates the resident's ability to perform facial expression, lift eyebrows, and control lips (smile).[21,41] The practitioner observes for bilateral facial symmetry. Asymmetry may indicate oral weakness or reduced tone. Working in the client's visual field helps to establish trust and facilitates understanding of assessment instructions.

The intraoral assessment (Table 12-6) examines oral structures, the tongue, and the swallowing mechanism. Like the extraoral assessment, it is important to note any weakness or deviation of the tongue to the stronger side or affected side. Manipulating the tongue forward and side to side from the oral cavity should result in a firm versus a mushy feel, which supports neuromuscular impairments.

TABLE 12-5 Examples of an Extraoral Assessment

Function	Instruction to Resident	Test Instruction
Facial expression	Lift your eyebrows Suck in your cheeks	Apply downward pressure to eyebrow Push air out in each cheek
Lip control	Smile Pucker your lips to make a kiss	Observe for symmetry
Jaw control	Open mouth as wide as possible	Observe head control; support under chin if needed

(Adapted from Jenks, K. L., & Smith, G. [2013]. Eating and swallowing. In H. Pendleton & W. Schultz-Krohn [Eds.], *Pedretti's occupational therapy: Practice skills for physical dysfunction* [6th ed., pp. 617-621]. St. Louis, MO: Mosby.)

TABLE 12-6 Examples of an Intraoral Assessment

Function	Instruction to Resident	Test Instruction
Tongue protrusion	Stick out your tongue	Apply slight pressure to the tip of the tongue
Lateralization	Move your tongue side to side	Resist side to side with tongue blade
Tipping	Touch your tongue to the roof of your mouth, front and back	Apply downward pressure to tip of tongue

(Adapted from Jenks, K. L., & Smith, G.[2013]. Eating and swallowing. In H. Pendleton & W. Schultz-Krohn [Eds.], *Pedretti's occupational therapy: Practice skills for physical dysfunction* [6th ed., pp. 617-621]. St. Louis, MO: Mosby.)

A resident who has neurologic involvement may have a delayed swallow or deficits in any of the four stages of swallowing. Primitive reflexes, such as rooting, bite, and suck-swallow, may reappear in older adults who experience damage to upper motor neurons, the brainstem, or other cortical structures. An intact gag, palatal, and cough reflex protects the airway.[32] Assessment of oral structures and the swallowing mechanism will aid the practitioner in selecting safe and appropriate methods and assistive technology for oral hygiene.

Occupational therapists also may use standardized assessments to quantify performance of oral hygiene. Common assessments include the Katz ADL Index, the Functional Independence Measure (FIM), the Barthel Index, and the Rivermead ADL Scale. Qualitative measures, such as the Canadian Occupational Performance Measure (COPM), may also be used.

The Katz Index of Activities of Daily Living (ADLs)[35] is a standardized assessment that evaluates level of independence or dependence in grooming, feeding, continence, transferring, toileting, dressing, and bathing. Although this assessment does not address oral care directly, similar motor and sensory performance skills are required for grooming and feeding. A score of "A" on the index indicates complete independence in feeding, and a score of "G" indicates dependence in the aforementioned ADLs.[35,59]

The FIM is similar to the Katz Index of ADLs in that seven performance areas are scored, using a scale of 1 to 7 instead of A to G. Thirteen motor and five cognitive skills are evaluated. A score of 7 is total independence; 6 equals modified independence (uses an assistive device for oral hygiene or grooming); 5 requires supervision; 4 and 3 indicate minimal to moderate assistance; 2 indicates maximal assistance; and 1 indicates complete dependence (Table 12-7). An advantage of using the FIM is that it is quick to administer; a disadvantage is that it does not provide information about body structures or environmental barriers that may affect the performance of oral hygiene. The FIM also assesses process skills, such as social interaction, memory, comprehension, and problem solving, required to perform oral hygiene.[5]

The Barthel Index is an assessment that scores improvements in rehabilitation of the chronically ill. Like the FIM, it is used to compare occupational performance upon admission and at the time of discharge. The assessment requires the client to perform 10 tasks while being observed. One of the tasks is performing oral hygiene. A score of 5 indicates independence in cleaning teeth; 0 indicates that the client requires assistance.[44]

The Rivermead ADL Scale (Revised) was designed to assess basic and instrumental activities of daily living. (Instrumental activities of daily living (IADLs) are more complex activities than ADLs and are related to independent living (i.e., using the telephone, shopping, cooking, housekeeping, laundry, managing medications, managing finances, driving, or using public transportation.) IADLs are very relevant to community-living older adults who can manage their own personal care but might require limited occupational therapy

TABLE 12-7 Functional Independence Measure (FIM) Scores and Oral Hygiene

FIM Level	Scoring
Complete independence	7: Cleans teeth or dentures
Modified independence	6: Requires an assistive device (large-handle toothbrush
Supervision	5: Standby assistance, remind to apply toothpaste to brush
Minimal assistance	4: (client performs 75%)
Moderate assistance	3: (client performs 50%)
Maximal assistance	2: (client performs 25%)
Total assistance	1: (client performs less than 25%)

(Adapted from Amundson, J., Brunner, A., & Ewers, M. [2012]. FIM scores as an indicator of length of stay and discharge destination in CVA patients: A retroactive outcomes study. *University of Wisconsin-La Crosse Journal of Undergraduate Research, III*, 263-270. Retrieved from http://murphylibrary.uwlax.edu/digital/jur/2000/amundson-brunner-ewers.pdf.)

on an outpatient basis for these more complex tasks. An advantage of this scale is that the total score reflects level of disability and problem areas. Inpatient scores are compared with discharge scores to determine the level of progress. A score of 3 is independent, 2 requires verbal assistance, and 1 is dependent. The higher the score, the more independent is the resident. Oral hygiene is assessed under the "clean teeth section," which requires the resident to manage the toothpaste, manipulate the toothbrush, and perform the task.[40]

The COPM uses an interview to help the client identify what he or she perceives to be problems with occupational performance. The client identifies the problems, prioritizes the problems in terms of importance, then sets a goal for each problem. For example, Mrs. Davidson reports her problems and rates the problems in terms of importance on a scale of 1 to 5, with 5 being the least important (Table 12-8). Brushing her teeth is important to Mrs. Davidson; she rates her performance as poor and she is not satisfied with her performance; she indicates that the size of the handle on the toothbrush is not important and that she may be able to initiate applying toothpaste.

Remember from earlier in the chapter that the following goals were set for Mrs. Davidson during the care plan meeting with her family members:
a. improve her ability to care for her own oral hygiene;
b. reduce her resistant behavior when staff try to provide assistance with daily oral hygiene;
c. improve her nutritional intake; and
d. request a referral to a dentist regarding the missing teeth, possible difficulty chewing, and sores found in Mrs. Davidson's mouth.

The occupational profile informs the practitioner about prior level of function, what the client wants to achieve in therapy, and which occupations have meaning and improve quality of life. Therapists listen to the client and discuss realistic and obtainable goals; as Zirkel notes, "Your client is a real person who very well might have a real solution."[86]

Mrs. Davidson realizes that she needs assistance to perform oral care but may not be aware of how her physical and cognitive limitations affect her performance. Mrs. Davidson's role has changed; her independence is compromised by having a degenerative disease and dementia. Low self-esteem and self-efficacy may hinder motivation and initiation of participation. Impaired memory may also compromise performance. Self-esteem may be restored by structuring participation in oral care such that she experiences success. Self-esteem may also be enhanced by fostering a sense of control over the task.[34] For example, giving her a choice as to when she prefers to perform this task may make her feel like she has control over the task. Although memory may not be restored, consistent environmental prompts, such as establishing a morning routine, may be an effective first step to restoring participation.[34]

Oral Hygiene Promotion

Lifelong oral health can be maintained with daily oral care. Health professionals who care for older adults have an important role in promoting oral hygiene practices, maintenance of dentures, and the need for referral to a dentist.

Oral sensory and motor performance may be improved through graded sensory input, oral exercise, or other preparatory methods. Persons with dementia or traumatic injury may exhibit oral hypersensitivity and may benefit from graded tactile or sensory input to the oral cavity and gums. Rubbing the gums or using a moist Toothette (Figure 12-6) to clean the oral cavity provides sensory stimulation, facilitates oral awareness, and desensitizes sensitive oral tissues. "Oral hygiene for the non-oral or oral client can be used as effective sensory stimulation of touch, texture, temperature and taste."[32]

Proprioceptive neuromuscular facilitation (PNF) head and neck patterns develop enhanced proprioceptive awareness, range of motion (ROM), and the strength necessary to achieve midline stability. Occupational therapists should evaluate the client's specific needs to determine which type of PNF to apply, as well as frequency and duration. When PNF is combined with Shaker exercise (also called the Head Lift), the swallowing mechanism is strengthened. Graded sensory stimulation, such as alternating texture, taste, and temperature, may be performed by speech pathologists or occupational therapists who demonstrate competency in this area. Cold sensations, such as Popsicles, may be used to improve

---

TABLE 12-8   Results of Mrs. Davidson's Canadian Occupational Performance Measure Interview

Activity Problem	Importance	Rates Her Performance	Satisfaction with Current Performance
Brush her teeth	1	5	5
Hold regular-sized tooth-brush	5	5	5
Apply tooth-paste independently	2	5	5

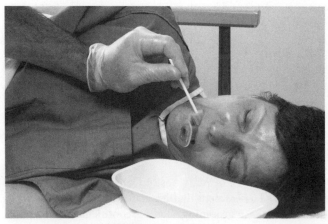

FIGURE 12-6   Toothette.

oral muscle tone and facilitate the lingual praxis required for bolus control (manipulating toothpaste, managing saliva, and rinsing the mouth with approved consistency of liquids).

Oral and facial exercise, such as opening and closing the lips, puckering or pursing the lips as if to make a kiss, whistling, and moving the tongue side to side (lateralization), also supports coordination and motor praxis. Oral and lingual exercise performed with graded resistance also facilitates inner and outer oral strengthening.

Occupational therapists prescribe strategies and low- and mid-technology devices for maintaining oral hygiene for a variety of health conditions. Low-technology devices include cylindrical foam to increase the size of the handle of the toothbrush; a mid-technology device would be a battery-operated or power toothbrush.

Osteoarthritis may result in joint pain; loss of range of motion, pinch, and grip; and disuse atrophy. Because of disuse atrophy and reduced shoulder strength (such as external rotators), it may be difficult for Mrs. Davidson to reach against gravity. Devices such as an overhead suspension sling or mobile arm support (Figure 12-7 A and B) eliminate gravity for those whose muscle strength is less than grade 3- out of 5 (Table 12-9).[37]

Toothbrushes are available in a variety of shapes and sizes based on consumer preferences; soft bristles are

TABLE 12-9 Muscle Testing/Grading

Grade	Strength	Movement
5	100%	AROM max resistance
4	Good 75%	Complete range of motion (ROM) Mod Res
3+	Fair+	Complete ROM Min Res
3	Fair (50%)	ROM against gravity
3−	Fair−	Some ROM against gravity
2+	Poor+	Initiates motion against gravity
2	Poor (25%)	Complete ROM gravity eliminated
2−	Poor−	Initiates motion if gravity eliminated
1	Trace	Slight contraction
0	None	No contraction palpated

(Adapted from Killingsworth, A., Pedretti, L. W., & Pendleton, H. [2013]. Evaluation of muscle strength. In H. Pendleton & W. Krohn [Eds.], *Pedretti's occupational therapy practice skills for physical dysfunction* [p. 529-574]. St. Louis, MO: Elsevier.)

recommended to prevent damage to the gingiva and abrasion of tooth enamel. Toothbrushes can be modified for clients who have dexterity limitations. A common low-cost and effective low-technology solution is to slide cylindrical foam tubing over the handle of the toothbrush.[80] The foam must be replaced often for infection control (due to the potential for bacterial growth). Scrap splinting material, such as Ezeform, may also be used to increase the handle circumference. Power toothbrushes facilitate brushing for both clients and caregivers and have been shown to decrease gingival bleeding and remove more plaque than manual toothbrushes.[13] Power toothbrushes may be contraindicated for clients who have neurologic sequelae, such as seizures secondary to the autonomic nervous system's hypersensitivity to vibratory response.

Superbrushes, such as the Collis Curve toothbrush, have bristles positioned at multiple angles so that a simple back-and-forth motion cleans all sides of the teeth at the same time, which again is helpful both for clients with dexterity challenges and for caregivers (Box 12-2). Toothbrush alternatives that have very small heads, such as the single-tufted brush, proxy brush, and interdental brush, are ideal for cleaning between teeth with large gaps. Moistened soft sponge swabs, such as the Toothette shown in Figure 12-6, can gently clean painful oral tissues and deliver glycerin or chlorhexidine (an antibacterial agent) to the tissues and teeth. For clients who require assistance in keeping their mouth open when receiving oral care, disposable mouth props are available (Figure 12-8).[79] To reduce bacterial transmission, allow toothbrush bristles to dry between uses, label and keep separate from other people's brushes, store far away from toilets, periodically clean by soaking in chlorhexidine or hydrogen peroxide, and replace every 3 to 4 months or after an illness.

Mrs. Davidson is unable to grip her toothbrush secondary to pain. The occupational therapist may recommend joint protection by using a universal cuff (Figure 12-9) to avoid the sustained finger flexion required to hold the toothbrush. A toothpaste

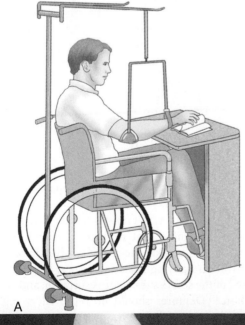

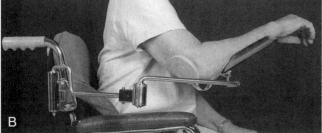

FIGURE 12-7 A, Overhead suspension sling. B, Mobile arm support.

BOX 12-2   Assistive Technology for Oral Care

Overhead Suspension Sling:
    http://www.wisdomking.com/product/suspension-
        arm-sling
Mobile Arm Support:
    http://www.rehabmart.com/category/Pediatric_Mobile_
        Arm_Supports.htm
Universal Cuff:
    http://www.pattersonmedical.com/app.aspx?cmd=get
        ProductDetail&key=070_921012442
Cylindrical Foam:
    http://www.wrightstuff.biz/cohafo.html
Suctioned Denture Brush:
    http://www.wrightstuff.biz/sudebr.html
Floss Holder:
    http://www.wrightstuff.biz/flossaid.html
Toothpaste Dispenser:
    http://www.wrightstuff.biz/eaouttusq.html
    http://www.pattersonmedical.com/app.aspx?cmd=get
        ProductDetail&key=070_921001563
Weighted Universal Holder:
    http://www.wrightstuff.biz/laweunho.html
Collis Curve Toothbrush:
    http://www.colliscurve.com/
Mouth Prop:
    http://www.nature.com/vital/journal/v7/n3/full/vital1186.
        html
Toothettes (Oral Foam Swabs):
    http://www.sageproducts.com/products/oral-hygiene/

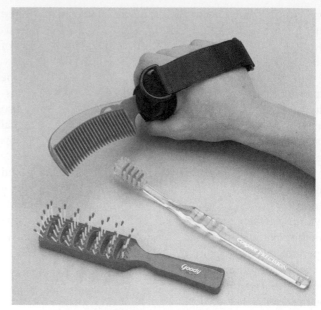

FIGURE 12-9   Universal holder.

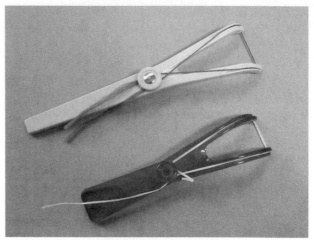

FIGURE 12-10   Floss holder.

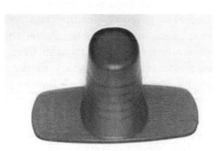

FIGURE 12-8   Mouth prop.

dispenser that has a pump handle can be activated using the base of the hand or palm for additional joint protection (Box 12-2).

Dental floss is available with pre-strung heads and extended handles to facilitate flossing for people or their caregivers with dexterity issues (Figure 12-10). Those with active and/or recurrent dental caries benefit from fluoride varnish applications and high-fluoride-containing toothpaste, both available by prescription.[8] Rinsing with a prescription 0.12% chlorhexidine gluconate mouthwash is effective against the bacteria that cause periodontal disease.[66] Frequent sips of water, stimulating saliva production with sugarless candy and gum, restricting caffeine intake, avoiding mouth rinses containing alcohol, using a vaporizer at bedtime, applying moisturizer to the lips, using commercial salivary substitutes, and

prescribing casein phosphopeptides toothpaste alleviate the symptoms of xerostomia.[66]

The occupational therapist must be aware of safety precautions when performing oral hygiene in clients who have dentures. Around-the-clock use of dentures causes inflammation of the underlying mucosal tissues, and can lead to overgrowth of the soft tissues, bone resorption, and candidiasis infection.[85] Dentures should be removed at night and placed in a container filled with water to prevent the acrylic from drying and possibly changing in dimension. Bacteria, stains, and calculus (tartar) collect on dentures and the oral tissues, and if not removed daily, can lead to odor, inflamed tissue, and candidiasis infection.[85] Dentures should be thoroughly brushed daily and rinsed after meals when possible. Dentures should be cleaned with a soft toothbrush and mild liquid soap over a basin partially filled with water or lined with a wet washcloth to prevent breakage if dropped. Toothpaste contains abrasives that will wear away the denture acrylic and should be avoided. The oral tissues, tongue, and any remaining teeth should also be brushed daily with a soft toothbrush. Soaking dentures daily in water with a commercial denture cleanser tablet will remove most stains; however, avoid using bleach, as it will tarnish the metal framework of partial dentures and leach the color of acrylic dentures. Calculus deposits can be removed by placing the denture in a plastic bag filled with cleanser and agitating in an ultrasonic cleaner. Loose or unstable dentures require a referral to a dentist for relining or replacement. Denture adhesives and home reline kits should be avoided, as their use can adversely affect the position of the denture on the supporting tissues and make it difficult to keep the denture clean. Many states require the owner's name to be incorporated in the denture. The occupational therapist may also provide a suctioned denture brush to compensate for reduced dexterity or for the use of one-handed cleansing.

Upper extremity incoordination (ataxia) inhibits the distal stability required for performing oral hygiene. Common clinical conditions associated with ataxia include multiple sclerosis, Parkinson's disease, and cerebral palsy. Existing literature recommends weighted handheld assistive technology. Weighted utensil holders (such as a toothbrush holder) provide some distal stability for clients who have intention tremor associated with multiple sclerosis. The literature is inconsistent regarding the use of weights to reduce rest tremors or the pill-rolling tremors associated with Parkinson's disease. Trail[75] recommends that the client reduce the degree of freedom of movement by holding the arms adducted and close to the body. Additional distal stability may be achieved by using one hand to hold the other wrist; a prefabricated wrist cock-up splint may also be used to reduce the effects of pronation and supination associated with the pill-rolling tremors observed in Parkinson's disease.[75]

The use of fluoride is critical for preventing dental caries. Daily brushing with fluoride-containing toothpaste is recommended for all older adults, and adding a commercial 0.05% sodium fluoride mouth rinse provides additional benefits to those with a dry mouth or higher risk for decay.[8] Toothpastes are also commercially available with additional ingredients, depending on the needs of the consumer. Pastes designed to reduce plaque buildup contain triclosan or zinc citrate; those designed to reduce calculus contain zinc citrate or pyrophosphate; those designed to reduce tooth sensitivity contain potassium nitrate, calcium carbonate, and arginine; and those designed to reduce dry mouth contain baking soda, lactoperoxidase, glucose oxidase, lysozyme, and lactoferrin. To reduce gagging and accidental swallowing, use only a small, pea-sized amount of toothpaste.

Care-Resistant Behaviors

Dementia is degenerative and progressive. Persons who have dementia need a consistent environment that provides structure and flexibility, and caregivers who realize that performance of oral hygiene is often slow and labored. Therapeutic interventions for ADLs focus on maximizing independence.

Clients with dementia may have decreased saliva, decreased denture use, and reduced dental access, and increased plaque, calculus, dental caries, mucosal lesions, and gingival bleeding and inflammation.[11] These clients may not be able to communicate their oral problems and instead manifest their discomfort or pain by not eating, pulling at the face or mouth, exhibiting aggression or restlessness, and chewing the lip, tongue, or hand.[11] Care-resistant behaviors, such as pushing away the caregiver, turning the face away from the care provider, or biting down on the toothbrush, are often invoked to oppose caregiving efforts. A successful pilot study of the Managing Oral Hygiene Using Threat Reduction (MOUTH) intervention found that using cues (polite one-step commands), bridging actions (older adult holds the same item as is being used in the mouth), and gestures (pantomimes of brushing) significantly reduced care-resistant behaviors and improved oral health.[30] Shanks[64] also recommends the technique of triggering. For example, once the client starts the task, verbal encouragement such as "You do it; no one can brush your teeth as clean as you can," followed by praise, is an effective triggering technique.[64]

There are four stages of dementia. (See chapter 15 for more detail on dementia.) The occupational therapist may use the following strategies to increase participation in oral hygiene for each respective stage of dementia reviewed in Table 12-10.[23,24,31,64]

Occupational therapists may employ the antecedent–behavior–consequences (ABC) model to understand the resistive behaviors associated with dementia. This model relies on the caregiver to identify the precipitating triggers of the resistant behavior (antecedent) and analyze the consequences. The caregiver determines and documents how long the behavior occurs (behavior), then plans an intervention.[43,45,48]

There are several strategies that caregivers may use for improving communication and reducing resistant behavior in a person who has dementia. First, gain eye contact, prepare the environment by minimizing distractions and clutter, identify yourself, and address the person by name. Avoid verbal expressions that may be taken literally. Don't speak in a childish manner. Speak to the person in a calm and moderately loud voice and state requests in a positive and supportive manner. Redirect or distract the person when he or she is agitated or distressed. Grade interactions from most to least complex (e.g., most complex: get ready to brush your teeth ["what do you need?"]; less complex: brush your teeth [use verbal cues, ask for specific information, e.g., "where is your toothbrush?"]; even less complex: help me brush your teeth [requires set up]; least complex: state the facts ["here is your toothbrush," perform with hand-over-hand guidance). In stages I and II of dementia, the occupational therapist may take step-by-step pictures of the client performing oral care. Picture instructions offer a nonthreatening means of enhanced triggering.[58,64]

Establishing an appropriate level of communication will reduce the possibility of resistant behavior. Use actual items with visual cues and hand-over-hand guidance. If there is resistance to hand-over-hand guidance, a mirror technique

TABLE 12-10 Stages of Dementia and Oral Care

Stage of Dementia	Signs and Symptoms	Intervention
Stage I	Early onset (< age 65 years) Absent-minded Mild short-term memory deficits Indecisive Decreased concentration Does not recognize familiar environments Misplaces objects Performs basic ADLs	Speak in a respectful manner Set up the task Perform oral hygiene in context Remind to select appropriate implement Standby supervision—slow performance
Stage II	More alert in morning after night's rest Aggressive and hostile Combative Expressive or receptive aphasia Agnosia (inability to recognize objects) Difficulty initiating motor planning (apraxia) Does not recognize written word Hyperorality—seeks increased oral stimulation Perseveration Hides items Safety is a concern	Plan ahead State your request clearly Lower the pitch of your voice Break tasks down into steps Use visual and tactile cues If the client is upset, distract and redirect Anticipate when to move to the next step Reduce distractions Expect agitation Maintain structure/follow routine Keep items in the same place
Stage III	Reduced oral intake Risk for dysphagia Does not recognize caregivers Maximum assistance for basic ADLs Impaired verbal communication	Perform oral care with moistened Toothette (Figure 12-6) Follow up with soft-bristle toothbrush
Stage IV	Bedbound Altered tone and posture Primitive reflexes Paratonia (automatic resistance to movement) Helpless Unresponsive Reduced oral intake Risk for dysphagia Dependent for oral care	Inhibitory strategies for bite reflex and rooting Perform oral care with moistened Toothette (Figure 12-6)

(Adapted from Fraker, J. [2007]. Dementia. In B. J. Atchison & D. K. Dirette [Eds.], *Conditions in occupational therapy* [3rd ed., p. 147]. Philadelphia, PA: Lippincott Williams & Wilkins; Gitlin, L. N., & Corcoran, M. A. [2005]. *Occupational therapy and dementia care.* Silver Spring, MD: AOTA Press; Jacobs, K., & Jacobs, L. Stages of Alzheimer's disease. [2009]. In K. Jacobs & L. Simon [Eds.], *Quick reference dictionary for occupational therapy* [5th ed., p. 406]. Thorofare, NJ: SLACK; Shanks, L. K. [1996]. *A caregiver's guide to Alzheimer's: Your name is Hughes Hannibal Shanks.* Lincoln, NE: University of Nebraska Press.)

may be used; the caregiver performs oral care step by step using the same utensils at the same time as the client.

The goal of behavior management is to respect the client's rights while delivering the necessary oral health services. Although the client may have difficulty in appropriately expressing his or her feelings, take the time to first know the client's preferences and responses. The client may be more cooperative with a particular caregiver, during a specific time of day, while listening to the television or radio, or when holding a comfort item. Additional suggestions include setting a routine time and place for oral care; identifying yourself and what you plan to do; using visual and verbal cues with short sentences and simple words; initiating tooth brushing but encouraging the client's participation by placing the brush in the client's hand and guiding it with your own; using positive reinforcement and maintaining a calm

demeanor; and, above all, attempting to provide oral care every day.[54]

The website Oral Care in Continuing Care Settings: Collaborating to Improve Policies and Practice provides a complete oral care manual titled "Brushing Up on Mouth Care."[54] Further information may be found in Box 12-1. This free resource includes tips for providing oral care for clients with dementia, tool kits, care cards, assessment forms, posters, fact sheets, information about products and aids, and a series of educational videos on personal daily mouth care.

Your recommendations to the interprofessional team regarding the care plan for Mrs. Davidson in Case Example 12-1 could include:

a. The diameter of the handle on her toothbrush could be increased with rubber tubing, making it easier for her to grip. If she can afford one, a power toothbrush would be easier for both her and a caregiver to use. If the facility can provide a superbrush, that would also be easier for her or a caregiver to use. Her missing teeth indicate that she may be at high risk for dental caries, so she should use a toothpaste containing fluoride, and, if cooperative, rinse with a fluoride mouth rinse. Providing her with pre-strung dental floss on an extended handle would facilitate either her or a caregiver's ability to floss.

b. Some observational trial and error is necessary to optimize Mrs. Davidson's cooperation. What are her preferences for and responses to a particular caregiver, during a specific time of day, while listening to the television or radio, or when holding a comfort item? Additional suggestions include providing a routine time and place for oral care every day, using visual and verbal cues with short sentences and simple words for each step of what you are doing, allowing Mrs. Davidson to hold a toothbrush while you are performing her oral care, initiating tooth brushing but encouraging her participation by placing the brush in her hand and guiding it with your own, using positive reinforcement, and maintaining a calm demeanor.

c. Her complaint of bland-tasting food could indicate that a diminished sense of smell is affecting her enjoyment of food. Mrs. Davidson's missing teeth make it challenging for her to adequately chew her food, and her medications may be causing xerostomia, resulting in difficulty in swallowing food. She requires some feeding assistance due to her arthritis, putting her at risk for aspiration pneumonia. A combination of the following suggestions could be employed:
- To stimulate her sense of smell and taste, add non-salt-containing spices to enliven the flavor, use more varied visual colors and textures of food, and add a daily multivitamin and mineral supplement.
- To address her xerostomia, actively encourage more water consumption during meals.
- To accommodate her compromised ability to chew, substitute fruit juices or canned fruits for fresh fruit and vegetable juices or cooked and mashed vegetables for raw vegetables; offer ground meat or protein alternatives such as eggs, milk, cheese, and yogurt; and replace uncooked or partially cooked high fiber whole grains with cooked grains (e.g., cooked cereals, rice, and bread pudding).
- To optimize her feeding assistance, slow the pace of eating and/or feeding and offer smaller-sized bites.
- To address her specific food interests, work with the dietitian to personalize her diet as much as possible.

REVIEW QUESTIONS

1. Describe client factors that affect oral hygiene.
2. Distinguish between upper motor and lower motor neuron lesions and lingual and oral performance.
3. How are aspiration pneumonia and oral hygiene related?
4. How does body righting and positioning influence oral hygiene?
5. What are some common low- and mid-technology devices used to enhance oral hygiene?
6. Which performance skills are required to perform oral hygiene?
7. List observations that indicate that a referral to a dentist is warranted.
8. What is an occupational therapist's role in educating other members of the interprofessional team about oral hygiene?

REFERENCES

1. Akpan, A., & Morgan, R. (2002). Oral candidiasis. *Postgraduate Medical Journal, 78,* 455–459.
2. American Geriatrics Society. (2009). *Clinical practice guideline: pharmacological management of persistent pain in older persons.* Retrieved from http://www.americangeriatrics.org/health_care_professionals/clinical_practice/clinical_guidelines_recommendations/2009/.
3. American Occupational Therapy Association. (2014). Occupational therapy practice framework: Domain and process. (3rd ed.). *American Journal of Occupational Therapy, 68*(Suppl. 1), S1–S48. http://dx.doi.org/10.5014/ajot.2014.682006.
4. American Physical Therapy Association. (2003). Nagi disablement model. In *Guide to physical therapist practice* (2nd ed., pp. 19–25). Alexandria, VA: American Physical Therapy Association.
5. Amundson, J., Brunner, A., & Ewers, M. (2012). FIM scores as an indicator of length of stay and discharge destination in CVA patients: A retroactive outcomes study. *University of Wisconsin-La Crosse Journal of Undergraduate Research, III,* 263–270. http://murphylibrary.uwlax.edu/digital/jur/2000/amundson-brunner-ewers.pdf.
6. Blaum, C. S., Xue, Q. L., Michelon, E., Semba, R. D., & Fried, L. P. (2005). The association between obesity and frailty syndrome in older women: The women's health and aging study. *Journal of the American Geriatric Society, 53,* 927–934.
7. Buchbinder, D., Currivam, R. B., Kaplan, A. J., & Urken, M. L. (1993). Mobilization regimes for the prevention of jaw hypermobility in the radiated patient: A comparison of three techniques. *Journal of Oral and Maxillofacial Surgery, 51,* 863–867.
8. Centers for Disease Control and Prevention. (2001). Recommendations for using fluoride to prevent and control dental caries in the US. *Morbidity and Mortality Weekly Report, 50* (RR-14), 1–42.
9. Centers for Disease Control and Prevention, Merck Institute of Aging and Health. (2004). *The state of aging and health in America 2004.* Washington, DC: Merck Institute of Aging and Health.
10. Centers for Medicare and Medicaid. (2012). *MDS2.0 information.* Retrieved from http://www.cms.gov/Research-Statistics-Data-and-Systems/Computer-Data-and-Systems/Minimum DataSets20/index.html?redirect=/MinimumDataSets20/.
11. Chalmers, J., & Pearson, A. (2005). Oral hygiene care for residents with dementia: A literature review. *Journal of Advanced Nursing, 52*(4), 410–419.
12. Chalmers, J. M., Levy, S. M., Buckwalter, K. C., Ettinger, R. L., & Kambhu, P. P. (1996). Factors influencing nurses aides' provision of oral care for nursing facilities residents. *Specialty Care in Dentistry, 16,* 717–719.
13. Davies, R. M. (2004). The rational use of oral care products in the elderly. *Clinical Oral Investigations, 8*(1), 2–5.

14. Dental, Oral and Craniofacial Data Resource Center. (2002). *Oral health US.* Bethesda, MD: NIDCR/NIH.

15. de Oliveira, C., Watt, R., & Hamer, M. (2010). Toothbrushing, inflammation, and risk of cardiovascular disease: Results from Scottish Health Survey. *British Medical Journal, 340,* c2451.

16. Domsic, R. T., & Medsger, A. (2011). Two scleroderma patients with differing patterns of muscle disease. In R. M. Silver & C. P. Denton (Eds.), *Case studies in systemic sclerosis* (pp. 251–258). New York, NY: Springer.

17. Dunn, W., Brown, C., & McGuigan, A. (1994). The ecology of human performance: A framework for considering the effect of context. *American Journal of Occupational Therapy, 48*(7), 595–607.

18. Dye, B. A., Tan, S., Smith, V., Lewis, B. G., Barker, L. K., Thornton-Evans, G., et al. (April 2007). Trends in oral health status: United States, 1988-1994 and 1999-2004. National Center for Health Statistics. *Vital Health Statistics, 11*(248), 1–92.

19. Dye, B. A., Thornton-Evans, G., Li, X., & Iafolla, T. J. (2015). Dental caries and tooth loss in adults in the United States, 2011-2012. In *NCHS Data Brief, No. 197.* Hyattsville, MD: National Center for Health Statistics.

20. Eke, P. I., Dye, B. A., Wei, L., Thornton-Evans, G. O., & Genco, R. J. (2012). Prevalence of periodontitis in adults in the United States: 2009 and 2010. *Journal of Dental Research, 91*(10), 914–920.

21. Everything Speech. (2010). *Dysphagia evaluation.* Retrieved from http://everythingspeech.com/evaluation/dyphagia/dysphagia-evaluation/.

22. Fox, P. C. (1997). Management of dry mouth. *Dental Clinics of North America, 41*(4), 863–875.

23. Fraker, J. (2007). Dementia. In B. J. Atchison & D. K. Dirette (Eds.), *Conditions in occupational therapy* (3rd ed., p. 147). Philadelphia, PA: Lippincott Williams & Wilkins.

24. Gitlin, L. N., & Corcoran, M. A. (2005). *Occupational therapy and dementia care.* Silver Spring, MD: AOTA Press.

25. Griffin, S. O., Griffin, P. M., Swann, J. L., & Zlobin, N. (2005). New coronal caries in older adults: Implications for prevention. *Journal of Dental Research, 84*(7), 715–720.

26. Griffin, S. O., Jones, J. A., Brunson, D., Griffin, P. M., & Bailey, W. D. (2012). Burden of oral disease among older adults and implications for public heath priorities. *American Journal of Public Health, 102*(3), 411–418.

27. Hunt, R. J., Slade, G. D., & Strauss, R. P. (1995). Differences between racial groups in the impact of oral disorders among older adults in North Carolina. *Journal of Public Health Dentistry, 55*(4), 205–209.

28. Institute of Medicine of the National Academies. (2011). *Relieving pain in America: A blueprint for transforming prevention, care, education, and research.* Retrieved from http://www.iom.edu/Reports/2011/Relieving-Pain-in-America-A-Blueprint-for-Transforming-Prevention-Care-Education-Research.aspx.

29. Jablonski, R. A., Munro, C. L., Grap, M. J., & Elswick, R. K. (2005). The role of biobehavioral, environment, and social forces on oral health disparities in frail and functionally dependent nursing home elders. *Biological Research for Nursing, 7*(1), 75–82.

30. Jablonski, R. A., Therrien, B., Mahoney, E. K., Kolanowski, A., Gabello, M., & Brock, A. (2011). An intervention to reduce care-resistant behavior in persons with dementia during oral hygiene: A pilot study. *Specialty Care Dentistry, 31,* 77–87.

31. Jacobs, K., & Jacobs, L. (2009). Stages of Alzheimer's disease. In K. Jacobs & L. Simon (Eds.), *Quick reference dictionary for occupational therapy* (5th ed., p. 406). Thorofare, NJ: SLACK.

32. Jenks, K. L., & Smith, G. (2013). Eating and swallowing. In H. Pendleton & W. Schultz-Krohn (Eds.), *Pedretti's occupational therapy: Practice skills for physical dysfunction* (6th ed., pp. 617–621). St. Louis, MO: Mosby.

33. Jones, J. A., Fedele, D. J., Bolden, A. J., & Bloom B. (1994). Gains in dental care use not shared by minority elders. *Journal of Public Health Dentistry, 54*(1), 39–46.

34. Kaplan, R. M. (2002). Quality of life and chronic illness. In A. J. Christensen & M. H. Antoni (Eds.), *Chronic physical disorders: Behavioral medicine's perspective* (pp. 27–39). Malden, MA: Blackwell Publishers.

35. Katz, S., Ford, A., Moskowitz, R., Jackson, B., & Jaffe, M. (1963). Studies of illness in the aged: The index of ADL: A standardized measure of biological and psychosocial function. *Journal of the American Medical Association, 21,* 914–919.

36. Kaz, M. E., & Schuhman, L. (1988). Oral health care attitudes of nursing assistants in long term care facilities. *Specialty Care Dentistry, 8,* 228–231.

37. Killingsworth, A., Pedretti, L.W., & Pendleton, H. (2013). Evaluation of muscle strength. In H. Pendleton & W. Krohn (Eds.), *Pedretti's occupational therapy practice skills for physical dysfunction* (pp. 529–574). St. Louis, MO: Elsevier.

38. Langmore, S. E., Terpenning, M. S., Schork, A., Chen, Y., Murray, J. T., Lopatin, D., et al. (1998). Predictors of aspiration pneumonia: How important is dysphagia? *Dysphagia, 13*(2), 69–81.

39. Laugerette, F., Passilly-Degrace, P., Patris, B., Niot, I., Febbraio, M., Montmayeur, J. P., et al. (2005). CD36 involvement in oro-sensory detection of dietary lipids, spontaneous fat preference, and digestive secretions. *Journal of Clinical Investigation, 115*(11), 3177–3184.

40. Lincoln, N. B., & Edmans, J. A. (1990). A re-validation of the Rivermead ADL scale for elderly patients with stroke. *Age and Aging, 19,* 19–24.

41. Logermann, J. (1998). *Evaluation and treatment of swallowing disorders.* Austin, TX: Pro-Ed.

42. MacEntee, M. I., Pruksapong, M., & Wyatt, C. C. (2005). Insights from students following an educational rotation through dental geriatrics. *Journal of Dental Education, 69*(12), 1368–1376.

43. MacLin, O. H., & Peterson, D. (n.d.). *ABCs of behavior modification. University of Northern Iowa.* Retrieved from http://www.uni.edu/~maclino/bm/book/sec1.1.pdf.

44. Mahoney, F. I., & Barthel, D. W. (1965). Functional evaluation: The Barthel index. *Maryland State Medical Journal, 14,* 61–65.

45. *Managing student behavior. Section I: Basic behavioral components (A-B-C model).* Project IDEAL, Texas Council for Developmental Disabilities. http://www.projectidealonline.org/basic-components-of-behavior.php.

46. Metcalf, S. S., Northridge, M. E., & Lamster, I. B. (2011). A systems perspective for dental health in older adults. *American Journal of Public Health, 101*(10), 1820–1823.

47. National Institute of Dental and Craniofacial Research. (2002). *A plan to eliminate craniofacial, oral, and dental health disparities.* Retrieved from http://www.nidcr.nih.gov/NR/rdonlyres/932B8B7D-E114-4491-BE85-ABA6F29663AE/0/hdplan.pdf.

48. National Institute of Dental and Craniofacial Research. (2004). Practical oral care for people with developmental disabilities. In *NIH Publication No. 04-5195.*

49. National Institute of Dental and Craniofacial Research. (2009). *Practical oral care for people with Down syndrome.* Retrieved from http://www.nidcr.nih.gov/OralHealth/Topics/Developmental Disabilities/PracticalOralCarePeopleDownSyndrome.htm.

50. Naylor, W. P. (1982). Oral management of the scleroderma patient. *Journal of the American Dental Association, 105,* 814–817.
51. New Jersey Education Association. (2010). *Antecedents, behaviors, consequences (ABC) (sample).* Retrieved from http://www.njea.org/PDFs/Review_Jan2010_autism_Table2.pdf.
52. Northridge, M. E., Glick, M., Metcalf, S. S., & Shelley D. (2011). Public health support for the health home model. *American Journal of Public Health, 101*(10), 1818–1820.
53. Nuttall, N. M., Steele, J. G., Pine, C. M., White, D., & Pitts, N. B. (2001). The impact of oral health on people in the UK in 1998. *British Dental Journal, 190,* 121–126.
54. Atlantic Health Promotion Research Centre. (n.d.). *Oral care in continuing care settings: Collaborating to improve policies and practice. Brushing up on mouth care: Complete oral care manual.* Retrieved from http://www.ahprc.dal.ca/projects/oral-care/default.asp.
55. Pace, C. C., & McCullough, G. H. (2010). The association between oral microorganisms and aspiration pneumonia in the institutionalized elderly: Review and recommendations. *Dysphagia, 25*(4), 307–322.
56. Palo Alto Medical Foundation. (2012). *Taste buds.* Retrieved from http://www.pamf.org/teen/health/skin/tastebuds.html.
57. Pedretti, L. W. (1996). Evaluation of sensation and treatment of sensory dysfunction. In L.W. Pedretti (Ed.), *Occupational therapy: Practice skills for physical dysfunction* (6th ed. pp. 222–224). Saint Louis, MO: Mosby.
58. Piersol, C. V., Earland, T. V., & Herge, E. A. (2012). Meeting the needs of caregivers of persons with dementia. *OT Practice, 17*(5), 8–12.
59. Poole, J., Conte, C., Brewer, C., Good, C. C., Perella, D., Rossie, K. M., & Steen, V. (2010). Oral hygiene in scleroderma: The effectiveness of a multi-disciplinary intervention program. *Disability and Rehabilitation, 32*(5), 379–384.
60. Pyle, M. A., Nelson, S., & Sawyer, D. R. (1999). Nursing assistants' opinions of oral health care provision. *Specialty Care Dentistry, 19,* 112–117.
61. Quagliarello, V., Ginter, S., Han, L., Van Ness, P., Allore, H., & Tinetti, M. (2005). Modifiable risk factors for nursing home-acquired pneumonia. *Clinical Infectious Diseases, 40*(1), 1–6.
62. Rahim-Williams, B., Tomar, S., Riley, J. L., & Blanchard, S. (2009). Influences of adult-onset diabetes on orofacial pain and related health behaviors. *Journal of Public Health Dentistry, 70,* 85–92.
63. Riley, J. L., Gilbert, G. H., & Heft, M. W. (1998). Orofacial pain symptom prevalence: selective sex differences in the elderly? *Pain, 76,* 97–104.
64. Shanks, L. K. (1996). *A caregiver's guide to Alzheimer's: Your name is Hughes Hannibal Shanks.* Lincoln, NE: University of Nebraska Press.
65. Shay, K., & Ship, J. A. (1995). The importance of oral health in the older patient. *Journal of the American Geriatric Society, 43,* 1414–1422.
66. Ship, J. A., & Mohammad, A. R. (Eds.). (1999, Winter). Clinician's guide to oral health in geriatric patients. *American Academy of Oral Medicine,* 1–57.
67. Simpson, T. C., Needleman, I., Wild, S. H., Moles, D. R., & Mills, E. J. (2010). Treatment of periodontal disease for glycemic control in people with diabetes. *Cochrane Database of Systematic Reviews, 12*(5), CD004714.
68. Sjogren, P., Nilsson, E., Forsell, M., Johansson, O., & Hoogstraate, J. (2008). A systematic review of the preventive effect of oral hygiene on pneumonia and respiratory tract infection in elderly people in hospitals and nursing homes: Effect estimates and methodological quality of randomized controlled trials. *Journal of the American Geriatric Society, 56*(11), 2124–2130.
69. Slade, G. D., Spencer, A. J., Locker, D., Hunt, R. J., Strauss, R. P., & Beck, J. D. (1996). Variations in the social impact of oral conditions among older adults in South Australia, Ontario, and North Carolina. *Journal of Dental Research, 75*(7), 1439–1450.
70. Smith, B. J., Ghezzi, E. M., Manz, M. C., & Markova, C. P. (2010). Oral healthcare access and adequacy in alternative long-term care settings. *Specialty Care Dentistry, 30*(3), 85–94.
71. Sollitto, M. (2012). *Loss of taste in the elderly.* Retrieved from http://www.agingcare.com/Articles/Loss-of-Taste-in-the-Elderly-135240.htm.
72. Taylor, G. W., Loesche, W. J., & Terpenning, M. S. (2000). Impact of oral diseases on systemic health in the elderly: Diabetes mellitus and aspiration pneumonia. *Journal of Public Health Dentistry, 60*(4), 313–320.
73. Terpenning, M. S. (2005). Prevention of aspiration pneumonia in nursing home patients. *Clinical Infectious Diseases, 40*(1), 7–8.
74. Terpenning, M. S., Taylor, G. W., Lopatin, D. E., Kerr, C. K., Dominguez, B. L., & Loesche, W. J. (2001). Aspiration pneumonia: dental and oral risk factors in an older veteran population. *Journal of the American Geriatric Society, 49*(5), 557–563.
75. Trail, M. (June 2004). An evidence-based approach to Parkinson's disease. *OT Practice,* 33–34.
76. Tumle forms image. (2012). Retrieved from http://www.nature.com/vital/journal/v7/n3/fig_tab/vital1186_F2.html.
77. Turnham, H. (n.d.). *Federal Nursing Home Reform Act from the Omnibus Budget Reconciliation Act of 1987.* Retrieved from http://www.ncmust.com/doclib/OBRA87summary.pdf.
78. Academic Geriatric Resource Center. (n.d.). *Module 4: Assessment of the geriatric patient: Oral and dental health.* San Francisco: University of California. Retrieved from http://gerigero-onlinecourse.ucsf.edu/modules/4/2.5.
79. U.S. Department of Health and Human Services. (2000). *Oral health in America: A report of the Surgeon General.* Rockville, MD: NIDCR/NIH.
80. U.S. Department of Health and Human Services. (2004). *Dental care everyday: A caregiver's guide.* Bethesda, MD: NIDCR/NIH.
81. Wardt, I., Anderson, L., & Sorenson, S. (1997). Staff attitudes to oral health care. A comparative study of registered nurses, nursing assistants and home care aids. *Gerontology, 14,* 28–32.
82. Wolf, L. S., Glass, R. P., & Carr, A. B. (1992). *Feeding and swallowing disorders in infancy: Assessment and management.* San Antonio, TX: The Psychological Corporation.
83. World Health Organization. (2001). *International classification of functioning, disability and health.* Retrieved from http://www.who.int/classifications/icf/en/.
84. Wyatt, C. C., So, F. H. C., Williams, P. M., Mithani, A., Zed, C. M., & Yen, E. H. K. (2006). The development, implementation, utilization and outcomes of a comprehensive dental program for older adults residing in long-term care facilities. *Journal of the Canadian Dental Association, 72*(5), 419–419h.
85. Zarb, G. A., Carlsson, G. E., & Bolender, C. L. (1997). *Boucher's prosthodontic treatment for edentulous patients* (11th ed.). St. Louis, MO: CV Mosby.
86. Zirkel, B. (2008). Who's calling the shots? *ADVANCE for Occupational Therapy Practitioners,* 15.

CHAPTER 13

Pharmacology, Pharmacy, and the Aging Adult: Implications for Occupational Therapy

Hedva Barenholtz Levy, PharmD, BCPS, CGP, Karen F. Barney, PhD, OTR/L, FAOTA

CHAPTER OUTLINE

OBJECTIVES

- Identify major environmental influences on medication use in older adults
- Define polypharmacy and explain its role in medication-related problems
- Define medication adherence and explain barriers to adherence that commonly affect older adults
- Describe the pharmacokinetic and pharmacodynamic changes that occur with age
- Define and provide examples of common medication-related problems
- Describe how the occupational therapy process integrates with various pharmacology and medication-use issues

Medication use is pervasive among older adults. Thirty-eight percent of Medicare beneficiaries age 65 years or older have four or more chronic medical conditions, such as diabetes, heart disease, and hypertension.[12] Treatment of these and other chronic conditions typically entails the use of multiple, long-term medications. However, medication use is not without consequences in this population. Understanding these consequences and related implications of medication use in older clients will enable the occupational therapist to incorporate appropriate interventions and management strategies into daily practice.

Medications have wanted and unwanted effects in the human body. Medications used today often are more potent in their actions, including both the desired actions as well as adverse effects, compared with earlier medications. Thus, one must consider the balance of benefit and risk for each medication prescribed. The benefit-risk balance is dependent on multiple factors that are distinctly affected by age, including pharmacologic, economic, and behavioral issues, as well as certain environmental influences that further impact medication use.

Setting the Stage for Medication Use

Private and public expenditures on health in the United States are the highest in the world. Health-care expenditures per capita in the United States in 2013 were $8700. Comparatively, per capita expenditures in Canada and Western European nations ranged from roughly $3000 up to $5600. Mexico and Eastern European nations spent less than $2000 per capita. Pharmaceutical spending per capita showed a similar imbalance: spending in the United States was $1034 compared with most European nations at $300 to $600 per capita. Per capita pharmaceutical spending in Mexico was $294; Canada $761.[41] Thus, clearly the United States leads global spending on medications. The 20 most commonly prescribed medications among Medicare beneficiaries are listed in Table 13-1, along with their category of use and drug class.[11]

Environmental Influences on Medication Use in Older Adults

Although chronic conditions are an important reason for medication use among older adults, other environmental and regulatory factors contribute to the high prevalence of medication use in the United States. Understanding these factors and how they affect older adults lays the groundwork to understand the bigger picture of why older adults are exposed to more medications than other age groups. Exposure to medications subsequently puts this age group at increased risk for medication-related problems, which are discussed later in the chapter.

TABLE 13-1 Twenty Most Commonly Prescribed Medications by Medicare Claims Data, 2013

Drug Name (Brand Name)	Category of Use	Drug Class
Lisinopril (Prinivil, Zestril)	Cardiovascular	ACE inhibitor
Simvastatin (Zocor)	Cholesterol	HMG-CoA-reductase inhibitor (statin)
Levothyroxine (Synthroid, others)	Thyroid	NA
Hydrocodone/acetaminophen (Vicodin, Norco)	Analgesic	Opioid combination
Amlodipine (Norvasc)	Cardiovascular	Calcium channel blocker
Omeprazole (Prilosec)	Gastrointestinal	Proton pump inhibitor
Atorvastatin (Lipitor)	Cholesterol	HMG-CoA-reductase inhibitor (statin)
Furosemide (Lasix)	Cardiovascular	Diuretic
Metformin (Glucophage)	Diabetes	NA
Metoprolol tartrate (Lopressor)	Cardiovascular	Beta blocker
Gabapentin (Neurontin)	Neurologic agent (seizures, atypical pain)	NA
Hydrochlorothiazide	Cardiovascular	Diuretic
Warfarin (Coumadin)	Anticoagulant	Vitamin K antagonist
Metoprolol succinate (Toprol XL)	Cardiovascular	Beta blocker
Losartan (Cozaar)	Cardiovascular	Angiotensin receptor blocker (ARB)
Clopidogrel (Plavix)	Antiplatelet/cardiovascular	$P2Y_{12}$ antagonist
Pravastatin (Pravachol)	Cholesterol	HMG-CoA-reductase inhibitor (statin)
Atenolol (Tenormin)	Cardiovascular	Beta blocker
Tramadol (Ultram)	Analgesic	Opioid
Carvedilol (Coreg)	Cardiovascular	Beta blocker

ACE = angiotensin-converting enzyme; HMG = hydroxyl-methylglutaryl; CoA = coenzyme A; NA = not applicable.
(From Centers for Medicare and Medicaid Services *Medicare Provider Utilization and Payment Data: Part D Prescriber CMS Claims Data.* Retrieved from http://www.cms.gov/Research-Statistics-Data-and-Systems/Statistics-Trends-and-Reports/Medicare-Provider-Charge-Data/Part-D-Prescriber.html). Accessed May 18, 2015.

Medical Advances

Adults are living longer as a result of advances in medical science and an improved understanding of and ability to prevent and treat many disease states. Similarly, more sophisticated developments in pharmaceutical research have led to new drug approvals. New pharmaceuticals are able to treat conditions that could not be treated in the past, such as cancer, stroke, and heart attack. Thus, adults not only are surviving previously devastating health conditions, but they are living longer to develop other medical conditions that require treatment, such as type 2 diabetes, heart failure, hypertension, neuropathy, and osteoporosis.

Multiple Physicians Prescribing Medications

Based on a sample from a Medicare population (greater than 65 years old), beneficiaries receive prescribed medications from an average of three different physicians. Eleven percent have five or more prescribing physicians. Notably, involvement of multiple prescribing physicians has been associated with an increased risk of adverse drug reactions.[27] Further research is needed to more clearly understand the nature of the association. Resultant fragmented care and lack of communication among physicians are potential factors that negatively affect client care. In addition, physicians may not ask about medications prescribed by other physicians, which can lead to drug interactions, duplication of therapy, and adverse drug events. Clearly, involvement of multiple prescribing physicians requires improved communication and cooperation among health-care providers. Until there is uniform

access to a client's health record, older adults and health-care providers need be diligent in creating, maintaining, and reviewing a complete medication list for each client.

Accessibility of Nonprescription Drugs and Dietary Supplements

The nonprescription and dietary supplement markets have burgeoned in the last few decades, with older adults commonly using these products in conjunction with their prescribed medications.[44] Nonprescription drug sales grew from approximately $3 billion in 1970 to over $19 billion in 2000.[28] In many cases, clients, including older adults, use these products without telling their physicians.[24] Many do not even consider these products as "medications." As such, clients may not include common and medically important medications such as aspirin, vitamins, or dietary supplements as part of their daily medication list. However, these nonprescription products indeed are drugs, with attendant adverse drug effects and potentially significant interactions with prescribed pharmacotherapy.

Nonprescription Products

Nonprescription products, such as antacids, cough and cold products, and laxatives, are regulated by the federal Food and Drug Administration (FDA). Since 1976, nearly 100 products have been reclassified from prescription to nonprescription status.[28] Notable switches include the proton pump inhibitors (PPIs) esomeprazole, lansoprazole, and omeprazole; the histamine$_2$-receptor antagonists (H$_2$RAs) cimetidine, famotidine, and ranitidine; the allergy medicines cetirizine, fexofenadine, and loratadine; and the nonsteroidal anti-inflammatory drugs (NSAIDs) ibuprofen and naproxen. Although now available for use without physician supervision, these over-the-counter (OTC) products still carry the risk of side effects and the potential to interact with other nonprescription and prescription therapies.

Pharmaceutical companies add further to the maze of nonprescription drug products by continuing to inundate the market with combination nonprescription drug products and brand-name extension products. Combination nonprescription products are a concern because of the potential for a client to unknowingly ingest a single medication from multiple sources. A prime example for older clients is acetaminophen. This common analgesic and antipyretic is contained in many cough and cold products (e.g., Alka-Seltzer Plus products), headache remedies (e.g., Excedrin), sleep products (e.g., Tylenol PM), and prescription pain medicines (e.g., Vicodin, Norco, Tylox). As a result of the widespread availability of acetaminophen and in response to increased reports of acetaminophen-related toxicity, the FDA in 2009 issued a ruling regarding labeling requirements for OTC acetaminophen products. Labels must now include a warning advising consumers to avoid concomitant use with other products that contain acetaminophen, as well as a warning about interaction with warfarin and revised wording about the potential for hepatotoxicity.[14]

Brand-name extension products are another source of confusion on pharmacy shelves.[28,43] Pharmaceutical manufacturers take advantage of well-known, trusted brand names and use these recognized names to market OTC products with different ingredients. Unknowing consumers may not realize they are choosing the wrong formulation of a well-known brand name product and end up consuming an ingredient different from what they or their physicians intended. Subsequently, adverse health outcomes can result. Examples of brand-name extension products are listed in Box 13-1.[43]

Other OTC products that have been reformulated and are coined as "improved," "advanced," or "maximum," leading to confusion. Choosing the right product is further compounded by similar packaging and placement adjacent to each other on the pharmacy shelves.

BOX 13-1 Brand-Name Extension Products

- Pepcid (famotidine) vs. Pepcid Complete (famotidine, calcium carbonate and magnesium hydroxide)
- Dulcolax (bisacodyl) vs. Dulcolax Stool Softener (docusate sodium)
- Mucinex (guaifenesin) vs. Mucinex Allergy (fexofenadine)
- Sudafed (pseudoephedrine) vs. Sudafed PE (phenylephrine)
- Tylenol (acetaminophen) vs. Tylenol PM (acetaminophen and diphenhydramine)

(From PL-Detail Document, OTC brand-name extensions. (2013). *Pharmacist's Letter/Prescriber's Letter*, June.)

Unintentional selection of OTC products can result in preventable adverse drug events, an area of great concern in older adults because of their increased susceptibility to medication effects. This is illustrated by reports of clients who chose the wrong Dulcolax product for a colonoscopy preparation and subsequently needed to reschedule the procedure. Thus, clients always should be encouraged to consult with their retail pharmacist when choosing an OTC product. Furthermore, it becomes increasingly important to identify the actual OTC product packaging when conducting a medication review or creating a medication list, so as to include the correct OTC medications a client is taking.

Dietary Supplements

Interest in dietary supplements has grown exponentially in recent years in the United States. Dietary supplements by definition include herbal products, minerals, vitamins, and other substances that supplement the diet.[51] Common examples of herbal products used by older adults include garlic, ginkgo, saw palmetto, and St. John's wort. Supplements often used by older clients include fish oil for the heart and glucosamine for osteoarthritis. Calcium is a commonly used mineral for bone health. Vitamin use ranges from single ingredient vitamin products, such as vitamin C or D, to combination vitamins, such as B-complex or a multivitamin. Dietary supplements commonly consume large sections of pharmacy shelf space, but unfortunately, "natural" does not always mean "safe," and presence on a store shelf does not always guarantee effectiveness. The cost of many dietary supplements is significant, as well. In the author's experience, older adults can be enticed by television advertisements for exotic products that promise overall improved health or a cure-all. Too often, the claims indeed are too good to be true, and the older adult has spent valuable money on a product with no proven health benefits.

The dietary supplement and herbal industry is vastly underregulated compared with the prescription industry. Since passage of the Dietary Supplement Health and Education Act (DSHEA) in 1994, dietary supplements have been regulated in a different manner by the FDA compared with the way prescription and nonprescription products are handled. New prescription and nonprescription drugs must be reviewed and approved by the FDA before being marketed, providing sufficient evidence to support that the new drug is safe and effective. In contrast, dietary supplements are not subjected to these strict safety and effectiveness requirements mandated for drug products. Manufacturers of dietary supplements are not required to prove their products are safe or effective before marketing them and require no premarketing approval. The FDA can take action only if a product is found to be unsafe once the supplement is on the market.[51] Furthermore, accuracy of product label information for dietary supplements has been called into question. Large variability and inaccuracies among herbal products marketed have been documented with regard to recommended doses, labeled ingredients, and inclusion of plant parts on the label.[25]

To combat the dearth of safety and effectiveness data for dietary supplements and herbal products, published research in this area is ongoing, with many federally funded studies completed or under way. Thus health-care providers have access to a growing database regarding mechanisms of action, effectiveness, interactions, and side effects for commonly used products. However, much information still is unknown for the majority of products being sold. The practice of combining herbal products with prescription medication use is a concern for which practitioners need to be vigilant. A more in-depth discussion about herbals and the herbal industry, although pertinent, is beyond the scope of this chapter, and readers are encouraged to consult other references. Suffice it to say that most consumers are unaware of the regulatory differences for dietary supplements. In addition, many do not perceive concerns regarding safety and effectiveness issues, including drug interaction concerns when combining supplements with prescription and nonprescription medications.

Regulatory and Cultural Influences

Regulatory and cultural changes have promoted medication use both directly and indirectly. Federal regulation in 1997 allowed direct-to-consumer advertising (DTCA) of prescription drugs on television and in print by pharmaceutical companies. As a result, spending by pharmaceutical companies to promote their products increased from $11.4 billion in 1996 to $29.9 billion in 2005,[15] with a subsequent increase in drug use in the United States. The change in DTCA has been controversial.

Critics are concerned that it encourages inappropriate use of medications, especially newer, higher-priced choices that may be unnecessary. Comparable treatments often are available at lesser cost for older adults, who so often live on a fixed income. Critics argue that the FDA does not adequately enforce DTCA regulations, and television advertisements may not present a balanced picture of the risks and benefits of therapy. Subsequently, DTCA might portray unrealistically positive outcomes of drug therapy through its imagery. Finally, critics state that greater attention needs to be given to drug safety issues in light of the lack of information known about rare, but serious adverse effects of new drugs.

On the other side of the controversy, proponents of DTCA argue that it has been associated with increased use of medicines to treat chronic diseases, something from which older adults can greatly benefit. Other purported benefits are that it increases consumer awareness about drug therapy options, and it helps clients initiate dialogue with their physicians about "delicate" subjects, such as incontinence, erectile dysfunction, or depression.

Growth of the World Wide Web and Internet access is another phenomenon that in recent decades has helped promote medication use, both via advertisements and myriad websites offering health advice and information. An abundance of health information—albeit of questionable reliability and accuracy—is now accessible to the general public. Clients often have greater awareness of diagnostic and treatment information, and subsequently might be more willing to self-treat with nonprescription or herbal products or ask their physicians to prescribe medications for them. The reliability, accuracy, and recency of the material found on the Internet remain a concern and a continual limitation of this source of health information. Undiscerning consumers are particularly vulnerable to the potential untoward effects of information gleaned from the Internet.

Polypharmacy

Polypharmacy is defined simply as the use of multiple medications. There is no standardized threshold to define what constitutes "multiple medications"; however, a threshold of at least five medications commonly is accepted. Using this definition, surveys estimate that polypharmacy occurs in roughly 20% to 30% of older adults, with half of older adults using nonprescription medications concurrently.[31,42] On average, community-dwelling older adults take four prescription medications daily.[27] Averages are higher in populations with more comorbidities and greater frailty. The average number of medications for residents in assisted living facilities is six,[5] and this number increases to eight medications daily for nursing home residents.[16]

The presence of polypharmacy itself does not denote inappropriate or incorrect use of medications, because older adults with more than one chronic medical condition typically require polypharmacy to manage their conditions. Indeed, three medications commonly are needed to manage symptoms of heart failure or control blood pressure to meet national guidelines. Clients with type 2 diabetes often require at least two medications for effective glucose control. Multi-ingredient combination tablets or capsules have been developed to address these and other examples of appropriate polypharmacy. In contrast, inappropriate polypharmacy can result from inattentive prescribing, lack of follow-up of medication use, or clients pressuring their physicians to prescribe a medication, for example.

Despite the cause of polypharmacy, the end result is that clients who take multiple medications are at higher risk of experiencing medication-related problems (MRPs), such as adverse drug reactions or drug interactions. Problems often result in increased utilization of health-care resources, from additional office visits to hospitalization or nursing home placement. Because of the potential for untoward outcomes related to polypharmacy, gerontology practitioners must be prudent in applying clinical guidelines to client care. In many cases, aggressive attempts to abide by clinical guidelines are not appropriate for certain gerontological clients. The frailty or robustness of each client must be taken into account as part of the risk and benefit assessment, along with consideration of the cost and complexity of the regimen. These latter two issues are addressed next.

The economic burden caused by polypharmacy presents a source of complications for older adults. Older adults who live on a fixed income often have difficulty affording their medications. They might choose not to fill a prescription or perhaps will cut tablets in half or skip doses to make the prescription last until the end of the month. The negative outcomes that can result from such behaviors are readily apparent.

Finally, polypharmacy makes it challenging for many clients to take their medications as instructed and continue to take medications over time. The more medications a person takes, the more complex the medication regimen likely becomes and the greater the risk of taking a medication at the wrong time, forgetting a dose, or otherwise skipping medication doses (i.e., increased risk of nonadherence to the medication regimen, discussed in the next section). Adherence is highest with once- or twice-daily dosing instructions, and decreases significantly with three or four daily doses.[13] Thus, medications that are dosed just once or twice daily are desirable. Pharmaceutical manufacturers wisely strive to develop long-acting formulations of existing drugs or new molecular entities with once-daily dosing properties for this reason. A common dilemma arises when there is a choice between a higher-cost, once-daily product and a less expensive generic drug that requires multiple daily doses and quite possibly has more side effects. The increased cost of the newer, once-daily product often is justified based on fewer side effects and greater likelihood of medication adherence.

The complexity of a medication regimen is further increased in the presence of polypharmacy, because of medications that must be taken at certain times of day or in a certain manner. For example, while most medications can be taken in the morning, some are more effective at bedtime. Some need to be taken 1 hour before a meal (i.e., on an empty stomach), others with food. When one adds to the mix the potential physical, psychological, or emotional medication adherence barriers faced by many older adults, it becomes easy to see how polypharmacy can adversely affect the ability of an older adult to adhere to his or her medication regimen. The important topic of medication adherence is discussed in more detail in the next section.

Aging and Medication Adherence

Medication adherence, formerly referred to as compliance, is defined as the extent to which a person takes medications as prescribed. "Compliance" has become a less preferred term because it conveys a passive client approach to medication use. In the compliance model, a client simply would be prescribed a medication and be told how to take it. In contrast, the term *adherence* implies a collaborative, cooperative approach between client and physician or pharmacist, in which the client mutually partakes in the treatment decision, negotiating the treatment regimen and discussing medication-taking behavior.[56]

Medication adherence has become an issue of national concern, with increased efforts to promote awareness of medication adherence as an issue significant to safe medication use.[38] The effects of nonadherence, especially on older adults, are significant. Nonadherence accounts for up to 30% of hospital admissions,[53] an estimated 23% of nursing home admissions,[49] and deaths. Unfortunately, medication adherence problems are not always obvious, and nonadherence

typically remains undetected until something unexpected or undesirable happens to a client. Most clients do not bring up adherence issues unless they are asked. Even then, they are reluctant to admit nonadherence.

Adherence problems can manifest in many ways, both overtly and covertly. Not all instances of nonadherence are easily detected. Box 13-2 provides examples to illustrate how nonadherence can be either purposeful or unintentional. Although the examples presented might seem straightforward, the reasons behind nonadherence rarely are.

The World Health Organization (WHO) has developed five factors or dimensions of adherence to help define the myriad contributors to nonadherence (Table 13-2):[56] health system, social/economic, therapy-related, client-related, and condition-related. Older adults typically experience multiple adherence barriers at once, further complicating attempts to improve adherence rates. For example, a client might be faced with multiple medications, a complex drug regimen, decreased memory, arthritis or poor vision, the need to take medications long term, and having at least one asymptomatic medical condition. Indirect barriers such as transportation issues or difficulty reaching one's health-care provider by phone similarly need to be considered. As a result, there is no one-size-fits-all approach to addressing adherence barriers in older adults. Success can be challenging. Approaches must be tailored to each client with ongoing support and reinforcement.

Remembering to take medications is one of the first barriers many clients need to address. There are many different types of memory adherence aids that can be recommended, depending on the specific barriers the client experiences. Reminder systems are some of the most common and accessible adherence tools. Calendars and medication charts posted on the refrigerator are simple and inexpensive reminder tools. Pill organizers come in a variety of styles, ranging from a one-strip organizer with one compartment for

---

BOX 13-2 Examples of Nonadherence

- Taking someone else's medication
- Taking more or less of a medication than prescribed
- Forgetting to take a dose or order a refill of a medication
- Skipping doses to make the supply last longer because of cost
- Skipping doses because of physical limitations (e.g., low vision, arthritis)
- Illiteracy that prevents the client from reading instructions on the pharmacy label
- Stopping a medication without physician's knowledge because of side effects or high cost
- Not ordering a refill of a medication because client does not know it needs to be continued
- Not filling a new prescription because of cost or because the client refuses to take additional medications
- Skipping by choice the evening dose of a medication because the client has a social engagement out of the house in the evening

TABLE 13-2 World Health Organization Five Dimensions of Adherence

Dimension	Examples
Health-system-related factors	• Ease of scheduling appointments • Drug formulary changes and restrictions • Quality of communication with health-care providers
Condition-related factors	• Asymptomatic chronic diseases that lack physical cues (e.g., high blood pressure or cholesterol, osteoporosis) • Mental health disorders (e.g., mood disorders, psychosis, dementia)
Patient-related factors	• Physical impairments (e.g., cognitive, vision, hearing, dexterity limitations) • Psychological/behavioral (e.g., anger, stress, alcoholism)
Therapy-related factors	• Complexity of medication regimen • Duration of therapy (usually life-long) • Inconvenient therapies that interfere with lifestyle • Medications with social stigma attached (e.g., for dementia) • Medication side effects
Social- and economic-related factors	• Low literacy; limited English language proficiency • Lack of health insurance • Cost of medications • Poor social support • Cultural beliefs and attitudes

(From World Health Organization. [2003]. *Adherence to long-term therapies: Evidence for action.* Retrieved from http://whqlibdoc.who.int/publications/2003/9241545992.pdf. Accessed May 18, 2015.)

each day of the week, to fancier weekly organizers that have four compartments for each day to accommodate medications that are dosed up to four times a day. Pill organizers should be checked to ensure a client is able to easily open the pill compartments, especially for clients with arthritis or tremor. Some organizers are easier to open than others. Other types of memory adherence aids include watches or "pagers" that can be programmed to beep on time, or phone call reminder systems that can record the voice of a family member or friend.

Other adherence aids address common adherence barriers. Clients with low vision can request large-print labels and written information from the pharmacy. Clients with arthritis can request prescriptions to be filled with non-childproof tops on the prescription bottles. Eye-drop squeezers are available for clients who have strength limitations, and eye-drop guides are available to facilitate the administration of eye drops for clients who cannot keep their eyes open or have difficulty aiming the eye drop accurately. Spacer devices that attach to metered dose inhalers can help clients who have difficulty using these inhalers properly (the spacer devices do

not work with newer dry powder or soft mist inhalers). Occupational therapists who identify specific medication-related adherence barriers with their clients are encouraged to discuss these or other options with the client's community pharmacist or a senior care pharmacist to develop an effective approach for each client.

The multifold nature of adherence issues for older adults makes nonadherence a uniquely challenging area for clients and practitioners alike. More detailed discussion of adherence is beyond the scope of this chapter; however, strategies to improve adherence often involve a collaborative and ongoing approach. Knowledge of the magnitude of the adherence problem will allow occupational therapists to be more alert to barriers their clients may face.

Age-Related Changes in Pharmacokinetics and Pharmacodynamics

Changes in pharmacokinetics and pharmacodynamics are an important contributor to medication-related problems in older adults. However, information on such changes and proper dosing of medications for seniors historically has been limited or unavailable. To address this safety concern, in 1989, the Food and Drug Administration issued guidelines to encourage routine evaluation of drug effects in older adults, especially clients 75 years and older.[52] Although the guidelines have been helpful in drawing attention to this issue, they are not mandatory, and in many cases, inclusion of older adults in clinical research trials remains inadequate. Subsequently, dosing information and pharmacodynamic data specific to the gerontological population may be based on only a few hundred clients and sometimes in none who are over 75 years. This section explains the nature of age-related pharmacokinetic and pharmacodynamic changes and provides examples of how these changes directly affect drug selection, monitoring, and, subsequently, safe use of medications in this population.

Pharmacokinetics

Pharmacokinetics is the study of how the body handles a medication introduced into its system. Pharmacokinetics is comprised of four components: absorption, distribution, metabolism, and elimination. Age-related changes can occur in any of these components, often necessitating modification of dose or choice of drug. Table 13-3 lists common age-related changes in pharmacokinetics that affect medication use.[8,50] Most commonly, drugs are taken orally and absorbed through the stomach, but drugs can be absorbed through the skin or mucosa, as with patches, rectal suppositories, or sublingual tablets. Drug absorption of some oral medications is affected by decreased acid production in the stomach and an increase in pH, leading to reduced absorption into the body. Examples of drugs that require an acidic environment include the antifungal drug ketoconazole and calcium carbonate supplements. In addition to the natural reduction in acid production that occurs, many older adults also take drugs that block acid production. PPIs or H_2RAs, for example, can further hinder absorption of drugs that require an acidic

TABLE 13-3 Effect of Aging on Pharmacokinetic Parameters

Pharmacokinetic Parameter	Common Age-Related Changes	Comments
Absorption	Decreased motility, blood flow Increased pH	Minimal clinical effects; extent of absorption typically not affected. Rate of absorption of drugs might be decreased. Certain drugs can further raise pH.
Distribution	Increased percentage of body fat Decreased percentage of muscle mass, total body water Changes in drug–protein binding (albumin and alpha₁-acid glycoprotein [AAG])	Drugs that distribute in fat tissue (e.g., diazepam, trazodone) are cleared more slowly from body, leading to more severe consequences. Drugs that distribute in water or muscle tissue (e.g., digoxin, lithium, alcohol) typically require smaller dosages. Albumin levels can decrease with age; no change or slight increase in AAG with age. Clinical implications of changes in protein levels are limited, but important in select situations.
Metabolism	Decreased hepatic mass, hepatic blood flow Decreased rate of certain metabolic pathways	Changes can lead to slower drug metabolism and higher concentrations of certain drugs. Hepatic changes are variable among patients of any age. Some hepatically metabolized drugs might require dose reduction.
Elimination	Decreased renal blood flow, renal mass, and secretion of drugs into the kidneys Decrease in kidney function estimated 1% per year after age 50, but variable	Approximately 30% of older adults have severe decrease in kidney function; 30% have moderate decrease; 30% have little change. Higher blood levels occur for drugs that primarily rely on the kidney for elimination (e.g., atenolol, digoxin, lithium, allopurinol, ranitidine) or whose metabolites are eliminated through the kidney (e.g., meperidine).

(From Bressler, R., & Bahl, J. J. [2003]. Principles of drug therapy for the elderly patient. *Mayo Clinic Proceedings, 78,* 1564-1577; and Stratton, M. A., & Salinas, R. C. [2003]. Medication management in the elderly. *Journal of the Oklahoma State Medical Association, 96,* 116-122.)

environment. The decreased gastric motility seen with age can affect the reliability of absorption of certain medications (e.g., variable effectiveness of furosemide in older adults is thought to be related to changes in gastric motility).[50]

Drugs distribute in the body based on their chemical characteristics and can be characterized as distributing mostly into the water compartment (i.e., plasma), muscle tissue, or fat tissue. With age, the percentage of total body water and lean muscle mass declines, and percentage of fat tissue increases. Thus, drugs that distribute primarily into lean muscle tissue or are hydrophilic are expected to be more "concentrated" in the aging body—that is, they have smaller volumes of distribution and thus smaller doses will be effective. Examples include digoxin, lithium, and angiotensin-converting-enzyme (ACE) inhibitors. In contrast, drugs that are lipophilic distribute into fat tissue, which is proportionately greater in older adults than in younger clients. The effect here is twofold: lipophilic drugs can take longer to reach equilibrium or constant levels in the body, and they can have a prolonged effect–therapeutic or adverse–because of increased accumulation in the fat tissue, which serves as a drug reservoir. Thus, "start low, go slow" with drug dosing in older adults is an important mantra. Amiodarone and diazepam are examples of lipophilic drugs that should be used selectively and with extreme caution in older adults. Examples of drugs that are highly protein bound include amiodarone, warfarin, and phenytoin. Changes in protein binding are of importance in clients with poor nutritional status.[50]

The liver is the main site of drug metabolism in the body. With age, there is reduced blood flow to the liver and reduced rate of drug metabolism. Many drugs rely on the liver to be transformed (i.e., metabolized) via enzymes into either inactive or hydrophilic molecules that are more readily eliminated from the body.[8,50] Age-related changes that affect drug metabolism can lead to reduced clearance of the drug from the body and increased duration of action and side effect risks. Examples of drugs that have slowed metabolism in older adults and prolonged effects include the benzodiazepines diazepam, chlordiazepoxide, and alprazolam; propranolol, diltiazem, and theophylline. The effects of these drugs can be prolonged by hours or up to days compared to younger clients. Metabolism of warfarin can be slowed in older adults, prompting lower doses; however, its disposition in the body is complicated by additional pharmacokinetic and pharmacodynamic issues.[8,50] Metabolism of verapamil and propranolol are examples of drugs that can be affected by slowed hepatic blood flow.[8]

Finally, the kidneys are one of the major routes of drug elimination from the body. Renal function decline is an important source of age-related pharmacokinetic change. It is estimated that kidney function decreases 1% for each year after 50 years of age. The effect is variable, though, and up to 35% of older adults may have little or no change in kidney function.[8] Drugs that are primarily excreted via the kidneys can accumulate in the body, leading to prolonged therapeutic as well as adverse effects. Examples of drugs that require dosage adjustment secondary to reduced renal elimination are plentiful. Ones that are used commonly in older adults include allopurinol, atenolol, digoxin, gabapentin, lisinopril, lithium, metformin, ofloxacin, and ranitidine. Importantly, lack of dose adjustment based on age-related changes in kidney function is a significant cause of preventable adverse drug events.[36]

Pharmacokinetic studies are required of every drug submitted for approval by the FDA. Pharmaceutical companies are encouraged to include more older adults in clinical trials; thus, information on changes in drug pharmacokinetics in gerontological clients is increasingly available. As a result, information typically is available to guide clinicians in making dosage adjustments for specific clients based on documented or anticipated changes in pharmacokinetic parameters. Once a drug is marketed, postmarketing data that include drug use among seniors can provide additional pharmacokinetic information. Sometimes this will lead to modifications of official geriatric dosing guidelines by the manufacturer.

Pharmacodynamics

Pharmacodynamics address the physiologic response of the body to a drug—for example, the ability of a drug to slow the heart rate, dilate blood vessels, or cause sedation. The study of pharmacodynamics helps us understand the relationship between drug dose and response. Changes that occur with aging can alter the response of the body to a drug. Typically, older adults are more sensitive to both the desired and adverse effects of medications. Pharmacodynamic changes are more difficult to study because of inherent interplay with pharmacokinetic issues and difficulty in quantifying medication effects (e.g., sedation from benzodiazepines). As a result, they are less well understood than pharmacokinetic changes. In addition, the effect of aging on pharmacodynamics is more variable among clients. Typically, age-related changes result in a smaller dose being needed to elicit the same clinical response compared with a younger population.

Common examples of pharmacodynamic changes that affect medication use in older adults are summarized in Table 13-4.[8,50] Because older adults generally are more sensitive to the effects of medications compared with younger clients, lower starting doses and more gradual adjustments of drug therapy are required (i.e., "start low, go slow").

Changes in receptor sensitivity mean that lower doses are needed to achieve the same therapeutic effect and minimize side effect risks. The starting dose of antidepressants and sleep medications typically is 50% of the dose for younger adults.[47] Decreased beta-receptor sensitivity has been documented, with a corollary reduced response to beta-blocker drugs in older adults. However, changes in pharmacokinetics of beta-blocker drugs typically offset changes in receptor sensitivity, making dose adjustment unnecessary.[50] The influence of baroreceptor function is clinically important for medications that can induce orthostatic hypotension—namely, diuretics, antihypertensives, and tricyclic antidepressant drugs. Increased risk of orthostasis is directly linked to fall risk and potential fractures.

An exaggerated response to certain medications is not uncommon in older adults. This is especially true for drugs that act in the central nervous system, such as sedatives and

TABLE 13-4 Effects of Aging on Pharmacodynamic Parameters

Examples of Changes with Aging	Examples of Clinical Effects
Increased receptor sensitivity	Increased sedative effect from benzodiazepines, antidepressants, alcohol, opioids analgesics, and other central nervous system depressants
Decreased receptor sensitivity	Decreased number of beta receptors; decreased heart rate response to beta-blocking drugs
Decreased baroreceptor function	Increased risk of orthostatic hypotension with diuretics, certain blood pressure medications (e.g., prazosin, doxazosin), and tricyclic antidepressants (e.g., amitriptyline, doxepin)
Increased response to medications	Increased risk of movement disorders or parkinsonism with antipsychotic agents; increased risk of anticholinergic effects; increased response to warfarin or hypoglycemic agents

(From Bressler, R., & Bahl, J. J. [2003]. Principles of drug therapy for the elderly patient. *Mayo Clinic Proceedings, 78*, 1564-1577; and Stratton, M. A., & Salinas, R. C. [2003]. Medication management in the elderly. *Journal of the Oklahoma State Medical Association, 96*, 116-122.)

hypnotics, antidepressants, opioid pain medications, and alcohol. Other examples of exaggerated response to medications in older adult clients include increased sensitivity to the anticoagulant effects of warfarin, hypoglycemia from certain types of oral diabetes agents, and movement disorders from antipsychotic medications. Older adults also are more sensitive to the anticholinergic side effects of medications. Anticholinergic side effects include peripheral effects like dry mouth, dry eyes, urinary retention, and constipation, and central nervous system (CNS) effects like confusion and decreased memory. Issues regarding anticholinergic drugs are discussed in greater detail later in the chapter.

In summary, pharmacodynamic changes, although more challenging to quantify, are extremely important in older adults. The aging body has less ability to adapt to changes, including the desired physiologic or adverse effects of medications. In turn, older adults become more susceptible to adverse drug events, as the body is less able to compensate for drug effects compared with a healthier or less frail population.[8]

Medication-Related Problems (MRPs)

Medication use, especially in older adults, is riddled with potential untoward events that are affected by the several factors discussed earlier: environmental influences, polypharmacy, medication adherence, and pharmacokinetic and pharmacodynamic changes in the body. Therefore, an important goal of prescribing medication is to minimize the potential for causing harm—that is, decrease the risk of experiencing a medication-related problem. This next section describes various types of MRPs and highlights specific issues in older adults.

An MRP is an event or circumstance involving drug therapy that actually or potentially interferes with an optimum outcome of therapy.[29] MRPs can involve an actual problem, such as a duodenal ulcer that develops in a client with arthritis taking an NSAID (e.g., naproxen, oxaprozin, ibuprofen, and others). MRPs also can involve a potential problem—something that could happen, given certain circumstances. An example is a client with atrial fibrillation who takes warfarin for stroke prophylaxis and then self-treats with high-dose acetaminophen for pain. A potential drug interaction can lead to an increased effect of warfarin and bleeding risks if blood work is not monitored more closely. Because the interaction is not predictable, not all clients will be affected similarly, and increased laboratory testing can prevent a potential problem. Eight categories of MRPs have been defined.[29] These categories are useful because they focus on outcomes that directly affect the client and, perhaps more importantly, identify potential sources of intervention to improve outcomes.

1. Untreated condition—The client has a medical problem that requires drug therapy, but is not receiving a drug for that indication.[29] Medical conditions might go untreated for several reasons. Clients might not tell their physicians about symptoms, such as incontinence, constipation, pain, or feelings of depression, and physicians might not ask. Clients might improperly try to self-treat a symptom, when actually treatment requires medical attention. In other examples, physicians incorrectly might attribute symptoms simply to the aging process without further evaluation. Omission of therapy also is an example of an untreated indication. Examples include absence of a beta blocker following a heart attack or absence of warfarin with atrial fibrillation. As discussed later in this chapter, explicit criteria for medication use recently have been developed to address omission of therapy for key conditions that arise in older adults.[40]

2. Improper drug selection—The client has a reason for taking the drug; however, a different drug is warranted because of safety or effectiveness issues. Explicit criteria are available regarding potentially inappropriate medication use in older adults and are discussed later in this chapter.[2,40] Use of medications on these lists generally is discouraged because harmful effects outweigh potential benefit in older adults. In most cases, safer alternatives are available that are preferred for this population.

3. Dose that is too low—The client has a medical condition that is being treated with too little of the correct drug.[29] As discussed earlier, older adults typically are more sensitive to the effects of drugs and require lower initial doses. However, doses need to be titrated to reach effective or therapeutic doses. Examples include a client receiving pharmacotherapy for blood pressure or cholesterol, but the client's blood pressure or lipid levels, respectively, remain elevated. Other examples are the Alzheimer's medications rivastigmine and galantamine, which need to be initiated at subtherapeutic doses to minimize stomach side effects. The doses ultimately need to be increased, yet prescribers may fail to increase to a therapeutic dose.

4. Failure to receive a medication—The client has a medical problem that is the result of his or her not receiving the drug.[29] In other words, medications cannot be effective if clients do not take them. There are a multitude of reasons why clients might not receive a medication: pharmaceutical reasons (e.g., drug was not absorbed in the bloodstream because of a drug interaction), psychological or sociologic reasons (client is afraid of side effects; poor health literacy; does not believe he needs the medication; caregiver withholds medication from client), economic reasons (client cannot afford to get a medication filled or refilled), system issues (drug not available at the pharmacy).

5. Dose that is too high—The client has a medical problem that is being treated with too much of the correct drug.[29] Excessive dosing is one of the more common MRPs in older adults. As described previously, age-related pharmacokinetic and pharmacodynamic changes often necessitate a lower dosage. Indeed, for many drugs, the initial gerontological dose is smaller than the usual adult dose, such as with warfarin or drugs used to treat insomnia, depression, or blood pressure. As discussed earlier, drugs that undergo renal elimination need to be dose adjusted. Failure to do so is a major source of preventable adverse drug events.

6. Adverse drug reaction (ADR)—The client has a medical problem that results from an ADR.[29] ADR refers to any harmful or unintended response to a drug that occurs with normally used dosages.[17] ADRs can be dose-related or non-dose related. Dose-related reactions tend to be predictable, common, and an extension of a drug's known pharmacologic effects. Examples include tremor from excessive albuterol inhaler use, sedation from benzodiazepine use, and dry mouth from oxybutynin. Note that drug interactions or reduced kidney function in older adults can cause higher than expected drug levels, even though the dose is considered in the usual range. In contrast, non-dose related reactions are unpredictable, uncommon, and unrelated to the pharmacologic effect of the drug. They are often more serious than dose-related reactions.[17] Examples of these more serious reactions include hypersensitivity reactions, agranulocytosis, and platelet dysfunction. Careful drug selection, monitoring drug therapy, and patient education can help reduce ADR occurrence. Unfortunately, ADRs in older adults might erroneously be attributed to aging or an existing medical condition. Examples of such nonspecific symptoms include weakness, loss of appetite, depression, and decreased memory or confusion. Unidentified ADRs can lead to a prescribing cascade, in which additional medications are prescribed to treat an ADR.

7. Drug interaction—Drugs can interact not only with other drugs, but also with disease states (e.g., pioglitazone and

NSAIDs can worsen heart failure) and foods and nutrients (e.g., grapefruit juice increases blood levels of diltiazem; metformin decreases absorption of vitamin B_{12}). Many drug-drug interactions result from inhibiting or inducing metabolism of other drugs in the liver. Amiodarone, calcium channel blockers, selective serotonin reuptake inhibitor (SSRI) antidepressants, and warfarin are just a few drugs that are metabolized by the liver and can affect metabolism of other medications metabolized by similar pathways. Another type of pharmacokinetic drug interaction is decreased effectiveness due to reduced absorption from the stomach; for example, antacids will bind to the antibiotic ciprofloxacin in the stomach, preventing its absorption. Pharmacodynamic drug interactions include orthostatic hypotension from taking multiple antihypertensive agents and bleeding that results from the combined use of aspirin and clopidogrel or an NSAID and warfarin. Although clinicians often are able to identify the possibility of a drug interaction based on pharmacologic characteristics, interactions are not always preventable. Namely, interactions that involve newer medications may not yet be known or fully understood. Some drug interactions are rarely clinically significant, but can be due to variable client response to medications. Thus, a client might unexpectedly be more susceptible to an interaction that would be detected only once it occurs and not preventable a priori based on population data. The science of pharmacogenomics will shed further light on such issues and improve drug safety.

8. Drug use without indication—The client is taking a drug for no medically valid indication.[29] Use of unnecessary medications increases a client's risk of drug interactions, ADRs, and other MRPs. Unfortunately, medications are more easily added to a client's regimen than discontinued. Medication use without an indication can occur in a variety of scenarios. Medications that were started during a hospitalization may no longer be appropriate upon discharge. For example, a PPI might be started for ulcer prophylaxis in a critical care unit, continued throughout the hospitalization, and inadvertently written as a discharge medicine. Iron or vitamin B_{12} replacement therapy might be continued once normal levels are restored or underlying cause is addressed. Medications intended for short-term use, such as treatment for reflux symptoms or insomnia, might be continued despite resolution of symptoms. Finally, a medication might have been appropriately started concomitant with another medication (e.g., a PPI with an NSAID for ulcer prophylaxis or folic acid with methotrexate to prevent toxicity), but continued once the other medication was stopped. These varied examples illustrate why older adults often take unnecessary medications and underscore the value of periodic medication reviews to detect this category of MRPs.

The importance of identifying, preventing, and/or correcting MRPs is paramount to promoting the safe use of medications in older adults. MRPs can negatively affect quality of life, clinical outcomes, and health-care costs. Notably, MRPs

can cause, aggravate, or contribute to a number of geriatric syndromes, such as confusion or delirium, depression, dizziness, falls, malnutrition, memory loss, and weakness. In turn, clients experience reduced quality of life due to increased health problems, stress, and difficulty maintaining one's independence. Negative clinical outcomes can result when MRPs cause a new medical condition or worsen symptoms of an existing condition. Finally, MRPs have been estimated to cost $177 billion in the United States, due to drug-related morbidity and mortality.[18] In this model, costs resulted from treatment failures, development of new medical problems, additional prescriptions (i.e., prescribing cascade), office visits, emergency department visits, and hospitalizations or nursing home admissions.[18]

It is incumbent on health-care practitioners to question the role of medications as a possible cause of new symptoms in older adults or when there is a lack of improvement of a treated condition. In doing so, MRPs can be identified and corrected to maximize the positive outcomes of therapy while minimizing risks.

High-Risk Medications in Older Adults

Certain medications are considered to be high risk for older adults because of their propensity to cause or contribute to adverse drug events. Identification of such high-risk medications is an area of active interest among geriatric and gerontology practitioners because of the importance of preventing or minimizing risk with regard to medication use. Drugs or drug classes that have been associated with increased risk of hospitalizations or emergency department visits include NSAIDs; medications that increase bleeding, such as warfarin, aspirin, and clopidogrel; certain cardiovascular agents; agents that increase the risk of hypoglycemia, namely insulin and certain oral antidiabetic agents; and centrally acting medications.[9,32,42,48,46] In addition, drugs that are associated with increased fall risk in older adults and drugs with anticholinergic activity deserve special mention. Each of these medications or categories is discussed next.

NSAIDs are considered high-risk medications in older clients because they carry a higher risk of ulcers, renal toxicity, and CNS side effects. The majority of NSAIDs also increase the risk of bleeding by inhibiting platelet function.[47] NSAID use is an important cause of emergency department visits and hospitalizations among older adults, mostly related to bleeding and ulcer complications. Age greater than 65 years is considered a risk factor for NSAID-induced ulcers. Subsequently, addition of a PPI is recommended to protect against ulcers in high-risk older adults.[34]

Warfarin, aspirin, and clopidogrel are considered high-risk medications because of their risk of bleeding. Aspirin increases the risk of peptic ulcer disease, especially when combined with an NSAID. Newer antiplatelet and anticoagulant medications should also be viewed as high-risk in older adults because of their shared potential to increase bleeding risk. At time of publication, evidence to support this concern awaits widespread use and epidemiologic studies of these newer agents. Until such evidence-based research becomes available, clinicians should be vigilant in monitoring bleeding risks in older adults. New antiplatelet agents include prasugrel (Effient®) and ticagrelor (Brilinta®). New oral anticoagulants include apixaban (Eliquis®), dabigatran (Pradaxa®), edoxaban (Savaysa®), and rivaroxaban (Xarelto®). Other drugs that increase the risk of bleeding, such as NSAIDs and SSRIs, that are used concomitantly with warfarin and/or aspirin further compound the risk of bleeding complications. Careful monitoring and client education are mandatory. Use of a PPI for ulcer prophylaxis is recommended in clients using an NSAID concomitant with aspirin.[34,40]

Among the cardiovascular medications, diuretics, blood pressure medications, and digoxin commonly are related to adverse events leading to emergency department visits and hospitalizations. Diuretics have the propensity to cause electrolyte disturbances if not monitored properly (namely, changes in potassium levels and cardiac conduction abnormalities) and to contribute to hypotension, dizziness, and falls. Similarly, blood pressure medications can lead to serious adverse events because of their potential to lower blood pressure too much, contribute to orthostatic hypotension, and increase the risk of a fall. Use of multiple cardiovascular agents that can increase potassium levels is another risk in older adults. For example, concomitant use of spironolactone and lisinopril or losartan can lead to severe hyperkalemia.[1] Finally, digoxin has been found to contribute to emergency department visits because it has a narrow window of safety, multiple drug interactions, and altered pharmacokinetics with age (discussed earlier).[9,32,48]

Insulin and oral hypoglycemic agents have been identified as high-risk medications in older adults because of the potential to cause significant hypoglycemia. Although insulin remains an excellent choice for controlling glucose levels—even in clients with type 2 diabetes—its use in older adults can be complicated by poor vision, decreased dexterity, or decreased cognitive function, which affect older adults' ability to safely measure and administer insulin. Oral hypoglycemic agents primarily refer to drugs from the sulfonylurea drug class, such as glyburide, glipizide, and glimepiride. These drugs have the propensity to cause hypoglycemia and need to be used cautiously in aging clients and avoided in clients with frequent hypoglycemia. When a sulfonylurea is needed, glipizide and glimepiride are preferred because of more desirable pharmacokinetic profiles in older adults. Clients receiving a sulfonylurea or insulin need to be carefully educated about the signs and symptoms of hypoglycemia. Older adults with diabetes who use beta blockers may experience unrecognized hypoglycemia because beta blockers mask common signs of hypoglycemia, such as increased heart rate and tremor.

Medications that consistently are identified with increased risk of falls in older adults include psychotropic drugs such as antidepressants, sedative/hypnotics, benzodiazepines, and antipsychotic agents.[55] Certain cardiovascular agents are associated with fall risk, namely, diuretics, nitrates, and digoxin. Other drug classes include opioids analgesics, NSAIDs, and anticonvulsants. The mechanism by which drugs contribute to

falls varies. Commonly, drugs implicated in fall risk act within the central nervous system and cause sedation, dizziness, or confusion. Multiple blood pressure medicines can lead to orthostatic hypotension or low blood pressure, thus causing dizziness and fall risk.

The concern with use of psychotropic drugs is significant. A retrospective case-control study found that the use of three or more centrally acting drugs in hospitalized adults aged 70 years and older was associated with almost a fivefold increase in fall risk.[22] Although the study may have limited generalizability to community-dwelling older adults, the increased fall risk is impressive. Guidelines state that polypharmacy with four or more drugs increases fall risk and should be evaluated.[3] Finally, an individual's frailty or robustness of health will ultimately influence a client's fall risk, despite what one might predict based on the literature and fall-risk medication data. Although stopping all fall-risk medicines rarely is an option, minimizing their number and educating the client about ways to decrease the risk of a fall is prudent.

Drugs with anticholinergic effects also are considered high-risk agents. The term *anticholinergic* refers to blockade or antagonism of receptors of the cholinergic system. The cholinergic nervous system relies on acetylcholine as its neurotransmitter. Figure 13-1 illustrates the autonomic nervous system in a very simplistic manner, showing the role of acetylcholine versus norepinephrine transmission.[26,54] Acetylcholine plays a role both centrally and peripherally via the parasympathetic system. Namely, peripheral cholinergic transmission affects the eye, salivary and lacrimal glands, heart rate, gastric motility, and bladder contractions.[26,54] Central cholinergic transmission plays a major role in memory and learning.[30] Consequently, blockade of acetylcholine activity by drugs that possess anticholinergic activity can result in an important

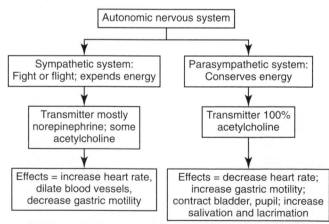

FIGURE 13-1 Schematic of autonomic nervous system. (Adapted from Westfall, T. C., & Westfall, D. P. [2005]. Neurotransmission: The autonomic and somatic nervous systems. In L. L. Brunton, J. S. Lazo, & K. L. Parker [Eds.], *Goodman & Gilman's the pharmacological basis of therapeutics* [11th ed.]. Retrieved from http://www.accesspharmacy.com/content.aspx?aID=956720 Accessed May 18, 2015.; and Goldberg, S. [1988]. *Clinical neuroanatomy made ridiculously simple* [14th ed.]. Miami, FL: MedMaster, Inc.)

constellation of side effects known as anticholinergic effects. Peripheral anticholinergic side effects include dry eyes, dry mouth, urinary retention, constipation, and blurred vision. Central anticholinergic side effects include dizziness, weakness, sedation, decreased memory, and confusion. Drugs that block acetylcholine receptors, therefore, can have a significant negative effect on older adults. Notably, these side effects can look like common changes of aging and may not be detected as reversible, drug-induced effects during a medical examination. Table 13-5 lists common medications and their relative anticholinergic activity.[33,37,45]

TABLE 13-5 Commonly Used Medications with Anticholinergic Effects

Generic Name	Brand Name	Use or Drug Category
Activity definite		
Amitriptyline	Elavil	Tricyclic antidepressant
Diphenhydramine	Benadryl, others	Antihistamine
Hydroxyzine	Vistaril	Antihistamine
Hyoscyamine	Levsin	Antispasmodic
Meclizine	Antivert	Antivertigo agent
Oxybutynin	Ditropan	Bladder antispasmodic (antimuscarinic)
Activity moderate		
Cimetidine	Tagamet	Histamine$_2$ receptor antagonist
Nortriptyline	Pamelor	Tricyclic antidepressant
Olanzapine	Zyprexa	Atypical antipsychotic
Paroxetine	Paxil	Selective serotonin reuptake inhibitor antidepressant
Quetiapine	Seroquel	Atypical antipsychotic
Risperidone	Risperdal	Atypical antipsychotic
Tolterodine	Detrol	Bladder antispasmodic (antimuscarinic)
Trazodone	Desyrel	Antidepressant
Activity small but measurable		
Alprazolam	Xanax	Benzodiazepine (anxiolytic)
Digoxin	Lanoxin	Cardiac glycoside
Furosemide	Lasix	Diuretic
Nifedipine	Procardia, Adalat	Calcium channel blocker (antihypertensive)
Prednisone		Corticosteroid
Ranitidine	Zantac	Histamine$_2$ receptor antagonist
Theophylline	Theodur, others	Asthma agent

(From Landi, F., Russo, A., Liperoti, R., Cesari, M., Barillo, C., Pahor, M., ... Onder, G. [2007]. Anticholinergic drugs and physical function among frail elderly population. *Clinical Pharmacology Therapy, 81*, 235-241; Mulsant, B. H., Pollock, B. G., Kirshner, M., Shen, C., Dodge, H., & Ganguli, M. [2003]. Serum anticholinergic activity in a community-based sample of older adults. *Archives of General Psychiatry, 60*, 198-203; and Rudd, K. M., Raehl, C. L., Bond, C. A., Abbruscato, T. J., & Stenhouse, A. C. [2005]. Methods for assessing drug-related anticholinergic activity. *Pharmacotherapy, 25*, 1592-1601.)

Anticholinergic drugs are considered high-risk medications in older adults because this age group is more sensitive to anticholinergic effects compared with younger clients and because the effects can be so problematic for older adults. Subsequently, anticholinergic drugs are recommended to be avoided in older adults when possible.[2,40] A growing body of literature furthermore supports that cumulative anticholinergic activity—that is, additive effects from taking several anticholinergic medicines—is associated with deceased memory and cognitive and physical functioning.* Undetected central anticholinergic effects that contribute to or worsen cognitive impairment are particularly concerning, as the number of clients with dementia in the United States is expected to increase in the coming decades. Thus, medication reviews to identify use of drugs with anticholinergic activity is critical in the older adult population, especially in those with suspected or diagnosed cognitive impairment or dementia.

High-risk medications cannot always be avoided in older adults, but they need to be used judiciously. Adequate monitoring and client education are needed. In other cases, safer alternatives or nondrug therapy should be used.

Explicit Criteria for Medication Use

Explicit criteria refer to a well-defined list of indicators that require minimal interpretation to apply. Explicit criteria for medication use identify specific drugs, drug classes, or other prescribing indicators that enable clinicians to easily identify high-risk or potentially inappropriate medication use. Because of growing awareness of the need to improve prescribing practices for older adult clients, there has been an increased interest worldwide to develop explicit criteria.[35] As a result, several sets of explicit criteria have been developed to identify medications that are potentially inappropriate in the older adult population.[35] Most well known among these are the Beers criteria[2] and the Screening Tool of Older Person's Prescriptions (STOPP).[40] STOPP is accompanied by a tool that uniquely addresses the absence of desired prescribing in older adults, called the Screening Tool to Alert Doctors to Right Treatments (START).[40] These criteria are introduced next.

The Beers Criteria initially were developed for use in a frail nursing home population.[7] The criteria were the first objective means to benchmark and address the critical issue of inappropriate prescribing in older adults. As such, they filled an important void and were quickly embraced by policymakers, clinicians, and researchers alike. In response to widespread use of the criteria in nonnursing home populations, the Beers Criteria subsequently were revised for the ambulatory setting.[2,6,19] The most recent update of the Beers Criteria was published in 2015.[2] The Beers Criteria consists of 36 drugs or drug classes that are recommended to be *avoided* or used only in certain clinical situations and 13 drugs or drug classes that should be used *with caution* in older adults. Examples of these criteria are provided in

*References 10, 20, 21, 33, 37, and 39.

Table 13-6. Drugs that are recommended to be used with caution in older adults often have plausible reasons for use in this age group; however, potential for harm or misuse warrants additional caution when prescribing them. The Beers Criteria also lists 14 diseases (e.g., heart failure) or syndromes (e.g., history of falls) for which certain medications should be avoided based on the medication's ability to exacerbate the disease state or syndrome. Examples of medications that are recommended to be avoided based on drug-disease or drug-syndrome interactions include the following:[2]

> Heart failure: NSAIDs; pioglitazone and rosiglitazone (agents for treating diabetes)
> Syncope: acetylcholinesterase inhibitors (agents for treating dementia)
> Delirium: anticholinergic agents (Table 13-5), benzodiazepines (BZDs), corticosteroids, H$_2$RAs
> History of falls or fractures: anticonvulsants, antipsychotic agents, SSRIs, BZDs, nonBZD hypnotics (eszopiclone, zaleplon, zolpidem)
> History of gastric or duodenal ulcers: NSAIDs (except for COX-2 selective agents) and aspirin (>325 mg per day)

The STOPP and START criteria were first published in 2008,[23] and revised in 2015.[40] They were developed in Europe to improve upon the perceived weaknesses of the 2003 U.S.-based Beers Criteria. Version 2 of STOPP consists of 81 criteria organized into 13 categories—for example, cardiovascular, renal, respiratory, drugs that increase fall risk, and analgesics. Examples are provided in Table 13-7.[40] START is the first tool to address prescribing omission (i.e., drugs that are recommended to be prescribed in older adults in certain situations). START consists of nine categories and 34 separate criteria that should be considered except for end-of-life or palliative care. Table 13-8 provides examples of criteria from START.[40]

The Beers Criteria, STOPP, and START draw much-needed attention to potential problems regarding drug selection in older adults. Due to the paucity of evidence-based medicine for gerontological clients, these sets of explicit criteria rely on expert consensus to determine risks of medications. Thus, these tools vary in their content, and no one tool can be considered universally acceptable. Nonetheless, the criteria fill a significant void regarding medication use in older adults and are important tools to guide clinicians in

TABLE 13-6 Examples of the Beers Criteria

Selected Potentially Inappropriate Medications in Older Adults with Recommendation to Avoid Use

First-generation antihistamines: (e.g., chlorpheniramine, diphenhydramine, hydroxyzine)
Antispasmodic (gastrointestinal) agents: dicyclomine, hyoscyamine
Alpha$_1$ blockers doxazosin, prazosin, terazosin
Antidepressants, highly anticholinergic (e.g., doxepin > 6 mg/day, imipramine)
Antipsychotic use for behavioral symptoms of dementia, unless other treatments have failed and patient is threat to self or others
Benzodiazepines for treatment of insomnia, agitation, or delirium: alprazolam, lorazepam, triazolam, clonazepam, diazepam, others
Estrogens (oral or topical patch; excludes vaginal cream)
Glyburide
Megestrol
Meperidine
Metoclopramide

Selected Potentially Inappropriate Medications in Older Adults with Recommendation to Use with Caution

Aspirin for primary prevention of cardiac events (caution if > 80 years of age)
Dabigatran (caution if ≥ 75 years of age)
Prasugrel (caution if ≥ 75 years of age)
Vasodilator drugs (can exacerbate episodes of syncope in patients with history of syncope)

(From American Geriatrics Society, Beers Criteria Update Expert Panel. [2015]. American Geriatrics Society updated Beers Criteria for potentially inappropriate medication use in older adults. *Journal of the American Geriatrics Society,* DOI: 10.1111/jgs.13702)

TABLE 13-7 Examples from STOPP: Potentially Inappropriate in Patients over 65 Years of Age

Item	Category	Sample Criteria
B2	Cardiovascular system	Verapamil or diltiazem with New York Heart Association (NYHA) Class III or IV heart failure
C2	Antiplatelet/anticoagulant drugs	Aspirin with a past history of peptic ulcer disease without concomitant proton pump inhibitor (PPI)
C10	Antiplatelet/anticoagulant drugs	NSAID and anticoagulant in combination
D8	Central nervous system and psychotropic drugs	Anticholinergics in patients with delirium or dementia
H2	Musculoskeletal system	NSAID with severe hypertension or severe heart failure
I1	Urogenital system	Antimuscarinic drugs (e.g., oxybutynin, tolterodine, others) with dementia or chronic cognitive impairment
K1, K2, K4	Drugs that predictably increase the risk of falls in older people	Benzodiazepines, neuroleptic drugs, hypnotic Z-drugs (e.g., zolpidem, zaleplon)

NSAID = nonsteroidal anti-inflammatory drug.
(From O'Mahony D., O'Sullivan D., Byrne S., O'Connor M. N., Ryan C., & Gallagher P. [2015]. STOPP/START criteria for potentially inappropriate prescribing in older people: version 2. *Age and Ageing, 44,* 213-218.)

TABLE 13-8 Examples of START Criteria: Therapy That Should be Considered in Most Situations

Item	Category	Sample Criteria
A1	Cardiovascular system	Warfarin or new anticoagulant drugs in the presence of atrial fibrillation
A3	Cardiovascular system	Antiplatelet therapy with documented history of coronary, cerebral, or peripheral vascular disease
C3	Central nervous system and eyes	Acetylcholinesterase inhibitor (donepezil, rivastigmine, galantamine) for mild to moderate Alzheimer's dementia
D1	Gastrointestinal system	Proton pump inhibitor with severe gastroesophageal reflux disease
E3	Musculoskeletal system	Vitamin D and calcium supplement in patient with known osteoporosis or previous fragility fracture
E5	Musculoskeletal system	Vitamin D supplement in older people who are housebound or experiencing falls with osteopenia
I1	Vaccines	Seasonal trivalent influenza vaccine annually

(From O'Mahony D., O'Sullivan D., Byrne S., O'Connor M. N., Ryan C., & Gallagher P. [2015]. STOPP/START criteria for potentially inappropriate prescribing in older people: version 2. *Age and Ageing, 44,* 213-218.)

choosing and evaluating drug therapy regimens for older adults. Importantly, the criteria do not offer a litmus test for good or bad prescribing. Rather, they are guidelines and educational tools, and require clinical judgment when being applied to a particular client's situation.

Principles of Safe Medication Use in Older Adults

Safe medication use in older adults most importantly should focus on limiting the number medications prescribed to older adults. When drug therapy is the treatment modality, drugs should be selected and dosed carefully, giving appropriate consideration to age-related pharmacokinetic and pharmacodynamic issues for each drug. Nonprescription and herbal products need to be included on every client's medication list, and one should be mindful that many clients may not consider these as medications and will need prompting to include them on their medication list. Clients need to be educated about proper use of all of their medications. Health-care professionals need to inquire about adherence issues and strive to remove or minimize barriers to adherence. Monitoring for the eight types of MRPs is fundamental to identify and correct actual or potential problems with pharmacotherapy and cannot be understated. Finally, familiarity with high-risk medications in older adults can prompt the need for client

education or communication with the physician or pharmacist to minimize their use when possible.

Role of Occupational Therapists in Promoting Safe Medication Use

The *Occupational Therapy Practice Framework* (OTPF)[4] includes developing, managing, and maintaining medication routines within the Instrumental Activities of Daily Living (IADL) Health Management and maintenance section of Table 1 (Occupations, p. S19). As part of the health-care team, occupational therapists can promote safe medication use among seniors by increasing awareness of both clients and caregivers about the risks and benefits of medication use. High-risk medications described in this chapter illustrate how medicines can cause serious adverse effects, such as bleeding and hypoglycemia, and contribute to drowsiness, dizziness, mental confusion or slowing, decreased memory, and fall risk. All of these potential drug side effects can hinder the occupational performance of activities of daily living (ADLs) and/or IADLs, thereby affecting overall quality of life. Should the individual be referred for OT assessment and intervention, side effects may impede progress and have a negative effect on the ability of the older adult to reach the goals for occupational therapy, as well as other positive health outcomes. By being attuned to the possibility of medication-related problems, occupational therapists can serve as advocates for their older adult clients.

Adherence is an important area in which occupational therapists can have a positive influence on health outcomes for the older client. Occupational therapists can be advocates for clients if they appear not to be adherent to their medications. In addition, they can promote and educate clients and their caregivers about adherence tools or adaptive devices. For example, occupational therapists can help older adults to find an appropriate pill organizer and teach them how to use it properly. Features need to match the client's functional abilities and needs, including proper size, ease of filling, and ability to open the pill organizer compartments. Other adherence tools can help clients handle eye drops, read prescription labels, or remind them to take medications on time, among other assistance, and the guidance of an occupational therapist can be invaluable.

The information provided in this chapter can serve as a foundation to help occupational therapy personnel identify potential high-risk situations or signals of a potential adverse drug events and also feel empowered to communicate such concerns to the client's physician or pharmacist, as appropriate. Keep in mind that OT personnel working with aging adults may play an important role in their clients' successful medication management, especially when special needs or problems are identified. Changes in cognitive function or occupational performance, excessive or easy bruising, decreased stability, or a fall, among other changes, all might indicate a medication-related problem. By bringing concerns to the attention of the primary care provider or the client's pharmacist, what might be a preventable problem can be corrected. Using observation skills and developing rapport with the client will allow the occupational therapist to determine whether any of the following medication management strategies are indicated:

- Reduce lack of adherence due to misinformation or misunderstandings about the need for medication use. Considerations include level of health-care literacy, cultural differences, and primary language (e.g., English as a second language).
- Bridge the information and understanding gaps between service providers and clients regarding medical terminology, medication names and uses, and potential or actual side effects.
- Facilitate removal of barriers to medication access.
- Collaborate with other disciplines to ensure advocacy and financial supports for affordable medication acquisition.
- Ensure transportation for client to pharmacy or delivery of medications.
- Develop strategies and routines to facilitate client independence in medication management whenever possible.
- Integrate medication use within the daily/weekly routine; Table 13-9 provides common dosage abbreviations used for prescription drugs, to indicate the appropriate medication usage. Note also that labels (e.g.,

TABLE 13-9 Medication Dosage Abbreviations

Term	Directions
QD	Every day
BID	Twice a day
TID	Three times a day
QID	Four times a day
QHS	Bedtime
ac	Before meals
pc	After meals
QOD	Every other day
Q2H	Every 2 hours
PO	By mouth
PRN	As needed

"Take with food," or those indicating potential side effects) may also appear on medication packaging.
- Organize areas in the client's home for ease of medication use, considering both low- and high-technology options (Table 13-10) and cost.

Recall that the overall role of occupational therapy is to ensure that the client's medications are taken in a manner that supports the client's health and well-being in accordance with the physician's and pharmacist's counsel.

TABLE 13-10 Occupational Therapy Strategies to Assist with Medication Use

Individual Guidelines	**General**
	• Use one pharmacy.
	• Use medication calendar or daily planner, including a log for doctor visits and contact information.
	• If taking from the pill bottle, add rubber bands as reminders for doses to be taken, and remove when taken per day (or week).
	• Store pills in the same location, which may vary by time of day, and organize carefully.
	• Use note cards, cell phone, or other electronic apps for quick references.
	Cognitive Simplification (for clients with limited health literacy, dementia, limited English proficiency, etc.)
	• Use pictures, word signs, and simple language.
	• Encourage questions:
	o What is each medication?
	o Why is each medication used?
	o When should the medication be taken?
	o What does the label say?
	o What happens if the pill isn't taken?
	o What are potential side effects?
	o Where does the client get medicines and refills?
	Upper Extremity Coordination
	o Use alternate forms of pill containers (easy-open tops, blister packaging).
	o Use assistive devices (syringe, weighted cups, pills in small paper cups).
	o Coordinate the time to take medication based upon side effects.
	o Use automatic dispensers for eye drops or medications.
	Swallowing Assistance
	o Crush or split pills (with pharmacist approval), using a pill crusher or splitter.
	o Use foods such as applesauce, pudding, or ice cream to ease ingestion of pills.
	o Alternate forms of medications: gummies, liquid, chewable, patches, injections.
	o Use swallowing techniques (tip head back or forward, whichever works best for the client).
	o Use a pop bottle for water.
	o Use pill glide swallowing spray.

TABLE 13-10 Occupational Therapy Strategies to Assist with Medication Use—cont'd

Request from Pharmacist	o Use blister packaging for pills if bottles are difficult to manage. o Remove child safety feature. o Provide information in Braille, native, or other languages. o Use different sizes or colors of bottles for pills that look similar. o Use generic equivalent medications. o Send reminders for refills, etc., via telephone, email, or text messaging.
Family Assistance	Set up medications by week or more, as indicated. Provide reminder strategies, if indicated.
Low-Technology, Low-Cost Options	Add large print with colorful labels (colored tape or paint) to pill bottles. o Use color-coded, weekly/monthly, Braille, or large-print containers; use containers with removable days for travel. o Provide medication prompts, such as text messages, emails, telephone calls, and cell phone reminders. o Use pill storage containers and weekly or monthly organizers. o Use a separate small bag for pills when traveling; store in carry-on bag. o Use a talking reminder clock. o Use a pill timer. o Use a pill splitter. o Use a pill dispenser or medication management wallet.

High-Technology, High-Cost Options	Glucose monitor and insulin pump
	Automatic pill dispensers
	Medicine cabinet with a light-emitting diode (LED) light and adjustable mirror
	Electronic medicine cabinet with medication management features
	Pill reminders:
	    Pill box that sets off alarm
	    Pager
	    Key chain alarm
	    Vibrating watch
	    Email
	    Text (Short Message Service [SMS])
	    Alarm watch
	    Glow cap
	Cell phone or tablet apps:
	    Remind client
	    Provide refill reminders and tracking
	    Record timing and dosing
	    Track missed and taken doses
	Ingestible sensor with accompanying skin patch that notifies caregiver (J,M,S US Patent 2007)
	Monthly medication system with reminder alarm
	Unit dose systems
	Home health services monitoring

CASE EXAMPLE 13-1   Medication Nonadherence

Subjective
LW is a 74-year-old female who requested a medication review because she had questions about the benefits and risks of lisinopril and lovastatin. Her brother had told her they were "not good for the body."

Past Medical History
Transient ischemic attack (TIA) about 5 years ago, hypertension (HTN), arthritis, back pain, type 2 diabetes mellitus (DM), osteoporosis; fell in shower a couple years ago and broke ribs, status post (s/p) wrist fracture within last year

Medications:
Prescription medications: amitriptyline 10 mg once daily at bedtime, atenolol 25 mg once daily, diazepam 5 mg once daily for anxiety (client takes around 7 p.m.), felodipine extended release (ER) 10 mg once daily, Forteo 20 mcg once daily (subcutaneous injection), furosemide 40 mg once daily, lisinopril 20 mg once daily (client currently not taking), lovastatin 20 mg once daily (client currently not taking), metformin 500 mg twice daily for diabetes, piroxicam 20 mg once daily, Plavix 75 mg once daily, potassium chloride ER 10 mEq once daily, zaleplon 10 mg once daily at bedtime

Nonprescription medications: calcium 600 + D (100 units) once daily; Vitality Calcium Complete (calcium 250 mg, vitamin D 100 units, magnesium 50 mg, phosphorous 33 mg) once daily; vitamin B$_{12}$ 1000 mcg once daily

Continued

CASE EXAMPLE 13-1 Medication Nonadherence—cont'd

Allergies: no known drug allergies (NKDA)

Social History

Client lives with spouse. Drinks about 4 oz of wine in the evening. No history of tobacco use. Client does light housework during the day; no regular exercise program.

Objective: height 5'1," weight 68 kg, blood pressure 147/83 mm Hg by client's machine at home (before taking morning medications).

Laboratory: Hgb A1c 6.1%; serum creatinine 0.69 mg/dL; total cholesterol 143 mg/dL, HDL 33 mg/dL, LDL 61 mg/dL, triglycerides 247 mg/dL; vitamin B_{12} 667 mcg/mL. Calculated creatinine clearance 61 mL/min.

Assessment

Adherence: Client stopped taking lisinopril and lovastatin because of incomplete or incorrect information about these medicines. Client's blood pressure is not controlled without her medications. Her triglyceride levels are high and high-density lipoprotein (HDL) levels are low; other lipids are within desired range. Client uses pill organizer for medicines, but sometimes forgets to take her medications in the evening because she has no set time to take them, just "around dinner time." Client's arthritis pain makes it difficult to open the pill organizer. Poor pain control is a barrier to medication adherence.

Fall risk: Medications that increase client's fall risk are amitriptyline, diazepam, zaleplon, hydrocodone/acetaminophen, furosemide, the three antihypertensives atenolol, felodipine, and lisinopril, and alcohol (wine in evening).

Unnecessary medicine: Client's B_{12} level is within normal limits; no history of pernicious anemia; re-evaluate need for long-term B_{12} therapy; duplicate therapy with two sedatives at bedtime and two calcium supplements

Insomnia: Client says she has difficulty getting to sleep and staying asleep. She takes amitriptyline and zaleplon at bedtime. Both of these drugs are considered to be potentially inappropriate medications in older adults based on explicit criteria.

Drug interaction/pharmacodynamic interaction: Plavix and piroxicam—piroxicam is an NSAID with higher potential for gastrointestinal (GI) ulcers compared with other NSAIDs. Taking both piroxicam and Plavix presents with increased bleeding risks.

Osteoporosis: Client not getting enough calcium; has very little calcium intake in diet. Guidelines recommend 1200 mg calcium and at least 800 units vitamin D per day through diet and supplements.

Plan

(Note: Occupational therapy personnel would especially reinforce the pharmacist's recommendations that are in italics.)

Adherence: Educate client about the risks and benefits of lovastatin and lisinopril. Advise client to continue both agents. Talk with physician about possibly switching from lovastatin to agent that will target triglycerides and HDL, such as fenofibrate. *Client agreed to*

purchase different type of pill organizer that is easier to open. To improve pain control, recommend alternative to piroxicam (see drug interaction below). *Client agreed to move evening medicine administration time to bedtime for increased consistency; she will keep reminder note in bathroom where she gets ready for bed to serve as reminder to take medications.*

Fall risk: *Educate client about fall-risk issues.* Recommend discontinuing diazepam and replacing it with lorazepam for anxiety as needed. Recommend discontinuing amitriptyline, which also is included in explicit criteria of potentially inappropriate medications in older adults. Educate client about interaction between lorazepam and alcohol in the evening. Suggest she not take lorazepam if drinking alcohol in the evening. *Encourage client to arise slowly from sitting or other lower position to minimize orthostatic hypotension risk.* Occupational therapy personnel can develop an occupational profile to determine if certain activities place the client at greater risk for falls, and also conduct a home/environmental safety assessment.

Unnecessary medicine: Recommend to discontinue vitamin B_{12} supplement. Suggest client stop the Vitality Calcium Complete (an expensive calcium product).

Insomnia: Recommend to discontinue amitriptyline and zaleplon for sleep and replace these two drugs with either zolpidem or temazepam—either will help client get to sleep and stay asleep; goal is to eventually discontinue nightly use of hypnotic due to risk of adverse events. Educate about risks of benzodiazepines and fall risk. *Provide client with occupational and sleep hygiene tips to help her minimize need for hypnotic medication. If OT follow up intervention determines that these tips are insufficient, the OT would recommend further consult with physician for other potential interventions.*

Drug interaction/pharmacodynamic interaction: Educate client about interaction between piroxicam and Plavix. Instruct her to monitor for signs of increased bleeding. Recommend to switch from piroxicam to meloxicam or celecoxib, NSAIDs with lower risk of ulcers and bleeding; or consider addition of PPI. Monitor for improved pain control; add acetaminophen as needed (PRN).

Osteoporosis: Increase calcium to twice daily. Discontinue Vitality Calcium Complete after using up current supply. Continue Forteo daily as instructed to build bone strength. Encourage increase in dietary calcium intake and provide information on variety of dietary sources of calcium. Continue calcium carbonate, once or twice daily, to achieve recommended amount of calcium per day. OT personnel would encourage the client to do the following: 1) maintain strength through desired activities and exercise, in order to reduce fall risk, 2) limit alcohol consumption, 3) quit smoking, if indicated, and 4) use protective measures to reduce stress on the client's skeletal framework. The latter includes limiting heavy lifting, sliding or pushing objects when possible, and/or delegating if the task will present risk to the client.

CASE EXAMPLE 13-2   OTC and Dietary Supplement Use

Subjective

MD is a 79-year-old female who requested a medication review to double check the use of several vitamins and supplements she takes on a daily basis.

Past Medical History

HTN, arthritis, type 2 DM, osteoporosis, glaucoma

Medications:

Prescription medications: Actonel 35 mg once weekly on Saturdays; brimonidine 0.2% eye drops twice daily; furosemide 40 mg once daily; lisinopril 20 mg, ½ tablet (10 mg) once daily; metformin 1000 mg twice daily; ibuprofen 400 mg twice daily; potassium chloride 20 mEq once daily; trazodone 100 mg at bedtime

Vitamins and supplements: aloe vera, twice daily in winter only; alpha-lipoic acid (ALA) 100 mg, once daily; cod liver oil (1250 units vitamin A and 135 units vitamin D) twice daily; multivitamin with minerals, one tablet twice daily (proprietary blend client orders by mail that contains gingko, cayenne, and basic vitamins; specific amounts per serving size of *three tablets* = vitamin A 10,000 units, vitamin D 240 units, and calcium 400 mg); Oscal (500 mg calcium and 200 units vitamin D) twice daily; red wine extract twice daily; Super Cayenne 450 mg, two tablets daily; vitamin D_3 1000 units once daily

Allergies: NKDA

Social history: Client lives alone. Client attends senior center most days of the week for social activities. Client gets lunch at the senior center. Drinks 1 to 2 glasses (8 oz) of milk a day. No history of alcohol or tobacco use. Client does minimal activity during day; no regular exercise program.

Objective: height = 5 ft, weight = 75 kg, body mass index (BMI) = 32

Laboratory: not available

Assessment

Vitamins: Client takes most of her supplements because she has heard they are "really healthy" for her. She does not have specific reasons for taking them, except calcium plus D supplement, which her physician told her to take. Her pharmacist had told her that aloe vera can interact with metformin.

Arthritis: Client takes ibuprofen for arthritis in right hip and back caused by degenerative disc disease. She still has pain and is unable to pull on her right stocking and feels the medicine is not helping enough.

Insomnia: Client has taken trazodone for sleep for a few years. She states she is not sure it is effective because on nights she does not take it, she sees no difference.

Diabetes: Client is obese, which has a negative effect on diabetes control. Client states she has not checked blood glucose levels at home "in a while." She takes metformin, the safe use of which is based on kidney function. Client has had diarrhea, which could be related to metformin. Aloe and ALA can lower glucose possibly (clinical significance variable).

Glaucoma: Client has arthritis and noticeable tremor (untreated), which can limit ability to instill eye drops.

Osteoporosis: Client takes Actonel and calcium supplement. Also gets vitamin D and calcium from other nonprescription products.

Plan

(Note: Occupational therapy personnel would include in the client intervention a discussion of the individual's medication, supplements, and vitamin use; especially reinforce the pharmacist's recommendations that are in italics; and encourage the client to obtain clarifying information as indicated).

Supplements and vitamins: Aloe vera has been reported to cause hypoglycemia. Check blood sugars regularly (every other day) when taking aloe vera in the winter. No information available to support *oral* use of aloe vera to help with dry skin. *Recommend that client discontinue this oral supplement. Apply topical moisturizers instead.*

Alpha-lipoic acid (ALA) is an antioxidant and might help diabetic neuropathy. It also can lower blood glucose. Client will want to monitor blood glucose changes if she stops ALA. *The supplement is not harmful, but not likely to be helpful.*

Client takes cayenne "for circulation." There are no clinical studies to support this, but product is not harmful. *Recommend to discontinue.*

Red wine extract (resveratrol) is purported to have health benefits; however, there are no data to support a benefit of this supplement in humans. *Recommend to discontinue.*

Cod liver oil is a source of vitamins A and D. Client also gets 10,000 units per day of vitamin A from her current multivitamin. Vitamin A is a fat-soluble drug and accumulation in the body can occur. Guidelines state maximum of 10,000 units vitamin A per day. *Client is getting too much vitamin A. Recommend to discontinue cod liver oil.*

Multivitamin from mail order company is expensive for client. It has no benefit over a multivitamin designed for older adults that can be purchased locally at much lower cost. *Switching to a generic of Centrum Silver, for example, would save client money and also decrease pill burden for this client (one tablet a day instead of two or three tablets with current proprietary multivitamin).*

Given the emphasis in gerontology on limiting the number of medications and supplements in aging clients, encouraging individuals to reduce their intake of these substances is recommended (J. Morley, personal communication, June 2, 2014).

Arthritis: Ibuprofen not effective for client's pain. Pain currently limits client's occupational performance of daily activities. Improved pain control would enable her to stay independent and would allow her to be more physically active. Recommend switching to different NSAID, for example, meloxicam or celecoxib, and monitor for improved effectiveness. If client is switched to any

Continued

CASE EXAMPLE 13-2 OTC and Dietary Supplement Use—cont'd

other NSAID or continues ibuprofen, client should also be prescribed PPI for ulcer prophylaxis. Add acetaminophen if needed for additional pain control. *The individual may also be encouraged to bathe before engaging in activities that are primarily physical, as the warm water will increase blood flow and frequently reduce or prevent pain associated with these activities.*

Insomnia: Trazodone no longer effective. Trazodone is approved by the FDA as an antidepressant, but at low doses it commonly is prescribed for sleep due to sedation as its major side effect. Other side effects include daytime drowsiness, dizziness, dry mouth, diarrhea or constipation, and blurred vision. *Recommend to discontinue trazodone; educate client about good sleep hygiene and optimal occupational performance in activities that may support improved sleep patterns.* If necessary, PRN zolpidem or temazepam could be prescribed for occasional use; both can increase fall risk, however.

Diabetes: Need to check serum creatinine (needs to be <1.4 mg/dL in women) to ascertain safe use of metformin. Evaluate if metformin might be contributing to diarrhea. Recommend physician to consider referral to dietitian or diabetes educator to *review meal-planning strategies.* Client encouraged to monitor blood glucose at home once a week and share results with physician at each office visit. Watch for signs/symptoms of hypoglycemia related to aloe vera and ALA. Monitor for

changes in glucose control if client discontinues these supplements. The occupational therapist would reinforce any recommended meal plan strategies and blood glucose monitoring.

Glaucoma: Review and confirm proper eye-drop administration technique with client. *Obtain eye-drop guide for client if needed in light of client's hand tremor. Also, lying on her back on her bed to administer drops might be helpful. Refer to occupational therapist to help with strategies for managing daily activities in light of hand tremor and any related low vision.*

Osteoporosis: Review and confirm proper administration of Actonel (take 1 hour before food or drink and other medications; stand or sit upright for at least 30 minutes). Client gets 1266 mg calcium through vitamins and supplement, plus 300 to 600 mg calcium from milk, and 1695 units vitamin D in supplements, plus 100 to 200 units per day from milk. Guidelines recommend 1200 mg calcium and at least 800 units vitamin D per day for postmenopausal women. Up to 2000 units of vitamin D daily is okay without physician supervision. Client therefore is meeting these requirements with her supplements and diet. Client can discontinue cod liver oil and switch to generic multivitamin and meet vitamin D recommendations. *Reinforce environmental and occupational performance fall-risk measures that client may implement to prevent falls and other injuries.*

REVIEW QUESTIONS

1. Discuss the pharmacokinetic and pharmacodynamic changes that occur with age, and how occupational performance may be affected.
2. Discuss how an older adult's environment may impact his/her medication use.
3. Describe common medication-related problems that may typically occur with age.
4. Explain how polypharmacy contributes to medication-related problems, and how occupational therapy personnel may appropriately intervene.
5. Discuss the relevance of medication adherence to the assessment and intervention process with older adults.
6. Describe interventions that assist older adults with their medication management.

REFERENCES

1. Abbas, S., Ihle, P., Harder, S., & Schubert, I. (2015). Risk of hyperkalemia and combined use of spironolactone and long-term ACE inhibitor/angiotensin receptor blocker therapy in heart failure using real-life data: A population- and insurance-based cohort. *Pharmacoepidemiology and Drug Safety, 24,* 406–413.
2. American Geriatrics Society 2015 Updated Beers Criteria for Potentially Inappropriate Medication Use in Older Adults By the American Geriatrics Society 2015 Beers Criteria Update Expert Panel Article first published online: 8 OCT 2015 | DOI: 10.1111/jgs.13702
3. American Geriatrics Society, British Geriatrics Society, & American Academy of Orthopaedic Surgeons Panel on Falls Prevention. (2001). Guideline for the prevention of falls in older persons. *Journal of the American Geriatrics Society, 49,* 664–672.
4. American Occupational Therapy Association. (2014). Occupational therapy practice framework: Domain and process (3rd ed.). *American Journal of Occupational Therapy, 68*(Suppl. 1), S1–S48. http://dx.doi.org/10.5014/ajot.2014.682006.
5. Armstrong, E. P., Rhoads, M., & Meiling, F. (2001). Medication usage patterns in assisted living facilities. *Consultant Pharmacist, 16,* 65–69.
6. Beers, M. H. (1997). Explicit criteria for determining potentially inappropriate medication use by the elderly. *Archives of Internal Medicine, 157,* 1531–1536.
7. Beers, M. H., Ouslander, J. G., Rollingher, I., Reuben, D. B., Brooks, J., & Beck, J. C. (1991). Explicit criteria for determining potentially inappropriate medication use in nursing home residents. *Archives of Internal Medicine, 151,* 1825–1832.
8. Bressler, R., & Bahl, J. J. (2003). Principles of drug therapy for the elderly patient. *Mayo Clinic Proceedings, 78,* 1564–1577.
9. Budnitz, D. S., Shehab, N., Kegler, S. R., & Richards, C. L. (2007). Medication use leading to emergency department visits for adverse drug events in older adults. *Annals of Internal Medicine, 147,* 755–765.
10. Carriere, I., Fourrier-Reglat, A., Dartigues, J. F., Rouaud, O., Pasquier, F., Ritchie, K., et al. (2009). Drugs with anticholinergic properties, cognitive decline, and dementia in an elderly general population, the 3-city study. *Archives of Internal Medicine, 169,* 1317–1324.

11. Centers for Medicare & Medicaid Services. (n.d.). *Medicare Provider Utilization and Payment Data: Part D Prescriber CMS Claims Data.* Retrieved from http://www.cms.gov/Research-Statistics-Data-and-Systems/Statistics-Trends-and-Reports/Medicare-Provider-Charge-Data/Part-D-Prescriber.html. Accessed 5.18.15.

12. Centers for Medicare & Medicaid Services. (2012). *Multiple Chronic Conditions HRR Report: All Beneficiaries by Age.* Retrieved from http://www.cms.gov/Research-Statistics-Data-and-Systems/Statistics-Trends-and-Reports/Chronic-Conditions/MCC_Main.html. Accessed May 18, 2015.

13. Claxton, A. J., Cramer, J., & Pierce, C. (2001). A systematic review of the associations between dose regimens and medication compliance. *Clinical Therapeutics, 23,* 1296–1310.

14. Department of Health and Human Services. (2009). Organ-specific warnings; internal analgesic, antipyretic, and antirheumatic drug products for over-the-counter human use; final monograph. *Federal Register, 74,* 19385–19409. http://edocket.access.gpo.gov/2009/pdf/E9-9684.pdf.

15. Donohue, J. M., Cevasco, M., & Rosenthal, M. B. (2007). A decade of direct-to-consumer advertising of prescription drugs. *New Engand Journal of Medicine, 357,* 673–681.

16. Dwyer, L. L., Han, B., Woodwell, D. A., & Rechtsteiner, E. A. (2010). Polypharmacy in nursing home residents in the United States: Results of the 2004 national nursing home survey. *American Journal of Geriatric Pharmacotherapy, 8,* 63–72.

17. Edwards, I. R., & Aronson, J. K. (2000). Adverse drug reactions: definitions, diagnosis, and management. *Lancet, 356,* 1255–1259.

18. Ernst, F. R., & Grizzle, A. J. (2001). Drug-related morbidity and mortality: Updating the cost-of-effectiveness model. *Journal of the American Pharmacists Association, 41,* 192–199.

19. Fick, D., Cooper, J. W., Wade, W. E., Waller, J. L., MacLean, J. R., & Beers, M. H. (2003). Updating the Beers Criteria for potentially inappropriate medication use in older adults. *Archives of Internal Medicine, 163,* 2716–2724.

20. Fortin, M. P., Rouch, I., Dauphinot, V., Gedeon, C., Genthon, S., Bonnefoy, M., et al. (2011). Effects of anticholinergic drugs on verbal episodic memory function in the elderly. *Drugs and Aging, 28,* 195–204.

21. Fox, C., Richardson, K., Maidment, I. D., Savva, G. M., Matthews, F. E., Smithard, D., et al. (2011). Anticholinergic medication use and cognitive impairment in the older population: the medical research council cognitive function and ageing study. *Journal of the American Geriatric Society, 59,* 1477–1483.

22. Gales, B. J., & Menard, S. M. (1995). Relationship between the administration of selected medications and falls in hospitalized elderly patients. *Annals of Pharmacotherapy, 29,* 354–358.

23. Gallagher, P., Ryan, C., Byrne, S., Kennedy, J., & O'Mahony, D. (2008). STOPP (Screening Tool of Older Person's Prescriptions) and START (Screening Tool to Alert Doctors to Right Treatment). Consensus validation. *International Journal of Clinical Pharmacology and Therapeutics, 46,* 72–83.

24. Gardiner, P., Graham, R. E., Legedza, A. T. R., Eisenberg, D. M., & Phillips, R. S. (2006). Factors associated with dietary supplement use among prescription medication users. *Archives of Internal Medicine, 166,* 1968–1974.

25. Garrard, J., Harms, S., Eberly, L. E., & Matiak, A. (2003). Variations in product choices of frequently purchased herbs, caveat emptor. *Archives of Internal Medicine, 163,* 2290–2295.

26. Goldberg, S. (1988). *Clinical neuroanatomy made ridiculously simple* (14th ed.). Miami, FL: MedMaster, Inc.

27. Green, J. L., Hawley, J. N., & Rask, K. J. (2007). Is the number of prescribing physicians an independent risk factor for adverse drug events in an elderly outpatient population? *American Journal of Geriatric Pharmacotherapy, 5,* 31–39.

28. Henderson, M. L. (2012). Self-care and nonprescription pharmacotherapy. In D. L. Krinsky, R. R. Berardi, S. P. Ferreri, et al. (Eds.), *Handbook of nonprescription drugs, an interactive approach to self-care* (17th ed., pp. 3–16). Washington DC: American Pharmacists Association.

29. Hepler, C. D., & Strand, L. M. (1990). Opportunities and responsibilities in pharmaceutical care. *American Journal of Hospital Pharmacy, 47,* 533–543.

30. Karimi, S., Dharia, S. P., Flora, D. S., & Slattum, P. W. (2012). Anticholinergic burden: Clinical implications for seniors and strategies for clinicians. *Consultant Pharmacist, 27,* 564–582.

31. Kaufman, D. W., Kelly, J. P., Rosenberg, L., Anderson, T. E., & Mitchell, A. A. (2002). Recent patterns of medication use in the ambulatory adult population of the United States; the Slone Survey. *Journal of the American Medical Association, 287,* 337–344.

32. Kongkaew, C., Noyce, P. R., & Ashcroft, D. M. (2008). Hospital admissions associated with adverse drug reactions: a systematic review of prospective observational studies. *Annals of Pharmacotherapy, 42,* 1017–1025.

33. Landi, F., Russo, A., Liperoti, R., Cesari, M., Barillo, C., Pahor, M., & Onder, G. (2007). Anticholinergic drugs and physical function among frail elderly population. *Clinical Pharmacology and Therapeutics, 81,* 235–241.

34. Lanza, F. L., Chan, F. K. L., & Quigley, E. M. M. (2009). Guidelines for prevention of NSAID-related ulcer complications. *American Journal of Gastroenterology, 104,* 728–738.

35. Levy, H. B., Marcus, E. L., & Christen, C. (2010). Beyond the Beers Criteria: A comparative overview of explicit criteria. *Annals of Pharmacotherapy, 44,* 1968–1975.

36. McDonnell, P. J., & Jacobs, M. R. (2002). Hospital admissions resulting from preventable adverse drug reactions. *Annals of Pharmacotherapy, 36,* 1331–1336.

37. Mulsant, B. H., Pollock, B. G., Kirshner, M., Shen, C., Dodge, H., & Ganguli, M. (2003). Serum anticholinergic activity in a community-based sample of older adults. *Archives of General Psychiatry, 60,* 198–203.

38. National Council on Patient Information and Education. (2007). *Enhancing prescription medicine adherence: A national action plan.* Retrieved from http://www.talkaboutrx.org. Accessed May 18, 2015.

39. Nebes, R. D., Pollock, B. G., Halligan, E. M., Kirshner, M. A., & Houck, P. R. (2007). Serum anticholinergic activity and motor performance in elderly persons. *Journal of Gerontology Medical Sciences, 62A,* 83–85.

40. O'Mahony, D., O'Sullivan, D., Byrne, S., O'Connor, M. N., Ryan, C, & Gallagher, P. (2015). STOPP/START criteria for potentially inappropriate prescribing in older people: version 2. *Age and Ageing, 44,* 213–218.

41. Organization for Economic Cooperation and Development (OECD). OECD Health Statistics 2015, Frequently Requested Data. Retrieved from http://www.oecd.org/els/health-systems/health-data.htm. Accessed 10/14/15.

42. Pirmohamed, M., James, S., Meakin, S., Green, C., Scott, A. K., Walley, T. J., Farrar, K., Park, B. K., & Breckenridge, A. M. (2004). Adverse drug reactions as a cause of admissions to hospital: Prospective analysis of 18 820 patients. *British Medical Journal, 329,* 15–19.

43. PL-Detail Document, OTC brand-name extensions. (June 2013). Pharmacist's Letter/Prescriber's Letter.

44. Qato, D. M., Alexander, G. C., Conti, R. M., Johnson, M., Schumm, P., & Lindaus, S. T. (2008). Use of prescription and over-the-counter medications and dietary supplements among older adults in the United States. *Journal of the American Medical Association, 300,* 2867–2878.

45. Rudd, K. M., Raehl, C. L., Bond, C. A., Abbruscato, T. J., & Stenhouse, A. C. (2005). Methods for assessing drug-related anticholinergic activity. *Pharmacotherapy, 25,* 1592–1601.

46. Samoy, L. J., Zed, P. J., Wilbur, K., Balen, R. M., Abu-Laban, R. B., & Roberts, M. (2006). Drug-related hospitalizations in a tertiary care internal medicine service of a Canadian hospital: A prospective study. *Pharmacotherapy, 26,* 1578–1586.

47. Semla, T. P., Beizer, J. L., & Higbee, M. D. (Eds.). (2011). *Geriatric dosing handbook* (16th ed.). Hudson, OH: Lexi-Comp.

48. Sikdar, K. C., Alaghehbandan, R., MacDonald, D., Barrett, B., Collins, K. D., Donnan, J., et al. (2010). Adverse drug events in adult patients leading to emergency department visits. *Annals of Pharmacotherapy, 44,* 641–649.

49. Strandberg, L. R. (1984). Drugs as a reason for nursing home admissions. *Journal of the American Health Care Association, 10,* 20–23.

50. Stratton, M. A., & Salinas, R. C. (2003). Medication management in the elderly. *Journal of the Oklahoma State Medical Association, 96,* 116–122.

51. Tsourounis. C., & Dennehy, C. (2012). Introduction to dietary supplements. In D. L. Krinsky, R. R. Berardi, S. P. Ferreri, et al. (Eds.), *Handbook of nonprescription drugs, an interactive approach to self-care* (17th ed., pp. 955–965). Washington DC: American Pharmacists Association.

52. United States Food and Drug Administration. (1989). *Guidelines for the study of drugs likely to be used in the elderly.* Rockville, MD: Food and Drug Administration/Center for Drug Evaluation and Research.

53. Vermeire, E., Hearnshaw, H., Van Royen, P., & Denekens, J. (2001). Patient adherence to treatment: Three decades of research, a comprehensive review. *Journal of Clinical Pharmacy and Therapeutics, 26,* 331–342.

54. Westfall, T. C., & Westfall, D. P. (2005). Neurotransmission: The autonomic and somatic nervous systems. In L. L. Brunton, J. S. Lazo, & K. L. Parker (Eds.), *Goodman & Gilman's the pharmacological basis of therapeutics* (11th ed.). http://www.accesspharmacy.com/content.aspx?aID=956720.

55. Woolcott, J. C., Richardson, K. J., Wiens, M. O., Patel, B., Marin, J., Khan, K. M., et al. (2009). Meta-analysis of the impact of 9 medication classes on falls in elderly persons. *Archives of Internal Medicine, 169,* 1952–1960.

56. World Health Organization. (2003). *Adherence to long-term therapies: Evidence for action.* Retrieved from http://whqlibdoc.who.int/publications/2003/9241545992.pdf. Accessed 5/18/15.

CHAPTER 14

Cognitive Executive Abilities in Aging and Everyday Life

Areum Han, PhD, OTR/L, Kathy Parker, MS, OT, Joan M. McDowd, PhD

CHAPTER OUTLINE

OBJECTIVES

- Describe the concept and structure of executive function
- Explain the relationship between executive function and functional status among older adults
- Select assessment tools and approaches for evaluating executive function
- Identify cognitive, physical, and social interventions for maintaining and improving executive function and functional abilities in daily activities among older adults
- Examine current best evidence for applying research on executive function to occupational therapy services for older adults

Understanding the factors that contribute to functional status in aging is essential for providing older adults with supports and services to maintain independence, as well as for care planning in the face of disability. Cognitive function is increasingly recognized as a critical factor in determining the functional status of older adults, particularly complex cognition such as executive function (EF) abilities. Occupational therapy (OT) is well positioned to play an important role in recognizing EF deficits and assessing their effect on daily-life functions, as well as for developing effective interventions to reduce or prevent functional declines. In this chapter, we present an overview of current conceptualizations of EF, existing data documenting the relationship between EF and functional independence among older adults, potential mechanisms that underlie this relationship, assessments designed to capture EF

in everyday context, and research designed to identify interventions that can maintain and improve EF and functional status among older adults.

Executive Function and Functional Status

EF is typically defined very broadly as "those capacities that enable a person to engage successfully in independent, purposive, self-serving behavior" (p. 35),[34] or as "a multidimensional construct referring to a variety of loosely related higher-order cognitive processes including initiation, planning, hypothesis generation, cognitive flexibility, decision-making, regulation, judgment, feedback utilization, and self-perception" (p. 171),[50] or a bundle of "general purpose control mechanisms that modulate the operation of various cognitive subprocesses" (p. 50).[40] Indices reflecting the status of these mechanisms appear to be better predictors of functional ability than are measures of overall cognitive status such as the Mini-Mental Status Exam (MMSE). For example, Grigsby et al.[24] found a significant association between executive functioning and seven functional status measures (self-report and observed performance in activities of daily living [ADLs] and instrumental activities of daily living [IADLs]) among 1158 community-dwelling older adults. By contrast, general mental status measured by the MMSE was not a significant predictor of functional status among this sample.

In a similar study, Johnson et al.[31] studied 7717 community-dwelling older adult women who completed cognitive and functional evaluations at an initial baseline testing and at a 6-year follow-up. They found that women with EF impairment at baseline were more likely to also have functional difficulty than women without EF impairment. In addition, women with EF impairment at baseline were more likely to experience either a new functional impairment or a worsening of an existing functional impairment over the 6-year follow-up period.

This pattern of results was observed regardless of their scores on the MMSE, and suggests that EF assessments may play an important role in assessing risk of functional decline among older adults. Similar findings of both cross-sectional and longitudinal relationships between EF and functional dependence have been reported in other studies as well.[11,13,46]

The findings just described are important for two reasons. First, these findings indicate that brief screening tests such as the MMSE are not sensitive enough to detect and assess more subtle but critical cognitive impairments in older adults. Second, they indicate that EF is a good predictor of functional status in normal aging, and should be included in assessments designed to gauge an individual's current and future care needs with the goal of supporting independence. However, to translate these findings into practical interventions, it is important to know more about the subcomponents of the broad construct of EF, and to understand which of these components are most closely related to functional status. Connor and Maeir[17] have made a similar point and provide a useful overview for understanding EF in the context of occupational performance. Additional work has been done in the field of psychology, also focused on a better understanding of the architecture of EF.

The Architecture of Executive Function in Relation to Functional Status

One of the fundamental questions about EF is whether it is best understood as a single construct, or as a multifaceted ability comprised of separable abilities. For example, Salthouse, Atkinson, and Berish[47] undertook an examination of the construct validity of EF in a sample of adults ranging in age from 18 to 84 years. Using factor analysis, they identified three factors, or component abilities, of EF: time-sharing (doing two things at once), updating (revising the contents of consciousness with the most recent relevant information), and inhibition (suppressing irrelevant information in favor of important goal-related information). These findings indicate that EF is made up of a set of separable subcomponents that are each differentially related to different functional tasks. However, Salthouse et al.[47] found evidence that these factors were highly correlated with one another. Thus, good performance on one component was associated with good performance on the other two components. In light of these findings, they concluded that EF was best characterized as a single construct.

Miyake and colleagues[23,40] have also addressed questions about the structure of EF. Based on a study sample of college students, Miyake et al.[40] reported evidence that the cognitive processes underlying EF performance were task shifting (switching between two or more tasks), mental updating of information, and inhibition of irrelevant information. Their analyses also showed a correlation between these three cognitive processes, but they concluded that EF is best described as involving both a general component and specific cognitive processes. Although a general ability seemed to be present across EF components, individual components also made unique contributions to task performance.

Vaughan and Giovanello[52] took the same approach as Miyake et al.[40] this time examining EF in a sample of older adults. They replicated Miyake et al.'s[40] findings, and identified the same three factors underlying EF: task shifting, information updating, and inhibition. They also reported that this three-factor model of EF provided a better fit to the data than

a single-factor model, supporting the notion of separable cognitive processes underlying the construct of EF. Overall, then, it seems reasonable to think of EF as having separate subcomponents, even though ability on one component may be related to ability on the others.

Why is it important to understand the structure of executive function? For the OT profession, knowing whether functional deficits are best attributed to an overarching ability to organize behavior or to one of the identified component processes of EF is important to make efforts to ameliorate such deficits.[17] Numerous researchers have attempted to identify specific EF components that are related to functional status. For example, Carlson et al.[13] assessed functional ability and what they called "executive attention" in a large sample of women from the Women's Health in Aging Study II. Their functional assessment included both ADLs (e.g., walking speed, dressing) and IADLs (e.g., dialing a phone, using a key in a deadbolt lock). Assessments of executive attention included measures of updating and flexibility in switching attention. In a series of regression analyses, they found that "executive tests of planning, organization, and flexibility were selectively associated with the performance of IADLs in a physically high-functioning, cognitively intact, community-dwelling sample of older women" (p. S268). Further, they found that the subtest of the Trail Making Test that requires attention switching accounted for the greatest proportion of variance among the cognitive tests. Thus, they concluded that "mental flexibility, rather than fine motor agility, is the attentional component critical to efficiently completing many complex, everyday activities" (p. S268).

Other studies have also identified switching as the EF component most related to functional status. Bell-McGinty et al.[7] examined multiple clinical EF measures to predict functional status among older adults. Their results indicated that measures of mental flexibility and novel problem-solving ability were significant predictors of performance in IADLs, as measured by the Independent Living Scales.[36] Vaughan and Giovanello[52] also found a strong relationship between task switching and performance-based IADLs. However, switching is not the only EF component that has been shown to be related to functional ability. For example, functional status has been shown to be related to inhibition[30,32] and updating.[9,28] As illustrated by these studies, it is difficult to summarize this work because different studies compared different executive functions and used different EF measures.

Measurement issues are complicated by the complexity of many EF tasks, some of which assess more than a single aspect of executive function. Vaughan and Giovanello[52] also point out that the population of older adults represented in these studies differs across studies, varying in health status or current living situation, for example. Although these discrepancies may frustrate the goal of identifying the single most important EF influencing functional status across individuals, from the point of view of the OT practitioner these discrepancies are much less troubling. If the therapeutic goal is to support independence for an individual, then the task is to identify the most important EF impairment *in that individual*. This is not to say that the therapist's task is without challenges, but it is different from the theoretical challenge of fully understanding the relation between EF and functional status. Presumably the identification of other individual difference variables such as physical health status that are important to the EF/functional status relationship will help round out the picture of the best EF predictors for functional independence.

Another issue in understanding the EF/functional status relationship is related to measures of functional status. Most studies measured IADLs by self-reported questionnaires;[30,37,46] relatively fewer studies used performance-based measures of IADLs.[7,13,39] Although task administration is more involved and time intensive, there is good reason to prefer performance-based assessments because they can remove informant bias through direct observation.[7,52] Also, performance-based measures of IADLs tend to be more highly related to EF than self-reported measures of IADLs.[43,46] Indeed, Vaughan and Giovanello[52] found no relation between measures of EF and self-reported measures of IADLs, but they did find significant relationships with performance-based measures.

Together, issues related to assessment validity and observed association with EF support the choice of performance-based measures of ADLs and IADLs as the best indicators of a person's functional ability.

Given the variations in measuring EF and functional abilities, it is difficult to summarize the findings relating specific EF components to functional status. Overall, however, it seems reasonable to conclude that the abilities captured by EF measures are important in determining an older adult's ability to maintain independence in daily living. Determining which of these abilities are most closely related to functional status remains to be determined. It may be the case that the EF abilities underlying functional deficits vary as a function of individual characteristics, such as brain health, physical fitness, or cognitive reserve. Because even minimal losses in EF ability can significantly affect participation and quality of life in older adults,[6] both accurate assessment and effective interventions are important to improve or maintain functional abilities among older adults.

Assessing Executive Function

Approaches to assessing EF can be grouped into three general categories: a neuropsychological approach, a cognitive approach, and a functional approach. The *neuropsychological approach* seeks to understand the relationship between impaired brain areas and behavioral outcomes on EF tests. However, neuropsychological assessments such as the Wisconsin Card Sorting Test or the Behavioral Assessment of the Dysexecutive Syndrome are complex tasks; impaired performance on these tasks might be due to a variety of underlying cognitive deficits, making intervention targets difficult to identify.[10,15] The *cognitive approach* aims to identify the specific cognitive processes that make up EF. Although researchers have had some success in identifying these processes,[52] to do so requires assessment tasks that measure a cognitive process in a limited context that may bear no resemblance to

everyday life, and the relation between these measures and functional ability has yet to be definitively established.

A *functional approach* to understanding EF typically involves performance-based assessments of everyday activities. For example, the Kettle Test[26] requires that a hot beverage be prepared; the Multiple Errand Test[48] requires that a series of tasks be accomplished, such as mailing a letter, using the phone, and gathering information about store hours; and the Executive Function Performance Test[5] requires that a cooking task be completed, along with assessments of using the telephone, managing medicines, and paying a bill. Observing task errors or amount of cuing necessary for successful task completion can provide a picture of a person's executive abilities. The developers of performance-based functional tasks are perhaps interested less in the specific brain areas or cognitive processes underlying performance as they are in identifying the strategies or supports that would help a person accomplish the task at hand.[21]

In a different taxonomy of EF assessments, Chan et al.[15] used the *International Classification of Impairments, Disabilities, and Handicaps* (ICIDH) terminology of pathology, impairment, activity, and participation[55] to describe approaches to measuring EF. They argue that the bulk of the evidence on EF relates to either the pathology or impairment level, characterizing functioning within the individual. Less attention has been paid to the activity and participation levels of functioning, although the functional approach to assessment described earlier represents a positive development. Chan et al.[15] argue that progress in assessment would be best served by a multifaceted approach that includes individual functioning as well as considerations of ecological and ethological validity. They suggest that the newly developing field of social cognitive neuroscience may provide a framework linking the separate approaches to assessing EF. Social cognitive neuroscience encompasses "the social level, which is concerned with the motivational and social factors that influence behavior and experience; the cognitive level, which is concerned with information-processing mechanisms that give rise to social-level phenomena; and the neural level, which is concerned with brain mechanisms that instantiate cognitive-level processes" (p. 211). Certainly this more holistic approach will provide a more complete picture of the strengths and weaknesses of an individual in a social-behavioral context, but further development of this approach awaits methodological and statistical development to support the integration of information from these various levels.

Interventions for Executive Function

Because cognitive ability has been closely tied to functional ability in everyday life, various intervention strategies have been developed to support independence among older adults, focusing on cognitive function in general[54] and EF in particular. The assumption underlying these interventions is that improving EF will in turn improve functional ability in everyday life. Although evidence is still accruing related to the effectiveness of interventions to improve EF, data are emerging in support of the beneficial effects of cognitive, exercise, and social interventions.

Cognitive Interventions to Improve Executive Function

Basak et al.[4] used an off-the-shelf video game called *Rise of Nations*[38] to train EF skills in older adults. *Rise of Nations* is a game of strategy in which the goal is to build cities and expand the borders of the player's nation. A player must "continually assess his or her available resources, plan and expend those resources, monitor his or her expanding territories and multiple cities, and introduce methods to generate revenues and improve technology" (p. 766).[4] Older adult participants played the game for 23.5 hours over 7 to 8 weeks. EF performance was assessed at the outset of training, midway, and after completion of all training. Basak et al.[4] reported that *Rise of Nations* performance improved significantly over the 8 weeks of training. In addition, video game improvement was found to transfer to improvements in other EF tasks that had not been practiced. Specifically, performance on tasks requiring switching and updating processes were found to benefit from training on the video game task, indicating that video game practice had a positive effect on other EF abilities. What remains to be seen is whether improvement on the video game task will generalize or transfer to everyday tasks; as noted by Basak et al., this question is particularly important in light of the fact that the commercial marketplace is being inundated by products and programs aimed at improving everyday function in older adults.

Wang, Chang, and Su[53] reported a similar study in which older adult participants were trained on a cooking task adapted from the work of Craik and Bialystok.[19] In the adapted-task version of Wang et al., participants watched a computer screen to monitor the cooking progress of four or six foods. Each food was to be cooked for a preset time, and all dishes were to finish cooking at the same time. Simultaneous with the cooking task was a computer-based table-setting task. The monitor displaying the foods also displayed an image of a table setting; participants had to drag and drop utensils, plates, bowls, and cups onto the table settings as quickly as possible while also monitoring the food as it cooked. The task required a variety of EF components, including shifting attention, updating information, and inhibiting irrelevant information; Wang et al.[53] had participants practice the task during one session per week for 5 weeks. They found that not only did participants improve on the cooking and table-setting tasks, but the improvement also generalized to other cognitive tasks that were not practiced over the 5 weeks. The authors did not assess the generalizability of their training task to real everyday tasks, and they acknowledge this as a limitation of their study. It remains to be seen whether the Wang et al.[53] findings indicating that EF processes can be improved in older adults will generalize to the functional activities of daily life.

Even the studies of commercial products designed to improve functional abilities have only indirectly measured everyday ability. For example, Nouchi et al.[42] had a sample of older adults practice Nintendo's *Brain Age* cognitive training game for at least 15 minutes a day, 5 days a week, for 4 weeks. A comparison group of older adults played the game *Tetris* for an equal amount of time. They were interested in whether other measures of cognitive function showed improvement after the 4 weeks of training on *Brain Age*. They found that several measures of EF and processing speed showed improvement after *Brain Age* training, but that global cognitive status (measured by the MMSE) was not affected by training. These results are encouraging in that a relatively simple and inexpensive training tool (*Brain Age*) led to significant improvement in EF measures in a fairly short period of time (4 weeks). However, whether these effects are maintained over time, and whether they will affect everyday function, remains to be addressed in future research.

Exercise Interventions to Improve Executive Function

The traditional distinction between cognitive and motor functions has broken down in recent years as increasing evidence points to significant relationships between the two domains. For example, Eggermont et al.[20] examined the relationship between physical activity and EF in a large sample of community-dwelling older adults. They were particularly interested in the possible mediating role that cardiovascular disease, cardiovascular risk factors, depression, and chronic pain might have in the relationship between cognition and physical activity. They measured physical activity using the Physical Activity Scale for the Elderly (PASE), a self-report measure that indexes type of activity and level of exertion across a selection of typical activities such as walking, yard work, housework, and so on. They assessed EF using the Trail Making Test, a clock-drawing test, and a verbal fluency test. After accounting for age, sex, and education, they observed a significant correlation between level of physical activity and performance on the EF tasks. In subsequent regression models adjusted for number of medications, cardiovascular disease, cardiovascular risk factors, depression, and chronic pain, most of the EF measures remained significantly associated with PASE score. This relationship was not observed for a measure of episodic memory included in this study, indicating that the relation between physical activity and EF "represents a specific biologically determined relationship" (p. 1754).

Eggermont et al.[20] conclude from their findings that physical activity may "contribute to the maintenance of executive function and thus independent functioning" (p. 1755). Their data, however, are cross-sectional and cannot implicate a causal relationship. However, various intervention studies have been conducted that do support causal relations between exercise and EF performance. Colcombe and Kramer[16] conducted an initial review of interventions studies; they addressed questions of dose-response in exercise interventions, and the role of individual difference variables in the effect of exercise interventions on EF performance. They found that moderate session duration (31–45 minutes) produced the largest effect on EF, larger than either shorter-duration or longer-duration sessions. In addition, their analysis revealed that although longer intervention programs (6 or more months) produced the greatest effect on cognition, shorter programs (1 to 3 months) also produced significant training effects, and these effects were greater than those of medium-length programs lasting 4 to 6 months. Colcombe and Kramer[16] also examined training effect sizes (i.e., improved cognition) as a function of the individual difference variables of age and sex. They reported that of adults aged 55 to 80 years, the group falling between 66 and 70 years showed the greatest benefit to cognition from the exercise intervention, significantly greater than either the younger or older groups. The evidence regarding sex was less direct; they compared effect sizes for studies with samples more than 50% male participants to samples with more than 50% female participants and found larger effects in studies with samples greater than 50% female. This suggests that cognition among women may benefit more than men from an exercise intervention, although females may also be less fit than males, contributing to the magnitude of the effect.

In a study examining race as an individual difference variable, Popa et al.[44] studied the relation between self-reported physical activity, cognitive function, and disability as measured by basic and instrumental activities of daily living in white and African American older adults. Using multilevel modeling techniques, they found that among white Americans, physical activity (regular exercise, gardening, walking, etc.) was significantly, directly, and inversely related to disability, and also indirectly related via positive effects on cognitive performance, which in turn were related to reduced disability. African Americans did not show this mediated relationship. In that group, physical activity was related to cognitive performance, and cognitive performance was related to disability, but physical activity was not directly related to disability. Popa et al.[44] hypothesize that racial disparities in health may result in less physiologic reserve capacity among African American older adults, reducing the effect of physical activity on disability. However, both whites and African Americans in their sample showed a positive relation between physical activity and cognition, suggesting that increasing physical activity to improve cognition may be a successful avenue for reducing disability and dependence in IADLs.

In a recent study of exercise and cognition in aging, Anderson-Hanley et al.[2] investigated the benefits of "exergames" in promoting exercise and improving cognitive ability. Exergames are exercise activities enhanced by virtual reality; in the Anderson-Hanley study they compared older adults who exercised on typical recumbent bikes to those who exercised on recumbent bikes fitted with three-dimensional (3-D) displays that showed scenery, bike courses, and potential competing cyclists. Although both groups improved their cognitive EF skills after the 3-month intervention, the virtual reality cyclists improved significantly more than did the group exercising with typical bikes. Interestingly, this difference could not be accounted for by differences in exercise frequency, intensity, or duration between groups because no such differences were observed. The authors suggest three possible accounts of the group differences in outcome. The first is that the virtual reality group actually experienced cognitive training in addition to physical exercise.

That is, the virtual reality display involved riders navigating a route, anticipating changes in direction or elevation, and competing with other riders on the course. Managing these additional cognitive demands may have functioned as "cognitive training" in a manner that was not anticipated by the investigators. A second, related account offered by the authors is that there may be some synergism or interaction between physical and cognitive exercise that produced the greater improvement in EF performance. And, finally, the investigators also observed a greater increase in brain-derived neurotropic growth factor (BDNF) among the group cycling in the virtual reality environment. BDNF is a biomarker that may indicate brain plasticity, and has been shown in previous studies to be associated with cognitive improvements following exercise. All three of these accounts are speculative at present, but point to some intriguing avenues for future research.

Another physiologic mechanism that has been hypothesized to underlie exercise effects on EF is heart-rate variability (HRV). HRV has been shown to be related to EF,[25] and both HRV and EF are associated with brain activity in the prefrontal cortex. Thus, it may be that HRV could serve as a measure of neural functioning that would in turn be reflected in EF. Albinet et al.[1] investigated this question in a 12-week intervention study comparing an aerobic exercise program to a stretching program. The outcome measure of interest was the Wisconsin Card Sorting Test (WCST), which requires shifting between stimulus dimensions, inhibiting irrelevant information, and updating the contents of working memory, all processes associated with EF. Following the intervention, members of the aerobic exercise group improved their WCST performance more than did those in the stretching group, and also increased their HRV. The authors conclude that these findings are consistent with the model of Thayer and colleagues,[1] positing a "unified structural and functional network linking HRV, prefrontal neural structures, and psychological processes such as executive functioning" (p. 622). Understanding the mechanism of the exercise/EF relation is important because it paves the way for developing effective interventions. If we understand how the physiologic, cognitive, and functional levels interact, we can intervene in ways that take advantage of these interventions and maximize the chances for positive outcomes.

In addition to exercise studies, other approaches have examined reciprocal relations between cognitive status and motor function as these abilities change over time, without intervention. For example, changes in walking speed have been reported to parallel changes in cognition,[45] and baseline EF has been shown to predict 3-year changes in walking speed.[3] Baseline walking speed has also been shown to be related to subsequent cognitive decline.[29] Liu-Ambrose et al.[35] reported an intervention study that used resistance training and stretching and toning exercises to improve gait speed. They also measured EF, using tasks assessing shifting, updating, and inhibition. They found that improvements in the inhibition component of EF were significantly associated with improvements in gait speed. The authors suggest that interventions designed to address EF in addition to physical functions may improve gait speed to a greater extent than those that target only one or the other.

Interestingly, Kuo et al.[33] had earlier suggested a mechanism to account for the observed relationship between cognition and motor function that would support the Liu-Ambrose[35] suggestion about maximally effective interventions. Kuo et al.[33] noted that pathways between cortical frontal regions and subcortical regions support both cognition for EF and gait and balance. Age- or disease-related damage to these pathways may affect both cognitive and motor function. In addition, interventions to improve EF may also affect motor function, and in so doing provide additional means for improving independence in functional tasks.

Overall, studies have suggested that older adults who engage in more physical activity or exercise show better performance on EF tests.* Even though there is not yet sufficient evidence to prescribe the dosage and intensity of exercise needed or determine what types of exercise programs are more beneficial to improve EF,[49] occupational therapists should recommend physically active lifestyles and regular exercise for older adults at risk of functional impairment. Physical activity appears to be a significant positive contributor to EF, which appears to have a critical role in independence, quality of life, and well-being of community-dwelling older adults.

Social Engagement Interventions to Improve Executive Function

A very different approach to improving EF is given by social engagement interventions. Instead of tightly controlled experimental designs, these approaches take advantage of real-life programs that promote cognitive and social engagement instead of explicit training activities. For example, Fried and colleagues[22] employed an intervention called Experience Corps® in an effort to promote healthy aging. Older adults volunteered their time in public grade schools, assisting with reading, library activities, and problem-solving abilities in children, along with promoting student attendance. These roles were designed to improve health by increasing physical activity, social engagement, and cognitive stimulation among the older volunteers. In particular, to have an effect on cognitive ability, volunteers participated in a 2-week, 30-hour training program that addressed each of the domains of involvement just listed. Each domain addressed different aspects of cognitive function, and switching between domains was assumed to increase mental flexibility and coordination. However, in this initial feasibility study the hypothesis under study related to cognition was only that study participation would not decrease cognitive activity outside of volunteer hours. Measures of books read per month and time spent in moderate- or high-intensity cognitive activity were not different before and after the school year in which participants volunteered. The authors did report that number of hours

spent watching television decreased for the volunteers relative to a comparison group that reported an increase in hours watched during this same time period. Volunteers also reported increased social activity and physical activity as a result of study participation, suggesting that an approach like Experience Corps may indeed be a fruitful one for promoting health among older adults.

Following the feasibility study of Fried et al.,[22] a larger study of Experience Corps[14] was undertaken. Older adult participants were randomized to either Experience Corps or a wait list control group. Participants in the intervention group volunteered in elementary schools as described previously. This study also included neuropsychological measures of EF; performance was compared before and after the volunteer experience. Results indicated that for those with impaired EF at the outset, the volunteer experience significantly improved performance on the EF measures. For those who were unimpaired at baseline, the volunteer experience did not affect performance on these EF tasks. Thus participating in Experience Corps has a positive effect on EF among older adults with impaired function, indicating significant potential for helping those who may be in most need of support.

Carlson and colleagues[12] have also examined the effect of Experience Corps on brain function, using functional magnetic resonance imaging (fMRI) to compare change in brain activity in a small number of Experience Corps participants with that of a group of matched controls. They also assessed EF using the Flanker Task, which is a speeded task requiring inhibition of irrelevant information. Carlson et al. reported improvements in inhibitory function on the Flanker Task in older adults who had participated in Experience Corps, but not in the comparison group, indicating that Experience Corps had a significant and positive effect on the inhibition aspect of EF. In addition, the Experience Corps group showed a significant increase in brain activity in the areas associated with EF on the Flanker Task (left and right dorsal lateral prefrontal cortex, the ventral lateral prefrontal cortex, and the anterior cingulate cortex). Together, these data suggest that "cognitive activity embedded within social settings" (p. 1280)[12] like that involved in Experience Corps may benefit older adults and reduce the risk of cognitive decline. Many questions remain, however, such as the intervention "dose" required to maximize benefits, whether individual difference variables other than initial EF affect the magnitude of the intervention effect (such as health status or physical abilities), and how long positive intervention effects are maintained once the Experience Corps activities are completed. Even so, the fact that the Experience Corps activity is "generative in giving meaning and purpose to one's life" (p. 1280)[12] may give it and similar interventions a motivational advantage in terms of engendering a sustained commitment to activity that can support healthy cognitive aging.

Another example of an engagement intervention is given by the work of Stine-Morrow and colleagues,[51] who adapted the Odyssey of the Mind program to engage older adults in cognitive and social activities with an eye toward preventing decline and maintaining or improving functional status.

---

*References 8, 13, 18, 20, 27, 41, and 45.

Odyssey of the Mind is a team-based activity; teams spend months working on a solution to a selected problem from science, literature, history, or engineering. Solutions are presented in an organized tournament competition that also includes on-the-spot problem-solving challenges. Stine-Morrow et al.'s[51] adaptation, called Senior Odyssey, allowed teams to choose the problem they would like to work on from among the domains just listed. According to Stine-Morrow et al.,[51] teams might be challenged to use balsa wood to design something to support a certain amount of weight, or to create and present a performance representing a well-known work from literature or event from history. Thus, there was no single solution to a given problem, and solutions could be revised and developed over time up until the time of the competition.

"Working toward the presentation of a solution to a long-term problem engages many basic cognitive skills in a creative and collaborative context" (p. 780); Stine-Morrow et al.[51] hypothesized that this work would lead to improved cognitive outcomes among participants. They put together a battery of cognitive tasks, some of which assessed EF, and administered them before and after the Senior Odyssey experience. Findings indicated a small but significant effect of Senior Odyssey participation on cognitive function; those in the Senior Odyssey program improved their cognitive scores more than those in the comparison group who did not participate. Like the Experience Corps study described earlier, the experience of Senior Odyssey was observed to positively affect cognitive performance, even without any explicit training of cognitive function.

The findings from Senior Odyssey and Experience Corps are an interesting parallel to functional activities that have become the hallmark of OT interventions. That is, rather than explicitly training a cognitive function through the repetitive and context-free practice of that function, these approaches provide a vehicle for improving cognition through an individual's behavior in context. The power of these approaches lies in their ability to sustain the motivation of the individual to participate in the "intervention," and also in their ability to achieve corollary goals such as improved self-efficacy and social support. Although their effects on functional status are yet unknown, these strengths would seem to merit further experimentation to assess their influence (Box 14-1).

BOX 14-1 **Combined Interventions for Executive Function: A Model Program**

The American Stroke Foundation (ASF) provides community-based wellness programs for stroke survivors in the Kansas City metropolitan area. Stroke survivors come to an ASF center several times a week to work on cognition, physical fitness, speech, and daily activities. The center becomes a home away from home for the survivors, resulting in a social context similar to that described by Carlson et al.[12] and Stine-Morrow et al.[51] The ASF is also an ecological learning laboratory for students in the area and from around the country. Level II occupational therapy (OT) students, from six OT programs, spend their 3-month fieldwork there; first- and second-year physical therapy students come with their department chairperson from a local university to teach a balance class; speech students from that same university volunteer two mornings a week to work with people with aphasia; and social work students spend their foundation year (first year of the master of social work program) at the center learning about stroke and community resources.

The program director at the ASF is an occupational therapist with many years of experience in university teaching. It is with her help that the OT students become the glue that makes the program a whole, because they are full-time workers for their 3-month experience and because the schedule of the center is in their hands. Along with a music therapist and a volunteer speech pathologist, these students work together to plan sessions that stretch the stroke survivors physically, cognitively, and socially. The students elicit ideas for classes and for off-site experiences from the stroke survivors. Some of those off-site experiences have included tours of a local brewery, lunch at a local Italian restaurant, and picnics and fishing trips to local parks.

The OT part of the program provides many activities to challenge the survivors both cognitively and physically. The group plays many different and unusual board games, some of which require no language (e.g., Qwirkle), and physical games that require motor planning, such as ladder golf or tarp Minesweeper (the game Minesweeper is played on a large gridded tarp). They also engage in many everyday activities such as cooking or simply eating a lunch that contains many small containers or zipped bags. Survivors have also participated in activities called "Give Back," where survivors plan activities to help other nonprofit organizations and benefit people who are in need (Figure 14-1).

Survivors provide each other with support and fill in for each other's weaknesses. All of these activities affect the survivors' cognitive and executive function. Carlson et al.[12] suggest that cognitive activity embedded within social settings may prevent cognitive decline, whereas others suggest that it may even improve cognition.[51] Anecdotal and preliminary empirical data suggest that improved cognition is also observable among ASF participants. As occupational therapists begin to develop sound performance-based assessments of EF to study the role of functional activity in supporting and improving cognitive function, evidence-based intervention design is not far behind.

Occupational therapists have tended to focus on acute stroke for many years. It is only recently that the field has begun to acknowledge that it might be beneficial to work with survivors for many years after their strokes. A program that includes fitness and classes that require different amounts of cognitive functioning will likely spell success for stroke survivors who otherwise would probably be sitting at home.

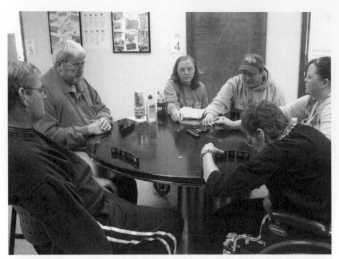

FIGURE 14-1 Participants at American Stroke Foundation Wellness Programs practice tasks that require executive function and cognition, fine motor abilities, and speech, while at the same time enjoying social support and camaraderie.

Summary

In summary, the literature on cognition and functional status indicates that EF is an important ability underlying successful ADL. The potential for intervening to improve EF and thus increase capacity for independence among older adults is great; a variety of intervention approaches has been presented here. The social engagement intervention approaches seem most consistent with occupational therapy, but the effect on daily life needs to be better articulated and supported by additional evidence. In addition, more work needs to be done to precisely specify the most beneficial approach for groups and individuals. The influence of this additional work will be broad and substantial; as the numbers of older Americans continue to grow, so will the costs of care unless reliable methods are identified to prevent disability and promote independence in the aging community.

CASE EXAMPLE 14-1   Phyllis

Phyllis is an 84-year-old widow and had been living by herself in her own home. She enjoyed watching television, playing solitaire on her computer, cooking, and gardening. She handled her own finances and prepared her own taxes. She drove and went to the movies with a neighbor and theater with her friends.

Things changed after Phyllis had a fall and fractured her ankle. The cause of the fall was not diagnosed by her physician, but it may have been due to seizure activity or a minor stroke. After the ankle fracture, it was necessary for Phyllis to have a caregiver come to her home for several hours a day. It seemed that cognitively she was not quite right. She had a lot of trouble maneuvering with her ankle brace and a walker, and she was unable to rise from the couch or toilet, which seemed odd because she had only fractured her ankle.

After 6 weeks her ankle brace was removed, and she was able to walk six houses down the block and did routinely get the mail. However, her cognition declined to a point where she could not be left alone. For example, she could not get to the bathroom on her own reliably. She could plan meals but couldn't organize the necessary steps

and had difficulty executing the plan. She made mistakes when paying bills and banking, and was easily distracted when trying to complete tasks. Her family arranged for 12-hour-a-day caregiving, but Phyllis was not happy with that. After several more weeks, her family placed her in an assisted living facility.

At that time the Mini-Mental Status Exam (MMSE) was performed, she scored in the normal range and so was considered "independent," and she received only minimal assistance. At this point she got herself to meals and did her laundry. She was able to use the TV, to record shows and watch recorded shows as was her custom, but became overwhelmed when trying to learn how to use the tablet computer that her daughter bought her for her birthday, thinking she might enjoy playing solitaire again or using email. She was unable to learn how to turn the tablet on and could not seem to get to the program even though it only required touching the screen to launch the app. She had a dog at the facility and became less and less able to care for her, not letting her out often enough. She does not participate in any of the activities at the assisted living facility.

REVIEW QUESTIONS

1. Why is understanding EF important for delivering OT services to older adults?
2. What are the concepts and components of EF?
3. How is EF related to functional status among older adults? How strong is the evidence supporting the relationship?
4. Which approaches and assessment tools fit best with OT services and your setting?
5. What intervention strategies are applicable to OT services and your setting?

REFERENCES

1. Albinet, C. T., Boucard, G., Bouquet, C. A., & Audiffren, M. (2010). Increased heart rate variability and executive performance after aerobic training in the elderly. *European Journal of Applied Physiology, 109*, 617–624. doi: 10.1007/c00421-010-1393-y.
2. Anderson-Hanley, C., Aciero, P. J., Brickman, A. M., Nimon, J. P., Okuma, N., Westen, S. C., & Zimmerman, E. A. (2012). Exergaming and older adult cognition: A cluster randomized clinical trial. *American Journal of Preventive Medicine, 42*(2), 109–119. doi: 10.1016/j.amepre.2011.10.016.

3. Atkinson, H., Rosano, C., Simonsick, E., et al. (2007). Cognitive function, gait speed decline, and comorbidities: The health, aging, and body composition study. *Journal of Gerontology: Medical Sciences, 62,* 844–850.

4. Basak, C., Boot, W. R., Voss, M. W., & Kramer, A. F. (2008). Can training in a real-time strategy video game attenuate cognitive decline in older adults? *Psychology and Aging, 23,* 765–777.

5. Baum, C. M., Morrison, T., Hahn, M., & Edwards, D. F. (2003). *Test manual: Executive Function Performance Test.* St. Louis, MO: Washington University.

6. Baum, C. M., Perlmutter, M., & Edwards, D. F. (2000). Measuring function in Alzheimer's disease. *Alzheimer's Care Quarterly, 1*(3), 44–66.

7. Bell-McGinty, S., Podell, K., Franzen, M., Baird, A. D., & Williams, M. J. (2002). Standard measures of executive function in predicting instrumental activities of daily living in older adults. *International Journal of Geriatric Psychiatry, 17*(9), 828–834.

8. Ble, A., Volpato, S., Zuliani, G., Guralnik, J. M., Bandinelli, S., Lauretani, F., et al. (2005). Executive function correlates with walking speed in older persons: The InCHIANTI study. *Journal of the American Geriatrics Society, 53,* 410–415.

9. Braver, T. S., Barch, D. M., Keys, B. A., Carter, C. S., Cohen, J. D., Kaye, J. A., et al. (2001). Context processing in older adults: Evidence for a theory relating cognitive control to neurobiology in healthy aging. *Journal of Experimental Psychology: General, 130,* 746–763.

10. Burgess, P. W. (1997). Theory and methodology in executive function research. In P. Rabbitt (Ed.), *Methodology of frontal and executive function* (pp. 81–116). East Sussex: UK: Psychology Press Ltd.

11. Cahn-Weiner, D. A., Malloy, P. F., Boyle, P. A., Marran, M., & Salloway, S. (2000). Prediction of functional status from neuropsychological tests in community-dwelling elderly individuals. *Clinical Neuropsychologist, 14*(2), 187–195.

12. Carlson, M. C., Erickson, K. I., Dramer, A. F., Voss, M. W., Bolea, N., Nielke, M., et al. (2009). Evidence for neurocognitive plasticity in at-risk older adults: The Experience Corps Program. *Journal of Gerontology Series A: Biological Sciences and Medical Sciences, 64*(12), 1275–1282. doi: 10.1093/gerona/glp117.

13. Carlson, M. C., Fried, L. P., Xue, Q. L., Bandeen-Roche, K., Zeger, S. L., & Brandt, J. (1999). Association between executive attention and physical functional performance in community-dwelling older women. *Journal of Gerontology Social Sciences, 54*(5), S262–270.

14. Carlson, M. C., Saczynski, J. S., Rebok, G. W., et al. (2008). Exploring the effects of an "everyday" activity program on executive function and memory in older adults: Experience Corps. *Gerontologist, 48*(6), 793–801.

15. Chan, R. C. K., Shum, D., Toulopoulou, T., & Chen, E. Y. H. (2008). Assessment of executive functions: review of instruments and identification of critical issues. *Archives of Clinical Neuropsychology, 23,* 201–215.

16. Colcombe, S., & Kramer, A. (2003). Fitness effects on the cognitive function of older adults. *Psychological Science, 14,* 125–130.

17. Connor, L. T., & Maeir, A. (2011). Putting executive performance in a theoretical context. *OTJR: Occupation, Participation and Health [Suppl.], 31*(1), S3–S7. doi: 10.3928/15394492-20101108-02.

18. Coppin, A. K., Ferrucci, L., Lauretani, F., Phillips, C., Chang, M., & Bandinelli, S., et al. (2006). Low socioeconomic status and disability in old age: Evidence from the InCHIANTI study for the mediating role of physiological impairments. *Journals of Gerontology Series A: Biological Sciences and Medical Sciences, 61*(1), 86–91.

19. Craik, F. I. M., & Bialystok, E. (2006). Planning and task management in older adults: Cooking breakfast. *Memory and Cognition, 34,* 1236–1249.

20. Eggermont, L. H., Milberg, W. P., Lipsitz, L. A., Scherder, E. J., & Leveille, S. G. (2009). Physical activity and executive function in aging: The MOBILIZE Boston Study. *Journal of the American Geriatrics Society, 57*(10), 1750–1756. doi: 10.1111/j.1532-5415.2009.02441.x.

21. Fitzgerald, S., & Baum, C. (2012). Executive functions. In L. M. Carey (Ed.), *Stroke rehabilitation: Insights from neuroscience and imaging* (pp. 208–221). New York, NY: Oxford University Press.

22. Fried, L. P., Carlson, M. S., Freedman, M., et al. (2004). A social model for health promotion for an aging population: Initial evidence on the Experience Corps model. *Journal of Urban Health, 81*(1), 64–78.

23. Friedman, N. P., & Miyake, A. (2004). The relations among inhibition and interference control functions: A latent-variable analysis. *Journal of Experimental Psychology: General, 133*(1), 101–135.

24. Grigsby, J., Kaye, K., Baxter, J., Shetterly, S., & Hamman, R. (1998). Executive cognitive abilities and functional status among community-dwelling older persons in the San Luis Valley health and aging study. *Journal of the American Geriatrics Society, 46*(5), 590–596.

25. Hansen, A. L., Johnsen, B. H., & Thayer, J. E. (2003). Vagal influence on working memory and attention. *International Journal of Psychophysiology, 48,* 263–274.

26. Hartman-Maier, A., Harel, H., & Katz, N. (2009). Kettle Test—a brief measure of cognitive functional performance: Reliability and validity in stroke rehabilitation. *American Journal of Occupational Therapy, 63,* 592–599.

27. Holtzer, R., Verghese, J., Xue, X., & Lipton, R. B. (2006). Cognitive processes related to gait velocity: Results from the Einstein Aging Study. *Neuropsychology, 20*(2), 215–223. doi: 10.1037/0894-4105.20.2.215.

28. Hull, R., Martin, R. C., Beier, M. E., Lane, D., & Hamilton, A. C. (2008). Executive function in older adults: A structural equation modeling approach. *Neuropsychology, 22*(4), 508–522. doi: 10.1037/0894-4105.22.4.508.

29. Inzitari, M., Baldereschi, M., Di Carlo, A., Di Bari, M., Marchionni, N., & Scafato, E., et al. (2007). Impaired attention predicts motor performance decline in older community-dwellers with normal baseline mobility: Results from the Italian Longitudinal Study on Aging (ILSA). *Journal of Gerontology Series A: Medical Sciences, 62,* 837–843.

30. Jefferson, A. L., Paul, R. H., Ozonoff, A., & Cohen, R. A. (2006). Evaluating elements of executive functioning as predictors of instrumental activities of daily living (IADLs). *Archives of Clinical Neuropsychology, 21*(4), 311–320.

31. Johnson, J., Lui, L., & Yaffe, K. (2007). Executive function, more than global cognition, predicts functional decline and mortality in elderly women. *Journal of Gerontology Series A: Biological Sciences and Medical Sciences, 62*(10), 1134–1141.

32. Jurado, M., & Rosselli, M. (2007). The elusive nature of executive functions: A review of our current understanding. *Neuropsychology Review, 17*(3), 213–233.

33. Kuo, H., Jones, R., Milberg, W., Tennstedt, S., Talbot, L., & Morris, J., et al. (2005). Effect of blood pressure and diabetes mellitus on cognitive and physical functions in older adults: A longitudinal analysis of the Advanced Cognitive Training for Independent and Vital Elderly cohort. *Journal of the American Geriatrics Society, 53*, 1154–1161.

34. Lezak, M. D., Howieson, D., & Loring, D. W. (2004). *Neuropsychological assessment*. New York, NY: Oxford University Press.

35. Liu-Ambrose, T., Davis, J. C., Nagamatsu, L. S., Hsu, C. L., Katarynych, L. A., & Khan, K. M. (2010). Changes in executive functions and self-efficacy are independently associated with improved usual gait speed in older women. *BMC Geriatrics, 10*, 25. doi: 10.1186/147-2318-10-25.

36. Loeb, P. A. (1996). *ILS: Independent Living Scales manual*. San Antonio, TX: Psychological Corporation, Harcourt Brace Jovanovich.

37. McGuire, L. C., Ford, E. S., & Ajani, U. A. (2006). Cognitive functioning as a predictor of functional disability in later life. *American Journal of Geriatric Psychiatry, 14*(1), 36–42.

38. Microsoft Game Studios. (2004). *Rise of nations: Gold edition*. [Video game]. Redmond, WA: Microsoft Corp.

39. Mitchell, M., & Miller, L. S. (2008). Prediction of functional status: The ecological validity of four Delis Kaplan Executive Function System tests. *Journal of Clinical and Experimental Neuropsychology, 30*(6), 683–690.

40. Miyake, A., Friedman, N. P., Emerson, M. J., Witzki, A. H., Howerter, A., & Wager, T. D. (2000). The unity and diversity of executive functions and their contributions to complex "frontal lobe" tasks: A latent variable analysis. *Cognitive Psychology, 41*, 49–100.

41. Nieto, M. L., Albert, S. M., Morrow, L. A., & Saxton, J. (2008). Cognitive status and physical function in older African Americans. *Journal of the American Geriatrics Society, 56*(11), 2014–2019. doi: 10.1111/j.1532-5415.2008.01938.x.

42. Nouchi, R., Taki, Y., Takeuchi, H., Hashizume, H., Akitsuki, Y., & Shigemune, Y., et al. (2012). Brain training game improves executive functions and processing speed in the elderly: A randomized controlled trial. *PLoS One, 7*(1), e29676. doi: 10.1371/journal.pone.0029676.

43. Pereira, F. S., Yassuda, M. S., Olieeira, A. M., & Forlenza, O. V. (2008). Executive dysfunction correlates with impaired functional status in older adults with varying degrees of cognitive impairment. *International Psychogeriatrics, 20*(6), 1104–1115. doi: 10.1017/S1041610208007631.

44. Popa, M., Reynolds, S., & Small, B. (2009). Is the effect of reported physical activity on disability mediated by cognitive performance in white and African American older adults? *Journal of Gerontology Series B: Psychological Sciences, 64*, 4–13.

45. Rosano, C., Simonsick, E. M., Harris, T. B., et al. (2005). Association between physical and cognitive function in healthy elderly: The Health, Aging and Body Composition Study. *Neuroepidemiology, 24*, 8–14.

46. Royall, D. R., Palmer, R., Chiodo, L. K., & Polk, M. J. (2004). Declining executive control in normal aging predicts change in functional status: The Freedom House Study. *Journal of American Geriatrics Society, 52*(3), 346–352.

47. Salthouse, T. A., Atkinson, T. M., & Berish, D. E. (2003). Executive functioning as a potential mediator of age-related cognitive decline in normal adults. *Journal of Experimental Psychology: General, 132*, 566–694.

48. Shallice T., & Burgess, P. W. (1991). Deficits in strategy application following frontal lobe damage in man. *Brain, 114*, 727–741.

49. Snowden M., Steinman, L., Mochan, K., Grodstein, F., Prohaska, T. R., Thurman, D. J., et al. (2011). Effect of exercise on cognitive performance in community-dwelling older adults: Review of intervention trials and recommendations for public health practice and research. *Journal of the American Geriatrics Society, 59*(4), 704–716. doi: 10.1111/j.1532-5415.2011.03323.x.

50. Spreen, O., & Strauss, E. (1998). *A compendium of neuropsychological tests* (2nd ed.). New York, NY: Oxford University Press.

51. Stine-Morrow, E. A., Parisi, J. M., Morrow, D. G., & Park, D. C. (2008). The effects of an engaged lifestyle on cognitive vitality: A field experiment. *Psychology and Aging, 23*, 778–786.

52. Vaughan, L., & Giovanello, K. (2010). Executive function in daily life: Age-related influences of executive processes on instrumental activities of daily living. *Psychology and Aging, 25*(2), 343–355.

53. Wang, M-Y., Chang, C-Y., & Su, S-Y. (2011). What's cooking? Cognitive training of executive function in the elderly. *Frontiers in Psychology (Cognition), 2*, 228. doi: 10.3389/fpsyg.2011.00228.

54. Williams, K., & Kemper, S. (2010). Exploring interventions to reduce cognitive decline in aging. *Journal of Psychosocial Nursing and Mental Health Services, 48*(5), 42–51. doi: 10.3928/02793695-2010331-03.

55. World Health Organization. (2000). *International classification of functioning, disability and health*. Geneva, Switzerland: Author.

CHAPTER 15

Cognitive Impairment, Dementia, and Occupational Therapy Interventions

Cindy Kempf, MA, OTR/L, Lauren R. Schwarz, PhD, ABPP-CN, Abhilash K. Desai, MD, Margaret A. Perkinson, PhD

CHAPTER OUTLINE

OBJECTIVES

- Define cognition
- Identify the effects of aging on cognition and identify atypical cognitive deficits in the older adult, with an emphasis on dementia
- Analyze the effects of cognitive impairment and dementia on occupational performance
- Identify assessment tools that can be used to evaluate cognitive impairment and dementia in the older adult
- Describe treatment options to help clients compensate for cognitive deficits
- Analyze case studies and suggest appropriate assessments, treatment approaches, and goals for clients with cognitive deficits and their family caregivers

In the United States the older adult population, those 65 years and older, is comprised of approximately 35 million individuals, a demographic that is projected to grow to over 70 million by the year 2030.[26] With the rising numbers of older adults, the identification and treatment of diseases that affect this population will assume significant importance and will affect health-care systems/providers, clients, and families. One such issue that affects older adults, and is the focus of the present chapter, is cognitive decline. Declining memory and other changes in cognition are common with age. This topic has been extensively researched, but perhaps initially dates back to the writing of V. A. Kral, who proposed that developmental changes in cognition can be divided up into those that are "benign" (or typical) and those that are "malignant" (or atypical).[33,34] To identify and intervene, it is essential for clinicians and researchers to have adequate knowledge of the continuum of cognitive aging, potential etiologies of cognitive change, and various treatments. Cognitive abilities are particularly relevant for occupational therapists, because they affect individuals' abilities to successfully complete activities of daily living (ADLs).

CASE EXAMPLE 15-1   Introduction to Cognitive Deficits in the Older Adult

Meet Ruth, an aging individual whose daily routine will provide a foundation for understanding the everyday translation of cognitive decline and how it affects occupational performance.

Ruth had recently moved into an independent living apartment complex for older adults due to increasing difficulty taking care of her large home. She had been living alone for the past 2 years since her husband's death, and Ruth's daughter observed that Ruth was having more difficulty keeping up with the housework and laundry and thought that it was because the house was too large. Ruth had always been a very social person but had recently stopped going out with friends because she said she was too tired. Ruth was an artist, and her watercolors could be found in the art galleries in her home town. However, she was no longer painting, despite the fact that she had multiple half-finished projects in the art room at her home.

In her new apartment, Ruth was able to take the facility van to the grocery store and she received two meals a day. However, her daughter found that Ruth was still too fatigued to participate in activities in the apartment complex or to clean her apartment. She took Ruth to the doctor and she received an order for occupational therapy to assess functional abilities. When the occupational therapist evaluated Ruth, she found deficits in her ability to initiate tasks. She also had impaired attention span, poor short-term memory, and moderately impaired problem-solving skills. She wore the same clothes over and over because she was overwhelmed by the amount of clothes in her overstuffed closet. Ruth hadn't showered because she couldn't figure out how to adjust the water in the shower. In her refrigerator, she had many containers of food from the dining room but couldn't determine which food was too old to eat and should be thrown away. She was not participating in facility activities because the monthly schedule was too complicated for her to follow. Finally, in her art room, her art supplies were scattered throughout the room, making them difficult to find, and Ruth was overwhelmed by the number of pictures that she had started but not finished. It was clear to the occupational therapist that Ruth's cognitive deficits were affecting her occupational performance.

Cognition, as defined by Abreu and Toglia,[1] is the method that the central nervous system uses to process and utilize information. It is the outcome of an ongoing dynamic interaction between person, activity, and the environment.[9] The ability to complete everyday tasks involves multiple cognitive skills. For example, when a client participates in a dressing task, his or her clothing selection is based on the knowledge of weather conditions, scheduled activities for the day, and an awareness of which clothes coordinate with others. The client has to sequence the dressing tasks and use problem-solving skills to compensate for any deficits. If the client has impaired balance, for example, he or she client may choose to dress from a seated position when putting on pants rather than attempting to don pants while standing.

Occupational therapy (OT) practitioners, through the use of occupation and activities, help people optimize their cognitive functioning skills. Cognitive skills impact all functional skills across the life course. Changes in cognition can be temporary or permanent, progressive or unchanging, demonstrated by sudden onset or caused by a gradual decline in cognitive ability. OT theory and research support the principle that cognition is essential to the performance of everyday tasks.[9,55]

Prevalence Rates of Dementia and Diagnoses with Cognitive Deficits

The prevalence of dementia in the United States in those individuals over the age of 71 years is 13.9%.[47] This number further increases with age, from 5.0% of those aged 71 to 79 years to 37.4% of individuals over the age of 90 years.[47] Alzheimer's disease (AD), vascular dementia (VaD), frontotemporal dementia (FTD), Parkinson's disease dementia (PDD), and Lewy

body dementia (sometimes referred to as dementia with Lewy bodies) (DLB) compromise approximately 90% of all diagnosed dementias.[27] Of this group, AD is the most common cause of dementia (50%), followed by mixed dementia (Alzheimer's with either vascular or Lewy body dementia) (20%) and vascular dementia (VaD) (10%).[27] For those individuals whose cognitive functioning is not intact, but do not meet dementia criteria, various categorizations have been proposed. More recently, the term mild cognitive impairment (MCI) is commonly used. For those diagnosed with MCI, Petersen et al. found that 12% convert to an AD diagnosis annually.[46]

In addition to working with clients with dementia, OT can benefit those with cognitive deficits caused by other diseases, such as Parkinson's, cerebrovascular accident (CVA), traumatic brain injury (TBI), and other neurological conditions. According to the Rotterdam study published in 2004, the incidence of parkinsonism increases with age, and incidence rates for Parkinson's disease are 0.3 per 1000 persons for adults 55 to 65 years of age and 4.4. per 1000 persons for adults over the age of 85 years.[17] Estimates by the National Institutes of Health Consensus Development Panel on Rehabilitation of Persons with TBI note that there are 5.3 million Americans living with TBI-related disabilities, including cognitive deficits.[14]

Types of Dementia from a Cognitive Perspective

To differentiate the various dementias, one must have a good grasp of the normal changes in cognition that accompany advancing age. Age-related cognitive decline (ARCD) involves subtle decline in many cognitive abilities, such as decline in episodic memory, reduced capacity to pay attention, and need for more time to do complex activities.[10,50] Individuals with ARCD may or may not have subjective memory complaints and objective cognitive deficits, and their ability to live independently is not compromised.[49] The mechanisms of cognitive aging have been extensively researched by cognitive aging psychologists for many years. Park and Schwarz[43] note that four main mechanisms have been hypothesized to underlie the age-related differences in cognition: reduced speed of processing, decreased working memory capabilities, declining inhibitory control (e.g., impaired complex attentional capabilities), and sensory changes (e.g., visual and auditory deficits). Not all older adults experience ARCD. Some older adults experience little or no ARCD, remain highly functional in their later years, and continue to be actively engaged in life well into very old age.[50]

Changes associated with MCI dementia are beyond what one would expect for the normal aging process. Although not entirely consistent across research investigations, specific neurocognitive deficits have been associated with MCI, AD, VaD, and FTD. In individuals with amnestic-type MCI, one of the earliest areas to decline is learning and memory in the context of well-preserved other abilities.[32] As previously mentioned, each year a percentage of those with MCI will progress to meeting criteria for a dementia, typically of the Alzheimer's type.[46] The hallmark neurocognitive feature of the disorder is an insidious onset of progressive forgetting. When compared with individuals with normal aging or other forms of dementia:

- When attempting to recall information, individuals with AD receive little benefit from the provision of recognition cues.
- Language functions are also affected and manifest as word-finding or word-naming difficulties.
- As the disease process progresses, other cognitive domains become affected, such as executive functions (e.g., reasoning, planning, problem solving, mental flexibility).

Older adults with age-related cognitive decline may forget where they put their car keys but will usually be able to retrace their steps to find the keys. In contrast, individuals with dementia are unable to use memory and problem-solving skills to locate their keys, and often the keys are not found in a logical location (e.g., they may be found in the freezer). Occasional word-finding problems occur among most older adults. However, a person with dementia has increasing difficulty recalling words and is unable to follow conversations.

The second leading cause of dementia, VaD, can develop as a result of a variety of vascular events (e.g., large- and/or small-vessel ischemic or hemorrhagic damage). The pattern and severity of cognitive dysfunction depend on the location of the damage as well as the size of the affected area. In general, clients with VaD present with the following characteristics:

- Clients with VaD show impaired working memory/attention, slowed speed of processing, and executive dysfunction.[13]
- Regarding memory functioning, clients with VaD typically have difficulties with free recall tasks, but their performances improve when provided with recognition cues. This suggests that the memory impairment

in VaD is retrieval based rather than the rapid forgetting seen in AD (Table 15-1).

Compared with the other dementias previously discussed, FTD has a neurocognitive profile that is less well studied and is less agreed upon.[52] In part this has to do with the low incidence of FTD. However, more important, traditional neuropsychological testing is less sensitive at detecting the hallmark feature of FTD—namely, behavioral change (e.g., changes in personality, personal preferences, judgment, attention to personal hygiene, and so forth). Therefore, clients with FTD may test within the normal range on cognitive measures typically employed when conducting dementia evaluations. When deficits do appear on formal testing, they are likely to be in the areas of executive functioning and word generation (e.g., naming or verbal fluency).[58]

Although the process of differentiating dementias may seem relatively clear, this unfortunately is not always the case, particularly when the question is of AD versus VaD. The explanation for this may lie in the potential overlapping pathologies, such as the following aspects:

- Vascular changes (by contributing to vessel wall thickening) reduce elimination of amyloid through the perivascular (lymphatic) system.
- Vascular changes (hypoxia, hypoperfusion) increase formation of Alzheimer's disease pathology (beta-amyloid and phospho-tau).
- Amyloid angiopathy contributes/accelerates vascular damage.

Another possibility to consider is that the diseases can in some instances be co-occurring (e.g., mixed dementia).

A final comment on the process of differential diagnosis has to do with the severity of the disease process. As the severity of the dementia increases, it becomes difficult to discern a pattern of impairment that is suggestive of a likely etiology due to the global nature of the neurocognitive impairment at such time.

Dementia is a progressive impairment in cognition and ability to reason that substantially interferes with abilities to perform daily activities and live independently and may eventually cause death. Cognition is a combination of skills, including attention, learning, memory, language, praxis, recognition, and executive functions such as decision making, goal setting, planning, and judgment.[30] Recent estimates

TABLE 15-1 Cortical versus Subcortical Dementias

Domain	Subcortical (e.g., vascular dementia)	Cortical (e.g., Alzheimer's disease)
Language	Typically no aphasia	Aphasia early
Memory	Recall < Recognition	Recall = Recognition (both impaired)
Visuospatial	Impaired	Impaired
Frontal/Executive	Disproportionately affected	To some degree affected
Mental Speed	Slow early in the trajectory	Normal until late stage

from the Alzheimer's Association indicate that more than 5 million Americans have AD and related dementias. The report indicates that between 200,000 and 500,000 people younger than 65 years of age have some form of early-onset (young-onset) dementia. This includes FTDs and rare forms of AD that affect people in their 30s, 40s, and 50s.[19]

Thirty percent of individuals with dementia are cared for in a long-term care facility; the other 70% live in their homes in the community.[12] A high proportion of people with dementia (80% to 90%) eventually require placement in a long-term care facility. Approximately 66% to 80% of the residents of long-term care facilities have dementia.[30] Some assisted living facilities (ALFs) and nursing homes are designed for and care exclusively for people with dementia. Accurate diagnosis of dementia, identification of its cause, and initiation of appropriate treatment in individuals with cognitive impairment are critical for improving their quality of life. OT can play a role in helping individuals with dementia to maximize their ability to complete functional tasks through activity analysis, modification of the environment, and simplification of the task, and through training of caregivers to provide appropriate support to individuals with dementia. Intervention can initially take place in an outpatient or home health setting while the client is in the early stages; as the disease progresses, continued therapy is indicated in assisted living and long-term settings to help the client and caregivers adjust to declining cognitive abilities.

The Causes of Dementia

There are many causes of dementia (Table 15-2.) Progressive, irreversible dementias account for more than 90% of all causes of dementia. The relative frequency of AD and VaD increases with age, whereas the relative frequency of FTD and DLB declines with age. Males are overrepresented among those with DLB, whereas females are overrepresented among individuals with AD with age of onset over 70 years.[56]

Probable Alzheimer's Disease

Alzheimer's disease is an age-related irreversible dementia that develops over a period of several years. AD is the most common cause of dementia in people aged 65 years or older, accounting for 60% to 75% of all causes of dementia.[4] Insidious onset and a slow but relentless decline in cognition that impairs ability to perform daily activities are the most striking features of AD. There is no cure for AD. It is estimated that 2% to 5% of people over 65 years of age and up to 33% of those over 85 years of age have AD. More women than men have AD. The longer life expectancy of women as compared with men may be the key factor in the preponderance of women with AD.[4] The loss of the protective effects of estrogen and less testosterone in women than men may also contribute to the increased prevalence of AD in women. (However, women are less likely to have cerebrovascular disease than men, hence their lower incidence of vascular dementia.)

TABLE 15-2 Potential Causes and Mechanisms of Cognitive Impairment

Causes of Cognitive Impairment	Potential Mechanisms of Cognitive Impairment
Age-related cognitive decline	Allostatic load, "wear and tear" due to a lifetime of physiological or psychological stresses and adaptations
Anemia	Neuronal hypoxia
Alzheimer's disease	Amyloid and/or tau-mediated neurotoxicity, neuroinflammation
Lewy body dementia and Parkinson's disease dementia	Alpha synuclein–mediated neurotoxicity, neuroinflammation
Frontotemporal dementia	Ubiquitin or tau-mediated neurotoxicity, neuroinflammation
Cerebrovascular disease	Neuronal ischemia and hypoxia, neuroinflammation
Vitamin deficiencies (e.g., B_1, B_{12}, folate, D)	Impaired neuronal and neurotransmitter function
Protein energy malnutrition	Impaired neuronal function
Drug-induced	Decreased cholinergic neurotransmission
Harmful alcohol use	Direct neurotoxicity and indirectly (e.g., malnutrition, head injury)
Depression, anxiety	Hippocampal dysfunction with or without atrophy
Obstructive sleep apnea	Neuronal hypoxia, neuroinflammation
Head injury	Neuronal and synaptic loss
Normal pressure hydrocephalus	Neuronal and synaptic loss due to enlargement of ventricles
Brain tumor	Direct tumor-cell-mediated neuronal and synaptic loss and/or blockage of cerebrospinal fluid caused by tumor

A definitive diagnosis of AD is possible only after death, during brain autopsy, when the characteristic plaques and tangles can actually be seen under the microscope in specific areas of the brain and correlated with clinical manifestations of AD.

The typical clinical syndrome of AD includes an amnestic type of memory defect, with difficulty learning and recalling new information, and progressive language disorder beginning with anomia and progressing to fluent aphasia.[16] Short-term memory deficit is a classic characteristic, with remote memory remaining intact until the severe stages. Some clients with incipient memory loss are aware of their declining abilities (especially in young-onset [onset before age 60 years] AD), but most clients with evolving AD never acknowledge that they have significant memory dysfunction. It becomes obvious over time to family and friends that persons with incipient dementia routinely forget recent events and conversations and repeat themselves. Behind the forgetfulness that appears benign may be more serious mistakes such as forgotten bills, missed appointments, improperly taken medications, and misdirected travels. Deficits in executive function and disturbances of visual-spatial skills manifested by environmental disorientation are generally absent or mild in early AD but become evident in more advanced stages. Sometimes, anomia (inability to name objects) or visual agnosia (inability to recognize familiar objects) can be nearly as prominent as the anterograde amnesia in AD. Individuals with Down syndrome have a high risk of developing AD by the time they are in their 40s or 50s. A knowledgeable informant should be interviewed because genuine memory failure should be evident to those who are close to the client.

Criteria for Probable Alzheimer's Disease

The diagnosis of AD is made by using criteria established by various authorities, such as the National Institute of Neurological and Communicative Disorders and Stroke and the *Diagnostic and Statistical Manual*, fifth edition (DSM V).[7] Probable AD is determined when a person has the following characteristics:

- Dementia confirmed by clinical and/or neuropsychological examination; problems in at least two areas of cognitive functioning (memory, language [aphasia], praxis [apraxia], recognition [agnosia], and executive function [e.g., impaired judgment])
- Progressive worsening of memory and other cognitive functions
- No disturbance of consciousness
- No other disorders that might account for the dementia

Areas of cognitive impairment besides memory that are typically impaired in people with AD and other dementias include aphasia, agnosia, apraxia, and executive dysfunction.

Executive function skills are the skills that enable individuals to initiate, plan, self-monitor, and correct their approach to goal-directed tasks. (See Chapter 14 for more detail.) Disorders in executive function are often exhibited by deficits in self-control, self-direction, and organization.

According to the Alzheimer's Association, there are 10 signs and symptoms of early dementia:

1. *Memory loss that disrupts daily life.* This may include forgetting recently learned information and important dates or events, and asking for the same information over and over.
2. *Difficulty with planning or problem solving.* Individuals with dementia may have difficulty keeping track of monthly bills, organizing daily schedules, or following a recipe. They may have difficulty attending to a task and become distracted, and may require longer time to complete a task.
3. *Difficulty completing familiar tasks.* Task difficulty may occur at home, at work, or in leisure activities, such as driving to a familiar location or remembering the rules of a favorite game.
4. *Confusion with time or place.* For many older adults, once they retire, the days of the week tend to run together, and they may have occasional difficulties recalling the exact date. However, using a calendar or contextual cues, they are able to determine the date. A person with dementia

may lose track of time and may forget where they are or how they got there.
5. *Trouble understanding visual images and spatial relationships.* Individuals with dementia may have difficulty with depth perception. When they pass a mirror, they may not recognize themselves in the mirror.
6. *New problems with words when speaking or writing.* Individuals with dementia may have difficulty following a conversation, especially if they are in a noisy environment. They may repeat themselves or have word-finding problems or anomias.
7. *Misplacing things and losing the ability to retrace their steps to locate the object.* Individuals with dementia may put things in unusual places and are unable to go back over their steps to find them. They may accuse others of stealing things from them because they can't find the objects.
8. *Decreased or poor judgment.* Individuals with dementia may make poor judgments in regard to money, or a woman who was always well dressed may stop wearing make-up and wear the same clothes over and over again, even though the clothes are torn or dirty.
9. *Withdrawal from work, hobbies, or social activities.* Individuals with dementia may isolate themselves due to difficulty keeping up with conversation or following the rules of their favorite card game.
10. *Changes in mood and personality.* Individuals with dementia can become suspicious, confused, fearful, or anxious, especially when they are in an unfamiliar environment.[5]

The Five Stages of Alzheimer's Disease

There are five stages of dementia due to AD: pre-dementia, mild, moderate, severe, and terminal. The clinical stages (mild, moderate, severe, and terminal) generally span 5 to 8 years on average (range of 2 to 20 years) after diagnosis. The length of survival depends on the age at onset of symptoms (the younger the age, the longer the survival) and comorbid conditions (especially cerebrovascular disease). For clients above the age of 85 years, survival after the onset of dementia may be much shorter (average of 3 years).[4]

Pre-dementia Stage

AD begins in the entorhinal cortex, which is near the hippocampus and has direct connections with it. It then proceeds to the hippocampus, the structure that is essential to the formation of short-term and long-term memories. Affected regions begin to atrophy and show synaptic loss. These brain changes start at least 10 to 20 years before any visible signs and symptoms appear. Memory loss, the first visible sign, is the main feature of the amnestic type of mild cognitive impairment (aMCI). Many experts think aMCI is often an initial, transitional phase between normal brain aging and AD. Change in mood (irritability, depression, anxiety) and personality (passivity) may predate cognitive symptoms by years in people with AD. This stage can last for 10 to 30 years.

In this stage, OT professionals can assess the client's ability to complete tasks such as medication and financial management, and driving ability. Therapy can help the client identify ways to cope with memory loss, such as keeping a notebook to write down important information and the use of a calendar to track all appointments. In the workplace, strategies can be put in place to help with time management and modification of the environment to facilitate ease of completing tasks. Therapy can also help identify those tasks that are too complex for the client to complete without assistance.

Mild AD

As the disease begins to affect the cerebral cortex, memory loss continues, and changes in other cognitive abilities (such as language or praxis) emerge. The clinical diagnosis of AD is usually made during this stage. Signs of mild AD can include memory loss, repetitive statements, taking longer to accomplish normal daily tasks, trouble handling money and paying bills, poor judgment leading to bad decisions, loss of spontaneity and sense of initiative, confusion about the location of familiar places (getting lost begins to occur), mood and personality changes, and increased anxiety. In mild AD, physical abilities do not decline. Thus, the individual seems to be healthy, but is actually having more and more trouble making sense of the world around him or her. At casual glance, these early symptoms can be confused with changes that accompany normal aging. With systematic inquiry, early AD can be reliably diagnosed. Agitation is seen in 20% to 45% of individuals in this stage, especially in the latter half. The prevalence of major depression in this stage may be up to 20%. Depressed mood and sadness may be seen in 50% to 60% of individuals in this stage, and anxiety symptoms are also common. This stage can last for 2 to 10 years.

Often, the client with mild dementia is still living at home but may be beginning to have more difficulty with functional tasks. OT can help the client by structuring ADLs to facilitate successful completion. For example, in the case of Ruth, who was wearing the same clothes every day, the clinician could enlist the assistance of a family member to help Ruth clean out her closet by removing clothes that are torn or that no longer fit. In addition, clothes can be placed together in outfits to ease Ruth's decisions regarding what clothes she will be wearing. A laundry hamper can be placed in the area where Ruth gets undressed at night so that she can place her clothes directly into the laundry hamper so that they can be laundered before she wears them again. At this stage in Ruth's disease process, it would probably be helpful for her daughter to take over financial management. Ruth may be able to still take her medications but might need her daughter to organize the medications in her pillbox to help her identify the medications that she takes in the morning, at noon, and in the evening.

Moderate AD

By the moderate stage, AD-induced cell death has spread further to the areas of the cerebral cortex that control language, reasoning, sensory processing, and conscious thought. More intensive supervision and care become necessary, and many individuals are admitted to a long-term care facility in the latter part of this stage. The symptoms of this stage include increasing memory loss and confusion; shortened attention span; problems recognizing distant friends and family members; difficulty with language; problems with reading, writing, and working with numbers; difficulty organizing thoughts and thinking logically; inability to learn new things or to cope with new or unexpected situations; occasional muscle twitches; loss of impulse control (shown through sloppy table manners, undressing at inappropriate times or places, or vulgar language); and perceptual-motor problems (such as trouble getting out of a chair or setting the table). Stored long-term memories may be relatively spared early in this stage, prompting family members' comments such as, "she remembers what happened a long time ago better than I do."

Behavioral and psychological symptoms of dementia (BPSDs) are often the most disturbing dimension of moderate AD. Individuals with AD evidence more severe BPSDs in the moderate stage compared with the mild stage.[4] The dominant behavioral and psychiatric symptoms in this stage are delusions, depression, anxiety, irritability, and agitation (restlessness, pacing, wandering). Delusions and hallucinations are much more likely in this stage than in mild stage or terminal stage. The incidence of delusions in this stage is reported as 37%, and the incidence of hallucinations is as high as 24%.[4] Paranoid delusions in AD are the most common type of false belief; commonly occurring delusions include "Someone is stealing my belongings" and "My spouse is having an affair." Psychotic symptoms frequently contribute to agitation and aggression. Depression is also seen in this stage and may contribute to physical aggression.[24] The prevalence of major depression is 10% in this stage, whereas the prevalence of depressed mood and sadness is approximately 58%. In moderate AD, depression often coexists with prominent anxiety symptoms. The leading features of depression in the later part of this stage may include inversion of day and night, agitation, and aggression. Aggression occurs in 20% to 30% of individuals in this stage and appears to vary with severity, correlating with frontal lobe dysfunction, decline in ADLs, and greater cognitive impairment. The frequency of agitation is 40% to 55%, and increases in prevalence from the early to later part of this stage. Agitation is associated with shouting, pacing, restlessness, and wandering. Shouting is also associated with the later part of this stage. Inappropriate shouting is a means to communicate emotions and discomfort. Problems of gait and movement in this stage contribute significantly to functional decline. Of individuals with moderate-stage AD, 30% to 60% may develop mild extrapyramidal symptoms such as amimia (inability to use gestures to communicate), bradykinesia, gait impairment, parkinsonism, and paratonic rigidity. Gait apraxia, ascribed to impaired frontal lobe function, occurs with increasing frequency in moderate AD. It includes a constellation of impaired trunk and leg movements, impaired postural reflexes, disequilibrium, dyskinetic movements, and problems with locomotion. Falls are associated with severity of AD; more than one third of individuals with moderate AD experience this problem. The ability to move themselves and other objects is impaired in moderate to severe AD. This stage can last for 1 to 8 years.

CASE EXAMPLE 15-2   Bill

Bill is a 72-year-old male who was previously employed as an accountant. He was diagnosed with Alzheimer's disease 3 years earlier. He is still living at home with his wife but she has become concerned about her ability to manage things at home. Last week while she was taking a shower, Bill left the house without a coat and tried to get into the car so that he could go to work. When his wife took away his keys, he became very agitated. He is having increasing incidents of incontinence and is resistant to showering. In addition, he has had two falls in the last month and is no longer able to dress himself without assistance. When his wife attempts to help him, he becomes upset and yells at her, telling her that he is "not a baby." Bill's physician has referred him for occupational therapy (OT).

OT in the earlier stages of moderate dementia may be done in the home environment through home health. At this point in the disease process, the client will require closer supervision, and the therapist can help train the caregiver to provide assistance for solving problems. For Bill, grooming supplies should be set out in front of him and

clutter should be removed. Through activity analysis, the steps of functional tasks can be broken down, and his wife can be instructed to cue Bill to complete one step at a time. The importance of maintaining a routine is critical in this stage, and the use of a routine will help facilitate independence. A toileting routine could be established, and Bill could be given pull-up-type incontinent briefs to wear instead of underwear. In addition, pants with elastic waistbands, pullover shirts, and slip-on shoes may make it easier for Bill to dress himself. By presenting Bill with one item at a time, Bill will be able to sequence dressing tasks. Adapted equipment such as grab bars in the bathroom and a raised toilet seat may help decrease Bill's fall risk. An alarm can be placed on the doors to the house to alert his wife if he tries to leave unaided. Because he became so upset when his keys were taken away, he could be given a set of "car keys" made from old keys that are no longer used. In addition, his wife can encourage Bill to engage in an activity that he enjoys when she needs to shower or leave Bill unattended for a period of time.

Severe AD

The hallmark of severe AD is profound cognitive impairment. In this stage, which can last for 1 to 4 years, the individual may not even know his or her own name or recognize his or her spouse or children. Verbal ability is restricted to answering yes or no to simple questions. Many clients, even with advanced dementia, will still have some fleeting memory of their loved ones, which can surprise family and staff. A person with dementia (PWD) who has not spoken for months may suddenly respond to his or her spouse's voice. A PWD who has not responded to the spouse's presence may suddenly pick up the spouse's hand, kiss the hand, and say, "love you." These moments of explicit residual continuity with the client's past may be most evident in the mornings after the individual has had a good night's rest. Such moments are also extremely meaningful to the family.

Both urinary and fecal incontinence frequently develop in severe AD. Incontinence is a major factor associated with the decision of caregivers to seek long-term placement.

In clients with severe dementia, OT may focus on positioning the client in a wheelchair with appropriate supports to promote upright posture. From this upright posture, the client will have increased ability to observe the environment. The client may be able to transfer with some assist and will sometimes be able to initiate self-feeding tasks or even simple grooming tasks. The OT professional may recommend the use of finger foods at mealtimes and adapted cups to allow the client to drink with decreased spillage. Often the client has delayed responses, and caregivers should be educated to allow adequate time for the client to respond.

CASE EXAMPLE 15-3   Adele

Adele is a 97-year-old female with dementia. Until recently she has been able to assist with transfers. If finger foods are placed in her hand and tactile cueing is provided, she is sometimes able to bring her hand to her mouth and feed herself. Adele sits in the wheelchair with both upper extremities flexed at the elbow and shoulders adducted. She keeps bilateral hands in a tight fist but she is able to open her hands with assistance. She responds well to the facility dog and will reach down to pet the dog when the dog is brought to her. When her family is present, Adele will smile and laugh, especially when her young great-granddaughter visits. Adele has had two falls in the past week, and staff members want to keep Adele in bed except for meals.

Occupational therapy can position Adele in the wheelchair to help decrease her fall risk. Considerations might be given to the use of a tilt-in-space wheelchair that will allow

her to be positioned at 90 degrees at meals to allow her easier access to the table and facilitate safer swallowing but will allow her to be tilted back in the wheelchair for a change in position and pressure points. A rest schedule should be implemented because it was determined that when Adele fatigues, she falls asleep in the wheelchair and falls forward. She may also benefit from comfort objects that she can manipulate in her hands to help maintain her range of motion and prevent the development of contractures. In addition, activity staff should be encouraged to bring the facility dog to visit Adele because she responds to the dog. Her diet should be changed to a finger-food diet, and she may benefit from a cup with a lid. Staff should be educated to initiate self-feeding when Adele is more alert by placing the finger foods or cup in her hand, and, with tactile cueing, to assist her to bring the food or the cup to her mouth.

End-Stage AD

In the last stage of AD, plaques and tangles are widespread throughout the brain, and large areas of the brain have atrophied further. Persons with dementia in this stage have lost all ability to communicate and are completely dependent on others for care. Other symptoms can include weight loss; seizures; skin infections; difficulty swallowing; groaning, moaning, or grunting; increased sleep; and lack of bladder and bowel control. At the end, clients may be in bed much or all of the time. As bedridden status develops, contractures commonly occur. Myoclonus (i.e., sudden, involuntary jerking), either focal or multifocal, transient or recurrent, may also occur. Even at this stage some individuals with dementia may have emotional moments of relational recollection. But by now all of these individuals are extremely feeble, have limited mobility, and will begin to die of such conditions as sepsis related to incontinence, aspiration pneumonia, or skin ulcer; cardiac arrest; or secondary to minimal oral intake and inanition. At this stage, they are in effect dying, and referral to hospice may be appropriate, especially after a superimposed new medical problem or sudden decline. This stage can last for 2 months to up to 2 years.

During this end-stage, OT can help minimize the risk of pressure ulcer development through positioning in bed and in the wheelchair. Proper positioning at mealtimes can also help to decrease the risk of aspiration. Caregivers or family members can be shown how to complete gentle range-of-motion exercises during ADLs. In addition, caregivers should be shown how to encourage the client's ability to interact with the environment and complete purposeful movements (such as encouraging the client to turn his or her head to the music while asking "Do you hear the music?").

Dementia with Lewy Bodies

Between 15% and 20% of all older-adult cases of dementia reaching autopsy show dementia with Lewy bodies (DLB), making it the most common cause of degenerative dementia after AD.[39] Lewy bodies are round collections of proteins in the brain that are considered a pathological hallmark of DLB. In DLB, Lewy bodies are found in the cortex as well as in an area of the brain stem called the substantia nigra.

The cognitive disorder in DLB may be characterized by prominent anterograde amnesia and may be indistinguishable from AD. In AD the first loss in thinking skills is in memory; in DLB the earliest loss appears to be with attention and visual perception. Hence, DLB has also been described as a visual-perceptual and attentional-executive dementia.[39] Symptoms vary a great deal more from one day to the next than do symptoms of AD. In addition, up to 81% of clients with DLB have unexplained periods of markedly increased confusion that lasts days to weeks and closely mimics delirium. Clients with DLB are typically more apathetic than are individuals with AD. Diagnosis and treatment of DLB is often complicated by a lack of information about the disease. DLB should be considered in clients if spontaneous features of parkinsonism, fully formed visual hallucinations, and fluctuating cognition with pronounced variation in attention and alertness are seen early in the course of dementia. When fluctuating cognition occurs, family or caregivers often describe the individual as "zoned out" or "not with us." Such fluctuation is often mistaken for delirium superimposed on AD. Other symptoms that may help differentiate DLB from AD include daytime drowsiness and lethargy despite getting enough sleep the night before, falling asleep for 2 or more hours during the day, staring into space for long periods and episodes of disorganized speech, rapid-eye-movement (REM) sleep behavior disorder (RBD), recurrent falls, and change in personality early in the course of dementia (especially passivity). RBD is often a precursor of DLB and is present in about half of individuals with DLB.

Cholinergic deficits in DLB occur early and are more widespread compared with those of AD. This may explain some of the clinical differences and somewhat better response to cholinesterase inhibitors (ChEIs) as compared with AD. Persons with DLB are more functionally impaired (due to extrapyramidal motor symptoms) and have more neuropsychiatric difficulties (such as visual hallucinations, seen in 80% of people with DLB) than those with AD with similar cognitive scores. Also, persons with DLB have extreme sensitivity to high-potency antipsychotic medications (e.g., haloperidol, fluphenazine, risperidone), and thus these medications should be avoided due to increased risk of morbidity and mortality.

OT can benefit clients with DLB. Due to the fluctuating nature of this disease, caregivers should be instructed to complete more complex or stressful tasks (such as bathing) when the client is in a period of higher functioning. The environment should be kept clutter free, and caregivers should be instructed to approach the client from the front due to the visual perceptual deficits found in clients with DLB. In addition, simplifying the environment will help reduce fall risk.[57]

Vascular Dementia

VaD is the third most common cause of irreversible dementia and generally occurs with another neurodegenerative process, such as AD or DLB.[31] In individuals with VaD, cognitive impairment is typically abrupt in onset with stepwise deterioration. Cognitive impairment has its onset or dramatic worsening typically in association with a stroke or clear neuroimaging evidence of infarctions. Physical exam reveals neurological signs typical of stroke (focal neurological deficits, motor and reflex asymmetry). Some stroke-related syndromes include the clinical phenotype of anterograde amnesia that is identical to that of AD. Slowing down of mental processing (bradyphrenia) and movement may be an early sign that helps differentiate VaD from AD. Memory function, although impaired in VaD, is not the principal and devastating feature that it is with AD. Impaired judgment, personality changes, frank aphasia, or visuospatial disturbances may predominate either alone or in combination.

Many individuals with VaD also demonstrate parkinsonian symptoms (retropulsion, shuffling gait, loss of postural reflexes) and early urinary incontinence. Depression is more common in VaD compared with its prevalence in AD.

As many as 30% of stroke survivors may have dementia by 6 months after the stroke. The risk of dementia increases ninefold compared with individuals of the same age and sex without a new stroke. There is a remarkably high rate of silent infarcts on imaging, perhaps as high as 20%. Silent infarcts increase the risk of subsequent dementia by 226%. Besides stroke, VaD is also caused by small vessel cerebrovascular disease resulting from either arteriolosclerosis or amyloid angiopathy. Individuals with this type of VaD generally have a subcortical pattern of dementia with psychomotor slowing and relative preservation of naming and other language skills. Magnetic resonance imaging (MRI) of the brain shows obvious evidence of severe cerebrovascular disease. White-matter hyperintensities (WMHs; leukoaraiosis) if severe are associated with three times the risk of subsequent dementia. WMHs are an independent predictor of cognitive decline, even more powerful of an indicator than the presence of lacunar infarcts. Infarcts may involve the hippocampus directly, and subcortical ischemic vascular disease can also affect hippocampal volume. Thus, although the presence of hippocampal atrophy is highly indicative of AD, it cannot be taken as proof that AD is the cause of dementia to the exclusion of VaD. Thus, differentiating VaD from AD through neuropsychological testing or neuroimaging is not as useful as determining the cerebrovascular disease burden in all clients with AD. Pure VaD in people with dementia older than 70 years is rare, and most older clients diagnosed with VaD also have some AD. In younger clients, the possibility of pure VaD is more likely.

OT interventions for clients with vascular dementia typically include interventions used for the treatment of a CVA. The OT professional can address wheelchair positioning, self-care activities, visual-perceptual deficits, mobility impairments, and strength and coordination deficits to help the client maximize functional skills.

Parkinson's Disease Dementia

The typical case of Parkinson's disease dementia (PDD) occurs in a person with well-established Parkinson's disease (8.5 years on average, but by definition Parkinson's disease symptoms should be present for at least 1 year before onset of dementia) who then develops progressive cognitive impairment.[29] The cognitive deficits of individuals with PDD are similar to those in clients with DLB. Rest tremors, hypokinesia (slowed movement), masked facial expression, soft voice (hypophonia), tiny handwriting (micrographia), cogwheel rigidity of the limbs, and gait problems, including asymmetrical or decreased arm swing and abnormal postural reflexes, may be found on neurological examination. Approximately 1.5 million Americans have Parkinson's disease (PD). Up to 80% eventually develop PDD. The pathological hallmark of PD is the collection of Lewy bodies in the substantia nigra (an area in the brain stem). Relatively rare

syndromes of progressive supranuclear palsy (prevalence of 1 in 50,000 persons in the general population) and corticobasal ganglionic degeneration (prevalence of 1 in 100,000 persons) are both "Parkinson disease–plus syndromes," in which clients typically have cognitive abnormalities and rigidity without tremor.

OT intervention with persons with PDD typically focuses on physical impairments.[41] Therapy can help address balance difficulties, rigidity, and coordination problems that affect the ability to complete functional tasks. If the client is still living at home, recommendations can be made to modify the home environment to decrease fall risk. Grab bars can be placed across from the toilet to allow the client to flex forward when standing, which will help compensate for the retropulsion found in clients with PD. To help increase independence with self-care, clients can wear clothing without fastenings, such as pants with an elastic waistband and pullover shirts. Adapted cups, plate guards, and special utensils can help the client compensate for coordination difficulties. OT professionals can also position the client in a wheelchair to break up extensor tone in the trunk, which will help improve the client's ability to maintain a midline position in the wheelchair.[28]

Frontotemporal Dementia

Frontotemporal dementia (FTD; also called frontotemporal lobar degeneration [FTLD]) is the second most common cause of progressive irreversible dementia, ranking behind AD in clients younger than 65.[48] FTD is associated with degeneration of the frontal and anterior temporal lobes. Three clinical groups of FTD have been described: (1) behavioral variant of FTD (FTDbv), characterized by changes in behavior and personality and associated with cortical degeneration predominantly in the frontal lobes; (2) semantic dementia (SD), a syndrome of progressive loss of knowledge about words and objects associated with anterior temporal cortical degeneration; and (3) progressive nonfluent aphasia, characterized by difficulty with language expression (e.g., effortful language output, loss of grammar, and motor speech problems). FTDbv is characterized by insidious onset of behavioral and personality changes, and, typically, initial presentation lacks clear neurological signs or symptoms. Core diagnostic criteria for FTDbv include personality changes, such as emotional blunting and lack of insight.

The clinical manifestations of FTDbv are variable but may include poor judgment (neglecting normal responsibilities), disinhibition (impolite behavior), loss of empathy and sympathy for others, compulsive or socially inappropriate behaviors, excessive eating and weight gain, apathy, substance abuse, or aggression early in the course of dementia. Social misconduct in the form of theft or offensive language may occur in nearly one half of persons with FTDbv. Behavioral symptoms such as rigidity, stubbornness, self-centeredness, and adoption of compulsive rituals typically occur with disease progression. Individuals with FTDbv may exhibit dramatic alterations in self-identity, such as changes in political, social, or religious values. Stereotyped behaviors, such as compulsive cleaning, pacing, and collecting, are also common in FTDbv. In later stages, hyperorality, repetitive movements, and mutism may occur. Memory loss is not prominent until later in the disease. Initially, individuals with FTD may be misdiagnosed as having a psychiatric disorder (such as major depression, bipolar disorder, antisocial personality disorder, or obsessive compulsive disorder) and may have been under the care of a psychiatrist for years. It is only when symptoms advance to the point of obvious cognitive (loss of speech, memory deficits) and physical deficits (stiffness and balance problems) that the correct diagnosis is made.

Up to one third of people with FTDbv exhibit euphoria, which can take the form of elevated mood, inappropriate jocularity, and exaggerated self-esteem that can be indistinguishable from hypomania or mania. Gluttonous overeating and an exaggerated craving for carbohydrates are also common in FTDbv.

People in the earlier stages of FTDbv, as compared with AD, often achieve higher scores on the Mini-Mental State Examination (MMSE) at baseline. Bedside cognitive testing (such as the MMSE) thus is often insensitive to the early and isolated executive and/or language deficits of individuals with FTDbv. Individuals with FTDbv often display echopraxia (repeating whatever the other person says), perseveration (giving the same answer to a new question), and motor impersistence. Neuropsychological testing is highly valuable when FTDbv is being considered because bedside testing of executive function is inadequate. Normal performance on neuropsychological testing does not rule out FTDbv, especially early in its course.

Survival is typically shorter with the FTD subgroups, with the possible exception of SD, where the duration of illness is similar to that of AD.

FTD describes a group of diseases characterized by neuronal degeneration involving primarily the frontal and temporal lobes. Up to 15% of clients with FTD have clinical and electromyographic findings consistent with amyotrophic lateral sclerosis.

There are no medications approved by the Food and Drug Administration (FDA) for the management of FTDs. Therapeutically, selective serotonin reuptake inhibitors (SSRIs) are common first-line agents, given the well-described serotonergic deficits in FTD. SSRIs are generally given for treatment of anxiety, depression, compulsive behaviors, and agitation in clients with FTD. Clients with FTD are particularly prone to developing extrapyramidal side effects with use of antipsychotics because of dopaminergic deficits seen in the brains of people with FTD. Thus, use of antipsychotics should be restricted to treatment of behavioral emergencies and severe persistent aggression. The cholinergic system in FTD appears to be relatively intact. Thus, the use of cholinesterase inhibitors (ChEIs) for clients with FTD is not recommended. Memantine may be judiciously considered for treatment of some clients with FTD because preliminary data suggest that glutamate may play a role in FTD and that memantine may produce modest benefits. Please note additional information on the use of pharmacological agents in Chapter 13.

The OT professional's role in the treatment of clients with FTD can primarily focus on the management of the physical deficits, and providing tips to help deal with the behavioral symptoms.

Mixed Dementia

Mixed dementia (coexisting AD and VaD or AD and DLB, AD and PDD and VaD and DLB) is also common, and should be considered in the differential diagnosis. Mixed pathology is common. Concomitant AD is present in 66% of DLB clients and 77% of VaD clients.[56] Most people with clinical VaD have low to moderate coexisting AD. Even those older adults with high burdens of cerebrovascular disease (CVD) may still have some AD. More clinical evidence of CVD implies greater likelihood of VaD as the dominant etiologic factor in people with dementia. AD can never be ruled out on clinical or imaging grounds. At autopsy, clients with PDD will frequently have pathologic findings of AD as well.

Potentially Reversible Causes of Dementia

In clients with cognitive decline, unexplained focal findings, and atypical presentations, including incontinence, seizures, or severe headache, early in the course of dementia, the so-called surgically treatable causes—normal pressure hydrocephalus (NPH), subdural hematoma, and brain tumor—should be considered, but these typically do not present as isolated dementia.[35] NPH manifests initially with gait apraxia (leading to falls) followed by urinary incontinence and eventually dementia. Neuroimaging shows dilated ventricles, and diagnosis can be confirmed by demonstrating improvement in gait after removal of some amount of cerebrospinal fluid through lumbar puncture. Treatment of NPH involves insertion of a ventriculo-peritoneal shunt. Subdural hematoma may produce headache and dementia-like symptoms (cognitive deficits, changes in mood and/or personality of subacute onset) because of mass effect or induction of nonconvulsive seizures. Treatment involves neurosurgical intervention (burr hole and removal of the blood clot). Tumors involving the parietal cortex may mimic AD. The parietal cortex is not directly connected with motor output systems, and paralysis and abnormal reflexes may be absent despite significant mass effect. Although other abnormalities (e.g., sensory, complex behavioral, and visual-focal deficits) may occur, clients with tumors involving the parietal lobe are usually unaware of these deficits (anosognosia), and they may be missed on a cursory examination. In general, individuals with dementia due to brain tumor are younger (less than 70 years) compared with the typical age group of individuals with AD (more than 70 years). Neuroimaging (especially MRI with and without contrast) confirms the diagnosis of brain tumor. Primary gastrointestinal disorders such Whipple disease and celiac disease may have central nervous system involvement without prominent gastrointestinal symptoms.

Paretic neurosyphilis, although rare in the general population, should be considered in individuals with past history of sexually transmitted disease and/or HIV infection. Clinical presentation is that of disinhibited frontotemporal dementia. If the clinical picture strongly suggests paretic neurosyphilis, a fluorescent treponemal antibody absorption test is recommended. The first-line treatment of paretic neurosyphilis is antibiotics (such as penicillin). All clients with dementia should be adequately screened for HIV infection risk factors.

Differential Diagnosis of Dementia

Dementia should be differentiated from age-associated memory impairment, mild cognitive impairment, delirium, and depression.

Age-Associated Memory Impairment

Short-term memory is the storage of information for a brief period of time. It can last from a few minutes to a few days. Short-term memory that is mentally manipulated and processed is termed working memory. Procedural memory is the ability to remember how to complete a particular task or procedure. A client's ability to complete ADLs is based on the client's ability to use procedural memory. Long-term memory is usually the strongest type of memory, and it consists of information that is stored from a few days to many years. Older adults will often have deficits with short-term memory, but long-term memory and procedural memory are often still intact early in the disease process.

A hallmark of normal cognitive aging is slowed speed of processing. Particularly after age 70 years, but most marked in the population over age 85 years, is a tendency to have increasing difficulty in accessing names of people and objects, difficulty processing information rapidly, and the need for additional time to learn new things or skills (such as using technology) or grasp new ideas (particularly complicated skills or ideas), and to think through problems.[21] Age-associated memory impairment (AAMI; also called benign senescent forgetfulness or benign forgetfulness) involves forgetting the name of someone, particularly someone whom the individual has not seen in a while; finding it difficult to recall the right word to express oneself; or even not remembering the name of an object, event, or some other item or concept, particularly something that is not completely familiar. None of these problems is sufficient to cause impairment in daily activities or the person's ability to live independently. Memory function as measured by delayed recall of newly learned material is not substantially decreased in older adults. People experiencing AAMI complain of memory loss but generally have normal scores on psychometric testing for their age group. Office-based memory testing results are generally in the normal range. Although there is absence of significant decline in memory or functioning over time (months to years) in most people with subjective memory complaints, new research suggests that subjective cognitive impairment (SCI) is not as benign as generally thought because in some clients (e.g., highly educated people) subjective memory difficulties may be the earliest symptom of future dementia.[23]

Mild Cognitive Impairment

Mild cognitive impairment (MCI) is a syndrome characterized by impairment in a single cognitive domain, usually memory (amnestic MCI), or moderate impairment in several cognitive domains, but clients with MCI do not have significant impairment in their abilities to perform ADLs and do not meet criteria for dementia.[46] Prevalence of MCI among individuals living in long-term care settings varies from 5% to 10% in many nursing homes to up to 30% in some ALFs. The most frequently encountered form of MCI is the amnestic type. Less common variants of MCI present with localized impairment of other cognitive domains (such as executive dysfunction in FTLD). Clients with amnestic MCI commonly progress to AD, converting from one diagnosis to the other at a rate of approximately 10% to 15% per year on average. Thus, for many clients with MCI, MCI represents the earliest manifestation of AD. Not all persons with MCI will convert to AD or other dementia. Although most persons who convert from MCI to dementia have AD, many others may convert to VaD, FTD, DLB, and other less common dementias. Depression is common in people with MCI, and its presence increases the chances of people with MCI converting to dementia in the next few years. Neuropsychological testing is needed to accurately diagnose MCI and differentiate it from AAMI and mild dementia.

Delirium

Delirium typically has an acute, dateable onset; fluctuating levels of alertness in which the individual may appear drowsy, hyperalert, or alternate between them; and difficulties with attention and concentration.[38] As well, any and all causes of delirium may be accompanied by behavior changes such as agitation or psychotic symptoms such as visual hallucinations. The quiet/apathetic subtype, often called acute confusion, is often missed by care providers. Depending on the cause, in some cases onset of delirium may be subacute. This is in contrast to typical insidious onset in degenerative dementia. Acute onset, impairment in awareness (hyperalert, drowsy, stuporous), inattention, and daily dramatic fluctuation in symptoms (especially cognition but also behavior) are four key clinical features of delirium that help differentiate it from dementia (except in individuals with DLB). Orientation is generally impaired and memory deficits are also seen. Thinking is disorganized. Delirium should always be assumed to be treatable or reversible until proven otherwise. By identifying and removing the cause, the individual should return to his or her premorbid cognitive and functional baseline.

Depression

Major depressive disorder (hence forth called *depression*) in older adults may be associated with complaints of memory impairment, difficulty thinking and concentrating, word-finding difficulty, and an overall reduction in intellectual abilities.[24] This condition used to be called *depressive pseudodementia*, but is more properly termed the *dementia syndrome of depression*. This is a recognition that older adults who are clinically depressed may look like and even believe that they have AD because the depression can impair cognition. However, if only depression is causing cognitive changes, once it is effectively treated, the person should return to the premorbid cognitive baseline. Unfortunately, depression may be an early marker as well as a risk factor for AD. Also, depression coexists with AD in 30% to 50% of people with AD. In people with dementia who exhibit acute cognitive or behavioral decline, comorbid depression (as well as delirium) needs to be suspected and aggressively treated.

A history of gradual cognitive decline predating depressive symptoms may help in the diagnosis of AD with depression. To clarify the diagnosis, it is sometimes helpful to use an assessment tool, such as the Geriatric Depression Scale (GDS), Patient Health Questionnaire–9 (PHQ-9), or Cornell Scale for Depression in Dementia (CSDD).[2,53] The latter is most useful as a depression assessment tool for clients with advanced dementia. Neuropsychological testing is one of the best ways to reliably differentiate between cognitive deficits related to depression from MCI, MCI with depression, mild dementia, and key mild dementia with depression. Neuropsychological testing may show executive dysfunction, but the typical neuropsychological profile of AD is absent in individuals with depression but no dementia (Table 15-3).

Tools for Diagnosing Dementia

Current tools for the diagnosis of dementia include:
- detailed history from client and from family or other reliable informant
- physical and neurological examinations and laboratory tests
- neuroimaging
- standardized tests to assess cognition, function, and mood (depression)
- neuropsychological testing by a neuropsychologist when diagnosis or etiology is unclear

TABLE 15-3 Differentiation between Delirium, Dementia, and Depression

	Delirium	Dementia	Depression
Onset	Abrupt	Slow and insidious	Recent; may be associated with loss
Duration	Hours to days	Months to years	Stable; may be worse in a.m.
Attention	Impaired	Normal (except in severe cases)	Usually normal
Consciousness	Reduced, fluctuating	Clear	Clear

(From Federal Interagency Forum on Aging-Related Statistics. [2012, June]. *Older Americans 2012: Key indicators of well-being.* Washington, DC: U.S. Government Printing Office; Silverstein, N. M. & Maslow, K. (Eds.) (2006). *Improving hospital care for persons with dementia.* New York: Springer.)

Tests to Clarify Diagnosis

To date, there are no definitive antemortem tests to definitively diagnose degenerative dementias. Blood tests such as complete blood count (CBC); basic metabolic panel (BMP); liver function tests (LFTs); calcium, vitamin B_{12}, and folate levels; and thyroid-stimulating hormone (TSH) are recommended to detect treatable causes of cognitive impairment such as severe anemia, malnutrition, hyponatremia, severe renal disease, hypercalcemia, vitamin deficiencies, and thyroid disorders. These conditions are generally comorbid with irreversible dementias, but correcting them may improve cognition and may slow future cognitive decline. Neuroimaging may be necessary for accurate diagnosis if clinical presentation suggests the possibility of vascular lesions, NPH, tumors, subdural hematoma, or brain tumor, and for any atypical presentation (e.g., young-onset dementia, rapidly progressive dementia). MRI is preferred over a computed tomography (CT) scan of the brain, generally without contrast, because MRI better detects most lesions. Neuroimaging may be avoided for individuals who have clinical features of degenerative dementia and are in advanced stages because obtaining a brain scan may be too burdensome for these individuals and any findings on neuroimaging may not influence treatment decisions. Sleep disorders such as obstructive sleep apnea are also associated with cognitive impairment and should be investigated, especially in individuals with obesity, excessive daytime sleepiness, and nighttime snoring. A sleep study may be warranted to confirm diagnosis of obstructive sleep apnea.

The prevalence of reversible dementias has been decreasing over the last few decades. In selected cases (such as a history of sexually transmitted disease or of intravenous drug abuse), a rapid plasma reagin test for neurosyphilis or an HIV test for central nervous system manifestations of AIDS may be warranted. A positron emission tomography (PET) scan may be considered for an individual to help differentiate between AD and FTD. Neither a CT nor an MRI scan can diagnose AD, but looking for degree of atrophy or focal atrophy and hippocampal atrophy may be useful in differentiating between FTD and AD. Atrophy out of proportion to age is also important in the diagnosis of degenerative dementias. Dementia diagnoses may be inaccurate for many individuals in long-term care.

Neuropsychological testing, if available, may be considered to diagnose dementia more accurately. Neuropsychological testing is a useful tool for clarifying the diagnosis in individuals with significant depression and dementia, to differentiate between MCI and dementia and to differentiate between AD and other neurodegenerative dementias. Neuropsychological testing is also an important tool to diagnose AD in individuals who, at baseline, had extremely high or relatively low levels of cognitive/intellectual function (such as individuals with mental retardation due to Down syndrome who have developed insidious onset and progressive cognitive and functional decline from their baseline).

Clients with unusually rapid symptomatic progression of dementia and presence of myoclonus, or other atypical presentations, may need spinal fluid examination to evaluate for Creutzfeldt-Jakob disease and infectious etiologies of dementia (such as neurosyphilis or herpes simplex encephalitis).

Genetic testing is recommended only in cases of familial AD (AD with an autosomal-dominant pattern of inheritance in individuals who typically have an age of onset of dementia in the 30s or 40s) and some cases of FTD that have an autosomal-dominant pattern of inheritance. Genetic counseling by a professional genetic counselor, clinical geneticist, or expert in memory disorders at an academic center is strongly recommended before any genetic testing. Testing for the APOE-4 genotype is generally not recommended for use in diagnosis. For additional information on assessments and their rationales, see Table 15-4.

Behavioral and Psychological Symptoms of Dementia

Point prevalence of behavioral and psychological symptoms of dementia (BPSDs) is approximately 60%, and lifetime prevalence is 90%.[22] Among the most validated syndromes of BPSDs are depression, psychosis, and sleep disturbance

of AD.[40] Apathy syndrome of dementia is also gaining increasing interest. Prevalence of BPSDs does not vary by setting, but prevalence of specific symptoms does vary by setting (higher prevalence of aggression in individuals in long-term care facilities compared with people with dementia in the community) and by stage. Apathy is the most common BPSD seen in all types of dementia and across all stages. Its prevalence increases with advancing cognitive impairment.

Agitation is the next most common BPSD, typically seen more commonly as the dementia progresses to moderate and severe stages. Disruptive behaviors (such as wandering, verbal outbursts, physical threats/violence, agitation/restlessness, and sundowning) predict cognitive decline, functional decline, and institutionalization. The prevalence of agitation and aggression is approximately 25% in persons with dementia residing at home and 45% in those residing in long-term care facilities. Prevalence of clinically significant depression is approximately 32% in the mild stage, 23% in the moderate stage, and 18% in severe stages. Lower premorbid agreeableness (a personality factor) is associated with agitation and irritability symptoms in AD and also predicts an "agitation/apathy" syndrome.

Psychotic symptoms such as delusions and hallucinations are also prevalent in individuals with dementia. Sleep disturbances and anxiety symptoms are also common in individuals with dementia and often occur along with depression, psychoses, and agitation. BPSDs, especially psychosis, agitation, and problem wandering (safety issue), are the leading triggers for placement of a person with dementia in a long-term care facility.

Although dementia itself generally causes BPSDs, most behavioral and psychological symptoms in individuals arise from the complex interaction of the various factors listed in Table 15-5.

TABLE 15-4 Proposed Testing of Older Adults with Subjective Cognitive/Memory Complaints

Assessments	Rationale
Routine:	
Neuropsychological testing	Delineation of cognitive syndromes (SCI vs. MCI vs. AD*)
Hematology (full blood count)	Screen for anemia
Biochemistry (electrolytes, renal function, liver function, thyroid function, B₁₂ and folate)	Screen for treatable causes of cognitive complaints
For Specific Indication Suggested by History, Physical Exam, and/or Neuropsychological Testing:	
Neuroimaging	Generalized and regional (e.g., hippocampal atrophy, space-occupying lesions)
Electroencephalography	Epilepsy/seizures (especially absence and complex partial seizures)
Cardiac (e.g., echocardiography)	May reveal cardiac arrhythmia or sources of emboli
Inflammatory markers (e.g., ESR**)	Screen for inflammatory process
Treponemal serology	Tertiary syphilis

*SCI = subjective cognitive impairment; MCI = mild cognitive impairment; AD = Alzheimer's disease and other dementias.
**ESR = erythrocyte sedimentation rate.

TABLE 15-5 Causes of Behavioral and Psychological Symptoms of Dementia

Cause	Example
Iatrogenic	Medications (e.g., anticholinergic medications [oxybutynin, diphenhydramine]), therapeutic diets, impatient and/or inappropriate caregiver approach
Recreational drugs	Even modest amount of alcohol may cause agitation and insomnia
Medical conditions	Urinary tract infection, constipation, dehydration, pain, sleep disorders
Psychosocial	Loneliness, boredom, feelings of insecurity, struggle maintaining self-esteem
Unmet basic need	Hunger, thirst, sexual expression, discomfort (e.g., tight clothing)
Environmental	Excessive noise, inadequate lighting, lack of access to outdoors, too hot or too cold
Psychiatric disorders	Major depression, psychotic and anxiety symptoms

Agitation

Agitation is a generic term that includes verbally aggressive behaviors (e.g., swearing, threats), verbally nonaggressive behaviors (e.g., repetitive vocalization, pleas for help), physically aggressive behaviors (e.g., hitting, biting, scratching, kicking, pushing), and physically nonaggressive behaviors (e.g., pacing, wandering).[15] Agitated behaviors should be considered an expression of an individual's unmet needs (e.g., need for food, drink, toileting, relief from environmental stress [impatient or angry caregiver approach, excessive noise, excessive demand], relief from discomfort [due to pain, constipation]). Medications, medical conditions (such as obstructive sleep apnea, pneumonia, urinary tract infection [UTI], onychomycosis), and psychiatric disorders (depression, psychoses, delirium) may also manifest as agitated behaviors. Catastrophic reaction is an acute expression of overwhelming anxiety and fearfulness experienced by some individuals with dementia, usually triggered by a frustrating experience (e.g., difficulty dressing self) or in anticipation of one. These spells are typically brief, lasting less than 30 minutes, and self-limited.

To help minimize agitation, OT professionals can help caregivers simplify self-care routines to help decrease frustration and anxiety. Breaking down activities into simple steps can also help keep the client from feeling overwhelmed.[42] In addition, establishing toileting routines, providing clothes that are easy to manage, clearly marking the door to the bathroom with a picture of a toilet, and adding adaptive equipment in the bathroom such as a raised toilet seat and grab bars will make it easier for the client to be able to complete toileting without assistance. Encouraging the client to take frequent drinks throughout the day and providing easy-to-eat snacks will also help meet the needs of clients, which will help decrease anxiety caused by unmet needs.

Wandering

Wandering is one of the most common behavioral problems found in persons with dementia, often resulting in their being placed in a long-term care facility that offers "locked" units or other safeguards (e.g., use of wander-guard alarm system). Wandering manifests as aimless or purposeful motor activity that involves leaving a safe place, getting lost, or intruding into inappropriate places or situations. Individuals with dementia often wander, with rates of 35% to 40% per year of reported elopements from facilities. Individuals with dementia who remain ambulatory and are in relatively good physical health are at high risk for wandering. Once an individual begins wandering, more than 70% will engage in repeated episodes. Management of wandering primarily involves psychosocial environmental interventions. For example, some individuals may wander due to need for socialization or stimulation, and may benefit from a structured individualized activity schedule (such as a daily walking plan) to prevent boredom. Availability of safe and aesthetically pleasing areas (for example, therapeutic gardens with walking paths) may allow clients to wander and explore without risk of elopement.

CASE EXAMPLE 15-4 Irene

Irene is a 72-year-old female living with her daughter. She was diagnosed with vascular dementia 18 months after she had a CVA. Irene was referred to occupational therapy because of a sudden decline in her ability to complete self-care tasks and increasing problems using her right hand. Irene has always been right-hand dominant. At the time of the evaluation, Irene's daughter told the therapist that her mom had begun wandering and was beginning to have anxiety and problem behaviors that were interfering with family schedules. Irene would get up early and start to get dressed. She always put on the same clothes and became upset when her daughter tried to make her wear a different outfit.

The occupational therapist determined that Irene became agitated in the later afternoon. Her daughter shared that her mother had raised five children. She also recalled that her mother always had dinner on the table at 5:00 when her father arrived home from work. It was theorized that Irene was becoming anxious because she thought that she should be preparing dinner. The occupational therapist identified some simple meal preparation tasks that Irene could complete that would help improve the function in her right hand while also meet her occupational need to prepare meals for her family. Irene's granddaughter was also encouraged to become involved with her grandmother when she returned home from school. Finally, the therapist suggested that Irene's daughter should purchase duplicate outfits that her mother liked to wear. Irene would then be able to wear the same clothes that she felt comfortable in, but her daughter would be able to wash the outfits so that Irene would have clean clothes. When the occupational therapist returned for a follow-up visit 2 weeks later, Irene's daughter reported that Irene's anxiety had decreased significantly. They had also begun taking a walk together in the afternoon, which also seemed to decrease her wandering.

Treatment of Dementia

Medical treatment of dementia is treatment of its cause. Thus, treatment of reversible dementia is to treat the cause (removing offending medication, correcting vitamin and nutritional deficiencies, etc.). The medical and interdisciplinary interventions and goals of treatment of irreversible dementias are listed in Table 15-6. Early and aggressive management of irreversible dementias can delay symptom progression and help to maintain the quality of life of both the client and caregiver. Dementia has a tremendous negative impact on a client's self-esteem and feelings of security, especially if the individual has insight (partial or full) relative to his or her cognitive and functional limitations. Thus, helping clients to maintain self-esteem through engagement in creative and meaningful activities and, if necessary, providing supportive psychotherapy (in mild to moderate stages) can be very helpful.

TABLE 15-6 Medical and Interdisciplinary Interventions and Goals for Clients with Dementia

Interventions	Goals
Discontinue unnecessary/harmful medications	Improve daily functioning and quality of life
Antidementia drugs	Slow cognitive and functional decline
Antidepressants for major depression	Improve depression and quality of life
Control of vascular risk factors (e.g., hypertension)	Slow cognitive and functional decline
Assessment for capacity to make decisions	Prevent harmful decisions by helping client seek appropriate surrogate decision maker for health care and finances
Assessment and treatment of excess comorbidity	Improve quality of life (e.g., depression, pain, obstructive sleep apnea)
Referral to adult day program	Improve quality of life, delay nursing home placement
Dietetic therapy	Address nutritional concerns (e.g., weight loss)
Occupational therapy	Home safety assessment, environmental adaptation, interventions to improve ability to complete activities of daily living and other activities meaningful for client, education of family members on how to deal with symptoms
Physical therapy	Reduce risk of falls, energy conservation
Speech therapy	Address cognitive and communication problems and swallowing problems if present
Recreation therapy	Improve quality of life
Music therapy	Improve quality of life
Art therapy	Improve quality of life
Assessment by law attorney specializing in older-adult issues	Help with documents such as power of attorney for health care and finances, living will, and for guardianship issues

Treatment for Cognitive and Functional Deficits

At present, no purely medical therapy has been shown to prevent, cure, or arrest the progression of AD, DLB, PDD, and FTD. Antidementia drugs currently available include cholinesterase inhibitors (ChEIs) and the N-methyl-D-aspartate (NMDA) receptor antagonist memantine. A trial of one of the ChEIs, such as donepezil, rivastigmine, or galantamine, is recommended for people with mild, moderate, and severe AD, DLB, and PDD. A trial of memantine with or without concomitant use of a ChEI is recommended for individuals with AD in moderate to severe stages. Preliminary evidence indicates potential benefits of memantine in clients with PDD and DLB. Combination therapy (e.g., adding memantine to

the regimen of the client who is already on a ChEI) may provide added benefits. Memantine may also be considered for individuals with mild AD, although is not approved by the FDA for treatment of mild AD. Whenever antidementia drugs are prescribed, persons with dementia and their families should be apprised of the modest potential benefits as well as the potential adverse effects and added costs of medications.

Common adverse effects of ChEI are nausea, vomiting, anorexia, weight loss, and diarrhea. These adverse effects tend to be mild to moderate in severity but in frail individuals with dementia, even mild adverse effects can significantly impair quality of life. In individuals with PDD, ChEIs may worsen tremors. Other uncommon adverse effects of ChEIs include muscle cramps, bradycardia (which can be dangerous in individuals with cardiac conduction problems), and dizziness. ChEIs increase gastric acid production, a particular concern for those with history of peptic ulcer. Preexisting bradycardia, sick sinus syndrome or conduction defects, undiagnosed nausea, vomiting and diarrhea, gastritis, or ulcerative disease should be considered relative contraindications for ChEIs.[8] Finally, ChEIs may induce or exacerbate urinary obstruction, worsen asthma and chronic obstructive pulmonary disease (COPD), cause seizures, induce or worsen sleep disturbance, and exaggerate the effects of some muscle relaxants during anesthesia. Thus, ChEIs should be used with extra precaution for individuals with cerebrovascular disease, seizures, and COPD.

A relatively high proportion of persons with dementia living in long-term care facilities and taking antidementia drugs may not be benefiting enough from these medications to warrant continuation. Psychosocial-environmental interventions such as regular physical exercise (aerobics, balance and strength training), healthy nutrition (fruits, vegetables, whole grains, food rich in omega-3 fatty acids and monounsaturated fatty acids), cognitively stimulating and meaningful activities (reading aloud, doing puzzles, playing card or board games, etc.), yoga, meditation, and stress management strategies (relaxation exercises, mindfulness training), along with pharmacological interventions (antidementia drugs) and aggressive control of cardiovascular risk factors, may help highly motivated individuals with mild dementia to achieve high levels of cognitive function and slow cognitive and functional decline.

Treatment of Behavioral and Psychological Symptoms of Dementia

Ensuring safety and security is crucial, because behavioral and psychological symptoms often may be severe and can potentially be life threatening to the client displaying the behaviors (such as suicidal attempt) and/or dangerous to others (such as hitting a caregiver, causing injury).[22] Those with dementia who wander may be particularly at risk of exposure to dangerous weather conditions, dehydration, and medical problems due to missing doses of needed medications. Identifying triggers is important because modifying triggers often ameliorates the behavioral disturbances. Medical disorders (such as untreated pain, UTI) and psychiatric disorders (major depression, generalized anxiety disorder) are common causes of agitation in individuals with dementia and are eminently treatable.

Psychosocial-environmental interventions are the first-line intervention for all BPSDs. Commonly employed psychosocial-environmental interventions include structured and unstructured activities, exercise, music, dance, reminiscence, massage therapy, aromatherapy, pet therapy (animal-assisted therapy), therapeutic gardens, simulated presence therapy (e.g., hearing family members taped recordings), painting, other activities that allow creative expression, and spirituality. Daily exercises (walking, resistance training, flexion and stretch exercises) improve functional fitness and are critical for maintaining muscle mass and slowing cognitive and functional decline. A typical psychosocial-environmental intervention can involve continuous activity programming tailored to the unique needs, strengths, and interests of each individual that can prevent and abort many agitated behaviors in clients with dementia. There is growing consensus that spirituality is of great importance for not only those who have dementia but also for their caregivers. Bright light has a modest benefit in improving some cognitive and noncognitive (e.g., mood, sleep) symptoms of dementia. Often, "agitation" is a way for clients with dementia to communicate their feelings of insecurity. Many behaviors are an attempt by clients to feel connected to their surroundings. In such situations, the client needs empathic mirroring responses from caregivers who can understand the symbolic meaning of such behaviors.

Pharmacological Interventions for Behavioral and Psychological Symptoms of Dementia

Although evidence to support the efficacy of ChEIs and memantine in BPSD treatment is limited, in the absence of safer and effective alternatives, their use is appropriate.[22]

Palliative Care for People with Advanced Dementia

Discussion of wishes of an individual with dementia regarding life-prolonging treatment during advanced dementia (moderate, severe, and terminal stages) should take place when the person is in the mild stages (preferably the first half of the mild stage) because in this stage, the person retains the capacity to make medical decisions for himself or herself, can fully participate in the discussion, and can express his or her wishes to the family.[20] In general, as the dementia progresses, the burdens of life-prolonging treatment (such as hospitalization for pneumonia) increase dramatically, and potential benefits (such as increased duration of survival) decrease considerably. Health-care practitioners should assure the family that there is no right or wrong answer, and help family members to understand what the client would have wanted and to keep any promises and respect the wishes of the client. Practitioners should also understand the tremendous grief

(and sometimes guilt) issues the family may be dealing with at that time, and that these issues can influence their decisions considerably. Addressing these complex feelings can also help the family make the decision regarding life-prolonging treatment that is in keeping with the wishes and values of the individual with dementia. Other aspects of palliative care such as when to forgo cardiopulmonary resuscitation, degree of pain control versus adverse effects of pain medications (such as severely compromised awareness), and feeding tube placement should also be discussed as early in the course of dementia as is possible and with the involvement of the family.

Medical Comorbidity in Persons with Dementia

More than 60% of clients with dementia have three or more comorbidities. Hypertension, cardiovascular disease, arthritis, chronic kidney disease, anemia, diabetes, and diminution of vision and hearing, among other conditions, can be expected in the typical individual with dementia. Individuals with dementia have a higher incidence of parkinsonism, seizures, infections, malnutrition, sensory impairment, hip fractures and other injuries, and pressure sores. Optimal diagnosis and treatment of comorbid medical illnesses are essential components of dementia management and are key to sustaining cognition in the client with dementia. Treatment of medical comorbidities in individuals with dementia should weigh the possible benefits for the individual against the burdens imposed by such treatment.

Also, the goals of treating medical comorbidity should be in keeping with the individual's overall goals of care (palliative [comfort only] versus life-prolonging treatment). Discontinuation of medications with potential for significant anticholinergic symptoms should be considered in every individual with dementia. Clients with dementia are frequently transferred to emergency rooms and hospitalized for medical conditions (such as pneumonia), putting such individuals at high risk for delirium, falls, need for restraints, and functional decline during and after hospitalization despite successful treatment of the medical condition. Hospitalization for clients with dementia (especially frail individuals and clients with severe and terminal dementia) is extremely stressful. All of these risks of hospitalization need to be discussed before making the decision to hospitalize. Psychiatric consultation (preferably by a gerontological psychiatrist) is recommended for the management of agitation in clients with dementia who have been hospitalized.

Pain in Persons with Dementia

Older adults with dementia are not less sensitive to pain. They may fail to interpret sensations as painful, are often less able to recall their pain, and may not be able to verbally communicate it to care providers. Hence, older adults with dementia are often undertreated for pain. A label of dementia may bias the interpretation of pain cues in clients with dementia, and thus may contribute to lower use of as-needed analgesics in individuals with dementia compared with cognitively intact individuals. Individuals with dementia, just as individuals without dementia, are at risk for multiple sources and types of pain, including chronic pain from conditions such as osteoarthritis and acute pain. Poorly treated acute pain is a common cause of chronic pain in clients with dementia. Untreated pain in individuals with dementia can reduce quality of life; cause depression, agitation, and aggression; delay healing; disturb sleep and activity patterns; reduce function; and prolong hospitalization. Pain influences behavioral disturbances among individuals with severe dementia more often than it influences those with moderate or mild dementia, and clients with chronic pain who have severe dementia exhibit more dysfunctional behaviors than clients with chronic pain and earlier dementia. Terminal-stage AD is associated with pressure ulceration, limb contractures, and pain that can be much more difficult to assess. There is no evidence that surgery for hip fracture improves pain in people with advanced dementia. The primary reason to consider a surgical approach over a palliative care approach is when gain in function (especially ambulation) is the primary aim. Palliative care (pain control, skin care, bed rest, deep vein thrombosis [DVT] prophylaxis, personal care) is recommended for treatment of hip fracture in clients with severe or terminal dementia because of their limited life expectancy and inability to participate in the postoperative therapy necessary to achieve gain in function. Use of as-needed pain medications is not recommended for pain management in clients with dementia because they will not ask for pain medications. Regular (scheduled) administration of acetaminophen raises levels of general activity, social interaction, and engagement with television or magazines in long-term care individuals with moderate to severe dementia. In general, if there is an expectation that the client might have pain (for example, after having surgery), the client should be given pain medications.

Other Treatment Issues

Sexuality can be a difficult and challenging issue for professional and family caregivers to address in clients with dementia. This is particularly the case in relation to responding to incidents of hypersexuality or inappropriate sexual expression as a result of dementia.[22] Health-care practitioners should incorporate a discussion of needs for sexual expression into the routine care of clients with dementia. The client's family may need education and guidance regarding how best to meet their own needs for intimacy as well as the needs of the client.

Early and aggressive management of dementia and BPSDs can increase the chances of the client aging in place (i.e., if the person is living at home, he or she can delay having to move into a long-term care facility for a few years). With the availability of hospice and slowly improving understanding of palliative care for people with dementia, many individuals may live the last years of life entirely in their homes or an assisted living facility without having to transfer to a nursing home or hospital.

Caring for Family Caregivers

Perhaps the greatest "cost" of dementia is the physical and emotional toll on family, caregivers, and friends. Caring for a loved one with dementia also increases the risk of death for the caregiver. Dementia puts a gradually increasing burden on caregivers as the dementia progresses. Caregivers commonly report poor self-rated health, increased levels of depressive symptoms, and greater use of psychoactive medications. Caregivers often experience a profound sense of loss as the dementia slowly takes their loved ones. The relationship as it once was gradually ends, and plans for the future must be radically changed. Caregivers must come to terms with "the long goodbye." Research has also shown that caregiving may have important positive effects for some carers, such as a new sense of purpose or meaning in life, fulfillment of a lifelong commitment to a spouse, an opportunity to give back to a parent some of what the parent has given to them, renewal of religious faith, and closer ties with people through new relationships or stronger existing relationships.

Occupational Therapy Assessments for Persons with Cognitive Impairment

The goal of an OT cognitive assessment is to assess the client's ability to complete functional tasks as a foundation for treatment activities. Selecting an assessment tool to evaluate cognition is dependent on many different factors. The client's cognitive abilities before onset of the disease process or before an injury will influence the test that is selected. For example, if the client had difficulties with reading and writing, he or she will have more difficulty with testing involving reading or writing. For a client with auditory processing deficits, tests with oral instructions may not lead to accurate results. The client and family members should be interviewed before the testing is begun to determine the baseline status. For example, Carol was a physician who suffered a mild traumatic brain injury in a car accident. She was referred to OT for testing of executive function. She reported having difficulty recalling the names of her clients and was having difficulty with time management and organization of her day. She told the therapist "before I never had to write anything down... I remembered everything. Now I have to make notes to remind me of things. My friends tell me that this is normal but it was not normal for me." Carol's baseline cognitive status before her car accident was higher than the cognitive status of most clients.

Many practitioners evaluate cognition based on clinical observations during the performance of functional tasks. For example, while the client was completing a toileting task: Did the client remember to lock the brakes on the wheelchair before the transfer? Was the client able to correctly sequence the task? Did the client exhibit adequate safety awareness during the task? Was the client able to scan the environment and locate the toilet paper? Did the client become distracted during the task and need cueing to return to the task? However, there are many formal assessments that will help the clinician to evaluate cognition (Box 15-1).

Occupational Therapy Interventions with Clients and Their Family Caregivers

Once the occupational therapist determines the client's (and family caregiver's) goals and the level of the client's function by conducting the appropriate cognitive functional assessments and completing a historical occupational profile, he or she develops an intervention plan that outlines goals and the means to attain them. Various researchers[11,45] have identified common transitions or stages that family caregivers tend to experience during their "caregiving career." These include:

1. Role acquisition: initial adjustment, learning the caregiver role, redefining family dynamics, planning for the future
2. Role enactment: learning and enacting direct-care skills, managing dementia-related behaviors, continuing to engage the individual with dementia in meaningful occupations, learning to access and use appropriate supplementary services
3. Role disengagement: relinquishing aspects of caregiving that are no longer sustainable, finding appropriate home health or residential care and serving as the individual's advocate with service providers, supporting end-of-life needs, dealing with grief and bereavement
4. Role reengagement: establishing new or former roles and social ties, transitioning to a new phase of life

Each stage presents its own challenges and needs for both the client and the family caregiver.[45] Client- and family-centered intervention plans should take into account and address these stage-related needs.

The therapist then implements the intervention plan through individual and/or group activities and interventions, evaluates the plan and implementation relative to achievement of client and caregiver goals, and modifies the plan as needed.[6]

Based on his review of OT-based interventions for individuals with dementia, Padilla[42] derived four basic principles to guide OT practice with this population:

1. Individualize programs for clients to maximize their interest and retained abilities.
2. Provide short and clear cues when directing clients in a given program.
3. Individualize modifications of the physical environment and selection of simple adaptive equipment to support the unique needs and abilities of the client.
4. Provide training to family caregivers and support their involvement in the implementation of the individualized programs; this principle is critically important.

Table 15-7 provides a list of interventions or strategies designed to support memory and cognition in clients with dementia.

An additional literature review of the effectiveness of educational and supportive programs for dementia caregivers[54] indicated that these programs are most successful when they are home-based programs and engage both the caregiver and the client. The best interventions for dementia caregivers reinforce problem-solving skills, technical skills, basic home modifications, and the use of appropriate support and community resources.

It can be emotionally and spiritually draining to watch as dementia takes the memory and sense of self from one's loved one. Family caregivers must be reminded that there is no "right" way to help their loved one with dementia. Even small interventions (referral to support group, expressing support) may translate into improvements in the quality of life or confidence of the family caregiver. Education of family members about dementia, its effects on the individual, how best to respond to symptoms, and how to access and use all available resources (such as involving other willing family members, contacting the local chapter of the Alzheimer's Association) is recommended. Many excellent books and online factsheets on dementia family

---

BOX 15-1   Occupational Therapy Assessments of Cognition

- Cognitive Assessment of Minnesota (CAM): Assessment of store of knowledge, manipulation of old knowledge, social awareness and judgment, and abstract thinking in a hierarchical manner in the adult population[36]
- Lowenstein Occupational Therapy Cognitive Assessment (LOTCA): Test of orientation, visual perception, spatial perception, praxis organization, visuomotor organization, and thinking operations[36]
- ADL Situation Test: Direct assessment of ADLs in clients with Alzheimer's disease[44]
- Direct Assessment of Functional Abilities (DAFA): Direct performance measure of instrumental activities of daily living (IADLs) for clients with mild to moderate dementia[44]
- Kitchen Task Assessment (KTA): Functional measure of the level of cognitive support needed by a client to complete a cooking task[44]
- Performance Assessment of Self-care Skills (PASS): Performance-based test to assess short-term functional changes in older adult clients after hospitalization[44]
- Executive Function Performance Test (EFPT): Top-down performance assessment of a simple cooking task, telephone use, medication management, and payment of bills[36]
- Large Allen Cognitive Level Screen (LACLS): Screening tool designed to provide an initial assessment of cognitive function[3]
- Routine Task Inventory–Expanded (RTI-E): Assessment of cognitive abilities in the context of routine daily activities[3]

TABLE 15-7 Interventions to Reinforce Memory and Cognitive Function

Strategy	Description
Mindfulness	Focus on one task at a time, rather than trying to multitask. Research shows that cognition is more efficient in this manner.
Cognitive methods	To improve memory, try using *mnemonics* (such as ROY G BIV for remembering the colors of the rainbow); try to *make associations* with information (such as when we meet someone new, relating his or her name to someone else we know well). *Use cues* such as memory notebooks to cue the client's recall of information. Engage in learning new and challenging cognitive activities (e.g., a new language, a new musical instrument, a new dance). Consider computer-based brain exercises.
Rehearsal	Practice the information that individuals want to remember (such as silently repeating the information several times or writing it down).
Be patient	Often when individuals have difficulties with memory, they become frustrated with themselves, and this serves to make it more challenging to remember the information.
Exercise: mentally and physically	Engage in mental activities such as reading and crossword puzzles. The important point here is to do something that individuals enjoy, rather than making it a chore. Research has demonstrated that physical exercise (such as walking) also aids with memory. Of course this should be done under the supervision of a physician.
Diet	What is good for the heart is good for the brain. Fruits, vegetables, foods rich in omega-3 fatty acids (e.g., fatty fish such as salmon), whole grains, spices (e.g., turmeric), and small amounts of tree nuts (e.g., walnuts) are recommended as part of a balanced diet, along with an adequate amount of water.

TABLE 15-8 Interventions for Families/Caregivers

Intervention	Goal
Education about the illness	Help family caregiver prepare for future decline
Education about community resources, including relevant technology and home environmental supports	Reduce stress and provide appropriate, supportive interventions
Referral to Alzheimer's Association	Access to services (e.g., support groups, caregiver training, safe return program)
Individual and family counseling	Reduce caregiver stress, prevent and treat caregiver depression
Antidepressants to treat major depression	Improve depression and quality of life
Respite services	Prevent and treat caregiver burnout
Education about palliative care	Help prevent futile and harmful care

the primary caregiver's needs and how best to be helpful are also recommended. Improving caregiver well-being delays nursing home placement of clients with AD living in the community. A structured multicomponent intervention (in-home sessions and telephone sessions over several months to address caregiver depression, burden, self-care, and social support and care-recipient problem behaviors) adapted to individual risk profiles is recommended to increase the quality of life of ethnically diverse dementia caregivers.

OT professionals can help caregivers adjust to the changing demands of caring for a loved one with dementia (Table 15-8). Suggestions can be made to modify the environment to help improve safety in the home and decrease fall risk. OT professionals can help establish routines, simplify self-care tasks, and facilitate ease of care.

Summary

Persons with dementia and other cognitive impairments have a right to receive competent, compassionate, stage-appropriate, and consistent care. With appropriate care, we can substantially reduce the number of persons with dementia who have depression and agitation, and also reduce the number of persons with advanced dementia who receive inappropriate medical treatment (hospitalizations, surgeries, medication) and futile procedures. Thus, although most dementias are incurable, occupational therapy along with other appropriate comprehensive treatment can substantially improve the quality of life for individuals with dementia and their family members.

caregiving have been written for lay audiences.[18,25,37] Counseling and ongoing support for the family members (including both individual and family counseling, and telephone counseling) and encouragement for caregivers to join support groups are also recommended, especially for caregivers with limited social support and caregivers experiencing depression. Improving social support and reducing family conflict to help the caregiver withstand the hardships of caregiving and to help family members understand

---

CASE EXAMPLE 15-5   Betty

Betty was referred to occupational therapy due to increasing pain in her right shoulder, which was affecting her ability to complete functional activities. Betty lived alone in an apartment and was responsible for preparing her own meals, completing laundry tasks, paying her bills, and managing her medications. At the time of the evaluation, she was asked about the medications that she used for pain management. Betty admitted that she had run out of her "arthritis pills" 2 months ago and had her physician call in a new order to her pharmacy. However, her car insurance had expired 2 months ago and she wasn't sure if her driver's license was still valid. In addition, she couldn't remember how to get to the pharmacy because her husband was the person who usually drove to the pharmacy. Betty's husband had recently been admitted to a skilled nursing facility following hospitalization for a CVA. Betty also reported that she hadn't been eating much lately because her daughter was out of town and her daughter usually did her grocery shopping.

1. What assessments should you use to evaluate Betty's cognition?
2. Write a functional treatment goal addressing Betty's cognitive deficits.
3. Are there other disciplines that should be involved in Betty's care? If so, name and provide the rationale and expected role for each discipline.

REVIEW QUESTIONS

1. Define cognition.
2. What interventions can be used to reduce wandering and the risk for elopement?
3. Describe the primary differences among dementia, delirium, and depression.
4. Identify the differences in clinical manifestation of Parkinson's disease dementia and frontotemporal dementia.

REFERENCES

1. Abreu, B., & Toglia, J. (1987). Cognitive rehabilitation: A model for occupational therapy. *American Journal of Occupational Therapy, 41,* 439–449.
2. Alexopoulos, G. A., Abrams, R. C., Young, R. C., & Shamoian, C. A. (1988). Cornell Scale for Depression in Dementia. *Biological Psychiatry, 23,* 271–284.
3. Allen, C., Earhart, C., & Blue, T. (1992). *Occupational therapy treatment goals for the physically and cognitively disabled* (pp. 51–68). Bethesda, MD: The American Occupational Therapy Association, Inc.
4. Alzheimer's Association. (2013). 2013 Alzheimer's disease facts and figures. *Alzheimer's & Dementia, 9,* 208–245.
5. Alzheimer's Association. (2015). *Know the 10 signs.* Chicago, IL: Alzheimer's Association. Retrieved 10/18/15. http://www.alz.org/alzheimers_disease_know_the_10_signs.asp.
6. American Occupational Therapy Association. (2014). *Occupational therapy practice framework: Domain and process* (3rd ed.). Bethesda, MD: AOTA.
7. American Psychiatric Association. (2013). *Diagnostic and statistical manual of mental disorders* (5th ed.). Washington, DC.: American Psychiatric Association.

8. American Psychiatric Association. (2014). *Guideline watch: practice guidelines for the treatment of patients with Alzheimer's disease and other dementias.* Arlington, VA: American Psychiatric Association.
9. Amini, D. (2013). Cognition, cognitive rehabilitation, and occupational performance. *American Journal of Occupational Therapy, 67,* S9–S31.
10. Anderton, B. (2002). Ageing of the brain. *Mechanisms of Ageing and Development, 23,* 811–817.
11. Aneshensel, C. S., Pearlin, L. I., Mullan, J. T., Zarit, S. H., & Whitlatch, C. J. (1995). *Profiles in caregiving: The unexpected career.* San Diego, CA: Academic Press.
12. Caselli, R. J., Beach, T. G., & Yaari, R. (2006). Alzheimer's disease a century later. *Journal of Clinical Psychiatry, 67,* 1784–1800.
13. Cato, M. A., & Crosson, B. A. (2006). Stable and progressive dementias. In D. K. Attix & K. A. Welsh-Bohmer (Eds.), *Geriatric neuropsychology: Assessment and intervention* (pp. 89–102). New York, NY: Guilford Press.
14. Centers for Disease Control and Prevention. (2014). *Severe traumatic brain injury.* Atlanta, GA: National Center for Injury Prevention and Control. Retrieved 3/10/13. http://www.cdc.gov/traumaticbraininjury/severe.html.
15. Cohen-Mansfield, J., & Billig, N. (1986). Agitated behaviors in the elderly: A conceptual review. *Journal of the American Geriatric Society, 34,* 711–721.
16. Cummings, J. L., & Cole, G. (2002). Alzheimer's disease. *Journal of the American Medical Association, 287,* 2335–2338.
17. de Lau, L. M. L., Giesbergen, P. C. L. M., de Rijk, M. C., Hofman, A., Koudstaal, P. J., & Breteler, M. M. B. (2004). Incidence of parkinsonism and Parkinson disease in a general population: The Rotterdam Study. *Journal of Neurology, 63*(7), 1240–1244.
18. Department of Social and Health Services. (2013). *Family caregiver handbook. DSHS 22-277(X) (Rev. 6/13).* Washington State: Aging and Long Term Support Administration.
19. Desai, A. K., & Grossberg, G. T. (2010). *Psychiatric consultation in long-term care: A guide for health care professionals.* Baltimore, MD: The Johns Hopkins University Press.
20. Desai, A. K., & Grossberg, G. T. (2011). Palliative and end-of-life care in psychogeriatric patients. *Aging Health, 7,* 395–408.
21. Desai, A. K., & Morley, J. E. (2011). The aging body and brain. In M. E. Agronin & G. J. Maletta (Eds.), *Principles and practice of geriatric psychiatry,* (2nd ed., pp. 3–13). Philadelphia PA: Lippincott Williams & Wilkins.
22. Desai, A. K., Schwartz, L., & Grossberg, G. (2012). Behavioral disturbance in dementia. *Current Psychiatry Report, 14,* 298–309.
23. Desai, A., & Schwarz, L. (2011). Subjective cognitive impairment: When to be concerned about "senior moments." *Current Psychiatry, 10*(4), 31–32, 39–44.
24. Enache, D., Winblad, B., & Aarsland, D. (2011). Depression in dementia: Epidemiology, mechanisms, and treatment. *Current Opinion in Psychiatry, 24,* 461–472.
25. Family Caregiver Alliance. (2004). *Caregiver's guide to understanding dementia behaviors.* San Francisco, CA: California Department of Health.
26. Federal Interagency Forum on Aging-Related Statistics. (June 2012). *Older Americans 2012: Key indicators of well-being.* Washington, DC: U.S. Government Printing Office.
27. Feldman, H., Levy, A. R., Hsiung, G-Y., et al. (2003). A Canadian Cohort Study of Cognitive Impairment and Related Dementias (ACCORD): Study methods and baseline results. *Neuroepidemiology, 22,* 265–274.

28. Foster, E. (2011). *Executive dysfunction among individuals with Parkinson's disease [Handout]*. Bethesda, MD: The American Occupational Therapy Association, Inc.
29. Galvin, J. E., Pollack, J., & Morris, J. C. (2006). Clinical phenotype of Parkinson disease dementia. *Neurology, 67*, 1605–1611.
30. Grossberg, G. T. & Desai, A. K. (2006). Cognition in Alzheimer's disease and related disorders. In C. G. Kruse, H. Y. Meltzer, C. Sennef, & S. V. van de Witte (Eds.), *Thinking about cognition: concepts, targets and therapeutics* (pp. 19–27). Amsterdam, The Netherlands: IOS Press.
31. Hebert, R., Lindsay, J., Verreault, R., et al. (2000). Vascular dementia: Incidence and risk factors in the Canadian Study of Health and Aging. *Stroke, 31*, 1487–1493.
32. Howieson, D. B., Carlson, N. E., Moore, M. M., Wasserman, D., Abendroth, C. D., Payne-Murphy, J., et al. (2008). Trajectory of mild cognitive impairment. *Journal of the International Neuropsychological Society, 14*, 192–198.
33. Kral, V. A. (1958). Neuro-psychiatric observations in an old peoples home: Studies of memory dysfunction in senescence. *Journal of Gerontology, 13*, 169–176.
34. Kral, V. A. (1962). Senescent forgetfulness: Benign and malignant. *Canadian Medical Association Journal, 86*, 257–260.
35. Larson, E. (2000). An 80-year old man with memory loss. *Journal of the American Medical Association, 283*, 1046–1053.
36. Law, M., Baum, C., & Dunn, W. (2001). *Measuring occupational performance: Supporting best practice in occupational therapy*. Thorofare, NJ: SLACK.
37. Mace, N., & Rabins, P. (2011). *The 36-hour day: A family guide to caring for people who have Alzheimer disease, related dementias, and memory loss* (5th ed.). Baltimore, MD: Johns Hopkins Press.
38. McCarty, E. F., & Drebing, C. E. (2001). Delirium in older adults: Assessment and clinical management. *Journal of Geriatric Psychiatry, 34*(2), 183–195.
39. McKeith, I. G., Dickson, D. W., Lowe, J., et al. (2005). Diagnosis and management of dementia with Lewy bodies: Third report of the DLB Consortium. *Neurology, 65*, 1863–1872.
40. Meeks, T. W., Ropacki, S. A., & Jeste, D. V. (2006). The neurobiology of neuropsychiatric symptoms in dementia. *Current Opinion in Psychiatry, 19*, 281–296.
41. Murphy, S., & Tickle-Degnen, L. (2001). The effectiveness of occupational therapy–related treatments for persons with Parkinson's disease: A meta-analytic review. *American Journal of Occupational Therapy, 55*, 385–392.
42. Padilla, R. (September/October 2011). Effectiveness of interventions designed to modify the activity demands of the occupations of self-care and leisure for people with Alzheimer's disease and related dementias. *American Journal of Occupational Therapy, 65*(5), 523–531.
43. Park, D., & Schwarz, N. (2000). *Cognitive aging: A primer*. New York, NY: Taylor & Francis.
44. Pendleton, H. M., & Schultz-Krohn, W. (2013). *Pedretti's occupational therapy practice skills for physical dysfunction* (7th ed.). St. Louis, MO: Elsevier.
45. Perkinson, M. A., Hilton, C., Morgan, K., & Perlmutter, M. (2011). Therapeutic partnerships: Occupational therapy and home-based care. In C. Christiansen (Ed.), *Ways of living* (4th ed., pp. 445–461). Rockville, MD: American Occupational Therapy Association.
46. Petersen, R. C., Smith, G. E., Waring, S. C., Ivnik, R. J., Tangalos, E. G., & Kokmen, E. (1999). Mild cognitive impairment: Clinical characterization and outcome. *Archives of Neurology, 56*, 303–308, 760.
47. Plassman, B. L., Langa, K. M., Fisher, G. G., Heeringa, S. G., Weir, D. R., Ofstedal, M. B., et al. (2007). Prevalence in dementia in the United States: The Aging, Demographics, and Memory Study. *Neuroepidemiology, 29*, 125–132.
48. Rabinovici, C. D., & Miller, B. L. (2010). Frontotemporal lobar degeneration: Epidemiology, pathophysiology, diagnosis and management. *CNS Drugs, 24*, 375–398.
49. Rodda, J., Morgan, S., Walker, Z. (2009). Are cholinesterase inhibitors effective in the management of behavioral and psychological symptoms of dementia in Alzheimer's disease? A systematic review of randomized, placebo-controlled trials of donepezil, rivastigmine, and galantamine. International Psychogeriatrics, 21, 813-824.
50. Salthouse, T. A. (2010a). Influence of age on practice effects in longitudinal neurocognitive change. *Neuropsychology, 24*(5), 563–572.
51. Salthouse, T. A. (2010b). Selective review of cognitive aging. *Journal of the International Neuropsychological Society, 16*, 754–760.
52. Smith, G. E., & Bondi, M. W. (2008). Normal aging, mild cognitive impairment, and Alzheimer's disease. In J. E. Morgan & J. H. Ricker (Eds.), *Textbook of clinical neuropsychology* (pp. 762–780). New York, NY: Taylor & Francis.
53. Spitzer, R. L., Kroenke, K., & William, J. B. (1999). Validation and utility of a self-report version of PRIMIE-MD: the PHQ primary care study. Primary Care Evaluation of Mental Disorders. Patient Health Questionnaire. *Journal of the American Medical Association, 282*, 1737–1744.
54. Thinnes, A., & Padilla, R. (September/October 2011). Effect of educational and supportive strategies on the ability of caregivers of people with dementia to maintain participation in that role. *American Journal of Occupational Therapy, 65*(5), 541–549.
55. Toglia, J., & Kirk, U. (2001). Understanding deficits in self awareness following brain injury. *Neurorehabilitation, 15*, 57–70.
56. Waldemar, G., Dubois, B., Emre, M., et al. (2007). Recommendations for the diagnosis and management of Alzheimer's disease and other disorders associated with dementia: EFNS guidelines. *European Journal of Neurology, 14*, e1–e26.
57. Weaverdyck, S. (2005; update 2010). *#12—Dementia with Lewy bodies: A summary of information and intervention: Suggestions with an emphasis on cognition. Dementia care series caring sheets: Thoughts & suggestions for caring*. Lansing, MI: Michigan Department of Community Health.
58. Welsh-Bohmer, K. A., & Warren, L. H. (2006). Neurodegenerative dementias. In D. K. Attix & K. A. Welsh-Bohmer (Eds.), *Geriatric neuropsychology: Assessment and intervention* (pp. 56–85). New York, NY: Guilford Press.

CHAPTER 16

Mental Health and Common Psychiatric Disorders Associated with Aging

Virginia C. Stoffel, PhD, OT, BCMH, FAOTA, Soo Lee, MD, Jaclyn K. Schwartz, PhD, OTR/L, George T. Grossberg, MD

CHAPTER OUTLINE

OBJECTIVES

- Understand occupational performance challenges associated with common psychiatric disorders, diagnostic criteria, symptoms, and aging
- Identify appropriate occupational therapy evaluations for use with older adults with psychiatric challenges and disorders

- Review occupational therapy interventions and strategies applied to older adults with psychiatric challenges and disorders
- Identify members of the interprofessional mental health team and the distinct value each brings to their professional roles

Occupational therapists have been enabling clients to have better mental health since the birth of the profession. In the early twentieth century, the founders of occupational therapy (OT) established the profession on the key belief that occupation can heal the mind and the body.[34] Today, OT practitioners continue to work to "promote mental health and well-being" and to "restore, maintain, and improve function and quality of life for people at risk or affected by mental illness"(pp. S30, 3) through participation in life and engagement in occupation.[3,5] Specifically, mental health is a positive state of functioning that includes (1) positive affective or emotional state, (2) positive psychological and social function, (3) productive activities, and (4) resilience in the face of adversity.[3,75]

Unfortunately, about 20% of adults age 55 years or older experience a mental health concern ranging from depression to severe cognitive impairment, meaning all OT practitioners working with older adults will see persons with mental illness on their caseload.[2] Almost 3% of OT practitioners work directly with persons with mental illness, and the 66% of practitioners who work in hospitals, nursing facilities, outpatient facilities, home health services, and community health services will see persons with mental illness as a secondary condition.[4]

The purpose of this chapter is to provide an introduction to the core mental health knowledge and skills OT practitioners need to work with older adults with mental illness, along with information on diagnostic medical assessment and intervention.[3] In addition to discussing foundations, or how mental illness affects participation in everyday occupations, this chapter will review OT evaluation and intervention as well as interprofessional roles.

Late-Life Mood Disorders

Depression

Depression, or a major depressive episode, is defined as a 2-week or longer period of depressed mood, anhedonia, disturbance in appetite, disturbance in sleep, poor concentration, poor energy, disturbance in psychomotor activity, and suicidality (Box 16-1).[6] Older adults are more likely to experience poor sleep, decreased energy, psychomotor retardation, and decreased interest in continuing life. They are less likely to report depressed mood, feelings of guilt, or worthlessness. A mnemonic commonly used by medical school students to recall the symptoms of depression is SIG-E-CAPS (Box 16-2).[17]

BOX 16-1   DSM-V Diagnostic Criteria for Major Depressive Episode

Five (or more) of the following symptoms have been present during the same 2-week period and represent a change from previous functioning; at least one of the symptoms is either depressed mood or loss of interest or pleasure:
- Depressed mood most of the day, nearly every day, as indicated by either subjective report (e.g., feels sad or empty) or observation made by others (e.g., appears tearful)
- Markedly diminished interest or pleasure in all, or almost all, activities
- Significant weight loss when not dieting or weight gain or decrease or increase in appetite
- Insomnia or hypersomnia
- Psychomotor agitation or retardation
- Fatigue or loss of energy
- Feelings of worthlessness or excessive or inappropriate guilt
- Diminished ability to think or concentrate, or indecisiveness
- Recurrent thoughts of death (not just fear of dying), recurrent suicidal ideation without a specific plan, or a suicide attempt or a specific plan for committing suicide

(American Psychiatric Association. (2013). *Diagnostic and statistical manual of mental disorders* (5th ed.). Arlington, VA: Author.)

BOX 16-2   Depression Diagnosis Mnemonic: SIG-E-CAPS

S: Suicidal thoughts
I: Interests decreased
G: Guilt
E: Energy decreased
C: Concentration decreased
A: Appetite disturbance (increased or decreased)
P: Psychomotor changes (agitation or retardation)
S: Sleep disturbance (increased or decreased)

(Caplan, J. P., & Stern, T. A. (2008). Mnemonics in a nutshell: 32 aids to psychiatric diagnosis. *Current Psychiatry, 7,* 27-33.)

Incidence and Prevalence

Depression is one the most common psychiatric illnesses in the gerontological population. Although depression may be a continuing diagnosis from earlier in life, more than 50% of older clients have their first depressive episode in later life.

Risk

Risk for depression is high among older adults living in long-term care settings. Depression can occur as a primary disorder and as a secondary disorder due to medications or general medical conditions, such as Parkinson's disease and Alzheimer's disease, or stroke. In particular, there is a growing interest in the study of vascular depression, in which late-onset depression is accompanied by vascular disease or multiple cerebrovascular risk factors or stroke.[33]

Late-onset depression is more likely to carry risk factors related to medical illnesses.[15] Risk factors may be social, psychiatric, and/or medical (Table 16-1).[28]

Medical Treatment

Treatment for late-life depression encompasses individual therapy, the use of antidepressants, and electroconvulsive therapy (ECT). Selective serotonin reuptake inhibitors (SSRIs) are the most common pharmaceutical intervention and may be known by the names duloxetine (Cymbalta), paroxetine (Paxil), or sertraline (Zoloft). Side effects include nausea, restlessness, dizziness, reduced sexual function, drowsiness, insomnia, weight gain or loss, headache, dry mouth, vomiting, and/or diarrhea.[47] Older adults may require a longer time to achieve response to medication, meaning that they may not see the effects for weeks to over a month after they have begun to take the medication. ECT is a medical procedure that may be used when clients have tried multiple medications without success, cannot tolerate medication, display severe self-destructive behavior, or previously had a good response to ECT.[28]

Many older clients may experience clinically significant depression but fail to meet the criteria in the *Diagnostic and Statistical Manual of Mental Disorders*, 5th edition (DSM-V) for major depressive disorder, but may benefit from similar treatment and management. Depression can be difficult to diagnose in older clients, because they may underreport depression, focus on somatic concerns, or have cognitive impairments posing a barrier to detection.[28]

Occupational Performance Deficits

Older adults living with depression may have difficulty with performance in all areas of daily life.[65] Depressed mood, diminished pleasure in activities, and loss of energy may reduce clients' motivation to engage in the activities they need and want to do. For example, clients may not feel up to engaging in community activities such as socializing with friends, or even activities of daily living (ADLs) such as showering and bathing. Changes in appetite may alter mealtime activities. Insomnia or hypersomnia may create maladaptive sleep and rest routines. Older adults with depression may also have declines in cognition and executive function, which then impair performance in complex ADLs.[72] Poor executive function is associated with difficulty in formulating and achieving goals, making decisions, self-correcting, and other areas, and may affect activities such as driving, cooking, and medication management.[8] Depression and associated medications are associated with significant impairments, which can affect all ADLs and instrumental activities of daily living (IADLs).

Bipolar Disorder

Bipolar disorder, historically known as manic-depressive disorder, is a mood disorder defined by the presence of one or more manic episodes with or without episodes of depression. The term *mania* comes from the ancient Greek word for a mood characterized by excitement and agitation. Today, mania is understood as a distinct period of abnormal mood, which may be irritable, elevated, or expansive. These moods are accompanied by inflated self-esteem, decreased need for sleep, pressured sleep, distractibility, hypervigilance, racing thoughts, and impulsivity (Box 16-3).[6] Symptoms can be recalled using the mnemonic DIG FAST (Box 16-4).[17]

TABLE 16-1 Risk Factors for Depression in Older Adults

Social factors	Unmarried status
	Living alone
	Lack of social support
	Negative life events: bereavement
Individual factors	Female gender (between ages 65 and 80 years)
	Caregiving role
	Negative views on aging
Psychiatric factors	Prior history of depressive episodes
	Substance abuse
	Prior suicide attempt(s)
	Family history of depression
	Anxiety disorders
	Cognitive impairment
	Dementia
Medical factors	Chronic comorbid medical illnesses
	• Cardiovascular disease
	• Cancer
	• Parkinson's disease
	• Lung disease
	• Arthritis
	Loss of hearing
	Prior stroke

(Ellison, J. M., Kyomen, H. H., & Harper, D. G. (2012). Depression in later life: An overview with treatment recommendations. *Psychiatric clinics of north america, 35,* 203-229.)

BOX 16-3 DSM-V Criteria for Manic Episode

A distinct period of abnormally and persistently elevated, expansive, or irritable mood, lasting at least 1 week (or any duration if hospitalization is necessary). During the period of mood disturbance, three (or more) of the following symptoms have persisted (four if the mood is only irritable) and have been present to a significant degree:
- Inflated self-esteem or grandiosity
- Decreased need for sleep
- More talkative than usual or pressure to keep talking
- Flight of ideas or subjective experience that thoughts are racing
- Distractibility
- Increase in goal-directed activity or psychomotor agitation
- Excessive involvement in pleasurable activities that have a high potential for painful consequences

(American Psychiatric Association. (2013). *Diagnostic and statistical manual of mental disorders* (5th ed.). Arlington, VA: Author.)

Mania Diagnosis Mnemonic: DIG FAST

D: Distractibility
I: Indiscretion
G: Grandiosity
F: Flight of ideas
A: Activity increase
S: Sleep deficit
T: Talkativeness

(Caplan, J. P., & Stern, T. A. (2008). Mnemonics in a nutshell: 32 aids to psychiatric diagnosis. *Current Psychiatry, 7*, 27-33.)

Incidence and Prevalence

Bipolar disorder is uncommon in the older adult population, with a prevalence rate of 0.1% to 0.5%, but it accounts for 17% of psychiatric emergency room visits by older adults in the United States. In the United States, the number of older clients suffering from bipolar disorder is expected to grow along with the increase in the older adult population, and more studies will therefore be necessary to address the needs of this population.[62]

Risk

Bipolar disorder occurs as a primary disorder but also secondary to medical conditions and substances (Table 16-2).[62]

Medical Treatment

Medical treatment of bipolar disorder consists of pharmaceutical intervention or psychotherapy. Medications prescribed may include mood stabilizers and second-generation antipsychotics. Mood stabilizers may be lithium or anticonvulsants (also known as Stavzor, Depakote, or Lamictal) and have the side effects of restlessness, dry mouth, digestive issues, weight gain, dizziness, and/or drowsiness.[47] Lithium also requires regular blood testing to ensure that the medication is not affecting the function of vital organs. Antipsychotics are available for persons who do not benefit from mood stabilizers and include aripiprazole (Abilify), olanzapine (Zyprexa), risperidone (Risperdal), and quetiapine (Seroquel).[47] Side effects of antipsychotic medication include weight gain, sleepiness, tremors, movement disorders, cardiac disturbances, and vision impairment. Psychotherapy may include cognitive-behavioral therapy (CBT), psychoeducation, family therapy, or group therapy. Counseling focuses on learning more about bipolar disorder and identifying unhealthy beliefs and habits. Older clients with bipolar disorder are disproportionately affected by secondary conditions of cardiovascular disease, diabetes, hypertension, hyperlipidemia, and obesity, and will likely receive medical treatment for these medical conditions as well.

Occupational Performance Deficits

Older adults with bipolar disorder may have occupational performance deficits across all ADLs.[65] Whereas symptoms can be disabling in middle adulthood, symptoms can be life threatening when combined with the disability associated

TABLE 16-2 Mood Disorder (Mania) Due to General Medical Conditions and Substances

Neurologic diseases	Tumors
	Cerebrovascular accidents
	Seizures
	Huntington's disease
	Wilson's disease
	Pick's disease
	Multiple sclerosis
Infectious diseases	Infectious mononucleosis
	HIV encephalopathy
	Meningoencephalitis
	Neurosyphilis
Endocrine diseases	Hyperthyroidism
	Pheochromocytoma
	Cushing's syndrome
Other conditions	Vitamin deficiency (e.g., B_{12}, folate)
	Carcinoid syndrome
	Uremia
Substance-induced mood disorders	Anabolic steroids
	Alprazolam
	Antiparkinsonian medications
	Antidepressants
	Cocaine
	Corticosteroids
	Dextroamphetamine
	Hallucinogens
	Hypericum perforatum (St. John's wort)
	Methylphenidate
	Opiates

(Sajatovic, M., & Chen, P. (2011). Geriatric bipolar disorder. *Psychiatric Clinics of North America, 34*, 319-333.)

with older adulthood. For example, psychomotor agitation, or unintentional and purposeless motions such as pacing around a room, may place older adults with poor balance at risk for falls. Similarly, inflated self-esteem or grandiosity may cause older adults to overestimate their abilities to complete ADLs and put them at high risk of engaging in unsafe behavior. As with depression, bipolar disorder can also affect sleep routines and cognitive tasks.

Suicide in Older Adults

Suicide is the taking of one's own life, but many individuals are brought into the health-care system after an unsuccessful suicide attempt. Attempts by older adults are more fatal because older adults are more likely to use lethal methods.[20] The leading method of completed suicide is firearms (approximately 70%), which is followed by poisoning and suffocation.[18] Aged adults are also more likely to live alone and less likely to be discovered promptly for potential intervention. With advancing age, clients have more chronic medical conditions and overall decreased physical health, resulting in increased risk of fatal outcomes from self-inflicted injuries. Although suicidal ideation is most prevalent in young adults, the completed suicide rate is highest among older adult males.

Incidence and Prevalence

Suicide in the older adult population is of growing concern. According to the Centers for Disease Control, in 2009 nearly 37,000 deaths in the United States were secondary to suicide, of which 5858 were completed by older adults aged 65 years and older.[18]

Risk

There are several risk factors identified for suicide in older adults, including age and psychiatric, medical, and psychosocial factors. In the United States suicide rates decrease with increasing age; however, the generation with the highest suicidality, the baby boomers, is now entering old age.[21] Although previous suicide attempt is a risk factor, many suicide completers do not have a previous history of suicide in the older adult population. Risk factors are listed in Table 16-3.[20,21,50]

Medical Treatment

Identifying suicide risk factors and minimizing such risk factors are current approaches to suicide prevention. Over 70%

TABLE 16-3 Risk Factors for Suicide in Older Adults

Psychiatric	Mood disorder (particularly major depressive disorder Substance abuse disorder
Personality traits	Low openness to experience Anxious traits Obsessive traits
Medical conditions	HIV/AIDS Huntington's disease Multiple sclerosis Renal disease Peptic ulcer disease Spinal cord injury Systemic lupus erythematosus Cancer Terminal illness Uncontrollable pain
Psychosocial factors	Loss of husband/wife Financial stressors Loss of social support Disconnectedness Living alone Lacking autonomy and personal control secondary to physical illness and impaired functioning
Other	Receiving home nursing/care services Use of hypnotics and sedative medication Access to lethal means

(Conwell, Y., & Thompson, C. (2008). Suicidal behavior in elders. *Psychiatric Clinics of North America, 31,* 333-356.
Conwell, Y., Van Orden, K., & Caine, E. D. (2011). Suicide in older adults. *Psychiatric Clinics of North America, 34,* 451-468.
Minayo, M. C., & Cavalcante, F. G. (2010). Suicide in elderly people: A literature review. *Revista de Saude Publica, 44,* 750-757.)

---

of older suicide completers suffer from a psychiatric condition, particularly depression.[50] For health-care providers, identification and treatment of depression would be the major means of intervention. Furthermore, recent studies have shown that social connectedness is associated with better overall health and is a protective factor for suicidality.[21] Increasing social connectedness would require entities beyond health-care settings, such as family, community members (e.g., churches, peer support) and community programs (e.g., case manager, counselor).

Unfortunately, there are many barriers to suicide intervention with aged persons. Older adults are less likely to report experiencing depression and suicidal thoughts. Mood disorders are more likely to manifest in physical symptoms. Clients seeking help for psychiatric illnesses often go to their primary care physicians rather than mental health providers. In the primary care setting, physicians lack the training to screen and treat gerontological depression and suicidality.[20] Education and awareness of all health-care providers may aid in recognition, treatment, and prevention of suicide among older adults.

Occupational Performance Deficits

As suicide attempts are often associated with other mental health conditions, suicidal older adults may have several occupational performance deficits. In the immediate period of time surrounding a suicide attempt, they may have trouble engaging in their daily activities with good safety. They may need assistance in becoming more independent in their ADLs in environments that are modified for optimal safety, such as through limited access or supervised use of sharp objects.

Late-Life Anxiety Disorders

Anxiety affects about 6% to 10% of older adults. Anxiety is a normal response to stressors and is characterized by fear and concern, which at times could help an individual to cope with problems.[63] Anxiety disorders that are excessive may cause great distress and lead to social and occupational dysfunction. Anxiety disorders include generalized anxiety disorder, panic disorder, posttraumatic stress disorder, obsessive-compulsive disorder, and phobic disorders. Each anxiety disorder is discussed in the following sections and summarized in Table 16-4.

Generalized Anxiety Disorder

Generalized anxiety disorder (GAD) is characterized by difficulty in controlling severe anxiety and worrying about activities and events. Anxiety occurs for at least 6 months with three or more of the following symptoms: restlessness, fatigue, difficulty with concentration, irritability, muscle tension, and/or sleep disturbances.[6] GAD is one of the most common anxiety disorders in older adults. Current prevalence is estimated to be almost 3%, half of which is late-onset GAD.[19] Overall, GAD decreases in prevalence with increasing age in the aged population. GAD is associated

TABLE 16-4 DSM-V Criteria for Anxiety Disorders

Generalized anxiety disorder	Excessive anxiety and worry (apprehensive expectation), occurring more days than not for at least 6 months, about a number of events or activities (such as work or school performance) exists. The person finds it difficult to control the worry. The anxiety and worry are associated with three (or more) of the following six symptoms (with at least some symptoms present for more days than not for the past 6 months): • Restlessness or feeling keyed up or on edge • Being easily fatigued • Difficulty concentrating or mind going blank • Irritability • Muscle tension • Sleep disturbance (difficulty falling or staying asleep, or restless and unsatisfying sleep)
Panic disorder	Recurrent unexpected panic attacks—a panic attack is an abrupt surge of intense fear or intense discomfort that reaches a peak within minutes, and during which time four (or more) of the following symptoms occur: • Palpitations, pounding heart, or accelerated heart rate • Sweating • Trembling or shaking • Sensations of shortness of breath or smothering • Feelings of choking • Chest pain or discomfort • Nausea or abdominal distress • Feeling dizzy, unsteady, light-headed, or faint • Chills or heat sensations • Paresthesias (numbness or tingling sensation) • Derealization (feelings of unreality) or depersonalization (being detached from oneself) • Fear of losing control or "going crazy" • Fear of dying At least one of the attacks has been followed by 1 month (or more) of one or both of the following: • Persistent concern about having additional attacks or their consequences (e.g., losing control, having a heart attack, "going crazy") • A significant maladaptive change in behavior related to the attacks (e.g., behaviors designed to avoid having panic attacks, such as avoidance of exercise or unfamiliar situations)
Posttraumatic stress disorder	Exposure to actual or threatened death, serious injury, or sexual violence in one (or more) of the following ways: • Directly experiencing the traumatic event(s) • Witnessing, in person, the event(s) as it occurred to others • Learning that the traumatic event(s) occurred to a close family member or close friend; in cases of actual or threatened death of a family member or friend, the event(s) must have been violent or accidental • Experiencing repeated or extreme exposure to aversive details of the traumatic event(s) (e.g., first responders collecting human remains; police officers repeatedly exposed to details of child abuse) Presence of one (or more) of the following intrusion symptoms associated with the traumatic event(s), beginning after the traumatic event(s) occurred: • Recurrent, involuntary, and intrusive distressing memories of the traumatic event(s) • Recurrent distressing dreams in which the content and/or effect of the dream are related to the traumatic event(s) • Dissociative reactions (e.g., flashbacks) in which the individual feels or acts as if the traumatic event(s) were recurring • Intense or prolonged psychological distress at exposure to internal or external cues that symbolize or resemble an aspect of the traumatic event(s) • Marked physiologic reactions to internal or external cues that symbolize or resemble an aspect of the traumatic event(s) Persistent avoidance of stimuli associated with the traumatic event(s), beginning after the traumatic event(s) occurred, as evidenced by one or both of the following: • Avoidance of or efforts to avoid distressing memories, thoughts, or feelings about or closely associated with the traumatic event(s) • Avoidance of or efforts to avoid external reminders (people, places, conversations, activities, objects, situation) that arouse distressing memories, thoughts, or feelings about or closely associated with the traumatic event(s)

Continued

TABLE 16-4 DSM-V Criteria for Anxiety Disorders—cont'd

	Negative alterations in cognitions and mood associated with the traumatic event(s), beginning or worsening after the traumatic event(s) occurred, as evidenced by two (or more) of the following: • Inability to remember an important aspect of the traumatic event(s) (typically due to dissociative amnesia and not to other factors such as head injury, alcohol, or drugs) • Persistent and exaggerated negative beliefs or expectations about oneself, others, or the world • Persistent, distorted cognitions about the causes or consequences of the traumatic event(s) that lead the individual to blame himself or herself or others • Persistent negative emotional states • Markedly diminished interest or participation in significant activities • Feelings of detachment or estrangement from others • Persistent inability to experience positive emotion Marked alteration in arousal and reactivity associated with the traumatic event(s), beginning or worsening after the traumatic event(s) occurred, as evidenced by two (or more) of the following: • Irritable behavior and angry outbursts (with little or no provocation), typically expressed as verbal or physical aggression toward people or objects • Reckless or self-destructive behavior • Hypervigilance • Exaggerated startle response • Problems with concentration • Sleep disturbances
Obsessive-compulsive disorder	Presence of obsessions, compulsions, or both: Obsessions are defined by: • Recurrent and persistent thoughts, urges, or images that are experienced, at some time during the disturbance, as intrusive and unwanted, and that in most individuals cause marked anxiety or distress • Attempts to ignore or suppress such thoughts, urges, or images, or to neutralize them with some other thought or action (i.e., by performing a compulsion) Compulsions are defined by: • The individual feels driven to perform repetitive behaviors (e.g., hand washing, ordering, checking) or mental acts (e.g., praying, counting, repeating words silently) in response to an obsession or according to rules that must be applied rigidly. • The behaviors or mental acts are aimed at preventing or reducing distress or preventing some dreaded event or situation; however, these behaviors or mental acts either are not connected in a realistic way with what they are designed to neutralize or prevent, or are clearly excessive.
Specific phobia	• Marked fear or anxiety about a specific object or situation (e.g., flying, heights, animals, receiving an injection, seeing blood) exists. • The phobic object or situation almost always provokes immediate fear or anxiety. • The phobic object or situation is actively avoided or endured with intense fear or anxiety. • The fear or anxiety is out of proportion to the actual danger posed by the specific object or situation and to the sociocultural context. • The fear, anxiety, or avoidance is persistent, typically lasting for 6 months or more.
Social anxiety disorder (social phobia)	• Marked fear or anxiety about one or more social situations in which the individual is exposed to possible scrutiny by others; examples include social interactions (e.g., having a conversation, meeting unfamiliar people), being observed (e.g., eating or drinking), and performing in front of others (e.g., giving a speech). • The individual fears that he or she will act in a way or show anxiety symptoms that will be negatively evaluated (i.e., will be humiliating or embarrassing; will lead to rejection or offend others). • The social situations almost always provoke fear or anxiety. • The social situations are avoided or endured with intense fear or anxiety. • The fear or anxiety is out of proportion to the actual threat posed by the social situation and to the sociocultural context. • The fear, anxiety, or avoidance is persistent, typically lasting for 6 months or more.

(American Psychiatric Association. (2013). *Diagnostic and statistical manual of mental disorders* (5th ed.). Arlington, VA: Author.)

with female gender, younger age, lower household income, depression and other anxiety disorders, personality disorders, and being widowed, separated, or divorced. Late-onset GAD usually presents with comorbid depression. GAD clients are at increased risk of cardiovascular disease, gastrointestinal diseases, and arthritis.[19,58]

Panic Disorder

Panic disorder is characterized by panic attacks that are recurrent. Clients continuously worry about the next panic attack and its consequences. Panic attacks are experienced as discrete periods of intense fear or discomfort during which four or more of the following characteristics are present: palpitations, diaphoresis, tremors, shortness of breath, suffocation, chest pain, nausea, dizziness, depersonalization, fear of loss of control, fear of dying, numbness, and chills.[6] Panic attacks are unexpected and symptoms peak rapidly, usually in 10 minutes. Panic disorder is uncommon in late life and rarely has an onset after age 55 years. Older adults with panic disorder experience fewer attacks and fewer symptoms, and are less distressed by symptoms, than younger individuals.[64]

Posttraumatic Stress Disorder

Posttraumatic stress disorder (PTSD) occurs in individuals who were exposed to traumatic events that resulted in responses of intense fear, helplessness, and/or horror. The trauma is persistently reexperienced, and individuals avoid trauma-associated stimuli and remain in a hyperarousal state.[6] PTSD may not be diagnosed in older adults due to underreporting of traumatic experiences secondary to forgetting and fear of stigmatization, and it may be mistaken for depression, anxiety, or a psychotic disorder.[11] PTSD is a common disorder in older adults despite lower prevalence compared with young adults. PTSD in older adults may be further differentiated by age of onset, which determines the course and symptom severity. In clients with late-onset PTSD precipitated by acute traumatic experience, the symptom severity is lower. Older adults exposed to traumatic experiences are also less likely to develop PTSD. Early-onset PTSD symptoms are more severe and decline with advancing age. Furthermore, with increasing age, there is decline in reexperiencing symptoms and an increase in avoidance symptoms.[11]

Obsessive-Compulsive Disorder

Obsessive-compulsive disorder (OCD) is characterized by obsessions, compulsions, or both. Obsessions are recurrent thoughts, impulses, or images that are recognized by an individual as senseless but are difficult to ignore, causing much distress. Compulsions are repetitive thoughts or behaviors that an individual performs in response to an obsession to avoid a dreaded consequence or reduce distress.[6] OCD occurs in less than 1% of the gerontological population and at a lower rate compared with young adults.[59] Disease onset is usually earlier in life, and symptoms are thought to remain stable with advancing age. OCD is associated with other anxiety disorders and depression. It is also associated with executive functioning impairment, particularly verbal fluency.[59]

Phobic Disorders

Phobic disorders are characterized by persistent and unreasonable fear of a specific object, activity, or situation, which is avoided by the individual. Phobic disorders include social phobia, specific phobia, and agoraphobia, among others. They occur less frequently in older adults compared with young adults. Although a person may have a phobia related to any specific thing or situation, agoraphobia, specific phobia, and social phobia will be discussed here.

Agoraphobia

Agoraphobia is anxiety and fear related to being in places or situations in which help might not be available and escape might be difficult. The places and situations are avoided and include crowds, bridges, traveling on buses, standing in line, and being outside the home alone.[6] Agoraphobia is one of the most common anxiety disorders in older adults, with late onset being associated with a traumatic event such as a fall.

Specific Phobia

Specific phobia is characterized by severe, persistent, and irrational fear due to the presence or anticipation of a specific object or situation. The individual recognizes that the fear is unreasonable but, with exposure, experiences symptoms similar to those of a panic attack and thus avoids the feared situations. The distress, anxious anticipation, and avoidance significantly interfere with individual's normal functioning.[6] Specific phobia in the gerontological population is associated with recurrent stressful life events, younger age, divorce or being single, female gender, and lower education level. Older clients with specific phobia are more likely to have lower health-related quality of life and to have medical illnesses, particularly cardiovascular disease.[19]

Social Phobia

Social phobia is characterized by severe and persistent fear of social or performance situations. Individuals fear possible humiliation and criticism by others. Social phobia can significantly impair one's social functioning and quality of life.

Medical Treatment

Anxiety disorders in older adults have effects similar to those of late-life depression, and research has shown them to be just as disabling.[29] Older adults are less likely to seek treatment for anxiety and more likely to use somatic health-care services. Late-life anxiety disorder treatment is largely unknown and is based on young adult treatment studies and guidelines. There are two treatment approaches, pharmacologic treatment and psychotherapy.[29,63]

Pharmacologic Approaches

Antidepressants, benzodiazepines, and buspirone are common pharmacologic approaches. Antidepressants, discussed in the depression section earlier in the chapter, include SSRIs, which are the preferred antidepressants for this population due to the high comorbidity with depression. Benzodiazepines are nervous system depressants used for panic disorder, and include alprazolam (Xanax) and lorazepam (Ativan).[47] Benzodiazepines are only used when current symptoms are severe and require immediate response because the medication may be habit forming. Older adults may also experience the side effects of dependence, respiratory drive suppression, cognitive impairment, psychomotor impairment, and gait instability with related falls. Buspirone, also known as BuSpar or Vanspar, is used for anxiety and has less serious side effects compared with benzodiazepines. Side effects may include confusion, depression, and weakness. Buspirone has delayed onset and decreased efficacy in individuals with previous benzodiazepine treatment.[29]

Psychological Treatment

Psychotherapy includes approaches such as cognitive-behavioral therapy (CBT) and exposure therapy.[29] CBT aims to identify and correct dysfunctional automatic thoughts, which involves cognitive reconstruction and education. Exposure therapy involves facing feared situations or objects in a graded fashion over an extended period of time. There are limited evaluations of the efficacy of CBT in older populations, and further studies are needed. These approaches may not be useful in older adults with cognitive impairment and physical limitations.[63] Treatment should be tailored to individual clients, taking into consideration any comorbid psychiatric and medical conditions, other medications, and cognitive functioning.

Occupational Performance Deficits

Anxiety may impair a person's physical, cognitive, and/or psychosocial functioning.[25] The presence of anxiety of any type hinders learning and may decrease memory ability, making it difficult to engage in cognitively complex activities.[14] Persons with PTSD or phobic disorders may avoid people, places, situations, and activities, which may cause them to not attend work or family functions, hindering essential relationships and roles. Research shows that individuals with an anxiety disorder have worse outcomes in education, employment, and developing/maintaining relationships with others.

Late-Life Psychosis

Psychosis is the loss of contact with reality that presents with hallucinations and/or delusions. A hallucination is a perception in the absence of a stimulus, such as seeing things that are not present. A delusion is a false belief that is strongly held despite contrary evidence.

Psychosis has multiple neuropsychiatric etiologies, including schizophrenia, delusional disorder, psychosis associated with dementias, psychosis associated with affective disorders, delirium, seizures, brain tumors, and substance intoxication or withdrawal.[37] In this section, we discuss psychosis in schizophrenia and psychosis associated with dementia.

Schizophrenia

Schizophrenia is a chronic, disabling psychotic disorder that affects behavior, thinking, and emotion. It manifests with at least two of the following symptoms: delusions, hallucinations, disorganized speech, disorganized or catatonic behavior, and/or negative symptoms. Negative symptoms of schizophrenia include affective flattening, alogia (lack of speech), and avolition (lack of motivation). In older adults, schizophrenia can be further divided by age of onset and includes early-onset (before age 40 years), late-onset (age 40-60 years), and very-late-onset (after age 60 years) types. Unlike early-onset schizophrenia, late-onset schizophrenia is seen more often in women and is characterized by fewer negative symptoms, less severe cognitive impairment, and treatment that requires lower doses of antipsychotic agents. In older adults, hallucinations are more likely to be visual, tactile, or olfactory compared with younger adults, who are more likely to experience auditory hallucinations. Clients with very-late-onset schizophrenia have better premorbid functioning, and illness is associated with more severe cerebral atrophy, which suggests a neurodegenerative process.[37] Impairment is found in executive functioning, attention, working memory, learning, and processing speed. Memory impairment is due to poor organization and registration, instead of poor retrieval of information as seen in Alzheimer's disease. In later life, the rate of cognitive decline is the same as that seen with normal aging, except for the rates in institutionalized clients.[37]

Incidence and Prevalence

In the gerontological population, the prevalence of schizophrenia is currently thought to be 0.55%, compared with 1% in younger adults. The decline in prevalence is thought to be secondary to recovery and to the high mortality seen in schizophrenia with advancing age.[49] In the next two decades, the number of clients with schizophrenia is expected to double as the current expansion of older populations continues.

Risk

Clients with schizophrenia have a higher mortality compared with the general population. The most common natural causes of death are respiratory and cardiovascular diseases. Accidental falls followed by suicide are the most common unnatural causes of death.[68] Suicide risk factors are depression, commanding hallucinations, and somatic delusions. Negative long-term prognosis is seen in clients with poorer premorbid psychosocial and overall functioning, prominent negative symptoms, gradual symptom onset, and early illness severity. The amount of time experiencing psychotic symptoms in the first 2 years of the illness is the strongest predictor of disability.[37]

Psychosis with Dementia

Psychotic symptoms are common in dementia and have characteristics different from those of schizophrenia. In psychosis of Alzheimer's disease, hallucinations are more likely to be visual than auditory. Hallucinations are associated with severe dementia, less formal education, and gait impairment. Delusions are more likely simple, nonbizarre, paranoid, and related to memory deficits. For example, an individual having difficulty recalling where an object was placed accuses others of stealing the object. Misidentification delusion is the most common type, followed by paranoid delusions. Psychotic symptoms in vascular dementia depend on the region of brain insult and not on dementia severity. In psychosis with Parkinson disease and Lewy body dementia, visual hallucination is the most common psychotic symptom.[37]

Incidence and Prevalence

In persons with Alzheimer's disease, psychosis occurs in 41% of cases, delusions occur in 36% of cases, and hallucinations in 18% of cases.[60] Psychosis increases progressively over the first 3 years after diagnosis and then plateaus.

Risk

Delusions are associated with older age, aggression, depression, and worse general health. Psychosis is associated with black ethnicity and more severe cognitive impairment.[60] Compared with clients without psychotic symptoms, Alzheimer's disease with psychosis is associated with increased cognitive impairment and greater rate of decline. Furthermore, clients have worse physical health, increased mortality, and poorer quality of life.

Medical Treatment for Late-Life Psychosis

Physicians may prescribe typical (first-generation) antipsychotics or atypical (second-generation) antipsychotic agents to combat the symptoms of psychosis.[67] Atypical antipsychotics, such as aripiprazole (Abilify), clozapine (Clozaril), olanzapine (Zyprexa), quetiapine (Seroquel), and risperidone (Risperdal), have fewer side effects than their first-generation counterparts and are used more frequently.[47] In Parkinson's disease, any antipsychotic use can worsen parkinsonism. Atypical antipsychotics carry black box warnings for cerebrovascular adverse events in older clients with dementia and are associated with increased mortality. Other significant side effects include orthostatic hypotension associated with falls, metabolic syndrome, sedation, extrapyramidal symptoms, and neuroleptic malignant syndrome.[37]

Psychological Treatment

Psychosocial interventions are available to improve level of functioning. Examples of these interventions are functional adaptation skills training and cognitive-behavioral social skills training. Education is also provided to family and caregivers. Community health-care providers help clients live in the community, maintain independence, and adhere to treatment. Many clients living in the community obtain employment, drive cars, and function independently for a portion of their adulthood. Clients with greater disability may require higher levels of support in group homes or nursing homes.[37]

Occupational Performance Deficits

Cognitive impairment is a core feature of psychosis and affects attention, working memory, and executive function.[13] Additionally, older adults with psychosis may have difficulty screening out irrelevant information and may be easily distracted during cognitive tasks. Cognitive impairment can

make it more difficult to complete daily activities such as going to the grocery store. Persons with psychosis may have difficulty in new or unfamiliar situations and may create rigid routines and return to the same places over and over again. Therefore, older adults with this condition may need assistance, particularly with complex and community-based IADLs, and subsequently have high utilization of nursing home care.[30] Additionally, persons with psychosis may have difficulty maintaining health and wellness routines, and as a result people with schizophrenia have a 20% shorter life expectancy and are more likely to die of heart disease. Finally, the stigma of living with a mental illness may create social barriers to community living and integration.

Delirium

Delirium is a common neuropsychiatric syndrome in the gerontological population and is characterized by acute onset of disturbance in consciousness and cognition or perception with a fluctuating course (Box 16-5).[6] Once delirium resolves, individuals may return to a premorbid level of functioning and personality; however, some changes are not completely reversible, particularly in older adults with preexisting dementia.[51]

The core diagnostic symptoms of delirium are disturbance in consciousness, attention, cognition (memory, orientation, and language), and perception. However, there are several other symptoms not mentioned in the DSM-V criteria that commonly accompany the core symptoms (Box 16-6).[38] The most common symptoms are disturbances in attention and sleep-wake cycles. The least common symptom is delusions, and the least common cognitive symptom is disorientation.[48]

BOX 16-5 DSM-V Criteria for Delirium

- A disturbance in attention (i.e., reduced ability to direct, focus, sustain, and shift attention) and awareness (reduced orientation to the environment) is noted.
- The disturbance develops over a short period (usually hours to a few days), represents a change from baseline attention and awareness, and tends to fluctuate in severity during the course of day.
- An additional disturbance in cognition (e.g., memory deficit, disorientation, language, visuospatial ability, or perception) is noted.
- The disturbances in attention and cognition are not better explained by another preexisting, established, or evolving neurocognitive disorder and do not occur in the context of a severely reduced level of arousal, such as coma.
- There is evidence from the history, physical examination, or laboratory findings that the disturbance is a direct physiologic consequence of another medical condition, substance intoxication or withdrawal (i.e., due to a drug of abuse or to a medication), or exposure to toxin, or is due to multiple etiologies.

(American Psychiatric Association. (2013). *Diagnostic and statistical manual of mental disorders* (5th ed.). Arlington, VA: Author.)

BOX 16-6	Delirium Symptoms

Cognitive

Orientation
Attention
Short-term memory
Long-term memory
Visuospatial ability

Neuropsychiatric and Behavioral Abnormalities

Sleep-wake cycle disturbance
Perceptual disturbances and hallucinations
Delusions
Lability in affect
Language
Thought process abnormalities
Motor agitation
Motor retardation

(Jain, G., Chakrabarti, S., & Kulhara, P. (2011). Symptoms of delirium: An exploratory factor analytic study among referred patients. *General Hospital Psychiatry*, 33(4), 377-385.)

BOX 16-7	Risk Factors for Delirium

- Age ≥ 65 years
- Male sex (if without premorbid dementia)
- Dementia/other cognitive impairment
- Previous history of delirium
- Depression
- Visual and hearing impairment
- Decreased intake (dehydration, malnutrition; in clients without dementia, low body mass index)
- Multiple-drug regimen
- Psychoactive drugs/alcohol abuse (more applicable to adult population)
- History of stroke, neurologic disease
- Chronic renal/hepatic disease
- Multiple coexisting medical conditions
- Severe medical illness/terminal illness
- HIV
- Decreased functional status (dependence, immobility, fragility, history of falls, pain, constipation)
- Prolonged sleep deprivation

(Lee, H. B., Mears, S. C., Rosenberg, P. B., Leoutsakos, J. M. S., Gottshalk, A., & Seeber, F. E. (2011). Predisposing factors for postoperative delirium after hip fracture repair in individuals with and without dementia. *Journal of the American Geriatrics Society*, 59, 2306-2313.
Mittal, V., Muralee, S., Williamson, D., McEnerney, N., Thomas, J., Cash, M., & Tampi, R. R. (2011). Review: Delirium in the elderly: A comprehensive review. *American Journal of Alzheimer's Disease and Other Dementias*, 26, 97-109.)

Based on psychomotor activity, delirium may be divided into four subtypes: hyperactive, hypoactive, mixed, and normal motor delirium. Hypoactive delirium is the more common type in older adults and is the most commonly missed or undiagnosed form of delirium. Hypoactive delirium has the following characteristics: slowing or lack of movement, paucity of speech with or without prompting, and unresponsiveness. In clients with premorbid dementia, hypoactive delirium has the worst survival rate.[76] Hyperactive delirium is more common in adults and is associated with medication side effects or substance withdrawal. Hyperactive delirium is characterized by restlessness, constant movement, and agitation. Mixed motor delirium has clinical features of both hyperactive and hypoactive delirium.[51]

Incidence and Prevalence

There is a high rate of delirium in medical and surgical settings and a much lower incidence in the community. Approximately 20% of all hospital inpatients acquire delirium, with proportions increasing to 25% at 50 years of age and 35% at 80 years of age.[61] In the community, however, the prevalence of delirium in older adults age 65 years and older decreases to about 1% to 2%.[43]

Risk

The risk factors for developing delirium are listed in Box 16-7.[44,51] Delirium is thought be a result of an aberrant response to a precipitating factor leading to an acute central nervous system failure. There are many causes of delirium, and it is usually a result of a multifactorial culprit. The precipitating factors may cause direct injury to the central nervous system or indirect insult via an aberrant stress response (Table 16-5).[55]

Medical Treatment

The goal of treatment in delirium is to treat the underlying medical condition (e.g., resolve infection; simplify polypharmacy). There are no drugs approved by the Food and

Drug Administration for the agitation, aggression, paranoia, and hallucinations that accompany delirium. However, psychotropic agents are commonly used to treat such symptoms, such as those discussed in the previous section on late-life psychosis. The first-generation antipsychotic haloperidol (Haldol) has the most data supporting its efficacy. High dosages of Haldol are associated with increased risk of developing extrapyramidal symptoms, primarily parkinsonism. All antipsychotic agents should be used with caution secondary to increased risk of cerebrovascular adverse events and death, which remains elevated months after use.[51]

Assessment involves obtaining thorough history, temporal onset, review of preexisting medical and psychiatric history, review of medications and substance use, behavioral observations, cognitive assessment, physical examination, and laboratory studies (Table 16-6). History and temporal onset may help differentiate delirium from depression or dementia. Review of preexisting medical conditions, medications, and physical examination may help determine risk factors as well as precipitating factors.[51] Modifications of risk factors may prevent delirium, decrease the duration of disease, and decrease the use of psychotropic agents.

Occupational Performance Deficits

Delirium affects all occupational performance areas due to cognitive, motor, and sleep impairments. Persons with delirium may experience impairments in orientation, attention, memory, and visuospatial abilities, which limits a person's

TABLE 16-5 Precipitating Factors in Delirium

Direct Injury	
Metabolic abnormalities	Hypoxia, hypercapnia
	Electrolyte disturbances
	Hypoglycemia, hyperglycemia
	Hyponatremia, hypernatremia
	Acidosis, alkalosis
	Hypothyroidism, hyperthyroidism
	Anemia
	Renal insufficiency
	Hepatic insufficiency
Iatrogenic	Anticholinergic medications
	Narcotics
	Sedatives
	Antiepileptic drugs
	Psychotropic agents
	Steroids
	Fluoroquinolones
	Oseltamivir
	Muscle relaxants
	Antiplatelets and anticoagulants
Central nervous system	Stroke
	Head trauma (e.g., subdural hematoma)
	Increased intracranial pressure
	Epilepsy
	Intracranial infection
Aberrant Stress Responses	
Infections	Urinary tract infection
	Pneumonia
	Cellulitis
Cardiovascular	Myocardial infarction
	Cardiac surgery
Environmental factors	Intensive care unit admission
	Physical restraints
Other	Orthopedic surgery

(Mittal, V., Muralee, S., Williamson, D., McEnerney, N., Thomas, J., Cash, M., & Tampi, R. R. (2011). Review: Delirium in the elderly: A comprehensive review. *American Journal of Alzheimer's Disease and Other Dementias, 26*, 97-109.)

TABLE 16-6 Laboratory Tests for Delirium Workup

Initial Laboratory Studies	
Blood urea nitrogen/Creatinine	
Electrolytes	
Blood sugar	
Liver function test	
Thyroid function test	
Other Studies Depending on Assessment	
Preexisting heart disease	Electrocardiogram
Suspect inflammatory disease	C-reactive protein
	Erythrocyte sedimentation rate
Suspect infectious etiology	Urine analysis, urine culture
	Blood culture
	Arterial blood gas
	Chest x-ray
Suspect illicit drug use	Urine drug screen
Suspect nutritional deficits	Vitamin B_{12}
	Folate
Rule out seizure	Electroencephalogram
Rule out stroke, cerebral disease	Magnetic resonance imaging—brain
	Computed tomography—scan head
Suspect meningitis	Lumbar puncture

(Mittal, V., Muralee, S., Williamson, D., McEnerney, N., Thomas, J., Cash, M., & Tampi, R. R. (2011). Review: Delirium in the elderly: A comprehensive review. *American Journal of Alzheimer's Disease and Other Dementias, 26*, 97-109.)

ability to engage in even simple ADLs. Poor orientation to place, for example, can lead older adults to be unable to find ADL equipment such as a toothbrush. Sleep disturbances, in addition to poor orientation to time, can disrupt regular routines, such as mealtimes. Motor agitation or retardation can limit older adults' physical abilities to complete daily activities and may place individuals at a higher risk for falls. Delirium may become so disabling that it results in an increased length of hospital stay and higher rates of nursing home placement.[45]

Late-Life Personality Disorders

Personality is understood as individual characteristics that manifest in one's attitude and behavioral and emotional responses to different situations. Personality is usually developed by young adulthood and remains stable throughout life. The DSM-V defines personality disorder as an inflexible, pervasive, stable pattern of inner experiences and behavior that begins in childhood or adolescence and remains stable thereafter. Personality disorders manifest in cognitive, affective, interpersonal function, and impulse-control patterns that deviate from cultural norms, leading to distress and impairment in social, occupational, and other areas of functioning.[6]

Personality disorders are divided into three clusters in the DSM-V. Cluster A personality disorders are characterized by odd, eccentric thinking or behavior and include paranoid, schizoid, and schizotypal personality disorders. Cluster B personality disorders are characterized by dramatic, overly emotional thinking and erratic behavior and include antisocial, borderline, histrionic, and narcissistic personality disorders. Cluster C personality disorders are characterized by anxious or fearful thinking and include avoidant, dependent, and obsessive-compulsive personality disorders. DSM-V criteria are listed in Table 16-7.[6]

Although personality disorders are common in the older population, they may be underdiagnosed due to the time-intensive history, going back many decades. Further, the diagnosis cannot be based on current symptoms alone, and older adults are more likely to hide symptoms, problems in behavior, and relationships they find to be shameful.[1]

TABLE 16-7 DSM-V Diagnostic Criteria for Personality Disorders

Personality Disorder Type	Brief Description
Cluster A	
Paranoid personality disorder	A pervasive distrust and suspiciousness of others such that their motives are interpreted as malevolent, beginning by early adulthood and present in a variety of contexts, as indicated by four (or more) of the following: • Suspects, without sufficient basis, that others are exploiting, harming, or deceiving him or her • Is preoccupied with unjustified doubts about the loyalty or trustworthiness of friends or associates • Is reluctant to confide in others because of unwarranted fear that the information will be used maliciously against him or her • Reads hidden demeaning or threatening meanings into benign remarks or events • Persistently bears grudges (i.e., is unforgiving of insults, injuries, or slights) • Perceives attacks on his or her character or reputation that are not apparent to others and is quick to react angrily or to counterattack • Has recurrent suspicions, without justification, regarding fidelity of spouse or sexual partner
Schizoid personality disorder	A pervasive pattern of detachment from social relationships and a restricted range of expression of emotions in interpersonal settings, beginning by early adulthood and present in a variety of contexts, as indicated by four (or more) of the following: • Neither desires nor enjoys close relationships, including being part of a family • Almost always chooses solitary activities • Has little, if any, interest in having sexual experiences with another person • Takes pleasure in few, if any, activities • Lacks close friends or confidants other than first-degree relatives • Appears indifferent to the praise or criticism of others • Shows emotional coldness, detachment, or flattened affectivity
Schizotypal personality disorder	A pervasive pattern of social and interpersonal deficits marked by acute discomfort with, and reduced capacity for, close relationships as well as by cognitive or perceptual distortions and eccentricities of behavior, beginning by early adulthood and present in a variety of contexts, as indicated by five (or more) of the following: • Ideas of reference (excluding delusions of reference) • Odd beliefs or magical thinking that influences behavior and is inconsistent with subcultural norms (e.g., superstitiousness; belief in clairvoyance, telepathy, or "sixth sense") • Unusual perceptual experiences, including bodily illusions • Odd thinking and speech (e.g., vague, circumstantial, metaphorical, overelaborate, or stereotyped) • Suspiciousness or paranoid ideation • Inappropriate or constricted affect • Behavior or appearance that is odd, eccentric, or peculiar • Lack of close friends or confidants other than first-degree relatives • Excessive social anxiety that does not diminish with familiarity and tends to be associated with paranoid fears rather than negative judgments about self
Cluster B	
Antisocial personality disorder	A pervasive pattern of disregard for and violation of the rights of others occurring since age 15 years, as indicated by three (or more) of the following: • Failure to conform to social norms with respect to lawful behaviors, as indicated by repeatedly performing acts that are grounds for arrest • Deceitfulness, as indicated by repeated lying, use of aliases, or conning others for personal profit or pleasure • Impulsivity or failure to plan ahead • Irritability and aggressiveness, as indicated by repeated physical fights or assaults • Reckless disregard for safety of self or others • Consistent irresponsibility, as indicated by repeated failure to sustain consistent work behavior or honor financial obligations • Lack of remorse, as indicated by being indifferent to or rationalizing having hurt, mistreated, or stolen from another

TABLE 16-7 DSM-V Diagnostic Criteria for Personality Disorders—cont'd

Personality Disorder Type	Brief Description
Borderline personality disorder	A pervasive pattern of instability of interpersonal relationships, self-image, and affect, and marked impulsivity, beginning by early adulthood and present in a variety of contexts, as indicated by five (or more) of the following: • Frantic efforts to avoid real or imagined abandonment • A pattern of unstable and intense interpersonal relationships characterized by alternating between extremes of idealization and devaluation • Identity disturbance: markedly and persistently unstable self-image or sense of self • Impulsivity in at least two areas that are potentially self-damaging (e.g., spending, sex, substance abuse, reckless driving, binge eating) • Recurrent suicidal behavior, gestures, or threats, or self-mutilating behavior • Affective instability due to a marked reactivity of mood (e.g., intense episodic dysphoria, irritability, or anxiety usually lasting a few hours and only rarely more than a few days) • Chronic feelings of emptiness • Inappropriate, intense anger or difficulty controlling anger (e.g., frequent displays of temper, constant anger, recurrent physical fights) • Transient, stress-related paranoid ideation or severe dissociative symptoms
Histrionic personality disorder	A pervasive pattern of excessive emotionality and attention seeking, beginning by early adulthood and present in a variety of contexts, as indicated by five (or more) of the following: • Is uncomfortable in situations in which he or she is not the center of attention • Interaction with others is often characterized by inappropriate sexually seductive or provocative behavior • Displays rapidly shifting and shallow expression of emotions • Consistently uses physical appearance to draw attention to self • Has a style of speech that is excessively impressionistic and lacking in detail • Shows self-dramatization, theatricality, and exaggerated expression of emotion • Is suggestible (i.e., easily influenced by others or circumstances) • Considers relationships to be more intimate than they actually are
Narcissistic personality disorder	A pervasive pattern of grandiosity (in fantasy or behavior), need for admiration, and lack of empathy, beginning by early adulthood and present in a variety of contexts, as indicated by five (or more) of the following: • Has a grandiose sense of self-importance (e.g., exaggerates achievements and talents, expects to be recognized as superior without commensurate achievements) • Is preoccupied with fantasies of unlimited success, power, brilliance, beauty, or ideal love • Believes that he or she is "special" and unique and can only be understood by, or should associate with, other special or high-status people (or institutions) • Requires excessive admiration • Has a sense of entitlement (i.e., unreasonable expectations of especially favorable treatment or automatic compliance with his or her expectations) • Is interpersonally exploitative (i.e., takes advantage of others to achieve his or her own ends) • Lacks empathy: is unwilling to recognize or identify with the feelings and needs of others • Is often envious of others or believes that others are envious of him or her • Shows arrogant, haughty behaviors or attitudes
Cluster C Avoidant personality disorder	A pervasive pattern of social inhibition, feelings of inadequacy, and hypersensitivity to negative evaluation, beginning by early adulthood and present in a variety of contexts, as indicated by four (or more) of the following: • Avoids occupational activities that involve significant interpersonal contact, because of fears of criticism, disapproval, or rejection • Is unwilling to get involved with people unless certain of being liked • Shows restraint within intimate relationships because of the fear of being shamed or ridiculed • Is preoccupied with being criticized or rejected in social situations • Is inhibited in new interpersonal situations because of feelings of inadequacy • Views self as socially inept, personally unappealing, or inferior to others • Is unusually reluctant to take personal risks or to engage in any new activities because they may prove embarrassing

Continued

TABLE 16-7 DSM-V Diagnostic Criteria for Personality Disorders—cont'd

Personality Disorder Type	Brief Description
Dependent personality disorder	A pervasive and excessive need to be taken care of that leads to submissive and clinging behavior and fears of separation, beginning by early adulthood and present in a variety of contexts, as indicated by five (or more) of the following: • Has difficulty making everyday decisions without an excessive amount of advice and reassurance from others • Needs others to assume responsibility for most major areas of his or her life • Has difficulty expressing disagreement with others because of fear of loss of support or approval • Has difficulty initiating projects or doing things on his or her own (because of a lack of self-confidence in judgment or abilities rather than a lack of motivation or energy) • Goes to excessive lengths to obtain nurturance and support from others, to the point of volunteering to do things that are unpleasant • Feels uncomfortable or helpless when alone because of exaggerated fears of being unable to care for himself or herself • Urgently seeks another relationship as a source of care and support when a close relationship ends • Is unrealistically preoccupied with fears of being left to take care of himself or herself
Obsessive-compulsive personality disorder	A pervasive pattern of preoccupation with orderliness, perfectionism, and mental and interpersonal control, at the expense of flexibility, openness, and efficiency, beginning by early adulthood and present in a variety of contexts, as indicated by four (or more) of the following: • Is preoccupied with details, rules, lists, order, organization, or schedules to the extent that the major point of the activity is lost • Shows perfectionism that interferes with task completion (e.g., is unable to complete a project because his or her own overly strict standards are not met) • Is excessively devoted to work and productivity to the exclusion of leisure activities and friendships (not accounted for by obvious economic necessity) • Is overconscientious, scrupulous, and inflexible about matters of morality, ethics, or values (not accounted for by cultural or religious identification) • Is unable to discard worn-out or worthless objects even when they have no sentimental value • Is reluctant to delegate tasks or to work with others unless they submit to exactly his or her way of doing things • Adopts a miserly spending style toward both self and others; money is viewed as something to be hoarded for future catastrophes • Shows rigidity and stubbornness

(American Psychiatric Association. (2013). *Diagnostic and statistical manual of mental disorders* (5th ed.). Arlington, VA: Author.)

Incidence and Prevalence

Personality disorders occur in about 10% of the general population, and recent studies show no change in prevalence with increasing age.[52] In older populations, Cluster A and Cluster C personality disorders are the most common, whereas antisocial personality disorder prevalence declines with age. The course of borderline personality disorder fluctuates, often with remission in middle age and possible reemergence later in life.[52]

Medical Treatment

Pharmacologic and psychotherapy approaches are used to treat personality disorders. There are no medications approved to treat personality disorders in the United States, but physicians may use antidepressants, mood stabilizers, antipsychotic medications, and antianxiety medications, depending on the client's symptoms.[56]

Psychological Treatment

Psychotherapy includes dialectical behavior therapy, cognitive-behavioral therapy, and psychodynamic therapy. In psychotherapy, persons with personality disorder learn about their condition, strategize, and discuss moods and feelings. The goal of this treatment is to gain insight and to develop healthy strategies to manage symptoms.

Occupational Performance Deficits

Occupational performance deficits vary by cluster of personality disorder and may affect social participation, emotional modulation, and coping skills.[71] Persons with a Cluster A personality disorder may be seen as odd or eccentric. In general they are suspicious and distrusting of others, resulting in decreased interest in social relationships. Older adults with Cluster A personality disorders may have difficulty maintaining interpersonal relationships. Persons with

Cluster B personality disorders experience a lack of empathy and unpredictable behaviors and may seem aggressive and narcissistic. Older adults with Cluster B personality disorders may have unstable relationships and desire to be the center of attention. Persons with Cluster C personality disorders often have trouble coping and may feel unable to function without the help of others. This may cause persons with Cluster C personality disorders to be dependent on others to care for their daily activities. Personality disorders often result from negative interactions or environments and may result in decreased trust in others. Issues can also be seen with modulating emotions, impulsivity, and coping. Together, these symptoms increase the risk of self-harming behaviors, such as cutting, and substance abuse. Persons with personality disorders may need assistance in developing positive coping strategies and learning to control their emotions and impulses.

Elder Abuse and Neglect

Elder abuse is an intentional or negligent act leading to harm or creating a serious risk of harm to a vulnerable older adult by a caregiver or other persons.[74] Elder abuse includes physical abuse, psychological abuse, financial abuse, sexual abuse, and neglect. Previously, elder abuse was considered a social problem and was understood as a result of "caregiver stress." It obtained formal recognition in the 1970s after recognition of child abuse and domestic violence as serious issues. In the 1980s, Adult Protective Services was established to receive and investigate elder abuse reports. A decade later, elder abuse was addressed as a criminal justice problem, and the United States pursued national education and training of law enforcement and judicial system professionals regarding this issue. Entering the twenty-first century, more grants were awarded to medical forensics research related to elder abuse.[66]

Physical Abuse

Physical abuse involves physical force that causes bodily harm, pain, or impairment. Physical force may involve striking, hitting, pushing, shaking, slapping, kicking, pinching, burning, use of physical restraints, and force-feeding. Clients may present with bruises, cuts, fractures, sprains, and untreated injuries in various stages of healing.[54] Unlike accidental bruising, intentional bruising is larger in size (greater than 5 cm) and located in the lateral right arm, posterior trunk, neck, and head.[73] Laboratory studies may show medication overdose or underutilization of prescribed drugs. Suspicious behaviors include an abrupt change in an older adult's behavior or a caregiver's refusal to allow visitors to see an older adult alone.

Sexual Abuse

Sexual abuse of older adults is any nonconsensual sexual contact with an older person or a person unable to give consent. Such contacts include rape, sodomy, coerced nudity, unwanted touching, and sexually explicit photographing. Victims may present with torn, stained, or bloody underclothing

and report being sexually assaulted or raped. Victims may display unexplained changes in behavior, such as aggression, withdrawal, or self-mutilation, or out-of-character sexual behaviors. Victims frequently complain of abdominal pain, and physical examination may reveal bruises around the breasts or genital area, unexplained venereal disease or genital infections, and unexplained vaginal or anal bleeding.[54]

Emotional or Psychological Abuse

Psychological abuse involves verbal or nonverbal acts that cause anguish, pain, or distress. Verbal emotional abuse includes verbal assaults, insults, threats, intimidation, humiliation, and harassment. Nonverbal emotional abuse includes treating an older person like an infant, enforcing social isolation, and "silent treatments." Victims present with changes in sleep or eating patterns, emotional disturbance, unusual behavior such as rocking and sucking, and may appear withdrawn. Victims also avoid physical, eye, or verbal contact with caregivers.[54]

Neglect

Neglect is characterized by refusal or failure to fulfill a person's obligations or duties to an older adult. Obligations and duties involve providing life necessities such as food, shelter, medicine, personal hygiene, and safety. Victims of neglect may present with dehydration, malnutrition, untreated bed sores, poor personal hygiene, and unattended or untreated health problems. Victims may live under hazardous, unsafe, unsanitary, or unclean living conditions.[54]

Abandonment

Abandonment occurs when an individual who has physical custody or assumed responsibility for providing care deserts an older adult. Victims may be deserted at a hospital, nursing facility, shopping center, or other public location.[54]

Financial Exploitation

Financial exploitation involves illegal or improper use of an older adult's funds, property, or assets. Examples of financial exploitation are listed in Box 16-8.[54]

Self-Neglect

Self-neglect is characterized by the actions of some older adults that may threaten their health or safety. Self-neglect involves refusal or failure to provide necessities, including water, food, clothing, shelter, personal hygiene, and necessary medications. Victims may present with inappropriate clothing, dehydration, malnutrition, unattended medical conditions, and poor personal hygiene. They may lack necessary medical aids such as eyeglasses, dentures, or hearing aids. Victims may live in unsafe or unsanitary living conditions or may be homeless.[54]

Incidence and Prevalence

Approximately 10% of older adults experience abuse.[55] Unfortunately, only one in 14 cases of elder abuse is reported to the authorities. Approximately 0.05% of older adults self-report financial abuse, which is a higher self-report rate than the rates for emotional, physical, and sexual abuse, and neglect.

Risk

Each category of abuse and neglect carries different risk factors.[32] Females are more likely than males to be victims of elder abuse, whereas males are more likely to commit elder abuse.[42] Female victims are more likely to be abused by their child or a spouse, and male victims are more likely to be abused by strangers or acquaintances.[42] Persons with disabilities, persons with dementia, and persons in institutions are at higher risk of abuse and neglect.[55]

Medical Treatment

When elder abuse is suspected, health-care providers, including OT practitioners, are mandated to report to state-specific agencies, such as Adult Protective Services, and ensure client safety.[42] Ensuring client safety may involve calling 911 or the police when a client is in immediate danger. Safety achievement may require hospitalization, obtaining a court protective order, or placing the client in a safe home.

Occupational Performance Deficits

Abuse and neglect of older adults affects all life functions, including ability to complete ADL and IADL. Injuries associated with physical abuse, such as bruises, breaks, and strains, can limit an older adult's ability to physically complete basic ADLs. Sexual abuse may result in physiologic impairment of an older adult's genitals, resulting in difficulty with bowel and bladder routines. Psychological abuse not only impairs psychosocial function but can impair performance in sleep/rest and eating. Persons with physical disabilities who are unable to independently complete their basic activities of grooming, dressing, and bathing are at risk of neglect. Persons in negligent situations may be forced to go without bathing, bed mobility, or even eating.

Occupational Therapy Evaluation

The OT evaluation seeks to understand what a client needs and wants to do, what a client can do, and what supports and barriers to participation are available.[5] All evaluations should consist of an occupational profile and assessment of occupational performance. This section discusses the occupational profile and some specific assessments available to evaluate occupational performance in mental health.

Occupational Profile

The occupational profile is a summary of a client's current manner of living in addition to interests, values, and needs.[5] Using an interview process, the OT practitioner should determine what a client used to do, what the client needs to do to return home, and the barriers and facilitators present when returning home with a change in health status. It is important to understand the client's prior level of function and the occupations the client must be able to perform to return home. For example, is the client responsible for all of the cooking and cleaning, or are those chores shared or completely taken care of by another person? Does the client drive or use public transportation?

An occupational therapist can conduct the occupational profile using an unstructured or semistructured interview that inquires about a client's perception of his or her ability to engage in daily activity. The Canadian Occupational Performance Measure (COPM) is a semistructured interview that measures a client's self-perception of occupational performance in the areas of self-care, leisure, and productivity.[41] A client identifies activities in daily life that are difficult and then rates the importance of each activity. The five most important activities are also rated on satisfaction. Similarly, the Occupational Circumstances Assessment and Interview Rating Scale (OCAIRS) is a semistructured interview that inquires about one's roles, habits, interests, values, goals, communication, and environment.[31] Using this tool, the evaluator will inquire about typical roles and how well one is able to complete the roles. Caregivers may also provide input on their loved one's daily occupational routines and past occupational performance.

Analysis of Occupational Performance

Whereas the occupational profile describes what a client used to do and what the client needs to do, the occupational performance evaluation describes what a client can currently do. During the occupational performance evaluation, the occupational therapist assesses the client's performance of everyday activities through tools designed to "observe, measure, and inquire about factors that support or hinder occupational performance (p. S14)"[5] An occupational therapist can administer an evaluation composed of any combination of assessments and screens. The therapist should be sure to choose measures that evaluate areas of need identified in the occupational profile in addition to areas of anticipated impairments often associated with a diagnosis. Various tools are available for OT practitioners, as discussed next.

Screens

Screens are a quick and easy assessment of one construct and serve to inform the medical team if the client will require more services in a certain area. For example, depression, anxiety, and altered cognition may all go undetected in the older adult population. If a therapist perceives that a client may be struggling with one of these issues, he or she may administer a screen, and use the results to share with the team, to inform the plan of care, and to refer the client to other professionals.

If the occupational therapist suspects a cognitive impairment, he or she may administer a cognitive screen. The Mini-Mental State Examination (MMSE) consists of 11 questions testing orientation, memory, language, and visuospatial skills. It requires less than 10 minutes to complete and has been standardized on older adults.[70] The Saint Louis University Mental Status Exam is an 11-item cognitive assessment measuring orientation, memory, attention, and executive function.[69] This tool has also been standardized on older adults and requires approximately 7 minutes to administer.

Similarly, if an occupational therapist suspects depression, he or she may administer a screen for depression. The Beck Depression Inventory is a 21-item self-report tool that asks about behaviors associated with depression.[9,57] Standardized in the acute and psychiatric settings, the tool is appropriate for use with many populations. The Geriatric Depression Scale was created specifically for older adults to evaluate not only depression but suicidal ideation as well.[57] This 30-item tool is free for health-care professionals to use and has been standardized on several older adult populations.

Anxiety screens may help occupational therapists to identify if a client has demonstrated excessive or unhealthy levels of anxiety. The Hospital Anxiety and Depression Scale is a 14-item tool that identifies depression and anxiety among adults who are physically ill. The tool only requires about 5 minutes to administer, but has not been standardized on an older adult population.[10] The Depression Anxiety Stress Scale is a 21-item tool that measures the fundamental symptoms of depression, anxiety, and stress.[35] The tool requires about 10 minutes to administer and has been standardized on persons at clinics for depression, anxiety, phobia, and stress (but not specifically on older adults).

Performance

Whereas a screen investigates a person's health and function in a specific domain, occupational performance tools measure how well a client is able to complete a series of tasks needed to accomplish specific occupations. Various tools quantify performance for different activities. There are a number of performance tests available, but in this section we will cover three OT evaluations appropriate for use with clients with mental illness. The Kitchen Task Assessment (KTA) investigates a client's ability to safely cook pudding.[7] Developed specifically for persons with Alzheimer's disease, this tool is appropriate for use with older adults and persons with cognitive impairment. The KTA can also describe how much assistance a client will need with meal routines. The Kohlman Evaluation of Living Skills (KELS) was initially developed for use in inpatient mental health settings, and is increasingly being used with older adults in the community.[16] During the assessment, the client is asked to write a check and balance a checkbook, purchase items and receive correct change, read a phone bill, identify hazards in a picture, make a phone call,

and balance a budget. Performance is graded on a scale of 0 to 16. In addition to determining performance in the aforementioned tasks, the KELS may also help in making a safe discharge determination. In the Executive Function Performance Test (EFPT), the client is asked to prepare a light meal, manage medications, use the telephone, and pay a bill.[8] During the evaluation, the EFPT helps indicate what the person can do and where additional supports are needed to facilitate independence. The EFPT has been used in physical rehabilitation and mental health settings.

Activity and Participation

Several of the diagnoses discussed earlier in the chapter mentioned symptoms that may cause one to withdraw from completion of regular occupations. Measures of activity and participation evaluate which activities clients engage in and how often. Here we provide two examples of activity and participation measures. In the Activity Card Sort, clients are shown 89 photographs of persons completing various activities (e.g., gardening) and are asked to identify the activities they currently do, used to do, and would like to do.[39] The tool is appropriate for use with older adults. The Modified Interest Checklist provides the client with a list of 68 activities, and clients are asked to identify if they currently complete the activity, have completed the activity in the past, or would like to complete the activity in the future.[40] The checklist focuses more on leisure activities.

OT practitioners have a variety of tools available to screen for specific impairments, assess occupational performance, and establish a client's quality of activity and participation. Different tools are appropriate for different settings and client populations. All of these tools assess deficits common among psychological impairments, but can be used in a mental health facility or in a physical dysfunction setting. Mental illness may not be a client's primary diagnosis, but ensuring good mental health is an important part of any OT evaluation. (See chapter 6 for guidelines for selecting appropriate screening and assessment tools.)

Occupational Therapy Intervention and Outcomes

OT practitioners help older adults with mental illness engage in occupations related to health, well-being, and participation. Intervention helps the client reach goals, and progress is established through the use of outcomes. This section elaborates on some treatment intervention ideas and outcomes for use with older adult clients with mental illness.

Occupational Performance

Interventions for occupational performance help persons with mental illness do the things they need and want to do in everyday life. Occupational performance can be improved, so that clients return to a higher prior level of performance, or enhanced, so that clients can complete a new functional activity they have never completed before. During the evaluation, the occupational therapist and client identify the occupations for which the client would like to improve performance. Skills training, engaging in occupations, changing the context, and tailoring the activity are all strategies that may be used to improve occupational performance.

Skills training is an intervention strategy to directly train clients to complete a task. During the training, a skill is broken down into component parts, and clients are trained on all of the tasks needed to complete an occupation.[12] For example, skills training on medication management would include an OT practitioner and the client reviewing tasks of (1) sorting medication, (2) refilling medication, and (3) taking medication.

Sometimes OT practitioners may want to improve a client's capacities for certain occupations through engagement in another occupation. For example, medication management requires concentration and executive function skills to complete the process. Occupational therapy personnel may work to improve concentration and executive function with a craft project, such as asking a client to follow a series of directions to create a finished product. Although the craft project and medication management are different occupations, both activities work to improve concentration and executive function.

Occupational therapists and assistants may adapt the environment to facilitate the client's completion of a desired occupation.[36] For instance, using the medication management example, a client may have difficulty due to poor concentration. The occupational therapist or assistant may coach the client to simplify the environment by turning off the television and radio. By removing extra environmental stimuli, the client may be better able to concentrate on the medication task.

OT practitioners may tailor the complexity of a treatment activity. Sometimes clients need to experience success with an occupation to feel safe and able to complete the activity independently. OT practitioners can help the client to increase skill confidence by providing clients with the just-right challenge.[36] Using this strategy, OT practitioners provide challenges that meet the client's ability level. For example, for a client with poor concentration working on medication management, the occupational therapist may ask the client to address only one or two medications.

Prevention, Health, and Wellness

Interventions for prevention, health, and wellness help clients become and remain in a positive state of physical, mental, and social well-being. Mental illness is a chronic disease, and individuals with mental illness are at risk for a variety of secondary conditions. Prevention, health, and wellness interventions are essential to ensure that clients stay in good physical and mental health. Self-management plans and developing healthy routines are two examples of interventions for prevention, health, and wellness.

To prevent mental illness relapse, persons with mental illness may learn strategies to self-manage their conditions. Several different standardized interventions are available, including the Wellness Recovery and Action Plan[22] and the

Illness Management and Recovery Program.[53] In these interventions, clients work to develop a variety of skills, such as understanding triggers, creating a crisis plan, and identifying coping skills.[27]

Many clients demonstrate unhealthy behaviors that contribute to secondary conditions; OT practitioners can contribute by enabling clients to create healthy routines. Smoking addiction, obesity, and related diseases are common health conditions in persons with mental illness. Occupational therapists and assistants can help clients to modify their daily lives to incorporate healthier habits.[27] For example, therapists and assistants may help clients learn how to make use of a nearby gym or incorporate time to exercise in a schedule.

Participation and Role Competence

Participation and role competence interventions ensure that clients are not only able to complete activities, but to do so in a way that is satisfying and effective. Engagement in occupation, peer support, and family psychoeducation are three strategies that may help clients to demonstrate good participation and role competence.

Sometimes just engaging in an occupation and being with others is an intervention in and of itself.[27] Engaging in occupations such as work can alleviate symptoms of mental illness, increase life quality, and develop life meaning.[23] Intervention activities that motivate clients to engage in occupation and to be a part of a group may have significant benefits for persons with mental illness.

Unfortunately in mental illness, symptoms may cause a client to withdraw from participating in his or her regular roles. Peer support, however, can help encourage a person with a mental illness to reengage.[46] Peer support services can be delivered directly in a facility, occur in a support group, or can even happen online. Peer support helps individuals to develop a larger social network, increase autonomy, and develop socially valuable active roles.[24] OT practitioners can support clients in building these peer relationships by referring clients to online or in-person support groups, and prompt them to use the support when needed.

The client's family can also help engage the client in satisfying and meaningful life activities. Family psychoeducation helps key family members to learn how to better support the client.[24] In this training, family members learn how to interact with each other and create supportive relationships. Occupational therapists may play a role in the family psychoeducation process through caregiver training.

Quality of Life and Well-being

Quality of life and well-being are the summative outcomes of occupational performance, participation, and health. These constructs reveal a client's satisfaction, hope, and self-concept in addition to contentment with one's health and security.[5] When clients are able to complete the activities they need and want to do in a meaningful and satisfying way without concern for health, they will live full and productive lives. OT interventions throughout domains may contribute to optimal life quality and well-being.

Interprofessional Role and Service Outcomes

Mental health interventions focus on enabling the person to participate in everyday life. OT practitioners play a significant role in the process, but clients often need the support of a team of health professionals. Each health professional has specific training in a particular area of expertise. OT practitioners in mental health should be aware of team members and the roles they play. Psychiatrists, psychologists, primary care physicians, mental health nurses, social workers, licensed professional counselors, peer specialists, and hospice staff are common professionals involved in the care of older adults with mental illness.[26] This section reviews each of the professional roles. (See chapter 27 for additional discussion of inter- and intraprofessional processes.)

Physicians

Psychiatrists are physicians who have completed medical school in addition to 4 or more years of training in psychiatry. Psychiatrists can diagnose clients with a psychological disorder, prescribe medications, and provide psychotherapy. Primary care physicians often recognize mental health issues as a part of an integrative assessment of health.

Pharmacists

Pharmacists typically have a doctoral degree and complete 4 years of pharmacy training. In addition to dispensing medication, pharmacists advise physicians and clients about medication side effects, promote disease prevention, and troubleshoot medication regimens.

Psychology Professionals

Psychologists typically have a doctoral degree in psychology. These licensed professionals may evaluate and treat emotional, behavioral, and mental disorders. Licensed professional counselors also derive from the field of psychology. These professionals have a master's degree and at least 2 years of supervised work experience. Counselors may assess and treat psychiatric conditions.

Nurses

Mental health nurses are registered nurses who often have an associate's or bachelor's degree. Nurses can provide a variety of services, including evaluation and treatment of psychiatric illness and case management, and may even provide psychotherapy. Nurse practitioners in mental health provide similar services, but have master's or doctoral degrees. Nurse practitioners may diagnose conditions, prescribe medications, and provide therapy.

Social Workers

Social workers can have a variety of degrees, from a bachelor's to a doctorate, and fill several functions on the team. The social worker provides case management and discharge planning, and helps clients find placement and enroll in needed services. Social workers with a master's degree and appropriate licensure may also provide treatment, including psychotherapy. Social work and OT often work closely together for discharge planning.

Therapeutic Recreation Professionals

Therapeutic recreation professionals typically have associate's or bachelor's degrees. Using recreation activities, such as creative arts, therapists work to improve clients' psychological and social functioning. Therapeutic recreation professionals may work with OT practitioners to develop daily programming and activities for persons in inpatient facilities.

Peers

Peers are persons with mental illness who are living in recovery. The peer specialist can provide support from the perspective of someone who has been through the process. Peer specialists are certified by the state, and therefore requirements differ by location.

Hospice Staff

Hospice staff are any health-care professionals serving the needs of the terminally ill. Staff help persons who are only receiving medical care to ease pain (comfort care) and often are actively in the process of dying. Many psychological conditions may be present in a client who is dying or the client's close family and friends. Staff are trained in interventions and techniques to enable the family to complete the process with peace, dignity, and good mental well-being.

Summary

Many adult psychiatric illnesses continue into old age. However, certain cases of late-onset psychiatric illnesses and conditions are more likely to occur in older adults, such as delirium and elder abuse. Psychiatric symptoms in older adults may have different clinical presentations and carry different risk factors. Generally, psychiatric illnesses in older adults are poorly recognized and therefore often untreated by health-care providers. This is likely a reflection of the limited literature and clinical guidelines available at this time. However, psychiatric illnesses in older adults are a growing concern with the anticipated increase in prevalence in the decades to come.

Occupational therapists and assistants can play an important role in the lives of older adults with mental health concerns. Practitioners can evaluate a client's health and function in everyday life. After determining a plan of care, OT practitioners work to improve clients' occupational performance, health and well-being, participation, and quality of life as part of a coordinated interprofessional team.

REVIEW QUESTIONS

1. List and describe occupational performance challenges that typically accompany psychiatric disorders in later life.
2. Explain the role of evaluation in the process of intervening with older adults with mental health conditions.

3. Describe commonly applied OT interventions and strategies provided with older adults who experience psychiatric challenges and disorders.

4. How may an interprofessional mental health team promote optimal outcomes with aging mental health clients?

REFERENCES

1. Agronin, M. E., & Maletta, G. (2000). Personality disorders in late life. Understanding and overcoming the gap in research. *American Journal of Geriatric Psychiatry, 8,* 4–18.
2. American Association for Geriatric Psychiatry. (2015). *Geriatrics and mental health—the facts.* http:// www.cdc.gov/aging/pdf/mental_health.pdf. Accessed 7/15/14.
3. American Occupational Therapy Association. (2010a). Specialized knowledge and skills in mental health promotion, prevention, and intervention in occupational therapy practice. *The American Journal of Occupational Therapy, 64*(Suppl. 6), S30–S43.
4. American Occupational Therapy Association. (2010b). *Workforce trends in occupational therapy. In Your career in occupational therapy* (pp. 1–2). Bethesda, MD: Author.
5. American Occupational Therapy Association. (2014). Occupational therapy practice framework: Domain and process (3rd ed.). *The American Journal of Occupational Therapy, 68*(Suppl. 1), S1–S48.
6. American Psychiatric Association. (2013). *Diagnostic and statistical manual of mental disorders* (5th ed.). Arlington, VA: Author.
7. Baum, C., & Edwards, D. F. (1993). Cognitive performance in senile dementia of the Alzheimer's type: The Kitchen Task Assessment. *American Journal of Occupational Therapy, 47*(5), 431–436.
8. Baum, C. M., Connor, L. T., Morrison, T., Hahn, M., Dromerick, A. W., & Edwards, D. F. (2008). Reliability, validity, and clinical utility of the Executive Function Performance Test: A measure of executive function in a sample of people with stroke. *American Journal of Occupational Therapy, 62*(4), 446–455.
9. Beck, A. T., Steer, R. A., & Brown, G. K. (1996). *Beck Depression Inventory.* San Antonio, TX: Pearson Education.
10. Bjelland, I., Dahl, A. A., Haug, T. T., & Neckelmann, D. (2002). The validity of the Hospital Anxiety and Depression Scale: An updated literature review. *Journal of Psychosomatic Research, 52*(2), 69–77.
11. Bottche, M., Kuwert, P., & Knaevelsrud, C. (2012). Posttraumatic stress disorder in older adults: An overview of characteristics and treatment approaches. *International Journal of Geriatric Psychiatry, 27,* 230–239.
12. Brown, C. (2011a). Activities of daily living and instrumental activities of daily living. In C. Brown & V. C. Stoffel (Eds.), *Occupational therapy in mental health: A vision for participation* (pp. 659–675). Philadelphia, PA: F. A. Davis.
13. Brown, C. (2011b). Schizophrenia. In C. Brown & V. C. Stoffel (Eds.), *Occupational therapy in mental health: A vision for participation* (pp. 179–191). Philadelphia, PA: F. A. Davis.
14. Brown, C., & Stoffel, V. C. (2011). *Occupational therapy in mental health: A vision for participation.* Philadelphia, PA: F. A. Davis.
15. Bukh, J. D., Bock, C., Vinberg, M., Gether, U., & Kessing, L. V. (2011). Differences between early and late onset adult depression. *Clinical Practice and Epidemiology in Mental Health, 7,* 140–147.
16. Burnett, J., Dyer, C. B., & Naik, A. D. (2009). Convergent validation of the Kohlman Evaluation of Living Skills as a screening tool of older adults' ability to live safely and independently in the community. *Archives of Physical Medicine and Rehabilitation, 90*(11), 1948–1952.
17. Caplan, J. P., & Stern, T. A. (2008). Mnemonics in a nutshell: 32 aids to psychiatric diagnosis. *Current Psychiatry, 7,* 27–33.
18. Centers for Disease Control and Prevention. (2014). *Web-based injury statistic query and reporting system (WISQARS).* Atlanta, GA: Author.
19. Chou, K-L. (2009). Specific phobia in older adults: Evidence from the national epidemiologic survey on alcohol and related conditions. *American Journal of Geriatric Psychiatry, 17,* 376–386.
20. Conwell, Y., & Thompson, C. (2008). Suicidal behavior in elders. *Psychiatric Clinics of North America, 31,* 333–356.
21. Conwell, Y., Van Orden, K., & Caine, E. D. (2011). Suicide in older adults. *Psychiatric Clinics of North America, 34,* 451–468.
22. Copeland, M. E. (2002). Wellness Recovery Action Plan: A system for monitoring, reducing and eliminating uncomfortable or dangerous physical symptoms and emotional feelings. *Occupational Therapy in Mental Health, 17*(3-4), 127–150.
23. Craik, C., & Pieris, Y. (2006). Without leisure "it wouldn't be much of a life": The meaning of leisure for people with mental health problems. *The British Journal of Occupational Therapy, 69*(5), 209–216.
24. Davidson, L., Chinman, M., Kloos, B., Weingarten, R., Stayner, D., & Tebes, J. K. (1999). Peer support among individuals with severe mental illness: A review of the evidence. *Clinical Psychology: Science and Practice, 6*(2), 165–187.
25. Davis, J. (2011). Anxiety disorders. In C. Brown & V. C. Stoffel (Eds.), *Occupational therapy in mental health: A vision for participation* (pp. 167–178). Philadelphia, PA: F. A. Davis.
26. Duckworth, G., & McBride, H. (1996). Suicide in old age: A tragedy of neglect. *Canadian journal of psychiatry. Revue canadienne de psychiatrie, 41*(4), 217–222.
27. Eklund, M. (2011). Occupation and Wellness. In C. Brown & V. C. Stoffel (Eds.), *Occupational therapy in mental health: A vision for participation* (pp. 649–658). Philadelphia, PA: F. A. Davis.
28. Ellison, J. M., Kyomen, H. H., & Harper, D. G. (2012). Depression in later life: An overview with treatment recommendations. *Psychiatric Clinics of North America, 35,* 203–229.
29. Flint, A. J. (1999). Anxiety disorders in late life. *Canadian Family Physician, 45,* 2672–2679.
30. Folsom, D. P., Lebowitz, B. D., Lindamer, L. A., et al. (2006). Schizophrenia in late life: Emerging issues. *Dialogues in Clinical Neuroscience, 28,* 45–52.
31. Forsyth, K., Deshpande, S., Kielhofner, G., Henriksson, C., Haglund, L., & Olson, L., et al. (2005). *The Occupational Circumstances Assessment Interview and Rating Scale.* http://www.cade.uic.edu/moho/productDetails.aspx?aid=35. Accessed 7/15/14.
32. Garre-Olma, J., Planas-Pujol, X., Lopez-Pousa, S., Juvinya, D., Vila, A., & Vilata-Franch, J. (2009). Prevalence and risk factors of suspected elder abuse subtypes in people aged 75 and older. *Journal of American Geriatrics Society, 57,* 815–822.
33. Gonzalez, H. M., Tarraf, W., Whitfield, K., & Gallo, J. J. (2012). Vascular depression prevalence and epidemiology in the United States. *Journal of Psychiatric Research, 46,* 456–461.
34. Gordon, D. M. (2009). The history of occupational therapy. In E. Crepeau, E. Cohn, & B. Schell (Eds.), *Willard and Spackman's occupational therapy* (11th ed., pp. 202–215). Philadelphia, PA: Lippincott Williams & Wilkins.

35. Henry, J. D., & Crawford, J. R. (2005). The short-form version of the Depression Anxiety Stress Scales (DASS-21): Construct validity and normative data in a large non-clinical sample. *British Journal of Clinical Psychology*, 44(2), 227–239.

36. Howells, V. (2011). Leisure and play. In C. Brown & V. C. Stoffel (Eds.), *Occupational therapy in mental health: A vision for participation* (pp. 724–735). Philadelphia, PA: F. A. Davis.

37. Iglewicz, A., Meeks, T. W., & Jeste, D. V. (2014). New wine in old bottle: Late-life psychosis. *Psychiatric Clinic in North America*, 34, 295–318.

38. Jain, G., Chakrabarti, S., & Kulhara, P. (2011). Symptoms of delirium: An exploratory factor analytic study among referred patients. *General Hospital Psychiatry*, 33(4), 377–385.

39. Katz, N., Karpin, H., Lak, A., Furman, T., & Hartman-Maeir, A. (2003). Participation in occupational performance: Reliability and validity of the Activity Card Sort. *OTJR: Occupation, Participation and Health*, 23(1), 10–17.

40. Kielhofner, G., & Neville, A. (1983). *The modified interest checklist*. Chicago, IL: University of Illinois.

41. Kirsh, B., & Cockburn, L. (2009). The Canadian Occupational Perfromance Measure: A tool for recovery-based practice. *Psychiatric Rehabilitation Journal*, 32(3), 171–178.

42. Krienert, J. L. (2009). Elderly in America: A descriptive study of elder abuse examining National Incident-Based Reporting System (NIBRS) data, 2000-2005. *Journal of Elder Abuse and Neglect*, 21(4), 325–345.

43. Lange, E. D., Verhaak, P., & Meer, K. (2013). Prevalence, presentation and prognosis of delirium in older people in the population, at home and in long term care: A review. *International Journal of Geriatric Psychiatry*, 28(2), 127–134.

44. Lee, H. B., Mears, S. C., Rosenberg, P. B., Leoutsakos, J. M. S., Gottshalk, A., & Seeber, F. E. (2011). Predisposing factors for postoperative delirium after hip fracture repair in individuals with and without dementia. *Journal of the American Geriatrics Society*, 59, 2306–2313.

45. Leslie, D. L., Marcantonio, E. R., Zhang, Y., Leo-Summers, L., & Inougye, S. K. (2008). One-year healthcare costs associated with delirium in population. *Archives of Internal Medicine*, 168(1), 27–48.

46. Lloyd, C., & Deane, F. P. (2011). Social participation. In C. Brown & V. C. Stoffel (Eds.), *Occupational therapy in mental health: A vision for participation* (pp. 711–723). Philadelphia, PA: F. A. Davis.

47. *Mayo Foundation for Medical Education and Research*. (2014). http://www.mayoclinic.org/diseases-conditions. Accessed 7/14/15.

48. Meagher, D. J., Moran, M., Raju, B., Gibbons, D., Donnelly, S., & Saunders, J., et al. (2007). Phenomenology of delirium: Assessment of 100 adult cases using standardized measures. *The British Journal of Psychiatry*, 190, 135–141.

49. Meesters, P. D., de Haan, L., Comijs, H. C., Stek, M. L., Smeets-Janssen, M. M. J., & Weeda, M. R., et al. (2012). Schizophrenia spectrum disorders in later life: Prevalence and distribution of age at onset and sex in a Dutch catchment area. *American Journal of Geriatric Psychiatry*, 20, 18–28.

50. Minayo, M. C., & Cavalcante, F. G. (2010). Suicide in elderly people: A literature review. *Revista de Saude Publica*, 44, 750–757.

51. Mittal, V., Muralee, S., Williamson, D., McEnerney, N., Thomas, J., & Cash, M., et al. (2011). Review: Delirium in the elderly: A comprehensive review. *American Journal of Alzheimer's Disease and Other Dementias*, 26, 97–109.

52. Morse, J. Q., & Lynch, T. R. (2004). A preliminary investigation of self-reported personality disorders in late life: Prevalence, predictors of depressive severity, and clinical correlates. *Aging and Mental Health*, 4, 307–325.

53. Mueser, K. T., Corrigan, P. W., Hilton, D. W., Tanzman, B., Schaub, A., & Gingerich, S., et al. (2002). Illness management and recovery: A review of the research. *Psychiatric Services*, 53(10), 1272–1284.

54. National Center on Elder Abuse. (2007). *Major types of elder abuse*. Alhambra, CA: U.S. Administration on Aging.

55. National Center on Elder Abuse. (2011). *Statistics and data*. Alhambra, CA: U.S. Administration on Aging.

56. Paris, J. (2008). Clinical trials of treatment for personality disorders. *Psychiatric Clinics of North America*, 31, 517–526.

57. Parmelee, P. A., & Katz, I. R. (1990). Geriatric depression scale. *Journal of the American Geriatrics Society*, 38(12), 1379.

58. Porensky, E. K., Dew, M. A., Karp, J. F., Skidmore, E., Rollman, B. L., & Shear, M. K., et al. (2009). The burden of late-life generalized anxiety disorder: Effects on disability, health-related quality of life, and healthcare utilization. *American Journal of Geriatric Psychiatry*, 17, 473–482.

59. Pulular, A., Levy, R., & Stewart, R. (2013). Obsessive and compulsive symptoms in a national sample of older people: Prevalence, comorbidity, and associations with cognitive functioning. *American Journal of Geriatric Psychiatry*, 21, 263–271.

60. Ropacki, S. A., & Jeste, D. V. (2005). Epidemiology of and risk factors for psychosis of Alzheimer's disease: A review of 55 studies published from 1990 to 2003. *American Journal of Psychiatry*, 162(11), 2022–2030.

61. Ryan, D. J., O'Regan, N. A., Caoimh, R. Ó., Clare, J., O'Connor, M., & Leonard, M., et al. (2013). Delirium in an adult acute hospital population: Predictors, prevalence and detection. *BMJ Open*, 3(1), pii: e001772. doi: 10.1136/bmjopen-2012-001772.

62. Sajatovic, M., & Chen, P. (2011). Geriatric bipolar disorder. *Psychiatric Clinics of North America*, 34, 319–333.

63. Schuurmans, J., & van Balkon, A. (2011). Late-life anxiety disorders: A review. *Current Psychiatry Reports*, 13, 267–273.

64. Sheikh, J. I., Swales, P. J., Carlson, E. B., & Lindley, S. E. (2004). Aging and panic disorder: Phenomenology, comorbidity and risk factors. *American Journal of Geriatric Psychiatry*, 12, 102–109.

65. Spangler, N. W. (2011). Mood disorders. In C. Brown & V. C. Stoffel (Eds.), *Occupational therapy in mental health: A vision for participation* (pp. 155–166). Philadelphia, PA: F. A. Davis.

66. Stiegel, L. (2006). Recommendations for the elder abuse, health, and justice fields about medical forensic issues related to elder abuse and neglect. *Journal of Elder Abuse and Neglect*, 18, 41–81.

67. Suzuki, T., Remington, G., Uchida, H., Rajji, T. K., Graff-Guerrero, A., & Mamo, D. C. (2011). Management of schizophrenia in late life with antipsychotic medications. *Drugs and Aging*, 28, 961–980.

68. Talaslahti, T., Alanen, H-M., Hakko, H., et al. (2012). Mortality and causes of death in older patients with schizophrenia. *International Journal of Geriatric Psychiatry*, 27(11), 1131–1137.

69. Tariq, S. H., Tumosa, N., Chibnall, J. T., Perry III, M. H., & Morley, J. E. (2006). Comparison of the Saint Louis University Mental Status Examination and the Mini-Mental State Examination for detecting dementia and mild neurocognitive disorder—a pilot study. *The American Journal of Geriatric Psychiatry*, 14(11), 900–910.

70. Tombaugh, T. N., & McIntyre, N. J. (1992). The Mini-Mental State Examination: A comprehensive review. *Journal of the American Geriatrics Society*, 40(9), 922–935.

71. Urish, C. (2011). Personality disorder. In C. Brown & V. C. Stoffel (Eds.), *Occupational therapy in mental health: A vision for participation* (pp. 143–154). Philadelphia, PA: F. A. Davis.

72. van den Kommer, T. N., Comijs, H. C., Aartsen, M. J., Huisman, M., Deeg, D. J., & Beekman, A. T. (2013). Depression and cognition: How do they interrelate in old age? *The American Journal of Geriatric Psychiatry, 21*(4), 398–410.

73. Wiglesworth, A., Austin, R., Corona, M., Schneider, D., Liao, S., & Gibbs, L., et al. (2009). Bruising as a marker of physical elder abuse. *Journal of the American Geriatrics Society, 57*, 1191–1195.

74. Wolf, R., Daichman, L., & Bennett, G. (2002). Elder abuse. In E. G. Krug, L. L. Dahlberg, J. A. Mercy, A. B. Zwi, & R. Lozano (Eds.), *World report on violence and health* (pp. 123–145). Geneva: World Health Organization.

75. World Health Organization. (2005). *Promoting mental health: Concepts, emerging evidence, practice: A report of the World Health Organization, Department of Mental Health and Substance Abuse.* Geneva: Author.

76. Yang, F. M., Marcantonio, E. R., Inouye, S. K., Kiely, D. K., Rudolph, J. L., & Fearing, M. A., et al. (2009). Phenomenological subtypes of delirium in older persons: Patterns, prevalence, and prognosis. *Psychosomatics, 50*(3), 248–254.

CHAPTER 17

Spirituality and Aging

James W. Ellor, PhD, D. Min, LCSW, DCSW, Judith E. Bowen, MPA, FAOTA

CHAPTER OUTLINE

Defining Terms
Relevant Theories
    Wholism
Perception of God
Experience and Expressions of Spirituality in Later Life
Multicultural Dimensions of Spirituality
Interprofessional Perspectives and Interventions
Summary

OBJECTIVES

- Assist the client in identifying his or her spiritual needs
- Understand spirituality as a domain of meaningful activities that may be enhanced by appropriate occupational therapy interventions
- Discuss the relevance of theories of occupational science, occupational therapy, and gerontology to the understanding of spiritual well-being
- Articulate aspects of religion or spirituality most useful for working with the older client
- Determine the appropriate use of spiritual/religious support for the individual client
- Identify the role of occupational therapy in the interdisciplinary team process for providing spiritual support

Occupational therapy (OT) was founded on the belief that client-centered practice reflects the integration of "mind, body and spirit."[19] When Mrs. Gonzales, age 72 years, had her stroke she was the full-time caregiver for her two grandchildren at home and held a job at a local retailer as a greeter that she had to keep to maintain her family. It is one thing to prepare her to address the physical challenges, yet still another to work with the emotional and spiritual questions and feelings that she is having that will affect her recovery. In many ways, healing the body is easier than walking with the client into an emotional and/or spiritual place that may involve unfamiliar religious beliefs or other intangibles. One way to address the emotional and spiritual aspects of the person is to refer the individual to the appropriate professional, if one is readily available. But what happens if the occupational therapist or OT assistant is the individual who is listening when the client says that he or she won't do the exercise for some spiritual reason? Sometimes the occupational therapist or OT assistant is the only person available to handle the situation.

The medical model is built on an interesting form of division of labor. In classical division of labor, each person has a separate job, with rules as to who does what carefully defined. In medicine, there are clear license-based rules for dealing with physical health, but when it comes to emotional and spiritual health, the situation is less clear. One would not, for example, call a social worker to perform surgery or even to provide adaptive measures for eating after the client has had a stroke. However, particularly in rural areas, clinics, and other settings outside of the major medical settings, there may not be someone to refer the client to for spiritual support. Whether the occupational therapist is the only provider in the clinic or even if there is a wide array of professionals available, wholistic client support is as much a mind-set as it is a specific task. In the *Occupational Therapy Practice Framework: Domain and Process*, 3rd edition,[1] a clear statement is made that " . . . occupational therapists recognize the importance and impact of the mind-body-spirit connection as the client participates in daily life. . . . a focus on the whole is considered stronger than a focus on isolated aspects of human function" (p. S4).[1] "The profession recognizes that values, beliefs, and spirituality influence a person's motivation to engage in occupations and give his or her life meaning" (p. S7).[1]

A similar statement is made in the *Occupational Therapy Guidelines for Client-Centered Practice* from the Canadian Association of Occupational Therapists (CAOT).[8] However, in the Canadian document, the occupational therapist is admonished to also "pay attention to your own spirit" (p. 101).[12] Both of these key documents refer to a holistic approach to practice. (NB: The difference between the terms holistic and wholistic is explained later in this chapter). The wholistic model does not mean that everyone must be cross-trained to do everything in medicine, which would be unrealistic. However, it does mean that everyone on the team needs to understand the person as having more than physical needs and be prepared when called upon to at least respond to him or her, to walk with that person through these challenges.

The focus of this chapter is on working with the spiritual needs of the older adult. There is a great deal of confusion as to what the term *spiritual* means in the literature, which makes it that much more challenging to address. This chapter offers some definitions as to what spiritual needs are and discusses tools that occupational therapy personnel can use to work with clients to address those needs.

Defining Terms

The challenge of working with the spiritual needs of clients starts with trying to understand what the term *spiritual* means. Numerous authors have noted confusion in regard to this term.[24,35] Few persons in North America have grown up employing the term in everyday life the way it has been framed in the last 20 years.[2] The term *spirituality* first entered the gerontological vocabulary in the United States in the form of *spiritual well-being* in 1971 at the White House Conference on Aging.[14] The term *spiritual well-being* was not actually defined in 1971, but rather in 1975 by what would become the National Interfaith Coalition on Aging (NICA), now a part of the Forum of Religion Spirituality and Aging, which is a constituent unit of the American Society on Aging. The NICA defined the term as follows: "The affirmation of life in a relationship with God, self, community and environment that nurtures and celebrates wholeness" (p. xiii).[30] A recent meta-analysis of the use of the terms *religion* and *spirituality*[16] indicates that the terms *religion* and *spiritual well-being* were the dominant terms in the 1970s and 1980s, eventually to be supplanted by the term *spirituality* in the late 1980s.

The term *spirituality* is defined in the *Occupational Therapy Practice Framework: Domain and Process* by the American Occupational Therapy Association (AOTA) as follows: "The aspect of humanity that refers to the way individuals seek and express meaning and purpose and the way they experience their connectedness to the moment, to self, to others, to nature, and to the significant or sacred" (p. 887).[1] This definition reflects the overwhelming contemporary understanding of the term *spirituality* as the development of some type of meaning in one's life, whether that includes reference to divinity or not.

Those who conceptualize spirituality in secular terms generally refer to the meaning of life as it is experienced in the world around us. Meaning comes from the environment, from other people, from all that makes up the world in which one lives. Often for such persons there does not need to be a divine being in this world to make it meaningful.

In a recent study by Ellor and McFadden of the membership of the American Society on Aging, gerontological practitioners who span the entire range of professions working with older adults suggested that their understanding of spirituality is linked with their self-understanding of being religious. In this study, 55.6% of the sample said that in their own self-perception, they are both religious and spiritual, 33.7% said they were only spiritual, 2.4% said they were only religious, and 8.1% said that they are neither religious nor spiritual.[15] If this sample is representative of the professional community in which the reader is working, this suggests that the largest group of people will relate spirituality to their sense of religion.

This continuum between the definitions of meaning when linked with spirituality relates to an understanding that some individuals find meaning in God, however they understand that God, and others find meaning in the world around them and through other people without needing God to be in their lives. It is helpful as one listens to clients as they begin to talk about religious or spiritual matters to listen to see if they are relating their definition of the spiritual to their religious faith in some way, or simply to their

self-understanding of a meaningful life that interacts with the world around them. In the case of the former, they will most often employ religious terminology, whereas the latter tend to utilize relationships to creation and the environment as their source of meaning. Either definition can offer important motivation for wellness. However, those who maintain a religious identity or affiliation with a religious tradition or institution may also be linked to a support system from the church, synagogue, temple, or mosque, along with more secular informal system, (e.g., neighbors, colleagues, friends, and family members).

For occupational therapy personnel in the United States, it is important to note that in the revisions of the *Occupational Therapy Practice Framework* (2nd and 3rd editions), the concept of spirituality has been moved from the domain of context, "a variety of interrelated conditions within and surrounding the client that influence performance," to the domain of client factor, which supports the concept of "spirituality residing within the client rather than as a part of a context" (p. 665).[1] The importance of this transition is that it moves from being an environmental context, which is often defined by culture and/or community, to being an individual client practice or preference. This suggests that occupational therapy personnel need to be conscious of listening to the individual's own understanding of what spirituality means in her or his life. Occupational therapists and assistants need to be conscious of both the client's understanding of spirituality as well as their own. It is easy to want clients to agree with the therapist's own views or to project one's own view onto the client. Both of these would be inappropriate. Proselytization of clients would be equally inappropriate. It may be of interest to note that other helping professions, including the fields of both psychology and social work, still emphasize spirituality as a part of the cultural context of the client. This is brought together in a helpful way by Griffith et al., who note: "Within the Canadian Model of Occupational Performance …spirituality resides in persons, is shaped by the environment and gives meaning to occupation" (p. 83)[21]

Peloquin writes in the *Canadian Journal of Occupational Therapy* that she has long argued "that meaningful occupation animates and extends the human spirit, that when occupational therapists help others with occupations that make or remake their lives, they engage in work that may be called spiritual. . . .When we help others engage in occupations with meaning, we engage their spirits whether we name that action spiritual or not" (p. 16).[32]

Malchiodi reflects a similar viewpoint. She states that although the word *transcendence* is often thought of as moving beyond the earthly life into some highly spiritual state of being, that "transcendence means finding a place within oneself where spirit resides and then carrying that spiritual self back into life, no matter what obstacles exist" (p. 175).[27] She then describes a woman in the final stages of metastatic breast cancer, who, despite the medical issues, medications, and pain, "was still motivated to express herself (through art) and, in that process, transcend her illness and heal her spirit even without hope of a cure" (p. 175).[27]

Myss, in her work as a medical intuitive and healer, discovered, when working with groups, that when individuals were able to see their problems within a spiritual framework their healing process was accelerated "because it adds a dimension of meaning and purpose to their crises" (p. 64).[29] Psychologist Kenneth Pargament refers to this as coping through the use of reframing, in which a human problem is reframed to become divine will.[31]

Meaning and purpose in the contexts just mentioned are linked with the spiritual. The act of guiding a client into connecting with occupations that give the client's life meaning allows the process by which the client ultimately finds that place where his or her spiritual self lives and then carries it back into the forefront, no matter how injured the body or mind may be.

As we bring the concepts of spirituality and religion into practice, one of the key connections is through work with client instrumental activities of daily living (IADLs). Religious observances are understood as an IADL. This IADL is linked specifically to "participating in *religion,* an organized system of beliefs, practices, rituals, and symbols designed to facilitate closeness to the sacred or transcendent" (p. 844).[28] Religious expression is often a strong motivator for the client.

The CAOT notes that the therapist can think of spirituality and its effects on IADLs in three areas.[9] First, spirituality can be thought of in relationship to one's self, such as finding hope, faith, and altruism. Second, it is found in relationship to other people in terms of tolerance for and caring about other people. Finally, spirituality can be found in reference to a supreme power as reflective of belief, higher authority, and unconditional love.[9] This multidimensional view of spirituality is helpful in terms of its influence on the client and the client's motivation for engaging in the IADL of religious practice. The wish to attend religious services can be motivation for the physical and social skills needed to attend. In the same way, caring about others reflects a movement away from the natural internal reflection that persons often have after a physical, emotional, or social assault. The *"I can't do this"* becomes *"I want to do it because I care about someone or something else."*

At the core of OT practice is the OT process of evaluation, analysis, intervention, and targeted outcomes. Although the *Occupational Therapy Practice Framework* emphasizes that the OT process "is fluid and dynamic, allowing occupational therapy practitioners and clients to maintain their focus on the identified outcomes, while continually reflecting on and changing the overall plan to accommodate new developments and insights along the way" (p. S11),[1] reimbursement realities often more strongly support and require attention to measurement and concrete goal setting.

Farah and McColl (p. 5) pose the following questions: "What does it mean to focus on the spiritual in occupational therapy? What interventions would qualify as legitimate spiritual modalities? What tools can we use to address the spiritual aspects of clients? Where do the boundaries lie between the professional and the personal?"[18] In an extensive discussion on the use of prayer as a spiritual modality, they

comment, "for a therapist to tend to a client's spiritual needs, he or she would have to do so in a way that was genuine, in accordance with his or her personal integrity, and that flowed naturally from the therapeutic relationship" (p. 10).[18]

A second influence of spirituality can be found in pain management. Ron Melzack, as quoted in Koenig et al., has proposed the "gate theory of pain," which suggests that "pain signals from an injured part of the body are modulated at the spinal cord level by other, simultaneous somatic inputs and by descending influences from the brain" (p. 348).[26] Koenig et al. go on to note that psychological influences such as religious belief or past experiences can affect somatic inputs and thus effectively influence the perception of pain and pain control.

However, the intent to connect spiritually with a client, if not carried out in relationship to that specific client's needs, may become problematic. In a commentary on the Farah and McColl article, Peloquin writes of a personal illness experience, describing how a well-intentioned nurse aide asked her, "Do you want to pray with me?" (p. 15).[32] It was not what Peloquin needed and she declined. The aide was offended and her ministrations suddenly became impersonal. How does a practitioner identify what might be an appropriate exploration of spiritual management in a given situation?

The scope of interactive settings in which occupational therapy personnel become engaged with the aging population is quite broad. It includes wellness and preventive care, life transitions, health behavior and lifestyle change, chronic illness care, and terminal illness.[10] Spirituality is present in older adults as it is present in all human beings. The question becomes one of learning to listen and to hear what individual spiritual needs might be.

Griffith, Caron, Desrosiers and Thibeault, in a study involving community-dwelling older adults, noted that "older adults have identities that are no longer tied to performing the occupations of self-care, productivity and leisure, but rather to a sense of being active in life despite physical limitations" (p. 88).[21] Weill[36] notes these prevalent concerns of older people: "(1) they don't want to suffer; (2) they don't want to be a burden to others; (3) they want the remainder of their lives to be meaningful" (p. 262). Depression and anxiety may accompany aging-related changes to the physical body as the changes begin to affect activities that were once so effortless in youth.

Relevant Theories

Two areas of theory seem to be important when examining the effects of spirituality in clients seen by occupational therapy personnel. The first is the concept of wholism. Wholistic care is reflected as a basis for the approach to care for occupational therapists.[25] A second relevant area is a new concept from the field of sociology that may be more helpful in understanding the religious or spiritual needs of older adults than either the traditional questions of denominational preference or spiritual identity. This is the approach to understanding the way that the client understands God.

Wholism

The terms "holism" and "wholism" are frequently confused. Holism is defined as "the theory that parts of a whole are in intimate interconnection, such that they cannot exist independently of the whole, or cannot be understood without reference to the whole, which is thus regarded as greater than the sum of its parts."[30] Wholism is in agreement with the basic notion that different parts of a system are interconnected and cannot be understood without understanding the entire whole. In terms of health, wholism expands the scope of the holistic focus on mind-body interactions to include consideration of spiritual factors. The following section offers additional clarifications and considers implications for OT practice.

The theoretical concept of wholism or holistic health has had a bumpy beginning in most medical circles. In psychology, the work of Sigmund Freud, who saw religion and spirituality as harmful and a part of a "universal neurosis," influenced two areas of this discussion.[2] First, the suggestion that religion was essentially related to pathology, not health, made it difficult for practitioners to embrace both good practice and religion. Second, Freud's own work reflected his work as a physician, constantly trying to tear apart the various emotional and physical aspects of any psychopathology, thus supporting a more divided and less wholistic approach to the needs of the client.

Counterforces were growing in the field of philosophy. In 1926 Jan Christian Smuts, a South African statesman, a friend of Winston Churchill, and an avid advocate for wilderness preservation, wrote his book *Holism and Evolution*. Although his text takes a decidedly naturalistic perspective on wholism, he writes, "this character of 'wholeness' meets us everywhere and points to something fundamental in the universe."[34] It is this concept of wholism that offered the basis for the use of the term *wholistic health* employed by Granger Westberg, best known as the founder of parish nursing. Dr. Westberg was a Lutheran chaplain and lecturer at the University of Illinois College of Medicine in Chicago. He frequently lectured his students on the spiritual needs of the whole person. As students came to appreciate the addition of the spiritual to the traditional physical, social, and emotional aspects of the person, they wanted a new way to speak of the person. Borrowing on the work of Jan Smuts, Granger Westberg added the "w" to *holism*. To be wholistic is to consider the needs of the entire person, including spiritual needs. It is easy enough to understand the thought that there are these four aspects to the person. Unfortunately, most authors at that time personified the concept of wholism by talking about the four pieces of the pie. For example, Larry Renetzky, writing in a *Christian Social Work Journal* article, refers to spirituality as the fourth dimension.[33]

In his original work, Smuts talks about the integration of the dimensions of the entire environment. Smuts warns against examining the whole through the mechanisms of the parts. Rather, he suggests that we need to see the whole person in terms of the individual's past, present, and future.[34]

When researchers and clinicians talk with an older adult they immediately encounter the person, not a part of that person. Similarly, to cut off my leg is a physical act, but because I have feelings about it, it also makes it an emotional act. Because having one leg, even with a prosthetic limb, has a social effect and that social effect will also affect the spiritual, cutting off a leg, whether it is due to trauma or, as is more likely in older adults, diabetes, will make a difference in every aspect of the person's life.

In many ways, occupational therapy is a naturally wholistic profession. Frequently, the work of the occupational therapist starts after the surgeon has completed the physical repair and the therapist must then draw together all of the aspects of the client. Often the spiritual aspect is the one where the client may well find her or his motivation for health and well-being. One can argue that on the potter's wheel, the occupational therapist and/or assistant blends and shapes clients in light of every aspect of who they are and who they are becoming.

Perception of God

Within the field of pastoral care, the need to understand the role of God, or the lack thereof, in the life of the person has been long understood.[22] Although many of the helping fields have focused on the more meaning-oriented concepts of spirituality, a new approach by Froese and Bader starts from the concept of the person's perception of God.[20] Froese and Bader, based on the longitudinal Baylor study of religion, suggest that starting from the person's view of God may be more useful for the practitioner than beginning by trying to understand the more amorphous concept of spirituality. They create four subgroups from the study data by creating a matrix of two opposing continua, judgment (more judgmental versus less judgmental) and engagement (more engaged versus less engaged). When Froese and Bader lined up the data in their study, they were able to create four useful subgroups, each with its own perception of God: the Benevolent God, the Authoritative God, the Distant God, and the Critical God (Figure 17-1).

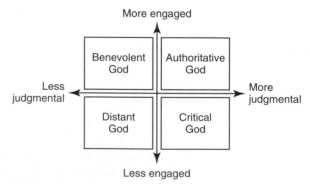

FIGURE 17-1 Four Views of God (From Froese, P., & Bader, C. (2010). *America's four Gods: What we say about God—and what that says about us.* New York, NY: Oxford University Press.)

The person who believes in the Authoritative God understands God to be more engaged and more judgmental than do persons in the other three groups. The Authoritative God is a highly judgmental God. Therefore a natural disaster such as Hurricane Katrina would be clearly seen as reflecting the wrath of God sent to the Gulf Coast, whose inhabitants are known for their "gambling, sin, and wickedness." According to Froese and Bader, the Authoritative God displays his wrath by allowing tragic events to occur in the hope that these occurrences provide us with a "wake-up call."[20] Persons who believe in the Authoritative God would see the amputation due to diabetes as the wrath of God for living a sinful lifestyle.

The Benevolent God is believed to be more engaged, but less judgmental. The Benevolent God would not send a disaster as a wake-up call, but will be there actively with the person to walk through the storm. Evidence of God's presence in times of trial or struggle is clear when talking to older adults after any sort of trauma. This person does not see God as the source of the trauma, but rather the source of healing from the trauma.

For those persons who believe in the Critical God, there is a strong emphasis on divine justice. This justice is mainly handed out in the afterlife, but it is clear that although those who believe in the Critical God perceive God to be highly judgmental, this perspective of God is low in engagement. When something bad happens to a person with this belief, the individual is often quick to suggest that the reason for the bad thing is not something she or he has recently done, but such actions are known by God and will be dealt with by God in God's time. In some ways this perception of God is similar to the concept of karma in Hinduism. Bad things can happen according to one's karma that are related to bad things from earlier existences. For Christians, the focus is on God's will, yet this perception of God is that God is not ready to be critical at the moment, but rather will even the score in the next life.

Finally, Froese and Bader discuss the Distant God. The Distant God is both low on judgment as well as low on engagement. Much like the understanding of God found in process theology, this perception of God emphasizes the creator God, who creates the universe, along with all of the various natural systems and forces of nature that drive the universe, but then pulls back and allows the creation to move forward based more on these natural forces than on direct intervention. For this person, bad things happen due to some combination of natural forces, possibly some that have gone astray from God's original intention. For this group, God is much more abstract and less active in the lives of everyday human beings.

Each of these conceptions of God is useful as one listens to the spirituality of clients to the extent that they believe in God. In the United States more than 80% of people believe in God, yet only around half attend a church, synagogue, temple, or mosque. Unlike most clergy, the average occupational therapist or assistant does not only encounter those whose spirituality is denominationally supported; rather, occupational therapy personnel see the entire range, from persons who do not believe in any sort of divine being, to atheists who are clear that God does not exist, to those persons who have a very full belief in the presence of a divine being. It turns out that persons who simply don't believe in God, or fully don't believe in anything, are a fairly small part of the total population. Most often occupational therapy personnel will encounter clients with some belief in God, albeit not necessarily a connection to any formal religion. Part of the utility of the four-God concept, which in some ways is the four-God-plus-no-God concept, is that it cuts across religions and denominations. When the therapist or assistant works with a client, the critical factor is the influence of the client's beliefs, not necessarily the need to fully understand the many nuances of each one of those beliefs. If the client needs someone to help sort out the finer aspects of his or her faith, it would be appropriate to call a chaplain. But if the client comes to you and says that the physical challenge that you are there to help with is the product of the wrath of God, it will have some influence on the client's behavior and conceivably on the client's recovery.

Experience and Expressions of Spirituality in Later Life

Let us return, then, to looking at "religion" versus "spirituality" in a treatment setting, remembering that religion is defined as an IADL. Farah and McColl remind us that our role as occupational therapists "is not that of a spiritual counselor or chaplain," and that although clinical judgment is important in knowing "when the client's spiritual needs go beyond their comfort level or competence," it is also important to not "make assumptions about the client's spiritual practices based on his or her affiliation with a particular spiritual or religious group." (p. 11).[18] The therapist's or assistant's understanding of that spiritual affiliation may be incomplete or misinformed. If the client appears to be struggling with issues of meaning, linking those issues to his or her particular religious beliefs in a way that blocks the client from re-engaging with meaningful occupation, referral to a spiritual counselor or chaplain is appropriate. A straightforward question, such as, "Do you have any spiritual beliefs or practices?" might be appropriate, or just letting the client know that spiritual care is available if necessary may be sufficient.

Unfamiliar beliefs might be encountered within clients' religious traditions, as illustrated in this occupational therapist's comments and observations (J. Bowen, personal communication, May 2008):

> In my 13 years of working in Deep South Texas I learned that there were, within this 88% Hispanic culture, religious biases that went beyond my previous understanding of what I knew as familiar religious groups. The Roman Catholic Church was the predominant denomination but there were established Protestant denominations as well, including Methodist, Pentecostal, Seventh Day Adventist, Jehovah's Witness, and Church of the Latter Day Saints. Added to this mix is *curanderismo*, a system of healing body, mind and soul, which is practiced in that culture. *Curanderismo* grew out of healing practices of indigenous Mexicans blended with Spanish and African approaches to healing.[3]

The *curandero* is seen as a highly spiritual person who has special powers. Such a healer may treat all of the familiar physical ailments, but in addition might treat rage, envy, bad air, the evil eye, bad luck, a hex, fright, or soul loss.[3] This is a healing tradition, but also a spiritual tradition and lives in and amongst traditional religious practice.

Over time, I learned from my Hispanic neighbors and friends, that members of Protestant denominations, in that culture, viewed Roman Catholics as devil worshipers because of their use of candles, incense, special garments, and worship of Saints (which could also be found within *curanderismo*). If I had not learned these shades of cultural beliefs, and had a client who was clearly experiencing spiritual distress, I might have referred that person to a spiritual counselor who was not appropriate for their needs, ultimately causing them even more distress. For some, the most appropriate spiritual counselor might be a *curandero*.

Now we must consider spirituality in practice, as compared with religion. Earlier, spirituality was defined as guiding a client into connecting with occupations that give his or her life meaning. Within this process, the client ultimately finds that place where his or her spiritual self lives and then carries it back into the forefront, no matter how injured the body or mind may be.

Spiritual connection in this way does not need to involve religion or spiritual language. When therapists and assistants talk with people about what is vital and sacred and meaningful to them, in their own words, therapists are engaging them on a spiritual level. Occupational therapists and assistants need to use language that connects with the client, such as "What keeps you going?" It is helpful to find a few questions that work for each client's culture and to pick up leads from conversation with clients. "The particular question is not as important as raising the subject of what matters in somebody's life" (p. 207).[10] Facilitating conversations that invite clients to reflect on what is vital and sacred to them, meeting clients where they are, and helping clients to reconnect with what has been most important to them in their lives is spiritual work.

Bowen has described a continuum of healing.[4] The occupational therapist must be able to identify where the client is in that process to effectively structure intervention. Immediately after a significant change in health or life circumstance there is a period of disruption. The capacity to absorb new information is diminished as the person struggles to deal with what has happened. It is important at this stage for the therapist to simply be able to hear the client's story or narrative—to be present with the client in his or her struggle. Richness of spirituality often resides in stories.[10] It is our role to allow the emotional and spiritual space for clients to tell the stories they need to tell.

Strategies that are useful in this time of disruption include paying attention, being aware, being empathetically in the present moment with the client, and listening without judgment and with acceptance. Occupational therapy personnel do not have to fix everything. It is caring and intention that are the bedrock for spiritual exchange.

Occupational therapists and assistants, as part of the OT process, often need to be "tellers" of information: giving instructions about exercises, home management, activity planning, and so forth. It is important to be a listener as well, as it is the client's truth that is paramount.

An elderly woman has just had her dominant hand crushed in an automobile accident. She says, "It was like a shock, a dream. I can't depend on me anymore. It tore my mind up. It was like my life was erased off the board.... I was always the strong one. I had been very independent, then had to turn everything over to someone else, including care of myself. This was worse than the injury" (p. 18).[4]

As the healing process continues so does a period of chaos. Turmoil persists, and all of the normal parameters once used to conceptualize the future are in disarray. "We cannot yet piece together what all the events mean in terms of the meaning of our lives" (p. 36)[5] Here, however, the therapist can guide the client into distancing from the effects, through "simple conversation, play, joking, talking about family... guiding persons into taking each task as it comes, attending to those matters that are still under their control, restoring a sense of competence by doing what they are capable of doing in the present moment, allowing what they cannot influence to run its course" (p. 16).[4] Questions useful during this period include the following: What do you care about? What is your goal? Are there times when you feel you are moving forward? What do you hope for?

Consider the following conversation:

Client: I took my problems to the Lord. There was nobody else. I feel like I am a bad person. My family is pushing me to get over it.
Therapist: OK...how would you put into words what is most important to you now?
Client: I just have to get through this somehow.
Therapist: Can you think of something that has been helpful to you in the past?
Client: I used to enjoy just sitting in my garden with my flowers and the birds singing.
Therapist: Is that something you can do now?
Client: Yes. I can just sit and be with the Lord there.

The final step in the healing process is that of reintegration. Finally, the person is able to begin putting pieces back together in the building of a new reality, "shaping a new meaning."[5] Essential aspects of reintegration include hope, faith, remembering, imagination, creation, and affirmation. "Hope is a vital component of survival. ... Hope is born of the kind of faith that makes us believe that our lives serve an ultimate purpose in the scheme of things" (p. 17).[6] Strategies available for the occupational therapist include guiding the client in remembering and using old strengths, affirming the emergence of a new self-perception, and encouraging creativity in new ways of thinking. Some appropriate questions might be: What are you trying to figure out, and is it something we can work on together? It looks like things may not change for you medically. How can you live your life fully given this situation?

Consider the following conversation:

Client: I felt that the therapists had hope too. My family said, "Why go on? Just accept it." They gave up on me. They said I didn't need help. I did not get hope at home. Your hope kept me going. If I had given up hope in the first few months…I don't know where I'd be. It gave me the time to gain enough emotional strength to take the reality. There are times when that's all I had.[4]

The occupational therapist then, may meet the aging client in any number of contexts and at any stage of the client's life journey. What do occupational therapists bring to these encounters? What skills do occupational therapy personnel have that prepare us to engage spiritually with our clients?

Craigie proposes an "embodiment" model: "Spirituality is embodied in everything that we do" (p. 26).[10] Occupational therapists are already familiar with the specialty model, such as pediatrics, neurology, mental health, and gerontology, but the embodiment model encompasses everything and anyone occupational therapy personnel might encounter.

Craigie would say that all the skills needed are already in place.[10] Occupational therapists and assistants are empathetic and flexible, and enjoy interacting with and establishing relationships with others. They already understand how to connect spiritually with clients. That understanding simply needs to be cultivated and developed.[10]

CASE EXAMPLE 17-1　Norma

In this case example, an "off-duty" occupational therapist brings communion to a parishioner as a lay server in her church. The parishioner has been hospitalized with metastatic breast cancer.

Therapist Commentary

Norma was elderly and had spent her entire work life as a teacher's aide. After completing the communion process, I asked her how she felt. She said, "I am afraid." I asked her if she was afraid of dying. She said, "Yes, but I've got to fight! I thought I was dying the other night." Then she looked at me and said, "There is no caring in this place." Her room was right across from the nurse's station and I could see people in white moving busily and hurriedly around in that space, but no one looked into her

room (p. 48).[6] Norma was unable to recline because of difficulty breathing, and was propped up in a sitting position with an assortment of pillows. She said sometimes at night the staff let her rest her head on their stomach for a minute. A brief touch. I asked her if she would like me to hold her and she said yes. I got up and reached around her and held her. She held onto my arm and after a few minutes let go, saying that was enough. She said, "It helps calm me to be held and I am okay now." She died 3 days later.[6]

It took so little to hear her need and meet it—the need for human touch and connection in a time of fear and vulnerability. My questions of her and my responses to her came from my intuitive self, my own spiritual self. It all began with my asking her how she felt.

CASE EXAMPLE 17-2　Helen

In this case example, Helen, a 78-year-old woman with a diagnosis of depression, was referred to the occupational therapist working in an outpatient gerontology clinic. The client was alert, lived alone, and managed all of her own self-care and IADLs; however, she had been losing weight and her physician and family were concerned. There was no medical reason for her loss of weight.

Therapist Commentary

Helen was pleasant and well dressed, but appeared frail and withdrawn. Her responses to my questions about her daily routine, habits, and so forth were short and to the point. I began to feel that the way things were going was not productive, so I just slowed down, waited, and gave her space just to be quiet. After a while, she said, "It's just been so hard." I asked her if she could tell me more. She began to tell her story. In the past 11 months, seven people very close to her had died, one of whom was her sister. She said, "Each time I started to feel like I was coming up from the blow, another hit. I just can't get up any more." I felt the enormity of her losses and I

acknowledged how deep her grief must be. I just allowed space for a while, did not talk. I felt that her grief needed to be honored.

Then I said, "Helen. You have lived a long time. I'm sure there have been other hard times in your life, times that have been very hard to deal with. Can you think of any?" She looked a bit surprised and thought for a minute, and then said, "Yes." I then asked her to think about how she handled those hard times. I asked her to remember how she coped. I told her that I wanted her to do that thinking as homework and to make notes for herself on her thoughts and then bring them back to me for our next session. Our next session focused on looking at her effective coping skills of the past. I asked her to choose one or two that she could use now. In that way, over a few sessions, she began slowly to reconnect with her own strength, which included her spiritual support system and eventually activities that she had found meaningful. She was much improved at discharge and had started gaining weight. She told me that she felt such a feeling of peace within our sessions. (J. Bowen, personal communication, November 1992)

CASE EXAMPLE 17-3   Thomas

In this case, Thomas, a 74-year-old African American gentleman, was admitted to a gerontological rehabilitation unit in a large, mid-South hospital system. He had been admitted to the hospital with terminal cancer and was referred to this unit because his wife wished to be able to take him home so that he could die there. He was a retired president of a church-affiliated university in that community. He was loved and respected for his leadership and commitment. Both occupational therapy and physical therapy (PT) were ordered.

Therapist Commentary

When I first meet Thomas, I was shocked at his condition. He was a tall man, but was frail and wasted. I introduced myself and said that we would work on improving his strength to a point where his wife would be able to manage him at home. He was alive, but there was no life in him. His eyes were open, but I could not find a place in them to connect. The feeling I had was that he had given up on life and was no longer engaged. I felt strongly that my first goal was to awaken his spirit—to find a spark of connection.

His wife was a gentle presence and her love for and pride in her husband was palpable. I came to feel she was a part of the treatment team, even though she just sat quietly in the room. I talked with them both about an activity that would be meaningful to him, a place to begin. His wife said that the first thing he did every morning was shave. She and I decided that was a place to start. He accepted

that. The PT goal was for him to be able to transfer with minimal assist.

Treatment sessions lasted only 10 to 15 minutes because of his weakness. I saw him twice daily. That was all he could tolerate. We used his electric razor, and in the beginning he could neither grip nor hold it. I fitted him with a universal cuff that held the razor, turned it on, and held his hand as I, in fact, shaved him. He could only tolerate partially shaving one side of his face in the beginning. I shaved the rest.

As the days went on, Thomas very slowly began to manage more of the task on his own, and at the time of discharge he was able to shave himself totally. The activity was never the goal. It was the means for him to re-engage with life. We did not talk a lot. His endurance did not allow. But I grew to know him well. I always came into his room with the belief that he was alive and well and whole in spirit. I saw him that way. Progress was incremental. First he began to make eye contact with me. Then I saw the hint of a smile. Then I saw life begin to appear in his eyes and we began to enjoy the interchange. I felt that I entered his space. It was a time we could share. I touched him every day and in my touch was the intention to heal. My time of knowing Thomas was sacred.

All of us knew he probably would not shave himself at home, at least not for long. They would have help and his wife was devoted and loving. But when he left, he was a person who was living. (J. Bowen, personal communication, September 1985)

There are numbers of ways that OT personnel might be involved with other professionals. Chaplains, spiritual leaders of all faiths, and those involved with specialty care situations such as hospice are available and usually easily accessible in traditional treatment settings. It is important as well for therapists and assistants to familiarize themselves with other resources in the community. For example, in a small southern Pennsylvania community, Pastor Fred has developed a wellness support system for those living with chronic illness. As was mentioned earlier in this chapter, older adults are not focused on traditional activities of daily living (ADLs), but on learning how to live full lives given the changes that come with aging and illness. Pastor Fred has organized a series of meetings, seminars, and discussion groups that focus on wellness and that are strongly faith based. Participants share stories and draw what they need from these encounters. Occupational therapists and assistants can be participants in such groups and can also refer individuals to the groups.

I was invited to such a group by my office manager. She knew I was an occupational therapist and interested in her situation. She is in her late 60s and has been on dialysis for 3 years, awaiting a kidney transplant. She comes to work every day, then goes home in the evening to plug herself into her home peritoneal dialysis unit for 9 hours. She is an effective and capable worker and I admired her courage. Within the group meeting she was a featured speaker, talking of how she has lived with her situation. She made a powerful statement

that reverberated for me, as applicable to all. She said, "*I am not my illness*" (J. Bowen, personal notes, March 2011).

The past two decades reflect an increased interest in spirituality and health care. A majority of American medical schools now include the area of spirituality in their educational curricula, and the Accreditation Council for Occupational Therapy Education (ACOTE) requires that all programs address spirituality in the evaluation and intervention process. A theme that surfaces is that all human beings are spiritual beings. Craigie writes, "for me, the most succinct statement of the overarching picture of spirituality comes from former Surgeon General, Dr. C. Everett Koop. Speaking in 1994 at the annual Maine symposium on spirituality and health…, he defined spirituality as 'The *vital center of a person; that which is held sacred*'" (p. 20).[10] Andrew Weill notes that although change is universal, some essence of everything is unchanging.[36] Bowen writes, "I remember a phrase from an article I read a long time ago, in which the author refers to our physical body as the sandal for our soul. The sandal may become tattered and worn and scuffed, and may even lose a strap or buckle, but until the leather is totally worn away it provides protection for what is within. When it has finally out-lived its usefulness, it falls away, leaving free that which it has protected" (p. 40).[7]

Effective spiritual care of our clients begins with us. Craigie suggests some exercises to discover and nurture our own spirituality:[10] journaling, identifying the qualities of character you wish to cultivate, writing your own origin story, stating your personal mission, attending retreats, and giving examples of how you stay connected to your purpose. Weill supports the writing of an ethical will, having to do with nonmaterial gifts: the values and life lessons that you wish to leave others.[36] This might also be a fine activity for a client.

The client and the practitioner each have their own wisdom to bring to an encounter. It is the awareness and honoring of this wisdom that allows collaborative engagement with the spiritual, particularly for those individuals who are concerned with making sense of their lives and the fact of aging.

Multicultural Dimensions of Spirituality

Spirituality affects culture and culture affects spirituality. Culture is often understood to be a multilayered concept with at least three dimensions.[11] The first dimension reflects the nurture of the natural capacities of the human being. Spirituality or religion offers a manageable ultimate understanding of life. At times this understanding of one's life is dominated by religious and spiritual concerns; at other times religion and spirituality are relegated to external influences to be accepted or rejected by the individual. End-of-life concerns provide an example. Funerals and the laws around funerals have been largely dictated by religions. Even if the client is not a spiritual or religious person, the dominant culture's ritualistic needs have often been converted into laws that must be followed.

A second layer reflects the intellectual and imaginative products of the civilization. Often best reflected in the art and music of the culture, studies have found that worship elements such as liturgical music engage persons with significant cognitive impairments in activities in ways that secular music would not achieve.[17] The influence of this area of culture can also be seen by looking around the room of an older adult. Often pictures and symbols of her or his faith are evident as symbols of support and comfort to the individual.

Finally, the entire way of life of the individual may be affected by her or his spirituality. Religious admonitions about food preparation, for example, among Jews and Muslims affect every aspect of mealtimes. Religious assumptions also affect how people relate to one another. At one time many Protestants were not allowed to dance. Even in later life, when these admonitions have been relaxed by most traditions, many Protestant older adults never learned to dance, so they think it is fruitless to try. It is important to talk with clients about their cultural assumptions concerning their faith traditions. Even persons who share the occupational therapist's own faith tradition may come from a different culture and thus interpret some rituals differently.

Possibly the most challenging part of working with the cultural aspects of religion and spirituality comes when the occupational therapist or assistant does not fully understand the religious tradition of the client. Although many aspects of religion are positive, it is also possible that a client might express religious beliefs in a pathological way. A familiar example is the hallucinating schizophrenic person who believes he or she is Jesus Christ, or the individual who does something because the Devil told him or her to do so. These are some of the more spectacular examples, but other examples come from food preparation, cleanliness, and even the way persons relate to one another. A recent conversation between the author and a resident in a nursing home found the resident explaining that she does not go to groups because her Armenian Church does not believe that women should meet in groups. A call to the priest of her tradition found that this is not at all true, just her way of avoiding what she understood to be an anxiety-prone situation. This sort of thing, however, is a challenge, because no one can know all of the appropriate rules of every tradition. It can be helpful to have an agency consultant from within the various traditions to help sort out some of these types of concerns.

Older adults may confront situations that prohibit participation in important rituals. For example, if an older adult finds it meaningful to have her Catholic priest hear her confession, yet she is bed bound and the local priest unavailable to come to the home, who will hear her confession? At other times persons may find themselves to be a minority in a nursing home (e.g., the situation of one elderly Jewish woman in a Roman Catholic facility). When she found that she could not find a rabbi willing to visit, she began to attend Catholic Mass. When asked by a staff member why she, a practicing Jew, would attend a Roman Catholic mass, she noted, "they are such nice people and they even serve a little snack at the end." In other cases where clergy are not available, staff members are tempted to substitute for meal preparations and even religious rituals. This phenomenon is referred to as *functional equivalence* in religious practice. For example, the Roman Catholic who cannot leave home to attend Mass can watch the *Mass for Shut-ins* program on television. This is generally considered an appropriate functional equivalent. However, inappropriate ones may include having a friend stand in for the priest to hear a confession or, as in one nursing home, having a nurse aide say the Mass because a priest is not available to come into the facility to do so.

Functional equivalents are substitute rituals, accessible fallbacks for times when a person is unable to participate in the original activity. It is important to note that they are generally not as emotionally satisfying as the activity they replace, in which clients have engaged for a lifetime. However, they become a substitute for this important activity.

In the case of a functional equivalence, the ability to get back to doing the original act, such as attending Mass rather than watching *Mass for Shut-ins*, can be a motivator to progress in therapy with the occupational therapist. At other times, the occupational therapist may hear about or even observe a client's substitute ritual that simply does not seem appropriate to the therapist. In such cases, consulting with clergy from the client's denomination and possibly having the clergyperson visit and offer a more appropriate substitute would be important.

Although religion can be misused, it can also be an incredible strength, emotionally and in terms of social supports. Ellor and Coates note that most religious organizations provide basic support services for seniors.[13] From transportation to and from various physicians' appointments to ad hoc meals, friendly visiting and even some formal social services, religious congregations are often informal caregivers for many older adults.

Interprofessional Perspectives and Interventions

At the heart of any intervention around religion and spirituality for occupational therapy personnel is whether religion and spirituality are the domains of clergy alone. Clearly, religion and spirituality are the cognate fields of the clergy. However, there are times when clergy are important and times when the occupational therapist or assistant is actually the more appropriate person to intervene. Chaplains vary in their preparation for their role. Many are both religious professionals as well as excellent counselors. In this case, when the client is clearly struggling with a religious or spiritual issue, the chaplain would be the appropriate person to be called. However, what if you are working in a facility that does not have a consistent presence from a chaplain? What if there are local clergy available, but none are trained counselors and you feel that they would be ineffective in helping? What if the person turns to you during a therapy session and asks a particularly pointed spiritual question—do you stop therapy and run for a chaplain?

When a chaplain or other religious professional is the appropriate person to respond to the client, then that person should be called. However, at other times the occupational therapist or occupational therapy assistant is also appropriate for certain interactions. It is not the role of either the chaplain or the OT personnel to try to tell a senior what to believe. Rather, as illustrated in the case studies, it is their role to listen to and focus on what the client is saying and feeling. When the client is looking for advice as to what persons in his or her faith tradition believe, then a clergyperson from the client's tradition would be the most appropriate professional. With this said, when the occupational therapist needs to be the one present for the client at a time of spiritual need, the following are intervention guidelines:

- Listen to the individual, try to understand the meaning of what the client is talking about, and support the client's right to believe whatever is under discussion. This does not mean that the occupational therapist needs to believe it—only that the occupational therapist or assistant affirms that he or she understands that the client believes it.
- Understand the role of religion and spirituality in coping with adversity. As noted earlier, often the way clients talk about their understanding of God will reflect how they understand the source and meaning of this adversity. If the religious or spiritual explanations given by clients seem to be helpful in dealing with the anxiety, then they are probably appropriate. Such explanations may further help occupational therapists to understand why clients react to some aspects of their motivation for wellness in the way that they do.

- Call religious professionals or chaplains when they are available and especially when the client is asking for a religious ritual or needs religious consultation. The occupational therapist can support the client's feelings about the client's beliefs, but should not try to interpret or tell the person how to believe. In most instances the chaplain will not do this either, but may be better equipped simply by the symbolism of his or her office to help the individual struggle with whatever issues are presented.

Chaplains are important members of the interprofessional team. However, there are numerous times when the occupational therapist or assistant is the best responder during therapy, as a fellow human being who can support the client in times of spiritual distress.

Summary

Spirituality affects the lives of both the client and occupational therapy personnel. As noted in the CAOT guidelines, the topic of spirituality is bidirectional between the occupational therapist and the client.[8] The spirituality of the client may or may not reflect the client's stated religious preference. No matter how it is defined, spirituality is understood to reflect the personal relationship with something larger than the person. Whether that is seen as God or as the environment, it is generally understood to bring meaning to the client. As occupational therapists and assistants work with their clients, they need to listen to the spirituality presented by each older adult. There may be a personal crisis hidden in the discussion, or there may be a real strength toward healing and wellness found within. By listening and supporting the client's spiritual needs, the occupational therapist or assistant walks with the whole person—body, mind, and soul.

REVIEW QUESTIONS

1. Discuss the mind-body-spirit connect from the perspective of the Occupational Practice Framework.
2. Describe the various ways that Occupational Therapy is naturally wholistic in its approach to working with clients.
3. Discuss the appropriate use of religion versus spirituality in OT practice.
4. Discuss spirituality as an IADL and the OT role in facilitating participation and performance in this domain.

REFERENCES

1. American Occupational Therapy Association. (2014). *Occupational therapy practice framework: Domain and process* (3rd ed.). Bethesda, MD: Author.
2. Aten J. D., & Leach M. M. (2009). A primer on spirituality and mental health. In J. D. Aten & M. M. Leach (Eds.), *Spirituality and the therapeutic process: A comprehensive resource from intake to termination* (pp. 9–24). Washington, DC: American Psychological Association.

3. Avila, E., & Parker, J. (1999). *Woman who glows in the dark: A curandero reveals traditional Aztec secrets of physical and spiritual health*. New York, NY: Penguin Putnam.

4. Bowen, J. (1999). Health promotion in the new millennium: Opening the lens-adjusting the focus. *OT Practice, 20*, 14–18.

5. Bowen, J. (2006). The process of healing. *OT Practice, 11*, p. 36.

6. Bowen, J. (2007a). Reflections from the heart. Connections. *OT Practice, 12*(3), p. 48.

7. Bowen, J. (2007b). The heart-healing connection. *OT Practice, 12* (20), p. 48.

8. Canadian Association of Occupational Therapists. (1991). *Occupational therapy guidelines for client-centered practice*. Toronto, Canada: CAOT Publications ACE.

9. Canadian Association of Occupational Therapy. (2003). *Spirituality in enabling occupation*. Ottawa, Canada: CAOT Publications ACE.

10. Craigie, F. (2010). *Positive spirituality in health care: Nine approaches to pursuing wholeness for clinicians, patients, and health care organization*. Minneapolis, MN: Mill City Press.

11. Culture. (1997). In J. Bowker (Ed.), *The Oxford dictionary of world religions* (p. 248). New York, NY: Oxford University Press.

12. Egan, M., & DeLaat, M. D. (1994). Considering spirituality in occupational therapy practice. *Canadian Journal of Occupational Therapy, 61*(2), 95–101.

13. Ellor, J. W., & Coates, R. B. (1986). Examining the role of the church and aging. In M. Hendrickson (Ed.), *The role of the church in aging*. Binghamton, NY: The Haworth Press.

14. Ellor, J. W., & Kimble, M. A. (2004). The heritage of religion and spirituality in the field of gerontology: Don Clingan, Tom Cook, and the National Interfaith Coalition on Aging. *Journal of Religious Gerontology, 17*(1/2) 143–153.

15. Ellor, J. W., & McFadden, S. H. (2011). Perceptions of the roles of religion and spirituality in the work and lives of professionals in gerontology: Views of the present and expectations about the future. *Journal of Religion, Spirituality, and Aging, 23*, 50–61.

16. Ellor, J. W., & McGregor, A. (2011). Reflections on the words "religion," "spiritual well-being," and "spirituality." *Journal of Religion, Spirituality, and Aging, 23*(4), 275–278.

17. Ellor, J. W., Stettner, J., & Spath, H. (1987). Ministry with the confused elderly. *Journal of Religion and Aging, 4*(2), 21–32.

18. Farah, J., & McColl, M. (2008). Exploring prayer as a spiritual modality. *Canadian Journal of Occupational Therapy, 75*(1), 5–13.

19. Farrar, J. E. (2001). Addressing spirituality and religious life in occupational therapy practice. *Physical and Occupational Therapy in Geriatrics, 18*(4), 65–85.

20. Froese, P., & Bader, C. (2010). *America's four Gods: What we say about God—and what that says about us*. New York, NY: Oxford University Press.

21. Griffith, J., Caron, C., Desrosiers, J., & Thibeault, R. (2007). Defining spirituality and giving meaning to occupation: The perspective of community-swelling older adults with autonomy loss. *Canadian Journal of Occupational Therapy, 74*(2), 78–90.

22. Hiltner, S. (1961). Psychoanalytic education: A critique. *Psychoanalytic Quarterly, 30*, 385–403.

23. Holism. (n.d.). In Oxford Dictionaries online. Retrieved from http://www.oxforddictionaries.com/us/definition/american_english/holism

24. Howard, B. S., & Howard, J. R. (1997). Occupation as spiritual activity. *The American Journal of Occupational Therapy, 51*(3), 181–185.

25. Kang, C. (2003). A psychospiritual integration frame of reference for occupational therapy. Part 1: Conceptual foundations. *Australian Occupational Therapy Journal, 50*, 92–103.

26. Koenig, H. G., McCullough, M. E., & Larson, D. B. (2001). *Handbook of religion and health*. New York, NY: Oxford University Press.

27. Malchiodi, C. (2002). *The soul's palette: Drawing on art's transformative powers for health and well-being*. Boston, MA: Shambhala.

28. Moreira-Almeida, A., & Koenig, H. G. (2006). Retaining the meaning of the words religiousness and spirituality: A commentary on the WHOQOL SRPB group's "A cross-cultural study of spirituality, religion, and personal beliefs as components of quality of life." *Social Science and Medicine, 63*, 843–845.

29. Myss, C. (1996). *Anatomy of the spirit: The seven stages of power and healing*. New York, NY: Harmony Books.

30. National Interfaith Coalition on Aging. (1975). *Spiritual well-being: A definition*. Athens, GA: NICA.

31. Pargament, K. I. (1997). *The psychology of religion and coping*. New York, NY: The Guilford Press.

32. Peloquin, S. (2008). Morality preempts modality: A commentary of exploring prayer as a spiritual modality. *Canadian Journal of Occupational Therapy, 75*(1), 15–16.

33. Renetzky, L. (1977). The Fourth Dimension: Applications to social services. *Paraclete, 4*, 2, Winter.

34. Smuts, J. C. (1999). *Holism and Evolution: The original source of the holistic approach to life*. Sherman Oaks, CA: Sierra Sunrise Publishing.

35. Thompson, B. E., & MacNeil, C. (2006). A phenomenological study of exploring the meaning of a seminar on spirituality for occupational therapy students. *The American Journal of Occupational Therapy, 60*(5), 531–539.

36. Weill, A. (2005). *Healthy aging: A lifelong guide to your well-being*. New York, NY: Anchor Books: Random House Publishing.

CHAPTER 18

Successful Aging

Kate de Medeiros, PhD; Shirley J. Jackson, MS, OTR/L, FAOTA,
Margaret A. Perkinson, PhD

CHAPTER OUTLINE

OBJECTIVES

In 2010, the first members of the baby boom generation turned 65 years old. In addition, the number of people aged 65 years and over in the United States is expected to increase by 44%, from around 310 million in 2010 to 440 million in 2050.[81] The growing population of older adults will also be more diverse; the percentage of minority older adults will increase from 20% of those 65 years old and over in 2010 to 42% in 2050.[81] Soon, one in five people will be aged 65 years or over; thus, it is important to consider ways in which older individuals can optimize their later years, or "age successfully." This includes paying particular attention to cultural diversity and challenging current assumptions about older age to meet the changing needs of tomorrow's older population.

As many have noted, aging is a global phenomenon. Kinsella and He[45] report that for the first time in history, people aged 65 years and over worldwide will soon outnumber children under 5 years. By 2050, one in eight inhabitants in the world (around 16% of the entire population) will be at least 65 years old.[59] The most rapid growth in the older population is occurring in developing countries.[59] With the growth of the older population come new challenges and considerations: larger proportions of people are "retired," leaving fewer people in the workforce to provide financial support for both children and older adults;[39] chronic, noncommunicable diseases are now the biggest causes of death and pose a heavy burden from a health care perspective; and changes in family structure have altered long-term care options for older people, moving from family-centered care to some form of paid caregiving. All of these make the goal of "successful aging" even more imperative.

Yet, what does it mean to age successfully? At first glance, "successful aging" seems self-apparent and likely includes the idea of aging in such a way as to maximize intellectual interest, physical function, sense of meaning, and capability to accomplish one's goals throughout life. However, upon further thought, one may ask, "How does one achieve maximum intellectual interest?", "What comprises physical function?", and other inquiries that call into question how successful aging can be defined so that is it is a meaningful, attainable concept across many disciplines, cultures, and setting.

Within the broad field of gerontology, the concept of successful aging has evolved over the last several decades; its definition is continually being debated and redefined. In this chapter, we aim to accomplish the following: (1) provide an overview of the strengths and critiques of "successful aging" and related theories and concepts linked to optimizing the experience of aging; (2) explore the role of culture and cross-national perspectives in influencing views of and expectations for older age; (3) propose a new definition of successful aging based on past research and recent changes in social life (e.g., increases in life expectancy at birth, retirement); (4) discuss and outline the relevance to occupational performance deficits and occupational therapy interventions; and (5) outline interprofessional perspectives and interventions.

The Evolution of the "Successful Aging" Paradigm

Although the concept of successful aging was introduced more than 50 years ago,[18,63] it has since taken on many meanings, models, domains, and correlate terms (e.g., "the good life",[47] productive aging,[17,32] comfortable aging,[29] optimal aging,[8] active aging,[84] healthful aging, aging gracefully, and others[7, 14, 34, 38, 63, 66, 67]). To reconsider and perhaps refine what is meant by successful aging, it is important to first consider how it has evolved.

The term *successful aging* was first formally used by Pressey and Simcoe,[63] who suggested that not all older people were subject to the same experience of aging, and that physiological and psychological differences played an important role in determining successful or problematic age.[75] Eight years later, Baker[7] was also interested in potential triggers that could lead one older person to be "successful" in later life while leaving another "unsuccessfully aged." Baker described the *unsuccessfully aged* as "those with the diagnosis of 'chronic brain syndrome with senile brain disease'" (p. 570), those who suffered from inadequate psychosocial reinforcement, and those who would benefit from positive stress adjustment.

Although components pertaining to genetics, lifestyle, and coping mechanisms such as social interactions were present in early definitions and conceptions of successful aging, missing was a subjective component in which the older person determined his or her own "success" in aging. Havighurst,[36] therefore, proposed a broader concept of successful aging that stressed the importance of life satisfaction indices as essential components of any measures used to determine "success." His concept of successful aging begins with the question, "What are the conditions of individual and social life under which the individual older person gets a maximum of satisfaction and happiness?" (p. 8). For Havighurst, the individual's subjective interpretation of his or her own aging experience must accompany any attempts of objective measurement.

Perhaps the most commonly used definition of successful aging currently in use, however, comes from Rowe and Kahn.[66,67,68] Rowe and Kahn set forth three criteria necessary to be considered successfully aged: "low risk of disease and disease-related disability, high mental and physical function, and active engagement with life" (p. 38).[67] This basic model formed the basis of the MacArthur Studies of Successful Aging, a multisite, longitudinal study that ran from 1988 to 1996.[69] In this series of studies, a subsample of highly functioning older adults, aged 70 to 79 years, was drawn from three ongoing Established Populations for the Epidemiological Study of the Elderly (EPESE) studies with the overall goal of differentiating between "normal" and "exceptional" aging.[9] Participants underwent a 90-minute battery composed of assessments of physical and cognitive function and performance (gait, memory, balance, strength, self-reported activity), "productive activities" (e.g., volunteer work, child care, paid employment), social and support networks (e.g., size of networks, perceived quality of support, proximity to networks), psychological characteristics (e.g., depression, mastery, happiness), biological and health status measurements, and physiological measurements obtained from blood and urine samples. There have been numerous papers based on findings from the MacArthur studies, such as discussion of the relationship between physical disability and depression and their effect on health and well-being,[12] the role of physical exercise and emotional support in predicting better physical performance over a 2.5-year follow-up period,[70] social relationships and cognitive decline,[71] and dozens of others. A recent study using data from four data points from the national Health and Retirement Study found that the percentage of people meeting Rowe and Kahn's criteria of successful aging ranged from 15.7% to 16.8% (for those aged 65 to 74 years).[55] The authors also reported that men, overall, had a higher percentage of successful aging than women, 11.5% to 12.8% and 10.5% to 11.4%, respectively. In addition, White study subjects were "successfully aged" in greater percentages (11.7% to 12.8%) than both Blacks (4.4% to 7.1%) and Hispanics (4.9% to 5.6%).[55]

Critiques of Rowe and Kahn's model include lack of reference to earlier definitions and studies of successful aging,[38] lack of any subjective components or self-rated "success" in aging,[83] no measure of "spirituality,"[28] and others.[51] Wong,[83] for example, defines successful aging as "an individually constructed cognitive system that is grounded in subjective values and capable of endowing life with personal significance and satisfaction" (p. 516). As Wong points out, many of the studies of successful aging have found that one's ability to cope with and adapt to changes in old age contributes to higher levels of psychological health and satisfaction. Coping and adaptation are present in one's "constructed cognitive system." Tapping into personal meaning may therefore be a strategy that leads to better coping and adaptation skills.

Crowther and colleagues[28] cite the importance of a fourth component to the Rowe and Kahn model, positive spirituality, which they define as involving "a developing and internalized personal relation with the sacred or transcendent that is not bound by race, ethnicity, economics, or class and promotes the wellness and welfare of self and others" (p. 614). Having a sense of being able to move beyond one's current circumstances or to be able to exert some positive effect beyond one's immediate physical condition may be an essential component of successful aging for some people.

In a meta-analysis of studies of successful aging in older adults, including but not limited to the MacArthur studies, Depp and Jeste[31] identified 28 successful aging studies and 29 different criteria used to define what comprised successful aging. They report that nearly all of the studies ($n = 26$) used some measures of physical function and/or disability; 13 of them included cognitive performance, nine included life satisfaction/well-being, eight included social/productive engagement, and six included presence of illness. Only two included any type of self-rating of successful aging, in response to the question, "I am successfully aged."

Recently, Martinson and Berridge[51] completed a systematic review of critiques of successful aging from 1987 through 2013. Of the 67 articles that met their inclusion criteria, the authors found four categories of critiques: (1) "add and stir" described articles that suggested that a model of successful aging was possible, but that there were missing pieces to the current models being used; (2) "missing voices," which described the need for subjective views from older people themselves, (3) "hard-hitting critiques," which suggested that the successful aging paradigm not be used at all due to its ageist and able-bodied assumptions and other fatal flaws; and (4) "new frames and names," which proposed new models of successful aging that integrate spiritual and other meaning-based qualities. All of these critiques point to general questions about what successful aging is and what it could be (or should not be).

Other Theories and Approaches to Successful Aging

In addition to successful aging, there have been several other terms aimed at describing the sense of somehow achieving or doing well as one grows older. These include *productive aging*,[17] *comfortable aging*,[29] and *active aging*.[84] Productive aging, unlike successful aging, is focused on economic return in terms of producing some service that has tangible, monetary value rather than on health and well-being outcomes. Babysitting grandchildren could be considered an activity of productive aging because there are costs associated with child care. Other forms of volunteering and civic engagement as well as part-time and full-time paid work are also under this umbrella. The overall emphasis in the productive aging concept is on rethinking how retirement years are spent, from a time associated with relaxation and potential withdrawal from responsibility to a time in which to continue contributing to economic well-being and production. Productive aging is the concept adopted by the American Occupational Therapy Association (AOTA) Centennial Vision[3] to support health, well-being, and quality of life in the key practice area of aging.

The term *comfortable aging* was coined by Cruikshank[29] to move away from the success/failure models implied in previous descriptions of aging outcomes and instead considers ways in which gender, class, and other factors affect what is possible in older age. For example, a lifetime lack of access to appropriate resources (e.g., medical care, healthy food) will likely have negative consequences in older age. Rather than attributing these consequences to some sort of personal failure, which Cruikshank argues is present in some successful aging models, comfortable aging places emphasis on the ease with which one grows old, rather than on external measurements.

The World Health Organization (WHO) uses the term *active aging*, defined as "the process of optimizing opportunities for health, participation and security to enhance quality of life as people age" (p. 12).[84] The word *active* extends beyond participation in the labor force and includes social, spiritual, civic, or other forms of personal contributions to family, friends, or the greater community. This definition of active aging is meant to counter other views of aging in which people with disabilities or restricted physical or cognitive abilities would not be fully considered, as in some of the successful aging definitions. In addition, this concept applies to individuals as well as communities, because aging occurs within the context of others (e.g., friends, families, co-workers, neighbors), thereby making active aging a societal objective rather than a personal mandate.

Culture, Cultural Diversity, and Successful Aging from a Global Perspective

Cruikshank's description of comfortable aging and WHO's active aging definition recognize that different opportunities and values play a role in how one ages and views old age. As such, aging is often described as a cultural construction of a biological phenomenon.[10, 37] What appears to be a universal experience—growing older—differs in the way it is defined, experienced, and viewed by members of a given society based on systems of values and meanings.[46, 48] Any definition of successful aging must therefore be considered with regard to cultural relevance. Rosal and Bodenlos[65] define culture as "what is learned, shared, transmitted intergenerationally and reflected in a group's values, beliefs, norms, behaviors, communication and social roles" (p. 39). Culture shapes meaning and provides the framework for what behaviors and activities are considered "normal" for categories of individuals (e.g., children, middle-aged adults, older adults) in a given cultural group. This framework in turn influences a variety of health behaviors. We note that "culture" should be considered within societies (i.e., a group of people who share a common national identity) and within subcultures, defined as "a group within a society that functions by its own distinctive standards of behavior, while at the same time sharing some standards in common with the general culture" (p. 41).[65]

In considering successful aging, it is important to consider ways in which the term has been used in the past, as described in the previous sections, and in light of subcultures, cultural diversity, and global perspectives, which will be described in this section. We begin by looking at subcultures within the United States (primarily studied from an epidemiological model) and then move to a global societal perspective.* We then move toward defining successful aging in light of modifiable behaviors that have been linked to evidence-based outcomes considerations.

Subcultures of Aging in the United States

Subcultures of older adults in the United States are often defined and studied through variables such as ethnic and racial minority status, socioeconomic level and social class, disability and mobility status, gender, and even age cohorts, such as the growing baby boomer population. For example, neighborhoods, often defined by income level, are one way in which economic status and class can influence aging in regard to access to medical care, preventive care such as walking (e.g., whether there is a safe place to walk), safe and reliable transportation, and freedom from stress due to crime or uncertainty. Disability and mobility status and level of environmental support can determine whether one is able to get to important locations such as physician appointments, church, visits with friends, grocery stores, and others. It also may determine whether a person can remain living at home without assistance, can live at home with assistance, or must move to a facility that provides assistance.

The important aspect of a subculture is that some feature(s) may cause one group of older adults to experience older age in a fundamentally different way than another. Understanding the structural differences that may affect different subgroups of older adults and how they age is therefore critical when considering strategies for successful aging.

Regarding ethnic and/or racial minority status as a subculture of older adults in the United States, currently, African Americans experience a shorter life expectancy at birth by 5.1 years compared with non-Hispanic Whites.[4, 79] Although life expectancy rates for Mexican Americans are similar to those for non-Hispanic Whites, their levels of disability and chronic disease (e.g., diabetes) in older age are much greater.

In addition to differences in life expectancy, the presence of chronic disease differs by race and ethnicity. According to the U.S. Census Bureau,[79] the majority of older African Americans reported at least one chronic condition. Eighty-four percent reported having hypertension (compared with 71% of all older people who reported this condition), 53% were diagnosed with arthritis (compared with 49% of all older people), and 29% were being treated for diabetes (compared with 18% of all older people). Women also can experience aging in very different ways than men. Women, worldwide, have longer life expectancies at birth than men. However, with longer life comes more years of disability and often economic challenges. Understanding differences in health outcomes and health expectations is critical to understanding what is possible in a successful aging paradigm.[1]

Aging and Health from a Global Perspective

As mentioned earlier, aging is a global phenomenon in developed and developing countries. In fact, over 80% of the net gain in older people from 2007 to 2008 occurred in developing countries such as Singapore, Columbia, India, and Malaysia, although Europe has the oldest populations overall.[45] This growth is coupled with declines in fertility, leading to overall population decline despite the increase in older people, which can in turn create a crisis of care. Maintaining optimal physical and cognitive functioning is therefore a worldwide imperative, and should be considered in the realm of successful aging.

Keeping potential criteria for successful aging in mind, it is helpful to examine statistics regarding physical and cognitive function and well-being from around the world. These data can inform what a model for successful aging might look like and what interventions and strategies could be implemented to achieve functional goals for later life. Drawing from the WHO data, Kinsella and He[45] make distinctions among three types of health data: total survival, disability-free survival, and survival without disabling chronic disease. In considering total survival in terms of cause of death, the broad category of heart disease (to include stroke and heart attack) and lung cancer are major causes of death, especially in men, around the world. In addition, disability in the aggregate has decreased among older people,[44] although the prevalence of disability has increased in several developing countries.

Disabling conditions include arthritis, depression, blindness and poor vision, and incontinence. Currently around 16% of people of all ages in the United States suffer from osteoarthritis (the most common type of arthritis) or rheumatoid arthritis.[64] For the former, the strongest risk factor is increased aged. According to Reginster,[64] over 50% of people aged 75 years and over reported some form of arthritis. Given data from other developed countries, one could expect similar prevalence rates. Consequences of arthritis include difficulty with mobility and pain, both of which can restrict one's ability to complete activities of daily living (ADLs), such as bathing and meal preparation; restrict participation in social encounters, which can lead to depression; and interfere with other qualities of life.

Blindness or low vision is another problem for older people around the world. WHO estimated that over 40 million people in the world were blind or suffered from low vision in the 1990s,[26] 90% (36 million) of whom lived in developing countries. Leading causes of blindness include cataracts, glaucoma, and macular degeneration.[26] As with arthritis, there can be serious consequences associated with low vision, including inability to care for oneself especially without caregiver support; reduced social contact, which could lead to isolation; and, depending on the country, inability to secure necessary financial support for basic living expenses. Finally, depression is the most common mental disorder in old age. Because depression has different meanings in different cultures (e.g., may be viewed as sadness, which in turn could be viewed as a consequence of old age), global statistics are not readily available.

---

*We define "societies" in terms of formally recognized countries for the sake of being able to report data that have been gathered according to these divisions. We recognize, however, that many subcultures exist within and across national boundaries, although it is beyond the scope of this chapter to fully explore them.

When considering successful aging from a global perspective, the idea of cultural relevance comes into play. Torres,[78] for example, questions cultural relevance and argues that the concept of "success" is an American paradigm that places value on the self-sufficiency of the individual. It would therefore not necessarily be applicable to other cultural groups that have different values and conceptions of old age. Torres uses the example of Chinese older adults who participated in a cross-cultural study of successful aging, Project AGE, who considered successful aging in terms of the willingness of one's family to provide care in later years or dependence on family support rather than in terms of individual independence.

Successful Aging and Retirement

The idealized notion of retirement as a time of rest and relaxation after years in the paid workforce is very central to the everyday concept of successful aging. Retirement and successful aging together suggest that one has achieved some means of support in older age to pursue personal goals, good enough health and cognitive function to appreciate and use leisure time as one chooses, and some sense of satisfaction at having arrived at that status. As with the discussion of successful aging earlier in the chapter, "retirement" requires a bit of background before its implications for successful aging and occupational therapy can be fully considered. In this section, we briefly discuss the short history of retirement; the physical, psychological, and financial tolls of retiring; retirement and the baby boom generation; cultural perspectives on retirement; global considerations; and opportunities and challenges that may contribute to or detract from successful aging.

History of Retirement

Luborksy and LeBlanc[50] define retirement in the Western cultures as "the age-fixed and socially mandated final phase in a career of employment in which a person is excluded from full time career jobs, is entitled to financial support without the stigma of dependency and is personally responsible for managing his or her own life" (p. 254). German Chancellor Otto von Bismarck is credited with initially setting the retirement age at 70 years in 1889, although this was later changed to 65 years after Bismarck's death.[82] Before this type of state support, individuals were often faced with drawing from their personal savings if they were fortunate to have some, formal agreements with children to grant transfer of property in return for care, or reliance on various charities if they had no other means of self-support. Many have argued that retirement was initially intended to last for only a few years, because the assumption was that people would not live much beyond age 65 years, and to provide support for basic living expenses, that is, to keep people housed and fed until death.

Although retirement is a relatively new concept, it has quickly "taken off" for various reasons. In 1900, one quarter of American men aged 65 years and older had stopped working. In the late 1990s, nearly 80% of men over 64 years were retired.[27] Part of the change can be attributed to a shift from agricultural work to industrialized jobs that are more suited to retirement. Participation in the paid labor force for people aged 65 years and over in the United States has declined by 40% since 1950. In the 1950s, one in three people aged 65 years or over worked. In 2000, only one in five did.[45]

People in many countries have experienced large gains in years of life expectancy after retirement due to longer life in general and younger retirement ages in many places. This is especially true for women, who have an average longer life expectancy at birth than men. In countries such as Portugal and France, life expectancy for women after retirement has doubled since the 1970s, giving women there, on average, around 26 years of life after retirement from paid labor.[45] Men in these countries have, on average, around 18 years of life after retirement.

Physical, Psychological, and Financial Tolls of Retiring

There is a comprehensive literature regarding health outcomes and retirement. The Health and Retirement Study (HRS) is one example of a national longitudinal study investigating various economic and health indicators of U.S. adults over age 50 years that has produced numerous findings.[41] Although it is beyond the scope of this chapter to provide a thorough review of the literature, a brief description of some key findings is helpful when considering successful aging, because how one experiences retirement can have a great effect on one's physical and mental health.

Although retired or separated from their primary paid occupation, many people who have withdrawn from the full-time paid workforce may take on part-time employment or volunteer work. Advantages include increased social interaction, sense of meaning and purpose, and, in the case of paid work, potential economic gain. Greater social interaction has been linked to lower mortality and morbidity rates,[76] whereas social isolation and loneliness have been found to increase passive death wishes[6] and lead to poorer overall cognitive and physical health outcomes.

Others, however, may find themselves leading more sedentary lives and/or experiencing greater social isolation in addition to having potential economic difficulties. These in turn can negatively affect health and well-being. Sedentary behaviors, for example, have been linked to increased weight and increased risk of diseases such as diabetes and heart disease.[52]

In a study on well-being among male and female retirees in the United States, Kim and Moen[43] found that men's retirement was more closely related to decreased well-being than was women's, using indicators such as increase in depressive symptoms. However, it is important to note that they also found that financial status and social relationships can greatly influence well-being. Not surprisingly, perceptions of having adequate financial resources and personal and social relationships contributed to greater well-being. Increased perceptions of control were also associated with decreased depressive symptoms and increased morale. Luborsky and LeBlanc[50] point out that although retirement is not synonymous with old age in the West, it can be in other societies, and, therefore, retirement may signal other important transitions in one's life course.

The opportunities and challenges of retirement also represent opportunities and challenges for successful aging. How well one can enjoy retirement depends on one's level of function (physical, cognitive, social, spiritual) and one's finances. Being able to live at a level that one is satisfied with is important. As mentioned earlier, considerations such as neighborhood characteristics (e.g., whether it is safe, whether stores are within walking distance or accessible by reliable transportation) are related to health and well-being. Having something meaningful to do is critical to mental health. Avoiding a sedentary lifestyle, maintaining social relationships, and finding purpose in life all are important considerations of retirement.

Toward a Revised Definition of Successful Aging

Given all of the background on successful aging as a concept; statistics on physical, cognitive, and social functioning in older age; perspectives on various cultural and subcultural differences in the United States and beyond; and the growing and relatively new phenomenon of retirement, we propose our own definition of successful aging, one that can provide a guideline for effective occupational therapy interventions. In Figure 18-1 we provide a conceptual schema for how to think about successful aging on an individual level.

On the *x*-axis in Figure 18-1 are the areas of function broken down into physical, cognitive, social, and spiritual. These areas are purposefully left vague, so that the individual can describe what he or she feels belongs in each of these. For example, physical function for one person may involve the ability to walk unassisted, without a walker or wheelchair. For another person who is unable to ambulate, physical function may refer to the ability to write a letter or knit a scarf. Cognitive function includes mental abilities, such as memory, language, critical thinking, and others. A person who is struggling with language difficulties because of a stroke may see language as a key area of function that needs attention. Others may consider keeping their minds active to be a main goal. Social function can include participating in social events (e.g., a holiday with family), meeting new people, and communicating in some way with others via email or other technologies—basically, any activity that suggests connectedness with another. As with physical and cognitive function, personal needs in this area will most likely differ. Finally, spiritual function refers to the sense of meaning that one has in his or her life. It can include religious beliefs, personal beliefs about one's own place in the world, and other notions tied to meaningfulness.

The *y*-axis is a subjective measure of function. Much like the current pain scale commonly used in the United States, where clients are asked to rate their level of pain from 0 to 10, with 0 being no pain and 10 being unbearable pain, individuals can describe their level of function in terms of "no function" to "optimal function." Rather than providing one value for each category, however, the individual can think about what level of function he or she believes is attainable in a given area and what level the individual thinks he or she currently has attained.

Bridging the distance between the two lines is the goal of successful aging (Figure 18-2). In addition, the lines can change over time. For example, what may have appeared to be an attainable level of physical function may turn out to be beyond reach, regardless of effort or desire. Rather than considering someone to be "unsuccessful," a new level of attainable function is obtained. This type of negotiation between attainable and current levels, coupled with the individual's definition of what areas are important to him or her, creates a model of successful aging that is individually tailored and that takes into account different abilities, desires, and outcomes.

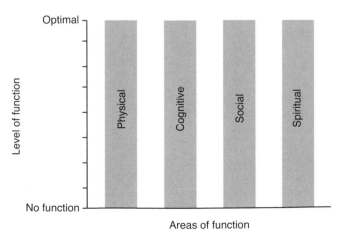

FIGURE 18-1   Conceptual schema for successful aging.

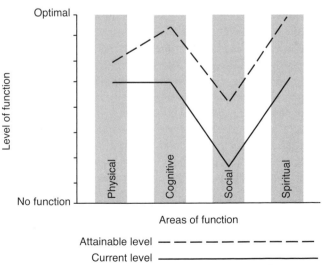

FIGURE 18-2   Self-anchored model of successful aging.

Relevance to Occupational Performance Deficits and Occupational Therapy Interventions

On a daily basis, occupational therapists come into contact with older persons whose identities have been threatened by performance limitations. These identity threats may occur as the result of normal aging, which often deprives a person of the sense of competence he or she once enjoyed, or result from injuries and diseases that leave lasting or progressive disability.

According to Christiansen,[19] if our identities are crafted by what we do and how we do it, then it follows that any threat to one's ability to engage in occupations and present oneself as competent becomes a threat to one's identity and thus to one's functional performance. Successful aging, then, encompasses how satisfied one is with having achieved desired and attainable levels of function and having sustained his or her identity throughout the aging process, and how important both of these aspects are to the individual.

Christiansen's[19] Eleanor Clarke Slagle Lecture described the concept of "selfing" as the lifelong process of how each person shapes his or her own identity through daily occupations. This concept has strong relevance to successful aging and continuity theory, which states that individuals, as they grow old, strive to maintain the self-identity that they have created over a lifetime.

Occupations, then, are more than activities or movements strung together, more than simply doing something; daily occupations create opportunities to express one's unique self and thus create one's unique identity.[19]

The extent to which occupational performance deficits and disabilities interfere with the competent (as self-defined) execution of tasks and roles can threaten one's sense of successful aging and thus the viability of sustaining one's lifelong identity. When disease, disability, or injuries result in bodily disfigurement, it further assaults the person's identity and increases the challenges associated with receiving social approval from family, friends, and associates.[19] Involuntary movements, paralysis, motor planning deficits, balance disorders, unwanted tics, forgetfulness, and moments of confusion are often among the many observable signs of disorders that gain unwanted public attention and increase the challenge of maintaining one's desirable social identity.[19] A central rehabilitation role for the occupational therapist becomes one of helping older aging adults use adaptive and compensation strategies to keep their identities intact by remaining as functionally independent as possible for as long as possible, regardless of the level of mental or physical dysfunction, and continually recalibrating the level of achievable function and criteria for functional independence as needed.

When older adults are able to make the essential adaptations and accommodations necessary to maintain a coherent sense of identity, successful aging is possible. Adaptations and accommodations may be necessary from a cognitive, social, physical, functional, and emotional perspective as one continues to age and find meaningful fulfillment in life. Adaptations and accommodations are essential to ensure the greatest level of safety, maximum independence in instrumental activities of daily living (IADLs), and self-management for the older adult. Adaptations and accommodations are necessary when there is clear evidence, based on cognitive and/or physical evaluations, of a decline in level of competence or a deficiency in any area of essential functioning. The role of an occupational therapist is to evaluate the client's performance strengths and deficits and develop intervention protocols, building on the strengths to address the deficits. Successful aging, then, is evidenced by being able to make the necessary adaptations and accommodations to maintain one's self-identity and to ensure optimum and achievable levels of functioning, safety, independence, and satisfaction with performance of meaningful occupations.

Research Related to Occupational Performance and Successful Aging

Evidence-based occupational therapy (OT) has become a part of the global OT professional psyche.[40] Numerous resources are now available to identify OT-relevant research. For example, the *American Journal of Occupational Therapy* (AJOT) hosts an online Evidence-Based Practice Forum, and OTseeker.com is a free online database that identifies relevant systematic reviews of critically appraised randomized controlled trials.[54] The following section describes several research studies relevant to OT practice to promote successful aging; some of these were conducted by investigators in other disciplines, but are nevertheless applicable to OT practice.

Social Participation and Quality of Life

Occupational therapists Stevens-Ratchford and Diaz[74] examined social participation, successful aging, and quality of life in a sample of 22 older Caucasians living in and around Baltimore, Maryland. Social participation was viewed as a lifelong engagement process in a variety of social occupations that included interactions and shared experiences with others that contributed to successful aging and quality of life. Participants were interviewed about their lived experience of social participation and its meaning in the context of successful aging over a 6-week period. They reported an overall positive quality of life, with the majority of responses ranging from being pleased to delighted. The two themes that emerged from the study were: (1) longstanding social occupation creates a network of social connectedness and active engagement with life, and (2) longstanding social occupations encourage habits for aging well. This study underscores the significance of occupational therapists' work to provide meaningful client-centered occupations of social engagement based on the client's interests and needs. Stevens-Ratchford and Diaz[74] showed how activities of engagement promoted health, well-being, social connectedness, aging well, and better functioning. For this sample, participation in social occupations contributed to their quality of life and successful aging.

Research on Successful Cognitive Aging

Daffner[30] conducted a comprehensive review of research on successful cognitive aging from four major lines of evidence: (1) epidemiologic/cohort studies, (2) animal/basic science studies, (3) human "proof-of-concept" studies, and (4) human intervention studies. Although there was no conclusive evidence from any one line of research showing how cognitive engagement practices promote successful aging, each approach had its advantages and limitations. The strongest case was made for physically and cognitively stimulating activities, both of which appear to enhance cognitive performance and reduce the likelihood of developing dementia. Epidemiologic studies suggest that regular exercise and participation in cognitively stimulating activities diminish the risk of dementia.[30] Animal studies showed that exercise was associated with upregulation of relevant neural growth factors such as brain-derived neurotropic factors (BDNF), and that environmental enrichment promotes neurogenesis, increasing one's capacity to compensate for cerebral insults and to augment cognitive functioning. Finally, the proof-of-concept studies highlighted the plasticity of the human brain, even in older adults. Randomized controlled intervention studies showed that aerobic exercise and cognitive training programs were associated with improved cognitive performance and could affect relevant biological markers.[30] Evidence from these studies can help occupational therapists design effective therapeutic interventions to support successful aging.

Research on Lifestyle Factors and Successful Aging

Many research studies have shown that chronic conditions and disability can be prevented, postponed, or diminished through positive lifestyle behaviors. For example, changes in exercise and diet, when used as a preventative intervention in older adults, can significantly reduce the risk of cardiovascular disease, osteoporosis, arthritis, diabetes, some forms of cancer, obesity, cognitive decline, and depression.[31] Studies have shown the positive correlations between levels of participation in social and productive activity and a range of health outcomes, including physical and cognitive function, self-efficacy, and quality of life.[33]

Peralta-Catipon and Hwang[62] examined personal factors that were predictive of health-related lifestyles among 253 community-dwelling older adults, aged 55 to 92 years, in Southern California. They examined demographic factors, number of chronic diseases and impairments, self-rated health status, and health-related lifestyle behaviors, using measures such as the Health Enhancement Lifestyle Profile (HELP) and a Rasch-based instrument that assessed health-promoting behaviors. The results showed that older adults who demonstrate more positive lifestyle behaviors may have fewer adverse health conditions in old age than those who do not. Self-rated health was also found to be a significant predictor for all aspects of the lifestyle measures.[62] Although cautioning about the generalizability of their findings, the authors offer the following possible relationships between demographic characteristics and different aspects of a health-related lifestyle, after taking personal health factors into account:

- Older men are more likely than older women to engage in exercise but less likely to participate in activities related to paid or volunteer work, social networking, stress management, and spiritual or religious participation.
- Employment, both full and part time, among older adults provides an opportunity for enhancing productivity and socialization; conversely, it may compromise the leisure participation of older adults.
- Compared with Whites, Asian and African American older adults are less likely to participate in paid or volunteer work as well as social and leisure activities.
- Compared with Whites, Asian, African American, and Hispanic/Latino older adults are more involved in spiritual or religious activities.
- A higher level of education correlates with a higher level of leisure participation as well as a higher frequency of health self-monitoring behaviors, such as checking blood pressure and body weight.
- The older the adult, the lower the frequency of health risk behaviors.[62]

The Harvard Study of Adult Development

The Harvard Study of Adult Development, a longitudinal study, represents the longest, most comprehensive examination of aging ever conducted[80] and provides further insight into successful aging. Beginning in the 1930s, researchers studied more than 800 men and women from adolescence to old age, looking for clues to behaviors that translated into happy, healthy longevity. The researchers reported many surprises, such as the fact that stressful events did not predict future health but how one deals with stress did. "Some people had a lot of stress in life but aged very well," noted Vaillant.[80] Vaillant also reported that people should not be obsessed with cholesterol or other genetic factors but instead focus on controllable lifestyle choices, such as avoiding cigarettes; making good adjustments and using good coping strategies; maintaining a healthy weight and exercising regularly; retaining strong social relationships, including a stable marriage; and continuing involvement in educational pursuits.[80] The book *Aging Well* describes the decades-long Harvard study and reports that it is "astonishing how many of the ingredients that predict longevity are within one's control".[80] Knowing this information can help therapists adopt supportive strategies to provide therapeutic intervention.

Research on "Quality Longevity"

Many other works on successful aging support the Harvard study findings. *The Longevity Bible*,[72] based on research conducted by Gary Small and G. Vorgan at UCLA, claims that only one third of what predicts how well we age is related to genetics, with the remaining two thirds being based on our personal lifestyle choices.

Small and Vorgan[72] parallels Vaillant's[80] work with the eight essentials that contribute to empowering oneself for future successful aging, or in his words, "quality longevity," the idea of living longer, younger, and healthier. To empower ourselves to remain healthy and fulfilled, Small and Vorgan's[72] eight essentials to quality longevity are: (1) maximize brain fitness with memory exercises to keep your mind sharp; (2) maintain a positive outlook on life; (3) maintain strong social relationships by remaining socially connected, thus boosting one's self-concept; (4) avoid and/or manage stress by reducing relationship clutter in your life; (5) personalize your immediate environment both at work and at home; (6) engage in a longevity fitness routine that covers cardiovascular conditioning, balance, flexibility, and strength training; (7) maintain a healthy diet plan that allows you to eat all of your favorite foods but incorporates the best scientific data on healthful eating for longevity and weight control; and (8) examine and use the latest medical options available to keep you looking and feeling healthy. An underlying principle of all eight essentials is *mindful awareness*, the subtle process of moment-to-moment awareness of one's thoughts, feelings, and physical states, which is key to sharpening memory and remaining mentally fit. By integrating mindful awareness into our daily lives, we not only enjoy ourselves more and live longer; we also take better care of ourselves, have a more positive outlook, and feel more empathy toward others.[72] Mindfulness often fosters a sense of spirituality, and several studies[53,56,77] have found that people who pursue some form of spirituality live longer. Increased longevity may result from many forms of spirituality, including religion, meditation, and a personal belief in God or a higher power.[72]

The longevity study showed that after 2 weeks, volunteers who followed the healthy longevity lifestyle program, compared with those in the control group who followed their normal routine, experienced improved memory performance and brain efficiency. They also reported greater levels of relaxation, lower levels of stress, significant weight loss, and decline in blood pressure and cholesterol levels. Scientific evidence indicates that adopting these lifestyle strategies may lower the risk for Alzheimer's disease and actually increase life expectancy—making us live longer and also adding to the quality of those years.[72]

Evidence-Based Community Health Promotion and Wellness Programs to Foster Successful Aging

Innovative and effective community-based interventions with the support of an evidence base are desperately needed.[57] Among the evidence-based programs that qualify are those dealing with OT interventions, creative arts, physical activity, falls management, nutrition, depression, and substance abuse. Not all of the programs discussed in the following sections were initiated by occupational therapists; however, they represent a sample of programs that OT professionals should find helpful in their work with older adults.

The Well Elderly Study 1 and 2

Although begun almost 20 years ago, this series of studies continues to stand as landmark work in gerontological OT practice. To investigate the complex and interlocking challenges faced by older adults, including the physical, psychological, economic, and social factors, Florence Clark and colleagues[20] conducted a 9-month randomized controlled study of 361 well older adults living in Los Angeles. Participants were men and women, 60 years and older, who had the capacity to benefit in multiple outcome areas from involvement in occupational therapy. The purpose of the study was to evaluate the effectiveness of primary prevention occupational therapy specifically targeting an urban, multiethnic, independent-living population. The researchers reasoned that because many of the principles of OT intervention focus on fostering meaningful and productive activity (occupation) to enhance function and maximize independence, this might prove to be an effective approach to promoting health in a vulnerable population. The researchers randomly assigned persons to participate in one of three research groups. The 120 people randomly assigned to the social control group participated in generalized group social activities designed to improve social interactions; the 122 people randomly assigned to the OT intervention group participated in specially designed OT protocols (i.e., Lifestyle Redesign®), including socialization activities, carried out by specialized occupational therapists; and the third randomized group of 119 persons received no specific treatment and served as the nontreatment control group. Participants in each group were encouraged not to share information about the study outside of their respective groups. Researchers hypothesized that participation in a social activity group alone would be less effective in positively promoting daily functioning and physical or psychosocial well-being as compared with participation in a well-designed primary prevention OT group carried out by experienced geriatric occupational therapists.

All 361 participants received pre- and posttest assessments of self-rated health, physical and social functioning, life satisfaction, and depressive symptoms, using well-validated self-administered surveys and scales. All test administration was conducted by independent paid research assistants who were blind to the group assignments and to the study hypothesis. The OT intervention focused on the central theme of "health through occupation," defined as grooming, exercising, shopping, and socialization activities. The goal of the 9-month OT intervention was to assist participants in gaining a greater appreciation for the role of meaningful activities in their lives, and to educate them to better select and perform activities to achieve a more satisfying lifestyle.

Participants in the OT intervention group also were asked to analyze how each activity affected their personal health and well-being. The occupational therapists developed modular unit protocols for intervention participants on topics such as transportation utilization, joint protection, personal safety hazards and preventive measures, energy conservation, exercise and nutrition, adaptive equipment, and overall home and community safety.

The Well Elderly Study 1 found significant benefits from the OT interventions across various health, function, and quality-of-life domains. This study provided the most comprehensive evidence and efficacy to date of the effectiveness of OT interventions with older adults. It had the largest sample population of all previous studies of older adults, incorporated a wider range of outcome domains, sampled for ethnic diversity, and due to the study design, demonstrated experimental control. Significant benefits from the primary prevention OT interventions emerged as improvements in functioning or a relative reduction in the extent of functional decline of individuals in this group, as compared with individuals in the control groups. These participants showed a more pronounced decline in daily functional status and primary response measures, even though there were no significant differences among the groups at baseline. The OT group demonstrated a significant gain in 10 of the 15 outcome measures studied, as compared with the control groups, providing solid evidence of the comprehensive effectiveness of a primary preventive OT intervention with well older adults.

Several years later, the team conducted a follow-up randomized control trial, Well Elderly 2, to replicate previous findings regarding the impact and cost-effectiveness of the activity-based intervention, Lifestyle Redesign®, and to understand the mechanisms underlying those effects. Relative to the controls, intervention participants showed more favorable change scores in regard to bodily pain, vitality, social functioning, mental health, composite mental functioning, symptoms of depression, as well as life satisfaction, and a significant greater increase in quality-adjusted life years.[21]

The Creativity and Aging Study

In 2001, the National Endowment for the Arts and the George Washington University Center on Aging in Washington, D.C., teamed with centers in New York and California to conduct a multisite national study of 150 older persons known as the Creativity and Aging Study. The goal of the study was to examine the effects of professionally conducted cultural arts programming on the general health, mental health, and social activities engagement of older persons between the ages of 65 and 102 years across three states.[25] The average age in the three program sites was 80 years, and 30% of the participants were racial and ethnic minorities. The groups were matched on level of functioning at the start of the study with a group of controls with similar physical health, mental health, and level-of-activity profiles. The intervention groups participated in intensive creative arts programs such as painting, singing in a chorale group, writing poetry, jewelry making, and creative crafts. The programs were held weekly for 9 months a year over a 2-year period. The positive outcomes across all intervention groups were reported as "staggering." Intervention groups across all three sites reported an increase in morale, a decrease in depressive symptoms, and a decreased sense of loneliness; better self-reported health, fewer physician visits, and reduced use of prescription and over-the-counter drugs; and increased involvement in activities.[24] The results of this research have direct implications for

OT practice, especially in the area of occupational engagement and participation. The study demonstrated that professionally run, community-based cultural arts programs for older adults reduce risk factors that drive the need for long-term care and promote successful aging.[22,23] Occupational therapists need to restore the effective use of occupation-based groups, using activity engagement, to promote successful aging.

Administration on Aging Health Promotion and Wellness Programs

The Administration on Aging (AoA) initiated programs to help older adults maintain health and independence within their homes and communities (see http://www.aoa.acl.gov/AoA_Programs/hpw/index.aspx for examples). Programs supported by the AoA Aging Network include those related to behavioral health, chronic disease self-management, diabetes self-management, disease prevention and health promotion services (Title IIID), falls prevention, HIV/AIDS, Medicare outreach, and oral health. (See also the Spring 2010 issue of *Generations* for additional examples of evidence-based community practices.)

The Stanford University Chronic Disease Self-Management Program

The Stanford University Chronic Disease Self-Management Program (CDSMP), a 6-week workshop conducted within community settings, is a model program for older adults with chronic conditions. The CDSMP covers the following topics: (1) techniques to deal with frustration, fatigue, pain, and isolation; (2) exercises to maintain strength, flexibility, and endurance; (3) appropriate use of medications; (4) techniques to improve communication with family, friends, and health professionals; (5) tips on proper nutrition; (6) decision-making strategies; and (7) guidelines for evaluating new medical treatments. Older adult participants quickly recognized that to achieve real benefits within this type of program they must willingly assume personal responsibility for managing their own chronic condition(s).[49]

The FallsFree™ Coalition

Three national organizations, the National Council on Aging, the Archstone Foundation, and the Home Safety Council, collaborated to create the national FallsFree™ Coalition. The Coalition's collaborative leadership now includes state departments of aging, public health departments, and healthcare providers. Since 2005 its membership has grown to include 64 national organizations. In 2005 the FallFree™ National Action Plan was released following presentations by leaders of successful national programs at the FallsFree Summit. The National Action Plan includes goals, strategies, and action steps that target physical mobility issues, medication management, and home and environmental safety. The document identifies and provides links to numerous resources that would be of interest to occupational therapists working with older adults. The National Action Plan continues to provide guidance for both state and local interdisciplinary programs. In addition, coalition members were instrumental in the passage of the Keeping Seniors Safe from Falls Act of 2007 (S845/HR5608) by the U.S. House of Representatives.

The Centers for Disease Control and Prevention Compendium of Effective Fall Interventions

The Keeping Seniors Safe from Falls Act continues to provide a focal point for identifying priorities in the ongoing efforts of states and localities to further reduce the occurrence of falls in older adults. Yet falls remain the largest cause of emergency room visits and hospitalizations, which are often followed by extended home health rehabilitation interventions. Data from 2008 from the National Center for Injury Prevention and Control of the Centers for Disease Control and Prevention (CDC)[58] rank unintentional falls in adults in the 45-54 years, 55-64 years, and the 65 years and older age ranges as the primary cause of nonfatal injuries. Within that time frame, 7,736,912 injuries occurred for adults within those age ranges. In response to these findings, the CDC developed a Compendium of Effective Fall Interventions,[73] which describes 22 evidence-based interventions for fall prevention for community-dwelling older adults.

Training the Health-Care Workforce—Present and Future

Currently, most health-care professionals do not receive the gerontological training necessary to respond to the unique and complex health needs of older adults and promote successful aging. Estimates have shown that proper gerontological care by *all* providers would reduce hospital, nursing home, and home care costs by at least 10% a year. By 2020 that could amount to a savings of $133.7 billion.[61] Improvement could occur if the following steps were taken:

- Provide all health-care professionals with education and training in gerontology and geriatrics.
- Remove policy barriers so older adults gain access to more timely and effective mental health services.
- Expand the Medicare reimbursement system to provide for better mental health coverage.
- Enable physicians to gain access to information that helps them better prevent and treat depression, falls, urinary incontinence, and other age-related conditions.
- Develop continuing education programs in gerontology and geriatrics based on effective models of practicing-physician education, interactive sessions, and evidence-based materials.
- Encourage physicians to routinely ask and counsel seniors about smoking, physical activity, diet, and other health risk behaviors.
- Target information and resources toward African Americans and Hispanics, because minority seniors remain at greater risk than Whites for several chronic conditions and health-damaging behaviors.

Future Trends

Given the demographic and accompanying socioeconomic and cultural changes described earlier, health-care providers and government agencies are tasked with being proactive in planning and preparing strategies to meet the mounting needs of older adults before they escalate beyond control.[15] They also need to recognize and value the strengths and talents that older adults have to offer. Therapists must successfully train and enable well older adults to become better self-managers of their chronic illnesses and enlist them as peer teachers to help others to facilitate their own successful aging.[42] The village-to-village model[35] of self-governing, grassroots, community-based organizations—developed with the sole purpose of enabling people to remain in their own homes and communities as they age—should be encouraged. Service providers increase their focus on community-based programs and interventions.[5]

Our Future Selves: A Virtual Glimpse into the Future

In 2011 and 2012, a team of Columbia University journalism students participating in the Carnegie-Knight Initiative on the Future of Journalism Education News21[16] program chose aging as their focal topic. Their online multimedia projects, titled "Brave Old World," aimed to convey the experience of aging in the contemporary United States and to help people acquire some perspective on how they might change with age. Freely available from the News21 Archives, these multimedia reports provide vivid video portraits of aging in a variety of settings and geographic locations. There are several subsections within the larger projects, and each deals with a different context or challenge for the aging adult, such as family caregiving, residential care, older workers, demographics of aging communities, and programs developed to allow people to age in place.

For example, the segment, "Aging Town" from the 2011 series, provides specific examples of strategies that older adults in a particular geographic area have used or found useful in their aging process in towns across the United States.

The "Our Future Selves" section may be particularly enlightening for those interested in demographics. It features an interactive tool that shows demographic, health, and economic changes over time, based on the user's data (age, sex, location, and marital status). The tool gathers available online data to present answers from economists, biostatisticians, and demographers to the following questions:

- How will the country's demographics change over the next 40 years?
- How do sex, race, and ethnicity affect our health?
- What does the financial picture look like for retirees?

By way of an example, consider Dorothy. She was born in 1930, lives in Virginia, is married, and has paid off the mortgage on her home. Population statistics for Virginia for 2014 indicate the following breakdown of its 323 million residents:

- 63% are White,
- 17% are Hispanic,
- 12% are African American,
- 5% are Asian, and
- 2% classified themselves as "Other."

By 2024, those demographics will have shifted for its now 354 million residents, resulting in the following breakdown:

- 58% will be White,
- 21% will be Hispanic,
- 12% will be African American,
- 6% will be Asian, and
- 3% will classify themselves as "Other."

As the program continues, it shows projections of demographics on aging by state, health forecasts, and predicted breakdowns of financial expenditures for an older adult with the user's characteristics.

Current and Future Practice Areas to Support Successful Aging

Occupational therapists and occupational therapy assistants must be committed to promoting successful aging by meeting current needs and creating new markets that address a progressively aging society. OT services must provide programs and interventions that sustain cognitive functioning, functional performance, social engagement, independence, and life satisfaction. The demand for OT consultant services for federal, state, and local agencies; community groups; and individuals will increase. OT and occupational therapy assistant students must be educated to meet the market demand as well as to advocate for future services. There will be a greater demand for evidence-based services consistent with research outcomes, and hence the need for resourceful educators, trained researchers of high quality, master clinicians, home modification specialists, and creative developers of effective assessment tools. Furthermore, training clients in the use of adaptive technology and providing services that improve daily functioning and help sustain independence will be essential skills for future occupational therapists and OT assistants.

The following are but a few of the OT-related programs and roles that may contribute to the quality of life of older adults and enable them to achieve successful aging:

- Older driver assessment services (e.g., CarFit, developed by the AARP [formerly the American Association of Retired Persons], American Occupational Therapy Administration [AOTA], and American Automobile Association [AAA])[2]
- Driving rehabilitation services
- Design, accessibility, and home modification assessments and consultant services[11]
- Low-vision assessment and services
- Lifestyle coaching and organized artistic and leisure service programs
- Health and wellness programs and consultant services (for corporations and individuals)[11]
- Consultant services for assisted living facilities
- Medicare consultant
- Guardian care consultant
- Falls prevention research and services
- Development of games and cognitive engagement programs

- Assistive technology development and consultant services
- Development of standardized assessments for older adults (especially in the areas of cognitive, social, and physical functioning)
- Professor and/or educational consultant on successful aging
- Private contract and consultant services for adult daycare programs, home health agencies, and nursing homes

The Bureau of Labor Statistics (2014–2015) reported that occupational therapists held about 113,200 jobs in 2012. The largest numbers of occupational therapist jobs (28%) were in state, local, and private hospitals. Other major employers included offices of other health practitioners, public and private educational services, nursing care facilities, community care facilities for older adults, home health care, and government agencies. During this same period, occupational therapy Assistants held 32,230 jobs, including significant numbers of positions in offices of other types of health practitioners, nursing care facilities, home health care services, continuing care retirement communities and assisted living facilities.

Employment of occupational therapists and assistants is expected to continue to increase by 29% through 2022, much faster than the average for all occupations. Job growth is, in part, being driven by the demand for services from the progressively increasing older adult population.[13]

Summary

We conclude with a poem that conveys an example of successful aging and the determination to live life to its fullest:

Excerpt from the poem, "When Death Comes" by Mary Oliver[60]

When it's over, I want to say: all my life
I was a bride married to amazement.
I was the bridegroom, taking the world
Into my arms.
When it's over, I don't want to wonder
If I have made of my life something
Particular and real
I don't want to find myself sighing and
Frightened,
Or full of argument.
I don't want to end up simply having
Visited this world.

REVIEW QUESTIONS

1. Case: Mrs. Briggs has been a successful accountant for 35 years at a major accounting firm in New York. She enjoys living alone, working independently to manage her own life, which is very important to her. She is a loner and primarily stays to herself. Her daily routine involved going to work on the subway very early every day, going to the opera occasionally, and watching lots of television every

night until about midnight. She has recently suffered a stroke which necessitates minimal to moderate assistance with her daily needs, and she can no longer live alone. Self-care independence and self-management were her highest areas of importance, as determined by the OT assessment. Determine an intervention plan to address her deficits and ideal successful aging profile.

2. Based on your understanding of this chapter, write a reflection paper on successful aging. What does successful aging look like? What does the role of a dynamic occupational therapist working to promote successful aging look like?

REFERENCES

1. Administration on Aging. (2012). *A profile of older Americans.* Retrieved 10/19/15. http://www.aoa.gov/Aging_Statistics/Profile/2012/docs/2012profile.pdf.
2. American Association of Retired Persons (AARP), American Occupational Therapy Association (AOTA), & American Automobile Association (AAA). (2008). *CarFit: Helping older drivers find their perfect fit.* http://elderlydrivingassessments.com/images/individ/carfitcheck.pdf/. Accessed 18.08.15.
3. American Occupational Therapy Association. (2007). AOTA's Centennial Vision and executive summary. *American Journal of Occupational Therapy, 61,* 613–614.
4. Angel, R. J. (2009). Structural and cultural factors in successful aging among older Hispanics. *Family & Community Health, 32*(10), S46.
5. Archstone Foundation News. (2011). *The village movement: A model for supportive communities for older adults.* Accessed 10/19/15. http://www.multihousingnews.com/news/west/archstone-foundation-awards-grants-for-villages/1004041182.html/.
6. Avalon, L., & Shiovitz, E. S. (2011). The relationship between loneliness and passive death wishes in the second half of life. *International Psychogeriatrics, 23*(10), 1677–1685.
7. Baker, J. L. (1958). The unsuccessful aged. *Journal of the American Geriatrics Society, 7,* 570–572.
8. Baltes, P. B., & Baltes, M. M. (1990). Psychological perspectives on successful aging: The model of selective optimization with compensation. In P. B. Baltes & M. M. Baltes (Eds.), *Successful aging: Perspectives from the behavioral sciences* (pp. 1–34). New York, NY: Cambridge University Press.
9. Berkman, L. F., Seeman, T. E., Albert, M., Blazer, D., Kahn, R., Mohs, R., & Rowe, J. (1993). High, usual and impaired functioning in community-dwelling older men and women: findings from the MacArthur Foundation Research Network on Successful Aging. *Journal of clinical epidemiology, 46*(10), 1129–1140.
10. Biggs, S. (2004). Age, gender, narratives, and masquerades. *Journal of Aging Studies, 18*(1), 45–58.
11. Brachtesende, A. (2005). New markets emerge from society's needs: The turnaround is here. *OT Practice, 23,* 13–19.
12. Bruce, M. L., Seeman, T. E., Merrill, S. S., & Blazer, D. G. (1994). The impact of depressive symptomatology on physical disability: MacArthur Studies of Successful Aging. *American Journal of Public Health, 84*(11), 1796–1799.
13. Bureau of Labor Statistics, U.S. Department of Labor. (2014-2015). *Occupational outlook handbook, 2014-15 edition.* Accessed 10/19/15. http://www.bls.gov/ooh/healthcare/occupational-therapists.html/.
14. Butler, R. N. (1974). Successful aging and the role of the life review. *Journal of the American Geriatrics Society, 22*(12), 529–535.
15. Carlson, M. Clark, F., & Young, B. (1998). Practical contributions of occupational science to the art of successful ageing: How to sculpt a meaningful life in older adulthood. *Journal of Occupational Science, 5,* 107–118.
16. Carnegie-Knight Initiative on the Future of Journalism Education. *News21 Archives.* http://news21.com/. Accessed 18.08.15.
17. Caro, F. G., Bass, S. A., & Chen, Y. P. (1993). Introduction: Achieving a productive aging society. In S. A. Bass, F. G. Caro, & Y. P. Chen (Eds.), *Achieving a productive aging society* (pp. 3–25). Westport, CN: Auburn House.
18. Cavan, R. S., Burgess, E. W., Havighurst, R. J., & Goldhamer, H. (1949). *Personal adjustment in old age.* Chicago, IL: Science Research Associates.
19. Christiansen, C. H. (1999). Defining lives: Occupation as identity: An essay on competence, coherence and the creation of meaning. *American Journal of Occupational Therapy, 53,* 547–558.
20. Clark, F., Azen, S., Zemke, R., Jackson, J., Carlson, M., Mandel, D., et al. (1997). Occupational therapy for independent-living older adults: A randomized controlled trial. *Journal of the American Medical Association, 278*(16), 1321–1326.
21. Clark, F., Jackson, J., Carlson, M., Chou C. P., Cherry, B. J., Jordan-Marsh, M., et al. (2012). Effectiveness of a lifestyle intervention in promoting the well-being of independently living older people: Results of the Well Elderly 2 Randomised Controlled Trial. *Journal of Epidemiology & Community Health, 66*(9), 782–790.
22. Cohen, G. D. (2005). National study documents beliefs of creativity programs for older adults. *The Older Learner, 13*(2), 1, 6.
23. Cohen, G. D. (2006a). *The Creativity and Aging Study: Executive summary. Final report.* Accessed 10/19/15. https://www.arts.gov/sites/default/files/CnA-Rep4-30-06.pdf.
24. Cohen, G. D. (2006b). *The mature mind: The positive power of the aging brain.* New York, NY: Basic Books.
25. Cohen, G., et al. (2006). The impact of professionally conducted cultural programs on the physical health, mental health, and social functioning of older adults. *The Gerontologist, 46*(6), 726–734.
26. Congdon, N. G., Friedman, D. S., & Lietman, T. (2003). Important causes of visual impairment in the world today. *Journal of the American Medical Association, 290*(15), 2057–2060.
27. Costa, D. L. (1998). The evolution of retirement. In D. L. Costa (Ed.), *The evolution of retirement: An American economic history, 1880-1990* (pp. 6–31). Chicago, IL: University of Chicago Press.
28. Crowther, M. R., Parker, M. W., Achenbaum, W. A., Larimore, W. L., & Koenig, H. G. (2002). Rowe and Kahn's Model of Successful Aging revisited positive spirituality—the forgotten factor. *The Gerontologist, 42*(5), 613–620.
29. Cruikshank, M. (2003). *Learning to be old: Gender, culture and aging.* Lanham, MD: Rowmann & Littlefield Publishers.
30. Daffner, K. R. (2010). Promoting successful cognitive aging: A comprehensive review. *Journal of Alzheimer's Disease, 19,* 1101–1122.
31. Depp, C. A., & Jeste, D. V. (2006). Definitions and predictors of successful aging: A comprehensive review of larger quantitative studies. *The American Journal of Geriatric Psychiatry, 14*(1), 6–20.
32. Doty, P., & Miller, B. (1993). Caregiving and productive aging. In S. A. Bass, F. G. Caro, & Y.-P. Chen (Eds.), *Achieving a*

productive aging society (pp. 143–166). Westport, CT: Auburn House.

33. Everard, K. M., Lach, H. W., Fisher, E. B., & Baum, M. C. (2000). Relationship of activity and social support to the functional health of older adults. *Journals of Gerontology, Series B: Psychological Sciences and Social Sciences, 55B*, S208–S212.

34. Fries, J. F. (2002). Successful aging—an emerging paradigm of gerontology. *Clinics in Geriatric Medicine, 18*, 371–382.

35. Greenfield, E. A., Scharlach, A., Lehning, A. J., & Davitt, J. K. (2012). A conceptual framework for examining the promise of the NORC program and Village models to promote aging in place. *Journal of Aging Studies, 26*(3), 273–284.

36. Havighurst, R. J. (1961). Successful aging. *The Gerontologist, 1*(1), 8–13.

37. Hazan, H., & Raz, A. E. (1997). The authorized self: How middle age defines old age in the postmodern. *Semiotica, 113*(3–4), 257–276.

38. Holstein, M. B., & Minkler, M. (2003). Self, society and the "new gerontology". *The Gerontologist, 43*(6), 787–796.

39. Howe, N., & Jackson, R. (2011). Global aging and the crisis of the 2020. 110, *Current History*, 20–25.

40. Ilott, I., Taylor, M. C., & Bolanos, C. (2006). Evidence-based occupational therapy: It's time to take a global approach. *British Journal of Occupational Therapy, 69*(1), 38–41.

41. Juster, F. T., & Suzman, R. (1995). An overview of the Health and Retirement Study. *Journal of Human Resources, 40*, S7–S56.

42. Kennedy, A., Rogers, A., Sanders, C., Gately, C., & Lee, V. (2009). *BMC Health Services Research article. Creating "good" self-managers: Facilitating and governing an online self-care skills training course?* Accessed 10/19/15. http://www.biomedcentral.com/1472-6963/9/93.

43. Kim, J. E., & Moen, P. (2002). Retirement transitions, gender, and psychological well-being a life-course, ecological model. *The Journals of Gerontology Series B: Psychological Sciences and Social Sciences, 57*(3), P212–P222.

44. Kinsella, K. (2000). Demographic dimensions of global aging. *Journal of Family Issues, 21*(5), 541–558.

45. Kinsella, K., & He, W. (2009). *US Census Bureau, international population reports*. Washington, DC: U.S. Census Bureau.

46. Lamb, S. (2014). Permanent personhood or meaningful decline? Toward a critical anthropology of successful aging. *Journal of Aging Studies, 29*, 41–52.

47. Lawton, M. P. (1983). The varieties of wellbeing. *Experimental Aging Research, 9*(2), 65–72.

48. Liang, J. & Luo, B. (2012). Toward a discourse shift in social gerontology: From successful aging to harmonious aging. *Journal of Aging Studies, 26*(3), 327–334.

49. Lorig, K. R., Ritter, P., Stewart, A. L., Sobel, D. S., Brown, B. W., Bandura, A., & Holman, H. R. (2001). Chronic Disease Self-Management Program: 2-year health status and health care utilization outcomes. *Medical Care, 39*(11), 1217–1223.

50. Luborsky, M. R., & LeBlanc, I. M. (2003). Cross-cultural perspectives on the concept of retirement: An analytic redefinition. *Journal of Cross-Cultural Gerontology, 18*(4), 251–271.

51. Martinson, M., & Berridge, C. (2015). Successful aging and its discontents: A systematic review of the social gerontology literature. *The Gerontologist, 55*(1), 58–69.

52. Matthews, C. E., George, S. M., Moore, S. C., Bowles, H. R., Blair, A., Park, Y., et al. (2012). Amount of time spent in sedentary behaviors and cause-specific mortality in US adults. *The American Journal of Clinical Nutrition, 95*, 437–445.

53. McCullough, M. E., Hoyt, W. T., Larson, D. B., Koenig, H. G., & Thoresen, C. (2000). Religious involvement and mortality: A meta-analytic review. *Health Psychology, 19*, 211–222.

54. McKenna, H. et al. (2004). Patient safety and quality of care: The role of the healthcare assistant. *Journal of Nursing Management, 12*(6), 452–459.

55. McLaughlin, S. J., & Connell, C. M. (2010). Successful aging in the United States: Prevalence estimates from a national sample of older adults. *The Journals of Gerontology Series B: Psychological Sciences and Social Sciences, 65*(2), 216–226.

56. Miller, W. R., & Thoresen, C. E. (2003). Spirituality, religion, and health: An emerging research field. *American Psychologist, 58*(1), 24–35.

57. Murphy, S. L. (2011). Update on geriatric research in productive aging. *The American Journal of Occupational Therapy, 65*(2), 197–206.

58. National Center for Injury Prevention and Control, Centers for Disease Control and Prevention. (2008). *National estimates of the 10 leading causes of nonfatal injuries treated in hospital emergency room departments, United States*. Accessed 10/19/15. http://www.cdc.gov/injury/wisqars/pdf/nonfatal_2008_bw-a.pdf.

59. National Institute on Aging (NIA). (2011). *Global health and aging*. NIH Publication no. 11-7737. Washington, D.C.: National Institute on Aging. Accessed 10/19.15. https://www.nia.nih.gov/research/publication/global-health-and-aging/preface.

60. Oliver, M. (1992). *New and selected poems* (Vol. 1, p. 10). Boston: Beacon Press.

61. O'Neill, G. (2003). *The state of aging and health in America*. Washington, DC: Merck Institute of Aging & Health and The Gerontological Society of America.

62. Peralta-Catipon, T., & Hwang, J. E. (2011). Personal factors predictive of health-related lifestyles of community-dwelling older adults. *American Journal of Occupational Therapy, 65*, 329–337.

63. Pressey, S. L., & Simcoe, E. (1950). Case study comparisons of successful and problem old people. *Journal of Gerontology, 5*, 168–175.

64. Reginster, J. Y. (2002). The prevalence and burden of arthritis. *Rheumatology, 41*(Suppl. 1), 3–6.

65. Rosal, M., & Bodenlos, J. (2009). Culture and health-related behavior. In S. A. Schumaker, J. K. Ockene, & K. A. Riekert (Eds.), *The handbook of health behavior change* (3rd ed., pp. 39–59). New York, NY: Springer.

66. Rowe, J. W., & Kahn, R. L. (1987). Human aging: Usual and successful. *Science, 237*, 143–149.

67. Rowe, J. W., & Kahn, R. L. (1998). *Successful aging*. New York, NY: Pantheon Books.

68. Rowe, J. W., & Kahn, R. L. (1999). Successful aging. In K. Dychtwald (Ed.), *Healthy aging: Challenges and solutions* (pp. 27–44). Gaithersburg, MD: Aspen.

69. Rubinstein, R. L., & de Medeiros, K. (2015). "Successful aging," gerontological theory and neoliberalism: A qualitative critique. *The Gerontologist.* 55.(1):34-42. doi 10.1093/geront/gnu79.

70. Seeman, T. E., Berkman, L. F., Charpentier, P. A., Blazer, D. G., Albert, M. S., & Tinetti, M. E. (1995). Behavioral and psychosocial predictors of physical performance: MacArthur studies of successful aging. *The Journals of Gerontology Series A: Biological Sciences and Medical Sciences, 50*(4), M177–M183.

71. Seeman, T. E., Lusignolo, T. M., Albert, M., & Berkman, L. (2001). Social relationships, social support, and patterns of cognitive aging in healthy, high-functioning older adults: MacArthur studies of successful aging. *Health psychology, 20*(4), 243.

72. Small, G., & Vorgan, G. (2006). *The longevity bible: 8 Essential strategies for keeping your mind sharp and your body young.* New York, NY: Hyperion Books.

73. Stevens, J. A. (2010). *A CDC compendium of effective fall interventions: What works for community-dwelling older adults* (2nd ed.). Atlanta, GA: Centers for Disease Control and Prevention, National Center for Injury Prevention and Control.

74. Stevens-Ratchford, R. G., & Diaz, T. (2003). Promoting successful aging through occupation: An examination of engagement in life: A look at aging in place, occupation and successful aging. *Activities, Adaptations and Aging, 27*(4), 19–37.

75. Strawbridge, W. J., Wallhagen, M. I., & Cohen, R. D. (2002). Successful aging and well-being: Self-rated compared with Rowe and Kahn. *The Gerontologist, 42*(6), 727–733.

76. Thomas, P. A. (2012). Trajectories of social engagement and mortality in late life. *Journal of Aging and Health, 24*(4), 547–568. doi: 0898264311432310.

77. Thoresen, C. E., & Harris, A. H. S. (2002). Spirituality and health: What's the evidence and what's needed? *Annals of Behavioral Medicine, 24*(1), 3–13.

78. Torres, S. (1999). A culturally-relevant theoretical framework for the study of successful ageing. *Ageing and Society, 19*(1), 33–51.

79. U.S. Census Bureau. (2012). Birth, death, marriages, and divorce. Accessed 10/19/15. https://www.census.gov/prod/2011pubs/12statab/vitstat.pdf.

80. Vaillant, G. E. (2003). *Aging well.* New York, NY: Little Brown and Company.

81. Vincent, G. K., & Velkoff, V. A. (2010). *The next four decades: The older population in the United States: 2010 to 2050* (No. 1138) U.S. Census Bureau: Washington, DC.

82. von Herbay, A. (2014). Otto von Bismarck is not the origin of old age at 65. *The Gerontologist, 54*(1), 5–5.

83. Wong, P. T. (1989). Personal meaning and successful aging. *Canadian Psychology/Psychologie Canadienne, 30*(3), 516.

84. World Health Organization. (2002). *Active ageing: A policy framework.* http://www.who.int/hpr/ageing/ActiveAgeingPolicyFrame.pdf/. Accessed 10.11.11.

CHAPTER **19**

The Physical Environment and Aging

Graham D. Rowles, PhD, Margaret A. Perkinson, PhD,
Karen Frank Barney, PhD, OTR/L, FAOTA

> *We now realize that how we design the built environment may hold tremendous potential for addressing many of the nation's greatest current public health concerns, including obesity, cardiovascular disease, diabetes, asthma, injury, depression, violence and social inequities (p.1382).*
>
> —**Richard J. Jackson**[66]

CHAPTER OUTLINE

OBJECTIVES

- Review alternative theoretical approaches to understanding the relationship between a person and their physical environment
- Understand older adults' use of and attribution of meaning to their physical environment
- Recognize the need for environmental modification and adjustment associated with relocation
- Provide approaches to effective occupational therapy practice that acknowledge the role of the physical environment in affecting well-being
- Understand how to conduct an occupational therapy assessment of physical environments

It has long been recognized that the behavior, physical and mental health, quality of life, and well-being of every individual is influenced—indeed, shaped—by the physical environment, and especially so in old age.[40,110,117] In this chapter we consider how the characteristics of the physical settings in which we live (both the natural and the built environment) interact with the changing capabilities of the aging adult to create personal patterns of behavior, lifestyles, and modes of "being in place" that are more or less adaptive for older adults. These patterns gradually evolve over time as individuals accommodate to changing personal capabilities and environmental challenges. We suggest that the normative trend in old age is for the dynamic homeostasis between the "press" exerted by the individual's environment and the individual's changing (generally reduced) capabilities to involve a constant process of adaptation and readaptation as the individual accommodates to changing circumstances. At first, such adaptation may occur through both subconscious and deliberate accommodation (e.g., environmental modification or lowered occupational performance motivations and expectations). Eventually, it may become necessary for the individual to relocate to a more supportive environment. Indeed, we may envision an array of possible trajectories of relocation along a continuum of supportive living options—perhaps from an independent residence to a congregate or assisted living facility and then to a nursing facility as the individual's circumstances change.

This general perspective on the changing relationship between the older individual and the physical environment has been expressed within a number of theoretical perspectives. We describe how these perspectives have evolved over the past three quarters of a century, beginning with Kurt Lewin's articulation of field theory[79] and the emergence of the basic $B = f(P.E)$ equation (where B = Behavior, P = Person, and E = Environment) and progressing through the classic ecological theory of Lawton and Nahemow,[76] to a series of comparable perspectives in occupational science. Such perspectives, including Person-Environment-Occupational Performance,[8,20] Person-Environment-Occupation,[74] and a Model of Human Occupation (MOHO),[70,71] have led to the expanded $B = f(P.E.A)$ conceptualization of Iwarsson[62] (where A = Activity), and to more recent transactional representations such as the Deweyan pragmatist perspective developed by Cutchin.[30,31,36] These models provide a foundation for occupational therapy (OT) intervention with aging adults, allowing for a variety of types of individual physical and socioemotional changes, and environmental changes, that typically occur over time.

Against this empirical and theoretical background we provide a contemporary perspective on the manner in which older people actually use their physical environments and develop implicit mental awareness of the settings of their lives. We suggest that, over time, the blending of habitual patterns of use and awareness imbues the environments of an individual's life with meanings that relate directly to his or her sense of well- or ill-being.

In the contemporary world, few people spend their entire lives in a single location. For most people, life involves relocation to new settings over the life course—a process over which, depending on age and circumstance, they exert a greater or lesser degree of personal control. This process involves a constant making and remaking of place that in old age becomes increasingly problematic as personal capabilities and resources decline. We present a model of the way in which, with respect to the re-creation of one especially important place in most people's lives, their home, the experience of relocation involves a continuous process of attempting to make or remake a place of meaning and identity. This process of making and remaking home is more problematic for some people than for others; in old age, it may become especially difficult. This is where planners, architects, interior designers, occupational scientists, physical therapists, and especially occupational therapists and gerontologists have a critical role to play.

The final portion of the chapter shifts to a focus on intervention. First, we consider contemporary approaches to creating optimal physical environments for older adults—from the micro scale of the individual dwelling to the macro level of neighborhoods and communities—that support and maximize the health and well-being not only of older adults, but all people. Second, we explore the role of OT environments and the interventions of occupational therapists as ways to proactively enhance quality of life through facilitating optimal adaptations to changing capabilities through maximizing the role of the physical environment in supporting a preferred lifestyle.

Aging and Environmental Press*

As we grow older, the configuration of the residence increasingly shapes and limits our behavior and use of space.

---

*The notion of "environmental press" is first credited to the psychologist Henry Murray, who coined the phrase in 1938.[88] The term was later adopted as a central tenet in M. Powell Lawton and Lucille Nahemow's ecological theory[76] described later in this chapter. The term refers to any environmental characteristic that influences behavior.

On a micro scale, getting in and out of the bathtub or the shower becomes more problematic. Even if there are convenient handrails, our aging bodies no longer have the strength to pull ourselves out of the tub, and the slipperiness of the shower floor becomes increasingly hazardous to an unsteady body. High shelves in the cupboards where we store occasionally used items become less safely accessible. We no longer use upstairs rooms because the stairs become a physical barrier. Indeed, the physical constraints of our residences lead to increasing "environmental centralization" as we confine ourselves to a more limited portion of the residence,[107] or "set up" within a single room.[100] Outside our dwelling, the physical environment of the immediate surroundings can be similarly constraining. The once easily traversed slope of a lengthy driveway may make it difficult to access a roadside mailbox, especially in inclement weather. The snow that we frolicked in as a child, in old age becomes a daunting physical barrier that may put us at risk for falls and related injuries. In the neighborhoods beyond our homes, we may find that the physical environment becomes increasingly hostile, with cracked sidewalks, poor lighting, dangerous slopes, lack of places to sit and rest, excessive noise, heavy traffic, crime-ridden areas, and other barriers that increasingly limit our lifespace.[4] There is some evidence that the physical setting of many neighborhoods discourages walking by older adults.[44,86] Growing concern with nurturing age-friendly neighborhoods and communities is a reflection of increasing recognition of the degree to which many current neighborhood environments are incompatible with the needs of older residents, lead to lifestyle constraints on environmental participation, limit options for maintaining a high quality of life, and constitute significant threats to well-being.[131]

Aging and Changing Environmental Competence

The effects of the physical environment are mediated by changes in individual capabilities that generally accompany the experience of growing old. Numerous normative changes limit environmental participation. Reduced lung capacity (caused by the tendency to lean forward as a result of the compression of the spinal column), calcification of ligaments, muscular atrophy and loss of strength, balance impairment (only partially compensated for by a widened gait), lowered "reserve capacity" of our physiologic systems, and slowed reaction times often act in combination to limit mobility and make environmental participation and occupational performance more difficult. (See chapters 8 and 9 for additional discussion.) Such changes are accentuated by sensory changes. With respect to sight, increasingly impaired depth perception, reduced peripheral vision, increased difficulties in distinguishing among colors (particularly in the blue-green end of the spectrum), increased susceptibility to glare, and the increasing opacity of the lens all make the physical environment seem more hostile and environmental negotiation more difficult. (See chapter 10 for additional discussion of low vision.) Such changes are often accentuated by hearing loss, including presbycusis, associated with growing difficulty in locating and distinguishing among sounds and filtering out background noise.

Normative physiologic and sensory changes are made more problematic by an array of primarily chronic health conditions ranging from arthritis to heart disease that often accompany old age. The combined effect of normative changes and health impairment is to reduce environmental participation and occupational performance by making older adults increasingly reluctant to venture forth from their homes, particularly at night and during busy times of the day.[93,109] As a result of the well-documented consequence of this—the tendency to spend a greater proportion of each day at home—the design and configuration of interior physical environments becomes increasingly important in sustaining well-being.[104]

Reconciling Environmental Press and Environmental Competence: Theoretical Foundations

Over the past century, the tension between the increased influence of environmental press and the limitations imposed by declining individual competence has been reflected in a series of theoretical perspectives that provide an important framework for interpreting the environmental participation potential of older adults. The seminal pioneering contribution of Kurt Lewin[79] in his development of field theory and the ecological equation (discussed earlier) has been complemented by increasingly sophisticated conceptualizations that have built upon his $B = f(P.E)$ formulation. The most influential of these conceptualizations is the ecological model developed by Lawton and Nahemow,[76] shown in Figure 19-1. The ecological model focuses on the individual's adaptation level, the point at which individual competence and environmental press are in a state of equilibrium. As indicated in Figure 19-1, at point A there is perfect balance between the press exerted by the environment and the competence of the individual to handle that level of press. However, person-environment adaptation is not static, and equilibrium—the fragile balance between individual competence (need) and environmental constraint (press)—is constantly evolving as either the individual's competence or the press of the environment changes.

It is useful to explain this process of dynamic equilibrium through an illustration. Imagine a 69-year-old individual, Mr. Fellows, living with his spouse in a suburban residence where he has successfully raised his family. The children have now left home. As he moves into his 70s, reduced physical strength, increasingly debilitating arthritis, a chronic heart condition, and impaired vision make mowing the lawn, climbing the stairs to the bedroom, and handling daily chores increasingly difficult. As his condition worsens, Mr. Fellows' competence level drops from point A to point B, where, as you will note, he is at the margin of maximum performance potential and close to moving into the zone of negative affect and

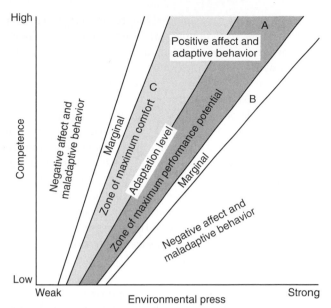

FIGURE 19-1   The ecological model. (From Lawton, M. P., & Nahemow, L. [1973]. Ecology and the aging process. In C. Eisdorfer & M. P. Lawton [Eds.], *The psychology of adult development and aging* [pp. 619-674]. Washington, DC: American Psychological Association.)

maladaptive behavior. At this point the level of environmental press is too strong for Mr. Fellows to function effectively. He has two options. The first is to attempt to effectively increase his level of competence by options that might include an exercise program to improve his strength or environmental or behavioral modifications (e.g., moving his bedroom downstairs or hiring a neighbor's son to mow his lawn). But there is often a limit to such in situ modifications. For many people the eventual outcome is the need to move to a more supportive environment (with less environmental press). So, Mr. Fellows may move to an assisted living facility, Point C in Figure 19-1, a location where he can establish a new adaptation level reflecting his level of competence. And so the process continues in an ongoing cycle of adjustment of his adaptation level within the framework of changing individual competence and environmental press.

Lawton and Nahemow's model has occupied center stage in environmental gerontology for several decades. However, it is being increasingly supplemented by new, more sophisticated perspectives generated in occupational science. One key perspective in this regard is the work of Iwarsson and her colleagues, which has elaborated on Lewin's classic equation by adding the notion of activity and presenting a transactional perspective.[11,62,64] This body of work indicated that the relationship between person and environment could be better understood by adding activity as a mediating variable. Thus, the equation now becomes $B = f(P.E.A)$. Expanding on Lawton's notion of environmental proactivity,[75] in this perspective the individual is regarded as having greater agency than in previous models and is explicitly viewed as being able to influence the nature of the person-environment interaction through his or her behavior or activity repertoire. So, with respect to the physical environment, the person is no longer viewed as a passive individual responding to environmental stimuli. For example, Mr. Fellows might purchase a riding lawnmower or, assuming a level of affluence, modify his home by installing an elevator to overcome the constraint of stairs, or even increase his environmental competence by beginning an exercise program.

Whereas the idea of a transactional perspective is an emergent element of Iwarsson's PEA model, it is the fulcrum of Cutchin's conceptualization of the human-environment relationship. Building on the pragmatism of John Dewey, Cutchin and colleagues develop the concept of place integration, in which the environment and the person are blended through action.[31,36] As a result, the person becomes integrated within a place through the very process of living within it. Within the notion of place integration, each of the elements of the PEA model is blended in a holistic view of the situation at any one time. This represents a complete shift from a simple sequential stimulus-response model in which the individual is influenced by the environment and the environment is modified by the individual to a model whereby person and place are fully blended in a manner that is dynamic and defined by the ongoing situation.

The notion of place integration is an implicit element within the most recent person-environment formulation, which blends significant aspects of previous conceptualizations within a dualistic experiential and developmental perspective on person-environment processes during later life.[91, 128,129] This model focuses on *belonging* and *agency,* dynamic processes considered to be motivational correlates of occupational behavior and lived experience (Figure 19-2). The developmental outcomes of these iterative processes, over time, are identity and autonomy and, ultimately, well-being.

Aging and Use of the Physical Environment

Theoretical perspectives offer an important superstructure providing alternative perspectives for understanding the person-environment relationship and the manner in which this relationship might relate to experienced dimensions of

identity, well-being, and autonomy, and to aging well. But, at a more pragmatic descriptive level, it is useful to provide an informational backdrop with respect to the fundamental dimensions through which individuals experience their physical environments.

At the most basic level, people of all ages experience an environment through its *use*, what many occupational scientists would term occupational performance. The infant rolls around in the limited space of her crib. The grade school child frequents the garden and the neighborhood (at least that component of the neighborhood that is sanctioned by the watchful parent); the teenager, particularly when he or she has received the geographic liberation of a driving license, travels more broadly and frequents an array of settings where typically he or she meets with peer-group friends. During their working lives, most people in Western cultures typically frequent a series of residential spaces as they move from an apartment to a first home to the dwelling where they will raise a family, and perhaps eventually to the place where they elect to retire. In each space and at each time of life, individuals trace an activity space that tends to become remarkably routine and repetitive. Activity spaces can be considered at a series of different scales.[130] There is a daily rhythm and routine to the manner in which residential space is utilized—the bedroom for sleeping, the living room or den in the evening for television watching, the kitchen at certain times of day for family gatherings or eating, and the dining room for special occasions. The use of this space may become so routinized that we may find ourselves on "automatic pilot" as we traverse familiar space without thinking, using the proprioceptive abilities that David Seamon termed *body awareness* of the environment.[113] Similarly, a regular temporal periodicity often evolves as we trace a daily route through physical space to work and back home again. Such patterns provide regularity in our use of the environment; often they are framed in relation to either moving away from or returning to our dwellings. As we use that limited portion of the physical environment that defines our pattern of daily activity, we gain a familiarity with its characteristics. For each individual, use of the physical setting is reflected in a unique imprint. And the reciprocity between person and environment in its use becomes habitual and generates a sense of comfort that in most cases evolves into a preference as we become more and more attuned to the familiar. Indeed, for most people, this process of habituation, on scales ranging from the residence through the neighborhood, to the community and beyond, results in a unique manifestation of relationship with the physical environment.[67,101] Inasmuch as our patterns of regular environmental use intersect with those of others whose lives are shaped by comparable space/time routines, we become part of a "place ballet" of intricately intertwined life worlds.[114]

Over time, use of the physical environment becomes taken for granted. We do not think about specific paths and physical locations (either within or beyond our residences). They become the places of life experience within which we are fully oriented. As people grow older, everyday physical activity

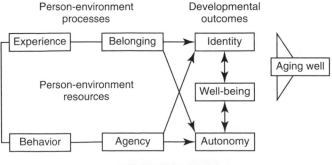

FIGURE 19-2   A model of person–environment processes in later life. (From Wahl, H-W., Iwarsson, S., & Oswald, F. (2012). Aging well and the environment: Toward an integrative model and research agenda for the future. *The Gerontologist, 52*(3), 306-316.)

spaces tend to become progressively more restricted both spatially and temporally.[57] Declining physical capabilities and the increased effort of maintaining a geographically extensive activity space, as well as loss of significant social roles (e.g., retirement, empty nest) and subsequent loss of economic wherewithal, mean that we tend to spend more time at home.[6,25,83] We become increasingly reluctant to drive at night and limit our excursions beyond the dwelling to those daytime hours when traffic on the roads is limited.[5,130] And as we grow older and become frail, our patterns of taken-for-granted use of the space within the residence may reflect an increasing medicalization of our homes as we gradually reconfigure the furniture and patterns of use and activity to accommodate disability and increasing medical need.[41]

Aging and the Meaning of the Physical Environment

Use of the physical environment is grounded in cognitive awareness of our environment on multiple scales (from the configuration of furniture and the rooms in our homes, through the layout of the neighborhood, to the street patterns of the larger communities in which we reside). Cognitive differentiation of the spaces we inhabit provides us with "mental maps" of the myriad spaces of our lives. These mental maps are images of known spaces that we can call to mind when we think of particular locations; they provide us with a cognitive atlas that we use for orientation and as a guide in successfully moving from place to place, whether it is crossing the living room without bumping into the furniture or successfully traversing the city to visit a friend or shop for groceries at a suburban mall.[99]

Over the life course, we develop countless mental maps of our lives that form a latent reservoir of environmental knowledge that can be resurrected at will to help us orient within and traverse our environments. Over time, mental maps of the physical environment are built and modified as the spaces we inhabit change and as our experience with the environment changes, either becoming more detailed with repeated use or increasingly vague and incoherent as a result of reduced use.[94] Our mental maps of specific neighborhoods may evolve over time as buildings are demolished and replaced by others or as the configuration of roads is altered during neighborhood transitions. As we grow older, reduced participation in environments beyond our homes and neighborhoods may lead to growing inaccuracy of our mental maps as our images of a particular space become increasingly based on recall of the way it was when we last visited. Indeed, we are often surprised and a little disoriented to discover, when visiting a location we have not visited for some time, how different it has become.

Both use and cognitive awareness are implicated in a third level of environmental experience, the emotional significance and meanings with which places are imbued as they are brought to life through lived experience. Over time we develop emotional affiliations (both positive and negative) with environments as they become increasingly embraced as a part of our personas. The locations where important life

events transpired may come to hold a special place in our consciousness and in our hearts as they become a part of the intricate tapestry of our relationships with the environments of our lives: the location where we were involved in a tragic motor accident; the park where we used to walk with the person who eventually became our spouse; the café where we were sitting when we learned we were to become a parent; or the gravesite of a close relative with the headstone and inscription that sustains them in our consciousness and links them to us even beyond their death. The mechanisms through which this transpires are beginning to be understood.[77,78] Over time, our environments become increasingly differentiated through repeated use, through selective incorporation within our mental maps of our world and through the assumption of meanings relating to our personal history of occupation.

For many people, the residence is the ultimate seat of meaning, a location that assumes increasing significance as it evolves from being merely a "house" or dwelling—the locus of activities—to a "home," a place that becomes the repository of one's identity and an expression of one's persona. There is a voluminous literature on the concept of home that identifies the plethora of interwoven meanings embraced in this construct. Whether the home is an arrangement of cardboard boxes under a freeway overpass, a tent in a refugee camp, a crude hut or cabin, a spacious apartment, or a suburban residence, the place that is home has been shown to embrace diverse dimensions of affinity.[1,18,80,103] These include the territoriality of a point of origin and centering[80,107]—the place from which we depart each morning and to which we return at night.[10,14,55,56,95] But home becomes imbued with an array of meanings beyond this: it becomes a source of identity,[82,108] self-expression,[121] security/safety,[34] privacy,[121] refuge,[98] continuity,[118] ownership,[90] social relationship,[118] belonging,[106] familiarity,[90,107] and freedom.[34] Overall, in the process of creating home, we transform a space into a place.[105]

An important feature of transforming spaces into places and both creating and maintaining a sense of home is the role that possessions play in shaping and reinforcing the meaning of the self in place.[19,29] An expanding literature explores the role of objects and treasured possessions as cues to personal identity. Many people surround themselves with personal objects and mementoes that both reflect and project their identity and provide them with a sense of being at home. The stuffed bear and security blanket of infancy and childhood may give way to the posters that adorn a dormitory room at college. As people move through life, there is a pattern of accumulation of artifacts that reflect the stories of their lives.[105] The growth of a family becomes expressed in an array of framed photographs on the side board. Statuettes and vases accumulated on holiday trips or received as gifts serve as reminders of important experiences. Rugs, furniture, and items gradually accumulated over time increasingly come to reflect the personality of a home and its residents. Indeed, some homes become museums of life. The importance of personal artifacts is clearly apparent in the angst that many people experience when, as they age, they find themselves having to divest themselves of some of these possessions as they move to progressively smaller living quarters.[38,39,87,116]

Aging, Relocation, and the Making and Remaking of Place

Consideration of a temporal perspective in the acquisition and divestiture of artifacts provides a useful segue to explicit consideration of the role of time in shaping the meaning of the physical environment as this evolves over the life course. For most people, and certainly for the average U.S. resident who relocates to a different residence more than 10 times over their life course,[125] life involves processes of constant adaptation to a changing physical environment, either through the necessity for in situ adjustments such as the need to close off an upstairs room or through the need to relocate to an entirely new setting as a result of failing health and environmental competence. This process is represented in Figure 19-3. Of course, moves may be temporary (e.g., the overnight stay at a motel where we are forced to re-create a very temporary semblance of a home) or permanent (the move to a new dwelling); however, the process is essentially the same, involving having to give up a familiar setting and create a new sense of being in place, or at home, in a different and initially unfamiliar physical space. Here, we focus on the process of permanent relocation.

Although the processes involved in environmental relocation are complex and multidimensional, relocation essentially involves three interwoven processes that are expressed differently and over which we have different levels of control at different points in the life course.[102] First, each relocation necessitates abandonment of a familiar mode of being in place; it requires abandoning familiar patterns in the use of space, the redundancy of well-established mental maps of the places we inhabit, and threat to the emotional affiliation of

places of meaning in our lives as we may no longer be able to frequent and experience these spaces and as they fade into memory. Second, relocation to a new physical setting necessitates *creation* of a new mode of being in place as we establish new patterns in our use of the environment, as we create new mental images to provide us with an orientation to the new setting, and as we develop new senses of emotional affiliation related to the events that transpire in the new setting. Each new setting provides constraints on establishing a familiar mode of being in place; our new residence may not have the fireplace that provided both physical and psychological warmth as we stared into the flickering flames; there may be no window sills for our plants. At the same time, there may be new opportunities—central heating may mean that we no longer have the chore of stepping out into the cold to gather logs from the stack on the back porch; a sun lounge may provide an even better setting for our African violets.

Both abandonment and creation are eased by a third process, transference—our ability to transport elements of our old and familiar environment into the new and unfamiliar setting as we engage in the process of making the unknown familiar. Such transference may involve the relocation of furniture and possessions. Indeed, we may "set up" in our new abode in a way that mimics, insofar as is possible in the new space, the arrangement of furniture and treasured artifacts in a configuration paralleling their placement in the home we have abandoned. Subject to the constraints of the new setting, we may also evolve a rhythm and routine in the pattern of daily life that reflects a continuation of the former lifestyle. We may rise at the same time, watch the same television programs, and attempt to establish relationships with our new neighbors comparable to the ones we have left behind. It is also possible to facilitate transference by retaining our links with former settings through return visits, ongoing contact with former neighbors, or retaining a vicarious affiliation as

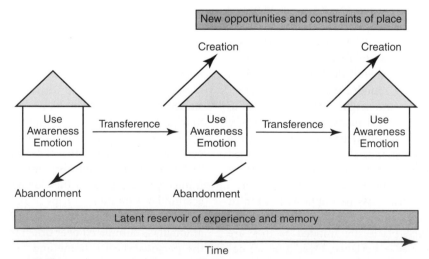

FIGURE 19-3 The experience of relocation: remaking home. (From Rowles, G. D., & Bernard, M. [2013]. The meaning and significance of place in old age. In G. D. Rowles & M. Bernard [Eds.], *Environmental gerontology: Making meaningful places in old age* [pp. 3-24]. New York, NY: Springer Publishing Company.)

we monitor events in our former neighborhoods or communities through the media. And, of course, unless we are cognitively impaired, our memories never leave us. We can always return to the places of our past by tapping the vast reservoir of experiences and memories that define who we are.

Over time, we are constantly making and remaking place as we move from environment to environment. Indeed, life entails an ongoing and never-ending quest for achieving a sense of being in place—being at one with the physical environment. Perhaps the most important factor in this process is the degree to which we have control over making and remaking place. During our early years, our autonomy and control are limited; the nature of our being in place and whether we relocate or not are shaped by our parents. As adults, our level of control and ability to shape our environments are generally much greater. We can decide where we want to live and the types of environments we wish to frequent according to our individual or family preference. Some people favor the vibrancy and excitement of a gentrifying inner-city neighborhood with a local deli, lots of bars and restaurants, frequent local festivals and events, and ready access to art galleries and concerts. For others, the more tranquil milieu of a rural setting with a slower pace of life, a focus on the pleasures of gardening, and the companionship of a few neighbors is preferred. But as the limitations of old age begin to have effect, generally not until our seventh and eighth decades, we become frail and may find ourselves with progressively less decisional autonomy and control over our physical environments as family members, physicians, and social services professionals have increasing input into the determination of our environmental circumstances.

It is in this context of changing environmental potential and what M. Powell Lawton, a founder of environmental gerontology, termed "environmental vulnerability" that we turn to consideration of the degree to which the physical environments we create, on scales from the entire neighborhood and community down to the design of an individual nursing home room, become so critical. Does society create environments that are conducive to the changing environmental experience of older adults and others who are environmentally vulnerable? And to what extent does the practice of occupational therapy facilitate and maximize environmental engagement and occupational performance? In the final two sections of this chapter, we turn to these issues.

Creating Physical Environments for Aging: Design Barriers and Opportunities

More than three decades ago, Joseph A. Koncelik[72] wrote "Thoughtless environmental design 'speaks' to people with sensory losses, telling them that they are incapacitated, senile, slow, weak, and perhaps too stupid to survive." Unfortunately, despite passage of the Americans with Disabilities Act in 1990, many community environments continue to speak the same way and to provide significant challenges to those who are environmentally vulnerable. In too many cities, traffic

lights remain timed too rapidly to facilitate safe pedestrian crossing.[73] Supplemental auditory prompts for walk lights are rare. There are still too few places to sit. Sidewalks remain uneven, in poor repair, or absent, and public spaces are poorly designed, precluding occupational participation and social interaction.[92]

There are some grounds for optimism. Initially facilitated by the World Health Organization's Healthy Cities Project of the 1980s and reinforced during the past decade by the Global Age-Friendly Cities and Communities Project, another World Health Organization initiative launched in 2005 in 33 cities around the world (including New York, NY, and Portland, OR), there has been a movement toward a more comprehensive approach to creating "livable" cities and communities. Increasingly, such highly publicized initiatives are being complemented by smaller-scale projects and programs in cities and communities throughout the world. In the United States, livable and age-friendly city initiatives are emerging in a plethora of locations at different scales. In a recent review, Andrew Scharlach identified 292 age-friendly initiatives representing four approaches: community planning, system coordination and program development, colocation of services, and the development of consumer associations.[115]

Some of these initiatives include a focus on enhancing the physical characteristics and accessibility of neighborhood environments. Scharlach notes that we are beginning to embrace the idea of "' . . .complete streets,' that enable multiple types of mobility, including walking, self-propelled and electric wheelchairs, golf-carts, bicycles, public transit, as well as automobiles."[115] There is also growing evidence of innovation to locate needed services on-site or in geographic proximity to naturally occurring retirement communities (NORCs).[115] These trends are reinforced by the development of measures to assess the physical characteristics of neighborhoods, including accessibility, amount of greenery, density, diversity, location, street pattern, block size, setback of dwellings from the street, and street topography, with respect to their ability to support the mobility and well-being of older residents.[9,24,97] We are rapidly developing an array of tools to assess older adults' needs and preferences with respect to their community environments.

Although these are all positive developments, it is important to temper optimism with a note of caution. As Scharlach[115] notes, few age-friendly or livable community initiatives have significant governmental support or command sufficient recurring resources from the private sector to instill confidence in their long-term sustainability or transformative effectiveness with respect to the physical supportiveness of neighborhood environments for environmentally vulnerable older adults.

Moving from the level of the community to the individual residence, there has been a parallel development of diverse initiatives in facilitating the optimal physical design of residential environments. Three trends in particular provide promise for the enhancement of occupational performance.

First is our increasing ability to measure the fit between an individual and his or her physical setting and to use such measurement instruments as a basis for both assessing need and designing effective intervention.[62] One important example here is the housing enabler concept, initially proposed by Steinfeld et al.[122] and operationalized by occupational therapist Suzanne Iwarsson and her colleagues in the Housing Enabler Instrument.[62,63] The housing enabler integrates assessments of functional limitations and physical barriers in the residence to create an accessibility score reflecting the unique outcome of the relationship between environmental needs and environmental press for a single individual. A second and often related tool, a "usability in my home" measure,[42,43] provides an approach to measuring the degree to which the physical environment is perceived by the individual to be supportive of activities of daily living (ADLs), including personal hygiene, getting dressed, grooming, and using toilet facilities, and instrumental activities of daily living (IADLs), such as cooking, doing laundry, washing dishes, and cleaning. With the more recent development of abbreviated versions of such instruments, we can anticipate continuing improvement in our ability to objectively measure the residential environmental needs and preferences of older adults.[12]

A second major development over the past several decades is the emergence of smart homes and the use of smart home technologies.[15] Efforts to improve housing accessibility and use through more sensitive design, such as the installation of ramps, the lowering of counter surfaces, and age-friendly bathroom design with grab bars and the introduction of surfaces to minimize slipping and the risk of falls, are now being supplemented by an array of innovations that involve the use of sophisticated technologies. Recently, body-worn sensors have been developed to monitor particular activities.[3] Motion-sensitive lighting is becoming increasingly common in contemporary dwellings. Monitoring from a distance is also an increasingly recognized option. It is now possible to use wireless sensors to monitor use of electrical devices, cabinet sensors, bed-use patterns, flow of water (indicating the use of facilities), and motion sensors to chart the use of individual rooms.[45,69] The basic idea is that the older individual is enabled to maintain independence at home because the occurrence of unusual patterns of use can trigger supportive intervention when needed. The use of camera-based surveillance systems of home monitoring has also emerged as an option for facilitating older adults' continuing ability to live alone. Finally, the frontier of technology in smart home design of the future lies in the use of robot technologies that are currently being developed in laboratories throughout the world. Additional information regarding technological supports for older adults may be found in Chapter 21.

The potential effects of smart technology are not limited to home environments, however. Future residential care facilities may offer "assisted cognitive systems" that are embedded in physical environments and are sensitive and responsive to residents' actions and needs.[27] A prototype dementia residential care facility, Oatfield Estates in Oregon, employs the concept of "layered architecture" to monitor all activities, doors, lights, and appliances within the building. Notable among its supports to residents are the "Activity Compass," which helps to direct residents to indoor destinations, and the "Adaptive

Prompter" that uses information from embedded sensor networks to guide a resident through selected activities, such as grooming or dressing.[68] A major issue in the introduction of smart homes, camera surveillance systems, and ambient intelligence alternatives is their acceptability to older adults. Research indicates reluctance of some older adults to be monitored in their homes by cameras, but there appears to be a surprisingly high level of acceptability of surveillance technologies by older adults provided that appropriate levels of privacy are maintained.[28,85,133] The tension between the need for surveillance invasiveness and the preservation of appropriate levels of privacy remains an ongoing challenge in the evolution of technologies that facilitate aging in place.[15,16]

Placing the changing environmental needs of older adults in the broader context of the life course leads to consideration of a third major development in the creation of physical environments conducive to the needs of older adults. One can make a strong argument that we should not be seeking to create environments for older adults but rather environments for all people at all stages of life. This is the fundamental premise of universal design, which focuses on incorporating a series of basic principles in facilitating the optimal design of environments for all users. There are seven broadly accepted principles of universal design (Table 19-1).[13,123] Each of these principles provides a template for design decisions that optimize the potential for older adults to be able to age in place.

A particular need in the evolution of universal design is for community-level change to accommodate intergenerational needs.[124] Recent estimates indicate an increase of more than 6% in the past decade in multigenerational housing—young adults returning home, and grandparents living with their children.[37] In addition, central cities in North America have grown faster in terms of both younger and older populations in comparison with surrounding suburbs, due to the attraction of being able to walk to shopping centers, restaurants, and other centrally located destinations. These factors may provide added impetus for the increased use of universal design principles in residential and other building construction.[37] The application of universal design principles enhances occupational performance for all generations; its implementation is intuitively attractive in community planning, new construction, and retrofitting housing.

An important issue with respect to the development of both smart homes and universal design is the availability of such options. There is a danger of developing many theoretical options but few pragmatic choices for the majority of older adults. Sophisticated smart home technologies are currently primarily to be found in the model smart homes that have been developed in research universities and experimental laboratories, such as the Georgia Institute of Technology "Aware Home," the "Gator Tech Smart House" at the University of Florida, and the "Place Lab" at MIT.[15] The costs of translating such innovative models into commercially viable housing options are likely to be considerable, and it may be many years before older adults are able to fully harness the power of such technologies.

TABLE 19-1 Principles of Universal Design

Universal Design Principle	Description	Example
(1) Equitable use	Useful and marketable to people with diverse abilities	Doors that automatically open
(2) Flexibility of use	Accommodates a wide range of individual preferences and abilities	Buttons on automated teller machines far enough apart to be pressed accurately
(3) Simple and intuitive use	Easy to understand, regardless of user's experience, knowledge, language skills, or current concentration level	Providing furniture assembly instructions in a series of clear illustrations instead of text
(4) Perceptible information	Communicates necessary information effectively to the user, regardless of ambient conditions or the user's sensory abilities	Computer software that relays information visually through text and pictures, and audibly through speakers
(5) Tolerance for error	Minimizes hazards and the adverse consequences of accidental or unintended actions	Hallways that return to common areas rather than stop in dead ends
(6) Low physical effort	Can be used efficiently and comfortably with a minimum of fatigue	Bottle caps that are easy to grip and require only a small range of motion to open
(7) Size/space for approach/use	Appropriate size and space is provided for approach, reach, manipulation, and use, regardless of the user's body size, posture, or mobility	Wall-mounted components (e.g., toilet paper) that are visible, easy to reach, and easy for all hand sizes to use

(Reproduced from Carr, K., Weir, P. L., Azar, D., & Azar, N. R. (2013). Universal Design: A step toward successful aging, *Journal of Aging Research*, Volume 2013 (2013), Article ID 324624, 8 pages. Accessed 10/20/15 http://www.hindawi.com/journals/jar/2013/324624/; Adapted from Story, M. F., Mueller, J. L., & Mace, R. L. [1998]. *The universal design file: Designing for people of all ages and abilities,* Raleigh, NC: North Carolina State University.)

The Role of the Physical Environment in Occupational Therapy with Older Adults

Although the use of sophisticated technologies offers a fascinating prospect for the future, most occupational therapists live in a world of the present as they confront the day-to-day challenges of older adults trying to accommodate to changing physical capabilities in home and community environments that seem increasingly hostile. No technology can replace an informed and caring practitioner. However, as environmental design and technology provide us with a widening array of alternatives, occupational therapists can enhance their contribution by being especially sensitive to the role of the physical environment in supporting effective therapy (Box 19-1).

The Influence of the Physical Environment on the Process of Occupational Therapy Assessment

Assessment of occupational performance outside of the older client's home and other familiar environments is likely to be a less accurate reflection of abilities in all areas of performance. Consider the physical environmental tenets

---

BOX 19-1 Fundamental Principles of Environmentally Sensitive Proactive Interventions with Aging Adults

1. When interacting with a new older client, whether in the community, office, clinic, or an institution, anticipate the client's physical environmental needs, so that if assessment processes are undertaken, the individual is not placed at a disadvantage:
   a. Ensure adequate lighting within the intervention space.
   b. Minimize or eliminate background noises.
   c. Provide the client with a chair with arms, if indicated.
   d. Ensure that any materials that the client may need or be asked to manipulate are within a distance of "easy reach." This includes seated tasks or those in bed.
   e. Facilitate cognition, time, and space orientation through use of clocks, signage, or additional visual cues.
   f. If the older client is away from home or other familiar environments when the occupational therapy intervention is conducted, include questions about the ease of use of the client's home and community environments, and arrange for a home visit, whenever indicated.
2. Conduct an environmental assessment in every intervention setting, whether community-based (agency or home) or institutional.
   a. Whenever possible, conduct a thorough review of the environment, noting strengths as well as areas in need of improvement or total change.
   b. If a thorough review is not possible, note the most obvious conditions in need of change.
   c. Make short- and long-term recommendations for additions and/or changes, based upon the needs of the aging clients served and the ability of the setting to comply. Wherever possible, advocate for aging-sensitive design of the environment, using the most current evidence to support recommendations for additions or changes.

introduced earlier. Typically, the older adult will find performance of activities more meaningful within a familiar space, such as the home, reflecting the older adult's "place integration." Therefore, motivation to perform is likely to be greater in such places than in unfamiliar spaces. In the client's home, the demonstration of performance skills is likely to be optimal, and reflect smooth, possibly rhythmic patterns of movement known as an individualized "place ballet" and "automatic pilot" that would be likely absent in different physical spaces. The occupational therapist will ideally be able to observe the client's implementation of his or her normal routines and habits that build upon well-established mental maps and physical function. If the client is unable to demonstrate fully, family members or others who are familiar with the individual's preferred routines may be sources of information critical to optimizing future occupational performance at home.

Physical Environment as Target of Occupational Therapy Interventions

At all levels of care, occupational therapy personnel are well positioned to facilitate the older adult's interactive relationship with the physical environment, to the extent that the individual's physical and psychosocial abilities allow. The *Occupational Therapy Practice Framework* (OTPF),[2] the conceptual schema that describes and guides the OT intervention process, pairs *Context* with *Environment*. The OTPF defines Contexts as referring to "a variety of interrelated conditions that are within and surrounding the client." These conditions include "cultural, personal, temporal, and virtual." The OTPF further defines Environments as referring to "the external physical and social conditions that surround the client and in which the client's daily life occupations occur" (p. S28). Thus, physical aspects of environments are viewed as circumstantial components that encompass the client and also mediate everyday living and lifestyle.

Older adults encounter the need for occupational therapy (OT) intervention for a variety of reasons, due to pressing physical and psychosocial problems as well as needs or problems that they have determined or of which they may be unaware. On behalf of aging adults, OT services are provided at three different levels: (1) directly with individuals and/or family/caregiver(s), (2) through consultation and administration with community organizations, and (3) through consultation and/or administration with governmental, nongovernmental, and/or international agencies.[7] Thus, occupational therapists may be direct providers of services, administrators, and/or consultants, depending on the nature of the setting. Historically, occupational therapists have conducted environmental assessments that consider the occupational competence of older clients living at home. Individually tailored recommendations, with short- and long-term goals, are established collaboratively with the client, and the occupational therapist assists the individual in remediating aspects of the physical environment that hinder occupational performance. For example, some of the most common adaptations for the

physical environment are grab bars and higher toilet seats that are recommended and installed in bathrooms to promote safety and compensate for diminished strength, coordination, or range of motion. Nevertheless, recommendations can cover all aspects of occupational performance within the physical environment, including the dwelling, yard, grounds, neighborhood, and/or community.

OT personnel may intervene as well on behalf of optimizing the physical environment across a range of settings within the medical continuum of care. Interventions may include consultations regarding the environmental design and retrofitting of health-related facilities, including primary care clinics and physician and dental offices, acute and subacute care settings, home health-care environments, long-term care settings such as residential and skilled care settings, and palliative and hospice care environments.

At the community level, occupational therapists and assistants conduct community-based wellness and injury prevention programs to facilitate the older individual's accommodation to the physical design of his or her current residential settings and neighborhoods. OT personnel are also involved in advocating and planning for livable communities and aging-in-place initiatives at the community, state, and national levels, to promote programs and developments that support a goodness of fit with the typical aging changes that older adults experience.

Clearly the nature of interactions and the extent to which OT personnel may facilitate older adults' environmental competence vary according to the amount of contact and the relationship that he or she has with each individual and with service-related administrative personnel. Occupational therapists and assistants need to be proactive in advocating for supportive environments that correspond with the service-delivery patterns in their settings and influence related administrative policies and procedures.

Beyond the macro-level contributions of informed advocacy, implementation of physical environment–sensitive OT interventions follows a similar process, whether the client is an individual, a setting within the established health-care system, or a community-based organization (Figure 19-4). Once the client is identified, an occupational profile, either a standardized version for individuals or one tailored to the setting, should be conducted to identify the occupational strengths, needs, problems, and priorities in completing occupational performance that is appropriate and meaningful to the client. (See Chapter 6 for additional discussion of assessment.) Once such a profile is established, an environmental assessment can be performed to determine the current level of environmental press on the client, and what, if any, appropriate measures might be taken to address revealed problems, deficiencies, and needs. A summary of both short- and long-term goals for remediation can then be completed, taking into consideration the feasibility and cost, if any, for recommendations made. Next, an occupation-oriented physical environmental intervention that addresses identified problems, needs, and deficiencies is designed, with ongoing consultation with the client, to ensure that the client's needs

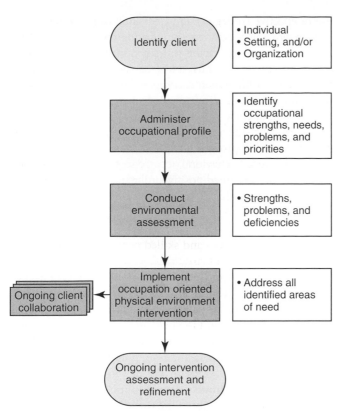

FIGURE 19-4 Universal occupational therapy physical environmental intervention process.

are met. Finally, an assessment process for determining the ongoing and potentially changing needs of the client should be operationalized, including integrated plans for continuous refinement, as needed. (See Chapter 7 for additional discussion of the intervention process.)

Physical environment–related OT interventions focus on supporting the client's age-related changes and/or comorbidities that affect the individual's ability to age in place and participate in desired activities/occupations. To be most effective, such interventions must address the aspects of being in place that have been identified earlier in this chapter. It is important to acknowledge and respect each individual's biopsychosocial occupational performance abilities together with his or her preferred habits and routines, and sense of being in place. Awareness of the rhythms and routines of daily life, processes of habituation, the place ballets that form the choreography of everyday life, the complex mental maps that constitute each person's orientation within his or her life space, and the emotional capital that is invested in the places of a person's life is an essential element of environmentally sensitive and meaningful intervention. Within this wider understanding of experiential and environmental context, interventions may often include not only adaptive accommodations but also the employment of appropriate assistive devices that compensate for occupational performance deficits.[7] Within this rubric, the aims of intervention become to (1) continually collaborate with the older adult to plan and

implement truly client-centered care, (2) tailor the approaches to meet the client's activity needs and potential, and (3) facilitate the maximization of the older adult's continued participation in society. Intervention must be appropriate and meaningful within the framework of the client's lived experience to ensure that he or she is enabled to maximize overall well-being and achieve the best possible quality of life.

Fundamental concerns of OT practitioners include supporting older adults' autonomy in setting priorities and making decisions regarding their participation, and maintaining a level of mastery and control over their environment and lifestyle. OT personnel, therefore, foster an enabling therapeutic relationship with older adults of all ability levels throughout the continuum of medical care or in community settings, together with clients' families and/or other support systems. The emphasis of OT intervention on the older adult's ability to participate in meaningful occupations promotes cost-effective care, individual competence, and optimal quality of life.[21,22,65] Acknowledging the role of the physical environment in this process is a critical component of this endeavor that is too often neglected. Frequently the constraints of therapists' and assistants' workload expectations in many health-care settings foster a limited approach to OT interventions, resulting in processes that emphasize improvement in components of older adults' physical function, without due consideration of environmental press or supports and related psychological well-being. Evidence-based OT interventions holistically include all components of well-being and quality of life, including the physical environments' meaning and level of support for older adults. Often in health-care settings, occupational therapists have the opportunity to recommend additionally supportive environmental features that can benefit all participants, as well as collaborate with older adults individually in maximizing their function and overall quality of life. Thus, the occupational therapist or assistant needs to view each setting and individual served as an occasion to evaluate and recommend physical environmental adaptations, wherever indicated.

Assessing the Effectiveness of Occupational Therapy–Based Environmental Interventions for Older Adults

Recent literature reviews[35,46,47,127] have identified a growing body of research on the effects of environmental interventions on the function and well-being of older adults in various settings, including hospitals,[61,84] assisted living facilities,[32] nursing homes,[26,33,89] dementia care facilities,[120,132] and home environments.‡ Iwarsson et al.[63] and Wahl et al.[127] both concluded that, compared with simple counts of total numbers of environmental hazards in a home, indicators of person-environment fit in home environments were stronger

---

‡References 23, 48, 51, 52, 59, and 81.

predictors of older adult function (e.g., frequency of falls), thus reinforcing our earlier discussion of the utility of the PE conceptual model.

A close examination of one "gold standard" OT-based environmental intervention for older adults, the Environmental Skill-Building Program,[53] underscores the power of the person-environment fit model to effectively guide research and inform practice related to the physical environments of older clients. The Environmental Skill-Building Program (ESP) was a randomized clinical trial of a home-based OT intervention that focused on the role of the physical environment in supporting dementia family caregiving and care receiver function. It was one of six longitudinal interventions supported by the National Institutes of Health (NIH) in the Resources for Enhancing Alzheimer's Caregiver Health (REACH) initiative, a multisite program designed to conduct social and behavioral research on interventions to enhance dementia family caregiving.[112]

The goal of the ESP intervention was to "help family caregivers reduce the disparity between environmental press and personal competence by providing skills to effectively manipulate dimensions of the home environment to manage daily problems associated with dementia care" (p. 536).[53, 54] After baseline assessments, caregivers were randomly assigned to either the experimental or control group. Members of the experimental group received the environmental intervention, six OT sessions that entailed: (1) caregiver training on Alzheimer's disease (AD) and on the effects (both supportive and detrimental) of the physical environment on their relatives' ADL functions and troublesome behaviors, (2) instruction on problem-solving strategies (including identification of triggers of problematic behaviors) that involved manipulating or modifying the physical and social environment, (3) implementation of individualized environmental strategies, and (4) the generalization of these strategies to emerging problems or issues (p. 536).[51] Strategies that modified the physical environment included installation of equipment (e.g., grab bars); removing, rearranging, or labeling objects; purposeful placement of objects (e.g., laying out clothing or hygiene products to facilitate dressing and grooming); and use of color contrasts. Other strategies addressed alteration of tasks (e.g., simplification techniques, cueing, planning routines, and providing graded activities) and alteration of the social environment (e.g., communicating with formal care providers, coordinating care tasks among family and friends). The interventions were individualized and client-based, based on OT needs assessments and assessments of the home to identify which of 11 caregiving domains the caregiver wanted to address. Occupational therapists continued training and reinforcement of strategies in subsequent sessions and continued to define attainable and concrete goals, assist in problem solving, and provide constructive feedback. Appropriate equipment and assistive devices were ordered and installed, and occupational therapists trained caregivers in their use. Three follow-up assessments were conducted at 6-month intervals.

At the 6-month follow-up, caregivers in the intervention group demonstrated significantly improved skills (i.e., greater use of effective strategies) and had significantly less need for help in providing daily care, indicating enhancement of the personal competence factor as defined in the PE model. They also reported significantly fewer behavioral occurrences by their relatives with dementia compared with the caregiver controls, thus reflecting diminished demands of environmental press on the caregiver. At the 12-month follow-up assessment, compared with the controls, caregivers in the intervention group reported improved affect and a trend for maintenance of skills and reduced behavioral occurrences.[50, 49] The researchers concluded the sustained positive influence of the intervention had a clinically significant effect, given the ongoing decline of the care receiver that is typical of the AD trajectory.

Summary

It is appropriate to conclude by envisioning a future agenda for a physical environment–sensitive occupational science that moves beyond the ideas presented in this chapter. Such an agenda would expand the field and enhance the effectiveness of occupational therapy. It would include greater consideration of the need to facilitate ongoing connections with nature—for example, through the design of sunrooms and modification of windows to maximize potentials for "setting up" and visual surveillance of the world beyond the threshold for those who are home or institution bound.[96,100] It would include more sophisticated understanding of design features such as the role of stairs—the paradox of steps as both an environmental barrier and beneficial to health.[117] It would include the design of ever-more-sophisticated personal and equipment-related technologies to facilitate continuing environmental participation.[126] It would include recognition and more refined understanding of the importance of abandonment, creation, and transference as elements of the making and remaking of home (Figure 19-3) and the development of OT strategies to facilitate minimally stressful relocation.[58,60] It would include exploration of "place therapy"[17, 111]—the manner in which physical environments and the places of people's lives may be therapeutic and used proactively as a focus of occupational therapy. Finally, increased recognition of the role of the physical environment may even extend to exploration of the role that the settings in which occupational therapy is conducted play in influencing the effectiveness of such therapy.[119] And so we end this chapter where we began, with words from Richard J. Jackson's important 2003 editorial:[66]

Whereas our generation may reap some benefits from the new field of the built environment and health, with a little vision and a lot of good science and hard work, our children and grandchildren will be able to walk or bicycle home from their workplaces through attractive communities designed to promote the physical and mental health of all people. (p. 1383)

To add to Jackson's words, our hope is that this sentiment can be extended to especially embrace those who are the most environmentally vulnerable—older adults and both older and younger persons with disabilities. Occupational science and occupational therapy have the capacity to make this so.

REVIEW QUESTIONS

1. Describe the theories regarding the relationship between a person and the physical environment that were discussed in this chapter.
2. What is "place ballet"? Provide an example.
3. Mrs. Traub, an 85 year-old widow, is moving into an assisted living facility because of failing vision. Using what you have learned from this chapter, how would you assist her in her relocation?
4. What is meant by the term "place integration"? Provide an example.
5. Mr. Braun's family has decided he should move to a dementia care facility. They are considering, one of the "smart homes" described in this chapter. How would you help them decide whether this would be a good place for their father?
6. With guidance from your faculty, select a standardized scale used by occupational therapy personnel to assess the safety and accessibility of physical environments. Use this scale to conduct an environmental assessment of the home of an older friend or relative. Write a report identifying the strengths and potential problems of this environment. Include in your report an occupation-supportive physical environment intervention to address the issues you discovered.

REFERENCES

1. Altman, I., & Werner, C. M. (1985). *Home environments.* New York, NY: Plenum Press.
2. American Occupational Therapy Association. (2014). Occupational therapy practice framework: Domain and process (3rd ed.). *American Journal of Occupational Therapy, 68*(Suppl), S1–S51.
3. Atallah, L., Lo, B., Ali, R., King, R., & Yang, G. Z. (2009). Real-time activity classification using ambient and wearable sensors. *IEEE Transactions on Information Technology in Biomedicine, 13,* 1031–1039.
4. Balfour, J. L., & Kaplan, G. A. (2002). Neighborhood environment and loss of physical function in older adults: Evidence from the Alameda County Study. *American Journal of Epidemiology, 155*(6), 507–515.
5. Ball, K., Owsley, C., Stalvey, B., Roenker, D. L., Sloane, M., & Graves, M. (1998). Driving avoidance and functional impairment in older drivers. *Accident Analysis and Prevention, 30*(3), 313–322.
6. Baltes, M. M., Maas, I., Wilms, H-U., Borchelt, M., & Little T. (1999). Everyday competence in old and very old age: Theoretical considerations and empirical findings. In P. B. Baltes & K. U. Mayer (Eds.), *The Berlin Aging Study: Aging from 70 to 100* (pp. 384–402). Cambridge: Cambridge University Press.
7. Barney, K. F. (2012). Geriatric occupational therapy: Achieving quality of daily living. In A. Sinclair, J. Morley, & B. Vellas (Eds.), *Pathy's principles and practice of geriatric medicine* (5th ed.). Chichester, West Sussex: John Wiley & Sons.
8. Baum, C., Christiansen, C., & Bass, J. (2014). Person-Environment-Occupational Performance model. In C. Christiansen, C. Baum, & J. Bass (Eds.), *Occupational therapy: Performance, participation, well-being* (4th ed., pp. 49–55). Thorofare, NJ: SLACK.
9. Burton, E. J., Mitchell, L., & Stride, C. B. (2011). Good places for ageing in place: Development of objective built environment measures for investigating links with older people's well-being. *BMC Public Health, 11,* 839.
10. Buttimer, A. (1980). Home, reach and the sense of place. In A. Buttimer & D. Seamo (Eds.), *The human experience of space and place* (pp. 166–187). London: Croom Helm.
11. Carlsson, G. (2002). *Catching the bus in old age. Methodological aspects of physical accessibility assessments in public transport. Doctoral dissertation.* Lund, Sweden: Department of Clinical Neuroscience, Lund University, Studentlitteratur.
12. Carlsson, G., Schilling, O., Slaug, B., Fange, A., Stahl, A., Nygren, C., & Iwarsson, S. (2009). Toward a screening tool for housing accessibility problem: A reduced version of the housing enabler. *Journal of Applied Gerontology, 28*(1), 59–80.
13. Carr, K., Weir, P. L., Azar, D., & Azar, N. R. (2013). Universal design: A step toward successful aging. *Journal of Aging Research, 2013,* 8. http://dx.doi.org/10.1155/2013/324624/. Article ID 324624.
14. Case, D. (1996). Contributions of journeys away to the definition of home: An empirical study of a dialectical process. *Journal of Environmental Psychology, 16,* 1–15.
15. Chan, M., Campo, E., Esteve, D., & Fourniols, J-Y. (2009). Smart homes—current features and future perspectives. *Maturitas, 64,* 90–97.
16. Charness, N., & Boot, W. R. (2009). Aging and information technology use: Potential and barriers. *Current Directions in Psychological Science, 18*(5), 253–258.
17. Chaudhury, H. (2003). Quality of life and place therapy. *Journal of Housing for the Elderly, 17*(1-2), 85–103.
18. Chaudhury, H. (2008). *Remembering home.* Baltimore, MD: The Johns Hopkins University Press.
19. Cherrier, H., & Ponnor, T. (2010). A study of hoarding behavior and attachment to material possessions. *Qualitative Market Research, 13*(1), 8–23.
20. Christiansen, C., & Baum, C. (1991). *Occupational therapy: Overcoming human performance deficits.* Thorofare, NJ: SLACK.
21. Clark, F. (2012). *Well Elderly 2, Los Angeles, California, 2004-2008. ICPSR33641-v1.* Ann Arbor, MI: Inter-university Consortium for Political and Social Research [distributor]. doi:10.3886/ICPSR33641.v1
22. Clark, F., Azen, S. P., Zemke, R., Jackson, J., Carlson, M., Mandel, D., et al. (1997). Occupational therapy for independent-living older adults: A randomized controlled trial. *Journal of the American Medical Association, 278*(16), 1321–1326.
23. Clarke, P. (2014). The role of the built environment and assistive devices for outdoor mobility in later life. *Journal of Gerontology B: Psychological and Social Sciences, 69*(Suppl. 1), S8–S15. doi: 10.1093/geronb/gbu121.
24. Clarke, P., & George, L. K. (2005). The role of the built environment in the disablement process. *American Journal of Public Health, 95*(11), 1933–1939.
25. Cohen-Mansfield, J., Shmotkin, D., & Hazan, H. (2012). Homebound older persons: Prevalence, characteristics, and longitudinal predictors. *Archives of Gerontology and Geriatrics, 54,* 55–60.
26. Cohen-Mansfield, J., & Werner, P. (1998). The effects of an enhanced environment on nursing home residents who pace. *The Gerontologist, 38,* 199–208.
27. Cook, D. J., Augusto, J. C., & Jakkula, V. R. (2009). Ambient intelligence: Technologies, applications, and opportunities. *Pervasive and Mobile Computing, 5*(4), 277–298.

28. Courtney, K. L. (2008). Privacy and senior willingness to adopt smart home information technology in residential care facilities. *Methods of Information in Medicine, 47*(1), 76–81.

29. Csikszentmihalyi, M. & Rochberg-Halton, E. (1981). *The meaning of things: Domestic symbols and the self.* Cambridge MA: Cambridge University Press.

30. Cutchin, M. C. (2003). The process of mediated aging in place: A theoretically and empirically based model. *Social Science and Medicine, 57,* 1077–1090.

31. Cutchin, M. C. (2004). Using Deweyan philosophy to rename and reframe adaptation-to-environment. *American Journal of Occupational Therapy, 58,* 303–312.

32. Cutler, L. (2007). Physical environments of assisted living: Research needs and challenges. *The Gerontologist, 47*(Suppl.1), 68–82. doi: 10.1093/geront/47.

33. Cutler, L., Kane, R. A., Degenholtz, H. B., Miller, M. J., & Grant, L. (2006). Assessing and comparing physical environments for nursing home residents: Using new tools for greater research specificity. *The Gerontologist, 46*(1), 42–51.

34. Dahlin-Ivanoff, S., Haak, M., Fange, A., & Iwarsson. (2007). The multiple meaning of home as experienced by very old Swedish people. *Scandinavian Journal of Occupation Therapy, 14*(1), 25–32.

35. Day, K., Carreon, D., & Stump, C. (2000). The therapeutic design of environments for people with dementia: A review of the empirical research. *The Gerontologist, 40,* 397–416.

36. Dickie, V., Cutchin, M. C., & Humphry, R. (2006). Occupation as transactional experience: A critique of individualism in occupational science. *Journal of Occupational Science, 13*(1), 83–93.

37. Duncan, R., & Levner, A. (2013). Better living design. In C. Starkloff (Chairperson) (Eds.), *Universal design summit.* St. Louis, MO: St. Louis University.

38. Ekerdt, D. J., Luborsky, M., & Lysack, C. (2012). Safe passage of goods and self during residential relocation in later life. *Ageing & Society, 32,* 833–850.

39. Ekerdt, D. J., Sergeant, J. F., Dingel, M., & Bowen, M. E. (2004). Household disbandment in later life. *The Journals of Gerontology: Series B, 59*(5), S265–S273.

40. Evans, G. W. (2003). The built environment and mental health. *Journal of Urban Health, 80*(4), 536–555.

41. Fange, A., & Ivanoff, S. D. (2009). The home is the hub of health in very old age: Findings from the ENABLE-AGE Project. *Archives of Gerontology and Geriatrics, 48,* 340–345.

42. Fange, A., & Iwarsson, S. (1999). Physical housing environment—development of a self-assessment instrument. *Canadian Journal of Occupational Therapy, 66,* 250–260.

43. Fange, A., & Iwarsson, S. (2003). Accessibility and usability in housing: Construct validity and implications for research and practice. *Disability and Rehabilitation 25*(23), 1316–1325.

44. Fisher, K. J., Li, F., Michael, Y., & Cleveland, M. (2004). Neighborhood level influences on physical activity among older adults: A multilevel analysis. *Journal of Aging and Physical Activity, 11*(1), 45–63.

45. Gaddam, A., Mukhopadhyay, S. C., & Gupta, G. S. (2011). Elder care based on cognitive sensor network. *IEEE Sensors Journal, 11*(3), 574–581.

46. Garin, N., Olaya, B., Miret, M., Ayuso-Mateos, J. L., & Power, M. (2014). Built environment and elderly population health: A comprehensive literature review. *Clinical Practice & Epidemiology in Mental Health, 10,* 103–115.

47. Gitlin, L. N. (2003). Conducting research on home environments: Lessons learned and new directions. *The Gerontologist, 43*(5), 628–637. doi: 10.1093/geront/43.5.628.

48. Gitlin, L. N., Corcoran, M., Winter, L., Boyce, A., & Hauck, W. W. (2001). A randomized, controlled trial of a home environmental intervention: Effect on efficacy and upset in caregivers and on daily function of persons with dementia. *The Gerontologist, 41,* 4–14.

49. Gitlin, L. N., Hauck, W. W., Dennis, M. P., & Winter, L. (2005). Maintenance of effects of the home environmental skill-building program for family caregivers and individuals with Alzheimer's disease and related disorders. *Journal of Gerontology Series A: Biological Sciences and Medical Sciences, 60*(3), 368–374. doi: 10.1093/gerona/60.3.368.

50. Gitlin, L. N., Hauck, W. W., Dennis, M. P., Winter, L., Hodgson, N., & Schinfeld, S. (2009). Long-term effect on mortality of a home intervention that reduces functional difficulties in older adults: Results from a randomized trial. *Journal of the American Geriatrics Society, 57,* 476–481. doi: 10.1111/j.1532-5415.2008.02147.x.

51. Gitlin, L. N., Hauck, W. W., Winter, L., Dennis, M. P., & Schulz, R. (2006). Effect of an in-home occupational and physical therapy intervention on reducing mortality in functionally vulnerable older people: Preliminary findings. *Journal of the American Geriatrics Society, 54,* 950–955.

52. Gitlin, L. N., Miller, K., & Boyce, A. (1999). Bathroom modifications for frail elderly renters: Outcomes of a community-based program. *Technology and Disability, 10,* 141–149.

53. Gitlin, L. N., Winter, L., Corcoran, M., Dennis, M. P., Schinfeld, S., & Hauck, W. W. (2003). Effects of the home environmental skill-building program on the caregiver-care recipient dyad: 6-month outcomes from the Philadelphia REACH initiative. *The Gerontologist, 43,* 532–546.

54. Gitlin, L. N., Winter, L., Dennis, M. P., Corcoran, M., Schinfeld, S., & Hauck, W. W. (2006). A randomized trial of a multicomponent home intervention to reduce functional difficulties in older adults. *Journal of the American Geriatrics Society, 54*(5), 809–816. doi: 10.1111/j.1532-5415.2006.00703.x.

55. Hagerstrand, T. (1970). What about people in regional science? *Papers of the Regional Science Association, 24,* 7–21.

56. Hayward, D. G. (1977). Psychological concepts of "home". *HUD Challenge, 8*(2),10–13.

57. Hendrickson, C. C., & Mann, W. C. (2005). Changes over time in community mobility of elders with disabilities. *Physical and Occupational Therapy in Geriatrics, 23*(2/3), 75–89.

58. Hertz, J. E., Rosetti, J., Koren, M. E., & Robertson, J. F. (2005). *Management of relocation in cognitively intact older adults.* Iowa City, IA: University of Iowa, Gerontological Nursing Interventions Research Center, Research Dissemination Core.

59. Horvath, K. J., Trudeau, S. A., Rudolph, J. L., Trudeau, P. A., Duffy, M. E., & Berlowitz, D. (2013). Clinical trial of a home safety toolkit for Alzheimer's disease. *International Journal of Alzheimer's Disease,* 2013, 913606. doi: 10.1155/2013/913606. Epub 2013 Sep 29.

60. Hunt, M. E., & Roll, M. K. (1987). Simulation in familiarizing older people with an unknown building. *The Gerontologist, 27*(2), 169–175.

61. Innouye, S., Bogardus, S., Charpentier, P., Leo-Summers, L., Acampora, D., Holford, T. R., et al. (1999). A multi-component intervention to prevent delirium in hospitalized older patients. *New England Journal of Medicine, 340,* 669–720.

62. Iwarsson, S. (2004). Assessing the fit between older people and their physical home environments: An occupational therapy research perspective. In H-W. Wahl, R. J. Scheidt, & P. G. Windley (Eds.), *Aging in context: Socio-physical environments. Annual review of gerontology and geriatrics* (Vol. 23, pp. 85–109). New York, NY: Springer Publishing Company.

63. Iwarsson, S., Horstmann, V., Carlsson, G., Oswald, F., & Wahl, H-W. (2009). Person-environment fit predicts falls in older adults better than the consideration of environmental hazards only. *Clinical Rehabilitation, 23,* 558–567.

64. Iwarsson, S., & Stahl, A. (2003). Accessibility, usability and universal design—positioning and definition of concepts describing person environment relationships. *Disability and Rehabilitation, 25,* 57–66.

65. Jackson, J., Carlson, M., Mandel, D., Zemke, R., & Clark, R. (1998). Occupation in lifestyle redesign: The Well Elderly study occupational therapy program. *American Journal of Occupational Therapy, 52*(5), 326–336.

66. Jackson, R. J. (2003). The impact of the built environment on health. *American Journal of Public Health, 93*(9), 1382–1384.

67. Kastenbaum, R. J. (1980/1981). Habituation as a model of human aging. *International Journal of Aging and Human Development, 12*(3), 159–170.

68. Kautz, H., Arnstein, L., Borriello, G., Etzioni, O., & Fox, D. (2002). An overview of the assisted cognition project. In *Proceedings of the AAAI workshop on automation as caregiver: The role of intelligent technology in elder care* (pp. 60–65). Edinburgh, Scotland: Information Science Reference (an Imprint of IGI Global).

69. Kaye, J. A., Maxwell, S. A., Mattek, N., Hayes, T. L., Dodge, H., Pavel, M., et al. (2011). Intelligent systems for assessing aging changes: Home-based, unobtrusive, and continuous assessment of aging. *The Journals of Gerontology, Series B: Psychological Sciences and Social Sciences, 66*(B)(Suppl. 1), 180–190.

70. Kielhofner, G. (1995). *A model of human occupation: Theory and application* (2nd ed.). Baltimore, MD: William & Wilkins.

71. Kielhofner, G., & Burke, J. (1980). A model of human occupation, part I: Conceptual framework and content. *American Journal of Occupational Therapy, 34,* 572–581.

72. Koncelik, J. A. (1979). Human factors and environmental design for the aging: Aspects of physiological change and sensory loss as design criteria. In T. O. Byerts, S. C. Howell, & L. A. Pastalan (Eds.), *Environmental context of aging: Lifestyles, environmental quality and living arrangements* (pp. 107–117). New York, NY: Garland STPM Press.

73. Langlois, J. A., Keyl, P. M., Guralnik, J. M., Foley, D. J., Marottoli, R. A., & Wallace, R. B. (1997). Characteristics of older pedestrians who have difficulty crossing the street. *American Journal of Public Health, 87*(3), 393–397.

74. Law, M., Cooper, B., Strong, S., Stewart, D., Rigby, P., & Letts, L. (1996). The Person-Environment-Occupation model: A transactive approach to occupational performance. *Canadian Journal of Occupational Therapy, 63,* 9–23.

75. Lawton, M. P. (1989). Environmental proactivity and affect in older people. In S. Spacapan & S. Oskamy (Eds.), *Social psychology of aging* (pp. 135–164). Newbury Park, CA: Sage Publications.

76. Lawton, M. P., & Nahemow, L. (1973). Ecology and the aging process. In C. Eisdorfer & M. P. Lawton (Eds.), *The psychology of adult development and aging* (pp. 619–674). Washington, DC: American Psychological Association.

77. Levy, L. (2001). Memory processing and older adults: What practitioners need to know. *OT Practice, 5,* CE1–8.

78. Levy, L. (2011). Cognitive information processing. In N. Katz (Ed.), *Cognition, occupation, and participation across the life span: Neuroscience, neurorehabilitation, and models of intervention in occupational therapy* (3rd ed.). Bethesda, MD: AOTA Press.

79. Lewin, K. (1951). *Field theory in social science: Selected theoretical papers.* In Dorwyn Cartrwrite, (Ed.). Oxford, UK: Harpers.

80. Mallett, S. (2004). Understanding home: A critical review of the literature. *The Sociological Review, 52,* 62–89.

81. Mann, W. C., Ottenbacher, K. J., Fraas, L., Tomita, M., & Granger, C. V. (1999). Effectiveness of assistive technology and environmental interventions in maintaining independence and reducing home care costs for the frail elderly. *Archives of Family Medicine, 8,* 210–217.

82. Marcus, C. C. (1995). *House as a mirror of self.* Berkeley, CA: Conari Press.

83. Marottoli, R. A., Mendes de Leon, C. F., Glass, T. A., Williams, C. S., Cooney Jr., L. M., & Berkman, L. F. (2000). Consequences of driving cessation: Decreased out-of-home activity levels. *Journals of Gerontology Series B: Social Sciences, 55*(6), S334–S340.

84. McCusker, J., Cole, M., Abrahamowicz, M., Han, L., Podoba, J. E., & Ramman-Haddad, L., (2001). Environmental risk factors for delirium in hospitalized older people. *Journal of the American Geriatrics Society, 49,* 1327–1334.

85. Meyer, S., & Mollenkopf, H. (2003). Home technology, smart homes, and the aging user. In K. W. Schaie, H-W. Wahl, H. Mollenkopf, & F. Oswald (Eds.), *Aging independently: Living arrangements and mobility* (pp. 148–161). New York, NY: Springer Publishing Company.

86. Michael, Y., Beard, T., Choi, D., Farquhar, S., & Carlson, N. (2006). Measuring the influence of built neighborhood environments on walking in older adults. *Journal of Aging and Physical Activity, 14*(3), 302–312.

87. Morris, B. (1992). Reducing inventory: Divestiture of personal possessions. *Journal of Women and Aging, 4*(2), 79–92.

88. Murray, H. A. (1938). *Explorations in personality: A clinical and experimental study of fifty men of college age.* New York, NY: Oxford University Press.

89. Namazi, K. H., & Johnson, B. D. (1992). Pertinent autonomy for residents with dementias: Modification of the physical environment to enhance independence. *American Journal of Alzheimer's Care and Related Disorders and Research, 7,* 16–21.

90. O'Bryant, S. L. (1983). The subjective value of "home" to older home owners. *Journal of Housing for the Elderly, 1*(1), 29–43.

91. Oswald, F., & Wahl, H.-W. (2013). Creating and sustaining homelike places in residential environments. In G. D. Rowles & M. Bernard (Eds.), *Environmental gerontology: Making meaningful places in old age* (pp. 53–77). New York, NY: Springer Publishing Company.

92. Peace, S. (2013). Social interactions in public spaces and places: A conceptual overview. In G. D. Rowles & M. Bernard (Eds.), *Environmental gerontology: Making meaningful places in old age* (pp. 25–49). New York, NY: Springer Publishing Company.

93. Persson, D. (1993). The elderly driver: Deciding when to stop. *The Gerontologist, 33*(1), 88–91.

94. Phillips, J. (2013). Older people's use of unfamiliar space. In G. D. Rowles & M. Bernard (Eds.), *Environmental gerontology: Making meaningful places in old age* (pp. 199–223). New York, NY: Springer Publishing Company.

95. Porteous, J. D. (1976). Home: The territorial core. *Geographical Review, 66*(4), 383–390.

96. Reynolds, L. (2011). *The perceived value of nature and use of gardens by older adults living in residential care. Doctoral dissertation.* Lexington, KY: University of Kentucky, Graduate Center for Gerontology.

97. Rosso, A. L., Auchincloss, A. H., & Michael, Y. L. (2011). The urban built environment and mobility in older adults: A comprehensive review. *Journal of Aging Research*, Volume 2011 (2011), Article ID 816106, 10 pages (online open access journal) Accessed 10/20/15. http://www.hindawi.com/journals/jar/2011/816106/. doi:10.4061/2011/816106.

98. Roush, C. V., & Cox, J. E. (2000). The meaning of home: How it shapes the practice of home and hospice care. *Home Healthcare Nurse*, 18(6), 388–394.

99. Rowles, G. D. (1978). *Prisoners of space? Exploring the geographical experience of older people.* Boulder, CO: Westview.

100. Rowles, G. D. (1981). The surveillance zone as meaningful space for the aged. *The Gerontologist*, 21(3), 304–311.

101. Rowles, G. D. (2000). Habituation and being in place. *Occupational Therapy Journal of Research*, 20(Suppl.), S52–S67.

102. Rowles, G. D., & Bernard, M. (2013). The meaning and significance of place in old age. In G. D. Rowles & M. Bernard (Eds.), *Environmental gerontology: Making meaningful places in old age* (pp. 3–24). New York, NY: Springer Publishing Company.

103. Rowles, G. D., & Chaudhury, H. (Eds.). (2005). *Home and identity in later life: International perspectives* (pp. 21–45). New York, NY: Springer Publishing Company.

104. Rowles, G. D., Oswald, F., & Hunter, E. G. (2003). Interior living environments in old age. In H-W. Wahl, R. J. Scheidt, & P. G. Windley (Eds.), *Aging in context: Socio-physical environments. Annual review of gerontology and geriatrics* (Vol. 23, pp. 167–194). New York, NY: Springer Publishing Company.

105. Rowles, G. D., & Watkins, J. F. (2003). History, habit, heart and hearth: On making spaces into places. In K. W. Schaie, H-W. Wahl, H. Mollenkopf, & F. Oswald (Eds.), *Aging independently: Living arrangements and mobility* (pp. 77–96). New York, NY: Springer Publishing Company.

106. Rubinstein, N. J. (2005). Psychic homelands and the imagination of place: A literary perspective. In G. D. Rowles & H. Chaudhury (Eds.), *Home and identity in later life: International perspectives* (pp. 111–142). New York, NY: Springer Publishing Company.

107. Rubinstein, R. L. (1989). The home environments of older people: A description of the psychological processes linking person to place. *Journal of Gerontology: Social Sciences*, 44(2), S45–S53.

108. Rubinstein, R. L., & de Medeiros, K. (2005). Home, self, and identity. In G. D. Rowles & H. Chaudhury (Eds.), *Home and identity in later life: International perspectives* (pp. 47–62). New York, NY: Springer Publishing Company.

109. Rudman, D. L., Friedland, J., Chipman, M., & Sciortino, P. (2006). Holding on and letting go: The perspectives of pre-seniors and seniors on driving self-regulation in later life. *Canadian Journal of Aging*, 25(1), 65–76.

110. Satariano, W. A. (1997). Editorial: The disabilities of aging—looking to the physical environment. *American Journal of Public Health*, 87(3), 331–332.

111. Scheidt, R. J., & Norris-Baker, C. (1999). Place therapies for older adults: Conceptual and interventive approaches. *International Journal of Aging and Human Development*, 48(1), 1–15.

112. Schulz, R., Burgio, L., Burns, R., Eisdorfer, C., Gallagher-Thompson, D., Gitlin, L., et al. (2003). Resources for Enhancing Alzheimer's Caregiver Health (REACH): Overview, site-specific outcomes, and future directions. *The Gerontologist*, 43(4), 514–520.

113. Seamon, D. (1979). *A geography of the lifeworld: Movement, rest and encounter.* New York, NY: St. Martin's Press.

114. Seamon, D., & Nordin, C. (1980). Marketplace as place ballet: A Swedish example. *Landscape*, 24, 35–41.

115. Sharlach, A. (2012). Creating aging-friendly communities in the United States. *Ageing International*, 37, 25–38.

116. Sherman, E. & Dacher, J. (2005). Cherished objects and the home: Their meaning and roles in late life. In Rowles, G. D. & Chaudhury, H. (Eds.), *Home and Identity in Late Life* (pp. 63–79). New York, NY: Springer Publishing Company.

117. Shipp, K. M., & Branch, L. G. (1999). The physical environment as a determinant of the health status of older populations. *Canadian Journal on Aging*, 18(3), 313–327.

118. Sixsmith, J. (1986). The meaning of home: An exploratory study of environmental experience. *Journal of Environmental Psychology*, 6(4), 281–298.

119. Skubik-Peplaski, C., Rowles, G. D., & Hunter, E. G. (2012). Toward a physical environmental continuum for occupational intervention in a rehabilitation hospital. *Occupational Therapy in Health Care*, 26(1), 33–47.

120. Sloane, P. D., Mitchell, C. M., Preisser, J. S., Phillips, C., Commander, C., & Burker, E. (1998). Environmental correlates of resident agitation in Alzheimer's disease special care units. *Journal of the American Geriatrics Society*, 46, 862–869.

121. Smith, S. G. (1994). The essential qualities of a home. *Journal of Environmental Psychology*, 14, 31–46.

122. Steinfield, E., Schroeder, S., Duncan, J., Faste, R., Chollet, D., Bishop M., et al. (1979). *Access to the built environment: A review of the literature.* Washington, DC: U.S. Government Printing Office.

123. Story, M. F. (1998). Maximizing usability: The principles of universal design. *Assistive Technology*, 10, 4–12.

124. Thang, L. L., & Kaplan, M. S. (2013). Intergenerational pathways for building relational spaces and places. In G. D. Rowles & M. Bernard (Eds.), Environmental gerontology: Making Meaningful places in old age (pp. 225–251). New York, NY: Springer Publishing Company.

125. U.S. Bureau of the Census. (2015). *Calculating Migration Expectancy using ACS data.* http://www.census.gov/hhes/migration/about/cal-mig-exp.html Geographic Mobility/Migration. 2007. Accessed June 12, 2015.

126. Verbrugge, L. M., Rennert, C., & Madans, J. H. (1997). The great efficacy of personal and equipment assistance in reducing disability. *American Journal of Public Health*, 87(3), 384–392.

127. Wahl, H-W., Fange, A., Oswald, F., Gitlin, L. N., & Iwarsson, S. (2009). The home environment and disability-related outcomes in aging individuals: What is the empirical evidence? *The Gerontologist*, 49(3), 355.

128. Wahl, H-W., Iwarsson, S., & Oswald, F. (2012). Aging well and the environment: Toward an integrative model and research agenda for the future. *The Gerontologist*, 52(3), 306–316.

129. Wahl, H.-W., & Oswald, F. (2010). Environmental perspectives on aging. In D. Dannefer & C. Phillipson (Eds.), *The SAGE handbook of social gerontology* (pp. 111–124). London: Sage.

130. Webber, S. C., Porter, M. M., & Menec, V. H. (2010). Mobility in older adults: A comprehensive framework. *The Gerontologist*, 50(4), 443–450.

131. Yen, I. H., Michael, Y. L., & Perdue, L. (2009). Neighborhood environment in studies of health of older adults. *American Journal of Preventive Medicine*, 37(5), 455–463.

132. Zeisel, J., Hyde, J., & Levkoff, S. (1994). Best practices: An environment-behavior (E-B) model for Alzheimer special care units. *American Journal of Alzheimer's Care and Related Disorders and Research*, 9, 4–21.

133. Zwijsen, S. A., Niemeijer, A. R., & Hertogh, C. M. (2011). Ethics of using assistive technology in the care of community-dwelling elderly people: An overview of the literature. *Aging and Mental Health*, 15(4), 419–427.

CHAPTER 20

Driving and Transportation: Dementia as a Model for Evaluation, Decision Making, and Planning

David B.Carr, MD, Linda Hunt, PhD, OTR/L, FAOTA

CHAPTER OUTLINE

OBJECTIVES

- Review how aging and disease may impair the ability to drive
- Discuss important related topics such as mobility counseling, which includes public and/or private options for transportation
- Examine mobility challenges within the context of dementia, given the ubiquitous nature of the disease, and knowing it is a common disease of aging and frequently encountered in driving evaluation clinics

This chapter reviews how aging and disease may impair the ability to drive and covers important related topics such as mobility counseling (which includes public and/or private

options for transportation). We focus on older adults with dementia as our model, given the ubiquitous nature of the disease, and knowing it is a common disease of aging and frequently encountered in driving evaluation clinics. Dementia offers unique challenges for evaluating cognitive and/or visual processing components of driving and unique challenges in regard to participation in community mobility options. The principles discussed in this chapter, however, may also be applicable for the myriad of chronic disorders that are associated with aging. The model or approach we outline in this chapter should assist the practitioner in determining best practices for community mobility. Furthermore, this chapter will explore client factors in the evaluation process that may be impaired by age-related diseases such as dementia, and include discussion of values and beliefs that need to be considered by the practitioner when making driving recommendations[9]. We also review additional common age-related illnesses that can affect driving and discuss their implications in the context of dementia and comorbidities.

Previously published chapters on older drivers' fitness to drive have focused on evaluating general disability and performance skills; recommendations for rehabilitation, including adaptive driving; and alternative solutions for community mobility.[35,61,100,101] This chapter offers a newer model for practice, one where health professionals may be able to apply to various comorbid states and diagnostic situations.

It appears driver evaluators have selected their preferred approaches for both off-road and on-road assessments, but may have difficulty with the decision-making process and weighing all the major components once data have been collected. It is our hope that health-care professionals will not only provide evidence-based driving evaluations, but also use appropriate decision making in regard to fitness-to-drive approaches. We propose a Multifactor Older Driver with Dementia Evaluation Model (MODEM) that may better guide fitness-to-drive decisions for our aging population. This chapter also discusses factors that affect older adults' abilities to use transportation options and offers a template to help guide accessibility to the community.[56] Health-care professionals must include the necessary guidance for community mobility once driving is no longer possible.

Overview of Driving, Aging, and Dementia

There are almost 40 million people aged 65 years and older living in the United States. Of these, over 30 million are licensed drivers.[120] The automobile is the most frequently used mode of transportation in the United States, accounting almost 90% of the trips that are made outside of the home.[77] Unfortunately, the presence of chronic disease may impair many older adults' abilities to operate a motor vehicle. Alzheimer's disease (AD), the most common dementing illness, currently afflicts over 5 million individuals in the United States.[6] With currently as many as 12% of individuals over age 65 years and half of individuals over age 85 years affected by AD, the economic and social effects of this disorder are already enormous. Eventually, as the disease progresses, individuals will no longer be able to operate a motor vehicle.

The literature on older adults with dementia indicates that some drivers with a dementing illness continue to drive, many well into the disease process.[24, 94] It has been estimated that 4% of current drivers over 75 years have a dementing illness.[41] Results from one study, in which researchers performed a cognitive screen on older adults during driver license renewal, found that almost 20% of those over 80 years were impaired.[117] Taken together, these studies probably underestimate the actual number of drivers with dementia on the road, because some older adults with memory loss may not renew their licenses and continue driving and/or are inaccurately reported as having stopped driving.

Although trends indicate that older adults are increasing the number of miles driven per year in comparison with previous cohorts,[62] data on the travel patterns of older adults with cognitive impairment are limited and, for obvious reasons, difficult to accurately assess. Some studies suggest that drivers with dementia have decreased yearly mileage in comparison with controls. For example, Trobe and colleagues found that individuals with AD drove an average of about 5000 kilometers annually in the 2 years before they stopped driving, compared with an average of 8000 kilometers driven for controls.[119] Other studies appear to confirm that, as a group, older drivers with dementia limit their driving exposure.[82,106] Despite data indicating that older adults with dementia may drive fewer miles, many studies (but not all) have demonstrated an increased crash rate compared with age-matched controls.[23] In one study, the crash risk for a driver with AD rose above that of the highest-risk group (teenage males) after the third year of disease.[33]

Aging Systems That May Impair Driver Performance

Vision

The prevalence of visual disability escalates with increasing age.[90] The risk of legal blindness at 20/200 in the best eye with correction, or visual fields of 20 degrees or less, is nearly 10 times greater for those older than age 65 years than for those who are younger.[102] The four major causes of vision loss are cataracts, glaucoma, macular degeneration, and diabetic retinopathy. All of these diseases increase in prevalence with aging.[93] (See Chapter 10 for additional information on vision and aging.)

The most common condition associated with aging is a change in the integrity of the crystalline lens of the eye, commonly referred to as cataracts. The lens also yellows, increasing the need for blue light to compensate for increased absorption of that portion of the spectrum.[89] Furthermore, the pupil becomes smaller and loses its ability to dilate in reduced illumination,[125] changes in the lens and capsule affect accommodation,[49] and neural pathways may be altered.[3,13] Not surprisingly, the prevalence of corrective lens use increases with aging as well, so that by age 75 years, over 90% of the population requires some optical correction to maintain visual function.[28] Furthermore, more than 25% of the population older than age 85 years has severe visual impairment,[91] defined as inability to read newsprint even when wearing corrective lenses. For such people, therefore, optical correction to near-normal vision is not possible. Those individuals who have visual acuity less than 20/70 in the best eye with correction are considered to have low vision.[38]

Visual acuity only describes a person's ability to resolve high-contrast detail and provides little information about the ability to detect the larger, low-contrast objects that are encountered in everyday life. The changes in the lens, pupil size, and accommodation, and reduced information received by the neural pathways, may all lead to decreased contrast sensitivity. Impairment in this functional ability has been correlated with unsafe driving in many studies.[98] Rubin and colleagues assessed the relationship between visual impairment, including contrast sensitivity, and functional ability in a sample of older adult American volunteers and found that impaired contrast sensitivity was the factor most strongly associated with self-reported difficulty in day and night driving.[119] Decreased contrast sensitivity makes driving difficult on overcast days. It is challenging to detect a gray car on an overcast day. In addition, a car the same color as the road, such as light brown or gray, may blend into the background of the road and, therefore, may not be detected by the older driver.

Aging and disease of the optical vision system may cause numerous problems that make driving unsafe. For example, poor vision may cause difficulty in reading signs, including street names. A reduced field of vision may impair search and the ability to detect approaching or merging vehicles, bike riders, or pedestrians. Poor night vision may impair orientation to objects and the ability to judge the distance between objects. A history of amblyopia with lowered visual acuity in one eye will impair depth perception. Although a driver is able to compensate during daytime driving by noting object size or the color of objects near and far, these depth-perception cues disappear during nighttime driving. Plus, glare from lights may temporarily impair vision altogether. Glare recovery time is often delayed in older adults. Keep in mind that all of these visual impairments, such as decreased acuity, decreased peripheral vision, prolonged glare recovery time, decreased contrast sensitivity, and a delay in processing speed and reaction time, may reduce the ability to respond to a traffic situation to prevent a crash.[58, 67]

Physical Frailty

Physical frailty is often a comorbid condition with dementia. There are scarce data on the association of physical frailty and motor vehicle crashes and/or performance-based road tests. However, we do know that many frail older adults continue to operate a motor vehicle.[21] Various studies have associated physical frailty with driving retirement. In one study, difficulty climbing stairs, the inability to walk 1/2 mile, or difficulty in performing heavy housework were associated with driving cessation.[17] Visual impairment, stroke, Parkinson's disease, arthritis, hip fracture, and memory loss were associated with driving cessation in a sample of community-dwelling older adults.[81] Approximately 50% of the study participants were still driving at the time of this study, suggesting that interventions may be supporting prevention of driving cessation in older drivers with frailty. Community-based interviews of older adults who have stopped driving indicate that medical conditions or health reasons were the most common reasons cited for driving cessation.

Older adults with cognitive impairment or dementia should be examined to rule out other diagnoses or comorbidities that can further reduce spare capacity. Two recent publications in this past decade summarize the extensive literature on driving impairment and medical conditions.[29,32] Medical conditions that have been associated with impaired driving ability include but are not limited to diseases affecting vision (e.g., cataracts, diabetic retinopathy, macular degeneration, glaucoma), cardiovascular disease, respiratory disease (e.g., sleep apnea, chronic obstructive pulmonary disease [COPD]), neurologic disease (e.g., dementia, multiple sclerosis, Parkinson's disease), psychiatric disease, metabolic disease, and musculoskeletal disease, along with medication side effects.[18]

Older adults with cognitive impairment are particularly susceptible to the adverse effects of medications on the central nervous system, which can result in delirium, dizziness, functional decline, injurious falls, anorexia, and disrupted sleep patterns. Criteria for potential driving impairment medication use in older adults have been described.[74] Classes of drugs to avoid or minimize include antihistamines, traditional antipsychotics, tricyclic antidepressants, bowel/bladder antispasmodics, benzodiazepines, muscle relaxants, and barbiturates. These classes include narcotics, benzodiazepines, antihistamines, antidepressants, antipsychotics, hypnotics, alcohol, and muscle relaxants.[50] Older adults may drive while intoxicated or under the influence of other medications.[53,64] Careful attention to these issues, not only in cognitively intact older drivers, but also in drivers with dementia, is warranted.

Diseases Common to Aging and the Effects on Driving

Cerebrovascular Accident

A cerebrovascular accident (CVA), or stroke, occurs when the blood supply to the brain in a specific area is diminished or occluded. Strokes are often classified into ischemic/infarcts or hemorrhagic/bleeds. Stroke is the fifth leading cause of death in the United States, where there are approximately 800,000 new strokes each year.[26] Stroke most heavily affects select groups, such as African Americans between the ages of 35 and 65 years.[26]

Research on the proportion of working-age stroke survivors who return to work shows mixed findings, with rates from 7% to 84% in 20 studies across a number of countries.[73] In 2012, the American Stroke Association noted that Americans will pay about $73.7 billion for stroke-related medical costs and disability.[47]

Symptoms of stroke are myriad and can include:

- Visual symptoms (e.g., visual field loss, inability to recognize objects)
- Motor impairment (e.g., weakness of the limbs, dysphagia or trouble swallowing)
- Sensory loss (e.g., numbness or loss of sensation)
- Cognitive impairment (e.g., neglect or hemispatial inattention)
- Deficits in gait/balance

Risk factors include:

- Hypertension
- Heart disease
- Diabetes
- Smoking
- Excessive alcohol use
- Hypercholesterolemia (possible risk factor)

The functional deficits from stroke that are relevant to driving include muscle weakness or paralysis; cognitive deficits such as memory loss, executive dysfunction, hemispatial inattention, or visual field cuts, and aphasia; and/or sensory loss.

Usually, the diagnosis is not difficult when symptoms and signs are obvious, and especially when they correlate with new findings from brain-imaging studies. However, small infarcts can escape initial detection, especially when they are asymptomatic or the symptoms are subtle. Definitions of stroke are usually based on the Trial of Org 10172 in Acute Stroke Treatment (TOAST) classification system, which has a high degree of interobserver reliability.[2] This stroke classification system provides for specific definitions of stroke and classifies the subtypes based on etiology.

Significant numbers of community-dwelling stroke clients continue driving (~42%),[71] yet most stroke clients (87%) do not receive any type of formal driving evaluation; they simply resume the operation of a motor vehicle.[39] The greater longevity after stroke suggests that health professionals will be faced with increasing numbers of clients who continue to drive. Crash studies related to stroke have been few, and results have not been consistent. One study did note an increase in crash risk in stroke clients compared with controls.[68] Of all of the areas in neurology (except for perhaps dementia), stroke has probably been the most studied disease in regard to fitness to drive or in determining the ability to pass a road test through off-road assessments.

Preliminary studies on fitness to drive in stroke clients note that those clients who fail road tests have worsening scores on measures of perception, cognition, and complex visual-perception/attention information.[37] One test, the Motor-Free-Visual Perception Test, appeared to have promise in a pilot study,[84] but was not found by itself to be predictive of failure on a road test with a larger validation study.[69] Lundqvist and colleagues[76] found that tests requiring high-order cognitive functions such as mental control, working memory, and attention provided the best differentiation of driving skills in clients with CVA. Work in Europe has tested the Stroke Driver Screening Assessment that includes a dot cancellation test (visual selective attention), compass test (divided attention, visuospatial orientation, reasoning), and road sign recognition (mental speed, working memory, and executive function). Using this battery the investigators were able to correctly classify 80% (pass/fail) of stroke clients who were administered an on-the-road test.[75,92] A summary of the evidence on psychometric tests and predicting fitness to drive in stroke was recently reviewed.[52]

Treatment of stroke usually includes both aggressive management of risk factors and rehabilitation. The latter can occur in a variety of settings, including inpatient rehabilitation, a skilled nursing center, or home. Clients may find themselves in more than one setting during their course of recovery. Cognitive rehabilitation has potential to improve those impaired domains that are crucial for driving. One promising study in this area was able to double the rate of stroke clients returning to driving by utilizing driving simulation training.[4] This study suggests that some stroke clients who retire from driving may be able to operate a motor vehicle, if only for the opportunity to receive remedial skills training.

Medications

Polypharmacy is often defined based on the number of medications that are routinely taken (e.g., five or more), but can also be defined simply as taking too many medications or unnecessary medications. Based on these definitions, polypharmacy is common in older adults. As many as 30% of older adults over age 65 years take five or more prescription medications.[114] Older adults represent 14% of the U.S. population, yet consume over 30% of prescription drugs.[103] Therefore, many older adults have multiple medical problems and are on numerous medications. As a group, they are at higher risk for adverse drug events, due to age-related changes in drug metabolism, the increased amount of routine medications taken and thus increased chances for drug–drug or drug–disease interactions, and the presence of comorbidities. For more detailed information on these topics, see Chapter 13: Pharmacology, Pharmacy and the Aging Adult.

Pharmacokinetics, or how a drug is metabolized in the human body, changes with aging. The proportion of adipose tissue increases with aging, so medications such as benzodiazepines (e.g., Valium, Xanax) will have a longer duration of action in older adults. Total body water decreases by 15% over age 80 years, so the volume of distribution for hydrophilic drugs, such as alcohol or cimetidine, is decreased, resulting in higher drug concentrations. Older adults have decreased lean body mass. Because digoxin binds to muscle, toxicity can occur at lower doses. The concentrations of plasma proteins such as albumin may decline in older adults. This results in a reduced bound form of many medications and greater free drug levels. Phase I (Cytochrome P450) oxidation generally declines with aging, and doses of medications that are metabolized through this pathway should be reduced. Many medications are excreted by the kidney and will often need to be adjusted by estimating creatinine clearance by age and body weight because kidney function declines with aging.

Pharmacodynamics describes the reaction or response to the specific drug. End-organ responsiveness to a drug at the receptor level may be altered with aging. Changes in receptor binding, a decrease in receptor number, or altered translation of a receptor-initiated cellular response into a biochemical reaction may be responsible. Findings in the literature include a decreased response to beta blockers and an increased sensitivity to benzodiazepines, opiates or narcotics, warfarin, and anticholinergics. It should be noted that many of the medications in the latter list have been implicated in driving impairment.

Certain drugs have a high likelihood of causing side effects in the gerontological population due to decreases in physiologic reserve in organ systems with aging or disease. There are published lists of medications that should be avoided (e.g., Beers criteria) in the older adult population, along with drug–drug and drug–disease interactions.[7] Many of these agents cause anticholinergic side effects or sedation, and have been associated with increased crash risk. The list of drug–drug or drug–disease interactions continues to grow as new agents are released, and it remains a difficult problem to stay up to date for many physicians and pharmacists. Most hospitals and pharmacies utilize computerized drug interaction software and may identify potential problems before they occur.

Many common medication classes have been studied and are associated with either increased crash risk or impaired driving skills when assessed by simulators or road tests. These include, but are not limited to, narcotics and barbiturates, benzodiazepines, antihistamines, antidepressants, antipsychotics, hypnotics, alcohol, antiepileptic agents, antiemetic agents, and muscle relaxants. One study focused on older drivers noted that long-acting benzodiazepines have been associated with increased crash rates.[51] Another report suggests that there may be a significant number of older adults driving while intoxicated or under the influence of other medications.[53,64]

Wang et al.[123] noted that any drug that can depress the central nervous system is associated with impairment in operating a motor vehicle. A new way to classify medications has been developed and classifies medications as to whether or not they are potentially driver-impairing (PDI) medications. As more PDI medications are prescribed and used, crash risk increases.[72] PDI effects may include sleepiness, fatigue, or sedation; light-headedness, dizziness, or low blood pressure; blackouts or syncope; or impaired coordination. One study suggested that impaired road test performance was associated with hypersomnolence as noted by higher scores on the Epworth Sleepiness Scale. Medications can affect eyesight in numerous ways, including blurred vision, impaired visual fields, and impaired nighttime vision. Some have noted that certain drugs have been found to delay central processing speed, leading to using inappropriate force with the steering wheel, or braking too late. However, it should be noted that many medication and driving studies are simply correlational in nature, and results may suggest increased crash risk but not necessarily prove causation. Whether it is the medication itself, the condition for which it is prescribed, the presence of other comorbidities, or some combination of these is difficult to sort out. Clinicians should be aware of the risk and attempt to use the safest class of medications based on the most recent evidence.

Older adults may have numerous physicians and multiple pharmacies. The primary care physician should write down all drugs by generic name and eliminate all unnecessary medications. Clinical indications should be identified and documented for all drugs, and those medications without a therapeutic benefit should be stopped. The side-effect profile of each drug should be known to the clinician. Safer medications should always be substituted, and lists in the medical record should be updated at each visit. Before a new drug is started, the clinician should identify risk factors for adverse drug reactions, including advanced age, liver or kidney disease, or multiple medications. The risk of medication errors increases dramatically with the number of medications taken by the client.

Compliance is another major issue with older adults. Drug regimens should be simple, utilize the same dosage schedule with other drugs, and be administered as part of a daily routine task, such as eating a meal. Instructing relatives and caregivers on drug regimens and monitoring by home health nurses and pharmacists may reduce adverse drug events. Aids such as pillboxes and calendars may increase compliance. Reviewing clients' knowledge of why they take medications, in addition to education about adverse drug reactions, is paramount.

Sleep Apnea

Sleep apnea can be referred to as a periodic cessation of breathing during sleep. It is commonly undiagnosed and often undertreated. It has been suggested that the prevalence rate may be as high as that for diabetes, with 4% of men and 2% of women affected.[126] It has been defined as cessation of breaths for at least a 10-second duration. This results in fragmentation of sleep, daytime sleepiness, and nighttime awakenings. Some clients have a reduction in their airflow or a hypopnea. The apnea-hypopnea index refers to the total number of episodes per hour during sleep. A value of 5 or greater is considered abnormal and is associated with impaired function.

There are many correlates of disturbed sleep, including high blood pressure and right-sided congestive heart failure,

and the disease is correlated with increased mortality. Two types of sleep apnea are often described: obstructive apnea, where there is resistance to airflow, and central apnea, where there is a reduced or diminished drive to breathe. Snoring is correlated with obstructive sleep apnea, and this occurs often during rapid-eye-movement (REM) sleep when the pharyngeal muscles are relaxed and the upper airway collapses. Risk factors include obesity, large neck circumference, male sex, and acromegaly. The other risk factors may be history of hypothyroidism and/or sedative or alcohol use.

Symptoms can be variable. They may include daytime sleepiness and snoring, but also there may be headache, memory loss, impaired concentration or coordination, irritability, depression, anxiety, sweating, dry mouth or drooling, and reflux. Detection may be reported by a bed partner who can provide information such as gasping, snoring, or breathing cessation during sleep.[95] Attempts have been made to predict a diagnosis of sleep apnea based on history or examination. These include questionnaires such as the Epworth sleepiness scale,[65] or using neck circumference size. Maycock[83] studied the Epworth scale and correlated impaired levels with crash risk. The gold standard for diagnosis is the overnight polysomnography. Based on an overnight sleep study, sleep clinicians will rate the presence and severity of the disease, usually in the mild, moderate, or severe category.

Drowsy driving is a common cause for a motor vehicle crash, and some authorities believe that 100,000 crashes a year attributed to fatigue may be a conservative figure. Crash risk is related to the amount of sleep that was previously obtained.[44] Sleep disorder crash risk may be confounded or enhanced by medication use, such as analgesic or antihistamine use.[55] Sleep apnea clients have been noted to have increased crash risk increase[36] and these drivers are also at risk for more serious injury.[86] These findings have been attributed to drowsiness and lack of concentration. Additional crash studies and driving simulator studies have found increased crash risk or impairment due to driver fatigue, and improvements in driver performance with treatment. These have been extensively reviewed elsewhere.[29] Thankfully, George[45] and other investigators have found that treatment reduces crash risk back to baseline levels.

Initial interventions may include weight loss (as little as 10% loss may be helpful), exercise, and behavioral therapy. There are oral devices that can assist clients with mild sleep apnea. Continuous positive airway pressure (CPAP) has been shown to improve cardiac function, reduce blood pressure, and improve quality of life.[78] Zozula and Rosen have documented that compliance rates are low.[127] Up to 40% of clients with untreated severe sleep apnea may die over an 8-year period.[48] Surgical procedures may be of benefit, and tracheostomy is performed in severe cases[5].

Muscle Weakness/Arthritis

It is probably accurate to state that musculoskeletal abnormalities (e.g., diseases that cause muscle weakness, physical frailty, or restricted joint range of motion) have been less studied in terms of driving outcomes. The different types of diseases that can affect musculoskeletal function are broad and include (but are not limited to) arthridities, amputation, spinal cord injury, trauma, surgery, and deconditioning and weakness. The prevalence of a common form of arthritis (osteoarthritis) is discussed in this section, and mobility issues in general that relate to driving impairment also are reviewed. See detailed information on the Musculoskeletal System in Chapter 8.

Osteoarthritis, in the category of degenerative joint diseases, is the most common form of arthritis in older adults and affects over 26 million people.[25] Cartilage is typically lost in this condition, causing bone-on-bone friction, deformities, pain, and restrictions in mobility. The joints that are usually affected are the large weight-bearing joints such as the hips, knees, and lower back, although the neck, hands, and feet are also commonly affected. Risk factors include family history, injury, obesity, and advanced age.

The major symptoms are pain, swelling, loss of joint mobility, restricted range of motion, and, if severe, diminished activities of daily living. Clinicians can assess muscle strength and joint range of motion by physical examination, but can also use devices such as dynamometers and goniometers for more specific measurements. However, these are less likely to be used in clinical practice and more commonly present in rehabilitation centers. The diagnosis of osteoarthritis is suggested by an insidious history of pain and discomfort along with common physical examination findings in typical joints, and is confirmed by radiographic findings.

Difficulties in driving an automobile that have been reported by clients with musculoskeletal disorders include problems in using seat belts and keys, adjusting mirrors and seats, steering, transferring in and out of the car, driving in reverse, and using the foot pedals. There have been several efforts to correlate functional abilities such as range of motion and muscle function with driving. However, it should be noted that these studies have not just focused on degenerative joint disease, but on general groups of older adults.

Older adults with physical disabilities or frailty may be at increased risk for a motor vehicle crash[80,112] and are more vulnerable to injury.[66] Walking less than one block a day, impaired left knee flexion, and the presence of foot abnormalities all correlated with an adverse driving event in one study.[80] Another study noted that crash-involved subjects were more likely to have more difficulty walking 1/4 mile than were controls.[113] The authors of that study also cite numerous references in the literature that have found an association between a history of falls and an increased risk for a motor vehicle crash. Diminished cervical range of motion and delayed rapid-pace walk have also been recently correlated with increased crash risk[12,115].

A diagnosis of arthritis and the use of nonsteroidal anti-inflammatory drugs (NSAIDs) were both associated with increased at-fault crash risk in a recent study.[85] This finding was also noted in a large study conducted in the state of Utah that examined medically impaired drivers and found an increased crash risk for drivers with musculoskeletal disorders, but not for muscle or motor weakness.[122] Conversely, clients with a specific diagnosis of osteoarthritis in one study[68] were found to be no more at risk for a crash than were controls.

Although the crash literature is incomplete, musculoskeletal abnormalities have been associated with driving cessation. In one study of an exercise intervention in which current and former drivers were compared, the current drivers had a lower rate of joint deformities, fewer sedating medications, faster cognitive processing speed, stronger grip strength, better joint range of motion, higher aerobic power, and faster walking.[20] Thus, arthritis, muscle strength, and range of motion may be important determinants of maintaining driving. The finding that weaker grip strength was an independent predictor of being a former driver also has been previously described,[105] and indicates that motor weakness may place older adults at risk for driving retirement.

Interventions for joint disorders include the use of various medications, ranging from acetaminophen to NSAIDs, narcotics, injections, steroids, and surgery. Nonpharmacologic interventions have met with various success in treating osteoarthritis and include exercise, weight loss, heat, cold, topical analgesics or anesthetics, transcutaneous electrical nerve stimulation (TENS) units, ultrasound, massage, and whirlpool. Many of these interventions are offered in pain clinics and/or rehabilitation centers. Early intervention in arthritic disorders has the potential to improve or maintain driving skills and decrease crash risk and driving cessation, although this still needs to be proven.

Dementia: A Disease That Offers a Model for Fitness to Drive

Various Types of Dementia

Dementia with Lewy bodies (DLB) is defined by cognitive impairment or dementia, hallucinations, parkinsonism, and fluctuations in attention. Unexplained falls, delusions, syncope, and neuroleptic sensitivity support the diagnosis of DLB. Frontotemporal dementia is less common, but should be considered if early loss of personal and social awareness (e.g., disinhibition, social inappropriateness) and/or pronounced language dysfunction is observed, especially in persons less than 70 years of age. Vascular disease often coexists with AD and other dementias, but can be the primary cause for cognitive impairment. Vascular dementia is characterized by an acute decline temporally related to an acute cerebrovascular event. The history of a stepwise decline in cognition and evidence of cerebral infarct by neuroimaging are generally required for the diagnosis of vascular dementia. The presence of infarcts on brain imaging alone, however, is insufficient for a vascular dementia diagnosis because infarcts often coexist with other dementias. Additionally, other vascular changes resulting in cognitive impairment, such as cerebral amyloid angiopathy and subcortical arteriosclerotic disease, may mimic dementia of Alzheimer's type (DAT), but present with more executive dysfunction (e.g., personality changes and problems in sequencing, abstract thinking, judgment, and organization). Note that chapter 15 provides additional information on dementia.

Depressive symptoms may be presenting features in individuals with cognitive impairment, and depression often coexists with dementia. Consequently, distinguishing depression from early dementia may be difficult. Although the majority of older adults with depression and cognitive impairment will continue to have cognitive impairment after depression is treated, some clients may improve. Using a screening tool such as the Geriatric Depression Scale or the Patient Health Questionnaire-9 in the early stages of the disease may also be helpful.

Vision and Alzheimer's Disease

Alzheimer's disease (AD) is viewed as a disorder primarily of memory loss. Yet researchers have long known that AD is characterized by impairments in several additional domains, including visual function. The neuropathology of this disease affects several brain areas that are devoted to processing visual functions, which in turn affect attention and cognition. Mapstone and Weintraub[79] discuss AD's spatial attention and navigation effects on driving behavior. Furthermore, Holroyd[54] points out that visual hallucinations are the most common type of hallucination in AD, with a prevalence rate between 12% and 53%. Holroyd[54] explains that the abnormalities of visual impairment may have multifactorial etiologies and include decrements in contrast sensitivity, stereoacuity deficits, and visual agnosia.

Vecera and Rizzo[121] argue that many of the attentional impairments evident in AD might be produced by limitations in visual short-term memory. They report that people with AD may exhibit impairments in searching when required to view a cluttered visual scene. Similarly, when driving, people are required to visually search the environment for information among an array of distracting objects and events, and AD may impair this ability. Visual short-term memory may be influenced by not receiving clear visual information at the initiation of the visual search. Hunt and Bassi[57] found that impairments in contrast sensitivity and visual acuity reduced participants' abilities to retain visual information. With vision slightly blurred and reduced contrast, healthy young and old participants copied initial information incorrectly and had trends toward reduced timed performance during the Digit Symbol test, a paper-and-pencil task of psychomotor speed. Impairments in visual short-term memory may contribute to a driver getting lost because lack of familiarity with or recognition of buildings or objects may not allow for adequate navigational orientation.[58] Mapstone and Weintraub[79] argue that less availability of visual spatial attention may lead to a reliance on object information for navigation, which is a memory-dependent strategy. Therefore the need for object memory and the deficits in visual memory may contribute to the impairments experienced by AD drivers.

Individuals with AD often present initially with complaints of visual loss, difficulties in recognizing objects, deterioration in eye–hand coordination, and topographic disorientation. These impairments in visual processing have been related to higher-order cognitive symptoms and a reduction in functional capacities.[46] A driver fitness-to-drive evaluation should include assessment of visual acuity, peripheral vision, contrast sensitivity, visual processing speed, figure–ground perception, and figure closure. A questionnaire and discussion regarding visual function may prove insightful for the person with dementia, helping with the understanding that driving is impaired. Everyone seems to understand the effects of vision on driving; however, the effects of cognition on driving may be less understood by impaired drivers.

Issues in the Evaluation and Decision-Making Process Regarding Fitness to Drive

Making decisions on fitness to drive may be difficult for health-care professionals. Often health-care professionals' goals are to prolong independence in community mobility. Driving is usually supported until the first incident occurs, such as getting lost, receiving a traffic violation citation, or causing an accident. Ideally, those who work in dementia care strive to prevent the first incident by deciding when the person with dementia should retire from driving. This difficult decision requires knowledge from a variety of sources. Ongoing conversations among occupational therapy (OT) personnel, physicians, and other health-related clinicians who practice in the area of driving and community mobility reflect the complexity of the evaluation procedures and the decision-making process. Past discussions have often focused on the road test as the sole determinant in clients' fitness- to-drive evaluations. Currently, there is a call for therapists to adopt evidence-based assessments for older clients with dementia.[116] Recently, models for driving evaluation have been discussed and promoted.[35,87] No standardized or universally accepted model exists for the decision-making process for clients with dementia, or, for that matter, any older adult with a chronic progressive disorder. Occupational therapists and assistants working in this area struggle with the decision-making process and still have difficulty answering the question of whether the client with dementia should continue to drive, and, if so, for how long.

Too often, therapists and assistants may base decisions on the results of one or two assessments, such as the performance-based road test, or individual psychometric tests such as Trail Making Part B or Useful Field of View. Therapists commonly struggle with the *professional reasoning* and *decision-making process* in regard to older drivers with dementia and the common comorbidities and/or myriad psychosocial issues that accompany these evaluations. Decisions on driving fitness may be made without the occupational therapist reviewing a medical record. This occurs during driving research evaluations where clients are asked to complete a series of assessments followed by a road test. The fitness-to-drive decision is usually based on the road test, and the results of a series of off-road psychometric assessments are later studied to determine whether they are significantly correlated or predictive of the road test results. Professionals using these research methods and outcomes usually are trying to develop predictive tools that can be used to replace the road test. However, they may not be the best practice or approach for the decision-making process in determining fitness to drive.

The objective of the next section of this chapter, therefore, is to put the spotlight on the evaluation, with a focus on the professional reasoning and the decision-making process that are involved in making final recommendations regarding fitness to drive in older adults with dementia. Occupational therapists and assistants are often responsible for providing appropriate guidance and decision making to all who seek their services.[9] The goal is to provide best practice to all clients, including older drivers, as well as caregivers, physicians, law enforcement, licensing agencies, and members of the general public, all of whom might seek guidance from OT personnel regarding the driving ability of individuals diagnosed with dementia. However, we would argue that this decision-making process as currently practiced needs to be more broadly based and comprehensive.

Toward this aim, this section of the chapter introduces the *Multifactor Older Driver with Dementia Evaluation Model* (MODEM), which illustrates the comprehensive components that should be considered to determine a driver with dementia's abilities to continue to drive safely (Figure 20-1). One unique aspect of this approach is that any specific component is not necessarily given more weight than other sources of information. This allows for an individualized approach to fitness-to-drive evaluation that does not rely solely on the performance-based road test. Nor does this model rely on one method of professional reasoning. Rather, it includes comprehensive data collection from many sources, filtered through a system of professional reasoning, to determine an ultimate decision regarding fitness to drive.

Background Research Progression: From Reports to Observed Performance

A body of literature discusses driving and dementia through the lens of trying to establish whether or not this population should be driving or at what stage in the disease process

driving is no longer safe. Moreover, the literature tries to identify one assessment that can be used to make this determination. Research includes caregiver observations and reports regarding crashes, licensing reports of accidents, and actual observations of driving behaviors.

Iverson and colleagues[63] published guidelines for the American Academy of Neurology to determine driving competence for the person with dementia, which include:

- Clinical Dementia Rating Scale (CDR)
- Caregiver report
- History of crashes or traffic citations
- Reduced mileage
- Mini-Mental State Examination scores of 24 or less
- Aggressive/impulsive personality

These guidelines offer information that the MODEM model includes under informant data and cognitive tests. However, MODEM also provides an interprofessional foundation that may provide caregivers and clients with dementia a better understanding of reaching a final decision for driving cessation. MODEM is a tool for making this decision, and, equally important, a tool for explaining driving cessation to impaired older drivers when they have been deemed unfit to drive

Major Categories to be Evaluated and Considered

The major categories that should be evaluated and considered in this fitness-to-drive model include informant data, cognitive status and dementia severity, client factors, the road test, and ethical construct. We cover these components and then embark on a discussion of the various models of professional reasoning and how they may apply to dementia and driving decisions. Case examples are provided to demonstrate the comprehensive aspects of MODEM. We stress that the final decision includes a reexamination of all critical information and may include details of transportation planning, ability to follow up for repeat testing and monitoring, psychosocial factors, and consultation reports from other professionals (e.g.,

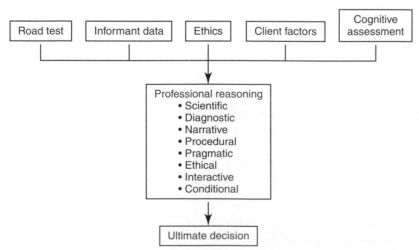

FIGURE 20-1 Multifactor Older Driver with Dementia Evaluation Model (MODEM). (From Schell, B. A. B., & Schell, J. W. [2009]. *Clinical and professional reasoning in occupational therapy.* Philadelphia, PA: Lippincott Williams & Wilkins.)

ophthalmologist, physical therapist) that may address additional problems noted during the evaluation.

Informant Data

The informant is defined as the client, caregiver, physician, or other individual who provides information that may lead to a better understanding of the client's fitness to drive. Informant data may begin with the client's perspective of the driver with dementia's abilities and the driver's beliefs about why he or she is required to participate in a fitness-to-drive evaluation. Some individuals with dementia will stop driving on their own and/or with family or physician encouragement. However, many individuals with dementia lack insight into their disease, and certainly their ability to drive safely. Impaired insight from dementia limits individuals' ability to recognize their limitations and, at times, their difficulties with ADLs. Furthermore, impaired insight often forms an obstacle for acceptance of driving cessation recommendations. Unfortunately, impaired insight may also result in a negative or confrontational interaction between clients and OT personnel during the driver evaluation.

Caregiver informant data includes the client's driving history, which has the potential to be helpful in the evaluation process. Past studies indicated that global measures of driving safety from the caregiver as informant may not be useful in determining who is fit to drive.[15] However, a recent questionnaire study of informants of drivers with dementia who were evaluated in a dementia subspecialty clinic documented that abnormal driving behaviors were observed over 75% of the time in traffic, and 50% of the time the driving of the older adult was rated as fair or poor.[30] Thus, the use of a standardized instrument such as the Driving Habits Questionnaire[99] or a checklist of driving behaviors as provided by Hartford[118] or the American Medical Association (AMA)[123] may be useful in raising concerns or red flags. Caregivers may provide invaluable information that the occupational therapist may have difficulty assessing, such as whether the client has a history of getting lost while driving.

Furthermore, caregiver informants may assist with global assessments of other ADLs. They may report clients' problems with sequencing a cooking activity or forgetting necessary hygiene ADLs. An exploration of instrumental and physical ADLs may serve several purposes. First of all, functional impairment in other ADLs may be a useful proxy to indicate that there could be impairment in the task of driving.[1] Second, some occupational therapists or assistants may be unsure whether their clients have dementia. The AD-8 screen,[43] which relies on a caregiver informant, also utilizes impairments in ADLs and may identify a client with the disorder. Importantly, to meet the criteria in the fifth edition of the *Diagnostic and Statistical Manual of Mental Disorders* (DSM-5) for dementia, impairment in function is usually a requirement and critical factor in making a diagnosis.[11]

The physician should also play a role in the diagnosis of a specific dementia, because subtypes of dementia may require

different approaches and/or follow different courses over time. For instance, the majority of the evidenced-based medicine in the field of dementia and driving is in the area of AD. The hallmark of this disorder is short-term memory loss, and in the very earliest manifestations of the disease, older drivers may still be deemed fit to drive. Eventually executive function, orientation, language, and other cognitive domains may be affected as the disease progresses. Some studies have indicated that the average time a client with AD drives an automobile is about 3 years from disease onset.[19] One recommendation for the average time to retest an AD client who passes a driving evaluation is about 6 months to 1 year, based on longitudinal studies.[34,101]

However, little is known about the clinical course or driving history of clients with vascular dementia (VD), dementia with Lewy bodies (DLB), and/or fronto-temporal dementia (FTD). DLB poses multiple issues because clients may have visual hallucinations, motoric impairment from an extrapyramidal disorder, fluctuations, and a rapid course of progression. Older adults with VD have been noted to have higher impairment rates on road tests in comparison with controls.[40] Similarly, FTD may result in early impairment in attention, impairment of executive function, disinhibition (e.g., road rage), and/or aphasia. A recent study of FTD drivers noted impairments such as improper speed, missing stop signs, and higher rates of crashes.[31]

Thus, the "normal" or "usual" approach to an Alzheimer's client in regard to the driving evaluation may need to be reconsidered in light of fluctuating cognitive and/or behavioral issues that are present in other types of degenerative dementias. These difficulties may not manifest problems during a one-time clinic evaluation or road examination, or present classically from a psychometric standpoint, and the clinician will need to use all available information in the history from the informant and the possibility of rapid progression to make a final decision in regard to traffic safety. This is where collaboration with a neurologist who specializes in dementia can be useful in directing final recommendations for OT personnel who do not have specific expertise in these disease subtypes.

Another area to consider is dementia severity. Some studies have correlated dementia severity with driving performance by using the Clinical Dementia Rating (CDR).[88] This scale rates dementia severity as very mild, mild, moderate, and severe. The CDR requires a reliable informant. Studies in the past have indicated that almost 50% of CDR = 1 (mild) clients with dementia will fail a performance-based road test,[60] and the majority will eventually fail when tested longitudinally.[34] A consensus statement from the Academy of Neurology stated that clients with AD and a CDR = 1 rating should no longer drive.[63] However, this finding was recently challenged by a recent study by Ott and colleagues, where CDR = 1 clients passed a road test and had a low prospective crash rate.[102] However, population-based studies indicate that not only do very few individuals in the community drive at the CDR = 1 or CDR = 2 level, many transition out of driving at the very mild level of CDR = 0.5.[41] We believe evaluation and education need to occur very early in the process once the diagnosis is made. We recommend the use of a standardized severity-rating instrument like the CDR to help guide recommendations.

Dementia can impair a variety of cognitive domains. These include and are not limited to short-term or episodic memory, working memory, orientation, language, visuospatial abilities, processing speed, visual search strategies, insight, executive function, attention, and behavior.

Many key cognitive domains appear to be important for driving and should be considered for measurement by the therapist. Cognitive abilities that have been associated with driving include divided attention/attention switching,[107] selective attention,[124] visual search,[97] visuospatial abilities,[104] verbal and working memory,[15,16] executive function,[42] geographic orientation,[30] and language.[22] Therapists should be most concerned with covering these important cognitive domains, then perhaps the specific type of test that is adopted for the clinic setting. OT assistants should refer to or consult with OTs for definitive evaluation and interpretation of findings if one or more of these cognitive domains are thought to be affected. Areas that appear to influence driving safety include speed of processing time, attention, working memory, judgment, and visuospatial ability. There is a consensus in the literature that tests of these abilities by themselves are not sufficient to determine driving recommendations, but may identify those individuals at increased risk in need of further assessment.[70] However, one should carefully consider whether to recommend driving cessation for drivers with dementia based only on extremely poor performance on a test or tests that are highly correlated with driving impairment (e.g., Trail Making Part B).

Informant data also include comorbidities. Because dementia occurs in an older population, this population may also have other chronic diseases such as diabetes, cancer, heart disease, eye diseases, arthritis, pain, and/or depression. It is necessary to screen for the presence of some of these factors and diseases that may relate to driving abilities. Information learned about these other conditions, such as unaddressed pain or depression, can be communicated back to the physician for treatment as part of the ultimate decision described in MODEM. Additionally, conditions such as limited motor function, balance problems, pain, depression, and decreased ADLs may be acknowledged and referred for follow-up to other health-care professionals. Interdisciplinary communication is a key component of MODEM.

Information about the use of sedating or potentially driver-impairing (PDI) medications may also come from reliable informant data. In older adults with dementia, certain medications may further reduce capacity and increase risk of poor functional performance. As noted earlier, many common medication classes have been studied and are associated with either increased crash risk or impaired driving skills when assessed by simulators or road tests,[74] including narcotics and barbiturates, benzodiazepines, antihistamines, antidepressants, antipsychotics, hypnotics, alcohol, antiepileptic

agents, antiemetic agents, and muscle relaxants. Older adults may have numerous physicians and multiple pharmacies. The occupational therapist should be aware of all routine and as-needed medications. The client and family should be encouraged to work with the pharmacist and/or the primary care physician to try to discontinue or substitute any drugs with the potential to impair driving.

Client Factors

It is essential to remind clients that gathering information is a method for assisting them. Here, questions can reflect clients' occupational profile, tapping into clients' occupational history and their patterns of daily living, interests, values, needs, spirituality, and bodily functions.[9] The therapist's use of therapeutic self during this data-collection process can help calm clients who are vulnerable or anxious. Therapists and assistants may acknowledge contrary viewpoints provided by physicians or caregivers while avoiding confrontation and minimizing confusion. Estimating one's abilities or being aware of one's own areas of deficit can be critical for acceptance of a recommendation to stop driving. Some drivers with dementia will never acknowledge their deficits, and clinicians and family members may reluctantly have to "agree to disagree." A lack of insight is another feature of the evaluation that factors into the ultimate decision about driver recommendations.

Road Test: The Activity Demand of Driving

Demands on attention, visuospatial abilities, motor programming, judgment, memory, sequencing, and speed of information processing make driving a motor vehicle a complex cognitive activity. It is assumed that the task of driving will certainly tap into all of these skills. Historically, occupational therapists have believed that the road test is the gold standard assessment for driving because it is ecologically valid and because they value having clients demonstrate their skills in a naturalistic environment. The road test also operationalizes the demands of driving.[9] A recent publication noted that individuals with dementia who passed a road test had a lower prospective crash rate compared with controls, suggesting that occupational therapists are able to identify safe drivers by this methodology.[97] However, some occupational therapists and assistants who evaluate drivers with dementia may rely exclusively on the road test to determine fitness to drive. Information provided by caregivers, physicians, state driving records, standardized cognitive assessments, or the driver themselves may be ignored because a driver passed a road test provided in an OT driver assessment. This pass (or fail) score usually means that a subjective rating of driving performance was assigned by a driving instructor or an OT practitioner. This score is deemed to equate to the likelihood of future safe (or unsafe) driving performance as measured by crash potential.[60] These global scores are subjective and may have only fair reliability or clinical stability[60] due to the demands and variability of the driving environment.[59]

Although the performance-based road test remains the gold standard for many, it is not without inherent difficulties, such as performance anxiety during testing, unfamiliarity with the testing car in some situations, and testing outside of familiar surroundings—all of which could result in an older adult who is a safe driver being directed to prematurely retire from driving.

Ethics

The *Occupational Therapy Code of Ethics*[8] has several principles that may assist therapists and assistants in this decision-making process. Principle 1 states that OT personnel shall demonstrate a concern for the safety and well-being of the recipients of their services. Therapists and assistants must consider a client's occupational profile and reflect on what strategies will be put in place to promote continuation of occupations and roles when driving is no longer an option. Interventions proposed need to be safe, meaning that transportation options cannot include being "dropped off" in an unfamiliar area or using public transportation independently.

Principle 2 states OT personnel shall take measures to ensure a client's safety and avoid imposing or inflicting harm. The informant data and cognitive assessments may provide a clear decision that the client should not drive. Therefore, we need to consider if it may be placing the client and/or the public in harm's way to require the client to perform a road test when it may not be necessary. For example, per state guidelines in Oregon, therapists do not evaluate individuals on road tests if there are clear indications that it may not be safe to do so. In addition, therapists and assistants who lean toward an unrealistically positive view of all of the data provided and try to prolong driving for impaired clients may be putting those clients and the public at risk. The desire to prolong driving may stem from therapists and assistants being professionally positioned to promote function and possibly to avoid confrontation with a difficult client or situation. Removing independent driving does not fit the profession's overall philosophy. Nevertheless, decision-making must be based on objective findings and reports, not on personal biases or unreasonable, illogical, or optimistic beliefs. Note that chapter 2 provides detailed discussion regarding ethical and legal aspects of OT practice with older adults.

Principle 3 states that OT personnel shall respect recipients and assure their rights. In the context of a driver evaluation, this means that the therapists and assistants must not prematurely discontinue driving when it is safe, be knowledgeable regarding state reporting laws, and educate clients and their families about these laws. Therefore, public policy and state laws may provide some guidance in the decision-making process. Equally important, actions in ensuring recipients' rights include being forthright before the evaluation of the possible outcomes, informing clients of where the results of the evaluation will be sent, and addressing any potential concerns in regard to confidentiality. Although this driver evaluation process can be very stressful, the clinician performing the evaluation needs to constantly remember the rights of the client as a person, which include fair and unbiased decision making and respect for the client throughout the entire process.

Further consideration must be given to the ethical issue of balancing independence and safety. Here, the driver evaluation outcome may be stressful on the occupational therapist or assistant. Russell et al.[109] suggest that a mismatch often exists between idealized and practice-based talk about independence and safety issues that may limit independence. They refer to this dilemma as the "safety clause." The OT practice area of driving and community mobility struggles with this safety clause with each evaluation. Therapists and assistants may believe they are not supporting independence and being client-centered when driving privileges are removed. They face internal ethical struggles in this practice area. Russell et al.[109] conclude that this may be an "inherently systemic" problem and that OT personnel need to take a leading position in the independence-versus-safety issue when providing ethical, client-centered care. Client opposition to therapists' and assistants' recommendations to cease driving may be tempered by jointly developing a plan for transportation options.

Professional Reasoning

Professional reasoning examines converging evidence and differences across assessment methods and attempts to integrate these in the final evaluation.[111] It starts when the therapist or assistant first meets the client and continues through every assessment and encounter with the client. Although Schell[110] describes several types of professional reasoning, we believe a mixed hybrid of approaches makes most sense for fitness-to-drive decision making. Here we describe some types of professional reasoning and how they apply to driving. However, we recommend reading Schell and Schell[111] for a deeper understanding of the various types that we have applied to MODEM.

Scientific Reasoning

This approach assists the therapist in identifying problems and guides the decision-making process. It considers the stage of the disease and evidence from research regarding individuals with dementia and their driver evaluation outcomes. It scientifically examines the results of evidence-based assessments[111] and how these influence the final decision. Scientific reasoning removes therapist individual biases associated with the decision-making process as it prioritizes the evidence and scientific reasoning in determining the final recommendations.

Diagnostic Reasoning

This perspective uses both personal and impersonal information from clients and their informants.[111] Here, all informant data are considered, plus clinical assessments and the results of the road test. This is sometimes the most common form of reasoning focused on the driving evaluation, but should not be the only method. Information gathered from informants through questionnaires and from performance on clinical assessments and the road test is certainly key in determining outcome. However, how we synthesize this information as clinicians to arrive at a final recommendation is based on not one type of reasoning, but in fact a combination of many facets.

Narrative Reasoning

How many therapists really listen to the client's particular story?[111] This not only takes time, but the ability to perceive the world clearly from differing viewpoints. OT personnel should develop a picture of how driving affects quality of life for each client and an understanding of which other forms of transportation are acceptable to the client. Therapists and assistants mentally consider options for support and networks as they listen to what individuals need to do in the community. Furthermore, clients may not be able to understand how scores on assessments relate to driving ability. Therefore, throughout the process, therapists should apply communication strategies to relate findings appropriate to each client's individual needs. When appropriate, the stage should be set to progress the client toward eventual acceptance of discontinuation of driving. This is vital because even if a driver with dementia is deemed "fit" in the early stages of the disease, the condition will progress and driving retirement becomes inevitable. Therefore, the initial evaluation can "prepare" the client and family that the "time is coming" and perhaps will allow for a higher degree of acceptability when driving cessation is recommended. In fact, there is some data to indicate that drivers with dementia who pass road tests appear to modify their driving with subsequent reduced crash rates.[96] Knowing and understanding the client and his or her viewpoints help this process develop in a more constructive and therapeutic manner.

Ultimate Decision

In many ways, drivers with dementia are in a category of their own in regard to driving evaluations and recommendations. The following specific constructs and theories pertain to establishing criteria for decision making in regard to driving ability for this particular population according to MODEM:

a. **Compatibility**: A review of the dementia and driving literature shows that the diagnosis of dementia contributes to knowing that the problems drivers demonstrate will progress to a point where functional performance is greatly impaired. We know that the diagnosis itself highlights memory loss in the early stages, and even mild memory loss may lead to drivers getting lost.[58] Caregiver report provides insight into how the person is driving outside the OT evaluation and may include information regarding getting lost and recent accidents. Cognitive and perceptual assessments used in the evaluation are evidence-based for dementia and contribute to information on the key functional domains that are necessary for driving. Finally, the road test is the part of the evaluation

that provides actual observable data in a realistic environment setting, not just in the clinical setting.

b. **Complexity**: The many factors described earlier are considered and included in an overall evaluation of determining fitness to drive. Other factors such as clients' roles, values, context, routines, quality of life, and caregiver issues assist with the recommendations provided in the final decision. For example, an evaluation that leads to assistance with transportation particular to a client is an example of one such outcome.

c. **Advantage:** MODEM is inclusive of all components of the *Occupational Therapy Practice Framework*, third edition.[9] MODEM provides therapists with the domains and a holistic process for providing excellent practice in regard to driving and community mobility. Not only is the evaluation in the model, but the therapist's decision, intervention, follow-up, and referrals to other services are emphasized. This model stresses a true client- and caregiver-centered approach, with a multitude of individual foci along the way that are considered as part of the decision-making and counseling process.

d. **Professional Reasoning**: All factors and assessment results must be guided by professional reasoning approaches (e.g., scientific, narrative, diagnostic). Professional ethics should play an equal role in the decision-making process, with the principle of "do no harm" being emphasized throughout. This means that clients, caregivers, and the public are protected as plans are made for continued community mobility. Driving cessation is never ideal, yet occupational therapists must use problem-solving skills and the therapeutic self to assist with developing the best transportation plan possible.

MODEM also requires an emphasis on follow-up with client, family, and physicians regarding transportation issues and psychosocial factors such as depression. It requires that OT personnel make the appropriate referrals and take the next step beyond assessment to providing actual recommendations that surface throughout the evaluation process.

After Driving Cessation

Driving cessation is particularly problematic for those individuals with dementia. Due to memory impairments and geographic disorientation, these individuals are not candidates for typical unescorted public transportation or other community mobility options. Even when transportation is set up to be door-to-door, meaning that someone will escort the individual from home to the destination and back home, problems may occur. For example, the client with dementia may not remember that these arrangements have been made. The client may refuse to allow the person into his or her home due to fear and forgetfulness that this person was designated to provide escorted transportation. In addition, the client may have comorbidities that may compromise physical endurance and the capabilities required for a community outing if the person providing the transportation is unfamiliar with these issues.

A pilot project at Pacific University's School of Occupational Therapy showed that escorted public transportation may be beneficial through the use of transportation coaches. In this project, four OT students partnered with Ride Connection. Ride Connection provides a wide array of transportation services to older adults and people with disabilities living in the Portland, Oregon, area, from door-to-door rides to teaching people how to use public transportation to vehicle-sharing programs. Students established rapport with older adults living in an assistive care facility in Washington County, Oregon, and together planned outings in the community using public transportation. The older adults were identified as having very mild memory problems; a diagnosis of dementia was not provided.

The older adults reported learning that public transportation was not "scary" when they were accompanied by someone they trusted. In addition, they reported looking forward to the scheduled outings with the students. Residents stated that they enjoyed the freedom of going to places of choice rather than trips planned by the assistive care facility. The students reported extensively researching the routes and noting walking distances from one place to the next, inclines of the walking routes, and whether or not there were benches to sit on while waiting for a bus; planning for increment weather; and planning for emergency transportation, such as a taxi when a bus failed to arrive as scheduled. Cell phones were a must.

Students also learned that older adults may try to exert themselves too much and that the students needed to request frequent breaks. Establishing trained transportation coaches may be a way for older adults living in assistive care facilities to gain individualized community mobility. The facility van may be used to take the resident and transportation coach to a bus or metro system stop where community outings may then be more personalized. Facility pickup arrangements follow at the end of the public transportation outing.

Occupational therapists and assistants must design reasonable transportation options with clients and caregivers. Hunt[56] used a template that listed all the destinations that the client needed and wanted to go to with corresponding individuals to help with each particular transportation outing. For example, the working adult son/daughter may take the parent out to the grocery store in the evenings or on weekends, as well as to physician appointments. The grandson/granddaughter may take the grandparent to the movies, out to lunch, or to the hair salon/barber. The place of worship might provide transportation for services, and a friend might provide transportation for social gatherings. Hunt[56] found, during follow-up phone conversations, that caregivers and the older adult spent more quality time together due to the "car time." Coming up with these options is more difficult when a spouse, family, and friends are not available. A brief list of some of the national organizations that provide community mobility options for older adults is as follows:

- Medical Transportation Management, Inc. (http://www.mtm-inc.net)—Provides nonemergency transportation for the disabled, underserved, and older adult populations through contracting with local, private, and public transportation providers.
- Area Agency on Aging (AAA; http://www.n4a.org)—Provides links to local AAA regarding transportation services in specific communities.
- Independent Transportation Network America (http://www.itnamerica.org)—Provides rides with door-to-door, arm-through-arm service to thousands of seniors nationwide by allowing older people to trade their own cars to pay for rides, and enabling volunteer drivers to store transportation credits for their own future transportation needs.

See Carr[20] for a discussion of driving cessation and community options.

CASE EXAMPLE 20-1   Mr. Miller

Bob Miller is a 63-year-old retired machinist, who requires services due to recently having had a transient ischemia attack (TIA). The physician determined that all signs of the TIA have resolved. However, Bob's family members have noticed changes because he now lives with his son and his son's family. For example, Bob was working on a project in the garage and it ignited into a small fire. Bob did not respond and instead his son who was present extinguished the fire. The family also noted that Bob had become more withdrawn. He went back to his physician, who determined that Bob was depressed and recommended medication. Bob refused. The family is now questioning Bob's ability to drive. He was referred for an occupational therapy driving evaluation. The occupational therapist noted that the mild depression and refusal to take medications were stated in the medical record, as were the family members' concerns about Bob's cognitive status.

The driver evaluation showed the following results:
- Score of 5 on the Short Blessed Exam
- Trail Making Test Part B completed in 115 seconds (at a level of concern)
- No impairments in visual acuity, field of view, proprioception, figure closure, Clock Drawing Test, visual memory, traffic sign recognition, muscle strength, and joint range of motion. The clinic does not have a road test.

Caregiver report stated that client has not driven in the 3 months since the mild stroke. Family members do not believe Bob should drive due to the garage fire incident. Additionally, he does not seem to have any energy or stamina. He rarely goes outside, sits around, and sometimes will go into the garage if his son is also there working on a project. Bob voiced that he wants to drive to visit an old friend who lives about 5 miles away. He became teary

Continued

CASE EXAMPLE 20-1 Mr. Miller—cont'd

eyed when he spoke about his pending new grandchild, an event he has been looking forward to experiencing.

Taking into account all the information present, the therapist believes that she needs to address the family's concerns and the wishes of the client. She also considers that there is no documentation of dementia in the chart. Bob passed all of the cognitive assessments and all scores were within normal ranges. However, depression may cause cognitive impairments and reduced reaction time. The therapist explains to the family that it may be the depression that is affecting Bob's abilities. The therapist counseled the client to follow his physician's advice and take the antidepressant medication. This would have the potential benefit of improving his affect, stamina, and alertness, and perhaps his functional abilities. The client and family agreed with this approach and to follow up with a repeat evaluation in 2 months. The therapist also suggested an exercise program of walking for the client. She explained the benefits of getting fresh air and exercise for cognitive well-being. She provided a schedule and goals that Bob could achieve in the area where Bob lives with his son—the area has neighborhood streets with sidewalks, providing a safe environment for the walking plan. Bob's son said that they have a dog that would love the walking as well.

The client and family returned in 6 weeks. His Short Blessed Exam score was a 4 and the Trail Making Test Part B was completed in 100 seconds. The client stated he had been compliant with his medication and that he was walking 20 to 30 minutes a day. His son reported that he bought his dad new walking shoes. Miller spoke about his new grandson without becoming teary eyed. The therapist recommended driving lessons to assist his traffic skills because the client had not driven for a while. The lessons would also serve as further evaluation of Bob's ability to drive. The family agreed. The client stated that he did not need lessons because he has driven all his life. However, he did finally agree when his son stated it would make everyone feel more confident in his ability to drive. The therapist stated that she would provide the information for contacting

an occupational therapist who is a driver educator. The therapist also noted that she would follow up with the client, family, and driver educator for a final recommendation after reviewing all of the information.

This case study reveals how the occupational therapist used the Multifactor Older Driver with Dementia Evaluation Model (MODEM). She problem solved beyond just the specific scores or components of a routine driver evaluation. Typically, a therapist would have examined the assessments and would have most likely passed this client, had a complete assessment that included road testing been performed. However, it is also possible that due to depression or perhaps unfamiliarity with the car, this client might have failed. Thus, his social mobility would likely have been worsened, his confidence further reduced, and, possibly, his depression or low mood further escalated. The therapist examined all of the information gathered from the client, family, physician, and assessments to design a specific lifestyle intervention. In this case, depression needed to be addressed. Ethical reasoning was applied by explaining to the client and his family that the depression may be creating some impairment in the client's thinking. Explanations of the benefits of antidepressive medications and the relationship between depression and impairment were provided. The client was therefore informed of all the possibilities.

The postponement of driving was explained, and the client and family seemed to agree that it was a fair decision. In addition, the therapist advocated for the client to engage in activities that would make him feel more in control. Exercise was recommended, and opportunities for the client to visit his friend were also emphasized. Not only was the driving issue addressed, but the client's depression and lack of meaningful activity engagement was also considered and improved. Using MODEM, the occupational therapist turned the driver evaluation into a multistep process that in this case did not even require an on-road test. Therapists must consider that decisions may proceed in steps or increments as information is received and reviewed.

CASE EXAMPLE 20-2 Mrs. Beck

Mrs. Beck is 74 years old. She lives alone. She has a daughter who lives 5 miles from her home and a son who lives out of town. She has been newly diagnosed with mild Alzheimer's disease. Her physician referred her to an occupational therapist for a driver evaluation because she has become lost while driving in familiar areas and has had a minor accident this past year. The circumstances of the accidents are unclear because the daughter noticed the rear light recently broken on Mrs. Beck's vehicle. Mrs. Beck does not recall what caused the broken light. All of this information was provided to the therapist before the evaluation through a physician report and a caregiver survey, which is mailed out to caregivers for completion.

On the day of the driver evaluation, Mrs. Beck arrives with a close friend and is not accompanied by her daughter.

Mrs. Beck explained that her daughter was busy and could not drive her to the appointment. The therapist excuses herself and calls the daughter on the phone. The daughter explains that her mother refused to allow the daughter to bring her and wanted her best friend to take her, probably to put her driving in a positive light.

The assessments showed the following important information: inability to complete Trail Making Part B; a score of 10 on the Short Blessed Test; and a score of 4 out of 7 on the Clock Drawing Test because she had numerous errors in the last quadrant and had difficulty identifying the merging traffic symbol sign, although she was able to identify the other traffic symbols such as stop, no right turn, and others. The therapist doubted the client's ability to drive. However, on the way out to take the in-car road test, the therapist decided to talk to Mrs. Beck's friend in private. The friend said she drives with Mrs. Beck all the time and is unaware of problems. "Sure, she has some forgetfulness, but she drives fine," the friend stated. When asked about the "accident," the friend stated that Mrs. Beck lives in a neighborhood where she has to parallel park on the street and she probably just got too close to the car behind her. "That could happen to anyone," the friend noted. "Her daughter is just too controlling."

The therapist then took Mrs. Beck for a 45-minute driving assessment. Although Mrs. Beck drove well below the speed limit and needed some prompting to proceed at intersections, she appeared to drive within the limits of what the occupational therapist believed to be reasonably safe, meaning she did not have a violation. She did need a verbal cue to check traffic before switching lanes, but there was no traffic present in the lane. The therapist assessed her parallel parking skills and gave her some tips about lining up the vehicle and when to use mirrors for cues.

The therapist concluded that she could only assess what the client presented to her while the client drove, and therefore passed Mrs. Beck on the evaluation. In addition, she believed that the friend's report mirrored what she experienced and observed during the driving assessment. The

therapist believed that the validity of the in-car road test showed that the client could drive. Decisions should be based on doing the actual activity, the therapist believed, and not based on a diagnosis. The next day the daughter called in anger and the physician called to question the report sent to him.

This is an example of a therapist basing the decision to drive only on one assessment, the in-car road test. Looking at MODEM, the informant information was not considered, such as the physician's diagnosis and concerns, and the daughter's report of her mother getting lost and having an accident. Furthermore, the therapist did not consider the implications of the cognitive assessments. All of these tests have research to support an association with driving fitness. Instead, the decision to continue driving was based on an in-car road test that may not have challenged Mrs. Beck's driving ability due to the nature of the traffic experienced at the time. Finally, the therapist believed the information from the friend, which may have been biased. Adult children may be more accurate reporters of driving ability than spouses, possibly because of less personal bias, but the reasons behind this discrepancy need further investigation.[14]

Summary

The decision that an occupational therapist makes to determine driving fitness for individuals with dementia is intricate and often involves complex decision making. MODEM attempts to assist therapists through this process. Dementia is a complicated and variable disease. Individuals may fluctuate and demonstrate variability on any given day, further reducing the reliability of psychometric and road testing. MODEM holds promise by providing occupational therapists performing driver evaluations with a tool that is comprehensive and holistic in nature. The MODEM approach offers professional reasoning using the many types of data collected during the driver evaluation. It is based on the main principle of the *Occupational Therapy Code of Ethics*[8], first do no harm. In addition, it captures the necessity of providing counseling to clients and caregivers, and referrals to other health-care providers, for optimal OT practice.[9]

Therapists voice a common heartfelt concern that they want the cognitive assessment results, physician reports, and caregiver reports to match the road test results. We emphasize the importance of improving how decisions are made for driver fitness when disparity exists in the evaluation findings. Our hope is that this model will guide the decision-making process and bring better satisfaction to our clients who seek driver-fitness information. It is our goal that MODEM will be supported by future research that empirically tests this approach. Correctly deciding if individuals with dementia should continue driving will only grow in importance with the rapidly increasing older population. Occupational therapists and assistants must partner with physicians and other informants to be prepared to help make the best decisions

possible for this group of individuals. Additionally, therapists and assistants with a passion for working with older adults regarding their driving skills may obtain Specialty Certification in Driving and Community Mobility, a process provided through the American Occupational Therapy Association.[10] This OT specialty practice area emerged in the past decade; with the projected increase in the number of older adults, many of whom drive, the potential for integration into an existing service, or developing this as a separate practice may be of particular interest.

REVIEW QUESTIONS

1. Explain why all occupational therapists working with older clients need to address the instrumental activity of daily living—community mobility.
2. Elaborate on how the diagnosis of dementia affects professional reasoning in determining fitness to drive.
3. The *Occupational Therapy Practice Framework: Domain and Process*, third edition, refers to an OT process that includes evaluation and intervention. Regarding a driver evaluation when using MODEM, what would the process look like?
4. An occupational therapist with no experience related to a driving evaluation receives a referral from a physician stating that he would like the client with frailty and possible dementia specifically evaluated for driving capacity. The client is presently being seen for a primary diagnosis of osteoporosis and post–hip surgery. The therapist decides to contact the hospital librarian for information regarding driving evaluations for clients with frailty. What

type of professional reasoning is the occupational therapist using?

5. Explain the dangers of driving with memory loss.

6. You are working in an acute hospital setting with a client who has had heart surgery and has a history of dementia. However, he was driving before his heart surgery. He is very weak and presently confused. He will be transferred to a skilled nursing facility in 2 days. You talk to his family about driving once he returns home to live with his daughter. You provide the name of an occupational therapist who specializes in driver evaluations. This is an example of what type of professional reasoning?

REFERENCES

1. Ackerman, M. L., Edwards, J. D., Ross, L. A., et al. (2008). Examination of cognitive and instrumental functional performance as indicators for driving cessation risk across 3 years. *The Gerontologist, 48*(6), 802–810.

2. Adams, H. P., Jr., Bendixen, B. H., Kappelle, L. J., et al. (1993). Classification of subtype of acute ischemic stroke. Definitions for use in a multicenter clinical trial. TOAST. Trial of Org 10172 in Acute Stroke Treatment. *Stroke, 24*(1), 35–41.

3. Ahmad, A., & Spear, P. D. (1993). Effects of aging on the size, density, and number of rhesus monkey lateral geniculate neurons. *Journal of Comparative Neurology, 334*(4), 631–643. DOI: 10.1002/cne.90334410

4. Akinwuntan, A. E., De Weerdt, W., Feys, H., et al. (2005). Effect of simulator training on driving after stroke: a randomized controlled trial. *Neurology, 65*(6), 843–850.

5. Alvi, A., & Lee, S. E. (2006). Putting sleep apnea to rest. Tailored therapy reduces fatigue-related risks. *Postgrad Med, 119*(3), 46–53.

6. Alzheimer's Association. (2015). *2015 Alzheimer's disease facts and figures.* http://www.alz.org/facts/overview.asp/. Accessed June 18, 2015.

7. American Geriatrics Society. (2012). American Geriatrics Society updated Beers Criteria for potentially inappropriate medication use in older adults. *Journal of the American Geriatric Society, 60*(4), 616–631.

8. American Occupational Therapy Association. (2000). Occupational Therapy Code of Ethics (2000). *American Journal of Occupational Therapy, 54*(6), 614–616.

9. American Occupational Therapy Association. (2014). Occupational Therapy Practice Framework: Domain and process. *American Journal of Occupational Therapy, 68*(Suppl. 1), s1–s48.

10. American Occupational Therapy Association. (n.d.) *Specialty certification in driving and community mobility.* http://www. aota.org/Education-Careers/Advance-Career/Board-Specialty-Certifications/Driving-Community-Mobility.aspx#sthash. K6LxfdEs.dpuf/. Accessed August 17, 2015.

11. American Psychiatric Association. (2013). *Major Neurocognitive Disorders, in Diagnostic and statistical manual of mental disorders: DSM-5. 2013.* Washington, D.C: American Psychiatric Association.

12. Ball, K. K., Roenker, D. L., Wadley, V. G., et al. (2006). Can high-risk older drivers be identified through performance-based measures in a Department of Motor Vehicles setting? *Journal of the American Geriatric Society, 54*(1), 77–84.

13. Bassi, C. J. & Lehmkuhle, S. (1990). Clinical implications of parallel visual pathways. *Journal of the American Optometric Association, 61*(2), 98–110.

14. Bixby, K., Davis, J. D., & Ott, B. R. (2015). Comparing caregiver and clinician predictions of fitness to drive in people with Alzheimer's disease. *American Journal of Occupational Therapy, 69*(3), 6903270030p1–6903270030p7.

15. Brown, L. B., Ott, B. R, Papandonatos, G. D, et al. (2005). Prediction of on-road driving performance in patients with early Alzheimer's disease. *Journal of the American Geriatric Society, 53*(1), 94–98.

16. Brown, L. B., Stern, R. A, Cahn-Weiner, D. A, et al. (2005). Driving scenes test of the Neuropsychological Assessment Battery (NAB) and on-road driving performance in aging and very mild dementia. *Archives of Clinical Neuropsychology, 20*(2), 209–215.

17. Campbell, M. K., Bush, T. L. & Hale, W. E. (1993). Medical conditions associated with driving cessation in community-dwelling, ambulatory elders. *Journal of Gerontology, 48*(4), S230–S234.

18. Canadian Medical Association. (2012). *CMA driver's guide: Determining medical fitness to operate motor vehicles,* (8th ed.). Accessed 10/22/15. http://www.cma.ca/En/Pages/drivers-guide.aspx/.

19. Carr, D. B, (1997). Motor vehicle crashes and drivers with DAT. *Alzheimer Disease and Associated Disorders, 11*(Suppl. 1), 38–41.

20. Carr, D. B. (2008). *Current knowledge on medical fitness-to-drive: The role of the clinician. Presented at the meeting of the AAA Foundation for Traffic Safety Conference.*

21. Carr, D. B., Flood, K., Steger-May, K., et al. (2006). Characteristics of frail older adult drivers. *Journal of the American Geriatric Society, 54*(7), 1125–1129.

22. Carr, D. B., LaBarge, E., Dunnigan, K., et al. (1998). Differentiating drivers with dementia of the Alzheimer type from healthy older persons with a Traffic Sign Naming test. *The Journal of Gerontology: Biological Sciences & Medical Sciences, 53*(2), M135–M139.

23. Carr, D. B., & Ott, B. R. (2010). The older adult driver with cognitive impairment: "It's a very frustrating life". *Journal of the American Medical Association, 303*(16), 1632–1641.

24. Carr, D., Schmader, K., Bergman, C., et al. (1991). A multidisciplinary approach in the evaluation of demented drivers referred to geriatric assessment centers. *Journal of the American Geriatric Society, 39*(11), 1132–1136.

25. Centers for Disease Control and Prevention. (2015a). *Osteoarthritis. prevalence.* http://www.cdc.gov/arthritis/basics/osteoarthritis.html/. Accessed June 18, 2015.

26. Centers for Disease Control and Prevention, (2015b). *Stroke.* http://www.cdc.gov/stroke/. Accessed June 18, 2015.

27. Centers for Disease Control and Prevention. (2015c). *Stroke Facts.* Accessed October 22, 2015. http://www.cdc.gov/stroke/facts.html/.

28. Centers for Disease Control and Prevention. (2015d). *Trends in vision and hearing among older americans.* http://www.cdc.gov/nchs/data/ahcd/agingtrends/02vision.pdf/. Accessed June 18, 2015.

29. Charlton, D. J., et al. (2010). *Influence of chronic illness on crash involvement of motor vehicle drivers.* Melbourne, Australia: Monash University, Accident Research Centre.

30. Croston, J., Meuser, T. M., Berg-Weger, M., et al. (2009). Driving retirement in older adults with dementia. *Topics in Geriatric Rehabilitation, 25*(2), 154–162.

31. de Simone, V., Kaplan, L., Patronas, N., et al. (2007). Driving abilities in frontotemporal dementia patients. *Dementia and Geriatric Cognitive Disorders, 23*(1), 1–7.

32. Dobbs, B. M. (2005). *Medical conditions and driving: Current knowledge, Final Report Association for the Advancement of Automotive Medicine. (DTNH22-94-G-05297).* Washington, DC: National Highway Traffic Safety Administration.

33. Drachman, D. A. & Swearer, J. M. (1993). Driving and Alzheimer's disease: the risk of crashes. *Neurology, 43*(12), 2448–2456.

34. Duchek, J. M., Carr, D. B, Hunt, L., et al. (2003). Longitudinal driving performance in early-stage dementia of the Alzheimer type. *Journal of the American Geriatrics Society, 51*(10), 1342–1347.

35. Ekelman, B. A., et al. (2009). Community mobility, in functional performance in older adults. In B. R. Bonder & V. D. Bello-Haas (Eds.), Philadelphia, PA: F. A. Davis.

36. Ellen, R., Marshall, S. C, Palayew, M., et al. (2006). Systematic review of motor vehicle crash risk in persons with sleep apnea. *Journal of Clinical Sleep Medicine, 2*(2), 193–200.

37. Engum, E.S, Lambert, E.W., Scott, K., Pendergrass, T.M., & Womac, J. (1989). Criterion-related validity of the Cognitive Behavioral Driver's Inventory. *Cognitive Rehabilitation, 7*(4), 22–31.

38. Faye, E. (1994). *Clinical low vision.* (2nd ed.), Boston, MA: Little Brown & Co.

39. Fisk, G. D., Owsley, C., & Pulley, L. V. (1997). Driving after stroke: Driving exposure, advice, and evaluations. *Archives of physical medicine and rehabilitation, 78*(12), 1338–1345.

40. Fitten, L. J., Perryman, K. M., Wilkinson, C. J., et al. (1995). Alzheimer and vascular dementias and driving: A prospective road and laboratory study. *Journal of the American Medical Association, 273*(17), 1360–1365.

41. Foley, D. J., Masaki, K. H., Ross, G. W., et al. (2000). Driving cessation in older men with incident dementia. *Journal of the American Geriatrics Society, 48*(8), 928–930.

42. Freund, B., et al. (2005). Drawing clocks and driving cars: Use of brief tests of cognition to screen driving competency in older adults. *Journal of General Internal Medicine, 20*(3), 240–244.

43. Galvin, J., Roe, C. M., Powlishta, K. K., et al. (2005). The AD8 A brief informant interview to detect dementia. *Neurology, 65*(4), 559–564.

44. Garbarino, S., Nobili, L., Beelke, M., et al. (2001). The contributing role of sleepiness in highway vehicle accidents. *Sleep, 24*(2), 203–206.

45. George, C. (2001). Reduction in motor vehicle collisions following treatment of sleep apnoea with nasal CPAP. *Thorax, 56*(7), 508–512.

46. Glosser, G. & Grossman, M. (2004). *Reading and Visual Processing in Alzheimer's Disease.* In: Cronin-Golomb A, Hof PR (eds): Vision in Alzheimer's Disease. Basel: Karger, pp 236-247.

47. Go, A. S., Mozaffarian, D., Roger, V. L., et al. (2013). Heart disease and stroke statistics—2013 update: a report from the American Heart Association. *Circulation, 127*(1), e6–e245.

48. He, J., Kryger, M. H., Zorick, F. J., et al. (1988). Mortality and apnea index in obstructive sleep apnea. Experience in 385 male patients. *Chest, 94*(1), 9–14.

49. Heron, G., Charman, W. N. & Gray, L. S. (1999). Accommodation responses and ageing. *Investigative Ophthalmology and Visual Science, 40*, 2872–2883.

50. Hetland, A. & Carr, D. B. (2014a). Medications and impaired driving. *Annals of Pharmacotherapy, 48*(4), 494–506.

51. Hetland, A. & Carr, D. B. (2014b). Medications and Impaired Driving, *Annals of Pharmacotherapy, 48*(4), 494–506.

52. Hetland, A. J., Carr, D. B., Wallendorf, M. J., et al. (2014). Potentially driver-impairing (PDI) medication use in medically impaired adults referred for driving evaluation. *Annals of Pharmacotherapy, 48*(4), 476–482.

53. Higgins, J. P., Wright, S. W. & Wrenn, K. D. (1996). Alcohol, the elderly, and motor vehicle crashes. *American Journal of Emergency Medicine, 14*(3), 265–267.

54. Holroyd, S. (2004). *Visual hallucinations in Alzheimer's disease* in: Cronin-Golomb A, Hof PR (eds): Vision in Alzheimer's Disease. Basel: Karger, pp 126-136.

55. Howard, M. E., Desai, A. V., Grunstein, R. R., et al. (2004). Sleepiness, sleep-disordered breathing, and accident risk factors in commercial vehicle drivers. *American Journal of Respiratory and Critical Care Medicine, 170*(9), 1014–1021.

56. Hunt, L. A. (2001). *G9: Remediation through adaptive equipment and training.* Washington, DC: National Highway Traffic Safety Administration.

57. Hunt, L. A. & Bassi, C. J. (2010). Near-vision acuity levels and performance on neuropsychological assessments used in occupational therapy. *American Journal of Occupational Therapy, 64*(1), 105–113.

58. Hunt, L. A., Brown, A. E., & Gilman, I. P. (2010). Drivers with dementia and outcomes of becoming lost while driving. *American Journal of Occupational Therapy, 64*(2), 225–232.

59. Hunt, L. A., Murphy, C. F., Carr, D., et al. (1997a). Environmental cueing may effect performance on a road test for drivers with dementia of the Alzheimer type. *Alzheimer Disease and Associated Disorders, 11*(Suppl. 1), 13–16.

60. Hunt, L. A., Murphy, C. F., Carr, D., et al. (1997b). Reliability of the Washington University Road Test: A performance-based assessment for drivers with dementia of the Alzheimer type. *Archives of Neurology, 54*(6), 707–712.

61. Hunt, L. A., & Weston , K. (1999). *Assessment of driving capacity.* In P. A. Lichtenberg (Ed.), *Handbook of geriatric assessment.* New York, NY: John Wiley & Sons, Inc.

62. Insurance Institute for Highway Safety and Highway Loss Data Institute. (December 2014). *Older drivers.* http://www.iihs.org/iihs/topics/laws/olderdrivers?topicName=older-drivers/. Accessed December 9, 2014.

63. Iverson, D. J., Gronseth, G. S., Reger, M. A., et al. (2010). Practice Parameter update: Evaluation and management of driving risk in dementia: Report of the Quality Standards Subcommittee of the American Academy of Neurology. *Neurology, 74*(16), 1316–1324.

64. Johansson, K., Bryding, G., Dahl, M. L., et al. (1997). Traffic dangerous drugs are often found in fatally injured older male drivers. *Journal of the American Geriatric Society, 45*(8), 1029–1031.

65. Johns, M. W. (1991). A new method for measuring daytime sleepiness: the Epworth sleepiness scale. *Sleep, 14*(6), 540–545.

66. Kent, R., Funk, J., & Crandall, J. (2003). How future trends in societal aging, air bag availability, seat belt use, and fleet composition will affect serious injury risk and occurrence in the United States. *Traffic Injury Prevention, 4*(1), 24–32.

67. Kline, D. W., Kline, T. J., Fozard, J. L., et al. (1992). Vision, aging, and driving: the problems of older drivers. *Journal of Gerontology, 47*(1), P27–P34.

68. Koepsell, T. D., Wolf, M. E., McCloskey, L., et al. (1994). Medical conditions and motor vehicle collision injuries in older adults. *Journal of the American Geriatric Society, 42*(7), 695–700.

69. Korner-Bitensky, N. A., Mazer, B. L., Sofer, S., et al. (2000). Visual testing for readiness to drive after stroke: a multicenter study. *American Journal of Physical Medicine & Rehabilitation, 79*(3), 253–259.

70. Langford, J. (2008). Usefulness of off-road screening tests to licensing authorities when assessing older driver fitness to drive. *Traffic Injury Prevention*, 9(4), 328–335.

71. Legh-Smith, J., Wade, D. T., & Hewer, R. L. (1986). Driving after a stroke. *Journal of the Royal Society of Medicine*, 79(4), 200–203.

72. LeRoy, A. A., & Morse, M. L. (2008). *Multiple medications and vehicle crashes: analysis of databases*. Final report. Washington, DC: NTSA

73. Lock, S. et al. (2005). Work after stroke: focusing on barriers and enablers. *Disability & Society*, 20(1), 33–47.

74. Lococo, K., & Tyree, K. (2003). *Medication-related impaired driving. Walgreen Health Services*. https://webapp.walgreens.com/cePharmacy/viewpdf?fileName=transportation_tech.pdf/. Accessed June 18, 2015.

75. Lundberg, C., Caneman, G., Samuelsson, S. M., et al. (2003). The assessment of fitness to drive after a stroke: the Nordic Stroke Driver Screening Assessment. *Scandinavian Journal of Psychology*, 44(1), 23–30.

76. Lundqvist, A., Gerdle, B., & Ronnberg, J. (2000). Neuropsychological aspects of driving after a stroke—in the simulator and on the road. *Applied cognitive psychology*, 14(2), 135–150.

77. Lynott, J., & Figuieredo, C. (2011). *How the travel patterns of older adults are changing: Highlights from the 2009 National Household Travel Survey*. http://assets.aarp.org/rgcenter/ppi/liv-com/fs218-transportation.pdf. Accessed June 18, 2015.

78. Mansfield, D. R., Gollogly, N. C., Kaye, D. M., et al. (2004). Controlled trial of continuous positive airway pressure in obstructive sleep apnea and heart failure. *American Journal of Respiratory and Critical Care Medicine*, 169(3), 361–366.

79. Mapstone, N., & Weintraub, S. (2004). *Closing the window of spatial attention: Effects on Navigational Cue Use In Alzheimer's Disease*. Cronin-Golomb A, Hof PR (eds): Vision in Alzheimer's Disease. *Interdisciplinary Topics in Gerontology*. Basel, Karger, 2004, vol 34, pp 290-304 (DOI:10.1159/000080014)

80. Marottoli, R. A., Cooney, L. M. Jr, Wagner, R., et al. (1994). Predictors of automobile crashes and moving violations among elderly drivers. *Annals of Internal Medicine*, 121(11), 842–846.

81. Marottoli, R. A., Ostfeld, A. M., Merrill, S. S., et al. (1993). Driving cessation and changes in mileage driven among elderly individuals. *Journal of Gerontology*, 48(5), S255–S260.

82. Marshall, S. C. (2008). The role of reduced fitness to drive due to medical impairments in explaining crashes involving older drivers. *Traffic Injury Prevention*, 9(4), 291–298.

83. Maycock, G. (1996). Sleepiness and driving: The experience of UK car drivers. *J Sleep Res*, 5(4), 229–237.

84. Mazer, B. L., Korner-Bitensky, N. A., & Sofer, S. (1998). Predicting ability to drive after stroke. *Archives of Physical Medicine and Rehabilitation*, 79(7), 743–750.

85. McGwin, G., Sims, R. V., Pulley, L., et al. (2000). Relations among chronic medical conditions, medications, and automobile crashes in the elderly: a population-based case-control study. *American Journal of Epidemiology*, 152(5), 424–431.

86. Medical News Today. (2007). *Risk of severe car crashes greatly increased in sleep apnea patients*. http://www.medicalnewstoday.com/articles/71543.php/. Accessed June 18, 2015.

87. Meuser, T. M., Carr, D. B., Berg-Weger, M., et al. (2006). Driving and dementia in older adults: Implementation and evaluation of a continuing education project. *The Gerontologist*, 46(5), 680–687.

88. Morris, J. C. (1993). The Clinical Dementia Rating (CDR): Current version and scoring rules. *Neurology*, 43(11), 2412–2414.

89. Morse, A. R. (1992). *Vision Problems and Vision Care in Nursing Homes*. In: B. P. Rosenthal & R. Cole (Eds.), Problems in optometry. Philadelphia, PA: J. B. Lippincott, 125-132.

90. Morse, A. R., & Rosenthal, B. P. (1996). Vision and vision assessment. *Journal of Mental Health and Aging*, 2, 197–212.

91. Nelson, K. (1987). Visual Impairment among elderly Americans: Statistics in Transition. *Journal of Visual Impairment and Blindness*, 81(7), 331–334.

92. Nouri, F. M., & Lincoln, N. B. (1993). Predicting driving performance after stroke. *British Medical Journal*, 307(6902), 482–483.

93. Nowak, M. S., & Smigielski, J. (2015). The prevalence of age-related eye diseases and cataract surgery among older adults in the city of Lodz, Poland. *Journal of Ophthalmology*, Published online, 2015, DOI: 10.1155/2015/605814.

94. Odenheimer, G. L. (1993). Dementia and the older driver. *Clinics in Geriatric Medicine*, 9(2), 349–364.

95. Olson, E. J., Moore, W. R., Morgenthaler, T. I., et al. (2003). Obstructive sleep apnea-hypopnea syndrome. *Mayo Clinic Proceedings*, 78(12), 1545–1552.

96. Ott, B. R., Festa, E. K., Amick, M. M., et al. (2008). Computerized maze navigation and on-road performance by drivers with dementia. *Journal of Geriatric Psychiatry and Neurology*, 21(1), 18–25.

97. Ott, B. R., Heindel, W. C., Papandonatos, G. D., et al. (2008). A longitudinal study of drivers with Alzheimer disease. *Neurology*, 70(14), 1171–1178.

98. Owsley, C. & McGwin, G. Jr. (2010). Vision and driving. *Vision Research*, 50(23), 2348–2361.

99. Owsley, C., Stalvey, B., Wells, J., et al. (1999). Older drivers and cataract: driving habits and crash risk. *The Journals of Gerontology, Series A: Biological Sciences & Medical Sciences*, 54(4), M203–M211.

100. Pierce, S. L . (2004). *Driving as an instrumental activity of daily living*. In G. Gillen & A. Burkhardt (Eds.), *Stroke rehabilitation: A functional-based approach*. New York, NY : Mosby, pp. 483– 513.

101. Pierce, S. L . (2007). *Restoring competence in mobility*. In C. A. Trombly & M. V. Radomski (Eds.), *Occupational therapy for physical dysfunction*. Philadelphia, PA : Lippincott Williams & Wilkins, pp. 665–693.

102. Pizzarello, L. D. (1987). The dimensions of the problem of eye disease among the elderly. *Ophthalmology*, 94(9), 1191–1195.

103. Rathore, S. S., Mehta, S. S., Boyko, W. L. Jr, et al. (1998). Prescription medication use in older Americans: a national report card on prescribing. *Family Medicine*, 30(10), 733–739.

104. Reger, M. A., Welsh, R. K., Watson, G. S., et al. (2004). The relationship between neuropsychological functioning and driving ability in dementia: A meta-analysis. *Neuropsychology*, 18(1), 85–93.

105. Retchin, S. M., Cox, J., Fox, M., et al. (1988). Performance-based measurements among elderly drivers and nondrivers. *Journal of the American Geriatric Society*, 36(9), 813–819.

106. Retchin, S. M., & Hillner, B. E. (1994). The costs and benefits of a screening program to detect dementia in older drivers. *Medical Decision Making*, 14(4), 315–324.

107. Rizzo, M., Reinach, S., McGehee, D., et al. (1997). Simulated car crashes and crash predictors in drivers with Alzheimer disease. *Archives of Neurology*, 54(5), 545–551.

108. Rubin, G. S., Roche, K. B., Prasada-Rao, P., et al. (1994). Visual impairment and disability in older adults. *Optometry & Vision Science*, 71(12), 750–760.

109. Russell, C., Fitzgerald, M. H., Williamson, P., et al. (2002). Independence as a practice issue in occupational therapy: The

safety clause. *American Journal of Occupational Therapy, 56*(4), 369–379.

110. Schell, B. A. B . (2009). *Professional reasoning in practice.* In E. B. Crepeau, E. S. Cohn, & B. A. B. Schell , (Eds.), *Willard & Spackman's occupational therapy.* Philadelphia, PA : Lippincott Williams & Wilkins.

111. Schell, B. A. B. & Schell, J. W. (2009). *Clinical and professional reasoning in occupational therapy.* Philadelphia, PA: Lippincott Williams & Wilkins.

112. Sims, R. V., McGwin, G. Jr, Allman, R. M., et al. (2000). Exploratory study of incident vehicle crashes among older drivers. *The Journals of Gerontology, Series A: Biological Sciences & Medical Sciences, 55*(1), M22–M27.

113. Sims, R. V., McGwin, G. Jr, Pulley, L. V., et al., (2001). Mobility impairments in crash-involved older drivers. *Journal of Aging and Health, 13*(3), 430–438.

114. Slabaugh, S. L., Maio, V., Templin, M., et al., (2010). Prevalence and risk of polypharmacy among the elderly in an outpatient setting: a retrospective cohort study in the Emilia-Romagna region, Italy. *Drugs Aging, 27*(12), 1019–1028.

115. Staplin, L. et al. (2003). Model driver screening and evaluation program, final technical report. Washington, DC: NTSA. Volume II: Maryland pilot older driver study.

116. Stav, W.B. et al. (2006). *Occupational therapy practice guidelines for driving and community mobility for older adults.* Bethesda, MD: American Occupational Therapy Association.

117. Stutts, J. C., Stewart, J. R. & Martell, C. (1998). Cognitive test performance and crash risk in an older driver population. *Accident Analysis and Prevention, 30*(3), 337–346.

118. The Hartford Financial Services Group. (2006). *A guide to Alzheimer's disease, dementia and driving* (3rd ed.), Hartford, CT: The Hartford Financial Services Group.

119. Trobe, J. D., Waller, P. F., Cook-Flannagan, C. A., et al. (1996). Crashes and violations among drivers with Alzheimer disease. *Archives of Neurology, 53*(5), 411–416.

120. U.S. Department of Transportation. *Highway statistics 2009-2010,* http://www.fhwa.dot.gov/policyinformation/statistics/2009/dl22.cfm/. Accessed June 18, 2015.

121. Vecera, S. P. & Rizzo, M. (2004) Visual attention and visual short-term memory in Alzheimer's disease. In A. Cronin-Golomb & P. R. Hof (Eds.), Vision in Alzheimer's disease: Interdisciplinary Topics in Gerontology. Basel, Karger, Vol. 34, pp 248–270.

122. Vernon, D. D., Diller, E. M., Cook, L. J., et al. (2002). Evaluating the crash and citation rates of Utah drivers licensed with medical conditions, 1992-1996. *Accident Analysis & Prevention, 34*(2), 237–246.

123. Wang, C. C, et al. (2014). *Physician's guide to assessing and counseling older drivers.* http://www.nhtsa.gov/People/injury/olddrive/OlderDriversBook/pages/Contents.html/. Accessed December 9, 2014.

124. Whelihan, W. M., DiCarlo, M. A. & Paul, R. H. (2005). The relationship of neuropsychological functioning to driving competence in older persons with early cognitive decline. *Archives of Clinical Neuropsychology, 20*(2), 217–228.

125. Winn, B., Whitaker, D., Elliott, D. B., et al. (1994). Factors affecting light-adapted pupil size in normal human subjects. *Investigative Ophthalmology & Visual Science, 35*(3), 1132–1137.

126. Young, T., Palta, M., Dempsey, J., et al. (1993). The occurrence of sleep-disordered breathing among middle-aged adults. *The New England Journal of Medicine, 328*(17), 1230–1235.

127. Zozula, R., & Rosen, R. (2001). Compliance with continuous positive airway pressure therapy: Assessing and improving treatment outcomes. *Current Opinion in Pulmonary Medicine, 7*(6), 391–398.

CHAPTER 21

Assistive Technology: Supports for Aging Adults

*Kimberly A. Furphy, DHSc, OTR, ATP, Debra Lindstrom, PhD, OTR/L,
David C. Burdick, PhD*

CHAPTER OUTLINE

OBJECTIVES

- Appreciate how population aging affects the need for occupational therapy services, and how the application of various assistive technologies will increasingly become part of and aid in those services
- Understand and be able to apply to occupational therapy practice some conceptual models linking humans to their environmental contexts, when various technologies are added

- Understand and appreciate other fields' conceptual models to improve one's interprofessional competencies
- Become more fully aware of various low- and high-technology devices and technologies that can aid in the provision of occupational therapy services to the aged and disabled
- Understand that despite the push for the latest gadgets and gizmos, several low-tech devices continue to best serve older clients
- Understand and be better able to practice in a care environment that will increasingly utilize automation, home and behavior monitoring, telehealth, and other smart technologies
- Be able to apply general concepts learned about the strengths and weaknesses of current technologies covered in this chapter to opportunities and threats posed by future technological developments
- Demonstrate increased ability to find additional information and resources on the topics addressed in this chapter

Readers of the other chapters in this book are now well aware of the important "megatrend" of population aging, and valuable paradigm shifts (e.g., successful aging, interdisciplinary collaboration/competencies, and aging in place), that will increasingly affect the provision of services, occupational therapy (OT) and otherwise, to older adults over the next several decades. This chapter builds upon this knowledge and presents technological innovation as another dramatic megatrend and potential "game changer" for the provision of OT services in diverse settings. Various technological tools, when properly designed, deployed, maintained, and used, can allow older adults to maintain independence longer and can contribute to a sense of empowerment, independence, and well-being. Technological tools that do not possess these characteristics can result in frustration, unnecessary expense, abandonment, and risks of higher morbidity and mortality. So, "buyer beware" is an appropriate caution in this discussion. A daunting array of products makes it difficult for consumer and provider alike to fully comprehend the variety of options. For example, Abledata.com (an excellent resource) lists nearly 40,000 products in 20 categories. Resources such as Abledata assist the consumer and practitioner alike in finding, selecting, and acquiring the appropriate technological tool (Table 21-1).

In this chapter, we first provide a brief introduction to the concepts of technology and gerontechnology to provide a conceptual framework and roadmap for what follows. Next we address effective low-tech devices that support activities

TABLE 21-1 Abledata Listing of Assistive Devices by Intended Function or Special Feature: Function, Description, and Major Categories

Device Function Type and Description	Major Categories
Aids for Daily Living: Products to aid in activities of daily living	Bathing, carrying, child care, clothing, dispenser aids, dressing, drinking, feeding, grooming/hygiene, handle padding, health care, holding, reaching, time, smoking, toileting, transfer
Blind and Low Vision: Products for people with visual disabilities	Computers, educational aids, health care, information storage, kitchen aids, labeling, magnification, office equipment, orientation and mobility, reading, recreation, sensors, telephones, time, tools, travel, typing, writing (braille)
Communication: Products to help people with disabilities related to speech, writing, and other methods of communication	Alternative and augmentative communication, head wands, mouth sticks, signal systems, telephones, typing, writing
Computers: Products to allow people with disabilities to use desktop and laptop computers and other kinds of information technology	Software, hardware, computer accessories
Controls: Products that provide people with disabilities with the ability to start, stop, or adjust electric or electronic devices	Environmental controls, control switches
Deaf and Hard of Hearing: Products for people with hearing disabilities	Amplification, driving, hearing aids, recreational electronics, sign language, signal switches, speech training, telephones, time
Deaf-Blind: Products for people who are both deaf and blind	
Education: Products to provide people with disabilities with access to educational materials and instruction in school and in other learning environments	Classroom, instructional materials
Environmental Adaptations: Products that make the built environment more accessible	Indoor environment, furniture, outdoor environment, vertical accessibility, houses, polling place accessibility, lighting, signs
Housekeeping: Products that assist in cooking, cleaning, and other household activities; adapted appliances	Food preparation, housekeeping, general cleaning, ironing, laundry, shopping
Orthotics: Braces and other products to support or supplement joints or limbs	Head and neck, lower extremity, torso, upper extremity
Prosthetics: Products for amputees	Lower extremity, upper extremity
Recreation: Products to assist people with disabilities with their leisure and athletic activities	Crafts, electronics, gardening, music, photography, sewing, sports, toys
Safety and Security: Products to protect health and home	Alarm and security systems, childproof devices, electric cords, lights, locks
Seating: Products that assist people to sit comfortably and safely	Seating systems, cushions, therapeutic seats
Therapeutic Aids: Products that assist in treatment for health problems and therapy and training for certain disabilities	Ambulation training, biofeedback, evaluation, exercise, fine and gross motor skills, perceptual motor, positioning, pressure/massage modality equipment, respiratory aids, rolls, sensory integration, stimulators, therapy furnishings, thermal/water modality equipment, traction
Transportation: Products to enable people with disabilities to drive or ride in cars, vans, trucks, and buses	Mass-transit vehicles and facilities, vehicles, vehicle accessories
Walking: Products to aid people with disabilities who are able to walk or stand with assistance	Canes, crutches, standing walkers
Wheeled Mobility: Products and accessories that enable people with mobility disabilities to move freely indoors and outdoors	Wheelchairs (manual, sport, and powered), wheelchair alternatives (scooters), wheelchair accessories, carts, transporters, stretchers
Workplace: Products to aid people with disabilities at work	Agricultural equipment, office equipment, tools, vocational assessment, vocational training, workstations

(From Abledata, Accessed 10/20/15. http://www.abledata.com.)

of daily living (ADLs) and instrumental activities of daily living (IADLs). We then turn to more high-tech devices (often electronic, involving computer and/or telecommunications technology; frequently called intelligent assistive technologies, or IATs) that support the work of occupational therapists and enhance the well-being of their older adult clients. These areas include telehealth, telemedicine, robotics, smart houses, and other computer assistive technologies.

Technology, Tools, and Gerontechnology

Our first order of business is to provide definitions, which should begin to guide the OT provider in understanding and applying materials to be subsequently addressed in this chapter. *Technology*, in its most general sense, refers to some sort of practical application of basic knowledge. It usually serves to extend our capacities or capabilities over space or time and increases our efficiency in carrying out various tasks. Earlier we used the term *technological tool*. A tool can be thought of as either "a handheld device that aids in the accomplishment of a task," "something used in performing an operation or necessary task in the practice of a vocation or profession," or simply "a means to an end."[54] Although the term *technological tool* may seem a bit cumbersome and redundant, we use it here to capture your attention and promote an important concept. That is, our gadgets and gizmos don't just appear out of nowhere, and they don't operate (effectively, at least) in a vacuum. Rather, we must understand and utilize them as part of a broader multidimensional and dialectic context: multidimensional because they involve individuals and groups (clients, caregivers, designers, manufacturers, distributors, salespersons, providers) within organizational, economic, and environmental contexts, and dialectic because the nature of these relationships is multidirectional, reciprocal, and ever-changing.[33]

Gerontechnology refers to the study of the complex relationship of biopsychosocial aspects of human aging and multiple forms of technology, primarily information/communication technology (computers and mobile devices), assistive devices, medical devices, and home modifications. This study involves scholars and researchers from a wide variety of basic and applied sciences, as well as those from the arts and humanities who, for example, consider ethical issues. Gerontechnology also refers to the application of this study to development and deployment of technological tools that assist with meeting the needs and fulfilling the wishes of older adults, and providing enhanced quality of life and life satisfaction, through support for aging in place, community/family engagement, and participation in ADLs.

Themes and Issues Concerning Gerontechnology and Occupational Therapy Practice

As you read the chapter and consider the technologies discussed, it will be helpful to keep in mind the following themes and issues that have bearing on the effective utilization of technological devices:

1. Cost and payment options: What does it cost to purchase a device? To maintain it? Are supplies needed that must be continually replenished? Will third parties pay the cost for purchase, maintenance, and supplies? Are "loan closets" that provide free use of recycled medical equipment available and accessible?

2. Barriers to use: Besides cost, are there other barriers to device use? For example, barriers could include emotional concerns such as stigmatization; cognitive barriers such as lack of awareness that a product/solution even exists; difficulty in use or lack of adequate instructions; ethical considerations, especially in terms of monitoring technologies; and access barriers such as limited vendors and limited, inefficient, or ineffective repair services.

3. Durability and adaptability: These two characteristics relate to cost and efficacy. Regardless of type (high tech or low), if the device is intended for long-term use, is it durable? If the person's condition worsens (or improves), is the device still fully or marginally useful? Where necessary, can it adapt to the changing needs of the user?

4. Evidence-based and best practice: Which devices are evidence-based interventions and "best practice" for specific conditions? Many businesses are bringing products of dubious quality and value to market. It is important, yet often difficult, to differentiate between appropriate/effective products and modern variants of "snake-oil" using "technobabble" to confuse and deceive unsuspecting older adults. Between the two extremes are devices and technologies that vary with respect to cost and effectiveness. Clearly, too, high tech is not necessary or appropriate when low tech or human assistance/intervention will suffice.

5. Enabling versus disabling: The provision of technological devices to an older person can have an array of outcomes based upon the specific interaction of that person's needs and abilities and the demand characteristics of his or her environment. Lawton and Nahemow's Ecological Model[34] (see also chapter 19) provides a useful way to predict these results. Individual competence in a given domain of functioning is compared with the demand (or press) characteristics of the proximal environment. When competence is slightly above press, the individual can complete a task with minimal effort and is described as being in a state of maximum comfort. If press is slightly above competence, the individual is in the zone called *maximum performance potential*. This is setting the bar just slightly above the person's capabilities. In this case, there is a rehabilitative opportunity. Whenever press and competence are widely mismatched, the result is commonly either negative emotions (ranging from frustration to boredom) or maladaptive behaviors (declining capacities, harmful or risky activities). Occupational therapists are accustomed to providing appropriate technologies to reduce the press, creating better balance between press and competence, and yielding desirable and therapeutic outcomes. Yet, client overdependence on assistive devices

can, for example, precipitate further declines in clients' abilities, make them more likely to fall when ambulating, or limit their ability to access multiple environments if the assistive devices are tied to the environments in which they are housed.

The demographic imperative presented by population aging in the United States, Europe, and elsewhere requires new care models and approaches. The number of Americans over 65 years of age is projected to double to 80 million by 2050, at which time there will also be an estimated 19 million people who are over 85 years of age.[31] Burgeoning numbers of people who are old, and old-old, and suffering from chronic conditions and impairments in ADLs and IADLs, coupled with a shortage of family caregivers, growing ethnic and cultural diversity, issues of health-care reform and the push for cost containment, and other social changes, have all enhanced the role of occupational therapists and the importance of assistive technologies.

Population aging and other secular trends (such as increasing obesity) have a clear influence on the prevalence and effects of ADL and IADL limitations. Although during the 1990s there were consistent findings of a slow, but consistent, decline in disability rates among older Americans (particularly in IADLs), more recent research may indicate that this trend has reversed. For example, one study reported a 9% increase in basic ADL disabilities among community-dwelling older adults between 2000 and 2005.[22]

The growing movement in North America and Europe toward the development of interprofessional competencies in gerontological care[24,30,48] is also a major paradigm shift that is effectively addressed and intertwined throughout this book, and that has enhanced importance in this chapter. Whereas a social worker's comfort zone for interdisciplinarity may often include teammates from nursing, medicine, psychology, and perhaps occupational or physical therapy, the modern occupational therapist involved in technological applications may need to work with the specialists just mentioned in addition to those in human factors/ergonomics, neuroscience, telecommunications, computer and industrial design, and others.

In considering the influence, or potential influence, of technologies in the care of the older adults and people who have disabilities, it is useful to include conceptual models and rubrics, such as the Lawton and Nahemow approach mentioned earlier. Lenker and Paquet[35] provide a useful review of conceptual models for assistive technologies, as does Burdick.[9] Other models for general provision of occupational therapy are also considered in chapter 4. The Humans, Activities, Assistive Technology (HAAT) Model is included in training by the Rehabilitation Engineering and Assistive Technology Society of North America (RESNA) for passing the RESNA Assistive Technology Practitioner Certification Exam. HAAT encourages human factors engineers and psychologists to consider the complex interactions of three variables: (1) a person, (2) acting or behaving, in (3) a context, especially when the use of assistive technology is part of that context.[11]

Another such rubric was provided by Fozard,[20] a major contributor to the study of gerontechnology. His useful classification matrix is designed to elucidate the array of domains in which technologies have potential influence as well as the nature of their influence.

The technologies discussed in this chapter can be recommended by occupational therapists and used by older adults to have multiple and spreading effects on physical, psychological/emotional, social, spiritual, and economic well-being. Fozard classifies human activity into five areas or domains and four effects.[20] The domains are as follows:

1. Health and self-esteem
2. Housing and daily living
3. Mobility and transport
4. Communication and governance
5. Work and leisure

The potential effects are as follows:

1. Prevention or delay of decline
2. Compensation for age-related loss
3. Care support and organization
4. Enhancement and satisfaction with respect to quality of life

It is important for the occupational therapist to always be mindful of the nature of the technology/device recommended or utilized, the potential domain(s) of its effects, and the scope or range of potential influence on the older adult user's life and well-being. Note that this taxonomy relates to both our earlier discussion of press/competence and to the categories of technology described next.

Although occupational therapists have their own taxonomies and professional jargon, and our approach in this chapter probably does not seem foreign, it is important to develop comfort with the models/methods of other professions that work with older adults, and that support interdisciplinary collaboration.

Low-Technology Devices

Housing and Activities of Daily Living

As people age, their abilities, needs, and desires may limit what they do, but taking care of themselves, their homes, and food preparation are often important occupational tasks for them to complete. Assistive technology can help improve their functional independence and safety for completing chosen/necessary tasks,[46] but their actual use of adaptive devices is very individualized.[27] Learning which occupational tasks the person wants/needs to complete is part of a discussion the occupational therapist must have to help determine the best method/device to complete that task safely and satisfactorily.

Although the self-care skills that many people need and want to complete are often very similar, the IADLs in which people choose to engage are more individualized. Which tasks the person chooses and needs to complete are established through collaboration among the older adult, family members/caregivers (when appropriate), and the occupational therapist.

What people need and want to do depends on their interests; their capacities in physical, perceptual/sensory, psychosocial, and cognitive domains; their living environment; and the type of assistance available to them. Adaptive equipment, or assistive technology, is readily available to both occupational therapists and consumers, and comparative pricing can be done by searching for a specific device in a search engine (e.g., Google). Companies also provide extensive web pages and catalogs that older adults and their families can browse through to see equipment that is available or to get ideas for making their own devices to help them do the tasks they want to do.

People's interest in and ability to use adaptive devices also varies depending on their perceptions of using the device and their satisfaction with how well they can complete the task when using the device (if they can indeed use the device effectively). Rogers, Mayhorn, and Fiske[50] found that failure to effectively use assistive technologies generally results from either poor design, unclear/overly complicated instructions, or a combination of both.

Basic Activities of Daily Living

Bathrooms are often found to be the most difficult place in the home for people with mobility limitations, and people who use a wheelchair or scooter throughout the rest of the house sometimes have trouble getting into the bathroom because of the width of the bathroom door. Many bathrooms would need to be remodeled or a door removed to widen the doors if a person is not able to safely use a more narrow or flexible device (e.g., turning the walker to get it through the door) but is still able to use the commode and shower/tub safely with assistance. Getting onto and off of the commode can cause difficulty, and a person may find that a raised toilet seat, strategically placed grab bars, and arm rests around the commode can improve safety without excessive cost or inconvenience. Very creative and functional methods are also used for low-cost, easy-to-make setups, such as a rope swing that could be used in the bathroom or bedroom after being securely attached to the ceiling.

Getting in and out of the bathtub can be very difficult if someone does not have good balance and the ability to lift his or her legs. Strategically placed grab bars are very helpful for getting into and out of the tub as well. A competent remodeler can carefully cut out a piece of the bathtub so that the person can step into the tub to sit on a bath bench and use a handheld shower while sitting in the tub. The lip left from the cut-out needs to be high enough to prevent the water from flowing out onto the floor during the handheld shower. The tub/shower combination can also be removed and a prefabricated no-step/low-step shower stall can be placed in the footprint of the original tub.

Cost and Payment Options for Durable Medical Equipment

Many of the assistive devices discussed so far—canes, walkers, wheelchairs, commodes, shower/bath benches, and so forth—are generally classified as *durable medical equipment* (DME). Such equipment is available for purchase from a wide variety of sources and vendors. If prescribed by a physician, 80% of the purchase cost could be paid for by Medicare in

2012, although recent policy changes have introduced new uncertainties. Due to extensive reports of fraud, and partly resulting from the Patient Protection and Affordable Care Act of 2010 (PPACA), the Centers for Medicare and Medicaid Services (CMS) began to require competitive bidding in nine markets in 2011, and extended bidding into the 91 largest U.S. markets in 2013.[10,25] Reportedly (personal communication with DME vendors) this new system means that a client will no longer be able to purchase all devices from one vendor because different vendors won different bids. Furthermore, device maintenance/repair (e.g., wheelchair repair or oxygen tank replacement), may become less convenient and more costly for the consumer. These costs were previously part of the purchase price.

Instrumental Activities of Daily Living
Cooking/Meal Preparation

Although some people choose to have others do much of their meal preparation for them (e.g., microwaving frozen meals, having prepared meals delivered to their home, or choosing to eat in restaurants or congregate meal sites), meal preparation is an important occupational task for some older adults. Osteoarthritis in the hands is very common among older adults and often impairs their ability to use their hands to do functional tasks.[58] Adaptive devices can often allow people with arthritis to complete tasks more easily and safely, and many universal-designed kitchen gadgets are available in department and kitchen stores to ease food preparation for everyone.

Having devices easily available for "touching/testing" in neighborhood stores or at a nearby mall simplifies the task of determining whether the device meets one's needs. When someone picks up a potato/carrot peeler that has a large soft handle, it is possible to determine whether or not the size or surface of the handle is actually more comfortable than the handle for the carrot peeler that the individual has used for the past 50 years. Even if the handle is more comfortable, some people still may not want to give up the device that is so familiar to them because they just want to continue peeling the same way that they have peeled for many years. Decisions about whether or not someone wants to use a device that might make things easier can be made by having someone "look and touch" in local stores before purchasing.

Some older adults also may feel "less handicapped" if their new device is sold in the local stores to everyone, not just "handicapped" people. Manufacturers, distributors, and stores selling these devices would do well to provide clear instructions on various device characteristics and information on how to choose the right product in sales displays and not just within packaging that cannot be opened until after purchase. Hammel[28] notes that "word of mouth" among older friends regarding useful assistive devices is often the most common catalyst for the decision of adoption by older adults.

A person's safety in the kitchen is an important component of meal preparation, and the ability to safely use the range, oven, microwave, and cutting utensils must be determined before making meal preparation recommendations (Case Example 21-1). Some examples of kitchen devices that

CASE EXAMPLE 21-1 Low-Technology Devices

Audrey and Sam have been married for 66 years and are living in the home that they moved into shortly after they wed. Audrey, who was a stay-at-home mother, is 86 years old and has moderately advanced Parkinson's disease. Her doctor has advised her to use a rolling walker both in the home and outside of the home because she recently fell— once at home and once at church. Sam, 88 years old, is a retired banker. He has some general health issues and seems to be getting progressively weaker.

Sam and Audrey are very active in their church. They have one grown daughter who is married and has a 20-year-old son. Their daughter and grandson try to help out as they are able. The home is a 1300-square-foot ranch-style home with the original breezeway converted to a family room; there is no step from the garage to the family room but an 8-inch step from the family room into the kitchen and the rest of the house. There are three steps leading into the front door.

The kitchen has the usual appliances and a kitchen table that seats four people; the door to the basement staircase is in the kitchen. The laundry is located in the basement and there is a railing on one side of the basement stairs; there is not a railing for the step from the family room to the kitchen.

The bedrooms and living room are typical of a small ranch home.

The bathroom is rather small, with the tub/shower combination straight ahead as you enter and the sink and commode on the left.

Sam had expressed concern that he was having trouble helping Audrey out of bed in the morning due to his lack of strength. After evaluation, it was determined that they needed one railing for the step from the family room to the kitchen and railings on both sides of the basement steps for safety, although it was recommended that Audrey not go to the basement at all. Laundry options were for Sam to do the laundry or, ideally, that someone else do laundry for them.

Versa-frame arm rests were placed on their commode to prevent falls. A higher commode was not recommended because Audrey is 4'11" and Sam is 5'3". Recommendations for alterations to the tub/shower were made but the couple did not consider that an option due to cost, so a clamp-on tub grab bar was recommended with another grab bar installed on the wall opposite the clamp-on grab bar. A shower chair and handheld shower were recommended and are being used for Audrey to bathe. A home bed assist handle was recommended so Audrey could help to pull herself out of bed.

These low-cost modifications were implemented, allowing Audrey and Sam to stay in their home for 3 more years before their physician suggested a move to a subsidized assistive living center due to cognitive and physical decline, to which they agreed.

are available to minimize the stress on the joints in the hand include tools with larger and softer handles, cutting utensils that use the whole hand instead of several fingers, choppers or food processors to minimize hand chopping, and electric mixers that stabilize and rotate the mixing bowl.

Other adaptations that can be made in the kitchen for food preparation and cleanup include accessible locations for the microwave or other appliances that are used frequently. Locating a microwave above the stove may have seemed like a great idea when someone was able to easily reach up and remove the hot dish, but as hand and shoulder strength diminish, and wrists become arthritic, the microwave may be safer at a waist-high level (on the counter or table) to make it safer to take hot dishes out and set them on a hot pad on the counter instead of lifting them down from a microwave at shoulder height.

A person's habits and routines in the kitchen can help determine the best location for appliances and storage locations for frequently used utensils/tools and foods for easy access. There are many appliance options available in kitchen departments to help users optimize their food preparation abilities if they have the financial resources to make changes, such as having a dishwasher drawer or small oven right under the counter. Home builders/renovators and kitchen designers are slowly becoming more aware of these issues. The National Association of Home Builders provides training and credentialing for Certified Aging in Place Specialists, who consider appropriate design in the kitchen, bathroom, garage, and other areas of the home. Nevertheless, the occupational

therapist may still be helpful in making such recommendations to older clients and following through with demonstration and/or training.

Forgetfulness in the kitchen can lead to spoiled food, or worse, to fire hazard. Door-open beepers on refrigerator/freezers that sound an alarm after 30 seconds and easily used timers and auto-shutoff or alarms on ranges and ovens can dramatically reduce risks and will become more common in newer models of appliances.

Cleaning and Laundry

As people age, their interest and ability in cleaning and laundry varies significantly. With all appliances, it is important to evaluate the older adult's ability to safely reach and use the controls before recommending independent completion of the task. The older adult's physical, sensory/perceptual, and cognitive abilities and safety must be incorporated into the plan for safe completion of these activities. If cleaning is considered an important occupational task for someone, and the person is determined to be safe in that task completion, the occupational therapist may be called on to assist with finding devices that will allow for safe and efficient completion of desired tasks. Devices available for making home management easier are also commercially available at many local stores.

A major barrier to an older adult independently doing his or her own laundry is the location of the washer and dryer. If they are on the main floor and controls are understandable and within reach, it may be a safe task. If the washer and dryer are in a basement, which is common in the older housing of most older adults today, the safety in going up and down stairs while carrying a basket of clothing must be determined when making recommendations for independently completing laundry. Stacked washer/driers, particularly near the master bedroom, may be a convenient space saver, but may create specific impediments for those with various handicaps. More-over, front- versus top-loading designs present different opportunities and hardships, based on the characteristic of each user. Recently, researchers at the University of Akron developed a height-modifiable laundry basket on wheels. The design allows users to scoop laundry from a separate front-loading washing machine and dryer into the basket rather than lifting and transferring the laundry.

When proper product placement and design are unable to overcome impediments to successful and safe use, options for having someone else complete these home management tasks may need to be explored. Also, when attempting to effectively fit a person to his or her environmental situation, appliances, assistive devices, fixtures, and so forth, it is important to project forward in time and accommodate further declines in the individual's capacity. Selecting a device that becomes obsolete within months due to a decline in the user's capacity can be expensive, frustrating, and dangerous.

Avocation

The location of vocational and avocational equipment and materials is critical to safe and efficient use as a person plans how to best stay actively engaged in meaningful activities and to age in place. This may mean, for example, moving a basement workshop to one stall of a two-stall garage, raising garden beds, moving a sewing machine to the ground floor, or changing the location and setup of the computer. Someone is more likely to stay engaged in a hobby if he or she can easily and safely get to the location where the equipment and materials are located.

A wide and growing variety of adaptive devices can make things easier for garden and outdoor work for people with osteoarthritis and limited strength or endurance. Gardening can be extremely rewarding and therapeutic for older adults, and encourages physical activity and stretching. Where capacity is limited or to minimize osteoarthritis pain, perennials are generally preferable to annuals. Raised beds and container gardening are also preferable (Figure 21-1), and there are various ways to simplify watering. The occupational therapist must understand each person's individualized interests, needs, and abilities to make recommendations for meaningful engagement and participation in avocational activities of clients' own choosing that will enhance their life satisfaction and personal well-being.

Functional Mobility

Mobility aids are assistive devices commonly used by older adults and, with the exclusion of wheelchairs, are often obtained without medical consultation or fitting.[19] Walkers and canes are much easier for people to use in homes, but if they are not fitted properly, they may actually increase the risk of falls.[37] Mobility aids can be purchased online or from local medical supply companies, where one of the clerks may be

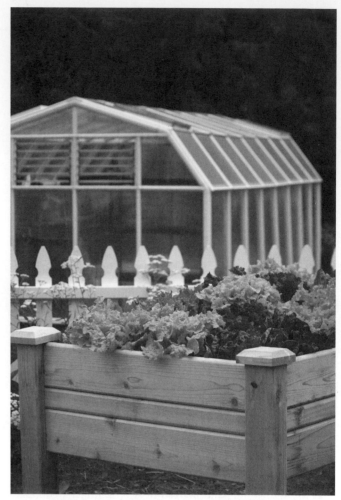

FIGURE 21-1   Raised garden bed. Photo © istock.com

able to help fit the device to the person. Wheelchairs are most often obtained through medical consultation and proper fitting, but they can also be purchased without a fitting for general mobility needs. The use of wheelchairs has been found to improve mobility, socialization, independence, a sense of freedom, and the ability to contribute to society among appropriate users.[19] It is often, however, difficult to get the wheelchair and the person into and out of homes, and move through narrow hallways within homes, and wheelchairs are more difficult to transport in private cars and vans than are walkers and canes. Many wheelchairs are manual models, but powered mobility devices, such as power wheelchairs and scooters, are also available for the use of older adults.

Getting into and out of Cars/Driving

Even if driving is no longer an option for some clients, the car is the most common and preferred method of transportation for more than 90% of older adults.[1] Rotation devices that the person sits on in the car seat can help the client swing his or her legs into and out of the car; a temporary grab handle placed into the latching mechanism on the door can help people get safely in and out of the car. Additionally, a limited number of car makes and models provide front driver and

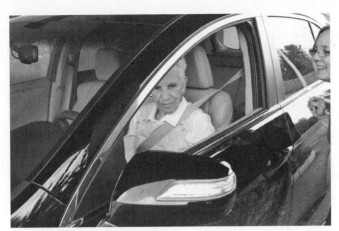

FIGURE 21-2   CarFit program assessment. Photo © istock.com

passenger seats that swivel toward the doorway to allow easier entry and egress. It is important for the occupational therapist to give recommendations for safe transfers for different types of vehicles because getting into a standard sedan is very different from getting into a sports car, pick-up truck, mini-van, or sport utility vehicle. The CarFit program, offered jointly by the American Occupational Therapy Association (AOTA), AARP (formerly the American Association of Retired Persons), and the American Automobile Association (AAA), is an educational program for older adults designed to maximize their safety, comfort, and mobility through making adjustments in their cars that facilitate optimal fit (e.g., seat position and mirror settings). (See chapter 20 for additional details on the CarFit program.)

Community Mobility

A person's ability to get around the community is critical for staying actively engaged in meaningful activities.[1] This may involve walking, bicycling for some, driving, or getting rides through privately arranged transportation, taxi services, community-provided passenger services, or public transportation. Even if public transit services are available/accessible, older adults who have never used public transit may be unwilling or unable to easily learn how to use it when they are no longer able to drive. Distance to bus stop, perceived cost, fear of crime, feelings of lost privacy, confusing bus schedules, and the need for transfers are all potential disincentives for older adults to use public transit. In an AARP transportation survey,[1] only 15% of people aged 50 to 74 years reported using public transit for their trips, and only 9% of people aged 75 years and older reported using the bus or train for their trips. The real and perceived shortcomings of public transit must be addressed, but it may still not be available or an acceptable option for some older adults. Some communities have reasonable transportation options for older adults through paratransit systems, local taxi services, faith-based organizational transportation services, and community services such as a transportation network that allows people to join the network and then receive car rides at a reasonable rate. One innovative network that is developing throughout the United States is the Independent Transportation Network,

in which older adults can receive ride vouchers in exchange for them donating their cars to the network's fleet of cars. Anyone with the specified age/disability status can join this network and use their vouchers to pay for rides to any location within the driving radius of the network. This type of system allows more safety, autonomy, and dignity because the participating older adults have bought into this network and can go wherever they want, not just to medical appointments and to buy groceries once a week. If they forgot something that they need and want to go back to the grocery store the next day, this is an option, just as it would be if they could drive.

Organizations such as the National Center for Senior Transportation and others are helping to improve accessible transportation for older adults and people who are disabled. The recent restructuring of the U.S. Department of Health and Human Services, incorporating the Administration on Aging, the Administration on Intellectual and Developmental Disabilities, and the Office on Disability into the new Administration on Community Living, may lead to many positive developments.

One of the options for older adults who live in communities where friends, stores, restaurants, community centers, and other places of destination are within walking distance is to get to desired locations by walking or by using their current ambulation devices. This walking/rolling is only possible if there are safe sidewalks and/or bike lanes that are barrier-free and safe crossings for streets that they need to cross. An innovative program being implemented throughout the United States called Complete Streets[42] helps communities focus on the safety in the streets for drivers, cyclists, parents pushing strollers, and pedestrians/rollers. Complete Streets focuses on safe access for all users and factors that allow buses to operate on time. This includes the provision of auditory and visual alerts and countdown indicators for crossing the street, the provision of enough time to actually get across during the walk sequence, and the implementation of curb cuts for motorized scooters, wheelchairs, and strollers.

Federal policy and initiatives will continue to hold promise for improved sustainable and livable communities for residents of all ages. For example, the U.S. Department of Housing and Urban Development (HUD) has partnered with the Environmental Protection Agency (EPA) and the Department of Transportation (DOT) to enhance the livability of communities. The guiding principles in this partnership include (1) providing more transportation choices, (2) promoting equitable and affordable housing, (3) enhancing economic development, (4) supporting existing communities, (5) coordinating policies and leveraging investment, and (6) valuing communities and neighborhoods.[55]

Communication

Older adults can have difficulties with communicating clearly due to various age-related changes or diseases that affect their ability to produce speech, to hear speech or to see someone communicating with them, or to read written words.

When people have difficulty producing words due to aphasia or a motor apraxia, or difficulty producing clear speech due to dysarthria or hearing difficulties, this can

CASE EXAMPLE 21-2   Augmentative Communication

Harold is a 70-year-old man who was diagnosed with a cerebrovascular accident (CVA) 1 year ago that resulted in significant declines in independence in self-care and mobility, and severe expressive aphasia. In the past year, he has improved in his functional ability in self-care activities and mobility but has not seen many improvements in his ability to speak so that others can understand him.

Harold is getting increasingly frustrated when trying to communicate his needs to others. His wife has asked for assistance in providing her husband with a means to communicate. After evaluation, it was determined that Harold had the ability to type and spell and was cognitively intact. Because of these characteristics, he was deemed a good candidate for a speech-generating augmentative and alternative communication (ACS) device. With a device that he can use to either spell out his needs or point to words to create sentences to indicate his needs, Harold will be able to communicate effectively with his family and friends.

significantly affect their quality of life. There are no-tech, low-tech, and high-tech assistive devices that can help individuals communicate by supplementing their current speech ability, replacing their difficulty in communicating verbally, or compensating for their sensory loss (vision or hearing). Devices that compensate for speech are called augmentative and alternative communication devices (Case Example 21-2).

Unaided speech options include the use of gestures, body language, and sign language, which enable the individual to get his or her meaning across without the use of devices. Low-tech options include writing on a tablet; pointing to items on a picture, phrase, letter, or word board; or choosing a word or phrase from a booklet that contains words and phrases most commonly used by the individual. It is important if the older adult has difficulty communicating that the occupational therapist consult with a speech and language pathologist to include the most appropriate communication words and symbols for that person's current capabilities. The speech and language pathologist would determine the words/pictures that are used for a low-tech communication board, and the occupational therapist would determine the access means to the device. There are a variety of ways that a person can access a communication device. The person conveying the message can use his or her finger or an alternative pointing device (e.g., a head pointer or laser pointer) to point to choices on the board. The individual could also use eye gaze to indicate his or her choice as the partner in the conversation watches where the individual's eyes are looking to determine the individual's choice.

Functional communication can also become difficult for older adults if they experience a loss of hearing or vision that is not corrected through traditional compensation devices such as glasses/contacts and hearing aids. Referrals to appropriate professionals (optometrists, ophthalmologists, or audiologists) are needed to find the best device or adaptation possible to maximize a person's functional communication in light of any sensory impairment. Hearing aids are expensive and unaffordable for many older adults because they are not currently a covered benefit for Medicare recipients. Not being able to hear what is going on around you is always frustrating, but older adults and their families can become extremely frustrated when hearing aids are purchased out of pocket and they do not totally compensate for a hearing loss and the older adult ends up not using them.

Other devices to compensate for a hearing impairment are adaptive alerting mechanisms such as alarm clocks that shake a bed, light-activated doorbells and warning systems, and telephone systems with extra-loud volume control. Most television sets that have been purchased in the last 10 years have settings to activate closed captions on television programs to allow someone with a hearing limitation to understand the content of programs by reading the closed captioning on the screen.

When you are communicating with people who have sensory impairments (visual or auditory), it is important to communicate in quiet environments with sufficient ambient lighting, while also reducing glare on the eyes of the older adult. Seating the client where the glare is to his or her back, rather than in the client's eyes, can dramatically improve the client's ability to pick up nonverbal cues and to use limited lip reading. (See chapter 10 for additional suggestions on dealing with low vision.)

Problems with communication due to vision loss may be compensated through enlarged print, colored overlays, brighter light, magnification (handheld magnifying glasses or increased magnification on a computer screen), and text-to-speech programs (simple programs are built into most computer operating systems, but much more sophisticated programs are also available commercially). These compensations are discussed in the following high-technology section of this chapter. Please refer to the websites in Box 21-1 for examples of available programs.

High-Technology Devices

Now that we have surveyed the many low-tech devices that can be used by occupational therapists and other professionals to assist older adults to maintain their independence, we will next turn to a review of high-tech alternatives. The following pages successively cover high-tech devices' potential to improve function in the areas of health and self-esteem, housing and daily living, communication and governance (including compensation for cognitive decline), and work and leisure. Please understand that we have not intentionally "saved the best for last." On the contrary, when a low-tech and low-cost alternative does a comparable or better job than the latest and greatest, we suggest that, particularly for the current older cohort, it is best to "keep it simple."

Activities of Daily Living

There are many high-technology devices that can help caregivers in the home as they provide care for older adults.

BOX 21-1 Technology Websites

Websites with a variety of assistive technology devices:
http://www.wisdomking.com/sammons-preston-adl-products;
http://www.wrightstuff.biz/getting-ready.html.
http://www.myspecialworld.net/
http://www.infogrip.com/
https://www.enablemart.com/
http://www.lighthouse.org/store/
http://www.maxiaids.com/

Equipment for assistance with activities of daily living (ADLs):
http://www.discountmedicalsupplies.com/store/commode-chair-fixed-arm-coated-steel-seat-lid-back.html
http://www.knobbrands.com/product/21623/delta-df565-grab-bar-white?gclid=CKHWuNKywMACFQqJaQodk7cANA
http://www.tubcut.com/
http://www.bathfitter.com/tub-to-shower-conversions/style1.aspx

Equipment for assistance with cooking/meal preparation:
http://www.arthritistoday.org/tools-and-resources/slide-shows/cooking-with-arthritis.php
http://www.easierliving.com/all-products/food-preparation-nutrition/food-preparation/
https://www.google.com/search?q=good+grips+potato+peeler
http://www.easierliving.com/health-conditions/arthritis-products/kitchen-dining-aids/default.aspx
http://www.thewright-stuff.com/one-handed-kitchen-products/
http://myhomeupgrades.com/wp-content/uploads/2010/08/myHomeUpgrades-Microwave-ventilation-microwave-and-stove-v2.jpg

Equipment related to avocations:
http://www.abc-med.com/sites/abc/files/gallery_ChicagoBotanicGarden_0146_47949_nmb_0.jpg
https://www.flickr.com/photos/gardeninginaminute/4999006101/in/photostream/

Equipment related to transportation and driving:
http://www.amazon.com/MTS-Car-Swivel-Seat/dp/B000J03SNM
http://www.dmesupplygroup.com/87501.html?gclid=CN-57tW3wMACFQkQaQod2goASA
http://pubs.aarp.org/aarpbulletin/201305_DC?pg=28#pg28
http://www.itnamerica.org/
https://www.flickr.com/photos/completestreets/sets/72157617261981677/
http://www.healthbydesignonline.org/documents/WalkabilitySurvey_HbD.pdf

Equipment related to communication:
http://www.sc.edu/scatp/aacsymbols.html
http://www.harriscomm.com/equipment/alarm-clocks.html
http://www.allaboutvision.com/lowvision/reading.htm

Equipment related to environmental control:
http://www.smarthome.com/_/index.aspx
http://www.x10.com/homepage.htm
http://www.innotechsystems.com/accenda/index.html
http://www.touchlesstrashcan.com/share/cgi-bin/site.cgi?site_id=touchlesstrashcan&page_id=mx
http://www.touchlesstrashcan.com/share/cgi-bin/site.cgi?site_id=touchlesstrashcan&page_id=ezfaucet

Equipment related to computer access:
http://www.enablemart.com/Catalog/Large-Key-Large-Print-Keyboards/Keys-U-See
http://www.aisquared.com/zoomtext_keyboard
http://www.logitech.com/en-us/mice-pointers/trackballs
http://www.evoluent.com/
http://www.imgpresents.com/smartclk/smc.htm
http://www.nuance.com/for-individuals/by-product/dragon-for-pc/index.htm
http://www.imgpresents.com/onscreen/onscreen.htm
http://www.imgpresents.com/wordcomplete/wordcomplete.htm
http://www.readingmadeez.com/products/TalkingCheckbook.html
http://www.aisquared.com/Products/Products.htm

Useful organization websites:
AOTA: http://www.aota.org/practice/work-industry/emerging-niche/new-technology-at-work.aspx
Abledata: http://www.abledata.com
Human Factors and Ergonomic Society: https://www.hfes.org/web/Default.aspx
American Society on Aging, NEST (Network on Environments, Services and Technologies): http://www.asaging.org/nest
LeadingAge: CAST (Center for Aging Services Technologies): http://www.leadingage.org/cast.aspx
Gerontological Society of America: GSA-TAG (Formal Interest Group on Technology & Aging): http://faculty.cua.edu/tran/gsa-tag/
LinkedIn (e.g. Gerontechnology) and Facebook discussion groups

Ceiling-supported transfer systems, bathtub lifts to get a person into and out of the tub (Figure 21-3), stairglides, elevators within the home, and outdoor lifts into a home are options that may be considered if the funding for those high-technology devices is available.

Mobility

Powered wheelchairs and scooters are often used when individuals are unable to walk on their own as well as unable to use their upper extremities to physically propel themselves in a wheelchair. Scooters are a popular choice for many older adults, with about 90% reportedly obtained without medical consultation. Scooters are reportedly easier to manage in homes[19] (once they are in the home and if there is enough space), but are very difficult to transport in private cars or vans without specialty lifts. With respect to best practice or outcome measures for the use of powered mobility devices, perhaps the best source of information is a 2008 review article by Auger and associates.[5] These authors systematically reviewed the literature over a 12-year period and

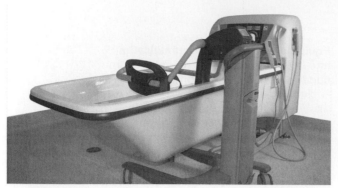

FIGURE 21-3 Bathtub lift. Courtesy of Geraldine B. Ellenberger

found 19 studies assessing effects in 52 domains. Their general conclusion was that the quality of research design was often marginal and that evidence supporting the use of such devices is therefore weak but improving.[5] Powered mobility devices can be extremely helpful for moving around inside the home and in the community, but the process to transport them requires a lift on a vehicle because of their size and weight.

Modern vehicles are providing more standard way-finding (e.g., global positioning system [GPS]) and collision avoidance devices that can make driving safer for the older or impaired driver. Some new vehicles (Lexus, Toyota, Ford, for example) have automatic parallel parking capacity (e.g., intelligent parking assist system [IPAS], advanced parking guidance system [APGS]), and it has recently been reported in the media that vehicles that "drive themselves" are not more than 10 years away. It is important to ensure that these devices do not increase the risk of accident via distraction or by giving a very impaired driver a mistaken sense of safety/security.

Augmentative and Alternative Communication

High-tech options for speech include electronic devices that produce speech as the individual points to pictures or types words on the device. Software for various tablet devices is becoming much more prevalent and useful. These devices are called augmentative and alternative communication (AAC) devices.

Communicating with friends and family can be accomplished through several media channels, such as Skype, video chats, smartphones, and cell phones. Skype can be used on a home computer, a tablet, or on a mobile phone. SkypePhones entered the marketplace in 2011, allowing "Skyping" without being connected to a computer. Although this service presents an inexpensive way to communicate through voice and video over the Internet, at least one review mentions that the audio quality in the early offerings was poor and had a noticeable hissing sound.[53] Because of normal age-related declines in hearing for high-pitched sounds (referred to as presbycusis) and the consequential difficulties in differentiating among similar consonants, the addition of an image to the small phone speaker is probably not a particularly useful feature. Further developments may mitigate this problem.

Cell phone technology, which sacrifices audio quality to carry more conversations on a given cell tower, presents a significant impediment for use by older adults, particularly in noisy environments.

Phones can be very simple, such as a specially designed flip phone that opens to answer and closes to hang up, or that has just one button to push for a live operator who connects the caller with predetermined contacts. The Jitterbug phone rates high in usability for older adults due to its larger buttons, brighter displays, and simplified operations as compared with many other phones on the market.

Many of even the very simple cell phones also have "reminder" features to allow someone to receive alarms and reminders to compensate for minor cognitive limitations. For more tech-savvy users, smartphones allow for voice calls and text messages, but they also can connect to the Internet and email, social networking pages, and global positioning devices, and can serve as AAC devices.

Developments in this domain are swift as the convergence of computer and telecommunication continues with mobile devices, so information provided here will become dated rather quickly. Samsung has currently taken the lead with a variety of services and peripherals available through its "Life Companion." For example, with easy-to-connect peripherals, it is possible to monitor sleep, ambulation, medication reminders/adherence, blood pressure, glucose levels, and similar parameters.

Many high-tech devices come with a touchscreen that the individual can touch to make a choice of words or phrases to speak. In fact, the development of tablets such as the Apple iPad has made access to AAC for many individuals a cost-effective reality because there are numerous apps that can be downloaded to aid in speech production for those with speech problems. Other devices come equipped with a camera that detects where the person is looking so that he or she can use eye gaze to choose words or phrases he or she wants to speak. Still others offer the individual the option of using switch scanning to choose letters, words, or phrases.

There has been some criticism of the use of AAC devices because it is feared that the individual will never develop or regain the ability to speak after suffering a disabling condition affecting speech, such as a cerebrovascular accident (CVA). However, studies have shown positive results regarding the use of AAC devices for individuals with dementia,[4,8] brain-stem strokes,[52] and Parkinson's disease.[7]

Control of Housing and Daily Living

Individuals are living longer, yet options for supported living environments for older individuals have not kept pace with this growth. In fact, the support available from and provided by family members has diminished in recent decades due to the need for family members to work, and will continue to decline because of fewer adult offspring born to baby boomers than among previous cohorts. In addition, many older adults choose to remain in their own homes due to the familiarity of the environment, the control afforded by living in their own homes, and their desire to remain independent for as long as possible.[13] Consequently, there is a growing need for supportive approaches, programs, and devices that encourage individuals to remain living independently in their own home and to "age in place."

Aging is associated with a variety of health disorders, conditions, and declines that jeopardize successful aging-in-place. For example, mobility issues, declines in sensory function, and falls all can inhibit an individual's ability to remain safe and independent in his or her own home. In recent years, technological advances in home automation have enabled individuals to age in place more safely and independently. Home automation options can range from standalone remotely operated lighting to smart homes in which functions can be accessed via the Internet to run lights and appliances in the home, monitor the residents' activity level, provide reminders for those with cognitive impairments, or assist with monitoring residents' health through blood pressure or blood sugar monitoring.[14] The following sections discuss some options to enable older adults to remain safe, independent, and healthy in their own homes.

Telehealth/Telemedicine Devices

Telehealth and *telemedicine* are two terms that have been used interchangeably to describe the exchange of health information, through video and audio technologies, between individuals in their homes and remote health-care professionals.[32] According to the American Telemedicine Association, the term *telemedicine* is more correctly used to describe the clinical services provided through electronic means to improve a client's health status. On the other hand, the term *telehealth* involves clinical services as well as medical education, administration, and research. In any case, the use of technology to remotely monitor an individual's health and safety has shown great promise in helping people to avoid diseases and injuries and to maintain their health.

There are various types of telehealth devices used in monitoring residents' health in their homes today.[14] Devices can monitor cardiac functions, blood sugar levels, weight, general activity, sleep patterns, and numerous other health-related parameters. Some of these telehealth devices are designed to measure only one item, such as blood pressure, whereas others are bundled to provide remote health-care providers with an overall picture of a client's health on a daily basis. Tracking and monitoring health measures on a daily basis has significant implications for keeping older adults healthy. For instance, information on weight gain in a client with congestive heart failure can provide the physician with information about the individual's heart function, enabling the physician to provide immediate intervention without the client having to wait for the next available appointment. Systems that do more than just transmit data, and instead gather and analyze data, show the greatest promise for cost-effective provision of care.

Home Automation/Electronic Aids to Daily Living

Home automation technology has significantly advanced in recent years, although home automation was seen as far back as the 1934 World's Fair in Chicago. Since then, availability in personal homes has been most possible since 1975 with the development of X-10 technology.[18] X-10 technology transmits and interprets signals sent from a remote control into functions such as "on" and "off" to control various devices in a person's home (Case Example 21-3). Today, X-10 technology remains the most popular means of communication with electronic devices for home automation, although there are alternatives with higher bandwidths.

Home automation devices have great implications for keeping older adults safe and independent in their own homes. Research demonstrates that home automation devices have reduced the prevalence of falls, have improved the quality of life of the older adults who use them, and have decreased the number of caregiving hours provided to those who require assistance with ADLs and IADLs.[16,17,38]

Virtually anything in a home can be automated. Devices that have only two functions, such as "on/off" or "open/close," are most easily automated and can be found in single, standalone controllers. Devices that require configuration of functions, such as temperature or volume control, often require a combination of technologies found in electronic aids to daily living (EADLs), once known as environmental control units (ECUs).

CASE EXAMPLE 21-3 Environmental Control

Anne Marie is a 62-year-old woman who was diagnosed with multiple sclerosis when she was 45 years old. She has progressively lost function in all of her extremities and at present can only control the movements in her neck. She is quite verbal, has no difficulty with projecting her voice, and is cognitively intact. She spends most of her day in her hospital bed because her personal care assistant finds it difficult to get her up and into in her wheelchair, and when up, Anne Marie fatigues after an hour or so.

Recently, Anne Marie has had more difficulty accepting her dependence upon her personal care assistant for simple tasks such as changing the channels on the television. She has asked for assistance in determining the best electronic aid to daily living (EADL) to allow her to control television functions, to turn her bedside lamp on and off, and to independently make and receive phone calls.

After evaluation, it was determined that the most appropriate device would be one that is controlled through voice-recognition technology. With an EADL that is controlled by voice, Anne Marie would be able to effectively control the devices she has identified. The recommended EADL device should be one that has infrared functions, which is the typical technology for control of television. The lights and telephone can also be controlled via infrared technology if an infrared receiver is integrated into the recommended system for the lights and the speakerphone recommended is one that is operated via infrared technology. With these items in place and with a little training of the unit to recognize her voice, Anne Marie is able to operate her television, make and receive telephone calls, and operate her bedside lamp independently.

Single, standalone controllers, such as "The Clapper," operate a single device and do not use X-10 technology. They can be operated via touch, sound, voice, or proximity. These simple control devices are most often used to operate appliances with two functions and are the easiest for older adults to set up and use. Similar standalone devices for control of the home allow older adults the ability to turn water on and off without having to turn faucets due to a weak grasp, but rather by proximity to the receiver. Some overhead lights and fans come standard with a remote control to allow the user to operate them without having to walk to a wall switch or reach for a pull string. This may reduce the number of falls an individual with mobility and balance problems could have during light and fan operation. Motion detectors for light operation and hallways and bathrooms can reduce the number of falls that older adults have during nighttime toileting activities.

Alternative television (TV) remote controls come with larger buttons for the visually impaired or are operated by voice commands for those with limited fine motor skill and strength that inhibits their ability to operate the buttons on a standard remote control device. Several cable TV operators now provide apps for iPads and other tablets that allow convenient viewing of program schedules and remote control.

EADL units help older adults to operate on/off devices such as lights, but also to control the temperature in their homes, operate telephones, open and close power-operated doors and drapery, and control TVs and other entertainment equipment. Virtually anything that is powered by electricity and does not require an outside force or function to operate it, such as vacuum cleaners and washing machines, can be automated and run by EADL units.

There are many options for EADL units. They can be freestanding and operate independent of a computer or be computer-based systems, which often allow many more functions. By installing EADL software on the individual's computer, when combined with peripheral EADL control devices running via X-10 (or other) technology, the individual can control a variety of devices in the environment. Both freestanding and computer-based EADL units can be wired, requiring the individual to be near where the control box is plugged in, or wireless, which essentially allows the individual to carry the controller throughout the home to operate devices from different rooms. Individuals can operate both freestanding and computer-based EADL units in various ways. Some offer operation through directly selecting the device and function that the individual wants to control by pushing a button on the controller. Others allow operation through voice commands or scanning selection. With scanning selection, the user hits a switch to turn a device on or off after being given an array of choices that are highlighted. Once the command the user wants to occur is highlighted, such as "turn light on," the user hits the switch and the light turns on. Computer-based EADL units offer the greatest number of options for control of devices because essentially any device used to control a computer, such as an eye-gaze system, can be used to control devices on a computer-based EADL unit. The advent of mobile devices has begun to radically change this, as described next.

Smart Homes

Smart homes were originally automated to allow individual control of items in the environment, such as heating/ventilation, security systems, and lighting, from a centralized in-home console. Today, with the advent of mobile devices, the notion of smart home has taken on a totally new meaning, with expansive implications for older adults' safety, security, and general well-being as they are increasingly allowed and encouraged to age in place. Due to the interest of four business sectors (utilities, home security, entertainment, and home health), it is estimated that by 2015 the average home in developed nations will have 16 connected devices, compared with four in 2012.[26] The Groupe Speciale Mobile Association (GSMA) further reports predictions of $44 billion in revenues by 2016 for utility company smart metering, home energy management, and home automation alone. Revenues including other smart home entertainment and telehealth/telemedicine will be considerably higher.

Recently, the idea of the smart home has expanded from simple control of devices in a home to also include remote monitoring. Monitoring of the resident's activities, specifically regarding falls, medication schedule management, and evening tracking of what a resident had to eat, can occur through smart home technology. Some smart homes also provide residents with memory deficits with alerts when medications need to be taken or even assist with sequencing tasks in which the individual needs to engage. Family members of residents in a smart home can monitor loved ones on several behavioral parameters from a remote setting through computer technology coupled with smart home technology and various sensor devices. Essentially smart homes combine telehealth technologies and home automation technologies to allow remote health-care professionals, family members, and caregivers the ability to know that their clients or loved ones are healthy and safe. In turn, these technologies allow older adults to remain living in their homes longer, which is a less expensive option than living in an assisted living or nursing home environment.

Smart home technology has been shown to reduce the burden on caregivers by reducing the cost of paid help, decreasing the amount of hands-on caregiving required, and essentially improving the quality life of the older resident.[3] However, smart home technology is not without its critics. Some research has shown that due to the lack of familiarity of many older adults with computers, the technology is actually viewed as more cumbersome than helpful. In fact, in some studies, people using the technology actually reported that their quality of life had declined since using the technology, but this was related to a variety of factors, such as age and perceived level of disability, in combination with the presence of the technology.[40] Smart homes also present security risks because computer hackers can access the home's network and turn off alarm systems to gain access to the home. Finally, many ethical issues have been debated surrounding the use of monitoring technology and its effect on the privacy of the homes' residents.[15]

Robotics

Robotics is the newest of the technologies that can be used to assist older adults with control over items in their environment and with completion of ADLs and IADLs. Although still in relative infancy, home robotic technology from around the world has been gaining interest as a form of assistance in keeping older adults in their homes longer. Research areas have included service robots that can help older adults with medication management; robotic garments that monitor activity level, breathing, and heart rate; and robotic devices that assist the older adult with transfers to and from various surfaces; to date, results indicate that these devices can have a positive influence on the physical and psychosocial functioning of older adults.[36,57] Researchers have recently found that older adults are likely to accept robotic care as opposed to human assistance for tasks such as housekeeping/cleaning, removing trash, and doing laundry, but prefer humans when they need assistance with bathing/toileting, dressing, and other more personal tasks. They are more likely to accept robotic assistance for these other tasks if it helps them to avoid institutional care.[23]

Although sophisticated multifunction robotic devices are cost prohibitive for most older adults to obtain, some simple robotic technologies are available on the mainstream market that can assist older adults with completing some home management tasks. A handful of commercially available robotic vacuums can help older individuals clean their carpets and floors despite balance, strength, and mobility issues. In addition, older adults wishing to maintain their own lawns, but unable to do so due to balance, mobility, or cardiac issues, can use a robotic lawn mower. Robotic pool and rain-gutter cleaners are other examples of robotic technologies that allow older adults to age in place. With the rapid pace of technological advances, it may not be long before robots are used more frequently to assist older adults in maintaining health, safety, and independence in their own homes.

Service Animals

Service animals are trained to assist people with disabilities in performing various tasks to help them to compensate for visual, sensory, motor, or cognitive deficits. Because these areas decline with age, it is appropriate to consider service animals as a viable alternative to human assistance at one end of a continuum and technological devices at the other end. People are most familiar with guide dogs that assist the visually impaired with mobility in different environments. Other types of animals, such as monkeys and miniature horses, have been trained and used to assist in accomplishing a variety of tasks. There are also animals that pull wheelchairs for those who are unable to push one independently or who fatigue easily. Some animals can assist with retrieving items from the refrigerator or picking up items from the floor for those who cannot reach those areas. Service dogs can be specifically trained to alert an individual to blood sugar changes or to alert and protect individuals affected by seizure disorders. Still others act as therapeutic companion animals.

The additional benefits of having a service animal in the life of an older adult have been well researched. Studies have shown that the presence of a service animal has helped to increase the independence of older adults in ADLs and IADLs, thereby allowing them to stay in their own homes longer.[49] Other studies have documented the psychological benefits of companionship afforded by the service animals to their older adult owners.[6,21]

Computer Assistive Technology

People use computers to accomplish many things in their daily lives. They use computers to communicate and socialize with family, friends, co-workers, and clients. People use computers to manage their homes, pay their bills, and shop online. They use computers to pursue recreational interests, for creation of videos and music, and for researching items of interest. When younger individuals think of computers, although ever present in today's society, they are seen as newer technology from which older adults usually shy away. Unlike younger generations, many older adults never used computers in the classroom or in their work environments and may not attempt to learn the technology out of fear of doing something wrong or not being successful.[51] However, as computers have become more prevalent in work environments, more people, including the baby boomers, have been exposed to computers and are comfortable with using them. In fact, the number of older adults actively using the Internet has increased by more than 55% from 11.3 million users in November 2004 to 17.5 million in November 2009.[43]

For novice and experienced older adult computer users, operating a computer may present certain challenges. Aging causes visual problems that may make seeing the computer screen difficult or may hinder an individual's ability to see the letters on the computer keyboard. Fine motor coordination problems may make operating a computer mouse difficult or may make hitting the correct keys on the keyboard impossible. Range-of-motion or strength limitations might make it difficult for an individual to reach all of the keys on a keyboard, move the computer mouse effectively, or click on icons to open files, folders, and Internet sites.

Fortunately, as computer technology has improved, so has the development of assistive technology devices and software as well as operating system modifications that make using the computer easier for older adults despite any deficits or disorders (Figure 21-4). The following are some examples of hardware and software devices that can enable an older adult to operate a computer more easily.

Computer Input Compensations
Mouse Modifications

Several standard tasks must be accomplished to operate a computer. First, an individual needs to be able to operate the computer mouse effectively enough to maneuver the pointer/cursor in all directions on the computer monitor to open icons, files, and folders. Some older adults have difficulty accomplishing this due to decreased strength and range of motion that occur due to various orthopedic and neurological conditions. Several devices are available that the older adult can use.

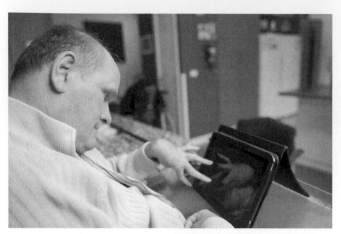

FIGURE 21-4   Using the computer. Photo © istock.com

Trackballs are perhaps the most common alternative to the standard mouse for those with limited upper extremity function. They allow the individual to move the cursor on the screen by moving a ball that sits on top of a base. Essentially, the individual can accomplish cursor movements without having the range of motion in the shoulder and elbow that is required with a standard mouse, because they can position the trackball close to the body and move the ball with minimal finger and wrist movement. There are many different types of trackballs, from ones with a larger base and ball to those that can be held in the hand and operated with thumb movement over the ball.

Another alternative to the mouse for moving the cursor on the screen is MouseKeys, a built-in accessibility feature in both Mac and Windows operating systems. Once enabled, this feature allows an individual to move the mouse cursor and perform all mouse functions via the number pad on the keyboard. This is a good option for people who cannot move the standard mouse due to range-of-motion or strength issues, but who have sufficient fine motor control to operate the keyboard keys.

People generally use computer joysticks for computer gaming, but these can also be used as an alternative to the standard mouse. Various alternative joysticks can be used by individuals with range-of-motion and strength issues to operate the cursor. These are also good alternative mouse options for people who are familiar with joystick operation on power wheelchairs, because they are comfortable with the control required to use these devices.

A final alternative to the mouse for individuals with compromised upper extremity function is the trackpad. Trackpads are commonly seen on laptop computers to allow portability of computer operation with little peripheral equipment. However, trackpads also can be added to desktop computers as well as to laptops to allow individuals with poor proximal upper extremity range of motion and strength to reposition the trackpad closer to compensate for their deficits and utilize their fingers to move the cursor by dragging them along the trackpad.

For individuals who have little to no upper extremity function, electronic head-pointing devices enable them to operate the computer mouse. These devices require the individual to wear a reflective dot or device on the head that transmits an infrared or ultrasound signal to a camera placed on the computer monitor. The camera detects the position of the individual's head and moves the cursor on the screen accordingly. Of course, to be able to operate this device effectively, the individual needs to have sufficient head and neck range of motion and strength.

A second skill an individual needs to operate a computer mouse is the ability to click the buttons on the mouse to open files, folders, and Internet sites. These tasks are usually accomplished by single or double click on the right or left buttons on the standard mouse. Sometimes individuals have difficulty with performing mouse clicks due to poor fine motor strength or coordination. There are numerous software and hardware solutions and devices, and operating system configurations, that will help individuals compensate for deficits in mouse-click operation. Changing mouse tracking sensitivity and required double-click speed can help, as can alternatives to double-clicking. Some software programs enable the individual to perform mouse-click, double-click, click-and-drag, and various other functions simply by holding the cursor over the item that needs to be opened or moved. That is, the individual needs to be able to activate a function such as double click by dwelling over the double-click icon on the program menu on the screen. Once double-click is activated, the individual moves the cursor to the icon of the program to be opened. Once there, the individual allows the cursor to dwell over the icon for a preset period of time, for instance, 3 seconds. Once the 3 seconds has elapsed, the program opens. The individual can use any pointing device described previously to move the cursor. People who operate the mouse with an electronic head-pointing device or those who are unable to isolate a finger to press the buttons on the standard mouse, trackball, or joystick often use this type of program.

Windows and Mac operating systems can be reconfigured easily to facilitate computer use by the individual who cannot perform the double-click or click-and-drag functions. By reconfiguring the settings, an individual can use a single click instead of the double click to open programs and can perform click-and-drag options without having to hold down the button while dragging and moving items. Instructions for doing this reconfiguration can be found on the help menu for the operating system, on videos on YouTube, and through Internet sites using a search engine.

A final way to perform mouse clicks is via use of a software program that enables the user to operate a switch to click on screen objects. In most cases, this is accomplished via a horizontal line that starts at the top of the screen and moves slowly downward. When the line reaches the desired object on the screen, the user hits the switch, thereby freezing the line. The user then presses the switch again to activate a pointer that moves horizontally along the line. Once the desired item is reached by the pointer, the user then hits the switch again, and the item is opened.

Older adults suffering from carpal tunnel syndrome and other repetitive stress disorders may have difficulty with operation of the computer mouse due to pain and discomfort. There are numerous types of ergonomic pointing devices available. These ergonomic pointing devices place the forearm and hand in a better position to reduce the strain placed on the upper extremity structures typically affected by overuse with mouse function.

Keyboard Modifications

Computer operation is further accomplished via keyboards to input letters, numbers, and symbols to create documents and perform Internet searches. Sometimes older adults have difficulty with hitting only one key at a time, releasing the keys quickly enough, reaching all of the keys on the keyboard, or isolating their fingers to hit keys due to upper extremity strength, range-of-motion, and coordination issues (Case Example 21-4).

Low-tech items such as typing sticks, mouth sticks, and head pointers allow individuals who cannot isolate their fingers due to coordination issues to hit individual keys. These devices offer individuals single-digit access to typing, which is a very slow means of typing. However, for individuals with little or no funding for devices, these are affordable options for many who want computer access at a low cost.

Individuals with range-of-motion issues due to orthopedic or neurological conditions often require the use of an alternatively sized keyboard to operate the keyboard most effectively. Smaller keyboards limit the individual's need to reach far from one side of the keyboard to the other to reach all of the keys. However, with the smaller keyboard size, the size of the keys is usually decreased. Therefore, good fine motor skill is usually necessary to use these keyboards.

An alternative to the smaller keyboard is an alternatively configured keyboard in which the layout of the keys is different from the standard QWERTY. These layouts place the most frequently used letters in the center of the keyboard and letters that are frequently used in combination, such as *t* and *h*, near each other. This reduces the amount of movement a person needs to make to type common words. This option for keyboarding is effective for one-handed keyboard users and for those who fatigue easily with standard keyboard use due to range-of-motion issues, but who cannot use a smaller keyboard due to fine motor issues.

For individuals who have poor fine motor control but good proximal range of motion and strength, a larger keyboard with larger keys is an option. This will eliminate the number of undesired characters appearing on the screen due to coordination deficits.

Older adults suffering from carpal tunnel syndrome and other repetitive stress disorders can benefit from the numerous types of ergonomic keyboards available. These keyboards place the keys in a more ergonomic position to reduce the stress placed on the upper extremity structures typically affected by overuse of computer operation.

Letter and number input can also be accomplished via the use of Morse code. Individuals using Morse code for letter input can use either a single or double switch to perform the series of dots and dashes used to produce letters. This is a nice option for computer input for individuals familiar with Morse code, but also for those who have little to no functioning in most of the body and cannot afford the eye-gaze systems discussed later in this section.

Computer keyboarding can also be accomplished via the use of an on-screen keyboard. These are images of keyboards that are projected onto the computer screen. Keys can be activated by clicking on individual letters, dwelling over individual letters for a predetermined period of time, or via switch scanning, in which the individual uses a switch or two to make letter choices as each row on the keyboard is scanned. Scanning is an extremely slow means of letter input, but may be the only option for some individuals with very little functioning in their bodies. With click-and-dwell options, users can point to the letters using any of the pointing devices discussed previously. Both Mac and Windows operating systems have on-screen keyboards in their standard accessibility features.

Speech-recognition programs allow the user to perform both mouse and keyboard functions via the use of the voice. The individual first needs to program the voice so that the computer recognizes what is being said. Once programmed, the user can dictate text and perform keyboard and mouse functions via voice. Both Mac and Windows operating systems offer speech-recognition features in their newer operating

---

CASE EXAMPLE 21-4   Computer Access

Andrew is a 68-year-old man with diabetes who was diagnosed with a cerebrovascular accident (CVA) 2 years ago. He is unable to use his left arm functionally, but has intact function in his right, dominant extremity. He has a history of diabetic retinopathy, which has caused his vision to decline enough that he has difficulty reading his pill bottles and the newspaper.

Andrew has used a computer over the last 10 years to communicate with family members and friends across the country via email and a videoconferencing software program he had used at work. He has noticed a decline in his ability to see items he has typed on the computer monitor, and he has indicated a desire to be able to type more efficiently using his right hand. He has asked for assistance in finding software and hardware that might allow him better access to his computer.

After evaluation, it was determined that Andrew would benefit from adaptations to his computer for input, processing, and output. For input, a keyboard with better one-hand access would be optimal. Often these keyboards are smaller in size to allow the one-handed computer user to access all of the keys more easily. Another recommendation would be for Andrew to use a word-prediction program to improve his typing speed by limiting the number of keystrokes he would need to make to produce text, making his typing more efficient. The final recommendation would be for Andrew to use a screen reader and magnifier software program to compensate for his declining visual function. With these adaptations, Andrew should be able to more effectively use the computer and continue to communicate with his family and friends.

systems. However, these programs do not allow the degree of functionality that is afforded by other commercial speech-recognition programs, such as Dragon Dictation. These speech-recognition programs are appropriate for individuals familiar with the standard keyboard functions because everything that was accomplished via the keyboard needs to be translated into voice command. Therefore, a fair degree of cognitive skill is required to learn how to use and operate these programs. Speech-recognition programs are a good alternative means of computer access for those with poor upper extremity functioning coupled with poor head control, but who have good respiratory function.

Eye-gaze systems are perhaps the newest option in computer input for those with no other options due to very little functioning of other body parts typically used for computer operation. With these systems, the individual simply needs to look at items on the screen to open them or to look at letters on an on-screen keyboard to input words and data. This is accomplished via a camera placed on the monitor that detects the position of the individual's eyes via reflection of light off of the retina. These systems are often cost prohibitive for many people because they are not covered by medical insurance for computer input, but are covered for access to electronic AAC devices.

Some computer users have difficulty with fine motor skill that causes them to hit two keys at a time, which places unwanted characters in the document. Keyguards are low-tech items that are placed on the keyboard to reduce the number of unwanted characters typed by hitting two keys at a time. Windows and Mac operating systems both have a feature called filter keys that can be configured to ignore the unwanted keystrokes by requiring the individual to hold down a key for a predetermined amount of time before it is recognized as a keystroke. Filter keys can also be configured for those who have difficulty with releasing keys quickly enough such that numerous repeated characters appear on the screen. To eliminate this problem, filter keys can be configured so that the individual must release a key and push it again before a repeat character can appear on the screen.

Computer Productivity/Processing Compensations

The computer access assistive technology described thus far can provide individuals with enhanced ability to operate the computer mouse and keyboard. However, in some cases, such as with character input via switch scanning, the ability to produce documents in a timely fashion is compromised. Speed and productivity are important not only in today's workforce, but also with other activities such as simply shopping online, because some sites limit the amount of time provided to individuals who are typing text into order forms.

Word Prediction

One way to speed up letter input is through the use of a software program that predicts the words an individual is trying to type based on the first few letters typed. These word-prediction programs give the individual a means to use fewer keystrokes to type the word. That is, when the person types

the letters *t* and *h*, for example, a menu of words that commonly begin with those letters is presented. If the desired word is in the list, the person chooses the word without having to type the entire word out. This is especially effective in reducing the time a person spends in typing longer words. For instance, if the person were trying to type *therefore*, this would require nine keystrokes or scanning phases to complete the word. With word prediction, once *th* is typed, *therefore* would appear in the list. The person chooses the word, thereby only requiring three keystrokes or switch hits—*t*, *h*, and *therefore*.

Abbreviation Expansion

Abbreviation expansion programs are another way to improve efficiency and productivity with computer input. With abbreviation expansion, the user simply needs to type in an abbreviation, such as *OT*, and once that combination of letters is recognized, the entire phrase *occupational therapy* will replace the *OT* originally typed. As you can see, the number of keystrokes required to type *occupational therapy* would be dramatically decreased, which would, in turn, speed up productivity.

Macros

A final way to speed up letter and number input is through the use of keyboard and mouse macros. Macros allow the individual to record common phrases or mouse actions and transform them from longer keystrokes or mouse movements into shorter sequences of keystrokes. For example, if an individual needed to type his or her name and address repetitively on multiple documents, he or she could record the name and address through the Macro Recorder, then apply a sequence of keystrokes, such as Alt-A, to represent the name and address. The next time the person needs to type the name and address, he or she simply hits the Alt and A key and the name and address will appear.

All of these productivity options can dramatically improve the efficiency of the computer user. In a world where speed and productivity are paramount, they are necessary accommodations for computer access for older adults with functional limitations due to age-related changes or various diseases. For older adults with repetitive stress disorders and arthritis, decreasing the number of times they need to press a keyboard key might allow them to complete keyboarding tasks with less pain and discomfort. For older people with progressive disorders, reducing the number of keystrokes can assist in keeping fatigue at bay.

Computer Output Compensations

For individuals with visual deficits, numerous low- and high-tech compensations and devices allow them to "see" what is present on the computer monitor. Perhaps the easiest compensations that an older adult with mild visual impairments can use are to enlarge the text size and increase the space between individual letters in web-browsing, word processing, and email programs while the individual is viewing materials or inputting text. This enables better visualization of the text being typed without having to pay for any other computer modifications because these options come standard in most software programs.

To compensate for more severe visual deficits, images on the monitor can be enlarged by other means. Low-tech screen magnifiers can be placed over the existing monitor to enlarge what is present on the screen. These are easy to obtain, but do not offer as much functionality as some of the other high-tech screen-magnification options. Both Mac and Windows operating systems offer an electronic screen-magnification option as a standard part of their accessibility options. There are also numerous commercially available screen-magnification software programs for purchase as well as several free programs available via Internet searches. These electronic magnification programs magnify either the whole screen or parts of the screen to enable those with visual impairments to see the screen better.

Two other options that allow individuals to "see" what is on the screen are screen readers and text-to-speech programs. These programs will read aloud icons and menus on the desktop and in programs, and read what is typed in a document via individual letters, whole words, full sentences, or any combination of these. Of course, to be able to use these programs the individual must be able to hear effectively, which may be a problem with some older adults. Also, environmental factors that might affect the use of these programs need to be considered. For example, such programs could not be used by older adults in a classroom situation or in libraries unless headphones are attached to the computer. There are several commercially available screen readers/text-to-speech programs as well as a few freeware programs available for download. Mac and Windows operating systems both offer a screen-reader option as a standard part of their accessibility features.

Psychosocial Effects

As stated previously, computers offer individuals the ability to manage their households, participate in leisure and recreational activities, create, communicate, and research information. This is true for older computer users, but computer use may also have added benefits for older adults. Research has shown that computer use for the older adult can have positive psychosocial value. Several studies have shown that computer use can have a positive influence in enhancing the quality of life of the older adult.[29,41,56] Opalinski[45] found that computer use allowed older individuals to acquire new skills and gain knowledge, thereby increasing their feelings of control, self-esteem, and self-efficacy. Other researchers found that by increasing the older person's interaction with others via the Internet, loneliness decreased, rates of suicide declined, independence in ADLs improved, and medication needs for ailments such as arthritis decreased.[11,39,44,47]

Options for compensating for functional deficits that affect the older individual's ability to use a computer are numerous, as shown in this discussion. These options, coupled with the fact that computers have proven benefits for the older user, make it clear that professionals working with the older adult population should not disregard the use of

computers with their older clients in trying to bring about functional gains. Unfortunately, most medical insurance plans will not pay for computer modifications that are not deemed medically necessary, and many older individuals are on fixed incomes and unable to purchase some of the technology discussed previously. It is important for the professional working with the older adult population to think "out of the box" for creative options for obtaining these devices. For example, grants are available that might finance a computer center in a senior housing complex, or OT professionals might search various online "freecycle" sites that provide gently used devices free of charge or for a nominal fee.

Mobile Devices

Mobile devices have become more mainstream in today's society, and they have taken on a greater role in the lives of older adults. Many options are available for providing older adults with mobile means for communication, health monitoring, environmental control, and cognitive stimulation.

Today, many older adults use mobile device technologies to communicate with family, friends, and community resources. Text messaging has become a popular way for older adults to communicate with their younger family members because this is often seen as the preferred method of communication of preteens and teens. Text messaging has its inherent difficulties for the older adult; for example, "text speak" or text jargon is often difficult for the older adult to understand. In addition, for older adults with arthritic hands, typing on the small keypads available on most mobile devices often inhibits the effective use of text messaging. Finally, the small screen and text fonts available often inhibit those with visual problems from effectively using this feature. Luckily, as mobile carriers have recognized the growing number of older-adult mobile technology consumers, there are more features being built into new devices to accommodate for these problems. In addition, numerous apps can be downloaded for free or for a nominal fee that can enlarge the keypad available on touchscreen devices, make the fonts larger, or read aloud what is being typed onto the screen. There are also devices, such as Jitterbug, that are designed specifically with the older adult user in mind.

Videoconferencing apps or video/voice communication apps have become popular with older adults to combat the effects of loneliness. According to a 2010 report by AARP,[2] loneliness is one of the biggest individual problems faced by older adults living alone; 25% of respondents aged 70 years or older, 32% aged 60 to 69 years, and 41% aged 50 to 59 years reported being lonely. AARP also found that loneliness is a significant predictor of poor health. Those who rated their health as "excellent" were less likely to report being lonely than those who rated their health as "poor."[2] One way to combat loneliness is to give the older adult a means to communicate face to face with friends and family who may not live close geographically. The use of apps, such as Skype or Facetime on mobile devices, has enabled the older adult to stay in touch with loved ones with minimal to no cost.

It is possible to monitor sleep, ambulation, medication reminders/adherence, blood pressure, glucose levels, and other health measures through the use of mobile technologies and apps and other peripherals that are both easy to use and often inexpensive. With the emphasis today on reducing health-care expenditures, the use of mobile monitoring devices that give physicians daily updates on client health can be at the forefront of the cost-saving measures that are necessary in reducing health-care costs. These technologies, such as the iHealth products and the Samsung Life Companion, have been shown to improve compliance with prescribed medical interventions as well as ensure that dietary and lifestyle changes are being implemented.

Mobile technologies have also provided older adults with alternatives to the traditional medical alert systems in the event that a fall or other medical emergency occurs. Mobile technologies have enabled active older adults to leave their homes where they may have previously been tethered to a medical alarm base station, such as that available from Lifecall. Services such as those offered by Great Call's 5 Star Urgent Response allow the older adult to leave the home, yet still be able to access help at any location with wireless coverage.

Control of electronic devices in one's home is also possible through the use of mobile technologies and apps. The apps enable the smartphone to be used as a remote control and offer access to devices in the environment that are connected to peripherals that interface with the app. This means that the older adult with mobility problems would not need to get up from bed to turn the lights on for those nighttime bathroom trips, or would be able to adjust the temperature settings in the home or remotely lock doors should the individual forget to do so before a long trip. Both Apple and Android operating systems offer numerous apps for environmental control. In addition, television and Internet service providers offer environmental control through their services, and most often allow for access to controls through a mobile app.

Age-related cognitive declines affect the older adult's ability to successfully age, but can be slowed, mitigated, or compensated for through mental stimulation and cognitive strategies. Mobile technologies and apps can be used to provide cognitive stimulation to the older adult, thereby reducing the effects of diseases such dementia and also providing for leisure outlets and social interaction. Research has shown that mobile technologies have improved the functioning of adults with dementia through the use of apps that target specific areas of cognitive functioning such as memory and problem solving (but recall that mobile technologies have inherent access problems for the older adult, as previously discussed).[12] Lumosity's Human Cognition Project conducted research into the effectiveness of the brain games it offers and found that individuals who are undergoing chemotherapy or who are recovering from strokes demonstrated improved mental awareness and information processing as benefits of daily participation in the brain games. In addition, apps such as "Words with Friends" provide the older adult with mental stimulation, and also the ability to engage in a leisure activity with family and friends or even complete strangers.

Just as with all of the technologies discussed in this chapter, it is best to match the technology with the needs of individuals based on their skills and desire to incorporate technology into their everyday lives. It is also important to note that as mobile technology becomes more prevalent in society, the incidence of "technophobia" will continue to decline. Mobile technologies offer the older adult more cost-effective, user-friendly options for communication, health monitoring, environmental control, and cognitive stimulation.

Summary

In this chapter we have attempted to provide the reader with fundamental and reasonably up-to-date information needed for occupational therapists to understand and effectively utilize assistive technology that supports overall well-being, life satisfaction, and quality of life among older clients. But, there's a catch. Some materials that are up to date as we complete this chapter may become obsolete by the time you read it. There are probably few other chapters in this book requiring this caveat, because the application of technology in occupational therapy practice is rapidly changing.

Constantly during our preparation of this manuscript, we authors were cognizant of new developments, products, services, research, and resources that would be appropriately covered in this book. So, it becomes important to ask, "How did we address this challenge, and how should the reader?"

First, we began with some fundamental guiding principles, paradigms, and models—from occupational therapy, but also from allied disciplines, from gerontology, from psychology, and from others. Your commitment to understand these principles will enhance your ability to apply them to your practice as a more effective occupational therapist, but it also enhances your interprofessional competencies. Yes, this may seem like a buzzword and fad to providers who have been in the field for some time. But, it is not! The ability to connect, communicate, and collaborate with specialists from other disciplines is crucial for your success and your clients' well-being. The ability to work as part of an interdisciplinary team is as important a tool in your toolkit as a paraffin bath for arthritic hands or a reaching stick in stroke rehabilitation.

After our coverage of some guiding principles, we then turned to a discussion of low-tech devices. To be sure, these are less likely to change as rapidly as the high-tech, electronic, mobile devices. There will be a never-ending push to always use the latest, greatest gadgets and gizmos. In a seemingly broken health-care system in search of enhanced outcomes and controlled costs, we definitely need our "early adopters" to continually push the envelope; just as NASA, Neil Armstrong, and the *Apollo* astronauts helped us to develop the technologies necessary to get to the moon, we need explorers in health-care delivery. Whether or not you are comfortable and effective as an early adopter has a lot to do with your personality, your training, your organization's leadership and risk-tolerance attitude, and your organization's financial resources. But, when deciding, please keep in mind the best interests of your clients. And from our gerontologist co-author, remind yourself that in gerontology, "old is good," and that this often also applies to the assistive devices that work best. The long-handled shoe horn sometimes works better than Velcro. The personal care robot that can effectively and efficiently clothe the client with a genuine smile and pat on the back is still years down the road. And down that road, the long-handled shoe horn should still have its place in your toolkit. The Luddites who feared the printing press and destroyed some along the way were as important as the early adopters. Sometimes old and low-tech options are not only effective, but are simply better than any new-fangled gadgets and gizmos the market throws at us. The lesson here, then, is to pay close attention to the tried-and-true technologies presented in the low-tech section of this chapter.

Our discussion next turned to high-tech options, circa 2015. We focused primarily on intelligent assistive technology (IAT), including environmental control devices for in-home care and support of daily living. We briefly covered the swiftly changing fields of telehealth, telemedicine, telehomecare, and personal care robots. Somehow, we snuck in service animals, and you may have asked, "What's this doing here" before you realized that the training of these animals and the array of services they provide are truly remarkable. Our high-tech section next discussed computer assistive technologies before concluding with mobile devices. For computers, we focused on input, output, and productivity/processing compensation issues.

As you think about the section on computer assistive technology, you may be thinking that computers are obsolete—the name of the game is mobile devices. This may be somewhat true, but the difficulties presented in computer use by older adults, and the technological adjustments made to overcome these difficulties, are perhaps even more pronounced and as yet poorly addressed, when it comes to supporting successful use of mobile devices by older adults. Small screen displays, glare on screens in bright/outdoor environments, limited bandwidth barriers to high-speed uploads/downloads, and other issues make mobile-enabled health deployment for older adults a work in progress.

How else should you prepare for continual change in your work with older adult clients, in collaboration with other occupational therapists and specialists from other fields? Get accustomed to knowing what organizations provide the best objective trustworthy information about new devices. The AOTA, of course, along with Abledata; the Human Factors and Ergonomic Society; the Network on Environments, Services, and Technologies (NEST) of the American Society on Aging; the Center for Aging Services Technologies (CAST) of LeadingAge; and the Technology and Aging Group of the Gerontological Society of America (GSA-TAG) are all useful sources. As well, there are useful discussion groups on LinkedIn (e.g., gerontechnology) and Facebook that can help you to effectively stay ahead of the curve.

REVIEW QUESTIONS

1. Gerontechnology
   a. refers to the study of the relationship of biopsychosocial aspects of aging with various forms of technology.
   b. involves researchers from a variety of basic and applied fields.
   c. refers to the application of research and deployment of technological tools designed to aid with successful aging.
   d. includes both a. and c.
   e. includes a., b., and c.

2. While technologies are intended to assist function and enable older adults to live more independently, if not properly deployed they can inadvertently lead to further disability. Which of the following is recommended for predicting outcomes and optimizing successful deployment?
   a. The HAAT Model (Humans, Activities, and Assistive Technology)
   b. Erikson's Theory of Psychosocial Development
   c. Lawton & Nahemow's Ecological Model
   d. Both a. & c.
   e. All of the above

3. Which of the following was **not** described by Fozard as a potential impact of gerontechnology?
   a. Prevention or delay of decline
   b. Compensation for age-related loss
   c. Care support and organization
   d. Enhancement and satisfaction with quality of life
   e. All of the above were described as potential impacts.

4. Learning which occupational tasks the person wants/needs to complete is part of a discussion the occupational therapist must have to help determine the best method/device to complete that task safely and satisfactorily.
   a. True
   b. False

5. Which of the following is *not* considered to be durable medical equipment?
   a. Pill dispensers
   b. Canes
   c. Walkers
   d. Shower/bath benches

6. The support of continued avocational Instrumental Activities of Daily Living is important for elder well-being and life satisfaction. Which of the following examples was cited in the chapter to support avocational IADLs?
   a. Moving a basement workshop to the ground floor or one bay of a two-car garage
   b. Providing a rope-swing to assist with toileting
   c. Providing container gardens and raised plant beds
   d. Both a. and c.
   e. None of the above

7. Adaptive alerting mechanisms for older adults with hearing impairments include
   a. alarm clocks that shake the bed.
   b. telephones with enhanced ringer and speaker volume.
   c. strobe-light fire/smoke alarms and doorbells.
   d. all of the above.
   e. none of the above.
8. The _____ rates high in usability for older adults due to larger buttons, brighter displays, and simplified operations, compared with many other phones on the market.
   a. skype phone
   b. jitterbug phone
   c. iPad phone
   d. Xfinity seniorphone
   e. POTS phone
9. Whereas *telehealth* may refer to clinical interventions, medical education, and research, *telemedicine* refers specifically to
   a. clinical services provided through electronic means to improve a patient's health status.
   b. call-in/online pharmacy and medications services.
   c. diagnostic, but not treatment, functions provided via telecommunications channels.
   d. clinical interventions, medical education, and research—telehealth and telemedicine are interchangeable terms.
10. Today, with the advent of mobile devices, the notion of smart homes has expansive implications for older adults' general well-being as they age in place. It is estimated that by 2015 the average home in developed nations will have _____ connected devices.
    a. four
    b. eight
    c. 16
    d. 32

ESSAY QUESTIONS

1. Describe the difference between the terms telehealth and telemedicine. Why is this delineation important when talking about technology that enhances independence with aging?
2. Describe ways in which a computer can be adapted to allow access for older adults. Consider the range of input, processing, and output devices/options when formulating your response.
3. Describe the range of home automation options that are available to older adults.
4. Discuss how mobile devices can enhance the independent living of older adults.

REFERENCES

1. AARP. (2005). *Beyond 50.05. A report to the nation on livable communities: Creating environments for successful aging.* Accessed 10/20/15. http://assets.aarp.org/rgcenter/il/beyond_50_communities.pdf/.
2. AARP. (2010). *Loneliness among older adults: A national survey of older adults aged 45+.* AARP the Magazine. Accessed 10/20/15. http://assets.aarp.org/rgcenter/general/loneliness_2010.pdf.
3. Alwan, M., Sifferlin, E. B., Turner, B., et al. (2007). Impact of passive health status monitoring to care providers and payers in assisted living. *Journal of Telemedicine and e-Health, 13*(3), 279–285.
4. Andrews-Salvia, M., Roy, N., & Cameron, R. M. (2003). Evaluating the effects of memory books for individuals with severe dementia. *Journal of Medical Speech-Language Pathology, 11*(1), 51–59.
5. Auger, C., Demers, L., Gelinas, I., et al. (2008). Powered mobility for middle-aged and older adults: Systematic review of outcomes and appraisals of published research. *American Journal of Physical Medicine and Rehabilitation, 27*(8), 666–680.
6. Banks, M. R., & Banks, W. A. (2002). The effects of animal-assisted therapy on loneliness in an elderly population in long-term care facilities. *The Journals of Gerontology: Series A: Biological Sciences and Medical Sciences, 57A*(7), M428–M432.
7. Beukelman, D. R., Fager, S., Ball, L., & Dietz, A. (2007). AAC for adults with acquired neurological conditions: A review. *Augmentative and Alternative Communication, 23,* 230–242.
8. Bourgeois, M. S., Dijkstra, K., Burgio, L., et al. (2001). Memory aids as an augmentative and alternative communication strategy for nursing home residents with dementia. *Augmentative and Alternative Communication, 17,* 196–209.
9. Burdick, D. C. (2007). Gerontechnology. In J. Birren (Ed.), *Encyclopedia of gerontology: Two volume set* (2nd ed., pp. 619–630). Boston, MA: Academic Press.
10. Centers for Medicare and Medicaid Services. (March, 2013). *The durable medical equipment, prosthetics, orthotics, and supplies (DMEPOS) competitive bidding program. ICN 900927.* http://www.cms.gov/Medicare/Medicare-Fee-for-Service-Payment/DMEPOSCompetitiveBid/.
11. Cody, M., Dunn, D., Hoppin, S., & Wendt, P. (1999). Silver surfers: Training and evaluating Internet use among older adult learners. *Communication Education, 48*(4), 269–286.
12. Coppola, J. F., Kowtko, M. A., Yamagata, C., & Joyce, S. (2013). *Applying mobile application development to help dementia and Alzheimer's patients. Proceedings of Student-Faculty Research Day.* CSIS, Pace University, New York, NY. Accessed on 10/20/15. http://csis.pace.edu/~ctappert/srd2013/a6.pdf.
13. Demiris, G., & Hensel, B. (2002). Smart homes for patients at the end of life. *Journal of Housing for the Elderly, 23*(1), 106–115.
14. Demiris, G., & Hensel, B. (2008). Technologies for an aging society: A systematic review of "smart home" applications. *Methods of Information in Medicine, 47*(Suppl. 1), 33–40.
15. Demiris, G., Parker-Oliver, D., & Courtney, K. L. (2006). Ethical considerations for the utilization of tele-health technologies in home and hospice care by the nursing profession. *Nursing Administration Quarterly, 30*(1), 56–66.
16. Demiris, G., Rantz, M. J., Aud, M. A., et al. (2004). Older adults' attitudes and perceptions of smart home technologies: A pilot study. *Medical Informatics and the Internet in Medicine, 29*(2), 87–94.
17. Demiris, G., Skubic, M., Rantz, M. J., et al. (2006). Facilitating interdisciplinary design specification of smart homes for aging in place. *Studies in Health Technology and Informatics, 124,* 45–50.
18. Driscoll, E. B. (2002). *A timeline for home automation.* Accessed 10/20/15. www.eddriscoll.com/timeline.html.
19. Edwards, K., & McCluskey, A. (2010). A survey of adult power wheelchair and scooter users. *Disability and Rehabilitation: Assistive Technology, 5*(6), 411–419.

20. Fozard, J. (November, 2005). Unpublished conference discussion. In D. C. Burdick & G. Lesnoff-Caravaglia (Chairs Eds.), *Technology and aging: Exemplars of interdisciplinary collaboration in diverse settings.* Orlando, FL: Annual Scientific Meeting of the Gerontological Society of America.

21. Friedmann, E., & Thomas, S. A. (1995). Pet ownership. Social support and one-year survival after acute myocardial infarction in the Cardiac Arrhythmia Suppression Trial (CAST). *American Journal of Cardiology, 76,* 1213–1217.

22. Fuller-Thompson, E., Yu, B., Nuro-Jeter, A., et al. Basic ADL disability and functional limitation rates among older Americans from 2000-2005: The end of the decline? *Journal of Gerontology: Series A Biological/Medical Sciences, 64-A*(12), 1333–1336.

23. Georgia Institute of Technology. (October 25, 2012). *Robots in the home: Will older adults roll out the welcome mat? ScienceDaily.* http://www.sciencedaily.com/releases/2012/10/121025161518.html/. Accessed June 9, 2013.

24. Goldberg, L. R., Koontz, J. S., Rogers, N, & Brickell, J. (2012). Considering accreditation in gerontology: The importance of interprofessional collaborative competencies to ensure quality health care for older adults. *Journal of Gerontology and Geriatrics Education, 33*(1), 95–110.

25. Goozner, M. (March 24, 2012). *New Medicare rule aims to curb waste and fraud in medical equipment business.* Washington Post. Accessed 10/20/15. http://www.washingtonpost.com/new-medicare-rule-aims-to-curb-waste-and-fraud-in-medical-equipment-business/2012/03/20/gIQARa0iYS_story.html.

26. Group Speciale Mobile Association (GSMA). (March, 2012). *Vision of smart home: The role of mobile in the home of the future.* Accessed 10/20/15. http://www.gsma.com/connectedliving/wp-content/uploads/2012/03/vision20of20smart20home20report.pdf.

27. Haggblom-Kronlof, G., & Sonn, U. (2007). Use of assistive devices—a reality full of contradictions in elderly persons' everyday life. *Disability and Rehabilitation: Assistive Technology, 2*(6), 335–345.

28. Hammel, J. (2004). Assistive technologies as tools for everyday living and community participation while aging. In D. C. Burdick & S. Kwon (Eds.), *Gerotechnology: Research and practice in technology and aging* (pp. 119–131). New York, NY: Springer Publishers.

29. Henke, M. (1999). Promoting independence in older persons through the Internet. *CyberPsychology and Behavior, 2*(6), 521–527.

30. Hyer, K., Flaherty, E., Fairchild, S., et al. (Eds.), (2003). Geriatric interdisciplinary team training: The GITT kit. (2nd ed.). New York, NY: John A. Hartford Foundation.

31. Jacobsen, L. A., Kent, M., Lee, M., & Mather, M. (2011). America's aging population. *Population Bulletin, 66*(1), 1–16.

32. Kaplan, B., & Litewka, S. (2008). Ethical challenges of telemedicine and telehealth. *Cambridge Quarterly of Healthcare Ethics, 17,* 401–441.

33. Kutzik, D., & Burdick, D. (2014). Technological tools in long term care: The state of the art and practical considerations for adopters. In D. Yee-Melichar, C. M. Flores, & E. P. Cabigao (Eds.), *Long-term care administration and management: Effective practices and quality programs in elder care.* (pp. 301–326). New York, NY: Springer Publishing Company.

34. Lawton, M. P. (1980). *Environment and aging.* Monterey, CA: Brooks/Cole.

35. Lenker, J. A., & Paquet, V. L. (2003). A review of conceptual models for assistive technology outcomes research and practice. *Assistive Technology: The Official Journal of RESNA, 15*(1), 1–15. doi: 10.1080/10400435.2003.10131885.

36. Libin, A., & Cohen-Mansfield, J. (2004). Therapeutic robocat for nursing home residents with dementia: Preliminary inquiry. *American Journal of Alzheimer's Disease and Other Dementias, 19*(2), 111–116.

37. Liu, H. (2009). Assessment of rolling walkers used by older adults in senior-living communities. *Geriatric Gerontology International, 9,* 124–130.

38. Mann, W. C. (1992). Use of environmental control devices by elderly nursing home patients. *Assistive Technology, 4*(2), 60–65.

39. McConatha, J. T., McConatha, D., Deaner, S., & Dermigny, R. (1995). A computer-based intervention for the education and therapy of institutionalized older adults. *Educational Gerontology, 21,* 129–138.

40. McCreadie, C., & Tinker, A. (2005). The acceptability of assistive technology to older people. *Age and Ageing, 2*(1), 91–110.

41. McMellon, C., & Shiffman, L. (2002). Cybersenior empowerment: How some older individuals are taking control of their lives. *Journal of Applied Gerontology, 21*(2), 157–175.

42. National Complete Streets Coalition. (2015). Smart Growth America. Accessed 10/20/15. http://www.completestreets.org.

43. Nielsenwire. (December 10, 2009). *Six million more seniors using the web than five years ago.* Accessed 10/20/15. http://researchive.weebly.com/uploads/4/2/2/8/4228265/six_million_more_seniors_using_the_web_than_five_years_ago.pdf. [Web log].

44. Ogazalek, V. (1991). The social impacts of computing: Computer technology and the graying of America. *Social Science Computer Review, 9*(4), 655–666.

45. Opalinski, L. (2001). Older adults and the digital divide: Assessing results of a web-based survey. *Journal of Technology in Human Services, 18*(3), 203–221.

46. Petty, L. (2003). Expanding environments through technology. In L. Letts, P. Rigby, & D. Steward (Eds.), *Using environments to enable occupational performance* (pp. 269–286). Thorofare, NJ: SLACK.

47. Philbeck, J. (1997). *Seniors and the internet. Cybersociology Magazine, 2.* Accessed 10/20/15. www.cybersociology.com/files/2_2_philbeck.html/.

48. Politynska, B., van Rijsselt, R. J. T., Lewko, J., et al. (2012). Quality assurance in gerontology and geriatric training programs: The European case. *Journal of Gerontology and Geriatrics Education, 33*(1), 39–54.

49. Raina, P., Waltner-Toews, D., Bonnett, B., et al. (1999). Influence of companion animals on the physical and psychological health of older people: An analysis of a one-year longitudinal study. *Journal of the American Geriatrics Society, 47*(3), 323–329.

50. Rogers, W., Mayhorn, C., & Fiske, A. (2004). Technology in everyday life for older adults. In D. C. Burdick & S. Kwon (Eds.), *Gerotechnology: Research and practice in technology and aging.* New York, NY: Springer Publishers.

51. Saunders, E. J. (2004). Maximizing computer use among the elderly in rural senior centers. *Educational Gerontology, 30,* 573–585.

52. Soderholm, S., & Meinander, A. (2001). Augmentative and alternative communication methods in locked-in syndrome. *Journal of Rehabilitation Medicine, 33*(5), 235–239.

53. Svensson, P. (2011). *Review: Skype phone not worth the hassle. USA Today Tech.* http://www.usatoday/tech/.

54. Tool. (2015). In *Merriam-Webster Dictionary online.* Accessed 10/20/15. http://www.merriam-webster.com/dictionary/tool.

55. U.S. Department of Transportation (2015). *Livability Initiative.* Accessed 10/20/15. www.fhwa.dot.gov/livability/index.cfm.

56. White, H., McConnell, E., Clipp, E., et al. (2002). A randomized controlled trial of the psychosocial impact of providing Internet training and access to older adults. *Aging and Mental Health, 6*(3), 213–221.

57. Wu, Y., Faucounau, V., Boulay, M., et al. (2011). Robotic agents for supporting community-dwelling elderly people with memory complaints: Perceived needs and preferences. *Health Informatics Journal, 17*(1), 33–40.

58. Zhang, Y., Niu, J., Kelly-Hayas, M., et al. (2002). Prevalence of symptomatic hand osteoarthritis and its impact on functional status among elderly: The Framingham Study. *American Journal of Epidemiology, 156*(11), 1021–1027.

ADDITIONAL READINGS

Agree, E., Freedman, V., & Sangupta, M. (2004). Factors influencing the use of mobility technology in community-based long-term care. *Journal of Aging and Health, 16*(2), 267–307.

Bewernitz, M., Mann, W., Dasler, P., & Belchior, P. (2009). Feasibility of machine based prompting to assist persons with dementia. *Assistive Technology, 21*, 196–207.

Cohen-Mansfield, J., Creedon, M., Malone, T., Kirkpatrick, M., Dutra, L., & Herman, R. (2005). Electronic memory aids for community-dwelling elderly persons: Attitudes, preferences and potential utilization. *Journal of Applied Gerontology, 2*(3), 3–20.

Colvin, J., Chenoweth, L., Bold, M., & Harding, C. (2004). Caregivers of older adults: Advantages and disadvantages of Internet-based social support. *Family Relations, 53*(1), 49–57.

Dishman, E., Matthews, J., & Dunbar-Jacob, J. (2003). Everyday health: Technology for adaptive aging. In R. W. Pew & S. B. Van-Hemel (Eds.), *Technology for adaptive aging* (pp. 179–208). Washington, DC: The National Academy Press.

Friederich, A., Bernd, T., & De Witte, L. (2010). Methods for the selection of assistive technology in neurological rehabilitation practice. *Scandinavian Journal of Occupational Therapy, 17*(4), 308–318.

Georgia Institute of Technology. (October 25, 2012). *Robots in the home: Will older adults roll out the welcome mat? ScienceDaily.* Accessed 10/20/15. www.sciencedaily.com/releases/2012/10/121025161518.htm.

Haigh, K. Z., & Yanko, H. A. (2002). *Automation as caregiver: A survey of issues and technologies. AAAI Technical Report WS-02-02.* Accessed 10/20/15. http://www.aaai.org/Papers/Workshops/2002/WS-02-02/WS02-02-007.pdf.

Hedberg-Kristensson, E., Ivanhof, S., & Iwarsson, S. (2007). Experiences among older persons using mobility devices. *Disability and Rehabilitation: Assistive Technology, 2*(1), 15–22.

Horowitz, A., Brennan, M., Reinhardt, J., & MacMillan, T. (2006). The impact of assistive device use on disability and depression among older adults with age-related vision impairments. *Journal of Gerontology, 61B*(5), S274–S280.

Johnson, K., Bamer, A., Yorkston, K., & Amtmann, D. (2009). Use of cognitive aids and other assistive technology for multiple sclerosis. *Disability and Rehabilitation: Assistive Technology, 4*(1), 1–8.

Karmarkar, A., Dicianno, B., Cooper, R., Collins, J., Matthews, J., Koontz, A., et al. (2011). Demographic profile of older adults using wheeled mobility devices. *Aging Research,* Volume 2011 (2011), Article ID 560358, 11 pages. Online free access journal. Accessed 10/20/15. http://www.hindawi.com/journals/jar/2011/560358/.

Kjeken, I., Darre, S., Smedslund, G., Hagen, K., & Nossum, R. (2011). Effect of assistive technology in hand osteoarthritis: A randomized controlled trial. *Annals of Rheumatic Disease, 70*, 1447–1452.

Kraskowsky, L., & Finlayson, M. (2001). Factors affecting older adults' use of adaptive equipment: Review of the literature. *American Journal of Occupational Therapy, 50*, 303–310.

Laforest, S., Pelletier, A., Gauvin, L., Robitaille, Y., Fournier, M., & Corriveau, H. (2009). Impact of a community-based prevention program on maintenance of activity among older adults. *Journal of Aging and Health, 21*(3), 480–500.

LaPlante, M., & Kaye, H. (2010). Demographics and trends in wheeled mobility equipment use and accessibility in the community. *Assistive Technology, 22*, 3–17.

Lung-Kai, P., Mann, W., Tomita, M., & Burford, T. (2010). An evaluation of reachers for use by older persons with disabilities. *Assistive Technology, 10*(2), 113–125.

Mann, W., Goodall, S., Justiss, M., & Tomita, M. (2002). Dissatisfaction and nonuse of assistive devices among frail elders. *Assistive Technology, 14*, 130–139.

Mann, W., Ottenbacher, K., Fraas, L., Tomita, M., & Granger, C. (1999). Effectiveness of assistive technology and environmental interventions in maintaining independence and reducing health care costs for the frail elderly: A randomized controlled trial. *Archives of Family Medicine, 8*, 210–217.

Resnik, L., & Allen, S. (2006). Racial and ethnic differences in use of assistive devices for mobility: Effect modification by age. *Journal of Aging and Health, 18*(1), 106–124.

Tomita, M., Mann, W., Fraas, L., & Stanton, K. (2004). Predictors of the use of assistive devices that address physical impairments among community-based frail elders. *Journal of Applied Gerontology, 23*, 141–155.

Wielandt, T., McKenna, K., Tooth, L., & Strong, J. (2006). Factors that predict the post-discharge use of recommended assistive technology (AT). *Disability and Rehabilitation: Assistive Technology, 1*(1-2), 29–40.

CHAPTER 22

Families and Aging: The Lived Experience

Shirley Kharasch Behr, PhD, FAOTA, Susan C. Tebb, PhD, MSW

> *"All we have to decide is what to do with the time that is given to us."*
> **J.R.R. Tolkien, *The Fellowship of the Ring***

CHAPTER OUTLINE

OBJECTIVES

- Identify societal contexts of aging, especially in regard to social roles and attitudes toward aging
- Appraise dynamics of older adults and their families as they are affected by social and cultural factors
- Discuss the lived experience of growing older within diverse family contexts
- Plan collaborative practices as an occupational therapist with older adults, families, and other health-care professionals

The information presented in this chapter offers current perspectives about the concerns, needs, challenges, expectations, and outcomes often experienced by aging individuals and their families. It includes several significant contributions that have been made to the field of gerontology, as well as insights that emerge from our own professional and personal experiences. The framework for presenting this information is organized around the following themes: the societal context of aging, aging individuals and their families, the dynamics of the lived experience, and future implications for collaborative practice and the occupational therapy (OT) profession.

The Societal Context of Aging

In 1961 Dr. Abraham Joshua Heschel presented the keynote address titled "The Older Person and the Family in the Perspective of Jewish Tradition"[24] to the first White House Conference on Aging. The insightful and discerning observations he shared 50 years ago continue to be relevant in the current environment. Dr. Heschel noted that although old age is something we are all anxious to obtain, many of us act as if it were a disease. White hair and looking old are often considered a defeat. Aged people are frequently assumed to be without ambition, and those who are considered as being no longer useful often experience an inner sense of emptiness, boredom, and a fear of time. Many worry that aging may mean the loss of status and rejection from their families. Dr. Heschel reminds us that the test of a people is their behavior toward the old, and that affection and care for the old, the incurable, and the helpless are the true gold mines of a people.

In 1968 the term *ageism* was coined by Dr. Robert N. Butler[7] and has become part of the English language. *Ageism* refers to the bigotry, systematic stereotyping, and discrimination that people experience simply because they are old. Ageism is considered the principal reason we fear growing older, becoming ill, becoming dependent, and approaching death. Members of the younger generation also fear growing old, and display ageist beliefs about older people when they categorize them as boring, stingy, cranky, demanding, bossy, dirty, and useless. The most extreme form of ageism is prejudice regarding the older person's capacity for work and sexual intimacy. Older people are frequently the victims of physical, emotional, social, sexual, and financial abuse. Dr. Butler noted that the two most profound forms of age prejudice are failing to validate work or purposeful activities, and demeaning the capacity for love.[7]

In 1997 Dr. Joan M. Erikson wrote "The Ninth Stage of Development,"[17] the final chapter in her husband Erik Erikson's last book, *The Extended Version of the Life Cycle Completed.* She identified 80- and 90-year-old individuals as those who are living in the final stage of the life cycle, noting that old age during this final stage brings with it new demands and difficulties. Those whose bodies have been in the best of condition begin to weaken and become less flexible; they may have less self-esteem and diminished autonomy; simple activities of daily living (ADLs) can be distressing, and even overwhelming. In regard to this stage, she writes:

> I do believe that in the ninth stage it is mandatory to lighten our load of possessions, especially those that call for supervision and care. If you hope to climb the mountain, whether or not meditation beckons you, travel must be light and unburdened. A lifetime of training is required for success. It's so easy to blame the terrain, the light, the wind for failures and backsliding. Moments of rest are mandatory, but there is no time for self-pity and weakening of purpose. Light too is necessary, for the way and the days are all too short. Song is joyous in the half-light. The dark offers release and dreams of those near and dear and much beloved.[17]

Challenges, conflict, and tension can be sources of growth, strength, and commitment. Dr. Erikson considered growing old a privilege that allows feedback on a long life that can be relived in retrospect. In contrast, the current model of aging that is most frequently embraced by our society has been one of "letting go." Letting go is a time of stagnation that promotes denial and a false old age, instead of encouraging aging individuals to seek a new model, a new life, and new roles. To date, attention in our culture has been focused on achieving perfection and measuring up to expectations, instead of going beyond the limits imposed by our world and seeking fulfillment. She suggests that because many of us are unprepared for old age, we need to revise our perceptions and attitudes about aging. Instead of focusing our efforts on achieving perfection and measuring up to expectations, we need to think about old age as the age of opportunities for inner growth, not as the age of stagnation. It should not be thought of as a defeat, but a victory; it is not a punishment, but a privilege. We need to remind aging individuals that every moment is an opportunity for greatness, and for eliminating resentments, bitterness, and jealousies. Time is our most important frontier.[3] It is the advance region of our age, a region where our true freedom lies. Despite the scientific and technological accomplishments made during their lifetime, aging individuals may consider themselves as belonging to the past.

Aging Individuals and Their Families

Aging individuals and their families often have multifaceted and challenging concerns that need to be addressed. These concerns may be individualistic in nature or associated with one or more of the following: caregiving, family relationships, social isolation, economic factors, social factors, psychoemotional and biophysical factors, coping with stress, and resilience.[10]

Caregiving

The demographics of the population in the United States are changing. In 1900, only 4.1% of Americans lived to age 65 years; in 2013 this age group numbered 44.7 million, equivalent to one in seven U.S. citizens. Projections for 2060 are for 98 million, more than twice the number in 2013.[47] Although advances in treatment are making it increasingly possible for people to survive medical crises they could not have been able to endure in previous years, they may need to continue living with a chronic condition. It is estimated that 50% of the U.S. population has at least one chronic condition, and represents more than 80% of spending on health care.[28] Furthermore, those with functional limitations and chronic conditions need more health-care services and assistance with ADLs. (See chapter 3 for more detailed discussion.)

The increase in numbers of older Americans has been well documented, particularly for people 85 years and older. Increasing numbers of people are living longer with chronic illnesses and disabilities, which may require complex care and sophisticated technology. In contrast, families are having fewer children, and the pool of available family caregivers is shrinking. With less help available, the stress on those who do provide care may increase, negatively affecting those individuals' physical, financial, and emotional health.

Informal Family Caregiving

Family caregiving is considered to be the act of providing assistance to family members or friends without being paid to do so; it is also referred to as informal (unpaid) care. It is a personal, economic, and public health issue. In the United States there are well over 50 million people who provide care for chronically ill, disabled, or aged family members during any given year; families provide 80% of all home health care to older adults.[38,46]

The average length of time spent on caregiving for a family member over the age of 50 years is about 8 years.[32] The value of services provided for "free" was estimated to be over $450 billion in 2009, based upon 42.1 million caregivers.[36]

The presence or absence of a family often determines how successfully an individual might grow older, but a study on caregivers of clients with dementia showed that the stress of family caregiving may affect a person's immune system for up to 3 years after their caregiving ends, thereby increasing the caregiver's chances of developing a chronic illness.[21] Older adult spousal caregivers who have a history of chronic illness and are experiencing caregiving-related stress have a 63% higher mortality rate than their noncaregiving peers.[37]

Family caregivers who provide care for 36 or more hours weekly are more likely than noncaregivers to experience symptoms of depression or anxiety. For spouses, the rate is six times higher; for adult children, the rate is twice as high. These caregivers have many unmet needs, including the following:

- Finding time for themselves
- Balancing their work and family responsibilities
- Keeping the person they care for safe at home and being able to manage the person's challenging behaviors
- Managing their own emotional and physical stress
- Knowing how to talk with doctors
- Making end-of-life decisions
- Managing incontinence or toileting problems

Approximately 50% of all caregivers assist their loved ones with personal care, yet less than one in five (18%) report having received formal training on how to care for this individual.[40]

Formal (Paid) Caregiving

Formal (paid) caregiving generally refers to paid assistance with activities of daily living (ADLs) and instrumental activities of daily living (IADLs). Care recipients may be of any age, and may receive either or both types of care.

Estimates vary on how many individuals are in the paid caregiving workforce. The Bureau of Labor Statistics,[48] indicates that personal care and home health care are among the fastest growing occupations in the United States. It should be noted that the ability to count caregivers becomes more blurred as more programs allow payment to family members for care.

The paid caregiving workforce is also facing challenges. High turnover, difficult work, and low compensation all contribute to difficulties in hiring quality staff, and this industry is subject to the same demographic influences as the pool of family caregivers. Strategies have been proposed to increase and sustain the pool of paid caregivers. One theory is that improving pre-employment training and continuing education reduces turnover by giving workers the competence and confidence they need to do the job well.[33] Training, including hand-on skills, safety (worker and client), infection control, communication, and behavior management, is required by the federal government for basic credentialing for certified nursing assistants (CNAs) and home health aides (HHAs). There may be a similar local requirement for personal care assistants (PCAs), but these vary by state. Ongoing training, according to federal law, must address weaknesses and provide the specialized knowledge needed to care for a particular client or resident population.[33] The need for basic and continuing education for paid caregivers may represent an opportunity for OT to contribute to the retention of competent paid caregivers, while also improving the quality of care provided to clients.[14]

Family Relationships

The relationship within the family provides several types of support: an emotional foundation (both positive and negative), resources, physical energy, and social contact. In a family we depend on other members for help in these areas of personal need. Family members try to reciprocate, and as individuals grow older the payback methods change. Often an individual must draw from an interpersonal "account" established many years before or contribute in other ways. This payback does not always work due to relationship issues brought on by death, re-partnering, or conflict within a family. Various ethnic groups view the obligations of family members to older adults differently.

Often as people grow older they place themselves or family members into the role of caregiver, depending on the physical and/or mental health needs of the older adults in the family unit. In families with older adults, the phrase "role reversal" is often used to describe the changing relations, but roles do not actually reverse:[18] Caring for an older adult is nothing like caring for a child. A parent prepares the child for leaving the support of the nuclear family, whereas caring for an older adult often involves changing the family structure in ways to accommodate a person who is becoming more dependent on the support of many. Families provide the majority of the support to older adults. For some individuals with strong, positive family networks, growing older can be a rewarding event, whereas for others, due to the type of family relationships, this process of change to older age is testy, but nonetheless typically families are part of each person's transition to old age. Often the family network serves as a system of support; and the majority of us will reach a point in our lives when we must rely on others, mainly family, for our everyday needs.

The longevity rates of older adults worldwide present stress to family systems. Many older adults live long enough to contract a chronic disease. With a pattern in the United States, Canada, and Western Europe of later marriages, and globally fewer children due to decreased birth rates, there are fewer family members to care for each other. Giving care to a family member is an awesome responsibility that has inherent risk and joy.[8]

Defining Roles

Becvar and Becvar[1] note that we do not relate to people; rather, we relate to a metaphor/role that we assign family members and ourselves. Our relationships within our families are identified by the complements to the metaphors/roles that have been assigned or selected (Box 22-1): "To define a role is to define a complementary role and thus a relationship, for their meanings are recursive" (p. 354).[1] A pathological perspective is to see roles in isolation and not in relationship to events in family life. Nothing has meaning by itself, only in

---

BOX 22-1 Family and Task Roles/Metaphors

Examples of Relationship Roles/Metaphors
Child
Adult child
Parent
Grandchild
Grandparent
Sibling
Friend
Neighbor
Lover

Examples of Task Roles/Metaphors
Caregiver
Breadwinner
Housekeeper
Yard maintenance worker
Social secretary
Driver

(From Becvar, D. S., & Becvar, R. J. (2009). *Family therapy: A systemic integration.* Boston, MA: Pearson Education)

context. Relationships are part of the balance necessary for each of the parts and thus of the whole—what an individual does is never independent of the whole but always within relationships. The roles of various family members thus change over the life of family, and all changes affect family relationships.[3,4]

Individuals play multiple roles and some overlap. Boundaries between roles can be ambiguous and thus the experiences in one role can spill over into other roles. Role spillover is two directional; events occurring in one role have the potential to affect experiences in other roles.[39] These roles can support or interfere with other roles, causing greater life satisfaction, conflict, strain, or the need to acquire resources to help manage the roles. For example, consider a parent and adult child who had an earlier strained relationship; when the parent suddenly has a stroke and now needs significant medical care, the child may be conflicted in how to proceed.

When Roles Begin to Shift

Nothing speaks better to defining family relationships than the saying "the whole is greater than the sum of its parts." Acknowledging this concept also brings the issue of complexity to the forefront because the more we add to the whole, the more complex it becomes. A person cannot be considered without considering the family to which the person belongs; we all are part or parts of a family or families. It is also important to note that when one part of a family changes, it affects all family members, because all family members are interrelated.[1]

It is possible to work with just one member of a family, but that work will affect the other members, as the family unit shifts into a pattern of stability, adapting to the change in one member. It was this discovery that led the first family therapists to begin to work with the whole family and not a lone family member in treating an issue. If an intervention doesn't consider and work with the family context, it fails to address the systemic issues.

Solutions need to occur in the larger context—within the "family relationship,"[1] for we are all in relationship with one another. Becvar and Becvar[1] found that all events should be looked at in terms of relationship: No event has meaning or identity by itself, only in its complement. What an event is called can make a difference in terms of the relationship implied by the particular metaphor/illusion. This refers to "family members" who aren't actually blood relatives. For example, an individual in her teens realized that "Grandma Jean" wasn't actually a blood relative; she was a childhood friend of her grandmother's. Grandma Jean did not have children of her own; thus the teen's sister and she became her "grandchildren."

When we have time to prepare for role changes, or models to use to guide role transitions, it is often easier to find homeostasis within the family, as opposed to when the role change comes suddenly without warning, such as with illness or death (see the discussion later in the chapter on coping with stress). The multiple roles that older adults hold contribute to the perception of well-being—or lack of it—thus, as noted earlier, it is the cognitive coping strategies that we as

health-care providers can most aptly assist with, to bring about positive contributions of growing older within family. Drawing on our own experiences of loss, OT practitioners can strengthen the team, building from strength and acceptance of ambiguity, and not suggesting closure but instead allowing the ambiguity of events to be part of the process of aging families.[6]

Family Dynamics

Familism is defined as the feelings of loyalty, reciprocity, and solidarity experienced among members within a family unit.[13] Familism can be significantly high or low depending on how members view family within different cultures. OT practitioners should consider familism as a cultural value that influences how roles are perceived within the family.

In serving families with older members, a greater appreciation for cultural differences is one step that we, as OT practitioners, can take in response to systemic oppression of the older family member. Oppression can play out in a number of ways. The following actions by all practitioners, for example, contribute to oppression:[9]

- Making decisions without consulting and including the family of a culture different from our own in the older adult's care decisions
- Assuming that race and ethnicity are linked to the behavioral and genetic differences that an older adult may be experiencing
- Being unwilling to explore the metaphors of race and ethnicity in our practice contexts
- Denying the historical, political, or economic effects of oppression on older adults, not seeing them as part of the larger social context (and thus denying older adults the dignity that each deserves)

To work effectively in diverse cultures requires us to work as a team with family and creatively integrate what we know with multiple perspectives—most especially the family's—into all parts of our work. The issues of diversity, cultural understanding, and appreciation are part of the social fabric as those living in this world grow older with each generation.

To provide health and wellness in a family-centered way we need to learn and know the cultural context of the older adults being served. A useful way to look at ethnic and cultural diversity in older adults in the United States is to examine the following domains:[34,51]

- Personal health perspective
- Care-seeking behaviors
- Unique genetic attributes (e.g., increased risk of osteoporosis for non-Hispanic whites)
- Living environment
- Barriers to processing information
- Trust in the health-care system and helping professions

As OT practitioners working with culturally diverse older adults, we must look beyond our knowledge and wisdom and focus on the perceptions of the family and family members, thus creating a person- and family-centered team, a team that develops competent ways of working with and appreciates the differences among people—in this case, older people. Our response often has not reflected this perspective, as exemplified by the disparities in health care seen in the United States among African Americans, Native Americans, Latinos, and other groups in regard to access to and quality of care; many within these groups have often have a shorter lifespan and more health disabilities. [14,51]

Isolation

Social isolation from relationships can be an unfortunate outcome of growing older. Physical and mental aging can bring about physical health, mental health, and economic issues, and when it does, older adults can become isolated from those around them. In working with older adults, isolation is generally seen as social isolation, often measured in the number of people the individual sees each week.[44] But when isolation is viewed as part of a process where people lose their perception of connection to others, it is a multidimensional process—not just the issue of the isolated older adult, but an issue regarding the relationships within family and community.

Rathbone-McCuan and Hashimi[35] conceptualized a framework for isolated older adults along two dimensions, with the first occurring at the individual level and the second at the family/community level. Both dimensions are divided into four areas of isolators:

1. Economic
2. Social
3. Biophysical
4. Psycho-emotional

Increased awareness of the levels of isolators is likely to increase OT staff ability to work and be part of a team with an older adult. Isolation additionally concerns a complex relationship with the economic, social, biophysical, and psychoemotional issues of the family. Isolation often cuts older adults off from potential support and assistance. Next addressed are possible isolators on the individual level and then on the family/community level.

Economic Factors

As an individual ages, the ability to continue to work and/or increase personal income often ceases; the individual retires, no longer is promoted, or is terminated to hire a younger person who can be paid less or who possesses different skills and experiences. This is a time when income can become inadequate, if it was not already; medical care, future long-term care needs, and the cost of basic needs in the future are all unknown and can exacerbate isolation. At the family/community level, inadequate policies and/or services to support family can serve as the economic isolator as family members become older; lack of services or the cost of these services may deter families from using support when it is needed.

Social Factors

One of the biggest isolators at the individual level is the loss of relationships with friends, spouses, and family members due to death, retirement, or health issues. At the family/community level, isolation is often due to society's stereotypical and often negative views on aging, or, as Robert Butler coined it, "ageism."[7] Shifts in roles and emotional health, such as depression

and anxiety, can also contribute to changes in an individual's coping strategies and thus isolate and cause fear. Additionally, societal expectations of family relationship roles and where and how an individual should live as an older adult can be an isolator to the family. For example, possible nursing home placement can be feared by many and can tear family members apart, should this become a choice they must consider; the decision around this choice can be isolating to the family.

Biophysical and Psycho-Emotional Factors

The physical aging of both the body and mind can isolate the individual, and, in turn, the resulting isolation can contribute to the physical decline of the mind and body. This can be experienced in several family members if multiple members are living in a household and growing old together. At the family/community level, lack of knowledge regarding the physical state of an individual or individuals in a family can isolate these individuals, because their family members or communities are unaware, or don't know how to assist them. Biopsychosocial changes are the primary isolator of individuals who are growing older.[44] An individual's physical health affects levels of isolation; social, economic, and psycho-emotional function; and well-being—as health declines, economic resources are used, and social contacts with others become difficult, potentially resulting in depression and anxiety. At the family/community level, the lack of knowledge about health issues affects policy, available resources, forms of assistance, and society's view of ageism.

Prevention or Mediation

To mediate isolation in relationships, OT personnel, as health/mental health care providers, need to recognize that isolation limits an individual's ability to seek help. Thus, we need to pay attention to isolating dimensions and reach out to families with older adults and listen for potential isolators. We can also educate family members and their communities about potential relationship isolator factors. A range of formal and informal supports is needed for older adults and families. Where formal services are available, they need to be culturally appropriate, affordable, and accessible. With informal supports, we need to build upon the strength of relationships with family members and friends and repeatedly offer support to the older adult and family to avoid or lessen isolation.

Adult Developmental Factors

Growing older is a highly individualistic and complex process that unveils itself in a number of dimensions—social, physical, emotional, and spiritual. We must be aware of these dimensions so that we can distinguish between so-called "typical" age-related changes and disease processes. Age-related developmental changes can speed up the aging process if they interact with disease. Underlying these dimensions is the premise that all individuals, regardless of age, have an inherent ability to learn and change. It is important to examine both typical and alternative ways of understanding adult development in the aging process.

Typically, adult development is viewed as being centered on chronological age or attainment of particular social roles. Weick[50] proposes an alternative perspective that views adult growth around tasks and life events, enabling the acknowledgment that the environment often prevents people from growth because of role expectations forced on them by society, and this is especially true for older adults. Personal growth and change, regardless of age, may also be inhibited because of the necessity to first meet survival needs. Beyond survival, other significant factors affect growth and change. Coping strategies appear to be a significant factor that may influence an individual's family life course. Given the belief that individuals have an inherent potential for growth, change can occur at any age. However, such change may be more difficult for older persons because the energy that could be directed toward growth may be consumed in coping with physical and interpersonal losses. Those interpersonal losses may include both intimate partnerships and family systems.

As previously discussed, a critical characteristic of human nature is that lives are lived in relationship to other people. This is played out explicitly within a family system in which all of us are a part. Family development, like individual development, is viewed as a series of tasks and events.[22] Placing the stressing event within the framework of current family tasks provides a vivid conceptualization of each family member's part in the event. Each event disrupts the homeostasis of the family and causes role shifts and realignment of family boundaries,[5] no matter what the event. Perception of the event, as gain or loss, is a significant coping response. These events can create the potential for learning new coping skills within the family and can help individuals adapt positively to the various tasks encountered in the family lifespan with older adults.[30]

Coping with Stress

Stressors are present everywhere in human existence; humans are required to cope all of the time. Coping with stress presents a complex process that involves changing conditions that have a history and a future. It involves role modification. A theoretical framework, the ABCX Family Crisis Model[25,26] was created to explain family adjustment to life stresses (Figure 22-1). This model proposes that factor A (a life-straining event), interacting with factor B (the family's existing resources and coping strategies) and also with factor C (the family's perception of the event), produces factor X (a crisis or reason for the homeostasis of the family to change). It is defined as a crisis by the family if the members see it as threatening and perceive their coping abilities and resources as inadequate to meet the demands of the event.

McCubbin and Patterson's[30] work on the interactions of the family event/crisis before and after its occurrence suggests that a family undergoes the initial event and over time experiences an accumulation of the stress and its daily demands. They expanded the Hill model to the Double ABCX Model,[30] introducing adaptation to three kinds of stressors: the initial event, the events resulting from the changes made to the events, and those events resulting from the family's attempt to adapt. Change and stress are viewed in this model as an ongoing

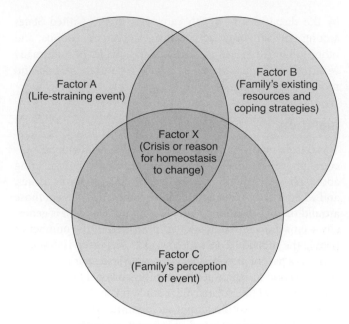

FIGURE 22-1 The ABCX Family Crisis Model.

process through which the family may begin to adapt to the event. Adaptive coping is a way families obtain necessary resources. The family is viewed as a resource exchange network, and coping, both cognitive and behavioral, is the action that assists this exchange within the family.

Taylor developed a cognitive adaptation theory of coping. In her work with family members experiencing cancer she found that with the event of cancer, families used three cognitive themes in coping: looking for the meaning of the event, attempting to master the event and find homeostasis in life again, and restoring self-esteem through self-enhancing evaluation.[41] Taylor maintains that the families that manage effectively in the threat of difficult events are those that develop a process of adjustment that involves the acquisition of these three cognitive themes. So our job as professional helpers is to help families find ways to bring resolution to these three themes when an event or change occurs that disrupts the homeostasis of the family. Taylor's later work[43] found that effective resolution of the themes relies on the ability of the individual and the family to develop what she terms "positive illusions," or positive perceptions/views of the event. She found that it is these positive perceptions that protect and buffer stressful life events. Resiliency can be learned. Research shows that resilient people have common qualities,[27,49] and these are qualities that practitioners can teach. Siebert[27] found that resilient families stay connected and help each other; they are optimistic and see the glass as half full; they are spiritual and playful; they like themselves; they give back, and in doing so receive and experience hope; they pick their battles; they are as healthy as nature allows; they seek solutions and are willing to learn; and they reframe events into strength from adversity.

To assist with positive coping strategies, families need to be helped to develop internal coping by reframing the event, which includes problem solving and attitude adjustment, especially in regard to anger, denial, and withdrawal around the initial event, and external coping by accepting formal, social, and spiritual supports.

The first author's work on positive family contributions[2] developed questionnaires that measure four perceptions of cognitive coping proposed by Taylor:[41] assigning a cause for the event(s), gaining a sense of control over the event, comparing one's family with others, and finding positive benefits from the event. She found that many families need to learn to cope in a positive manner, and as health-care helpers we can work as a team with the family to learn positive coping strategies. We can offer interventions that emphasize the coping techniques of control and mastery; this includes information on available resources, learning to ask for help, and using available help. Coping strategies must be realistic for the family, not geared at changing a situation over which one has little control. The perception of the event can serve as a mediator between the event and how the event affects the family. Helping families take control of the perceptions and the loss they experience may help them cope in a more positive manner. Interventions that look at the change in the relationships between family members over time help the members to develop perceptions of control and positive adaptation. Older adults often cannot problem solve as they have in the past, but they can be helped to develop cognitive coping strategies that allow them to accept assistance and take control over their thinking processes. So much of our work as health-care providers to families with older adults should be to help them develop and accept cognitive coping methods as the primary method in addressing events that occur within the family unit. Because adaptation to events is an ongoing and evolving process, help needs to be available at all stages of family life with older adults.

Resilience

Resilience is a term used to describe the psychological and biological strengths that are required to successfully master change.[19] The more resilient an individual is, the more quickly he or she establishes trusting, collaborative relationships. Attributes that describe resilient individuals include the following:
- Have the motivation to make things better
- Search for solutions
- Have a strong sense of self-esteem and independence of thought
- Have a high level of personal discipline and sense of responsibility
- Are open-minded and receptive to new ideas
- Are willing to dream
- Have a wide range of interests
- Demonstrate a keen sense of humor
- Exhibit high tolerance of distress
- Are committed to life
- Interpret their personal experiences with meaning and hope

Family members draw on relationships with extended family and their social networks to gain resilience, a sense of meaning, and strength. The importance of relationships in promoting resiliency within the family circle, between family members, and within the social network of the community is a consistent theme among many cultures. The

contextual nature of a family's community has a strong influence on the nature of the family's problems, the risk factors, and the types of resources available to promote resiliency. It is important to balance our knowledge about the nature of the family membership against the information we may acquire from individual members in terms of what fits the family members.

Culture

The United States is a country with diverse languages, religions, cultures, and ethnicities as a result of past and current immigration and political and economic refugees. As OT practitioners, our question is how we come to terms with these differences among the families as we work to support them in our work with older adults. We also must ask ourselves how we work as practitioners while not continuing to add to the disparities families undergo due to their ethnicity, language, or religion. We need to work with ourselves to accept, not just tolerate, differences in the older families we work with. This involves the following behaviors:
- Acknowledging the barriers that many have to our services and working to break down these barriers
- Looking within and seeing what barriers we might put in place that do not allow us to work effectively with older adults and their families
- Being willing to accept that we might not know about another's culture and being willing and open to learning

This requires lifelong learning on the part of the OT practitioner. We cannot go to a workshop to learn how to be culturally competent; we must be willing to learn from the families with whom we work, be tolerant of being uncomfortable, and be willing to ask for help.

Capitman[9] notes that three tasks for practitioners are: "(1) meeting the needs of current elders from diverse groups; (2) managing an eldercare workforce that is quite different in race and ethnicity and life experiences from the aging boomers; and (3) supporting the economic achievements of younger people from diverse backgrounds while promoting their sense of social solidarity with elders so that they will continue to be willing and able to support elder-care programs" (p. 9).[9] Where this type of diversity is present, it can be a strength that we celebrate.

Characteristics of Diversity

The following are general family dynamics examples within the United States. OT personnel should spend some time with each family to ascertain what is appropriate and relevant regarding that family's particular dynamic.

African American families tend to participate in supportive social networks that facilitate their adaptation to the demands and challenges of the environment. They rely on flexible relationships within the family unit, a strong sense of religiosity, and a strong identification with their racial group. Native American and First Nations families belong to a large number of groups that have distinct cultural heritages. Potentially relevant interventions are based on a relational model that has a holistic perspective and emphasizes balance. Interventions are organized to establish or restore a balance model that incorporates the mind, body, spirit, and context, which includes the culture, work, community, history, and environment. The body includes all physical aspects; the spirit includes teaching and practice (both positive and negative) and metaphysical and innate forces. Family resiliency is supported by stories told within the family circle.[51]

Latino families represent the largest racial/ethnic group in the United States. This population faces a wide range of circumstances, ranging from great wealth to poverty. Because there are important differences among Latino groups, it's important to understand the historical context of the groups in general and the individual families. Although the groups vary on a number of dimensions, they all have important values that are sources of resiliency. These sources include respect, involving the entire extended family, and spirituality. The extended family and the church are very important sources of informal supports.

Unity of the person, family, nature, and the spiritual world is an essential basis of resiliency among Native Hawaiian families. They experience themselves as united with the larger social, natural, and spiritual forces of the world. They typically believe that harmony and health can be restored by acting with loving kindness, caring, and responsibility to the family, nature, and society. The combination of social responsibility and reciprocity maintains the community context that is important for families. Social support is an important buffer.

Asian families represent a wide variety of individual national and cultural groups with different histories and religions. Conceptualization of family may include ancestors as well as current family members, and typically family members are expected to contribute to the family unit as a whole. Some families have experienced major trauma due to war. Family situations can be complicated, and individuals may vary widely in their adherence to national values and ways of life. The immediate and extended family unit is central, and loyalty to and respect for the family is very important. Family members are expected to uphold the honor of the family and to avoid bringing shame to the family. A series of studies on how families deal with older adult members revealed that Asians have a powerful sense of filial obligation to care for their older adult parents; however, this expectation is beginning to change with the times. Historically, however, it has been important for older family members to preserve and transmit their processes to the younger generation.

The Lived Experience

Aging has been changing throughout much of the world, and has become both an individual and a social process. New experiences of aging have transformed the options available for families. Over the past decade studies have provided us with a greater understanding of the important connection between families and aging. Some studies emphasize the need to conceptualize families more broadly, and to emphasize the importance of connections between family members. They call attention to the value of recognizing that the wishes and capabilities of individuals change as they grow older, and that family relationships need to change as well.[3,4]

Narrative accounts of important events in our lives provide insights about how we and others have been affected. Narratives become our "personal stories" to illustrate sequences of events, the positive and negative challenges we encountered, how individuals responded to these challenges, and the dynamic interactions that took place.[12] Narratives also provide retrospective perspectives about the purpose lived experiences have in developing meaningful growth experiences, as in the following examples of Mary, who cared for her aging mother, and Susan, whose mother was diagnosed with Parkinson's disease. These narratives present authentic information provided by two professional colleagues. These individuals offered to share their narratives with our readers to illustrate the dynamics of "real" lived experiences with aging parents and their families.[42,43]

CASE EXAMPLE 22-1 Mary's Lived Experience

Mary, a single woman, has been a practicing occupational therapist and an OT educator throughout her adult life. Mary's mother, Pat, became a widow at the age of 40 years and subsequently raised her two children (Mary and her younger brother John) as a single parent. Pat earned a master's degree in education shortly after her 65th birthday. She was a trained musician, a reading specialist, and a music educator for piano, organ, cello, and singing lessons. Pat was also a lifelong scholar and, despite her unremitting physical decline due to diabetes, she remained mentally alert until just a few days before her death at the age of 97 years. Pat owned a duplex home that made it possible for Mary to live in the separate adjacent apartment. Their physical proximity and positive relationship allowed Mary to meet most of Pat's needs as her primary caregiver for 20 consecutive years. Throughout that time Mary held several demanding administrative positions with multiple obligations that required extensive travel. Mary's brother John, his wife, and their children were helpful and caring family members with a keen understanding of the demands made on Mary by her role and responsibilities as Pat's caregiver. They were especially mindful of the performance demands and expectations made by Mary's professional position, and by the needs imposed by matters related to her personal life. John, a physician, was Pat's medical power of attorney and was responsible for communicating with medical staff. He was always supportive of Mary's needs and was her advocate and advisor at all times. John, his wife, and their children made it possible for Pat to visit with their family members and to be in contact with their children and grandchildren.

The opportunity to reflect on the many issues associated with her role as Pat's caregiver for those 20 years made it possible for Mary to develop new insights about the difficult issues she encountered. The most difficult issue was the challenge caused by Pat's ongoing physical and sensory decline. Pat's hearing loss, restricted vision,

CASE EXAMPLE 22-1   Mary's Lived Experience—cont'd

and limited mobility had an increasingly negative effect on her ability to move about, listen to music, and read. The loss of her musical acuity was particularly difficult, and the cumulative effect of all of her losses became the loss of her roles and her identity. It was as though she had lost both her voice and her credibility. Professionals began directing their questions to Mary instead of to Pat, who began to feel like a nonentity. Pat came to recognize that these individuals had very little interest in her past life, or in her current interests and abilities.

Mary recognized it was time to consider a different continuum of care that would better serve Pat's changing needs. A suitable assisted living facility was selected with Pat's approval, and she lived there in comfort during the last few years of her life. Pat developed new friendships with other residents, and took part in and enjoyed the social activities. Pat also welcomed the opportunities to spend time with all of her family. Family relationships had even greater meaning to Pat during those last few years. In the last 3 months of her life, Pat's health issues made it necessary for multiple emergency visits to the hospital. Immediately after Pat's last emergency visit, 10 days before her death, she requested never to be returned to the hospital. The reason

she gave was "they throw me around like a sack of potatoes." The insensitive nature of the staff and the lack of understanding about her personal needs were extremely difficult for her to cope with, even more difficult than the pain intervention indicated by her health status.

Mary still reflects on her lived experience and the influence it had on her life. She recognizes that the most rewarding outcomes were the many opportunities she had to deal with challenges and conflicts, to become much closer to her mother, and to know her mother and herself much more deeply. Mary has ongoing concerns about current issues that shape care for aging individuals and their families. Those include respite support, role reversal, finances, roles of siblings, job obligations, friendships, finances, work, family relations, co-workers, physical and psychological limitations, and communication. Mary considers her caregiving journey to have been a dynamic, constantly changing experience. It has been through her own lived experience that Mary appreciates the reality of each person's journey being distinct. Each journey reflects the traits and relationships among those involved, the circumstances of each person's life, the nature of the care that is needed, and the resources available to meet those needs.[43]

CASE EXAMPLE 22-2   A Family's Lived Experience: Lessons Learned and Gifts Received through Caregiving

The following narrative* provides a family member's account of her mother's experience with Parkinson's disease. She includes descriptions of how her family coped with the changes in function and needs over time resulting from the diagnosis and disease progression.

Twenty years ago we became a "family with Parkinson's disease." That is how my father describes it. My mother, diagnosed with Parkinson's at the early age of 58 years, was now 10 years into her diagnosis and no longer able to function on her own. By that time Dad, principal caregiver, had framed some guidelines for his personal use in that role. Here they are as he shared them with my sister, my brother, and me:

• Attend directly and fully to those things that must be done and that only you can do. If time and energy permit, do whatever else can be comfortably done; otherwise seek additional help.
• Share with your loved one, at whatever level she can function, the ongoing relationship of you two people on a life path together. Memories, family stories, family activities, celebratory moments, special events, sometimes even frank discussion of the disease process and what together can be done about it—these and other ways of sharing create the context within which meaning for everyday living can be preserved and extended.
• For you, the caregiver, look through, beside, and beyond the confines of the illness. Define and seek activities and relationships that are nurturing to your own sense of self.

The "Servant Self" must also be the "Growing Self," or else burnout will cancel all hopes, all joys, and all meaning for both parties to the journey.[23]

In retrospect, as Mom's illness progressed and Dad's daily challenges became increasingly demanding, those guidelines became woven into the fabric of his living. However vaguely they were recognized in his mind before, now they became a lifeline for him, 10 years into her illness.

Some months after Dad really began living these daily directions, Mom fell and broke her hip. Realization of the responsibility for her care at this new level came to Dad while she was recovering in the hospital. He knew he could no longer provide the full daily care she needed, and thus she was moved to the extended care unit in the retirement center where Mom and Dad lived. There she stayed, for 8 1/2 years, until her death, and Dad continued his daily caregiving, although now with the help of the nursing unit.

In honor of Mother's death at the 10-year point, I asked Dad to reflect on the care our family (especially Dad) provided over those 20 years of caring. He responded with the following lessons of learning that came to him through efforts to perform the caring role. All are important, even though some came to him too late to be of help to any great extent. Perhaps they can provide insight to others as they embark on the role of caregiver.

Lessons learned by the family from caring:
• Although it is the patient/client who bears the chronic problem, the entire family suffers the problem and is inescapably its victim also.

*This narrative is adapted from Tebb, S.S., & Steiger, R. (2008). Time Taken as a Caring Family. *Reflections: Narratives of Professional Helping, 14*(3), 1-11.

Continued

CASE EXAMPLE 22-2 A Family's Lived Experience: Lessons Learned and Gifts Received through Caregiving—cont'd

- The caregiver could truly "die of the loved one's disease," if he or she permits burnout to occur.
- Don't take negatives personally when expressed by the patient/client.
- Your loved one is a fractured person. You may not be hearing from the person with whom you once shared life and love.
- Live your life anyway, even when you must serve your loved one in crucial ways. Take regular and special breaks.
- Find and/or create events/settings where your loved one is included in group experiences. Help your loved one continue to belong.
- Do not lay expectations on your loved one that he or she cannot fulfill, even if your loved one has carried that item all his or her life before becoming very ill.
- Teach yourself the art of silent grief—dispose of grief, day by day, as losses occur.
- Project your own life not only "with," but also "aside from" and "beyond" the stresses of everyday caring.
- Seek all the help you can get as caregiver. Call on every resource you can unearth. Even then it will never seem enough. Few primary caregivers are as fortunate as we were, having in the family both a social worker and a nurse as helpers, consultants, and supporters. Still, there were times when even more insight and assistance could have been helpful.

As I reflect again and again on these thoughts Dad shared, I realize the numerous gifts the caregiving experience has brought to our family. Let me share four of them here:

1. The experience has helped our family understand and be touched by the pains and problems of other caregivers.
2. Because of what we shared as a caregiving family, Dad especially is able to help many of his neighbors and residents in his community to live "with," "aside from," and "beyond" the everyday care they are giving their loved ones.
3. My siblings, our children, and I have grown from the caregiving experience. We are more aware of the possible changes that occur in families and how families need to continue to work, grow, and support each other through these times.
4. We also are very aware that we will more than likely be caregivers in our lifetime, and we hope we can be as gracious at it as our dad/grandpa was.

The following quote by Olympia Dukakis describes what we as a family came to learn, believe, and support as a family giving care: "Whether the illness is cancer or Alzheimer's (or whatever) there can be no hard-and-fast rules about life after diagnosis—except that you need to be honest and flexible. It's an inherently personal process, and I doubt that caregiving decisions are ever easy. But made conscientiously—as is the case of the Edwards family (Senator John and Elizabeth Edwards), the fictional Fiona (a character in the movie *Away From Her*) and, I believe, my own family—those decisions should be respected" (p. 35).[15]

Importance of Family-Centered Collaborative Practice

OT personnel typically partner with parents, families, and caregivers of individuals with disabilities and chronic illness. That partnership develops in a variety of settings across all stages of the life cycle, ranging from early intervention with very young children, to school-based programs for older students, to client education and discharge planning for adults in health-care settings. It also includes working with aging individuals in the community, whether in their own homes, long-term care settings, or hospice, and has contributed significantly to the gerontological and caregiving literature.

The OT literature addresses the challenges of providing family-centered services and the role of environmental influences on occupational performance for caregivers and care recipients.[20] As key professionals who promote client function, safety, and community living, occupational therapists and assistants can be identified in practice settings as primary professionals whose contributions can provide targeted caregiver education, training and skill-building, and psychosocial support, to reduce "excess disability" among care recipients, reduce caregiver burden, and promote safety, health, and well-being for both caregivers and care recipients. Health-care professionals need to become collaborative partners in the delivery of these services and to help families learn how they can best contribute to the healing process. They need to recognize that families are also "experts" about the problems of their loved ones. They also need to understand and appreciate the needs of families and include them in treatment/intervention planning. In today's health-care environment we increasingly depend on families to carry out a variety of procedures at home—a responsibility that formerly was done primarily by licensed professionals.

Implications for Occupational Therapy

In 2005 the Executive Board of the American Occupational Therapy Association (AOTA) commissioned an Ad Hoc Committee to develop a strategy for advancing the profession's involvement with and commitment to families and caregivers across the lifespan. Following are several recommendations presented to the AOTA Executive Board that have relevance to our current concerns about aging individuals and their families. These recommendations also have implications for our collaboration with other professions.

1. Recognize families and caregivers across the lifespan as an essential and significant domain of OT practice, and assess the effects, over time, of efforts to establish the practice domain of families and caregivers.
2. Provide workshops and special forums for practitioners, educators, families, and caregivers to share and examine

the most/least promising approaches and benefits of intervention for aging individuals and their families.

3. Examine the nature of collaborative partnerships among researchers, educators, and practitioners that have been established to support enhancement of this practice area, and partner with universities and other associations to obtain grants to fund research on these efforts.

4. Develop materials for legislators to explain the unmet needs of caregivers and families and the potential cost-benefits of supporting them in their roles at various life-cycle stages, including aging.[31]

5. Collaborate with other professional entities to explore potential applications of technology for providing services and disseminating data.

6. Identify researchers, educators, and practitioners to collaborate with AOTA to provide support for further development of this practice area.

7. Conduct a survey among the educational institutions to identify the current teaching strategies used to address this topic in professional training programs.

8. Expand partnerships with community-based organizations that serve aging families and their caregivers.

Summary

Most, if not all, of us belong to families and hope to have long, healthy, and productive lives. Many, if not all, of us concur with Heschel's and Erikson's convictions that it is a great privilege to grow old. We may also acknowledge that the information, concepts, and concerns presented in this chapter have professional and personal relevance, and that they offer opportunities to apply our understanding of current aging issues. We should consider the positive contributions we can make to our aging clients and their families, the development and implementation of collaborative efforts with our professional colleagues, and the creation of a plan that can enable us to have a more positive influence on our own lived experiences. One approach to addressing these considerations is to reflect on the following issues:

- As your family member (or client) experiences physical and/or cognitive decline, who do you think will be that individual's primary caregiver, and what burdens would this likely impose?
- How would you want the health professionals to interact with you and your family (or your clients and their families)?
- What conflicts do you anticipate having with the health-care system and care providers, and how do you think those conflicts can be resolved?
- What supports would be available to you?
- How might relationships change in your family (or among your professional colleagues)?
- What additional roles may you need to assume (in your family or in your professional role)?

In addition to the contributions made to aging families and aging clients, consider introducing the following

developmental agenda designed for individuals who are approaching midlife:[11]

- Get to know and be comfortable with yourself
- Learn how to live well
- Have good judgment
- Despite loss and pain, learn to feel whole—psychologically, interpersonally, and spiritually
- Live life to the fullest, right to the end
- Give to others, to your family, and to your community
- Learn to tell your story
- Continue the process of discovery and change
- Remain hopeful, despite adversity

Finally, the most prevailing message inherent in this chapter is that aging represents one of our newest and most important frontiers. Thus, we must revise our prior perceptions and attitudes about aging. We need to recognize that positive change and making a significant difference will require our collaborative efforts as professionals and as individuals.

REVIEW QUESTIONS

1. Discuss how you believe older adults are viewed in North America and how that varies globally.

2. Think about whether you have any prejudices about growing older and/or older adults. Discuss what they might be.

3. How do you think family caregiving might change roles within a family?

4. How might race, ethnicity, and cultural contexts affect family caregiving?

5. What factors might play a role in isolating an older adult?

6. Considering Taylor's cognitive adaptive theory of coping, discuss how you might, as a health-care professional, help a family move toward homeostasis after assuming the role as family caregiver to an older adult.

7. How might you, as an occupational therapist, assistant, and/or health-care professional, develop a collaborative practice with older adults, families, and other professionals?

8. Share your reflections on the issues posed in the chapter summary.

REFERENCES

1. Becvar, D. S., & Becvar, R. J. (2009). *Family therapy: A systemic integration.* Boston, MA: Pearson Education.

2. Behr, S. (1990). *The underlying dimension of positive contributions that individuals with developmental disabilities make to their families: A factor analytic study.* Ann Arbor, MI: University Microfilms International.

3. Berg-Weger, M., Burkemper, E., Rubio, D. M., & Tebb, S. (2002). The well-being of siblings who share care: A case study. *Journal of Gerontological Social Work, 35*(1), 89–106.

4. Blieszner, R. (2009). Who are the aging families? In S. H. Qualls & S. H. Zarit (Eds.), *Aging families and caregiving* (pp. 1–18). Hoboken, NJ: John Wiley & Sons.

5. Boss, P. (1980). Normative family stress: Family boundary changes across the lifespan. *Family Relations, 29,* 445–450.

6. Boss, P. (2006). *Loss, trauma, and resilience.* New York, NY: W. W. Norton.

7. Butler, R. N. (1980). Ageism: A foreword. *Journal of Social Issues, 36,* 8–11. doi: 10.1111/j.1540-4560.1980.tb02018.x.

8. Butler, R. N. (2008). *The longevity revolution: The benefits and challenges of a long life.* Washington, DC: PublicAffairs.

9. Capitman, J. (2002). Defining diversity: A primer and a review. *Generations, 26*(3), 8–14.

10. Chambers, P., Allan, G., Phillipson, C., & Ray, M. (2009). *Family practices in later life.* Bristol, UK: The Policy Press.

11. Cohen, G. D., Perlstein, S., Chapline, J., Kelly, J., Firth, K. M., & Simmens, S. (2006). The impact of professionally conducted cultural programs on the physical health, mental health, and social functioning of older adults. *The Gerontologist, 46*(6), 726–734.

12. Connidis, I. A. (2010). *Family ties and aging* (2nd ed.). Thousand Oaks, CA: Pine Forge Press.

13. Crowther, M., & Austin, A. (2009). The cultural context of clinical work with aging caregivers. In S. H. Qualls & S. H. Zarit (Eds.), *Aging families and caregiving* (pp. 45–60), Hoboken, NJ: John Wiley & Sons.

14. Dooley, N. R., & Hinojosa, J. (2004). Improving quality of life for person with Alzheimer's disease and their family caregiver: Brief occupational therapy intervention. *American Journal of Occupational Therapy, 58*(5), 561–569.

15. Dukakis, O. (May, 2007) Heartfelt decisions. *AARP Bulletin, 48*(5), 35.

16. Dymski, J. D. (2002). *Aging gracefully: The keys to holier, happier golden years.* Chicago, IL: ACTA Publications.

17. Erikson, E. H., & Erikson, J. M. (1997). *The life cycle completed: Extended version with new chapters on the ninth stage of development.* New York, NY: W. W. Norton.

18. Fingerman, K. L., Miller, L. M., & Seidel, A. J. (2009). Functions families serve in old age. In S. H. Qualls & S. H. Zarit (Eds.), *Aging families and caregiving* (pp. 19–43), Hoboken, NJ: John Wiley & Sons.

19. Flach, F. (1988). *Resilience: Discovering a new strength in the times of stress.* New York, NY: Ballantine Books.

20. Gitlin, L. N., & Corcoran, M. (2005). *Occupational therapy and dementia care—the home environment skill building program for individuals and families.* Philadelphia, PA: Jefferson Elder Care Publications, Thomas Jefferson University Press.

21. Glaser, R., & Kiecolt-Glaser, J. (2005). Stress induced immune dysfunction: Implications for health. *Nature Review Immunology, 5*(3), 243–251.

22. Goldernberg, I., & Goldernberg, H. (1980). *Family therapy: An overview.* Belmont, CA: Wadsworth.

23. Hasselkus, B. R. (2011). *The meaning of everyday occupation.* Thorofare, NJ: SLACK.

24. Herschel, A. J. (1961). *The older person and the family in the perspective of Jewish tradition.* Washington, DC: Presentation at the initial White House Conference on Aging.

25. Hill, R. (1949). *Families under stress.* New York, NY: Harper and Row.

26. Hill, R. (1958). Social stresses on the family. Social casework. *The Journal of Contemporary Social Work, 39,* 139–158.

27. Howard, S., Dryden, J., & Johnson, B. (1999). Childhood resilience: Review and critiques of literature. *Oxford Review of Education, 25*(3), 307–337.

28. Lewin Group. (2010). *Individuals living in the community with chronic conditions and functional limitations.* http://www.aoa.acl.gov/site_utilities/Search.aspx?cx=017781414769350254827:fyjzvqtz0su&cof=FORID:11&q=chronic%20conditions%20data.

29. McCubbin, H. I., & Patterson, J. M. (1983a). Family transitions: Adaptations to stress. In H. I. McCubbin & C. Figley (Eds.), *Stress and the family: Coping with normative transitions* (Vol. 1, pp. 5–25). New York, NY: Brunner/Mazel.

30. McCubbin, H. I. & Patterson, J. M. (1983b). The family stress process: The Double ABCX Model of Adjustment and Adaptation.

Marriage & Family Review, 6(1-2), 7–37. DOI:10.1300/J002v06n01_02.

31. MetLife. (1995). *Study of employer costs for working caregivers.* Washington Business Group on Health. http://www.caregiving.org/data/employercosts.pdf.

32. MetLife Mature Market Institute. (2006). The Metlife study of Alzheimer's Disease: The caregiving experience. www.metlife.com/assets/cao/mmi/publications/studies/mmi-alzheimers-disease-caregiving-experience-study.pdf.

33. Paraprofessional Healthcare Institute (PHI). (2005). *The role of training in improving the recruitment and retention of direct-care workers in long-term care.* http://phinational.org/research-reports/role-training-improving-recruitment-and-retention-direct-care-workers-long-term.

34. Phillips, C. (2008). Cultural sensitivity: A wellness program necessity. *Aging Well: The Magazine for Professionals Promoting Positive Aging, 1*(4), 8–9.

35. Rathbone-McCuan, E., & Hashimi, J. (1982). *Isolated elders: Health and social intervention issues.* Rockville, CO: Aspen Systems, Inc.

36. Reinhard, S., Feinberg, L.F., Choula, R., & Houser, A. (2015). Valuing the Invaluable 2015 update: Undeniable progress, but big gaps remain. AARP Public Pokicy Institute. www http://www.aarp.org/ppi/info-2015/valuing-the-invaluable-2015-update.html Accessed October 21, 2015

37. Schulz, R., & Sherwood, P. R. (2010). Physical and mental health effects of family caregiving. *Journal of Social Work Education, 44*(3), 105–113.

38. Stephen, M., Crowther, J., Hobfoll, S., & Tennenbaum, D. (1990). *Stress and coping in later-life families.* New York, NY: Hemisphere.

39. Stephens, M. A. P., & Franks, M. M. (2009). All in the family: Providing care to chronically ill and disabled older adults. In S. H. Qualls & S. H. Zarit (Eds.), *Aging families and caregiving.* (pp. 61–83), Hoboken, NJ: John Wiley & Sons.

40. Talley, R. C., & Crews, J. E. (2007). Framing the public health of caregiving. *American Journal of Public Health, 97*(2), 224.

41. Taylor, S. E. (1983). Adjustment to threatening events. *American Psychologist, 38,* 1161–1173.

42. Taylor, S. E. (1989). *Positive illusions.* New York, NY: Basic Books.

43. Taylor, S. E. (1991). Asymmetrical effects of positive and negative events: The mobilization-minimization hypothesis. *Psychological Bulletin, 110*(1), 67.

44. Tebb, S., & Jivanjee, P. (2000). Caregiver isolation: An ecological model. *Journal of Gerontological Social Work, 34*(2), 51–72.

45. Tebb, S. S., & Steiger, F. R. (2008). Time taken as a caring family. *Reflections: Narratives of Professional Helping, 14*(3), 1–11.

46. *U.S. Department of Health & Human Services. Agency for Healthcare Research and Quality, Research Activities, November-December 2013. Individuals living with chronically ill household members have lower health-related quality of life.* http://www.ahrq.gov/news/newsletters/research-activities/13nov-dec/111213ra15.html.

47. U.S. Department of Health and Human Services Administration for Community Living. (2013). *Administration on Aging: Aging Statistics.* http://www.aoa.acl.gov/Aging_Statistics/index.aspx.

48. U.S. Department of Labor. (2013). *Bureau of Labor Statistics Employment Projections—2012-2022.* http://www.bls.gov/news.release/pdf/ecopro.pdf.

49. Van Hook, M. P. (2008). *Social work practice with families: A resiliency-based approach.* Chicago, IL: Lyceum Books.

50. Weick, A. (1983). A growth-task model of human development. Social casework. *The Journal of Contemporary Social Work, 64,* 131–137.

51. Yee, D. (2002). Introduction: Recognizing diversity, moving toward cultural competence. *Generations: Journal of the American Society on Aging, 26*(3), 5–7.

CHAPTER 23

U.S. Health Care System Overview and the Occupational Therapy Services Interface

Louise A. Meret-Hanke, PhD, Karen Frank Barney, PhD, OTR/L, FAOTA

CHAPTER OUTLINE

OBJECTIVES

- Differentiate and describe the U.S. medical health-care and public health systems
- Describe the continuum of care within the medical health-care system
- Discuss occupational therapy health promotion strategies throughout the continuum of care
- Explain the significance of access to care
- Define utilization, overutilization, and underutilization
- Discuss sources of reimbursement for health care, and their relevance to services for older adults

The U.S. health-care system is large, complex, and multifaceted. An apt analogy for it is an ecosystem. Like an ecosystem, the U.S. health-care system is made up of interdependent components that are affected by external forces (e.g., economic)

and events occurring in other components. The key components of the U.S. health-care system are health-care professionals, provider organizations, clients and families, insurance companies, employers, and government. The health-care system is also made up of geographically based subsystems that function at the local, state, regional, and national levels. The organization and delivery of health-care services often differ substantially from one geographic area to another. These differences reflect the unique needs, resources, and characteristics of the area when the local health-care system historically began to develop.

The U.S. health-care system faces many challenges, including high costs, unequal access, and quality concerns. Current health reform efforts are intended to address these challenges. In 2013 the United States spent $2.9 trillion, or an average of $9,255 per person, on health care; this spending represents 17.4% of U.S. gross domestic product (GDP)—the total monetary value of all the goods and services produced in the country.[11] Other developed countries spend an average of 9.5% of GDP and $3,268 (USD) per capita on health care.[7] Despite the high level of spending, access to health care and quality of care are problematic. In 2013, before the start of the major provisions of the Affordable Care Act (ACA) of 2010, more than 41 million Americans, or 16.7%, of the non-older-adult population lacked health insurance and had limited access to medical care.[32] Clients and providers are concerned about the quality of medical care.[35] The World Health Report ranks the United States as 37th in terms of overall health outcomes,[40] and the nation failed to meet most of the health goals of the *Healthy People 2010* initiatives.[14]

This chapter provides an overview of the U.S. health-care system. It begins with a discussion of health and health care, occupational therapy (OT) roles and interventions within the health-care system, and access to health care. It then discusses the history and current structure of the U.S. health-care system and ways in which health care is financed. Occupational therapists provide services to aging adults throughout the U.S. health-care system. Therefore, OT professionals who work within the system need to be informed of related administrative structures, organization, and policies to effectively participate as professional providers with aging adults.

Health and Health Care

Health can be defined narrowly as the absence of illness or disease or more broadly as "a state of physical and mental well-being that facilitates the achievements of individual and societal goals" (p. 1382).[52] The latter definition reflects the growing body of research showing that every aspect of a person's life affects health.[48] Thus, health is increasingly seen as a multidimensional concept incorporating physical, mental, social, and spiritual well-being. This broader definition is consistent with OT's focus on engagement in occupations and life.[2]

Health is a result of a number of different factors, including lifestyle and behavior, heredity, social and physical environments, and access to health care. According to the Centers for Disease Control and Prevention (CDC), lifestyle and behavior are directly related to 50% of premature mortality.[8] Biology and genetics account for 20% of premature mortality, as do social and physical environmental factors. Health care is responsible for only 10% of premature mortality. Ideally, health-care expenditures would address lifestyle and behavioral factors, which can be modified through health education and promotion. However, 97% of national health expenditures is spent on medical health-care services.[48]

Health care is the prevention and treatment of illness or disability. According to Leavell and Clark, prevention occurs at three levels: primary, secondary, and tertiary. *Primary prevention* seeks to prevent a disease or condition before it happens.[36] Primary prevention services include facilitating health education and immunizations, enforcing regulations regarding hygiene and sanitation, and protecting against environmental and occupational hazards. *Secondary prevention* seeks to maintain health through early diagnosis and prompt treatment. Secondary prevention services include screening for disease, limiting the spread of communicable disease, and shortening the period of disability. *Tertiary prevention* attempts to halt or minimize the disease process or disability once it has started. These services include specialized treatments and rehabilitation interventions. (See chapter 3 for a detailed discussion of the Leavell-Clark model.)

Occupational Therapy Interventions within the Health Care System

Occupational therapy is, fundamentally, a profession that supports quality of life and can play a significant role within the health promotion and medical care system continuum with aging adults. "Leavell's levels," as the prevention levels noted by Leavell and Clark[36] are known, provide a conceptual framework for designing OT prevention services that support the health-related quality of life of our aging clients seen within the community in both medical and community wellness settings.

Consider that in all interventions, whether they occur at the primary, secondary, or tertiary care level, OT should promote the optimal health of the individuals served. Shortell,[49] promoted "bridging the divide between health and health care," and OT is optimally positioned to contribute to that effort. Note that chapter 3 on the continuing increasing numbers of aging adults with diseases also identifies opportunities for OT to address health promotion needs among aging adults. Thus, health promotion is the emphasis throughout all types of interventions despite the level of client and/or caregiver function, including interventions with terminally ill individuals in hospice care. Figure 23-1 explicates the levels of care, where they occur, and whether diagnosed disease is present or absent.

Primary Care

The purpose of primary care is to maintain optimal individualized health and protect individuals from diseases, conditions, and dysfunction. Should early signs of ill health occur, ideally immediate support is provided to prevent deterioration, so that a potential disease is prevented. Ordinarily, the client resides in the community and interventions are provided at a physician's office, a wellness clinic, the individual's workplace, or other community venues.

Historic examples of occupational therapists working in primary care are worker health initiatives within businesses and industries in which OT professionals conduct worksite evaluations and production line worker interventions to prevent musculoskeletal deterioration, including repetitive motion injuries. With an aging workforce, the potential need for

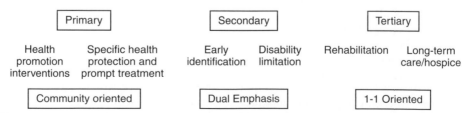

FIGURE 23-1 Levels and forms of OT services. (Adapted from Leavell, H. R., & Clark, E. G. [1965]. *Preventive medicine for the doctor in his community. An epidemiologic approach* [3rd ed.]. New York, NY: Blakiston-McGraw Hill.)

increased physical and/or mental health interventions for workers in many types of employment is readily apparent.

Within the past decade, the OT profession initiated efforts to partner with physicians in primary care clinics to enhance services, advance health promotion efforts, and promote cost-effective medical care.[16,34,37,39] At the present time, a few models of OT services in primary medical care offices exist in the United States. To date, the most receptive physicians have been family medicine practitioners[39] and geriatricians. These individuals capitalize on the presence of an occupational therapist to assess clients through screening to address fundamental daily quality-of-life issues related to activities of daily living (ADLs) and instrumental activities of daily living (IADLs); age-related vision, hearing, or other sensory changes; coping with emerging or long-term mental illness, diminished cognition, or dementia; transitions in life, such as retirement; risk assessment for falls and other injuries; and related spousal and caregiver needs.

The role of the occupational therapist may include screening as well as mitigating occupational performance deficits about which the physician may be unaware. For example, an older female client who has difficulty with dressing due to degenerative joint changes in her shoulders may not report this problem to her doctor. However, when an occupational therapist is present, any problems with ADLs or IADLs, along with psychosocial and leisure activity limitation concerns, are routinely queried and addressed. In this example, the occupational therapist collaborates with the client in implementing an acceptable adaptive dressing routine and clothing recommendations to minimize shoulder pain and discomfort.

Typically, because neither physicians nor the general public have an understanding of what occupational therapists can provide to add value to the client visit, occupational therapists need to be proactive in communicating the relevant highly educated, yet practical and holistic approach that is inherent in interventions that support and enhance these individuals' lives.

Secondary Care

The occupational therapist or OT assistant may play a role in identifying diminished cognitive, psychosocial, or physical occupational performance and/or related symptoms that lead to an early identification of a disease or condition—the aim of secondary care. Additionally, limiting disability is a further goal of this level of service, which may also be provided in the home, community, or physician's office or clinic. For example, historically, occupational therapists and OT assistants have provided community education programs in collaboration with arthritis organizations. Either newly diagnosed clients or individuals who have been living for years with various forms of arthritis, including rheumatoid and osteoarthritis, attend these educational programs. Weekly, biweekly, or monthly sessions provide information on the differentiation among the types of arthritis, related etiology, and principles and practices that they can apply to their everyday lives. Recommendations are provided for joint protection, energy conservation, and work simplification approaches, along with

strategies to assist them to maintain an optimal quality of life, despite their diagnosis. These older adults are encouraged to be proactive in advocating for assistance, wherever relevant. For example, when grocery shopping, requesting that items be placed in more bags, to lighten the weight and resulting stress on joints, is recommended. Requesting assistance with carrying heavy purchases could also promote joint protection and energy conservation, wherever needed. OT personnel work to empower these older adults to adapt their lifestyles, emphasizing the individual's priorities and needs for meaningful activities. Occupational therapists may not traditionally identify with secondary care, but should recognize the importance of disability limitation within any area of practice with aging adults.

Tertiary Care

Occupational therapists and OT assistants are typically associated with and well known for their interventions in tertiary care. Since the profession's founding nearly 100 years ago, occupational therapists have provided rehabilitative services to wounded veterans in hospitals after World War I, and to individuals living in the community. In subsequent years, OT personnel occupational therapists have delivered most of their services in tertiary care, in acute, subacute, and rehabilitation hospitals, and long-term care settings such as skilled nursing care facilities. OT interventions in community-based centers for aging persons with developmental disabilities and hospice care facilities are not well publicized, but have existed for decades. A skilled nursing facility example includes a holistic approach to the setting. First, the occupational therapist conducts an environmental assessment, beyond what is considered "up to standards." Is the setting not only meeting the safety standards, but tending to the holistic needs of the community of typically aging residents? The environmental assessment includes the nature of the context—is it supportive to the psychosocial well-being of the residents, supporting a culture of enhancing each aging adult? The occupational therapist's responsibility goes beyond the cognitive, physical, psychosocial, or ADL process prescribed for the resident and includes examining which contextual elements are supporting (or not) the optimal occupational performance of this resident, and her or his health-related quality of life. Note that chapter 25 on long-term care further describes current and potential roles for OT practitioners.

Access to Health Care

Access to health care is the ability to obtain needed, affordable, accessible, and acceptable health services. A perceived need for health care does not always result in access to health care. Individual and societal factors play a substantial role in whether someone seeks out and uses health-care services. Andersen's Behavioral Model of Health Services Utilization,[3] illustrated in Figure 23-2, is commonly used to describe how a need for health care can be translated into access and use of health-care services. It also considers personal health behaviors as a factor in determining overall health.

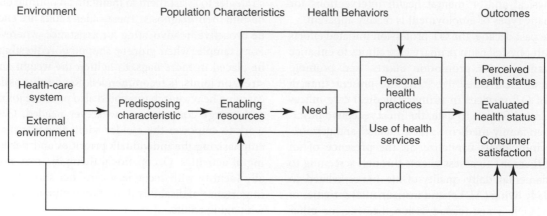

FIGURE 23-2 Behavioral Model of Health Care Utilization. (From Andersen, R. [1995]. Revisiting the behavioral model and access to medical care: Does it matter? *Journal of Health and Social Behavior. 36*[1],1-10.)

According to this model, the environment, including the health-care system and the broader societal factors, affects the availability and distribution of health-care resources that individuals could access. The likelihood that an individual will seek out and use health services is also strongly influenced by the type and amount of health-care resources available in the community (e.g., number of OT professionals or hospital beds per 1000 persons).

Use of health services is influenced by predisposing characteristics, enabling resources, and need for care. These factors help explain why individuals respond differently to symptoms. Perceived need for care has the largest effect on demand for care. However, the demand for care is also influenced by predisposing characteristics (e.g., health beliefs, culture, socioeconomic status, and demographic characteristics) and enabling resources (e.g., income, health insurance, having a regular source of care).

Enabling resources affect an individual's ability to access health care in response to a perceived need. Individuals with health insurance and other personal resources are more likely to be able to afford health services, and therefore access them. The availability of public insurance, such as Medicaid and the Children's Health Insurance Program (CHIP), makes health services affordable even to low-income families. By expanding eligibility for Medicaid and subsidizing private insurance for low-income individuals and families, the ACA provides even more low-income Americans with the ability to obtain needed health care. Safety-net clinics and hospitals provide health services at fees that are geared toward low individual and family income. Proximity to these services improves access for individuals and families with low incomes. The availability of transportation, flexible service hours, and accommodations for disabilities also greatly affects access to health care, especially among the working poor.

Environmental, population, and individual characteristics influence personal health practices and the use of health-care services. Ultimately, each of these factors influences health outcomes, including perceived and evaluated health status and satisfaction with the health-care system. These characteristics are described via a widely used conceptual framework known as the Behavioral Model of Health Services Utilization. This model is frequently used in health care needs assessment, service planning and evaluation, and health service research.[3]

Who Are the Uninsured?

The lack of health insurance is the most substantial financial barrier to accessing needed health services. In 2013, 41 million people, or 16.7% of the non-older-adult population, lacked health insurance.[32] The number of uninsured in the United States increased steadily between 1999 and 2010.[13] Expansion of health insurance under the ACA resulted in a decline of 1.3 million in the number of uninsured people between 2010 and 2011.[12,13]

Evidence shows that, as predicted by the Behavioral Model of Health Services Utilization, lack of health insurance negatively affects individuals' health. One quarter of people without health insurance go without needed care due to cost, as compared with only 4% of the insured. The uninsured are also less likely to receive preventative screenings.[27] Self-reported health, mortality rates, and outcomes from acute and chronic illnesses are worse among the uninsured as well.

The lack of health insurance is a problem that disproportionately affects families with low incomes and racial and ethnic minorities. Over 80% of the uninsured are non-white. Two thirds of the uninsured are from families with incomes less than 200% of the federal poverty level (FPL), or approximately $47,100 for a family of four in 2011.[30] Of employers, 61% offer health insurance; however, those who employ low-wage workers are the least likely to offer it. Even when employers offer health insurance, many low-income individuals may not be eligible or be able to afford their share of the premiums.

Underuse, Overuse, and Misuse of Health-Care Services

The U.S. health-care system is faced with the triple problem of underuse of recommended and appropriate services, overuse of services performed even though the risk of harm exceeds its likely benefit, and misuse through medical errors, incorrect diagnoses, and other sources of avoidable complications. Underuse is a common problem. Research has shown that all clients in the United States receive approximately half of all recommended services, including preventive care, treatment of acute conditions, and treatment of chronic conditions.[42]

Overuse increases the likelihood of both harm and costs. Retrospective review of medical records by independent panels of physicians found that significant numbers of delivered health services were either clinically inappropriate or of equivocal value.[38] Overuse is also found in the extent of geographic variation in use of the same health service without evidence of differences in outcomes.[42]

Misuse refers to medical errors and other events that could lead to serious outcomes. Since 1996 the Institute of Medicine (IOM) has issued several reports documenting the extent of medical errors and their consequences.[4] Medicare and other insurers have begun efforts to reduce medical errors and improve health care quality through financial incentives and penalties.

U.S. Health-Care System

The foundations of the existing health-care system were laid in the mid- to late 1800s. Before this time, health care was extremely limited and medical practice played a very small role in society. Acute illnesses and injuries were common. However, treatments typically were ineffective, and care was provided by families.[48] Early government action focused on protecting the public from infectious diseases introduced by travelers. This involved inspecting ships arriving at harbors and the quarantine of persons suspected of carrying contagious diseases. By the late 1800s, advances in medical sciences, the establishment of medical research in the United States, and surgical techniques developed during the Civil War expanded the scope of health services.[24]

At this time, the health-care system developed into two distinct branches: public health, which addresses population-wide health concerns, and personal health-care services, which deliver care to individuals. Both provide services at each level of prevention; however, their emphasis is different.

The public health system's largest role is in delivering primary prevention services; it also provides some secondary services and has a minor role in tertiary prevention. The personal health-care system focuses more on secondary and tertiary prevention, although it provides primary prevention such as immunizations.

Ideally, public health and personal health-care services would have multiple linkages and work in tandem to address health threats.[20] Regulations specify what information must be provided to the public health services. However, few other connections were developed. Barriers to communication between public health and personal health-care services include different sources of funds and separate governance structures. In particular, public health is directly funded and delivered by government agencies,[23] whereas personal health-care services are delivered predominantly by numerous private entities. In the past decade, both branches have begun to recognize the need for coordination of efforts. A dialogue has begun to address specific issues, including emergency response management, and will hopefully grow to cover more areas.[20]

Public Health

U.S. public health efforts date back to the 1700s and are responsible for substantial improvements in the population's health in the subsequent centuries. *Public health* is the science and art of preventing disease, prolonging life, and promoting health and efficiency through community effort.[15] It helps communities to cope with health problems that arise when people live in groups. A health problem becomes a public health problem if and when it is amenable to systematic social actions.

Public health problems can affect a small group of people and have severe outcomes (e.g., severe food poisoning at a restaurant) or a large group of people with less severe outcomes (e.g., herpes).

The government is involved in public health at the federal, state, and local levels. The federal government's primary public health function is to provide funding to state and local public health entities.[22] The lead federal agency responsible for public health is the U.S. Public Health Service, part of the Department of Health and Human Services (DHHS). Other federal agencies also have a role in public health, including the Environmental Protection Agency and Department of Homeland Security. State governments contribute funding and disperse federal funds to local public health departments. States also set standards and regulations for public health, collect public health information, and provide support (e.g., laboratory services) to local governments. Local governments' main responsibility is to deliver public health services.[24]

Advances in medical science expanded the ability of public health efforts to control the spread of infectious disease. Safer vaccines (e.g., for smallpox) enabled widespread immunization. The identification of several microbes that caused infectious disease led to the "great sanitary awakening".[15] With the recognition that sanitation problems were sources of disease, public health efforts focused on improving social and environmental conditions (e.g., sewage disposal). These efforts substantially improved population health and almost doubled life expectancy at birth during the century.

The structure and responsibilities of public health have changed vastly since that time. In 1988 the CDC adopted a set of three core functions of public health: assessment, policy development, and assurance.[24] Each core function has a set of essential public health services; the core functions and essential services are listed in Table 23-1. Assessment involves monitoring community health status and diagnosing and

TABLE 23-1 Public Health Core Functions and Essential Services

Core Function	Essential Public Health Service
Assessment	Monitor health status to identify community health problems
	Diagnose and investigate health problems and health hazards in the community
Policy development	Inform, educate, and empower people about health issues
	Mobilize community partnerships to identify and solve health problems
	Develop policies and plans that support individual and community health efforts
Assurance	Enforce laws and regulations that protect health and ensure safety
	Link people to needed personal health services and assure the provision of health care when otherwise unavailable
	Assure a competent public health and personal health-care workforce
	Evaluate effectiveness, accessibility, and quality of personal and population-based health services
	Conduct research for new insights and innovative solutions to health problems

(From Centers for Disease Control and Prevention. [2013]. *10 Essential public health services*. Retrieved from http://www.cdc.gov/nphpsp/documents/factsheet.pdf. Accessed May 9, 2012.)

investigating health problems. Policy development includes informing and educating the public about health issues, mobilizing community partnerships to identify and solve health problems, and developing polices and plans that support these efforts. The function of assurance is to enforce laws, link people with needed services, develop a competent healthcare workforce, evaluate the effectiveness of public health and personal health-care services, and conduct research into solving health problems.[24]

Public health efforts suffer from inadequate funding and a wide variation in the amount of resources and infrastructure available at the local level.[22] Consequently, not all of the 10 essential public health services are delivered by all local departments of public health. The services delivered vary considerably from state to state and among local health departments. However, more than two thirds of local health departments provide the following core services: adult and childhood immunizations; communicable disease control; community outreach and education; epidemiology and surveillance; and environmental health regulation, such as food safety services and restaurant inspections.[22]

In *The Future of Public Health*, the IOM proposed six actions that are necessary for assuring the population's health.[22] First, public health needs to adopt a population health approach that incorporates multiple determinants of health rather than just biological threats. Second, governmental public health infrastructure has suffered and needs to be strengthened to address current and future threats. Third, public-private partnerships are needed to address the diverse needs of communities. Fourth, systems of accountability need to be established to assure the quality and availability of public health services. Fifth, evidence based public health practices should inform all decision making. Finally, enhanced communication is needed within the public health system, with other government agencies responsible for health, and with the community. The success of public health efforts to improve the population's health is dependent on adequate funding and sufficient resources to implement these actions.[22]

Personal Health-Care Service

Personal health-care services include acute care and long-term services and supports. By the early 1900s, health-care professionals and hospitals emerged to take advantage of medical advances.[48] The institutions, organizations, and professions that formed at this time focused on treating episodes of acute illness and injury. These were the dominant health threat at the time. The nature of personal health-care services has evolved over time in response to advances in medical science and technology. Nevertheless, the personal health-care system remains largely geared to delivering services that focus on episodes of acute care rather than a continuum of care.[48]

Personal health-care services include primary care, secondary care, tertiary care, and long-term services and support (formerly known as long-term care).[48] Occupational therapists historically have worked in the areas of secondary care, tertiary care, and long-term care. Primary care is often the "first contact" with the medical system and involves delivery of preventative care, screening, and treatment of acute and chronic illnesses that do not require specialized care. The primary care provider (PCP) can be a physician, advanced practice nurse, or physician's assistant. Primary care is long term, frequent, and less intense than secondary and tertiary care. Increasingly, OT is entering primary care to support or improve daily quality of life and overall well-being.[51]

Secondary care includes hospital care, routine surgery, specialist consultations, and rehabilitation. This type of care is used to address more advanced and serious health problems than those covered by primary care. It is usually short term and episodic. Tertiary care is the most complex level of care. Tertiary care provides highly specialized and technologically advanced care for less common but serious diseases.[51] Examples include organ transplants, advanced treatment for acute and chronic illness, and so forth.

Inpatient Care

Inpatient care is provided in hospitals and skilled nursing facilities where the client stays overnight. Hospitals primarily provide short-term acute care, whereas skilled nursing facilities provide rehabilitative and long-term care.[48] Hospitals must be licensed, have an organized physician staff, provide continuous nursing services under the supervision of registered nurses, have a governing body that is responsible for hospital conduct, and have a chief executive officer with responsibility for operations. In addition, the hospital must also maintain medical records on each client, have pharmacy services available, and provide food services to meet the nutritional and therapeutic requirements of the clients. Hospitals are regulated by federal, state, and local laws. To participate in Medicare and Medicaid, hospitals must meet the standards to be certified or accredited by The Joint Commission.[48]

In 2011 there were over 5700 hospitals in the United States, the majority of which—over 4,900—were community hospitals.[1] Community hospitals provide short-term care to the general public and are not federal government hospitals. Community hospitals include specialty hospitals (e.g., rehabilitation), academic medical centers, and other teaching hospitals. The remaining institutions are federal hospitals, psychiatric hospitals, and long-term care hospitals. Hospitals are often classified according to ownership. Of community hospitals, 58% are not-for-profit entities, 20% are for-profit, and 20% are state and locally owned.[1]

Nursing homes provide rehabilitation and personal care. Rehabilitation is provided by skilled nursing facilities and typically follows a hospital stay. The goal is to help the individual regain capacity lost as a result of illness or injury.[48] Personal care in these facilities provides assistance with daily activities such as dressing and bathing to individuals who are unable to perform these tasks themselves. These services will be discussed at length in the section on long-term services and supports later in the chapter. In 2004 there were over 16,000 nursing facilities with 1.7 million beds and 1.5 million residents in the United States.[9] Despite the increase in the aging population, the number of facilities identified as nursing homes has decreased to 15,700 with the same number of licensed beds, and 1.4 million residents..[10] Since many older adults prefer to remain in their homes versus residing in nursing homes, the changes appear to be related to an increase in the number of adult day services, home health care services, residential care facilities, and hospice services.

Outpatient or Ambulatory Care

Outpatient or ambulatory care refers to a wide range of services, including physicians' services, diagnostic services, day surgery, and rehabilitation services.[48] The development of new technology has led to less invasive procedures, shorter-acting anesthetics, and faster recovery time, allowing many procedures to be performed without an overnight stay. Consequently, the volume of outpatient services is increasing, whereas inpatient care is decreasing. Initially, outpatient services were provided primarily in hospitals. However, outpatient services are increasingly available in other settings.

Long-Term Services and Supports

Long-term services and supports (LTSSs), previously referred to as *long-term care*, provide ongoing assistance with ADLs and IADLs to people who, because of a physical, cognitive, or chronic health condition, are unable to perform these activities independently.[43] The term *long-term services and supports* is replacing *long-term care* (LTC) because it better reflects the wide array of noninstitutional options available today. The goal of LTSSs is to maximize an individual's physical and cognitive functioning. To maximize functional independence, LTSSs must address the recipient's social and environmental needs along with physical needs. A person's living situation can either enhance or impede his or her physical and cognitive functioning. Consequently, the recipient's living conditions are an essential component of services.[33]

In 2011 approximately 11 million Americans needed LTSSs, and the majority (7 million) are aged 65 years and over.[43] The need for these services increases with age. People over the age of 85 years are seven times as likely to need LTSSs as those aged 65 to 74 years. The demand for LTSSs is expected to continue increasing as the population ages. The number of individuals aged 65 years and over is expected to increase from 40 million (13% of the population) in 2010 to approximately 72 million (19% of the population) by 2030.[18] On average, people turning 65 years can expect to require three years of LTSSs.[33] In addition, the number of people aged 85 years and over, 70% of whom have long-term care needs, is expected to increase from 5.5 million in 2010 to 8.7 million in 2030, and to 19 million by 2050.[18] These demographic factors are expected to dramatically increase the number of older adults requiring LTSSs.

With its client-centered approach, OT helps individuals maximize their ability to perform daily activities, and therefore has a large role to play in LTSSs.[2] Importantly, research has shown that high-intensity OT increases the likelihood that clients will regain some of their ability to perform ADLs.[25] In the United States, the number of occupational therapists needed is expected to grow by 33% between 2010 and 2020, in large part because of the increased need for LTSSs.[7] Therefore, more occupational therapists who are knowledgeable and skilled in gerontological interventions will likely be in demand.

LTSSs are provided in different settings, including nursing homes, residential care facilities (e.g., assisted living), continuing care retirement communities, and private homes. In some areas, naturally occurring retirement communities (NORCs) are evolving with residents' desire to age in the homes where they have lived for many years. In all of these settings, occupational therapists provide both individualized and group/community services to proactively support meaningful occupational performance to sustain these aging individuals at optimal functional levels for as long as possible. The range of long-term services and supports has increased over the past several decades.[33] The level of assistance available in each setting varies. Skilled nursing care is a medically oriented service provided by a licensed nurse in a nursing home. Care is based on an individualized treatment plan developed through a multidisciplinary assessment and authorized by a physician. Treatment includes rehabilitation (including OT), therapeutic diets and nutritional supplements, and other clinical services.

An important issue in serving older adults and others who need LTSSs stems from the fact that this population also has high acute care needs. Care is typically received from multiple providers. Coordination of care is often lacking as a result of fragmentation of the health-care system and the absence of incentives to encourage collaboration between providers.[33] Without effective care coordination, clients experience delays in receiving needed services, confusing and conflicting care plans, duplication of diagnostic testing, polypharmacy, and high rates of readmissions shortly after discharge.[5,19] Several policy initiatives are attempting to address this problem. The Medicare Prescription Drug, Improvement, and Modernization Act of 2003 (MMA) introduced a new Medicare Advantage plan category called Special Needs Plans (SNPs), which serve individuals with high need for acute and long-term services and supports.[29,44] Medicare Advantage SNPs were designed to complement state Medicaid programs and to improve coordination of care for older adults who are dually eligible for both Medicare and Medicaid.[44]

Integrated Delivery Networks

Until the 1980s, the majority of health-care organizations were standalone entities. However, in response to external pressures, health-care organizations consolidated into integrated delivery networks (IDNs) beginning the 1990s. Although the composition of IDNs varies, they provide a continuum of health care ranging from inpatient and outpatient services to diagnostics, pharmacy, skilled nursing facilities, LTSSs, and insurance. The first IDNs developed during the early to middle 1900s from the merger of multispecialty practices and hospitals. Examples of early IDNs include Kaiser Permanente, Geisinger Health, Mayo Clinic, and Cleveland Clinic, among others. During the 1990s, health-care organizations rapidly consolidated in response to external forces. These included the dominance of managed care (discussed later), federal health reform efforts, and the increased focus on the continuum of care rather than episodic care.

Furthermore, Medicare's adoption of a prospective payment system (PPS) in 1983 changed hospital reimbursement of charges billed to a PPS based on clients' diagnoses and necessitated developing efficiencies and economies of scale.[48] The result was that Medicare clients were discharged more quickly and had more need for post-acute care—skilled nursing care and home health. Hospitals found it advantageous to merge or acquire standalone skilled nursing facilities and home health agencies. This allowed them to facilitate moving clients from hospital to post-acute care. These services continued to be paid on a cost-plus basis. Medicare's expenditures for post-acute care increased rapidly until a PPS was introduced for skilled nursing facilities and home health in 1998 and 2000, respectively. The PPS proved successful at controlling the growth of Medicare hospital spending. Consequently, private payers followed suit and adopted PPSs as a way to reimburse hospitals.

Innovations in Personal Health-Care Delivery

By the 1980s, it became apparent that chronic disease and long-term disability were a greater threat to health than acute disease. The increased prevalence of chronic disease called for a different approach to delivering health care. The episodic approach developed to treat acute illness did not allow for the coordination and continuity of care needed to address chronic disease. The Chronic Care Model (CCM), illustrated in Figure 23-3, was developed to address the need for an ongoing, holistic approach to chronic disease treatment.[54]

The CCM is built around six key components: community resources, organization of the health-care system, self-management support, a proactive delivery system, evidence-based decisions, and a clinical information system. This combination of care elements leads to improved client outcomes and cost savings.[6] New models of health-care delivery are being adopted to take advantage of the CCM, including patient-centered medical homes (PCMHs) and accountable care organizations (ACOs).

Patient-Centered Medical Homes

A patient-centered medical home (PCMH) is a clinical system providing comprehensive, client-centered, ongoing, and

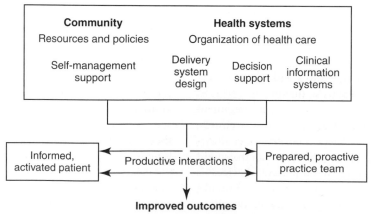

FIGURE 23-3 The Chronic Care Model. (From Wagner, E. H. [1998]. Chronic disease management: What will it take to improve care for chronic illness? *Effective Clinical Practice, 1*[1], 2-4.)

coordinated care.[41] The goals of the PCMH are to refocus the health system on primary care, improve access to primary care, and improve client health literacy. The personal physician leads a team of other health professionals in delivering ongoing care and prevention services. Each client has a personal physician who provides first-contact, continuous, and comprehensive care. Care is coordinated across medical subspecialties, hospitals, home health agencies, and nursing homes, and also with the client's family and public and private community-based services. Health information technology is an important component of a PCMH. It facilitates care provision and allows for client tracking, clinical monitoring, and specialist follow-up. Access is facilitated by open scheduling, which may offer increased evening and/or weekend hours with service providers, as well as expanded and after-hours access to personal physicians and practice staff by telephone and through secure email. Providers receive financial incentives, thus achieving cost savings and meeting quality improvement targets.[53] However, PCMHs face several challenges, including the shortage of primary care providers, the difficulty of implementing such a radical change in care delivery, and issues of how to activate client involvement in the process.

Accountable Care Organizations

An ACO is a group of providers (e.g., hospitals, physicians, and others involved in client care) that work together to coordinate care and manage chronic disease for Medicare beneficiaries.[17] ACOs should be client-centered and involve patients in making decisions about their care. ACOs are expected to control the growth of costs and improve the quality of care.

The ACA of 2010 provided funding for ACOs to serve Medicare beneficiaries. Currently, there are over 250 Medicare ACOs and an equal number under private insurance. An ACO can operate within one health-care organization (e.g., an integrated delivery system) or across several organizations. ACOs receive higher payment if they achieve quality goals, and they share in the savings if costs are controlled. The payment received by an ACO is shared across all providers.

ACOs are expected to face several challenges.[50] First, ACOs made up of separate organizations will need to negotiate responsibilities and payment and information exchange processes. ACOs within an integrated delivery network will have fewer difficulties with this aspect of implementation. Second, payments are based on outcomes, not on volume, as has been the case. Therefore, ACOs will need to change their focus from treatments to the overall health of their clients. Third, the metrics for evaluating ACO performance will likely need to be modified as we gain better understanding of the processes. Finally, ACOs are a new form of health-care delivery, and providers will need to learn how to work within the system. Because we have limited experience with this form of delivery, the learning curve is likely to be steep.[50]

Health-Care Expenditures

The $2.9 billion in total expenditures for the U.S. health-care system comes from several different sources.[21] As shown in

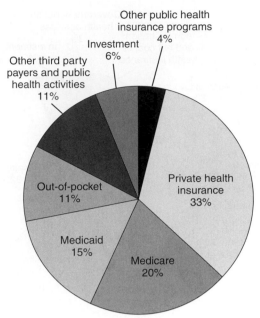

FIGURE 23-4   Sources of health-care financing, 2013. (From Centers for Medicare and Medicaid Services, Office of the Actuary, National Health Statistics Group [2013]. Health Spending by Major Sources of Funds. Retrieved from http://www.cms.gov/Research-Statistics-Data-and-Systems/Statistics-Trends-and-Reports/NationalHealthExpendData/nationalHealthAccountsHistorical.html)

Figure 23-4, the largest source is private health insurance, which accounts for one third of the total national health expenditures. The next largest sources are Medicare (20%), Medicaid (15%), and out-of-pocket expenditures (12%). Figure 23-5 shows the distribution of health-care costs. Inpatient care in hospitals accounts for 32%, the largest portion. Physician and clinical services account for 20% of costs, and pharmaceuticals account for 9% of total costs. OT services are included in other professional services, which account for only 3% of the total cost. Private health expenditures account for 51.8% of the $2.9 billion in total health expenditures, and public expenditures account for the remaining 48.2%.[48]

Private Financing of Health Care

Private financing of health care in the United States is mainly comprised of employer-sponsored insurance (ESI), individual private health insurance, and out-of-pocket spending. Unlike in many countries in Europe, efforts to develop a national health insurance did not succeed in the United States. Instead, a system of voluntary health insurance developed. The largest source of private payment is ESI, which covered approximately 60% of Americans in 2008.[48] The ESI system was established during World War II in response to wage and price controls and a tight labor market.[48]

Until the 1990s, the majority of private health insurance (ESI and individual) reimbursed the insured for a portion of the "usual and customary" charges. This payment approach is referred to as *fee-for-service* (FFS) and pays providers more for doing more. FFS payment resulted in a rapid increase in

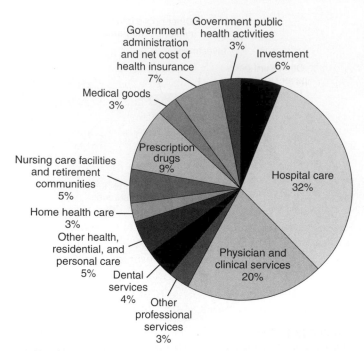

Government public health activities 3%

Government administration and net cost of health insurance 7%

Investment 6%

Medical goods 3%

Prescription drugs 9%

Hospital care 32%

Nursing care facilities and retirement communities 5%

Home health care 3%

Other health, residential, and personal care 5%

Dental services 4%

Physician and clinical services 20%

Other professional services 3%

FIGURE 23-5   Distribution of health-care expenditures. (From Centers for Medicare & Medicaid Services, Office of the Actuary, National Health Statistics Group [2014]. Retrieved from http://www.cms.gov/Research-Statistics-Data-and-Systems/Statistics-Trends-and-Reports/National-HealthExpendData/nationalHealthAccountsHistorical.html)

volume of health-care services delivered. Managed care developed in response to the resulting rapidly growing health-care costs and demands from payers for greater accountability from providers.[48]

Managed care refers to a variety of approaches used to integrate the financing and delivery of health care that seeks to contain costs and improve quality of care through contractual arrangements with providers.[48] After slow initial growth, managed care became the primary vehicle for financing and delivering care to the majority of Americans. Managed care organizations would either deliver health care directly to insured members or contract with providers to deliver a set of services for a predetermined price. Managed care was able to reduce the rate of growth in health-care expenditures. It did so through increased administrative and clinical efficiency, restricted client choice of providers, and utilization review.[28] Comprehensive studies found that quality of care was similar in managed care plans and FFS plans.

There are two main types of managed care organizations: *health maintenance organizations* (HMOs) and *preferred provider organization* (PPOs).[28] The first type of managed care organization was HMOs, which require members to choose a primary care provider (PCP) from a network of providers. The PCP acts as a gatekeeper in deciding whether a member should be referred to see a specialist. Providers are paid a fixed monthly payment per enrolled member, known as *capitation* and often referred to as *per member, per month* payment. Providers must deliver the contracted services in

exchange for the capitated payment. Capitation creates incentive for providers to reduce utilization of unnecessary services. Managed care organizations also review service utilization to ensure the services are medically necessary. Utilization review includes an expert evaluation of what services are medically necessary, determination of how services can be provided in the most inexpensive manner (e.g., outpatient versus inpatient), and review the course of medical treatment (e.g., when a client is in the hospital).[48]

PPOs emerged because members of HMOs complained about their limited choices and utilization review, and providers were unhappy with capitated payments and restrictions on how they practiced medicine.[48] PPOs give members the option of receiving care outside of the network at a higher out-of-pocket cost. Providers are paid on a discounted FFS basis, and the use of utilization review was curtailed. Typically, fees are discounted at 25% to 35% off providers' regular fees. Premiums and cost sharing are higher in PPOs than in HMOs because of the added cost of greater choice. PPOs are now the most common form of managed care.[28]

Public Financing of Health Care

Medicare (Title XIX of the Social Security Act), Medicaid (Title XVIII of the Social Security Act), and the Children's Health Insurance Program (CHIP; Title XXI of the Social Security Act) are the largest publicly funded health programs.[46] Medicare provides health care for older adults and people with disabilities. Medicaid provides health care to low-income people, including older adults and people with disabilities. CHIP provides health care to uninsured children in families with incomes that are modest but too high to qualify for Medicaid.

In 1965 the federal government passed Medicare and Medicaid to provide health insurance to older-adult and low-income Americans.[48] Medicare and Medicaid represented comprehensive health-care reform that expanded access to millions of Americans. The next expansion of public health insurance did not occur until CHIP was passed in 1997.[48] This was followed by the Medicare Modernization Act of 2003, which created a prescription drug program within Medicare. Most recently, the ACA expanded eligibility for Medicaid, effective 2014.

Medicare

Medicare is a federal health program for older adults and people with disabilities. It is funded through payroll taxes, general revenue, and premiums. Because it is a federal program, benefits and services are consistent across the country. Medicare covers approximately 41 million people and finances 20% of national health expenditures.[21]

To be eligible for Medicare, an individual or his or her spouse has to contribute to Medicare for 40 quarters (10 years) or pay monthly premiums to buy into the program. Beneficiaries also must be age 65 years or older, or disabled, and entitled to Social Security benefits (after a 2-year waiting period), or have either end-stage renal disease or amyotrophic lateral sclerosis (Lou Gehrig's disease). Medicare eligibility is not based on income or assets.[29] Eligible individuals can receive benefits when they reach age 65 years.

There are four parts to Medicare. Medicare Part A is known as hospital insurance; it covers inpatient care such hospital, skilled nursing facility, and hospice care. It is financed through mandatory payroll taxes levied on the employer and employee. Medicare Part B is known as Supplemental Medical Insurance (SMI) and covers outpatient services, including physician care. Part B is a voluntary program financed through premiums and general tax revenue.[29]

Medicare Part C, known as Medicare Advantage, provides several alternatives to traditional Medicare. Beneficiaries can choose from a number of HMOs, PPOs, or private FFS plans. The plans are financed by payments from Medicare and may require an additional premium. In exchange, these plans can provide additional benefits not covered by traditional Medicare.[29,31]

Medicare Part D provides prescription drug coverage. It was established by the Medicare Prescription Drug Improvement and Modernization Act of 2003 and implemented in 2006. It is a voluntary program and enrollees can choose between a standalone plan for prescriptions or a Medicare Advantage plan that provides prescription drug benefits. Premiums are subsidized for low-income beneficiaries.[29,31]

Medicaid

Medicaid is a joint federal-state program that provides health care for low-income people. In 2013 Medicaid covered 62 million people. Total Medicaid expenditures by state and federal governments totaled $432 billion in 2011.[26] Medicaid is administered by state governments. States operate Medicaid under general guidelines set by the federal government. To participate, states must provide a mandatory set of benefits. In addition, states can adopt optional Medicaid benefits. The federal government provides matching funds to states on an open-ended basis. The amount of matching funds varies from 50% to 76% depending on how wealthy the state is relative to the rest of the country.[26]

Medicaid eligibility originally covered welfare recipients. However, the Personal Responsibility and Work Opportunity Reconciliation Act of 1996 separated Medicaid eligibility from welfare eligibility. Currently, Medicaid eligibility is based on a categorical requirement and financial limits. The eligible categories include parents with dependent children, pregnant women, and individuals who are aged, blind, or disabled and whose income and assets do not exceed the maximum set by the state. Income eligibility varies by category, ranging from a low of 37% of the FPL for jobless parents to 235% of the FPL for children; states have the option to set higher income eligibility levels.[26] The ACA expanded Medicaid eligibility by raising the income eligibility level to 138% of the FPL.[30]

However, not all states have elected to adopt the new income eligibility levels. In 2014, 28 states (including Washington, D.C.) had adopted Medicaid expansion. An additional seven states were considering expanding Medicaid, and 16 had decided against Medicaid expansion at this time.[32]

Children's Health Insurance Program

When passed into law in 1997, CHIP was the largest expansion of publicly funded health insurance for children since the 1960s.[47] It covers uninsured children up to the age of 19 years in families with incomes too high to qualify them for Medicaid. The CHIP legislation provides block grant funds to states to cover low-income children and allows states to set eligibility requirements and policies within broad federal guidelines. Every state has an approved CHIP plan. Some states have used waivers of CHIP statutory provisions to cover the parents of children receiving benefits.

In 2013, CHIP covered 5.7 million children.[47] Although CHIP expands health insurance access to more low-income children, it is estimated that over 5 million additional children are eligible but remain uninsured. The Children's Health Insurance Program Reauthorization Act of 2009 (CHIPRA) expanded funding to states and requires states to develop effective strategies to identify and enroll uninsured children who are eligible for Medicaid or CHIP but are not enrolled.

In 2011 the Pew Research Center found that 7.7 million children one in 10 were living in their grandparents' homes. These children often are poor and thus may be eligible for CHIP.[45] In such instances, occupational therapists serving older adults with occupational performance needs at any level of care should consider lifestyle factors that include childrearing.

Summary

This chapter provided an overview of the U.S. health-care and public health systems and how occupational therapy personnel may interface with any aspect of either formal or informal service delivery with aging clients. As a primary quality-of-life-supporting profession, OT has much to offer throughout the continuum of care to support optimal occupational performance and overall well-being in aging adults. By collaborating with clients and other providers in systems of care, the profession has the capability to profoundly affect optimal service utilization, health-care cost containment, and health-related quality of life for all ages.

REVIEW QUESTIONS

1. Discuss differences between the U.S. medical care system and the public health system.
2. List the three levels of services provided within the continuum of care, and provide an example of an OT intervention with older adults for each level.
3. Explain the relationship of access to care and the health status of aging adults.
4. Discuss sources of reimbursement for health care, and their relevance to OT services for older adults.
5. Explain utilization of medical care services and how OT may effectively support cost-containment needs within the systems of care.

REFERENCES

1. American Hospital Association. (2013). *TrendWatch chartbook.* Washington, DC: Author.

2. American Occupational Therapy Association. (March/April, 2014). Occupational therapy practice framework: Domain and process (3rd ed.). *American Journal of Occupational Therapy, 68*(Suppl. 1), S1–S48.

3. Andersen R. (1995). Revisiting the behavioral model and access to medical care: does it matter? *Journal of Health and Social Behavior, 36*(1), 1–10.

4. Aspden, P., Wolcott, J. A., Bootman, L., & Cronenwelt, L. R. (Eds.) (2007). *Institute of Medicine, Preventing Medication Errors, Quality Chasm Series.* Washington, DC: National Academies Press.

5. Bodenheimer, T. (2008). Coordinating care—a perilous journey through the health care system. *New England Journal of Medicine, 358*(10), 1064–1071.

6. Bodenheimer, T., Wagner, E. H., & Grumbach, K. (2002). Improving primary care for patients with chronic illness: The chronic care model, part 2. *JAMA, 288*(15), 1909–1914.

7. Bureau of Labor Statistics. (2013). *Occupational outlook handbook: Healthcare occupations.* Retrieved on March 31, 2013 from http://www.bls.gov/ooh/healthcare/home.html/.

8. Centers for Disease Control and Prevention. (1979). *Healthy people: The Surgeon General's report on health promotion and disease prevention.* Washington, DC: U.S. Department of Health and Human Services.

9. Centers for Disease Control and Prevention. (2006). *2006 nursing facilities.* http://www.cdc.gov/nchs/data/nnhsd/nursing-homefacilities2006.pdf Access date April 6, 2013.

10. Centers for Disease Control and Prevention. (2013). *10 Essential Public Health Services.* http://www.cdc.gov/nphpsp/documents/factsheet.pdf/.

11. Centers for Medicare and Medicaid Services. (2014). *National health expenditures by type of service and source of funds: Calendar years 1960 to 2011. Research statistics data and systems.* http://www.cms.gov/Research-Statistics-Data-and-Systems/Statistics-Trends-and-Reports/NationalHealthExpendData/downloads/tables.pdf/.

12. Claxton, G., Rae, M., et al. (2012). *Employer health benefits 2012.* Menlo Park, CA: Henry J. Kaiser Family Foundation & Health Research & Education Trust.

13. DeNavas-Walt, C., Proctor, B. D., & Smith, J. C. (2012). *U.S. Census Bureau, Current Population Reports, P60-243 Income, poverty and health insurance coverage in the United States: 2011.* http://www.census.gov/prod/2012pubs/p60-243.pdf/.

14. Department of Health and Human Services. (2013). *Healthy people 2010.* Washington, DC: Author.

15. Department of Health and Human Services. (2014). *History: Commissioned Corps of the U.S. Public Health Service.* http://www.usphs.gov/aboutus/history.aspx.

16. Donnelly, C., Brenchley, C., Crawford, C., & Letts, L. (2013). The integration of occupational therapy into primary care: A multiple case study design. *BMC Family Practice, 14*(1), 60-71 doi: 10.1186/1471-2296-14-60.

17. Epstein, A. M., Jha, A. K., Orav, E. J., Liebman, D. L., Audet, A. M., Zezza, M. A., & Guterman, S. (2014). Analysis of early accountable care organizations defines patient, structural, cost, and quality-of-care characteristics. *Health Affairs, 33*(1), 95–102.

18. Freundlich, N. (2014). *Long-term care: What are the issues?* Princeton, NJ: Robert Wood Johnson Foundation.

19. Fuji, K. T., Abbott, A. A., & Norris, J. F. (2012). Exploring care transitions from patient, caregiver, and health-care provider perspectives. *Clinical Nursing Research, 22,* 258–274.

20. Glasgow, R. E., Vinson, C., Chambers, D., Khoury, M. J., Kaplan, R. M., & Hunter, C. (2012). National Institutes of Health approaches to dissemination and implementation science: Current and future directions. *American Journal of Public Health, 102*(7), 1274–1281.

21. Hartman, M., Martin, A. B., Lassman, D., & Catlin, A. (2014). National health spending in 2013: Growth slows, remains in step with the overall economy. *Health Affairs, 34*(1), 150–160.

22. Hernandez, L. M., Rosenstock, L., & Gebbie, K. (Eds.), (2003). *Who will keep the public healthy? Educating public health professionals for the 21st century.* Washington, DC: National Academies Press.

23. Honore, P. A., & Amy, B. W. (2007). Public health finance: Fundamental theories, concepts and definitions. *Journal of Public Health Management and Practice, 32*(2), 89–92.

24. Institute of Medicine. (1988). *The future of public health.* Washington, DC: National Academy Press.

25. Jette, D. U., Warren, R. L., & Wirtalla, C. (2005). The relation between therapy intensity and outcomes of rehabilitation in skilled nursing facilities. *Archives of Physical Medicine and Rehabilitation, 86,* 373–379.

26. Kaiser Commission on Medicaid and the Uninsured. (2013a). *Medicaid: A primer.* Menlo Park, CA: Kaiser Family Foundation.

27. Kaiser Commission on Medicaid and the Uninsured. (2013b). *The uninsured: A primer—key facts about health insurance on the eve of coverage expansions.* Washington, DC: Kaiser Family Foundation.

28. Kaiser Family Foundation. (2008). *How private health insurance coverage works: A primer 2008 update.* Menlo Park, CA: Author.

29. Kaiser Family Foundation. (2010). *Medicare: A primer.* Menlo Park, CA: Author.

30. Kaiser Family Foundation. (2013). *Summary of the new health reform law.* Washington, DC: Author.

31. Kaiser Family Foundation. (2014a). *Medicare Advantage fact sheet.* Menlo Park, CA: Kaiser Family Foundation; 4.

32. Kaiser Family Foundation. (2014b). *Status of state action on the Medicaid expansion decision.* http://kff.org/medicaid/state-indicator/state-activity-around-expanding-medicaid-under-the-affordable-care-act/.

33. Kaye, H. S., Harrington, C., & LaPlante, M. P. (2010). Long-term care: who gets it, who provides it, who pays, and how much? *Health Affairs, 29*(1), 11–21.

34. Killian, C., Fisher, G., & Muir, S. (2015). Primary care: A new context for the scholarship of practice model. *Occupational Therapy in Health Care, 29*(4):383-96

35. Kohn, L. T., Corrigan, J. M., & Donaldson, M. S. . (2001). *Crossing the quality chasm: A new health system for the 21st century.* Washington, DC: National Academies Press.

36. Leavell, H. R., & Clark, E. G. (1965). *Preventive medicine for the doctor in his community. An epidemiologic approach* (3rd ed.). New York, NY: Blakiston-McGraw Hill.

37. Letts, L. J. (2011). Optimal positioning of occupational therapy. *Canadian Journal of Occupational Therapy, 78*(4), 209–219.

38. McGlynn, E. A. (1998). *Assessing the appropriateness of care: How much is too much? RAND research brief.* Santa Monica, CA: RAND.

39. Muir, S. (2012). Health policy perspectives—Occupational therapy in primary health care: We should be there. *American Journal*

of Occupational Therapy, 66, 506–510. http://dx.doi.org/10.5014/ajot.2012.665001.

40. Murray, C. J. L., & Frenk, J. (2010). Ranking 37th—measuring the performance of the U.S. health care system. *New England Journal of Medicine, 362*(2), 98–99.

41. Nutting, P. A., Crabtree, B. F., Miller, W. L., Stange, K. C., Stewart, E., & Jaen, C. (2011). Transforming physician practices to patient-centered medical homes: Lessons from the national demonstration project. *Health Affairs (Millwood), 30*(3), 439–445.

42. Orzag, P. R. (2008). *The overuse, underuse, and misuse of health care: Testimony before the Committee on Finance United States Senate*. Washington, D.C: Congressional Budget Office.

43. O'Shaughnessy, C. (2013). *National spending for long-term services and supports (LTSS), 2011*. Washington, DC: National Health Policy Forum, George Washington University.

44. Peters, C. P. (2005). *Medicare Advantage SNPs: A new opportunity for integrated care? Issue brief*. Washington, DC: National Health Policy Forum, George Washington University.

45. Pew Research Center. (2013). *At grandmother's house we stay: One-in-ten children are living with a grandparent*. Washington, D.C: Pew Research Center.

46. Prima Hyman, D. N. (2008). *Public finance: A contemporary application of theory to policy*. Mason, OH: Thomson South-Western.

47. Rudowitz, R., Artiga, S., & Arguello, R. (2014). *Children's health coverage: Medicaid, CHIP and the ACA*. Menlo Park, CA: Kaiser Family Foundation.

48. Shi, L., & Singh, D. A. (2015). *Delivering health care in America: A system approach* (6th ed.). Burlington, MA: Jones and Bartlett.

49. Shortell, S. M. (2013). Bridging the divide between health and health care. *JAMA, 309*(11), 1121–1122.

50. Shortell, S., Casalino, L., & Fisher, E. (2010). How the Center for Medicare and Medicaid Innovation should test accountable care organizations. *Health Affairs, 29*(7), 1293.

51. Smith, M., Saunders, R., Stuckhardt, L., & McGinnis, J. M. (Eds.), (2013). *Best care at lower cost: The path to continuously learning health care in America*. Washington, DC: National Academies Press.

52. Society for Academic Emergency Medicine. (1992). An ethical foundation for health care: An emergency medicine perspective. *Annals of Emergency Medicine, 21*(11), 1381–1387.

53. Stewart, E. E., Nutting, P. A., Crabtree, B. F., Stange, K. C., Miller, W. L., & Jaen, C. R. (2010). Implementing the patient-centered medical home: Observation and description of the national demonstration project. *Annals of Family Medicine, 8*(Suppl. 1), S21–S32, S92.

54. Wagner, E. H. (1998). Chronic disease management: What will it take to improve care for chronic illness? *Effective Clinical Practice, 1*(1), 2–4.

CHAPTER 24

The Role of Occupational Therapy in Acute and Subacute Care with Aging Adults

Heather Turek Koch, MS, OTR/L, Joseph Flaherty, MD

CHAPTER OUTLINE

OBJECTIVES

- Identify the role of the occupational therapist working with older adults in both acute care and subacute care settings
- Explain the evaluation process in the acute care setting and the post acute (subacute) care setting while working with older adults
- Describe the occupational therapy intervention process in acute and subacute care
- Explain the role occupational therapy plays in determining the next best level of care for older adults once they are discharged from the hospital
- Describe the role that falls play in acute care admissions and their effects on the health and well-being of older adults
- Discuss the financial implications of falls

Introduction

The acute care hospital in the United States serves people of many different races and cultural backgrounds. Based on the Emergency Medical Treatment and Labor Act (commonly referred to as "EMTALA"),[7] which was passed in 1986, hospitals that accept payment from the Department of Health and Human Services' Centers for Medicare and Medicaid Services (CMS) under the Medicare program must provide care to anyone needing emergency health care treatment (including women in labor), regardless of citizenship, legal status, or ability to pay. In 2006, hospitals provided care to people in need at a cost of over $31 billion for which no payment was received.[1] Together Medicare and Medicaid represent 55% of payments for care provided by hospitals.

Definitions of Acute and Subacute Care

Acute care refers to care given in the general hospital setting to medically manage an individual following an injury, an exacerbation of a chronic illness, a new illness, or an accident. Acute care hospitals address the needs of multiple ages with multiple diagnoses, although hospitals will often "specialize" in one or more particular areas; it is a matter of finding the right hospital for the right individual. Pediatric hospitals primarily address the needs of children up to the teen years, whereas most general hospitals, if not identified as a pediatric hospital, serve adults. In the past two decades, acute care for the elderly (ACE) units have been developed, particularly in academic medical centers, to address the unique comorbidities and syndromes that older adults experience and that require highly specialized gerontological care.

Subacute care is comprehensive care provided for someone who has an acute illness, injury, or exacerbation of a disease process. It is goal-oriented treatment provided immediately after, or instead of, acute hospitalization to treat specific active complex medical conditions or to administer complex treatments, in the context of a person's underlying long-term conditions. Ideally applied via an interprofessional team, with highly interrelated processes, it may be provided in a specialized hospital unit or separate facility. *Postacute care* is defined as short-term skilled nursing and therapy services for individuals recovering from acute illness, usually following a hospitalization. This care is provided by home health agencies, skilled nursing facilities (SNFs), inpatient rehabilitation hospitals, and long-term care hospitals.

Medical Terminology

To be an effective therapist in the hospital setting, one must understand the language. In the case examples provided in this chapter, some of the terminology includes *echocardiogram*, *carotid Dopplers*, and acronyms such as *tPA* and *MRI*. Table 24-1 includes a list of common acronyms and abbreviations used in the hospital setting.

TABLE 24-1 Common Acronyms and Abbreviations Used In Acute Care

Abbreviation	Definition	Abbreviation	Definition
A&O	Alert and oriented	ETOH	Ethanol (alcohol)
A.Fib.	Atrial fibrillation (arrhythmia of the heart)	f/u	Follow-up
A/P	Anterior-posterior	FTT	Failure to thrive
AAA	Abdominal aortic aneurysm	FWB	Full weight bearing
AAROM	Active assistive range of motion	fx	Fracture
ACL	Anterior cruciate ligament	GAD	Generalized anxiety disorder
ADLs	Activities of daily living	GCS	Glasgow Coma Scale
AFO	Ankle foot orthosis	GERD	Gastroesophageal reflux
AICD	Automatic implantable cardio-defibrillator (pacemaker)	GYN	Gynecology
		H&P	History and physical
AKA	Above the knee amputation	h/o	History of
ALS	Amyotrophic lateral sclerosis	HA	Headache
AMA	Against medical advice	HD	Hemodialysis
AROM	Active range of motion	HEENT	Head, eyes, ear, nose, throat
AVR	Aortic valve replacement	HOB	Head of bed
B	Bilateral (both sides)	HR	Heart rate
B/S	Bedside	HTN	Hypertension (high blood pressure)
BID	Twice a day	Hx	History
BKA	Below the knee amputation	I&O	Intake and output
BM	Bowel movement	ICP	Intracranial pressure
BP	Blood pressure	ICU	Intensive care unit
BPH	Benign prostatic hypertrophy	IDDM	Insulin-dependent diabetes mellitus
BSC	Bedside commode	IM	Intramedullary (nailing)
CA	Cancer	IV	Intravenously
CABG	Coronary artery bypass graft	IVC	Inferior vena cava
CAD	Coronary artery disease	L	Left
c-diff	Clostridium difficile	LBP	Low back pain
CHF	Congestive heart failure	LE	Lower extremity
CHI	Closed head injury	LLQ	Left lower quadrant
CN	Cranial nerves (there are 12)	LOC	Loss of consciousness
COPD	Chronic obstructive pulmonary disease	LOS	Length of stay
COTA	Certified occupational therapy assistant	LP	Lumbar puncture
CPAP	Continuous positive airway pressure	LTAC	Long-term acute care
CPR	Cardiopulmonary resuscitation	LUQ	Left upper quadrant
CRF or CKD	Chronic renal failure or chronic kidney disease	MBS	Modified barium swallow
		MCA	Middle cerebral artery
CSF	Cerebrospinal fluid	MI	Myocardial infarction
CT scan	Computed axial tomography (type of x-ray that shows two-dimensional images of the parts of the body)	MRI	Magnetic resonance imaging
		MRSA	Methicillin-resistant *Staphylococcus aureus*
CVA	Cerebrovascular accident (stroke)	MS	Multiple sclerosis
CXR	Chest x-ray	MVA	Motor vehicle accident
D/C	Discharge	MVP	Mitral valve prolapse
d/t	Due to	MVR	Mitral valve replacement
DM	Diabetes mellitus	N & V	Nausea and vomiting
DME	Durable medical equipment	NG	Nasogastric tube
DNR	Do not resuscitate	NICU	Neonatal intensive care unit
DOB	Date of birth	NIDDM	Noninsulin-dependent diabetes mellitus
DOE	Dyspnea on exertion	NKA	No known allergies
Dx	Diagnosis	NOS	Not otherwise specified
ECT	Electroconvulsive treatment	NPO	Nothing by mouth
ED	Emergency department	NSAID	Nonsteroidal anti-inflammatory drug
EEG	Electroencephalogram	NWB	Non-weight bearing
EKG	Electrocardiogram	O_2	Oxygen
EMG	Electromyography	OA	Osteoarthritis
ENT	Ear, nose, and throat	OB/GYN	Obstetrics and gynecology
EOB	Edge of bed	OOB	Out of bed
ESRD	End-stage renal disease	OR	Operating room

Continued

TABLE 24-1 Common Acronyms and Abbreviations Used In Acute Care—cont'd

Abbreviation	Definition	Abbreviation	Definition
ORIF	Open reduction internal fixation (typically used in orthopedic clients; may consist of screws and nails to correct a bone fracture)	RN	Registered nurse
		ROM	Range of motion
		RT	Respiratory therapy
		RUQ	Right upper quadrant
OT	Occupational therapy	s/p	Status post (following something)
PA	Physician's assistant	SCI	Spinal cord injury
PE	Pulmonary embolism (blood clot in the lung)	SDH	Subdural hematoma
		SLP	Speech-language pathology or pathologist
PEG	Percutaneous endoscopic gastrostomy (used if adequate nutritional intake not being obtained due to malnourishment or dysphagia)	SLR	Straight leg raise
		SNF	Skilled nursing facility
		SOAP	Subjective, objective, assessment, plan
PET	Positron emission tomography (used for cancer screenings and follow-up)	SOB	Shortness of breath
		SROM	Self range of motion
PID	Pelvic inflammatory disease	ST	Speech therapy
PMH	Past medical history	STD	Sexually transmitted disease
POD	Post-op day (usually stands for number of days after a surgical procedure; e.g., "Mrs. Anthony is pod #3 following her r thr")	SW	Social worker
		sx	Symptoms
		TAH	Total abdominal hysterectomy
		TB	Tuberculosis
		TBI	Traumatic brain injury
PRBC	Packed red blood cells (used for a blood transfusion)	THA	Total hip arthroplasty
		THR	Total hip replacement
PRN	As often as necessary	TIA	Transient ischemic attack
PROM	Passive range of motion	TKR	Total knee replacement
PT	Physical therapy	TLSO	Thoracic lumbosacral orthotic (typically a back brace)
PTA	Prior to admission		
PTCA	Percutaneous transvenous coronary angioplasty (balloon angioplasty)	TMJ	Temporomandibular joint
		tPA	Tissue plasminogen activator
PUD	Peptic ulcer disease	TPN	Total parenteral nutrition
PVD	Peripheral vascular disease	TURP	Transurethral resection of the prostate
PWB	Partial weight bearing (sometimes given with a percentage, e.g., 50% WB, 33% WB)	UA	Urinalysis
		US	Ultrasound
q	Every	UTI	Urinary tract infection
qid	Four times a day	VRE	Vancomycin-resistant enterococci
R	Right	w/u	Workup
R/O	Rule out	WBAT	Weight bearing as tolerated
RA	Rheumatoid arthritis	WBC	White blood cells
RBC	Red blood cell	WDL	Within defined limits
RCA	Right coronary artery	WFL	Within functional limits
RLQ	Right lower quadrant	WNL	Within normal limits

The Acute Care Trajectory

There is a typical flow of care by which an individual enters into acute care: The individual arrives in the emergency department (ED) and is seen and evaluated by an emergency medicine physician, procedural tests are run, and in some instances the individual is admitted. The length of stay is typically short, ranging from 3 to 5 days, and discharge planning often happens immediately after the individual is admitted. In 2008, there were over 35,000,000 inpatient hospital admissions in the United States, with an average length of stay of 5.5 days.[1] The number of discharges from nonfederal short-stay hospitals totaled 13.1 million for those 65 years and older.[5]

The workup in the ED helps determine to which medical floor the client will be admitted. Different types of medical floors include the general medicine unit, medical/surgical unit, orthopedic unit, telemetry unit, and intensive care unit (ICU). Table 24-2 provides a list of typical acute care medical units; and figures 24-1 and 24-2 provide images of telemetry equipment and a typical ICU. Older adults are admitted to the hospital for many reasons, although falls and other injuries, dizziness, abdominal pain, and weakness are common. The types of symptoms each individual presents are usually treated following protocols established for each condition. Case Examples 24-1 and 24-2 help to illustrate this point.

TABLE 24-2 Hospital Departments

Types	Description	Common Client Diagnoses/Conditions
Medical unit	Provides hospitalist (a designated hospital staff physician provides medical oversight for client if client does not have primary care physician or if primary care physician does not come to the hospital); provides noninvasive monitoring	Pneumonia, asthma, or chronic obstructive pulmonary disease (COPD) exacerbations; weakness (due to fever, cough, diarrhea, dehydration); exacerbations of multiple sclerosis (MS); admissions due to pressure ulcers; new diagnosis of stroke (if telemetry monitor is found unnecessary)
Medical/ surgical unit	Monitors clients following major surgery	Colectomy or other abdominal surgeries, hysterectomy, pressure ulcer debridement surgery, mastectomy
Orthopedic unit	Monitors clients following orthopedic injury that may also include surgery	Total knee replacement, total hip replacement, hip fracture repair, humeral fracture repair, conservative upper or lower extremity management following injury
Telemetry unit	Continuously monitors clients' heart rate with the use of telemetry equipment (Figure 24-1)	Syncope, dizziness, atrial or ventricular fibrillation, myocardial infarction, congestive heart failure
Intensive care unit	Closely monitors patients because of intensity of illness; cares for clients who need mechanical ventilation (Figure 24-2)	All diagnoses that may have been complicated by respiratory failure, heart failure, or kidney failure

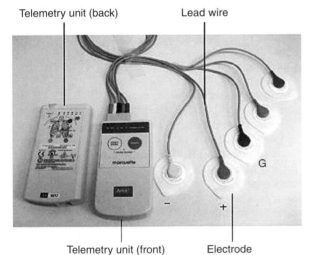

Telemetry unit (back)   Lead wire

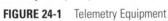

Telemetry unit (front)   Electrode

FIGURE 24-1   Telemetry Equipment

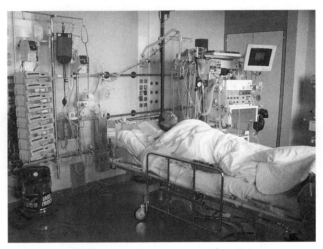

FIGURE 24-2   Typical Intensive Care Unit

CASE EXAMPLE 24-1   Stroke (Cerebrovascular Accident)

Mr. Thomas, an 85-year-old white male living at home, went to bed at 9:00 PM. He awoke at 1:00 AM to use the bathroom and fell when getting out of bed. He felt weakness in his right arm and leg and could not get himself off of the floor. His wife of 60 years heard him hit the floor. She suddenly got out of bed to tend to her husband. She noticed his speech was quite garbled and she could not understand what he was saying. Thanks to earlier discussions with their granddaughter, Olivia, an occupational therapy student, Mrs. Thomas recognized her husband's symptoms as a stroke. She raced to the phone to call 911. Paramedics soon arrived and rushed him to the nearest emergency department, at St. Joseph's Hospital, which was about a 15-minute drive from their home. Upon arrival, the following sequence of events occurs:

1. Mr. Thomas is taken to Room 7 of the Emergency Department (ED).

2. He is then examined by Dr. Sloan, an emergency medicine physician.

3. Dr. Sloan recognizes Mr. Thomas' condition as a stroke and initiates St. Joseph's stroke protocol.

4. The stroke protocol includes completing a computed tomography (CT) scan of the head, and calling the neurologist to see if Mr. Thomas is eligible for administration of tissue plasminogen activator (tPA; a clot-busting drug that can decrease the debility caused by a stroke). tPA can be administered up to 4.5 hours after the last well-known time of the onset of symptoms.

5. Dr. Lolly, the neurologist on call, states Mr. Thomas is not eligible for tPA but finds it necessary to admit him to the hospital.

6. Mr. Thomas is admitted to the designated stroke unit of the hospital, which is a telemetry unit. On the

Continued

CASE EXAMPLE 24-1 Stroke (Cerebrovascular Accident)—cont'd

telemetry unit individuals wear a heart monitor 24 hours/day, 7 days a week, (24/7) and the heart rhythm is closely observed.
7. Dr. Lolly orders further tests, including an echocardiogram, carotid Dopplers, and a magnetic resonance imaging (MRI) scan of the brain.
8. Dr. Lolly also orders physical therapy, occupational therapy, and speech therapy to evaluate and treat this individual.

9. The team, which includes the neurologist, the internist, the nurse case manager, and the therapists, collaborates to determine the next best level of care for Mr. Thomas.
10. The team's options include discharge to home with home health care services, discharge to an acute rehabilitation hospital, or discharge to a skilled nursing facility.

CASE EXAMPLE 24-2 Hip Fracture

Mrs. Anthony, a 75-year-old female living independently in a two-level home, arose from her chair to go to the bathroom. She suddenly tripped on her area rug and fell. She noticed she had a great deal of left hip pain. She was able to crawl to the phone to call 911. Emergency medical services (EMS) arrived and transported her to the St. Joseph's Hospital emergency department (ED), where the following sequence of events occurs:
1. Mrs. Anthony is taken to Room 6 of the ED.
2. She is examined by Dr. Sloan, and he orders an x-ray of the left hip and pelvis.
3. He finds that she has a left displaced femoral neck fracture.
4. Dr. Sloan notifies Dr. Shaeffer, the on-call orthopedic surgeon.
5. Mrs. Anthony is taken to surgery and has a left total hip replacement performed to treat the injured hip.
6. She is then taken to the orthopedic unit.
7. Dr. Shaeffer orders physical therapy and occupational therapy to start the day after surgery.
8. According to the orders, Mrs. Anthony is on hip precautions and is weight-bearing as tolerated on her left lower extremity.

9. Mrs. Anthony verbalizes to Dr. Schaeffer that she would like to return home alone upon discharge from the hospital.
10. Dr. Schaeffer communicates this in the client's medical record.
11. The occupational therapist teaches Mrs. Anthony how to safely transfer from bed to chair and how to use various types of adaptive equipment, including long-handled reachers, sock aids, canes, and other devices to assist with dressing and ambulation.
12. The team's options include discharge to home with home health care services, discharge to an acute rehabilitation hospital, or discharge to a skilled nursing facility.
13. The physical therapist and occupational therapist both agree that Mrs. Anthony is not safe or able to return home alone and both recommend continued therapy at the acute (rehabilitation) hospital.
14. The case manager alerts the social worker about placing Mrs. Anthony in another facility following discharge, after observing the occupational therapist's and physical therapist's initial evaluations of Mrs. Anthony.

Overall Role of Occupational Therapy in Acute Care

The occupational therapist's role in the acute care setting is a vital one. There are three primary roles the therapist may play in the hospital: educator, rehabilitator, and consultant. Occupational therapy assistants are less likely to provide services at this level of care, due to the critical status of many clients.

The educator role includes instructing the client on safe and necessary adaptations that need to be made to carry out all personal activities of daily living (ADLs) independently. In the previous case example of Mrs. Anthony, who sustained a hip fracture and needed a total joint replacement, the occupational therapist's role is to educate the client on hip precautions related to occupational performance and positioning; relevant adaptive equipment; safe toilet transfers; and appropriate durable medical equipment, such as a raised toilet seat, grab rails and bars, and bath benches; and to provide family education. Individuals who have sustained hip fractures requiring joint replacement or internal fixation, must follow strict hip precautions during the

rehabilitation phase of recovery. Figure 24-3 provides precautionary measures to be taken by the client following hip surgery. The occupational therapist's role may also include educating the medical team, so that they fully understand what occupational therapy (OT) can do to help their clients.

The second role of the occupational therapist is that of rehabilitator. OT should be started in the hospital for those clients who require post-discharge therapy.[2] The therapy started in the acute care hospital could potentially be the first phase of rehabilitation that the client will experience. The client could then possibly continue on to an acute rehabilitation hospital or a skilled nursing facility, where the client will continue therapy until it is determined by the overseeing therapist that the client is ready for a safe discharge to home. Occupational therapy assistants may provide services in these settings, since the clients' health status is less severe than in acute care settings.

The third role of the occupational therapist is that of consultant. This is a very important role within the health care team because it provides the therapist's insight regarding the next best level of care for the client. The therapist's assessment of the client is considered along with the findings of other

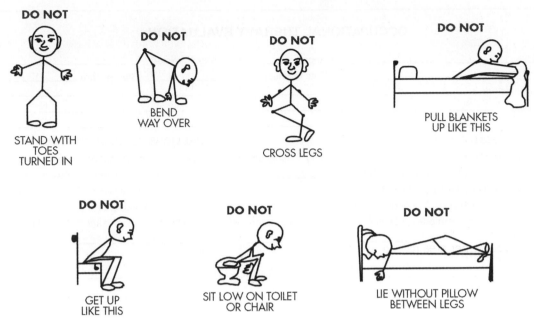

DO NOT
STAND WITH TOES TURNED IN

DO NOT
BEND WAY OVER

DO NOT
CROSS LEGS

DO NOT
PULL BLANKETS UP LIKE THIS

DO NOT
GET UP LIKE THIS

DO NOT
SIT LOW ON TOILET OR CHAIR

DO NOT
LIE WITHOUT PILLOW BETWEEN LEGS

FIGURE 23-3   Client Precautions Following Hip Surgery. From Christensen B. L., Kockrow E. O. [2011]. Foundations and adult health nursing, (6th ed.). St. Louis, MO: Elsevier.

members of the health care team to help determine the next optimal level of care. Because of the pressure for short hospital stays directed by insurance carriers and other reimbursement systems, the sooner a discharge plan can be put in place, the better.

Occupational Therapy Evaluation Process

The OT evaluation process in the acute care setting is typically quick. As stated earlier, a client might be in the hospital for only a few days. In some cases, the occupational therapist may only get one visit with the client before discharge. Because of this, and because of productivity demands in the hospital setting, the occupational therapist has to be efficient with his or her time, covering all important points when completing an evaluation. (Please see chapter 7 for an expanded discussion of the overall OT evaluation process)

Figure 24-4 shows an example of a typical acute care evaluation form. Documentation of the evaluation is typically structured as a SOAP note, in which S = subjective, O = objective, A = assessment, and P = plan; Box 24-1 provides an example of this format.

The evaluation usually starts with an occupational profile. This information helps the occupational therapist to understand how functional the client was before admission to the hospital; it is the "S" portion of the evaluation. Typical questions asked include:

- Do you live alone? If not, who lives with you?
- What type of home do you live in? Is it on one or more levels?
- Do you live in an apartment, condominium, loft, farm, or other dwelling? Do you have stairs, and if so, how many must you climb to get into your home? Does it have an elevator?

- Did you need any assistance with your ADLs (e.g., bathing, toileting, feeding, dressing, functional mobility) before admission to the hospital?
- Did you use any sort of equipment at home? A walker? A cane? A shower bench?
- Did you participate in any instrumental activities of daily living (IADLs) (e.g., cooking, laundry, driving, grocery shopping, household management, paying the bills, etc.)?

This information helps the occupational therapist to understand the client's level of function before the hospital admission. While obtaining this information the occupational therapist can also get an idea about the client's level of cognition if the family has not reported that information. As stated earlier, some older adults in the hospital setting may have a history of memory problems such as dementia, or develop confusion while in the hospital, also called delirium. (See chapter 15 for more information on dementia and delirium.) This may or may not be noted in the client's chart. If a cognitive problem is noted during the evaluation, the occupational therapist should document this in the medical chart to let the team know of the findings.

The evaluation continues with the objective ("O") portion—what the occupational therapist observes. This will include assessing the client's upper body function, range of motion, and strength using the manual muscle test (MMT); assessing sitting-to-standing transfers, bed-to-chair transfers, and toilet transfer; and examining the client's balance during the transfer. The evaluation then continues on to the core of the occupational therapist's intervention role: evaluation of the client's ADLs. The occupational therapist will observe feeding, grooming, bathing, dressing, and toileting. Most of the time, clients will be wearing a hospital gown and will not be using their own clothes in the hospital setting. In these instances, it is best to

OCCUPATIONAL THERAPY EVALUATION

Name _____ Room _____ Referring physician _____

Diagnosis _____ Date of onset _____ Start of care _____

Previous medical history _____
_____

Precautions _____

PREVIOUS SOCIAL HISTORY

Living: ☐ Home alone ☐ With others ☐ Assisted living ☐ Nursing home

Tub/shower: ☐ Combo ☐ Walk-in shower ☐ Other _____

Employment: ☐ Actively employed ☐ Retired

Activity: ☐ Driving ☐ Active ☐ Sedentary ☐ Confined to bed

Equipment owned: ☐ 3 in 1 commode ☐ Shower bench ☐ Tub transfer bench ☐ Wheel chair ☐ Grab bars ☐ Hand held shower head

Patient goal: _____

PREVIOUS LEVEL OF FUNCTION

ADLS: ☐ Independent ☐ Assist dependent

Mobility: ☐ Independent ☐ Assist dependent

☐ No device ☐ Cane ☐ Walker

☐ Wheelchair

OBJECTIVE INFORMATION

COGNITION _____ VISUAL-PERCEPTUAL _____

UPPER EXTREMITY FUNCTION

ROM   R _____   Coordination R _____

L _____   L _____

Strength R _____   Sensation R _____

L _____   L _____

OVERALL ENDURANCE/THERAPY TOLERANCE   ☐ Poor   ☐ Fair   ☐ Good

<15 minutes   30-60 minutes   >60 minutes

ADL	Ind	SBA	Min	Mod	Max	Dep
Feeding						
Grooming						
UE dressing						
LE dressing						
Bathing						
Toileting						

Mobility/transfers	Ind	SBA	Min	Mod	Max	Dep
Bed mobility						
Sit to stand						
Commode						
Chair/wheelchair						
Shower						

ASSESSMENT:

Primary limitations ↓ ADLs ↓ Transfers/mobility

Due to: ↓ Endurance ↓ UE strength/coordination

Orthopedic restrictions ↓ Safety/cognitive impairment

Other _____
_____

RECOMMENDATIONS:

1. Continue OT _____ visits towards following goals
2. DME _____
3. No OT indicated at this time
4. Other _____
_____

Therapist signature: _____

PLAN OF CARE:

Adaptive equipment/DME training

Energy conservation/work simplification

Education/training   Home exercise program

Total hip precautions   ADL training

UE AROM/strengthening   Coordination

Positioning/splinting   Transfer training

Other _____

GOALS:

1. ↑ ADLs (_____) to _____
2. ↑ _____ transfers to _____
3. _____
4. _____
5. _____

Date: _____

Name: _____

D.O.B. _____ Medical record # _____

FIGURE 24-4 Sample Acute Care Occupational Therapy Evaluation Form

BOX 24-1   SOAP Format

- *Subjective: Information the client or family member is providing to the therapist.* This discussion should include how the client was functioning before admission, especially regarding activities of daily living (ADLs).
- *Objective: What is observed by the therapist.* This description includes the client's upper and lower extremities, trunk control, and ADL assessments.
- *Assessment: What the therapist concludes from the evaluation.* What barriers, if any, are present that keep the client from returning to the previous environment, such as the client's own home?
- *Plan: The occupational therapist's recommendations.* Given the example of Case Example 24-2 (Mrs. Anthony, with a hip fracture), the occupational therapist may find that the client is not safe or able to return home alone. The occupational therapist may document, "Plan to continue seeing the client once daily for adaptive equipment and ADL training." The occupational therapist may also document his or her recommendation in the client's chart: "Client does not appear safe or able to return home alone. Recommend continued OT services upon discharge" (e.g., discharge from the acute care hospital).

simulate dressing tasks, if possible, with their own clothes if they are to be discharged to home. Again, the occupational therapist checks mobility and upper extremity function, assesses standing balance, and evaluates whether or not the client can reach his or her feet to don shoes and socks/stockings. In some cases, the client may not be allowed to attempt reaching the feet due to hip precautions, back surgery, or other factors. Occupational therapists must use their best judgment to help determine the client's level of mobility and function and what assistance, if any, the client requires: no assistance, minimal assistance, moderate assistance, or maximal assistance.

The "A" (assessment) and "P" (plan) sections go somewhat hand in hand. Following administration of the objective portion, the occupational therapist can then make an informed decision about the client's next best level of care. The occupational therapist needs to identify any barriers that are limiting the individual, and decide what level of care may be most appropriate for the client. This process may determine whether or not the client is able to return home.

The Context of Occupational Therapy Work in Acute Care: The Interprofessional Health Care Team

The occupational therapist in acute care works as a vital member of a coordinated health care team. The following is a list of the typical health care providers in the acute hospital setting with whom the occupational therapist often works; all can equally contribute to the determination of the next best level of care (see chapter 27 for further discussion of the interprofessional health care team).

- Case manager: In acute care the case manager is usually a registered nurse. It is the case manager's job to oversee the client's length of stay in the hospital and to document the justification for reimbursement purposes. This may include talking with physicians regarding tests that may be ordered, negotiating with insurance companies to cover specific tests, and talking with clients and their family members to coordinate a discharge plan that ensures the client is going to a safe and appropriate environment upon discharge.
- Nurses: Nurses administer the medical care that physicians prescribe. They also play a key role in symptom management and in the identification of any new problems that arise with the client. Occupational therapists can educate nurses about client-specific safety concerns before clients return home, discuss medical concerns with nurses, advise them about recommendations for the client (e.g., how many people will be needed to help transfer the client to bed), and communicate safety needs to the physician and family if they are not present when the occupational therapist is treating the client.
- Certified Nurse Assistants (CNAs): CNAs, also referred to as "nurse techs" or "care partners," among other names, are responsible for helping clients with basic care such as toileting, transferring, and bathing. They also check the vital signs sometimes.
- Physical therapist: The occupational therapist tends to work closely with the physical therapist. They may discuss what they think is the best next level of care for the client they may be co-treating. In some complex cases, the occupational therapist and physical therapist may not agree with each other as far as next level of care, but it is beneficial to have a working relationship with the aim of returning the client to as high of a level of functioning as possible while ensuring the client's safety—always the number one priority.
- Physician: The physician oversees all of the medical care the client receives in the hospital. It is the physician's duty to order all appropriate tests, including magnetic resonance imaging (MRI), x-rays, blood work, and therapies. It is also the physician's job to call on a specialist to help care for the client if deemed necessary. Typical specialties utilized include neurology, nephrology, cardiology, pulmonology, and surgery. If a client is older and has multiple problems, a geriatrics consultant can be helpful, if available.
- Social worker: The social worker typically maintains a close relationship with the case manager. The social worker's job is to help ensure an individually appropriate discharge plan. Duties include talking with family members about their preferences for discharge (e.g., going home with home health care services, discharge to an acute rehabilitation facility, or discharge to an SNF) and making the necessary phone calls to transport the client to the intended destination upon discharge. This also includes providing the necessary documentation to the insurance company for reimbursement of services.

- Speech therapist: The speech therapist also collaborates on assisting the client to maintain or regain function, and regarding any safety concerns. The speech therapist is typically called in to evaluate the client's swallow for safety with eating and drinking, and for further cognitive testing. The occupational therapist can discuss cognitive concerns with the speech therapist and relies on the speech therapist for recommendations of appropriate diet modifications, if necessary.

Hospitalization Sequelae: Deconditioning

All members of the teamwork to prevent and limit the deconditioning that can accompany hospitalization. When older adults are hospitalized, there is a great sense of loss: loss of independence, loss of ability, and loss of familiar environment. Many older adults in the hospital experience *deconditioning*, which is defined as the multiple changes in organ system physiology that are induced by inactivity, but that may be reversed by a return to activity.[15] Deconditioning can be caused by the individual's being bedbound and not participating in normal daily routines while dealing with an illness, which may not even be disabling, but that limits the client's activity level. This can contribute to a decreased level of occupational performance.

Humans need to complete their occupations to feel productive in society. When typical activities are not pursued during hospitalization, the outcomes can be devastating. According to research done by Eyres and Unsworth,[8] a therapy program that provides opportunities to make decisions about, and participate in usual occupations can help "minimize poorer client outcomes associated with bed rest, inactivity, lack of engagement in occupation and loss of control over the environment."[8] These researchers completed a randomized controlled study to measure the effectiveness of an additional OT program to maintain occupational performance in hospitalized older adults. This pilot study evaluated 15 medically stable individuals within a 72-hour period upon hospital admission. For each individual, functional status was measured with the Functional Independence Measure (FIM), confidence level was evaluated with the Self-Efficacy Gauge, and quality of life was assessed with the Life Satisfaction Index. The experimental group consisted of individuals participating in a daily additional OT program that included the following elements:[8]

1. A self-care program
2. A set of IADL tasks (e.g., cooking, laundry, café visits)
3. Functional and community mobility activities (walking outdoors; accessing the café, garden, or park)

The control group may or may not have received traditional OT services. The individuals were then evaluated again on all three measures, and the results demonstrated that although the outcomes for both groups were not statistically significant regarding the three factors measured because of the small number of study participants, "many benefits to the program were found clinically and from participant feedback. Several clients reported feeling more confident in their ability to manage required occupations, such as self-care and mobility upon discharge."[8] Many also reported a greater feeling of well-being, and families and caregivers expressed appreciation

for the program. Helping older adults to realize that they can return to their preadmission "former selves" can be very empowering for them and rewarding for the therapist.

Subacute or "Postacute" Care

Several terms are used to describe the care that occurs after individuals leave the acute care hospital. *Subacute care* is the most commonly used term, but the terms *postacute care* and *aftercare* are also found in the medical literature for the same or similar care following the acute care hospitalization period.

The occupational therapist has much to consider regarding the acute care discharge plan and the transition to the next stage of intervention (if any is necessary). Input from occupational therapists offers much to the health care team, because occupational therapists not only determine what they feel is best and safe for the client and what the individual can tolerate, but ultimately also consider the client's goals and priorities. Most clients are very determined to return home and yet may not realize the scope of their impairments that will affect occupational performance. Determining the appropriate next level of care can be a tough decision to make; it helps to obtain opinions from the other members of the health care team. This decision-making is a collaborative process, and responsibility should not be left to only one team member. As previously stated, there are many options to consider after acute care hospitalization (Table 24-3).

Appropriate clinical reasoning on the part of the occupational therapist is essential in acute care discharge planning, to determine the best option for the client and the family. Taking into account the OT evaluation can help the team to determine the next best level of care. In discharge planning, the occupational therapist must ask him- or herself: What can I offer this client at this level of care? What do I think is going to be the next best step in this client's recovery process for the client to regain his or her prior level of function? Do I think the client can handle this next level of care, both emotionally and physically? If involved in the client's life what is the family's/support system's perspective regarding care? It is best to discuss the options with the health care team, because the decision-making process is difficult to complete independently and should be a collaborative effort. Thus the occupational therapist collaborates with the team in deciding on the next best level of care for the client, whether additional medically supervised care is needed, and whether the individual may be safely discharged to home. When the individual is discharged to another care provider, the medical chart or electronic system of records and documentation maintained by the team accompanies the client.

In the next section we provide an in-depth look at the five subacute or postacute care options for clients after hospitalization, so that the reader can appreciate the difference between acute care and subacute care.

Long-Term Acute Care Hospital

The long-term acute care hospital (LTACH) is a possible option for discharge for an older adult after a stay in an acute medical hospital. LTACHs "provide specialized acute care for medically complex clients who are critically ill with

TABLE 24-3 Subacute Care Options

Facility	Admission Parameters
Long-term acute care hospital (LTACH)	The client still has significant medical needs that need to be addressed (such as clients with tracheostomies or intensive wound care needs). The client can also participate in therapy, but the participation amount can vary depending on the severity of the medical illnesses.
Acute rehabilitation hospital	The client must be able to participate in 3 hours of therapy per day in order to be a candidate for acute rehab. A more intense program like this may lead to faster recovery.
Skilled nursing facility	The client will receive up to 1 to 2 hours of therapy per day. The client may improve, but it may not be a short process as in acute rehab.
Home health care	The client will return to his or her prior living situation and have a therapist come to the home three times a week. It may also be necessary, in some cases, to have a 24-hour caregiver, depending on the circumstance.
Long-term care (at a nursing facility, also called a nursing home)	The client is typically dependent in activities of daily living or has a significant cognitive impairment, either of which is unlikely to improve.

CASE EXAMPLE 24-3   A Client Discharged to a Long-Term Acute Care Hospital: Occupational Therapy Intervention Process

Margaret is a 60-year-old female admitted to the acute hospital with abdominal pain. Workup revealed diverticulosis. Margaret then underwent a hemicolectomy (partial removal of the colon). Following the surgery, Margaret did not have a smooth recovery. She was immediately transported to the intensive care unit because she was ventilator dependent (unable to breathe on her own). About 10 days after the surgery, Margaret was conscious and the team considered removing the ventilator. After about 12 hours being off of the ventilator, the team decided to place her back on the ventilator. She was otherwise stable from the surgery and other medical conditions. The team allowed occupational therapists and physical therapists to start working with her even though she was still on the ventilator. Margaret worked very hard and wished to return home once she was able. The team members agreed that it was no longer appropriate for Margaret to stay in the acute medical hospital because all systems were stable except for the ventilator dependence, and thus they decided to send Margaret to an long-term acute care hospital (LTACH). When team members at the LTACH facility received the client, they determined the goals were to get her off of the ventilator and slowly help her to begin to regain her strength following her hospitalization.

---

multi-system complications or failures and required long hospitalizations."[6] Clients in these facilities still receive therapy services, but their conditions are much more medically complex than those of clients typically seen in a rehabilitation facility or a skilled nursing facility (SNF). Clients may be ventilator dependent, have wounds, or simply be extremely debilitated due to a long hospitalization, and may be unable to tolerate what is expected at a rehabilitation hospital or SNF (Case Example 24-3). Although a client may be released to an LTACH, the goal is usually still for the client to return home. The client may very well be transferred to a rehabilitation hospital or SNF once discharged from the subacute setting.

The length of stay and course of treatment for clients admitted to an LTACH facility are highly individualized based upon need and dependent on many factors. The typical length of stay is 20 to 30 days.[10] As noted by the Medicare Payment Advisory Commission, "In 2008, in the U.S. Medicare spent $4.6 billion on care furnished in an estimated 386 LTACHs nationwide. About 115,000 beneficiaries had almost 131,000 LTACH stays."[10,11] Some facilities have a protocol that is followed to determine the optimal level of therapy for each client. There may be some individuals who receive very little therapy each day, and some who require extensive treatments. Let us return to the example of Margaret, who arrived at the ED and then was admitted to acute care. The receiving team at the LTACH has a record of what Margaret was able to do at the hospital during her stay. The OT report from the hospital states:

This individual was independent with all ADLs, ambulation, driving, and cooking before her illness. She was seen for the first OT visit 12 days following surgery. Although she was awake, alert, and appeared to be cognitively intact, she was unable to vocalize, due to her ventilator. Margaret demonstrated active range of motion in upper extremities bilaterally, yet was unable to hold against gravity: 2-/5 strength on bilateral upper extremities while supine in bed. She demonstrated difficulty in reaching to attempt washing her face and in attempts at oral care. Active assistive range of motion and passive range of motion to bilateral upper extremities was performed. On day 2, the occupational therapist and physical therapist co-treated to attempt to sit her on the edge of the bed. She moved to the edge of her bed dependently with a two-person assist, and she sat on the edge of the bed for 3 minutes with total assistance required. She then became somewhat anxious and her heart rate increased, at which time she was returned to a supine position.

In the following days, therapists continued to sit Margaret on the edge of her bed, and her time up generally increased daily, reaching up to 6 minutes over 5 days of trying. From this information, the occupational therapist at the LTACH decided to evaluate the client and see if she had improved. The therapists worked together to get the client up to a wheelchair; a client lift was required. The client was still somewhat anxious, but displayed 3-/5 on bilateral upper extremities. The treating therapists then decided the client would be appropriate for three to four units per day of therapy. The treating therapists knew, though, that it would be a day-by-day case with Margaret to build her endurance to eventually be able to tolerate greater than five units of therapy per day.

The evaluation in the LTACH is not much different from that conducted in the acute hospital. The big difference is that the therapist has much more time to treat the client. The goal is still to obtain the client's prior level of function, gather the ADL information, and determine a treatment plan, which is frequently a month-long plan. The occupational therapist should be conscientious in writing both short- and long-term goals, whereas in the acute hospital, short-term goals are the most appropriate to write due to the short length of stay. Clients may or may not be wearing their own clothes at this point. The goal is to start practicing skills using their clothes; however, with many different pieces of medical equipment or severe wounds that may not be possible. Again, occupational therapists must use their best judgment to determine the ideal approach.

Acute Rehabilitation Hospital (Acute Rehab)

Acute rehabilitation facilities help clients experiencing a loss of function from injury or illness that results in limited ability to care for themselves. The aim of treatment is for clients to become as independent as possible in ADLs so that they may return home and reenter the community. Presenting limitations upon admission include impaired mobility, balance, and coordination; decreased strength and range of motion; sensory loss or visual/perception problems; cognitive problems (issues with memory, problem solving, etc.); difficulty with speech and communication; and swallowing disorders.

The acute rehab unit provides comprehensive rehabilitation for clients across a wide variety of diagnoses, including but not limited to amputations, arthritis, traumatic brain injury, burns, cerebrovascular accident, hip fractures, neurological disorders, spinal cord injury, and chronic conditions made worse by illness, such as chronic obstructive pulmonary disease and cardiovascular disease.

The acute rehab hospital ideally utilizes an interprofessional team approach toward successful rehabilitation. Occupational therapists are part of the rehabilitation team whose members are dedicated to meeting clients' physical, psychological, and social needs in an environment that promotes wellness, confidence, and independence. Team members develop individualized treatment plans to maximize each client's functional abilities. They also provide information about community resources to help smooth the transition to home and community. Additional team members typically include a medical director, a physician (often a specialist called a physiatrist), rehabilitation nurses, physical therapists, speech/language therapists, social workers, psychologists, and dietitians. The interprofessional team process implies highly coordinated communication and intervention approaches.

In addition to daily OT, physical therapy, and/or speech therapy, clients in an acute rehab unit are encouraged to get out of bed each day, participate in daily care such as dressing and grooming to promote independence in ADLs, join in individual and group leisure activities to help resume their normal occupations, and eat meals with other clients in the dining room to encourage socialization. Typically, participation of family and friends in treatment and educational programs is encouraged.

Skilled Nursing Facility

Skilled nursing facilities (SNFs) provide inpatient health care with the same types of staff and equipment necessary to provide skilled care, rehabilitation, and other related services to individuals who need nursing care but not at the level of intensity as acute rehabilitation. (see Table 24-3)

The care of every client is under the supervision of a physician, who usually sees the clients once or twice a week and is available by telephone. In the United States SNFs are the most common settings for providing subacute care.[12]

Home Health Care

The goals of home-based services are to assist older adults who are recovering after a hospital stay or need additional support to remain safely at home and avoid an unnecessary rehospitalization. These services may include short-term nursing, rehabilitative, and assistive care. Skilled services are provided by registered nurses, occupational therapists, physical therapists, speech-language pathologists and medical social workers. In addition to the skilled services, other personnel such as home health aides or chore workers may assist the individual with ADLs, cleaning the home, and/or meal preparation. For terminally ill individuals, services may include hospice care.[12]

Falls and the Older Adult

Falls happen all too frequently among older adults. Consider the following findings:

- Every year, one out of every three adults aged 65 years and older will suffer a fall.[3]
- Falls are the most common cause of injury deaths, trauma injuries, and hospital admissions for trauma in those 65 years of age and older.[13]
- Older adults are five times more likely to be admitted to a hospital for injuries sustained from a fall than from an injury of another cause.[3,13]

- The rate of fall injuries in 2009 for those 85 years old and over was almost four times that of adults aged 65 to 74 years.[3]
- In 2007, over 18,000 older adults died from unintentional fall injuries.[3]
- One in five older adults who have suffered a hip fracture die within 1 year of the injury.[4]

Physical Effects of Falls

Injuries sustained from falls include head trauma from striking the head (which in turn may cause bleeding in the brain) and fractures of bones such as the hip, spine, pelvis, shoulder, arm, wrist or leg. Falls are the most common cause of traumatic brain injuries (TBIs); in 2000, TBI accounted for 46% of fatal falls among older adults.[3]

Some falls can be fatal, but most are not. Although bleeding in the brain can be serious enough to cause death (for e.g., if the bleeding causes a large amount of pressure on the brain), death related to head trauma among older clients often is due to other complications, such as those associated with immobility: pneumonia, aspiration, deep vein thrombosis, and pulmonary embolus.

Similarly, although death during the surgery for surgical repair of fractures is rare, death after surgery is generally due to the complications associated with immobility. It is important to note that bed rest is no longer an acceptable part of treatment for either fall-related head injuries or fractures. Although partial-weight-bearing activity or non-weight-bearing activity might be ordered for the specific extremity with the fracture, getting out of bed is essential to maintaining function and optimal recovery. (Please see chapter 8 on Muscoskeletal System Changes for more information on recovery from fractures.)

Those 75 years and older who fall and sustain an injury may spend up to a year in a long-term facility before they can be released back home.[3] Most clients, however, spend a brief time (e.g., weeks) in a subacute care facility or are discharged to home with supportive home care services.

Psychological Effects of Falls

In 2010, Rochat et al.[14] found that a "fear of falling was independently associated with gait performance in a population of community dwelling, well-functioning older persons aged 65-70 years."[14] Participants were given a gait assessment and a questionnaire that assessed fear of falling. They were asked, "Are you afraid of falling?" and given the choice to rate their responses as no fear, moderately fearful, and very fearful. If they answered fearful at any level, it was then followed up with questions regarding whether they restricted their activities in any way. Out of the sample size of 860 participants, responses were as follows:[14]

- 70.3% (605) reported no fear of falling,
- 24.4% (210) reported fear of falling without activity restriction, and
- 5.2% (45) reported fear of falling with activity restriction.

To the knowledge of the authors, this study is the first to demonstrate the association between gait variability and fear of falling "in relatively young elderly persons without specific gait impairment."[13]

Not only do falls create a detrimental shift in a person's life, they are also costly events. "In 2000, the total direct medical costs of all fall injuries for people 65 and older exceeded $19.2 billion; $0.2 billion for fatal falls and 19 billion for non-fatal falls. By 2020, the annual direct and indirect cost of fall injuries is expected to reach $54.9 billion (in 2007 dollars)."[3] In 2006, Stevens et al.[16] conducted a study that examined the incidence and direct costs of fatal and nonfatal fall injuries among adults aged 65 years and older. Table 24-4 illustrates their findings.

The authors concluded that to reduce the amount of costs related to falls among older adults, the implementation of cost-effective fall prevention programs is critical. Fall prevention programs can be initiated by hospitals and subacute care facilities, with the additional input of occupational therapists.

Fall-related monetary costs can include hospitalization (medications, doctors, therapy services) and subacute (post-hospitalization) services, including home health services; rehabilitation services, including skilled nursing services; and long-term acute care hospital services. The ultimate goal is to reduce falls and fall injuries among older adults. Some hospitals take on that initiative by providing fall prevention programs. Haines et al.[9] conducted a randomized controlled trial that provided a falls education program using multimedia materials. The study focused on hospitalized clients, 65 years and over, admitted to acute and subacute wards at two Australian hospitals. The participants were divided into three groups: (1) the control group (traditional care provided by the hospital staff), (2) the complete intervention group (provided with a multimedia client education program including video and written materials, and additional one-on-one follow-up with a physiotherapist), and (3) the materials-only group (educated simply with video and written materials and no follow-up with a therapist provided).[9] The authors found that the rates of falls did not differ significantly among the three groups, yet they did find "a significant interaction between the intervention and presence of cognitive impairment."[8] They found that "cognitive impairment can limit the ability of patients to adhere to the planned safety promoting behaviors and is a reason why an education program might not be beneficial to these patients."[8] Health professionals in the acute care setting typically encounter older adults with cognitive impairments. Some may ask, why educate them if they don't understand? The key is to educate the appropriate caregivers. The caregivers can be family members or nursing staff, depending on the next level of care once clients leave the hospital.

Preventing falls in this older population is vitally important. The occupational therapist in the acute hospital will likely be consulted to see an older adult client to help determine the next best level of care; additionally, the occupational therapist can offer tips in preventing falls (Box 24-2).

TABLE 24-4 Incidence and Costs of Fatal Fall Injuries by Sex, Age, Body Region, and Type of Injury, United States, 2000

Age (years)*	Incidence n = 10,300	Incidence (%)	Cost (millions) n = $179	Cost (%)
65-74	1700	17	30	17
75-84	3800	37	64	36
85+	4800	47	85	47
Sex				
Men	4700	46	81	45
65-74	1000	21	18	40
75-84	1900	40	32	40
85+	1800	38	31	38
Women	5600	54	97	55
65-74	700	13	12	12
75-84	1900	34	32	33
85+	3000	54	53	55
Body region				
Traumatic brain injury	4700	46	82	46
Lower extremity	3300	32	60	34
Torso	800	8	13	7
Other head/neck	300	3	5	3
Other region†	600	6	9	5
Unspecified	600	6	10	6
Type of injury				
Fracture	4300	42	78	44
Internal organs	2900	28	52	29
Systemic/late effects	200	2	2	1
Superficial/contusions	100	1	1	0
Other type‡	100	1	1	1
Unspecified	2800	28	44	25

*Column totals may differ slightly due to rounding.
†"Other region" includes injuries of the upper extremity, vertebral column, spinal cord, and systemic/late effects.
‡"Other type" includes dislocation, strain/sprain, amputation, blood vessel, crushing, burns, and nerves.
(From Stevens, J. A., Corso, P. S., Finkelstein, E. A., et al. [2006, October]. The costs of fatal and non-fatal falls among older adults. *Injury Prevention, 12*(5), 290-295.)

BOX 24-2 Fall Prevention Tips

- Do not walk and talk at the same time. Trying to multi-task adds risk to walking. Therefore, concentrate on the task of walking and continue the conversation after you have reached a safe place.
- Wear appropriate footwear. When walking long distances, on stairways, or in unfamiliar areas, wear flat, nonslip shoes. Also wear shoes that fit well and are comfortable.
- Arrange furniture so that there is plenty of room to walk freely. If you use a walking aid, ensure that doorways and hallways are large enough to get through with any devices you may use.
- Install railings in hallways and grab bars in the bathroom and shower to prevent slipping.
- Be sure you have adequate lighting throughout your house.

- Install nonslip strips or a rubber mat on the floor of the tub or shower.
- Remove throw rugs or secure them firmly to the floor.
- Remove clutter from your home.
- When items are out of reach, use a reacher or a safety ladder; do not stand on chairs.
- Use caution when carrying items while walking.
- Use nightlights on the pathway to the bathroom when getting out of bed at night.
- Stay active, including exercise, to maintain overall strength, balance, and endurance.
- Know your limitations. If there is a task you cannot complete with ease, do not risk a fall by trying to complete it.

(Adapted from the American Occupational Therapy Association. [2012]. *Fall prevention for older adults.* Retrieved from http://www.aota.org/-/media/Corporate/Files/AboutOT/consumers/Adults/Falls/Falls-Prevention-Tip-Sheet-LARGE-PRINT.pdf)

BOX 24-3   Occupational Therapy Fall Prevention Resources

1. American Occupational Therapy Association. (2001). *After your hip surgery: A guide to daily activities.* Rockville, MD: Author. [SKU: 1110B; ISBN: 978-1-56900-175-2]
2. Centers for Disease Control and Prevention. (2005). *Check for safety: A home fall prevention checklist for older adults.* Retrieved from http://www.cdc.gov/HomeandRecreationalSafety/Falls/CheckListForSafety.html.
3. Falls Community of Practice website (https://sites. google.com/a/slu.edu/cop/): Funded by a grant from the U.S. Health Resources and Services Administration received by the Saint Louis University Geriatric Education Center (director: John Morley, geriatrician), this website provides educational programs about falls for health care professionals who work with older persons. Both Karen Barney and Margaret Perkinson have been core faculty for these programs.
4. Cochrane Review. (2012). *Interventions for preventing falls in older people in care facilities and hospitals.* Retrieved from http://onlinelibrary.wiley.com/doi/10.1002/14651858.CD005465.pub3/abstract.
5. Public Health Agency of Canada. (2011). *The safe living guide: A guide to home safety for seniors.* Ottawa, Canada: Author.
6. Robnett, R. H., Hopkins, V., & Kimball, J. G. (2003). The SAFE AT HOME, a quick home safety assessment. *Physical and Occupational Therapy in Geriatrics, 20,* 77–101. Available at http://informahealthcare.com/doi/abs/10.1080/J148v20n03_06.
7. Tomita, M. R., Saharan, S., Rajendran, S., Nochajski, S. M., & Schweitzer, J. A. (2014, November/December). Psychometrics of the Home Safety Self-Assessment Tool (HSSAT) to prevent falls in community-dwelling older adults. *American Journal of Occupational Therapy, 68*(6), 711-718. Retrieved from http://agingresearch.buffalo.edu/hssat/
8. Westmead Home Safety Assessment (WeHSA): The WeHSA was developed by Dr. Lindy Clemson of the University of Sydney, Australia. The WeSHA can be ordered online (http://www.therapybookshop.com/coordinates/) or at the following address:
   Coordinates Therapy Services
   PO Box 59
   West Brunswick, Victoria, Australia 3055
9. World Health Organization. (2012). *Falls.* Retrieved from http://www.who.int/mediacentre/factsheets/fs344/en/.

Additional resources for OTs to assist in fall prevention are identified in Box 24-3.

Summary

Occupational therapy plays a vital role in working with older adults in both the acute care setting and subacute, longer-term acute care settings. OT evaluations and assessments can be important factors in determining the most appropriate next level of care, if indicated, as well as fall prevention strategies. As occupational therapists, we want to be sure we are offering our clients many alternatives, yet we need to find those that best suit them and will help to increase their level of independence, which can in turn increase their quality of life.

REVIEW QUESTIONS

1. Describe the typical stages of entry into a hospital for an older adult who needs acute care.
2. Discuss deconditioning as a likely syndrome that accompanies hospitalization, and explain how OT can intervene to limit this outcome.
3. Describe the OT evaluation and intervention process in acute care, including the interprofessional team process.
4. Discuss at least two options for discharge following acute care, describing the type of medical supervision provided in each example.
5. Explain the importance of fall prevention in supporting aging adults' physical, psychological, and economic well being.

REFERENCES

1. American Hospital Association. (2008). *Hospital facts to know.* http://www.aha.org/aha/content/2008/pdf/08-issue-facts-to-know-.pdf.
2. Belice, P., & McGovern-Denk, M. (April 29, 2002). Reframing occupational therapy in acute care. *OT Practice,* 21–27.
3. Centers for Disease Control and Prevention. (September, 2013). *Costs of falls among older adults.* http://www.cdc.gov/HomeandRecreationalSafety/Falls/fallcost.html.
4. Centers for Disease Control and Prevention. (2013). *Hip fractures among older adults.* www.cdc.gov/HomeandRecreationalSafety/Falls/adulthipfx.html.
5. Centers for Disease Control and Prevention. (2013). *Falls among older adults.* www.cdc.gov/HomeandRecreationalSafety/Falls/adultfalls.html.
6. Connecticut General Assembly. (2004). *Long term acute care hospitals.* www.cga.ct.gov/2004/rpt/2004-R-0966.html.
7. Emergency Medical Treatment and Labor Act (EMTALA), 42 USC §1395dd.
8. Eyres, L., & Unsworth, C. (2005). Occupational therapy in acute hospitals: The effectiveness of a pilot program to maintain occupational performance in older clients. *Australian Occupational Therapy Journal, 52,* 218–224.
9. Haines, T., Hill, A., Hill, K., et al. (2010). Patient education to prevent falls among older hospital inpatients. A randomized controlled trial. *Archives of Internal Medicine, 171*(6), E1–E9. doi:10.1001/archinternmed.2010.444.
10. Kasprak, J. (2004). *Long term acute care hospitals (LTACHs). Connecticut General Assembly.* www.cga.ct.gov/2004/rpt/2004-R-0966.html.
11. Medicare Payment Advisory Commission. (2010). *Report to the Congress: Medicare payment policy. Long-term care hospital services*

(section D, pp. 241–255). http://medpac.gov/documents/Mar10_EntireReport.pdf.

12. Mosby. (2013). *Mosby's medical dictionary* (9th ed.). St. Louis, MO: Author.

13. National Academy on an Aging Society. (2007). *The state of aging and health in America.* http://www.agingsociety.org/agingsociety/pdf/state_of_aging_report.pdf.

14. Rochat, S., Bula, C., Martin, E., et al. (2010). What is the relationship between fear of falling and gait in well-functioning older persons aged 65 to 70 years? *Archives of Physical Medicine Rehabilitation, 91,* 879–884.

15. Siebens, H., Aronow, H., Edwards, D., et al. (2000). A randomized controlled trial of exercise to improve outcomes of acute hospitalization in older adults. *Journal of the American Geriatrics Society, 48*(12), 1545–1552.

16. Stevens, J. A., Corso, P. S., Finkelstein, E. A., et al. (2006). The costs of fatal and non-fatal falls among older adults. *Injury Prevention, 12*(5), 290–295.

CHAPTER 25

Long-Term Care: The Role of Occupational Therapists in Transformative Practice

*Sherylyn H. Briller, PhD, Amy Paul-Ward, PhD, MSOT,
Mirtha M. Whaley, PhD, MPH, OTR/L*

CHAPTER OUTLINE

OBJECTIVES

- Provide an overview of long-term care
- Describe the history of long-term care in the United States
- Discuss current occupational therapy education for long-term care practice
- Envision innovative, transformative long-term care practice

Introduction

Long-term care has been historically part of the medical/health-care continuum frequently highlighted as needing significant reform to properly serve the vulnerable individuals who rely on its services. Because journalists and others reported extensively for decades on serious flaws in long-term-care delivery, it is not surprising that conversations about real problems as well as some persistent myths about long-term care abound in the public imagination. It is well known that many people fear needing long-term care, especially that provided in a nursing home, for a wide variety of economic, social, and personal reasons. In conversations about growing older, people may express related worries about aging and wonder what the odds are that they will need long-term care. It is not surprising that there is ever-increasing discussion in the public domain and among health-care professionals about how to improve long-term care.

In this chapter, we will discuss long-term care in a rapidly aging world and the need to transform this health-care sector and the education of practitioners for cutting-edge care. We primarily focus on long-term care in the United States, who is likely to use it, and its predicted growth in the future. A historical overview of some of the ideas that shaped American long-term care and what it looked like in different eras is provided. Our discussion mainly centers on the U.S. context because there are numerous factors that influence how long-term care is conceptualized, funded, and implemented cross-culturally. Additionally, most of our own experience as occupational therapy (OT) educators, gerontological researchers and practitioners, and medical anthropologists relates to U.S. long-term-care settings. In the latter part of the chapter, we will use our multidisciplinary perspectives to consider the current state of OT education and how occupational therapists should be prepared for key roles in providing client-centered long-term care. Finally, we will contemplate how to further enrich OT education to produce truly innovative long-term-care practitioners.

Overview of Long-Term Care

Long-term care (sometimes referred to as long-term services and supports) aims to provide support for individuals who need assistance with health, personal care, or social services. In some cases, individuals using long-term care may need such assistance due to acquired chronic illnesses or disabilities; in other cases individuals may have never been able to function entirely independently. Oftentimes these individuals may need help with activities of daily living (ADLs) such as dressing or using the toilet. Although many people associate long-term care with institutional settings such as nursing homes, this category is actually broader because long-term care could happen in the home, in assisted living settings, or in nursing homes. In fact, much ongoing discussion today focuses on promoting the idea that it would be advantageous to offer more long-term care in community settings versus institutional ones.[24] Although it is often assumed that those served by long-term care are older adults, long-term-care services are actually used by people of different ages, depending on their needs.

With advanced aging, the likelihood of needing long-term care increases considerably. An important report published by the Institute of Medicine[24] titled "Retooling for an Aging America: Building the Health Care Workforce" addresses some of these demographic issues and care provision concerns. This report states that from 2005 to 2030, the number of U.S. older adults aged 65 years and over is predicted to nearly double (from 37 million to more than 70 million). The report also highlights that U.S. older adults use more health-care services, have more complex health-care needs, and are more likely to need long-term-care services. In 2012 approximately 9 million older Americans needed long-term care, and this number is estimated to rise to 12 million older adults by 2020. The U.S. Department of Health and Human Services[56] projects that 70% of people who reach 65 years may need long-term care, and nearly 40% of people may enter a nursing home at some point in their lives. It is estimated that 10% of people who enter a nursing home will remain there for over 5 years.[39] For many others, they may enter long-term care temporarily, such as when someone needs rehabilitation services after a hip fracture or continuing care after an acute illness.

It is increasingly recognized that a growing aspect of long-term care involves providing sensitive and humane end-of-life care. The oldest old, those over age 85 years, are significantly more likely to live in a long-term-care setting than other older adults—more than four times more likely, in fact, than those aged 75 to 84 years.[25] Older adults living in nursing homes and other residential care settings typically have more serious health needs than community-dwelling older adults; these needs often relate to areas like symptom management and palliative care.[24] Other critical areas besides frailty and health needs that can impact long-term care placement are age, gender, disability, living arrangements, and availability of informal support.[56] A major national study that identified where U.S. older adults with dementia were most likely to die found that 70% died in nursing homes.[42] It is not surprising that much animated discussion revolves around how to best offer compassionate end-of-life care in these settings.[5,6,19,20,27,37,53]

History of Long-Term Care in the United States

The historical roots of American long-term care go back to earlier forms of institutions developed centuries ago for those who would not be able to care for themselves and were typically impoverished. (Please also refer to chapter 23.) In prior times, these institutions that housed those who were aged, frail, disabled, and without sufficient support to sustain themselves in their homes were often sponsored by religious institutions such as monasteries. The seventeenth-century Elizabethan Poor Laws in England further structured ideas about how sick and poor older adults should be cared for in institutional settings, if they lacked adequate familial support.[46] These patterns carried over to colonial America, where similar institutions were then set up in newly established American cities. In the eighteenth and nineteenth centuries, these types of institutions continued to grow as American cities expanded and people lived longer, with increased health-care needs in later life.[33,37]

Winzelberg[57] provides an informative history of how nursing homes in the United States continued developing over the course of the twentieth century, largely devoid of national policymaking for the long-term-care sector. Before the Great Depression, the poorhouse model still prevailed, in which these institutions provided only for residents' most basic needs. Having low overall

quality maintained the idea that the public should find it undesirable to live in these settings, unless absolutely necessary. Winzelberg then traces how over time poorhouses changed into public old-age homes and eventually nursing homes.

Some key legislation in the 1930s influenced how the American long-term-care sector developed over time.[33,37,57] The Social Security Act of 1932 aimed to help older adults stay out of the almshouses by providing monies that would enable them to remain living in the community. The thinking was that if it were prohibited to use these monies for almshouses, older adults would use these funds to pay instead for private care. Restrictions in how funding from the Social Security retirement program and the Old Age Assistance program could be used eventually resulted in the collapse of the almshouses and a shift to other types of care-related institutions. Private boarding homes that were the precursor to nursing homes increased because federal monies could be used to pay for care in these settings. However, this informal care sector remained highly variable in terms of both the arrangements for and quality of care at that time.

The trend toward more private and for-profit long-term-care settings continued over the next few decades as the numbers of older adults needing such forms of residential care grew. In the 1950s, the very influential Hill-Burton Act put into place building and operational policies that made long-term-care settings much more like hospitals and prioritized an institutional and highly medical model of care. In a few respects, this step can be viewed as an improvement in that long-term-care settings were supposed to be similar to acute care hospitals because the need for higher standards in providing clinical care was now recognized. Some positive aspects, such as a greater emphasis on rehabilitation services over time, also accompanied this increased medicalization. For the most part, however, it must be emphasized that many long-lasting negative consequences occurred when it became the norm to have an institutional environment in long-term settings versus a residential ambiance. Indeed, current long-term-care reform efforts now center largely on reducing the institutional character and related operational policies of these settings.

In the 1960s and 1970s, long-term care continued to rapidly grow. Much of this growth was in the for-profit sector, and many nursing homes that were built were part of corporate chains. The development of the Medicare and Medicaid programs in 1965 was a major new source of income for nursing homes. Despite the large amount of monies that these programs began to put into the long-term-care sector, this infusion of funding was not initially coupled with increased governmental oversight of these facilities. Over the next two decades, though, there were greater efforts to link overall long-term-care quality within nursing homes to federal funding entitlements. During this initial time period regulatory problems persisted, resulting in numerous exposés widely reported by the media regarding issues with poor care, dangerous settings, fraud, and abuse. These nursing home scandals in the 1970s provoked public outrage and congressional investigations into the lack of adequate oversight in the long-term-care sector.

In light of these ongoing and very significant problems in many nursing homes, the Omnibus Budget Reconciliation Act of 1987[44] (OBRA-87) was passed. This major federal law was designed to make sweeping reforms in the long-term-care sector. Nursing homes now had to "attain or maintain the highest practicable physical, mental, and psychosocial well-being of each resident"(p. 1330).[44] Evaluation of overall quality of care was meant to be linked with this vision. A resident-assessment instrument called the Minimum Data Set (MDS) was created to help with measuring quality.[12] However, the MDS instrument still mainly focused on medical care issues and was limited in its ability to more holistically assess quality of life for residents in these settings. A very important result of the implementation of OBRA-87 was the overall reduction in the use of both physical restraints (e.g., belts, vests restricting motion) and chemical restraints (e.g., sedative drugs) in nursing homes. Other key elements of OBRA-87 were additional staff training, individualized care plans, and regular comprehensive assessment of resident status. Associated documentation with these care practices was also now required.

Another significant occurrence after the passage of OBRA-87 was the development of special care units (SCUs) for residents with dementia.[35,49,50,52] These were specially designed environments that were meant to be more supportive in terms of their physical, social, and organizational characteristics. They were typically separate spaces that were meant to take a holistic approach to therapeutic dementia care. In such settings, much more attention was now paid to how physical environment, organizational policies, and staff care practices were intertwined with residents' needs and how excess disability could be better prevented in these settings.[10]

Although OBRA-87 provided better federal guidelines for regulating care, subsequent developments went even further in considering how to move away from a medicalized model and to a more person-centered form of care. The social psychologist Kitwood's landmark 1997 book, aptly titled *Dementia Reconsidered: The Person Comes First,*[29] was enormously influential in popularizing person-centered care. In this paradigm, a central point was the "person should be the focus of care delivery and not the disease or illness (p. 834)."[15] Consequently, new emphasis was placed on the uniqueness and worth of each individual and the necessity to be respectful and reflective of individuals' distinct histories, values, and preferences in designing long-term-care environments and in providing care.[56] Long-term-care practices that were considered depersonalizing and disempowering received new scrutiny. The idea also came into vogue that residents should guide their own care whenever feasible. Even if people had significant cognitive impairments or other types of disabilities, it was encouraged that they participate in personalizing and tailoring their care to the extent possible. A series of new comprehensive models for long-term care incorporating some of these ideas about personhood were tried out, including the Wellspring Model, Eden Alternative, Green House Project, and others.[56]

There is no doubt that the person-centered care movement was a very important development in reforming the long-term-care sector during the last two decades. However,

some working in the areas of dementia care research and practice have argued that we must now move beyond only using the concept of personhood.[3] The personhood movement in long-term care affirmed important ideas such as the intrinsic worth of people with dementia and emphasized improving individual-level care interventions; yet current critiques suggest personhood is too much of an individual-focused and apolitical notion. As such, it has been argued that personhood does not take into account the larger societal context in which long-term care is delivered and must be reformed.[3] A result of this emergent discussion is closer examination of how ideas about aging, disability, long-term care, and broader notions of citizenship are entwined. Thus, the interconnection of biological, psychological, cultural, and sociopolitical dimensions of life is now a central focus.[3,4,11]

The contemporary culture-change movement represents another significant development in the transformation of the current long-term-care sector. In 1997 a key umbrella organization called the Pioneer Network was formed to take an active leadership role in long-term care reform.[30] Some positive steps, such as promoting resident-centered care and decision making more broadly, developing team-based work practices and processes designed to deliver that care, and creating resident-friendly, homelike living environments, have occurred.[14,30] The culture-change movement is well recognized and positioned to create advances in the long-term sector by further exploring and developing linkages between higher quality in long-term care and regulatory processes. Some of the movement's recent projects include sponsoring large-scale survey research to better understand perceived barriers to both initial and sustained culture change[41] and developing training materials to aid long-term-care staff in taking steps toward making clinical and cultural changes.[7] Most of the educational initiatives that the culture-change movement has promoted so far are aimed at current long-term-care practitioners; however, in latter sections of this chapter we will discuss how to introduce culture change earlier in the education of health-care practitioners, specifically OT education.

Based on the chronologic account just provided, one can see how the philosophy and models of long-term care in the U.S. context evolved over time. Discussions about improving quality of care and quality of life changed greatly from the days of the almshouse to the private boarding house, to the medical institutional model, to the rehabilitation center, to person-centered care, to political models of citizenship, to the culture-change movement. It is important to know this history to avoid repeating mistakes of the past and to contemplate what innovative long-term-care practice could look like nowadays and in the near future.

Now that we have provided the historical context of long-term care in the United States, we will turn our attention to the role of occupational therapists in this setting. In the next sections we seek to accomplish two tasks: (1) to briefly discuss the current state of OT education for long-term care and (2) to discuss what additional critical thinking skills, in our opinion, such practitioners must have to advance the context and quality of long-term care.

Preparing the Occupational Therapy Practice Workforce

Similar to the sequence of events presented earlier for long-term care, the history of occupational therapy moved from a socially oriented to a more medically oriented model over the course of the twentieth century. Early OT practice was predicated on Adolph Meyer's[40] views of: (1) humans as occupational beings, (2) *occupation* as central to health, (3) the unity of mind and body, (4) the effect of occupational disruption on the individual's health and quality of life, and (5) the role of the physical, temporal, and social environments in the individual's ability to engage in organizing behavior.[28] As occurred in long-term care, we saw a major paradigm shift in occupational therapy in the 1950s in response to the profession's perceived need to become more scientifically and medically oriented.[28] The trend has now shifted back from the predominance of a medical model to taking a more holistic approach toward both OT education and OT practice.

Because most readers of this book are likely to be familiar with the history of occupational therapy, we will not dwell on that subject here. For those who wish a more complete account of this history, see Kielhofner,[28] which presents a detailed overview of the profession's development. What is important to recognize for our discussion of transformative trends in long-care practice is the following. The focus of a more medically oriented occupational therapy was largely to correct and/or to cure. As such, OT was heavily concerned with physiologic, individual-level barriers to performance and to correcting deficits through specific therapeutic interventions and through assistive devices that compensate for lost function without always full consideration of other aspects of an individual's environment. Reflecting this orientation, occupational therapists received a strong foundational grounding in the biological sciences (e.g., anatomy, kinesiology, pathology, neuroscience, etc.). Armed with this medical mindset, occupational therapists learned about "normal" development and "atypical" circumstances in individual health and functioning. In terms of "hands-on" skills, they learned to perform a range of assessments (e.g., physical, sensory, cognitive) to identify conditions adversely affecting individual health and functioning and develop treatment plans to address these conditions. Learning these skills took up much of the curricular time in many OT programs.

Although some clinical and academic settings continue to prioritize the medical educational model, today's practitioners are becoming more aware of the influence of cultural, contextual, economic, and political factors on health and functioning. Practitioners in long-term care need to understand these factors and how they affect the design and delivery of care for older adults at all levels of function. An ongoing discussion at both the broader disciplinary level and at the local educational program level today involves how to best include these issues as part of adequate professional preparation. A related conversation centers on how to empower occupational therapists to act as agents of change in these settings. The interconnection of social and rehabilitative issues and whether occupational therapy personnel should be empowered to act as agents of change within their settings of care are very salient issues in occupational therapy at this time. (Note also the approaches reported in chapter 29.)

Potential variability in preparing occupational therapy personnel for practice in these areas is mitigated by the OT education accreditation process, which is defined by the Accreditation Council for Occupational Therapy Education (ACOTE). The Council is charged with providing the "blueprint" for accreditation of all educational programs in the United States in the form of accreditation standards that outline the minimum competencies that students must have to obtain a master's or doctoral degree and sit for the licensure examination. In a nutshell, the standards provide the overarching philosophic framework for what level entry therapists should know for practice. The nuts and bolts of the assessment and treatment process are reflected in the *Occupational Therapy Practice Framework*.[2]

According to ACOTE, practitioners should be able to "plan and utilize occupational therapy interventions through addressing performance skills in a variety of contexts so as to support engagement in everyday activities that affect health, well-being, and quality of life."[1] For long-term care, this idea is relevant to ensure that people are able to participate in meaningful occupations that support their well-being and add to their perceived quality of health, even in circumstances such as frailty, dementia, or late life. To achieve this goal, occupational therapists need to analyze how the systems and structures within many long-term-care settings today limit engagement in occupations, thus contributing to declining health and poor quality of life.

As a profession, OT is moving in the right direction for transformative long-term care, but the process is far from over. There are still many issues related to long-term care that need to be considered more fully. Too often the curricula provide somewhat cursory discussions of client settings, focusing more on the individual-level diagnostic and intervention skills that therapists will need when working with clients with specific treatment needs. As mentioned already, this focus may be related to the amount of foundational knowledge that students need to acquire to be entry-level practitioners. Although some may consider this "generalist" training as adequate, students also need to be trained to understand the influence of contextual factors on one's ability to engage in meaningful occupations. Such education is more likely to occur in doctoral-level OT educational programs. Yet, by preparing OT students at all levels to better understand how social and rehabilitative issues intersect, they will be better prepared to act as advocates for clients and change agents in the profession.

Innovative Education for Occupational Therapy Practice in Long-Term Care

Culture and Context

Health-care practitioners should receive adequate training on the interrelated parts of the larger cultural system of long-term care. A critical gerontology education for long-term-care practice should include an understanding of both structural issues relating to social and occupational justice, and cultural values and beliefs that shape what people think and do in these settings. Occupational therapists should consider the long-term-care settings in which they work as a community of interacting cultures (e.g., resident, staff, organizational cultures, etc.). They should be sensitive to the cultural construction of long-term-care settings and how social order is made there.

Nursing home ethnographies are excellent tools to illustrate how health-care practice is enacted and perceived by a variety of actors in long-term care, including residents, families, and health-care providers. Nursing home ethnography began with the publication of a classic ethnography called *Culture against Man*,[23] in which Jules Henry movingly discussed the predicament of older adults in three hospitals for the aged. Since then many ethnographies have contributed significant cultural insights to understanding institutional order and its meanings, the professional socialization of health-care personnel working in long-term-care settings, and the cultural construction of health-care experiences.[13,17,21,26,34,37,47,48] In addition to these full-book-length ethnographies, several key edited volumes have been published containing chapters that ethnographically examine specific aspects of social life in long-term care from a variety of vantage points.[22,51]

Nursing home ethnography illustrates the relevance of context and culture for improving long-term-care practice. Many discuss in a very detailed and nuanced way how those in particular roles go about delivering care in these settings. For example, McLean and Perkinson's chapter on a head nurse as key informant systematically analyzes "a nurse's beliefs about dementia as they entered into her construction of good care, her work history on the unit as that affected her supervisory approach, and the institutional constraints within which she had to structure the delivery of care."[38] Reading ethnographies can help occupational therapists to gain skills in feeling comfortable in consistently noticing and interpreting the social life and organizational practices of long-term-care settings.

Based on these benefits, it would seem a given that long-term-care practitioners could benefit from exposure to nursing home ethnographies and ethnographic training. Yet the collaborative teaching and practice relationships between fields such as anthropology and occupational therapy are still not as fully developed as they could be. Although the ACOTE standards call for students to be knowledgeable in the social sciences, including anthropology, there is variability in how that material is handled in preparing OT practitioners to most fully understand long-term care as a social type of institution as well as a medical one.

Further collaboration with social scientists for some of the formative education on how culture shapes and drives the running of long-term-care institutions, their specific organizational policies and practices, and the design of future long-term care could be very exciting in OT education. Working across disciplinary lines, it should be possible to develop curriculum in which detailed ethnographic case studies are regularly used in teaching this subject matter, even if the time constraints of the curriculum do not permit space for extensive reading of full-length ethnographies. Teaching partnerships for providing such integrated training could also help with working across disciplinary lines for developing truly transformative care. For example, anthropologists have much to say about how the term "culture" is used within and by the culture-change movement to ensure that it is well understood in its deployment to improve long-term care.

Social and Occupational Justice

Health care does not take place in a vacuum. However, for much of occupational therapy's history, the educational curriculum focused mainly on the "mechanics" of practice. Students often were not taught the role that politics and economics play in shaping the health-care settings where they would practice, beyond what it meant in terms of reimbursement by third-party payers. Over the last 10 years there has been a growing recognition of the need to become advocates not only for the profession but also for our clients. This advocacy movement has grown out the work of a series of scholars (see Townsend and Wilcock;[54] Kronenberg, Algado, and Pollard,[31] and Pollard, Sakellariou, and Kronenberg[45]) who posit that occupational injustices occur when individuals are barred from participating in meaningful occupations. (See also chapters 28 and 29.)

The growing social justice literature in OT demonstrates how the complex relationships between the government and society affect not only poverty but also access to health care across the life course. The concept of social justice is not new; historically, we can trace the roots of social justice concepts to the work of the early philosophers (e.g., St. Thomas Aquinas, John Locke, David Hume, and Jacques Rousseau), when the focus was on "the moral and philosophic meaning of individual rights, free society and free will."[9,8] Over time, social justice evolved into a study of the complex relationships between government, society, access, and poverty. The National Conference of Catholic Bishops advocates a vision of social justice that implies that people "have an obligation to be active and productive participants in the life of society and that society has a duty to enable them to participate in this way."[43] Social justice can also be viewed as the process of giving voice and participation to people regarding the decisions that affect their lives. This tradition emphasizes the individual's responsibility to control his or her own life and resources while recognizing that people in positions of power (e.g., government, agencies, and organizations that hold resources) can facilitate opportunities for people to control their own lives.[9,16]

As mentioned earlier, occupational scientists and occupational therapists have increasingly recognized the need to incorporate a social justice perspective into research, curricula, and practice. This recognition is apparent in many forms, especially the growing body of OT-based literature that addresses issues of politics and economics, and how these affect clients both in and out of the therapeutic arena. Significantly, many official documents from the American Occupational

Therapy Association (AOTA)[2] incorporate social justice constructs. Moreover, as discussed earlier, many goals of social justice are implicitly embedded in occupational therapy's philosophy, core competencies, recognized professional beliefs, and responsibilities. The AOTA *Occupational Therapy Practice Framework* stresses the importance of social participation, which is defined as "organized patterns of behavior that are characteristic and expected of an individual in a given position within a social system" (p. S21). It is noteworthy that no less than 16 of the ACOTE standards[1] address factors and issues that promote or correct social injustice, occupational deprivation, and disparities in the receipt of care.

Inherent in the OT discourse on social justice is the belief that more critical work is needed to sufficiently address the larger societal issues that ultimately affect OT practitioners' ability to advocate for and with clients. Although social justice is an interdisciplinary movement, OT has offered its own occupation-based language for a discussion of justice-related issues, namely, "occupational justice." Within occupational therapy, occupational justice is viewed as related to the "rights, responsibilities, and liberties of enablement (p. 78)."[54,55] Furthermore, it has been argued that occupational injustice occurs "when participation in occupation is barred, confined, restricted, segregated, prohibited, undeveloped, disrupted, alienated, marginalized, exploited, excluded, or otherwise restricted (p. 78)."[54] Integral to this notion of occupational justice is an emerging area of scholarship in the area of occupational apartheid. Proponents of occupational apartheid argue that some people are deemed by society as being of different economic and social value than others.[32] This value distinction leads to some groups being pushed to the periphery of mainstream society, affecting their social and occupational participation. This notion is relevant to the area of long-term care in that, by design, these systems tend to devalue and marginalize their "members" by labeling them as different from other individuals living and aging in the community. Further, the system disrupts occupational engagement; residents are often limited in access to their former social networks and experience loss of their valued occupations and life roles.[36]

Viewing the world with a social justice lens presents new ways of thinking about access, engagement, empowerment, participation, and meaning. This lens provides the necessary focus to consider the role that external forces play in the daily lives of clients, challenging the profession "to move beyond advocacy" to identifying strategies for transforming societies.[18] There are many occupational justice lessons to be learned from long-term care, including, but not limited to, the many systemic issues that promote the occupational deprivation and social injustices among residents in long-term care (e.g., loss of roles, loss of meaningful occupations, and loss of autonomy in making key decisions, such as how to use their time). It also is useful to apply a social/occupational justice perspective when thinking about how to reframe end-of-life experiences in long-term-care settings. Incorporating an occupationally just perspective in how we conceptualize good care, and acting as advocates for this type of care will enable occupational therapists to provide opportunities for clients to maintain valued roles, engage in meaningful occupations, and participate more successfully as full, equal members within their long-term-care communities. As OT practitioners, it is both an individual and a collective responsibility to use the knowledge obtained from population-focused research efforts as well as from clinically learned lessons to effect positive social change for individuals in long-term-care settings so they can live out all, including their final, days with dignity.

Finally, it is important to draw attention to social and occupational justice issues for those who work as well as those who live in long-term-care settings. Clearly, the organizational aspects of different kinds of long-term-care environments and their related policies and procedures affect the ability of workers to participate in and provide transformative care. The training that various workers receive and how they are empowered or disempowered from acting to make positive change in these settings are issues that merit further thought. These ideas should be central in the education of occupational therapists who are preparing to work in the long-term-care sector.

CASE STUDY 25-1   Mrs. M's Story: How to Think about Loss of Identity and Meaningful Occupations

What would educating occupational therapists for transformative practice in long-term care look like? The curriculum would further reflect both the art and science of the profession.

Knowing more about how social, medical, and rehabilitative issues are intertwined should be emphasized in this professional preparation. Occupational therapists' roles as agents of change in these settings ought to be emphasized. Let us consider the case of Mrs. M.

This is how a typical, medically oriented history given for a nursing home resident often starts today. Mrs. M was a married Hispanic woman with a medical history of high blood pressure, two significant strokes with full physical recovery, a history of transient ischemic attacks (mini-strokes) with resultant multi-infarct dementia (dementia resulting from multiple mini-strokes), a myocardial infarction (heart attack), and late-life onset of diabetes. Within progressive occupational therapy (OT) curricula, however, an effort would be made to show how these medical attributes do not fully define her, nor did the 5-year period during which Mrs. M's recovery was less than complete until, at age 83 years, her condition required long-term admission to a nursing home as a resident.

OT students must also think closely about how Mrs. M, a seamstress for most of her life, had created magic with her hands—everything from baby layettes, designer

---

CASE STUDY 25-1   Mrs. M's Story: How to Think about Loss of Identity and Meaningful Occupations—cont'd

dresses, gowns for entire wedding parties, beaded formals for society events, prom gowns, and more. Her family would help her reminisce and engage her in conversations about fabrics and styles and dresses she had made for her daughters and clients, sometimes taking trips to local fabric stores just to look and elicit memories. Transformative OT practice should involve engaging her at this level. OT students would be cautioned about how therapists had mainly focused on Mrs. M's physical rehabilitation, missing cues of her cognitive difficulties. Nursing home staff had tried to promote attendance to activities that were neither interesting nor suitable for her abilities. Often, craft projects would be "done for" Mrs. M, a sign of the poor match between task and abilities. Importantly, students would also learn that, at age 85 years, Mrs. M suffered a heart attack unattended during the night because no one on staff could communicate with her in Spanish, the only language she

spoke fluently. Nor was her family called at that time to notify them of her "agitation" and allow them to visit her and intervene. Instead she was left in her room with the door closed, fearful, alone, and in pain.

This brief account of Mrs. M's time as a nursing home resident is extreme—but also unfortunately a true story. It sheds light on why a more holistic approach to OT education is needed for transformative long-term care practice. As we discussed in this chapter, such an approach involves thinking about cultural, contextual, economic, and political factors and how these factors affect how care is delivered and received by a long-term care resident such as Mrs. M. This case helps show how advanced interdisciplinary fieldwork education will involve developing a series of critical thinking skills, knowledge and attributes that can be applied holistically within transformative long-term care practice.

A View from the Bridge: Enhancing Occupational Therapy Education for Long-Term-Care Practice

Some practitioners have the opportunity to view long-term care from the additional vantage point of family caregiver, both actually connected, both providing a bridge from one perspective to another. This chapter's third author, Mirtha Whaley, was fortunate to have the opportunity to enhance teaching and practice of occupational therapy by drawing upon both vantage points to better understand what should change in long-term-care settings. This section describes in her own words how these experiences influenced her thinking as an OT practitioner and educator and recommends necessary skills and knowledge for practicing in long-term-care settings.

As a practicing occupational therapist, I have experienced the tension of wanting to be truly client centered and yet too often encountering situations where "efficiency" and "productivity" trumped client-centered care. I have felt the frustration many therapists feel when treatment recommendations are disregarded by other personnel and when use of my skills and knowledge is restricted by facility regulations and reimbursement patterns. With that in mind, I emphasize in my teaching the necessity of not losing sight of what is important in client-centered care.

My belief in client-centered care was heightened during the time my mother was a resident in several different long-term-care settings. During the last 5 years of her life, I experienced the distress of watching her live through repeated incidents of poor care, diminished dignity, and the obliteration of her "self." My mother, as too often happens in long-term-care settings, experienced a spiral of decline and losses mistakenly attributed to age and/or to progressive medical or mental conditions. My current work is informed by seeing how these types of health disparities arise for those who reside in long-term care. It is also informed by how she and others residing in that setting were treated as agents of their

own decline and labeled as lacking motivation; being manipulative, combative, and uncooperative; or not being suitable candidates for rehabilitation. All too often clinicians failed to look beyond the immediate, so they could not realize how systemic and structural problems served to promote dependence and excess functional and cognitive disability through lack of social stimulation, engagement in daily routines, and provision of appropriate activities.

Not surprisingly, my experiences as a family caregiver influenced my clinical practice. Over time I became even less able to look the other way when I noticed instances when the long-term-care system was not set up to best serve the interests of the residents. I was even more outraged when I saw that happen to the most vulnerable residents, whose quality of life and dignity were negatively affected.

Take-Home Lessons

The following list summarizes some of the beliefs that most influence my work with older adults.

1. The most important tool at our disposal is how we use ourselves in the treatment context with our clients and their families.
2. There is a huge difference between using clinical judgment and being judgmental; the latter always should be avoided.
3. For the most part, what separates us from our clients and their caregivers is but a very thin line, and that we should treat our clients as we would want someone else to treat our loved ones.
4. What sets us apart as a profession is our understanding of human beings as whole entities and occupational beings.
5. "Contexts" or environments (cultural, social, religious, economic, political, and regulatory) play an integral part not only in an individual's development, but in the health care he or she receives and in the outcomes of that care.

6. We are but a small part of a system of care, including public health.
7. Collaborating with other professionals and keeping the client at the very center of our efforts improve care, outcomes, and satisfaction.
8. We should practice with our eyes and ears open, looking at the whole person and listening, rather than engaging in rote exercises or other activity just to meet productivity quotas.
9. There are public health implications of our clinical practice (i.e., that what we do or fail to do for our clients really does affect the health of the nation).
10. Our clients' stories, their narratives, are important to understand who they really are and what has shaped their lives, personally, culturally, and contextually.
11. We must advocate for our clients, for their caregivers, and for better care overall.
12. Our role should be to "do with" our clients, rather than to "do to".
13. Interventions are not always geared at fixing or curing the person, but that they may be designed to tweak the task, and/or to modify the physical and social environment so that the individual can participate safely in life and in valued occupations.
14. If care is going to change and improve, it starts with us.

Transformative occupational therapy is more than basic skills and techniques. Some in the field of OT call the things that I am really interested in the "soft skills." Perhaps many see these as more difficult to impart, perhaps because we have fewer guidelines for them. Entering this profession carries a degree of responsibility to our clients and to improving care, not just the assurance of job stability or a reasonable income. When it comes to issues of long-term care, to the occupational deprivation that many residents experience, to social injustices promoted or simply sustained by our current system, we must prepare our students and ourselves so that we do not become desensitized and blinded to these conditions.

As practitioners, we need to recognize social and occupational injustices for what they are, rather than blaming the individual and personalizing these incidents by repeatedly complaining about others' failure to follow our professional recommendations. As therapists, we must always put the care of our clients before the task at hand. We must remember the occupational nature of human beings, our need to be engaged and to experience a sense of mastery regardless of the quality of the end product. Our clients need to be valued and be loved, including the need for continuity, so that they may maintain their sense of self and their self-esteem. We must remember that "doing" is only possible when the demands of the task and the support from the social and physical environment match the individual's abilities; we must remember that "correcting" problems is only part of our job, and that real healing takes place through a relationship of mutual trust, respect, and personal engagement with our clients and their caregivers. We must live up to our perceptions of being a holistic practice, with full understanding that individuals function as entities within the context of a culture and a sociopolitical system that influence our beliefs about health and wellness, about who is entitled to care and to what extent.

As faculty, we must remember that teaching the science and skills without engaging in the art of occupational therapy turns out incomplete practitioners and perpetuates delivery of services that fosters continued social injustice and occupational deprivation and promotes excess disability among long-term-care residents. We must strive to ensure that emerging therapists understand that families are frequently as much in need of our services as are their loved ones who have been referred to us. We must know the difference between value judgment and critical reasoning to avoid stigmatization and labeling that ultimately cause excess disability.

Summary

In this chapter we initially defined long-term care and then traced the history of the development of this care sector in the United States. In doing so, we outlined a series of important philosophic shifts that influenced how models of care were structured and how care was delivered at different moments in time. This history was provided as a backdrop for our subsequent discussion of innovative education for occupational therapists in long-term care.

Our perspectives on educational reform and how it can possibly lead to transformative long-term care came from our own lengthy experiences in these settings. Progressive education in this area can lead to real change in local long-term-care practice as those with different kinds of knowledge embark on providing new forms of truly client-centered care in these settings. For us, much interesting discussion stemmed from considering how the holistic orientations of occupational therapy and anthropology are powerful and complement one another. We are trying to expose our students in the classroom and in practice settings to some of these same kinds of discussions. At the moment, a perception by some in the field of occupational therapy is that there is mainly room for such critical thinking and these types of discussions in doctoral programs, where there is the luxury of more time to reflect on these issues. Understanding the fundamental interconnection between social and rehabilitative areas must be brought up earlier in the education of all therapists. For long-term-care practitioners, that understanding will enable them to demonstrate growth in knowledge, skills, abilities, and dispositions to make real change in these settings. Although it would be possible to end a chapter on the topic of long-term care with a pessimistic view of where things are now, we prefer to look ahead, envisioning a time when occupational therapists, sensitized to the issues of social justice, can help to bring about transformative care in this sector. Occupational therapists can indeed have a vital role to play as change agents in reforming long-term care.

REVIEW QUESTIONS

1. Long-term care is exclusively a service for older adults, due to specific physical and cognitive needs. (True/False)

2. In person-centered care, a key principle is
   a. a lot of family and friends should visit the resident on a regular basis.
   b. it is important to speak kindly to a long-term care resident all of the time.
   c. the resident should guide his or her own care to the extent possible.
   d. a resident in rehabilitative care should have the highest priority for services.

3. Scholars and practitioners interested in social and occupational justice are concerned about people being denied access to meaningful participation in occupations on the basis of
   a. disability.
   b. ethnicity.
   c. country of origin.
   d. all of the above.

4. Nursing home ethnography can be used to instruct healthcare practitioners because these books
   a. teach about context and culture.
   b. discuss the belief systems of long-term care staff.
   c. analyze social life and organizational practices in long term care.
   d. all of the above.

5. Transformative occupational therapy education requires that students learn
   a. basic clinical skills and techniques.
   b. a holistic approach to care.
   c. critical thinking skills for understanding how long term care is set up today.
   d. all of the above.

REFERENCES

1. ACOTE. (2011). *Accreditation Council for Occupational Therapy Education (ACOTE®) standards and interpretive guide. American Occupational Therapy Association.* Accessed 10/21/15. http://www.aota.org/-/media/Corporate/Files/Education Careers/Accredit/Standards/2011-Standards-and-Interpretive-Guide.pdf.
2. American Occupational Therapy Association. (2014). Occupational therapy practice framework: Domain and process (3rd ed.). *American Journal of Occupational Therapy, 68*(Suppl. 1), S1–S48. http://dx.doi.org/10.5014/ajot.2014.682006.
3. Bartlett, R., & O'Connor, D. (2007). From personhood to citizenship: Broadening the lens for dementia practice and research. *Journal of Aging Studies, 21*(2), 107–118.
4. Behuniak, S. M. (2010). Towards a political model of dementia: Power as compassionate care. *Journal of Aging Studies, 24*(4), 231–240.
5. Bern-Klug, M. (2010). *Transforming palliative care in nursing homes: The social work role.* New York, NY: Columbia University Press.
6. Bern-Klug, M. (2011). Rituals in nursing homes. *Generations, 35*(3), 57–63.
7. Bowers, B., Nolet, K., Roberts, T., & Esmond, S. (2009). *Implementing change in long-term care: A practical guide to transformation.* New York, NY: Commonwealth Fund.
8. Bowring, W. (2002). Forbidden relations? The UK's discourse of human rights and the struggle for social justice. *Law, Social Justice and Global Development Journal, 1*, 1–17.
9. Braveman, B., & Suarez-Balcazar, Y. (2009). Social justice and resource utilization in a community-based organization: A case illustration of the role of the occupational therapist. *AJOT: American Journal of Occupational Therapy, 63*(1), 13–23.
10. Briller, S., Proffitt, M., Perez, K., & Calkins, M. (2001). Maximizing cognitive and functional abilities. In M. P. Calkins (Series Ed.), *Creating successful dementia care settings (Vol. 3).* Baltimore, MD: Health Professions Press.
11. Castillo, E. H. (2011). Doing dementia better: Anthropological insights. *Journal of Aging Studies, 27*(2), 273–289.
12. Centers for Medicare and Medicaid Services. (2015). *Long term care minimum data set (MDS).* http://www.cms.gov/Research-Statistics-Data-and-Systems/Files-for-Order/Identifiable DataFiles/LongTermCareMinimumDataSetMDS.html/. Accessed 04.06.2015.
13. Diamond, T. (1992). *Making gray gold.* Chicago, IL: The University of Chicago Press.
14. Doty, M. M., Koren, M. J., & Sturla, E. L. (2008). *Culture change in nursing homes: How far have we come? Findings from the Commonwealth Fund 2007 National Survey of Nursing Homes.* New York, NY: Commonwealth Fund.
15. Edvarsdsson, D., & Innes, A. (2010). Measuring person-centered care: A critical comparative review of published tools. *The Gerontologist, 50*(6), 834–846.
16. Fawcett, S. B., White, G. W., Balcazar, F. E., Suarez-Balcazar, Y., Mathews, R. W., Paine-Andrews, A., et al. (1994). A contextual-behavioral model of empowerment: Case studies involving people with physical disabilities. *American Journal of Community Psychology, 22*, 471–496.
17. Foner, N. (1994). *The caregiving dilemma: Work in an American nursing home.* Berkeley, CA: University of California Press.
18. Frank, G., & Zemke, R. (2005). What is occupational science and what will it become? *Paper presented at the Society for Applied Anthropology and Society for Medical Anthropology Joint Meeting.* Vancouver, British Columbia.
19. Fulton, A. T., Rhodes-Kropf, J., Corcoran, A. M., Chau, D., & Castillo, E. H. (2011). Palliative care for patients with dementia in long term care. *Clinics Geriatric Medicine, 27*, 153–170.
20. Gelfand, D., Raspa, R., Briller, S., & Schim, S. (Eds.). (2005). *End-of-life stories: Crossing disciplinary boundaries.* New York, NY: Springer.
21. Gubrium, J. (1975). *Living and dying in Murray Manor.* New York, NY: St. Martin's Press.
22. Henderson, J. N., & Vesperi, M. D. (1995). *The culture of nursing home care: Nursing home ethnography.* Westport, CT: Bergin & Garvey Publishers.
23. Henry, J. (1963). *Culture against man.* New York, NY: Random House.
24. Institute of Medicine. (2008). *Retooling for an aging America: building the healthcare workforce.* Washington, DC: National Academy of Sciences. Accessed 10/21/15. http://www.nap.edu/catalog/12089/retooling-for-an-aging-america-building-the-health-care-workforce.
25. Jones, A. (2002). *The national nursing home survey: 1999 summary.* Hyattsville, MD: National Center for Health Statistics.
26. Kayser-Jones, J. (1990). *Old, alone and neglected: Care of the aged in Scotland and the United States.* Berkeley, CA: University of California Press.

27. Kayser-Jones, J., Schell, E., Lyons, W., Kris, A. E., Chan, J., & Beard, R. L. (2003). Factors that influence end-of-life care in nursing homes: the physical environment, inadequate staffing, and lack of supervision. *The Gerontologist, 43*(Suppl. 2), 76–84.

28. Kielhofner, G. (2004). *Conceptual foundations of occupational therapy*. Philadelphia, PA: F. A. Davis.

29. Kitwood, T. (1997). *Dementia reconsidered: The person comes first*. Buckingham: Open University Press.

30. Koren, M. J. (2010). Improving quality in long term care. *Medical Research and Review, 67*(Suppl. 4), 141S–150S.

31. Kronenberg, F., Algado, S., & Pollard, N. (2005). *Occupational therapy without borders: Learning from the spirit of survivors*. London: Elsevier.

32. Kronenberg, F., & Pollard, N. (2005). Overcoming occupational apartheid: A preliminary exploration of a political nature of occupational therapy. In F. Kronenberg, S. Algado, & N. Pollard (Eds.), *Occupational therapy without borders: Learning from the spirit of survivors* (pp. 58–86). London: Elsevier.

33. Lacey, D. (1999). The evolution of care: A 100 year history of institutionalization of people with Alzheimer's disease. *Journal of Gerontological Social Work, 31*(3/4), 101–131.

34. Laird, C. (1979). *Limbo: A memoir about life in a nursing home by a survivor*. Novato, CA: Chandler & Sharp.

35. Lawton, M. P., Fulcomer, M., & Kleban, M. H. (1984). Architecture for the mentally impaired elderly. *Environment and Behavior, 16*(6), 730–757.

36. Magasi, S., & Hamel, J. (2009). Women with disabilities' experiences in long-term care: A case for social justice. *American Journal of Occupational Therapy, 63*(1), 35–45.

37. McLean, A. (2007). *The person in dementia: A study of nursing home care in the US*. Toronto: Broadview Press.

38. McLean, A., & Perkinson, M. (1995). The head nurse as key informant: How beliefs and institutional pressures can structure dementia care. In J. N. Henderson & M. D. Vesperi (Eds.), *The culture of long term care: Nursing home ethnography* (pp. 127–148). Westport, CT: Bergin & Garvey Publishers.

39. Medicare. (2012). *Long term care*. Accessed 10/21/15. http://news.morningstar.com/articlenet/article.aspx?id=564139.

40. Meyer, A. (1922). The philosophy of occupational therapy. *Archives of Occupational Therapy, 1*, 1–10.

41. Miller, S. C., Miller, E. A., Jung, H. Y., Sterns, S., Clark, M., & Mor, V. (2010). Nursing home organizational change: The "culture change" movement as viewed by long term care specialists. *Medical Care Research and Review, 67*(Suppl. 4), 65S–81S.

42. Mitchell, S. L., Teno, J. M., Miller, S. C., & Mor, V. (2005). A national study of the location of death for older persons with dementia. *Journal of the American Geriatric Society, 53*(2), 299–305.

43. National Conference of Catholic Bishops (NCCB). (1986). *Economic justice for all. Pastoral letter on Catholic social teaching and the U.S. economy*. Washington, DC: United States Catholic Conference. Accessed 10/21/15. berkleycenter.georgetown.edu/publications/economic-justice-for-all-pastoral-letter-on-catholic-social-teaching-and-the-u-s-economy.

44. Omnibus Budget Reconciliation Act of 1987. *Public Law No. 100-203, subtitle C: Nursing Home Reform (101 Stat 1330)*.

45. Pollard, N., Sakellariou, D., & Kronenberg, F. (2008). *A political practice of occupational therapy*. London: Elsevier.

46. Quadagno, J. (1999). *Aging and the life course: An introduction to social gerontology*. Boston, MA: McGraw Hill.

47. Savishinsky, J. S. (1991). *The ends of time: Life and work in a nursing home*. New York, NY: Bergin & Garvey.

48. Shield, R. R. (1988). *Uneasy endings: Daily life in an American nursing home*. Ithaca, NY: Cornell University Press.

49. Sloane, P. D., Matthew, L., Scarborough, M., Desai, J. R., Koch, G., & Tangen, C. (1991). Physical and chemical restraint of dementia patients in nursing homes: Impact of specialized units. *Journal of the American Medical Association, 265*, 1278–1282.

50. Sloane, P. D., Mitchell, C. M., Preisser, J. S., Phillips, C., Commander, C., & Burker, E. (1998). Environmental correlates of resident agitation in Alzheimer's disease special care units. *Journal of the American Geriatrics Society, 46*, 862–869.

51. Stafford, P. B. (2003). *Gray areas: Ethnographic encounters with nursing home culture*. Santa Fe, NM: School of American Research Press.

52. Teresi, J., Holmes, D., & Ory, M. (2000). The therapeutic design of environments for people with dementia: further reflections and recent findings from the National Institute on Aging Collaborative Studies of Dementia Special Care Units. *The Gerontologist, 40*(4), 417–421.

53. Thompson, S., & Oliver, D. P. (2008). A new model for long term care: balancing palliative and restorative care delivery. *Journal of Housing for the Elderly, 22*(3), 169–194.

54. Townsend, E., & Wilcock, A. (2004). Occupational justice and client-centered practice: a dialogue in progress. *Canadian Journal of Occupational Therapy, 71*, 75–87.

55. Urbanowski, R. (2005). Transcending practice borders through perspective transformation. In F. Kronenberg, S. Algado, & N. Pollard (Eds.), *Occupational therapy without borders: Learning from the spirit of survivors* (pp. 302–312). London: Elsevier.

56. U.S. Department of Health and Human Services. (2015). *National clearinghouse for long term care information*. Accessed 10/21/15. http://www.healthinaging.org/resources/resource:national-clearinghouse-for-long-term-care-information/.

57. Winzelberg, G. (2003). The quest for nursing home quality: learning history's lessons. *Archives of Internal Medicine, 163*, 2552–2556.

CHAPTER 26

Home: An Evolving Context for Health Care

Laura N. Gitlin, PhD, Catherine Verrier Piersol, PhD, OTR/L

CHAPTER OUTLINE

OBJECTIVES

- Recognize the value of home care for older adults
- Distinguish the potential funding sources for home care services
- Describe conceptual models that guide home care practice
- Explain cultural considerations when working with older adults in their homes
- Describe the relevance of using a problem-solving approach with older adults in home care

Mrs. M, a 94-year-old white Irish Catholic woman in good health, fell while walking outside to buy groceries and broke her femur. After surgery and a month's stint in subacute rehabilitation, she returned home with a walker and other adaptive equipment. She needed further rehabilitation at home, where she lives alone, to help her learn how to ambulate and carry out self-care, meal preparation, and home management activities in that environment.

Mr. B, a 79-year-old African American, has dementia and lives with his wife. His physician provided a prescription for occupational therapy (OT) for a home safety evaluation and to evaluate ways of supporting his daily function at home and helping his wife, the primary caregiver, manage day-to-day tasks.

Mrs. M and Mr. B illustrate the important reasons why older adults receive care at home from occupational therapists. Although historically the home was the initial setting for providing health care, with the rise of organized systems of care, health-care delivery shifted to specialized environments. However, the home is emerging once again as one of the most important contexts for delivering a wide range of health-care services, including episodic, short-term, and long-term care, to older adults. A confluence of multiple and critical societal trends has conspired to bring health care back into the home. These include rising hospital and nursing home costs spurring physician acceptance of alternative care approaches, increased risks of infection and mortality with hospital-based care, a soaring aging population seeking to age in place, rising incidence of chronic disease and its functional consequences requiring home management and care, development of accountable care organizations seeking to minimize hospital readmissions and associated costs, significant gaps transitioning from hospital to home leading to increased risks of health declines and hospital readmissions and hence increased costs, and evidence suggesting better recuperative outcomes with care at home.[1,2,20] The home as epicenter of aging, well-being, and health-care provision, particularly in very old age, is a persistent trend that is anticipated to only increase now and into the future.[7,25]

This chapter provides a broad overview of home health care and the role of occupational therapists. It briefly examines the system and structure of home care; explores the benefits and challenges of delivering care in homes, including the home as a work environment; and discusses the clinical reasoning processes essential to successful home care delivery.

The Home Care System

Although homes are unique and personal, the delivery of health care in the home is a highly regulated industry. The largest single payer for home care services is Medicare, with Medicaid and other for-profit insurance companies following Medicare's requirements for coverage of services.[22]

Home health agencies (HHAs) provide home care services under the Medicare Part A benefit. Approximately 12 million individuals currently receive home health care from 33,000 providers, with annual expenditures for home health care projected at $72.2 billion.[18] Most (70%) clients receiving home health care are 65 years and older; 55.7% have Medicare, 22.4% have Medicaid, 12.3% pay through private health insurance, 5.8% pay out-of-pocket, and 3.0% have another payment source.[3]

According to the Centers for Disease Control and Prevention (CDC), most home health-care clients receive medical care and skilled nursing, followed by personal care and therapeutic services. Additionally, most home health-care clients receive help with one or more activities of daily living, primarily bathing. Home health care is a growth industry with an average of 5.05% annual growth from 2007 to 2012 and revenue of about $69 billion.[11]

Therapy services can also be provided in the home under the Medicare Part B, or outpatient, benefit. The conditions of participation under which HHAs are regulated do not apply under Medicare Part B; for example, the client does not need to be homebound. This venue offers therapists the opportunity to work with clients within the comfort of their homes and in the community, rather than in the clinical outpatient setting.[22]

Role of Occupational Therapy

Occupational therapists may serve as independent contractors or employees of home care agencies. To provide OT in the home, therapists must be licensed in the state and have a physician's prescription indicating the need for OT evaluation and treatment, according to the state's practice act. Occupational therapists have numerous roles in home care, including but not limited to evaluating clients for home safety, making home modification and adaptive equipment recommendations and training in their use, providing restorative interventions, and helping clients learn new or modified ways of performing self-care and instrumental activities of daily living (IADLs). Occupational therapists also provide education and strategies for managing the functional consequences of chronic illness, and can offer caregiver skills training in managing daily care challenges.[9] Because treatments are restricted to reimbursement regulations, end-of-life care, activity-based therapies, stress reduction strategies, and preventive interventions are services that therapists could provide but that may not be funded.

Benefits of Providing Care in the Home

In contrast to health care provided in facilities (e.g., outpatient clinic, inpatient hospital or rehabilitation unit), providing care in the client's home has many important advantages.[5] First, therapists are able to more fully evaluate the person's best functioning in his or her own, familiar context versus that of a sterile, unknown setting such as a clinic or rehabilitation facility. Concomitantly, clients may feel more relaxed and motivated to participate in therapy at home. They may be able to more clearly and easily discern their own capabilities and areas for improvement and personal goals than in a foreign setting devoid of their personal artifacts and the meanings associated with living at home. Second, therapists are able to teach skills and new techniques within the context in which they will be used, a critical principle in adult learning. Contextual learning minimizes the challenges clients may confront in translating new skills or techniques learned in a standardized setting, such as a hospital, for use in their own life spaces. For example, learning to transfer to the left when getting onto a tub transfer bench may work in the hospital, but may not work in a person's home where the bathroom configuration requires the person to transfer to the right. Without home care intervention, older adults may find it difficult to generalize the directionality of steps involved. Third, providing care in the home enables therapists to observe that environment for clues as to how best to quickly relate to and work with the client and family members (if relevant) and to more easily form a therapeutic

relationship.[16] A therapeutic alliance is essential for promoting motivation and adherence to rehabilitative techniques.[4] Additionally, providing care in the home provides invaluable firsthand knowledge about the capacity of the client and the supports and barriers in his or her environment from which to derive an effective treatment plan. Finally, a home evaluation can reveal more safety hazards and unhealthy environmental conditions as well as disentangle what an older adult can do from what he or she is actually doing more so than relying on self-report in a clinic or physician's office.

Challenges of Delivering Care in the Home

In contrast to structured, routinized care environments of hospitals, nursing homes, physician's offices, or outpatient clinics, homes are highly individualized, uncontrolled, diverse, imbued with personal preferences and cultural attributions, personalized, and potentially a contaminated context.[6] There is wide variation in homes, including their location, size, physical condition and features, safety, and the presence of others, that can affect the type of care needed and how it is provided.[17] Solutions such as installation of adaptive equipment, home modifications, or telemedicine technology suitable for one client and his or her home environment may not work in another due to the physical and social features of the living space. For example, recommending a stair glide may not be possible if an older adult is obese, children live in the home, or the walls and staircase are in poor condition.

Homes as well as neighborhoods can help or hinder an older adult's ability to carry out various household, personal, and self-care tasks. Additionally, older adults and families differ in their knowledge of and willingness to engage in the home care process, their preferences for where health-related and adaptive equipment can be set up and care tasks performed, and how and where the therapy session will transpire in the home.[6,17]

Another challenge in home care is that many older adults live in homes that may adversely affect their health, the health of the care provider, and the delivery of home care. For example, over 6 million households have significant home repair needs, including heating, plumbing, and electrical deficiencies.[17] These problems are more prevalent for persons living below the poverty line, who may also be at risk of exposure to lead paint, vermin and pest infestations, water leakage, and exposed wiring and electrical problems,[17] and may more adversely affect vulnerable populations such as older adults. Moreover, physical hazards affect the ability to install, maintain, and use adaptive equipment and may make it challenging or impossible for home care therapists to work effectively and safely in the home environment. The interface of home repair needs with everyday functioning at home is often not considered but is clearly evident in home care.[24]

The social environment is another consideration. The presence of children and/or other adults in the home may influence delivery of home care services, particularly in regard to privacy during therapy or for a client's performance of self-care, the client's motivation level and adherence to the therapy plan, and the appropriateness of equipment recommendations, which may have to fit with the needs, preferences, and expectations of the client's social context. Involvement of family members in a home care session may be relevant yet pose challenges. For example, conflict between the older adult and family member(s) or poor quality of relationships may interfere in home care participation and progress. Therapists must seek a balance between preserving the autonomy of the older adult in view of what may be limited cognitive and/or functional capacities and family involvement.[10]

Home care also poses distinctive challenges as a work environment. First, home care requires strong clinical and time management skills, and the ability to work independently and without direct supervision.[22] Being a home care therapist may not be right for everyone. Second, home environmental conditions may present a hazard to not only the older adult but to the therapist as well. For example, extreme clutter, confined spaces to work in, infestation, inadequate sanitation, exposed infectious or hazardous materials, poor air quality, poorly regulated heat or air conditioning, excessive noise, poor lighting, presence of aggressive dogs or other pets, presence of firearms or other weapons, smoking or drug use in the home, extreme home repair needs, inadequate electrical capacity and outlets, and lack of privacy all may place a therapist at risk and/or cause discomfort and significantly compromise treatment planning and execution.

Where to Sit and Other Cultural Considerations

Consistent across surveys of older adults is the importance of aging in place at home.[12] Home is a key cultural symbol imbued with many meanings, including independence, autonomy, comfort, security, control, protection, and history and family remembrances.[19,20,21,23] Often conceptualized as an extension of oneself, the home has many meanings to older adults and reflects the intersection of objective social and physical conditions and subjective appraisals, personal goals, values, and emotions.[19] As such, the home care therapist must be sensitive to the client's cultural beliefs and values. For example, when introducing changes to the way a client takes a bath or shower, an activity that is very personal, a therapist needs to take into account the client's (and family's) preferences and long-standing routines.

The home as a culturally complex setting is evident the moment the therapist enters this setting. Unlike the clinic, which has clear directives as to where clients sit and the pace of the visit, the home is uncharted. Rules of engagement are implicit and mostly directed by the resident. Each home care situation is unique and the therapist must be flexible and open to going with the flow as established by the client in his or her own setting. It may be the client, for example, who dictates where the home care session occurs, where the therapist will sit, and how long the session will last.

With age and reduced functional capacity, older people spend more time in the home.[20] As such, the home takes on increasing importance as the principal context for socialization,

leisure participation, and health-care delivery.[2] In that capacity, the home also assumes new meanings as the principal location for safety, security, familiarity, and support of daily function.[14] (See chapter 19 for additional discussion on the meaning of home in later life.) The presence of health professionals and specialized equipment, medications, and other medical or rehabilitative artifacts may not be readily acceptable because these items serve as visual and concrete reminders of declining abilities and threaten the meanings attributed to the home. Home care represents the interface between the home as a private and personalized space, the aging process and its associated health declines, and medical and rehabilitative objectives and societal demands. This tension may be intimately experienced by an older adult and influences acceptability of therapist recommendations for equipment or compensatory strategy use.

Conceptual Models Guiding Home Care Practice

Lawton's competence-environmental press framework[14] and its expansion in occupational therapy to include occupation[13] provide a broad, overarching framework to understand an older client's levels of competencies and types of losses (e.g., sensory, physical mobility, or cognitive), environmental factors (e.g., housing features, social characteristics, and neighborhood conditions), and the interface with chosen activities or occupations. The model suggests the need to strive for the most optimal combination of environmental circumstances in view of changing competencies. It also suggests that a just-right fit leads to the highest possible behavioral and emotional functioning for that person.[5,15,26] Yet another tenet of this model is that older adults with lower levels of competence become the most susceptible to their environments, such that low competence in conjunction with high environmental press, negatively affects autonomy, affect, and well-being. A related point is that as competencies decline, the zone of adaptation for promoting well-being narrows such that environmental choices become increasingly more limited. The competence-environmental press framework, and its expansion to include an occupational framework, continues to provide the basic mechanism of person-environment relations as people age and has been supported by a considerable body of empirical research. The model represents a broad, overarching framework for understanding the role of occupational therapy in home care and effectively frames the compensatory perspective relevant to therapies used in the home context. (See chapters 4 and 19 for additional discussion of the competence-environmental press model.)

Using a Problem-Solving Approach in Home Care

Problem solving is a core feature of clinical reasoning processes used by all health and human service professionals in any care context. However, when working with older adults in the home, and particularly for individuals with complex health conditions requiring symptom management and family involvement, it is especially relevant. For the home care therapist, problem solving begins immediately upon entering the neighborhood, parking the car, and walking to the front door of the home of an older client. All of this information, gathered through keen observation, provides foundational knowledge and the backdrop from which the older client will be approached and assessed, and needs identified.

Approaches to problem solving vary. They can range from broad thinking and action processes to a highly structured and manualized approach such as problem-solving therapy, a formal therapeutic modality developed in psychology that teaches problem-solving skills. Here we refer to a broad problem-solving approach that is central to caring for older adults with complex conditions.[8]

Although approaches to problem solving vary, shared basic characteristics include the purposeful engagement of individuals with chronic illness and/or their family members in a set of thinking and action processes that move through problem identification to implementation of concrete, practical solutions. The first step involves clearly identifying and defining the client's key problem to target; the identification process should involve the client, family, and therapist perspective. Problem identification can be complex and a multifaceted process. Next is to establish specific and realistic goals for managing or eliminating the identified problem. Some individuals may engage in wishful thinking and develop a goal that is unrealistic (e.g., seeking a cure for the disease, or being able to drive), requiring redirection and guidance as to what is realistic and appropriate. The third step involves systematic questioning to identify the characteristics or nature of the problem (e.g., when it occurs, frequency of occurrence) to uncover potential contributing factors. By understanding the dimensions of a problem (e.g., lack of adherence to medication regime) and contributory factors (e.g., complexity of medication directions, poor planning), clients and families learn ways to prevent its occurrence or minimize its effects. The fourth step is to identify specific solutions or alternative approaches that are realistic for managing the identified problem. One approach is to engage individuals in brainstorming such that they become actively involved in generating possible solutions. Once solutions are proposed, each one should be reviewed for feasibility and acceptability to client and family, if appropriate. This is in contrast to a prescriptive approach, in which solutions are provided by health-care providers without input from the client. Although occupational therapists may have the requisite knowledge concerning the health problem and specific ideas for its management, involving older adults in this process reinforces and validates the need for their active role in their own self-management. It also demonstrates problem solving and builds their skills in being able to use this process independently. Additionally, individuals may perceive greater ownership of solutions they help generate and be more likely to implement and adhere to them. The fifth step involves implementing agreed-upon solution(s), and the final, sixth step involves evaluating whether implemented solutions improved or worsened the problem and modifying them accordingly. (See chapter 7 for additional discussion of the intervention process.) Problem solving has important advantages in helping older adults cope with chronic illnesses and its functional consequences. Its use reflects a movement toward consumer-directed health care that relies on informed consumers to direct their own health-care choices and participate in disease management.

Summary

Home care is gaining prominence in the health-care system as an approach that may prevent hospitalization, readmissions, and nursing home placement, and enable aging in place. Funding sources for home care include Medicare Part A and Part B, as well as private health insurance. As a work environment, the home poses unique challenges; every home is distinct and unique—reflecting the intersection of broad socioeconomic and cultural influences and individuation, personal preferences, histories, and values and beliefs. The occupational therapist is thrust in the mix of these factors with the goal of helping older adults gain, regain, maintain, or improve their functional foothold and well-being in that environment. For many older adults, the home, imbued with historical and personal meanings and social connectedness, may offer recuperative opportunities possibly not afforded in other settings. Embracing the challenges of home care and helping older adults and their families achieve the outcomes they desire is a noble and most rewarding endeavor.

REVIEW QUESTIONS

1. What are the major challenges in providing home care to older adults?
2. Why is home care important for promoting the health of older adults?
3. What is a problem-solving approach to home care therapy?
4. What are conceptual frameworks that can guide home care therapies, and how can they be applied in practice?

REFERENCES

1. Benjamin, A. E. (1992). An overview of in-home health and supportive services for older persons. In M. G. Ory & A. P. Duncker (Eds.), *In-home care for older people* (1st ed., pp. 9–52). Newbury Park, CA: Sage Publications.
2. Binstock, R. H., & Cluff, L. E. (2000). *Home care advances: Essential research and policy issues.* New York, NY: Springer.
3. Centers for Disease Control and Prevention. (2004). *Home health care patients: Data from the 2000 National Home and Hospice Care Survey.* Accessed 10/21/15. http://www.cdc.gov/nchs/pressroom/04facts/patients.htm.
4. Chee, Y., Gitlin, L. N., & Dennis, M. P. (2005). Provider assessment of interactions with dementia caregivers: Evaluation and application of the therapeutic engagement index. *Clinical Gerontologist, 28*(4), 43–59.

5. Gitlin, L. N. (2000). Adjusting person-environment systems: Helping older people live the good life at home. In R. Rubenstein, M. Moss, & M. Kleban (Eds.), *The many faces of aging: Essays in honor of M. P. Lawton* (pp. 41–51). New York, NY: Springer.

6. Gitlin, L. N. (2003). Conducting research on home environments: lessons learned and new directions. *Gerontologist, 43*(5), 628–637.

7. Gitlin, L. N. (2007). The impact of housing on quality of life: Does the home environment matter now and into the future? In H.-W. Wahl, C. Tesch-Romer, & A. Hoff (Eds.), *New dynamics in old age: Individual, environmental, and societal perspectives* (pp. 105–125). New York, NY: Baywood.

8. Gitlin, L. N. (2015). Problem solving: A teaching and therapeutic tool for older adults and their families. In I. Söderback (Ed.), *International handbook of occupational therapy interventions* (2nd ed., pp. 415–431). New York: Springer. Media and Science. doi:10.1007/978-3-319-08141-0_27.

9. Gitlin, L. N., Jacobs, M., & Earland, T. V. (2010). Translation of a dementia caregiver intervention for delivery in homecare as a reimbursable Medicare service: Outcomes and lessons learned. *The Gerontologist, 50*(6), 847–854. doi:10.1093/geront/gnq057.

10. Gitlin, L. N., & Schulz, R. (2012). Family caregiving of older adults. In T. R. Prohaska, L. A. Anderson, & R. H. Binstock (Eds.), *Public health for an aging society* (pp. 181–204). Baltimore, MD: John Hopkins University Press.

11. Ibis World. (2015). *Home care providers in the US: Market research report*. Accessed 10/21/15. http://www.ibisworld.com/industry/default.aspx?indid=1579.

12. Keenan, T. A. (2010). *Home and community preferences of the 451 population*. Washington DC: AARP.

13. Law, M., Cooper, B., Strong, S., Stewart, D., Rigby, P., & Letts, L. (1996). The Person-Environment-Occupation Model: A transactive approach to occupational performance. *The Canadian Journal of Occupational Therapy, 63*, 9–23.

14. Lawton, M. P. (1990). Residential environment and self-directedness among older people. *American Psychologist, 45*(5), 638–640.

15. Lawton, M. P., & Nahemow, L. (1973). Ecology and the aging process. In C. Eisdorfer & M. P. Lawton (Eds.), *The psychology of adult development and aging* (pp. 619–674). Washington, DC: American Psychological Association.

16. Levine, R. E., Corcoran, M., & Gitlin, L. N. (1993). Home care and private practice. In H. L. Hopkins & H. D. Smith (Eds.), *Occupational therapy* (8th ed., pp. 822–842). Philadelphia, PA: J. B. Lippincott.

17. National Academy of Science. (2011). *Health care comes home: The human factors*. Washington, DC: The National Academics Press.

18. *National Association for Home Care and Hospice*. Basic statistics about home care. (2010). Accessed 10/21/15. http://www.nahc.org/assets/1/7/10HC_Stats.pdf.

19. Oswald, F., & Wahl, H.-W. (2005). Dimensions of the meaning of home. In G. D. Rowles & H. Chaudhury (Eds.), *Home and identity in late life: International perspectives* (pp. 21–45). New York, NY: Springer.

20. Oswald, F., Wahl, H.-W., Naumann, D., Mollenkopf, H., & Hieber, A. (2006). The role of the home environment in middle and late adulthood. In H.-W. Wahl, H. Brenner, & H. Mollenkopf (Eds.), *The many faces of health, competence and well-being in old age* (pp. 7–24). Netherlands: Springer.

21. Oswald, F., Wahl, H.-W., Schilling, O., & Iwarsson, S. (2007). Housing-related control beliefs and independence in activities of daily living in very old age. *Scandinavian Journal of Occupational Therapy, 14*(1), 33–43. doi: 10.1080/11038120601151615.

22. Piersol, C. V., & Ehrlich, P. L. (2009). *Occupational therapy in home health care*. Austin, TX: Pro-Ed.

23. Rubenstein, R. L. (1989). Culture and disorder in the home care experience: The home as sickroom. In J. F. Gubrium & A. Sankar (Eds.), *The home care experience: Ethnography and policy* (pp. 37–57). Newbury Park, CA: Sage Publications.

24. Szanton, S. L., Thorpe, R. J., Boyd, C., Tanner, E. K., Leff, B., Agree, E., et al. (2011). Community aging in place, advancing better living for elders: A bio-behavioral-environmental intervention to improve function and health-related quality of life in disabled older adults. *Journal of the American Geriatrics Society, 59*(12), 2314–2320.

25. Wahl, H.-W., & Gitlin, L. N. (2003). Future developments in living environments for older people in the U.S. and Germany: Potential and constraints. In K. W. Schaie, H.-W. Wahl, H. Mollenkopf, et al. (Eds.), *Aging independently: Living arrangements and mobility* (pp. 281–301). New York, NY: Spring Publications.

26. Wahl, H.-W., & Gitlin, L. N. (2007). Environmental gerontology. In J. E. Birren (Ed.), *Encyclopedia of gerontology* (2nd ed., pp. 494–502). Oxford: Elsevier.

CHAPTER 27

Intradisciplinary and Interdisciplinary Processes in Gerontological Care

Nina Tumosa, PhD, Helen Lach, PhD, RN, GCNS-BC, Linda Orr, MPA, OTR/L, Karen Frank Barney, PhD, OTR/L, FAOTA

CHAPTER OUTLINE

OBJECTIVES

- Identify the value of the interdisciplinary team model as it relates to older adults
- Discuss and differentiate the different types of teams and the significance of each
- Explain the occupational therapist/occupational therapy assistant intraprofessional role delineation process and expectations in geriatric/gerontologic settings
- Identify the most common goals of health-care teams
- Identify and discuss the stages of team development
- Identify five components of behavior necessary to create effective health-care teams
- State how "good" teams develop and remain relevant
- Discuss team communication and its importance as it relates to effective and efficient teaming
- Discuss leadership roles of working with health-care team change
- Discuss conflict as it relates to teams
- Discuss the characteristics of effective teams outlined by Geriatric Interdisciplinary Team Training
- Discuss how health-care teams are assessed

Older adults typically have complex health problems affecting all aspects of their lives, including physical, psychological, and social issues. As a result, it takes an interdisciplinary team of health professionals to ensure that a holistic approach is used to identify and address the many challenges older adults may face. For example, an older woman may be recovering from a wrist fracture from a fall. Because she lives alone and has no family nearby, this seemingly small injury is affecting her ability to get her groceries or medications, and cook. She worries a lot about falling now, and so she is concerned about leaving her home. Besides addressing her medical condition, she needs help adapting to her current condition, assistance with her daily activities, and psychological support. Similar to this case, most older people have multiple chronic conditions, which are compounded by any acute health-care event. The skills, expertise, and collaboration of a variety of health professionals are essential to provide optimal care. As a result, an interdisciplinary team approach is the gold standard for high-quality, client-centered gerontological care.

Throughout this book an effort has been made to frame and explain occupational therapy (OT) processes in terms of participating personnel, which may include occupational therapists, occupational therapy assistants, and/or other supporting staff. Regardless of type of setting, whether institutional or community based, OT personnel typically relate to other health and additional types of professionals, such as business and law. Division of labor is typically made on the basis of the profession's credentialed expertise expectations and licensing standards. Role delineation expectations are clarified for whatever type of teamwork is appropriate in gerontological practice settings.

Over the past decade, increasing emphasis has been placed on ensuring that health professionals develop competence in working on health-care teams, and that this is included in professional education. Since the Institute of Medicine's 2003 report[12] on health professions education, interdisciplinary collaboration has been considered a key to addressing issues in health-care quality and safety. This position is endorsed by numerous health-care organizations concerned with quality gerontological care.[2] For those already in practice, or working on teams, continuing education can provide this training and improve team functioning. Ability to function on interdisciplinary teams is a core competency for all health professionals (Table 27-1).

Increasingly, evidence supports the effectiveness of interdisciplinary teams in improving quality of care and client outcomes,[19,21] especially for older adults. In a recent review of the literature on interdisciplinary care of older adults,[1]

TABLE 27-1 Team Members Overview

Members	Practice Roles/Skills	Education/Training	Licensure/Credentials[1]
Nurse	Licensed vocational nurse (LVN)—basic nursing skills that are dictated by the facility; registered nurse (RN)—associate degree, BA, or higher; increased scope of practice for associate degree in nursing (AN), including planning for optimal functioning, coordination of care, teaching, and direct and indirect patient care	LVN—1 year of training AN with associate degree—2 years of training, usually in a community college BS, AN—4 years of college MS, AN—2 years of postgraduate specialty study PhD, AN—3 to 4 years of postgraduate studies	LVN examination required for licensing Continuing education unit (CEU) requirements: AN; BS,; APN; MS, GNP, or other specialty ANs PhD, AN: must pass the national licensure examination and required to have 20 hours of CEUs per year
Nurse Practitioner	Health assessment, health promotion, histories and physicals in outpatient settings; orders, conducts, and interprets some laboratory and diagnostic tests; teaching and counseling	Master's degree with a defined specialty area, such as gerontology (GNP)	In addition to AN licensure, must pass a National Certification Examination in the appropriate specialty area (e.g., gerontology or family practice), CE requirements
Physician	Diagnoses and treats diseases and injuries, provides preventive care, does routine check-ups, prescribes drugs, and does some surgery	Medical school (4 years) plus 3 to 7 years of graduate medical education	State licensure required for doctor of medicine degree; examination required and possible examinations required for specialty areas; CE requirements
Geriatrician	Physician with special training in the diagnosis, treatment, and prevention of disorders in older people; recognizes aging as a normal process and not a disease state	Completion of medical school, residency training in family medicine and internal medicine, and 1-year fellowship program in gerontological medicine	Completion of fellowship training program and/or passing examination for Certificate of Added Qualifications in Geriatric Medicine (CAQ); recertification by examination required every 10 years and begins in the 8th year, as it is a 2-year process
Physician Assistant (PA)	Practices medicine with the supervision of a licensed physician; exercises autonomy in medical decision making and provides a broad range of diagnostic and therapeutic services; practice centered on patient care	Specially designed 2-year program at medical colleges and universities; bachelor's degree and over 4 years of healthcare experience typical before entering a PA program	State licensure or registration plus certification by the National Commission on Certification of Physician Assistants (NCCPA); recertification every 6 years by examination; 100 hours continuing medical education (CME) every 2 years
Social Worker (SW)	Assessment of individual and family psychosocial functioning and provision of care to help enhance or restore capacities; can include locating services or providing counseling	BSW—4-year college degree MSW—BSW plus 2 years of graduate work PhD—15 hours of continuing education required every year	State certification required for clinical social workers; LMSW (or master's level) or LSW (BS level); social work associate (SWA) with a combination of education and experience; ACP signifies licensure for independent clinical practice
Gerontological Psychologist	Assessment, treatment, and management of mental disorders; psychotherapy with individuals, groups, and families	Graduate training: 5 years beyond undergraduate training; most coursework includes gerontology and clinical/practice experience	PhD, EdD, or PsyD degree; state licensure for Clinical Psychologists; the American Psychological Association ethical code and state ethical codes

[1] Licensed health professionals in the U.S. have continuing education (CE) requirements; with license renewal, one must record, and, if requested, provide documentation of having completed CE in the amount required by state licensing laws.

Continued

TABLE 27-1 Team Members Overview—cont'd

Members	Practice Roles/Skills	Education/Training	Licensure/Credentials
Psychiatrist	Medical doctor who treats patients' mental, emotional, and behavioral symptoms	Medical school and residency specializing in psychiatry; residency includes both general residency training and 2 to 3 years in area of specialization (e.g., geriatrics, pediatrics)	State examination to practice medicine; Board of Psychiatry and Neurology offers examination for diploma in psychiatry, although not required for psychiatric practice in Texas
Pharmacist	Devises and revises a patient's medication therapy to achieve the optimal regime that suits the individual's medical and therapeutic needs; information resource for the patient and medical team	BS—5-year program Doctorate degree (PharmD) Requirements for annual continuing CEUs ranging from 10 to 15 hours	State examination required; national examination (NABPLEX), given every quarter, used in Texas; "RPh" used as title for a registered pharmacist in Texas; board certifications in specialties available (pharmacotherapy, nuclear pharmacy, nutrition, psychiatric, and oncology in near future)
Occupational Therapist (OTR)	Evaluation, prevention, and/or correction of physical, mental, or emotional dysfunction; maximization of function in the life of the individual through therapeutic goal-directed activity/occupation	BS, MS, MOT, or OTD degree in OT with a minimum of 6 months of fieldwork	National board examination for credential of OTR (occupational therapy registered); state licensure where applicable; continuing education
Occupational Therapy Assistant (COTA)	Delivers services under the supervision of and in collaboration with the OTR	AS, AAS, or certificate in OTA with a minimum of 4 months of fieldwork	National board examination for credential of COTA (certified occupational therapy assistant); state licensure where applicable; continuing education
Physical Therapist (PT)	Evaluation, examination, and utilization of exercise, rehabilitative procedures, massage, manipulations, and physical agents, including but not limited to mechanical devices, heat, cold, air, light, water, electricity, and sound, in the aid of diagnosis or treatment	MSPT, MPT, or DPT degree in physical therapy	National board examination for credential of PT; state licensure where applicable; continuing education
Physical Therapy Assistant (PTA)	Works under the direction and supervision of a PT	AS degree in physical therapy assistant	National board examination for credential of PTA; state licensure where applicable; continuing education
Chaplain	Provides visits and ministry to patients and family	Master's degree in theology, plus a minimum of 1 year of clinical supervision, if fully certified; can work in some settings without being fully certified	Certification through the Chaplaincy Board of Certification; however, credentials not normally used; most are ordained ministers, but not all; 50 hours per year CEUs required

TABLE 27-1 Team Members Overview—cont'd

Members	Practice Roles/Skills	Education/Training	Licensure/Credentials
Dietitian	Evaluates the nutritional status of patients; works with family members and medical team to determine appropriate nutrition goals for patients	BS degree in food and nutrition and experience required to be eligible for examination; CEUs required for both the licensed dietitian (LD) (6 clock hours/year) and registered dietitian (AD) (75 clock hours every 5 years); MS degree available also	AD is credential for a registered dietitian in Texas; must pass the national examination of the American Dietetic Association; LD is credential for a licensed dietitian Texas: same national examination required but processing of paperwork differs
Recreational Therapist	Plans, directs, and coordinates recreational programs for people with disabilities or illnesses using a variety of techniques, such as arts and crafts, drama, music, dance, sports, games and field trips; programs help to improve a client's physical and emotional well-being	BS in recreational therapy	National certification examination

Note: Continuing education requirements vary by state, and licensing and certification titles vary (e.g., LVN or LPN; LISW or LMSW; CSW, CISW, or CICSW).
(Adapted from Hyer, K., Flaherty, E., Fairchild, S., Botrell, M., Mezey, M., Fulmer, T., et al. [2003]. *Geriatric Interdisciplinary Team Training program [GITT]: Curriculum guide.* New York, NY: GITT Resource Center, New York University.)

outcomes such as improved chronic disease and medication management, better functional outcomes, and decreased hospitalizations were reported. Additional support was noted for teams to address issues related to older adults who are frail and hospitalized. Additionally, teams are needed to address issues relevant for older adults living at home through home health and outpatient care. Thus, the following sections provide an overview of key factors important for good interdisciplinary teamwork, and skills that health professionals need to assure effective team care for older clients.

Types of Teams

Ideally, gerontological health-care teams consist of small groups of professionals with complementary skills, committed to working closely together to improve client care. Each person is accountable for the work of the entire team and therefore for the work of the other persons on the team. For this to work, excellent communication and shared decision making are essential to the success of the team. An effective team works synergistically so that the team's overall performance exceeds that of the individual inputs of the members. This is how teams are able to solve problems that individuals cannot.

Teams can be of different types. Drinka and Clark[6] describe the classic team styles: ad hoc, unidisciplinary, multidisciplinary, and interdisciplinary (often called interprofessional). An ad hoc team is a group of health professionals who come together to solve a single, short-term problem. For example, an occupational therapist and physician may

work together to help an older client improve access to his or her home. Unidisciplinary teams include people from one profession who may have different kinds of expertise. An older client may have a gerontologist, orthopedist, and urologist helping address various medical conditions. Multidisciplinary teams include multiple disciplines, but they do not necessarily communicate or collaborate with one another. A true interdisciplinary team collaborates with a common purpose and shares leadership, information, and responsibilities.

All teams need a mission statement that describes the approach that will be used by the team and that lays the foundation for interdisciplinary teamwork. The mission describes the common purpose of the team for the members and keeps everyone focused on long-term goals. This is important for keeping team spirit alive when short-term failures interfere with those goals. The most common goals of health-care teams are to:

- Improve client function or maintain maximum client independence.
- Enhance client well-being.
- Increase client satisfaction.
- Reduce use of hospital services.
- Reduce health-care costs.
- Optimize work satisfaction of all team members.

However, no team should be totally defined by that mission statement. Rather, teams should be defined by the actions of all of the members of the team. The role of the team is to complete tasks that result in the accomplishment of a goal, usually an improved client outcome. More and more, funding

BOX 27-1 Tips for Effective Teamwork

- Teamwork is not something that arises naturally. It is something you have to PRACTICE:
- Play and laugh together.
- Recognize your role on the team and how it synergizes with those of the other team members.
- Accept roles and responsibilities according to skills, strengths, and weaknesses.
- Communicate positively.
- Trust each other.
- Improve the weakest link, thereby improving the team.
- Celebrate team successes together.
- Evaluate by measuring team outcomes and continuously make improvements.

and accreditation are dependent on facilities being able to document improved client outcomes. This documentation can be quantitative (decreased number of hospitalizations and rehospitalizations) or qualitative (increased satisfaction with services). Therefore, all tasks should be measurable and able to be easily communicated to all members of the team.

Teams and Teamlets

Teams come in all sizes, but for this discussion the concept of teams will be divided into small (two to five members), medium (six to 12 members), and large (more than 12 members). In general, large teams are not very effective. Communication is too unwieldy when many people are included. It is difficult for all members to be involved in the decision-making process or to reach a consensus. Large teams must be broken down into medium teams, small teams, or teamlets that can address specific issues or components of larger projects.

A teamlet (little team) is a model of care used in primary or other aspects of care to provide a higher quality of care for clients beyond that of the typical 15-minute physician visit.[3] Typically, a teamlet will consist of a clinician and two health coaches. In addition, teamlets from two or more sites may coalesce to collaborate on a problem that crosses sites, such as creating a plan of care for an older adult who returns home after hospitalization and continues to receive care at home, or to create a policy to provide better care during an emergency such as a hurricane or widespread power loss.

Small-sized teams often form the core of medium-sized and large teams. These small teams commonly consist of a social worker, a nurse, and a physician. Other members, who are added to meet the specific needs of clients, especially in transition-of-care situations, are often pharmacists, dieticians, physical therapists, occupational therapists, and pastoral care. Other members tend to be more site-specific. For example, community living centers (or nursing homes) often rely on peripheral team members such as maintenance or laundry workers to offer insights and/or solutions to problems. Optometrists and audiologists are often consulted to address vision and hearing issues. Home care teams may consult with lawyers, elder abuse experts, or police officers. Teams in assisted living facilities often rely on bus drivers to provide warnings about changing care needs. When the small

teams take on several such "consultants" they become medium teams, at least temporarily.

Medium teams can function efficiently as long as communication is carefully handled for the team. Also, they may serve as a pool of experts who work well together and who readily spin off into smaller temporary teams to handle specific short-term issues, such as addressing a quality improvement concern or acute rehabilitation need, or monitoring a health promotion project such as smoking cessation or diabetes management programs. Medium teams also result when small teams consult with teams from other facilities. This often leads to the development of virtual teams.

Occupational Therapist-Occupational Therapy Assistant Team

Many settings, both medical and community based, provide excellent opportunities for occupational therapist and occupational therapy assistant (OTA) team service implementation. As defined above, these role pairings are "teamlets" and optimally represent the best in intradisciplinary/professional processes. Currently, in the United States interprofessional processes are considered to be "state of the art," and the OTR–COTA intraprofessional process optimally represents a positive and highly productive relationship.

The advantages to intraprofessional collaboration in service provision are many, with the ability to maximize intervention impact through optimal skills use at each level. Well-matched teams represent highly complementary roles and high motivation to apply the best practices about which they are both educated and passionate. The American Occupational Therapy Association guidelines for intraprofessional role delineation are provided in Figure 27-1. The occupational therapist is held responsible for all OT services that are provided, whether or not the professional is present onsite. As such, in teaming with the COTA, it behooves the occupational therapist to have good communication and coordination processes established to ensure appropriate collaboration in service provision. Both the OTR and the COTA are responsible for appropriate supervision and implementation processes and are expected to respect and support the role of the other. Since the 1970's, many skilled nursing facilities (SNFs) across the U.S. have hired COTAs who are supervised by consulting and direct service OTRs who cover several facilities. Thus, effective OTR-COTA teamwork is imperative in providing quality services. In these instances, within settings with fulltime COTAs, they may take on a team leader role, while maintaining the required supervision relationship with the OTR. Utilization of an OTR–COTA team in either health care or community-based settings may favorably impact cost containment, and more importantly, focused and appropriate interventions with older adults. The team process components depicted in Figure 27-2 can be implemented to maximize the roles of both the OTR and COTA, so that more individuals may be treated or receive services in cost-effective ways. This figure presents the reciprocal, transactional relationship between the OT team members. The occupational therapist should consider all relevant sociocultural factors and client needs

Occupational Therapist (OTR)	Occupational Therapy Assistant (COTA)
Autonomous	**Must Receive Occupational Therapist Supervision**
• Responsibility for **all aspects** of occupational therapy service delivery	• Deliver services **under supervision of and in partnership with** OTR
• Accountable for safety and effectiveness of services and process	• Equally responsible for developing a **collaborative plan for supervision**
• Ultimately responsible for implementation of appropriate supervision	• Responsibility for **seeking and obtaining** appropriate supervision
BOTH	
Equal responsibility for developing a collaborative plan for supervision	

FIGURE 27-1   Intraprofessional Role Delineation: OTR & COTA. Ceranski, S., & Black, T. (October, 2014). Vision: Gear up to provide cost effective services that achieve outcomes of value to all stakeholders. Presentation conducted at the Wisconsin Occupational Therapy Association Annual Conference, Appleton, Wisconsin.

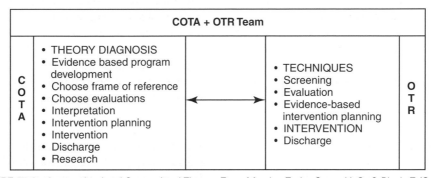

FIGURE 27-2   Intraprofessional Occupational Therapy Team Member Tasks. Ceranski, S., & Black, T. (October, 2014). Vision: Gear up to provide cost effective services that achieve outcomes of value to all stakeholders. Presentation conducted at the Wisconsin Occupational Therapy Association Annual Conference, Appleton, Wisconsin.

prior to program development and implementation. OT practitioners must adhere to the discipline's ethical standards, policies, and guidelines; as well as state, federal, and other regulatory and reimbursement guidelines that may apply to their service delivery or program. The OTR identifies the theoretical and evidence base upon which the program is developed, selects screening and evaluation tools to be utilized, interprets results, plans and conducts interventions, and oversees discharge or discontinuation of services, as well as any research conducted within the program. The OTA conducts delegated screening, evaluation, and reevaluation processes and provides verbal and written reports of observations and older client capacities, plans and conducts interventions, contributes to discharge/program discontinuation planning, and may assist in collecting research data.

OTR/COTA teams play important roles in medical settings that include acute care, rehabilitation, hand therapy, out-patient, mental health, and skilled nursing facilities. Both medical- and community-based programs are increasing the utilization of these teams gradually, in part due to changes in how health care is delivered. With the projected demographics regarding global aging and the emphasis on cost containment, we can expect an increase in the need for these teams in both traditional medical and nontraditional community-based services. Note that chapter 30, The Future of Gerontological Occupational Therapy, offers insight regarding areas of need and opportunity for the development of services and programs within which the use of these teams may be considered.

Virtual Teams

With the advent of modern communication techniques (electronic records, text messages, tweets, and blogs, to mention only a few), more teams are becoming virtual teams. That is, the team members do not need face-to-face meetings to communicate effectively. In fact, virtual teams are becoming the norm in such settings as hospice care, home care, and rural health care.

The electronic health record (EHR) can often be accessed from different workstations and even from different work sites. This means that pertinent client information can be communicated to a central repository as the data are collected. It then becomes the responsibility of team members to routinely access all of the information and to comment appropriately for the benefit of other team members. It is incumbent upon the team to act synergistically. To do this the members must spend time together as a team to communicate new information and to make shared decisions. For virtual teams this may be done online or on the phone, rather than in face-to-face meetings. Telemedicine and computer video capabilities offer opportunities for virtual face-to-face discussions.

Team Development and Effective Functioning

Gerontological interdisciplinary health-care teams consist of persons who meet frequently to exchange information about a client, to develop a treatment/intervention plan, and to oversee its implementation. This simple description masks the reality of team development. All teams go through a development phase. When a team first meets, personal attributes such as gender, age, personality, race, and stereotypical images of professions usually play a part in shaping informal roles that members adopt.[7] This informal role differentiation may diminish in later stages of team development when good leadership encourages the team to develop its own culture of trust and understanding. However, these roles can also persist, resulting in conflicts among team members. Tuckman[22] described the classic process of team development that includes stages where different challenges and interventions to improve team performance may be important:

- Forming: Team members are identified and join the group and begin getting to know each other.
- Norming: Members integrate goals and values of the team and the group process as they learn to work together.
- Confronting: Conflicts are identified as team members work together, and effective teams learn to resolve these conflicts in a positive way.
- Performing: Members achieve a level of performance focused on the client, rather than on the process or individual.
- Leaving: Members leave and may or may not be replaced with new members, or teams may be disbanded.

The process of developing teams can be painful, but the experience of working on a team consistently results in an increased understanding of the value of the interdisciplinary/ interprofessional team[10,17] although some disciplines are more sanguine than others about the team's rights to develop care/ intervention plans.[15]

The stage of team development will affect its performance. It is in the best interest of the client that the team works at the performing level as much as possible. Many team training programs have been developed to encourage understanding and appreciation between team members.[6,11] As new members arrive, time needs to be taken to learn about their strengths and weaknesses, their skills and expertise, and their expectations about their roles on the team. They in turn need to learn about the other team members. Socialization must be encouraged between team members in order for them to identify themselves as a team and to work more effectively together.[9] Studies in the past several years suggest the efficacy of narratives as a pedagogical tool of team building.[8]

Through synergism, teams can produce results that individuals cannot, but teams are only as strong as their weakest link. They are susceptible to dysfunctional team behavior.[5] This challenge is particularly true of teams that consist of mixed skills and expertise,[18] such as health-care teams comprised of medical and nonmedical persons. Conflict, low morale, and poor task management may result. Several components of behavior must be present to allow a team to be effective. These components include:

- Collaboration between persons with relevant expertise
- Communication based on mutual respect and congeniality
- Dually trained members
- Frequent meetings
- Leadership

Failure of any of these components can mean failure of the basic purpose of the team: to provide the best care possible to the client. The composition of interdisciplinary teams should reflect the needs of the client. Composition should be different for a client with acute care needs versus one with chronic needs. A team in a community living center will have different members than one providing hospice services. However, the one thing all interdisciplinary teams should have in common is that they are comprised of persons with relevant expertise to the problem being addressed. This makes them effective and efficient, because each member has a contributing role. The blurring of roles between some disciplines can cause role ambiguity, and these issues must be addressed.[24]

There are many opportunities for teams to fail. Therefore, it is essential to emphasize the strengths of all members and to work around their weaknesses. Good teams share both successes and failures, and every team has plenty of both. Therefore, it is necessary for teams to have social events to promote team building and team spirit. Such events promote good attitudes and help to develop cohesiveness. Persons who go into gerontology are persons who want to do "good." Such persons are not unlike Mark Twain, who reported "I can live for two months on one good compliment." Good teams result from hard work.

This hard work has several critical components. They include developing trust, defining expectations, assigning roles and tasks, and measuring outcomes. Trust is developed when the team members get to know and respect each other, as they share their skills, their personal goals, and their dreams. A good team leader helps team members define the team's goals and mission statement. Every time a team meets, its members must be given an opportunity to express confidence and/or doubts about their abilities to accomplish their assigned tasks. Potential ethical issues can result from poor team performance, including overwhelming clients with a large team, taking a long time to work through group issues while the client waits, or falling into "groupthink" and excluding new approaches to solve problems.[13] Quality assurance data need to be made available in a timely manner to the team to evaluate performance and consider potential problems. Finally, success of the team has to be recognized. This allows the team to celebrate its successes and address its failures. The team must be made aware of the customer service component of its work. Without the client and the family, the team would not have a job.

Communication

Collaborative discussion, the most positive form of team communication,[4] occurs when team members ask questions and exchange ideas to reach the best decision for the client. The ability to communicate well is more often learned than it is innate. Different members of the team may communicate in different ways during an interdisciplinary team meeting. In a study of interpersonal communication dynamics during hospice interdisciplinary team meetings,[23] the majority of communication time spent was aimed at gaining control of the information exchange, rather than focusing on client goals. Many of these attempts were made by persons new to the team. This finding suggests that, no matter how well a team has performed in the past, there is a constant need for vigilance on the part of the team to ensure good communication and group process. There is also a role for supplemental team training in communication even for established teams. One barrier to communication among members who have different roles is that they sometimes speak different languages. Finding a common language is important for effective communication.

In any group attempting to communicate, there often needs to be an interpreter, someone who speaks more than one language. Members of an interdisciplinary team represent multiple disciplines that address different areas of a client's life, and so they may not all speak the same language. The languages may represent clinical, social, psychological, or spiritual approaches, and team members need to take time to clarify information. It is important to remember that the client and/or family are part of the team, so the team needs to be able to communicate to them, addressing any health literacy or language barriers.

Communication does no good unless all members of the team receive the same information. The most effective manner to convey complex information is through meetings. Traditionally these meetings have been face-to-face encounters. Such meetings convey to all the members that each participant believes that this meeting is sufficiently important to stop multitasking and converge on a single point to work on this single problem. Table 27-2 provides a description of key components of effective meetings. With the advent of telemedicine, videoconferencing, and Skype, however, teams now have more freedom to interact effectively from different locations as well as face-to-face. Certainly the introduction of such processes as distance education programs and telemedicine is priming younger providers to a higher comfort level with multisite interactions. It is possible that future research will show that professionals have the skills and experience to show a higher comfort level with such meetings.

Leadership

With the advent of new modalities through which teams interact and the need for different team members to address unique client issues, effective leadership of teams becomes critical. Leadership should be organized in such a way that team members know how to work together and how decisions will be made in the group. Ideally, anyone on the team should be able to lead the team. This is because all members have relevant expertise and everyone shares the same goal. This shifting leadership role is particularly applicable as the client's health improves. During a health crisis, a primary care clinician may be the natural leader, but during recovery leadership might shift to an occupational or physical therapist, and near the end of treatment, a social worker may take the lead. Leadership should flow from the needs of the client. This can be formal or informal. As team members learn each other's strengths and expertise, there may be shifting of leadership based on the changing needs of the client.

Again, it takes a cohesive, well-trained team to put the needs of the client first and to shift leadership as the client's needs change. Team training and discussion can help in addressing issues related to leadership and to make sure everyone understands how the team process works. The variety of leadership "tasks" that individuals can play on a team are outlined in Table 27-3. Each team member should consider which roles come most naturally, which are covered within the membership of the team, and which ones need further development.

TABLE 27-2 Effective Team Meetings

Regular meeting times	Team members need to be able to plan to attend and arrange their calendars.
Agenda	Distribute an agenda with a list of clients, preferably before the meeting (of who or what is to be discussed).
Reporting format	Identifying an order of when and how team members will report can help the meeting flow smoothly. Team members should give informative reports and ask questions when appropriate.
Goal-setting process	Determine how decisions will be made as to goals for care, identification of problems, and strategies for addressing issues. Opinions should be solicited and given.
Time frame	Allocate time for the meeting and discussion of individual clients or issues.
Assignment of tasks	Tasks should be distributed evenly and by skill set of team members. Team members should come away from the meeting with a clear idea of their assignments.
Recording of information	Documenting the plan of team decisions about care and assignments helps everyone remember what decisions were made at the meeting.
Managing distractions	There are often distractions, from cell phones to off-topic discussions. Discuss and agree as a team how best to minimize these.
Planning time for evaluation	Some time should be included periodically to evaluate team functioning, discuss process issues, and provide for team training.

(Adapted from Lach, H-W. [2007]. Team work: Interdisciplinary geriatric care. In A. D. Linton & H-W. Lach [Eds.], *Matteson & McConnell's gerontological nursing: Concepts and practice* [3rd ed., pp. 759-776]. St. Louis, MO: Saunders/Elsevier.)

TABLE 27-3 Interdisciplinary Health-Care Teams: Leadership Tasks

Organizer/Mover	Finisher	Expert
Initiate team development	Impose time constraints	Provide special expertise
Identify team tasks	Focus on outcomes (clients treated,	Offer professional viewpoint
Identify strengths and weaknesses	goals achieved)	Identify interdisciplinary client
Call meetings	Seek progress	problems
Provide structure	Show high commitment to task	Use expertise of other disciplines
Review team needs	Manage projects	Understand client needs
Identify appropriate clients		Know team's expertise and limits
Ambassador	**Diplomat**	**Supporter**
Build external relationships	Build understanding between members	Build team morale
Promote awareness of the	Negotiate	Put team members at ease
team's work	Mediate	Ensure job satisfaction
Build bridges	Facilitate decision making	Help client work with team
Show concern for external team		
environment		
Judge/Evaluator	**Process/Analyzer**	**Mediator**
Listen critically	Identify team problems	Identify member conflicts
Evaluate clinical process	Analyze team problems	Help team members find ways to
Evaluate clinical outcomes	Consult with team members	resolve conflicts
Help team reflect	Offer observations	Help implement solutions
Promote appropriate treatment	Offer potential solutions to team problems	
Act logically		
Seek truth		
Creator	**Innovator**	**Challenger**
Generate new ideas	Discover resources	Offer skepticism
Visualize new programs/projects	Identify opportunities	Look in new ways
Visualize new alliances	Transform ideas into strategy	Question accepted order
	Propose new methods	
Renewer	**Quality Controller**	**Conformer/Follower**
Observe	Check output alignment	Seek agreement
Review team performance	Act as conscience regarding team goals	Fill gaps in teamwork
Promote review of process	Inspire higher standards	Cooperate
Give feedback	Ensure team reviews outcomes	Help relationships
Mirror team's actions		Avoid challenges
		Maintain continuity
Guard	**Teacher**	**Learner**
Protect team from too much	Help new members learn the norms and	Raise questions to enhance
output	values of the team	understanding across
Protect team from too much input	Teach shared leadership skills to other	disciplines or areas
	members	Raise questions regarding need
	Reorganize members' leadership potential	for interdisciplinary input
	Teach others when to seek specialty advice	

(Adapted from Hyer, K., Flaherty, E., Fairchild, S., Botrell, M., Mezey, M., Fulmer, T., et al. [2003]. Geriatric Interdisciplinary Team Training program [GITT]: Curriculum guide. New York, NY: GITT Resource Center, New York University.)

Management of Conflicts

Conflict is a natural part of teamwork, and some of the reasons for this have been described earlier in the chapter. A healthy team is aware of this and can address conflicts by either resolving them or comfortably "agreeing to disagree" without negatively influencing the team performance. Three types of conflict are common. The first is intrapersonal conflict, where an individual experiences role conflict with other job responsibilities or with his or her role on the team. Intra-team conflicts can involve two or more team members and may develop from disagreements about care, personality differences, or different styles of working or communicating.

Inter-team conflict occurs when the team has conflict with entities outside the team, such as other provider groups.

To address conflicts, ideally issues can be discussed openly and some kind of solution reached.[14] Some issues may be best addressed by the whole group, and others should be discussed just by the parties involved. Group leaders should help facilitate appropriate ways to address and solve team problems.

Assessing Team Performance and Training

Although team members often identify challenges when working together, there are some resources for evaluating team performance. The Geriatric Interdisciplinary Team

Training (GITT) program of the John A. Hartford Foundation provides evaluation materials and training exercises to help foster good team development (see http://www.gittprogram.org). The website offers information, pre- and posttests, a team observation tool, audio-visual materials, and case studies to use for evaluation and training your team. You can ask if your interdisciplinary team has the following characteristics of effective teams outlined for GITT:[11]

- Purpose, goals, and objectives are known and agreed upon.
- Roles and responsibilities are clear.
- Communication is open, sharing, and honest. There is disagreement without tyranny and constructive criticism without personal attack.
- Team members listen to one another.
- Team members are competent, professional, and personally effective, and make appropriate contributions.
- Team members cooperate and coordinate activities. Decisions are made by consensus.
- When decisions are made, assignments are made clearly, accepted, and carried out.
- Leadership shifts, depending on the circumstances.
- Team members support each other and act as different resources for the group.
- Team members trust one another, minimize struggles for power, and focus on how best to get the job done.
- The team evaluates its own operations.

Exemplars of Interdisciplinary/Interprofessional Care Teams

To provide optimal gerontological health care, interdisciplinary teams must be effective across the continuum of care. At no time are older persons more vulnerable than when they are ill and seeking health care outside of the home environment. And, of course, the older and more frail a person is, the more vulnerable he or she is. When a team works well together, health care improves. Two examples of successful interdisciplinary team models are illustrated next: the Program of All-Inclusive Care of the Elderly (PACE) and an acute care fall-prevention team.

Program of All-Inclusive Care of the Elderly (PACE)

A community-based program called the Program of All-Inclusive Care for the Elderly (PACE) provides primary, acute, and long-term care to older adults who are frail. A central component of the PACE model is the interdisciplinary care team.[16] In the PACE model, team members include nonprofessional as well as professional health-care workers. In this study, individuals' health, functional status, and mental status were reviewed in 26 PACE programs with 3401 enrollees to determine whether the interdisciplinary teams were associated with better risk-adjusted health outcomes for survival, both short-term and long-term functional status, and urinary incontinence. All of the PACE teams included the physician; the director of nursing; the physical, occupational, and recreational therapists; the social worker; the dietician; the day center coordinator; the personal care attendant; and

the driver. Other team members included the pharmacist or the chaplain. PACE teams are large; some have had as many as 50 members, although it was more usual for subgroups of 10 team members providing current care to meet formally, at least weekly, and informally as needed. Team leaders receive facilitator training and ensure that all team members provide input at the meetings. Results of the study show that short-term and long-term functional outcomes as well as long-term urinary incontinence outcomes are better for older adults who are frail and receive interdisciplinary team care. This suggests that for PACE programs to remain successful at providing good health care, they need to focus on keeping their teams working at the performing level.

Acute Care Fall-Prevention Team

The following study description illustrates the types of interaction between team members that are necessary to produce good health care in a hospital setting. Falls are a constant threat to the well-being of older clients. Many studies have looked at the causes (of falls), and many programs have attempted to reduce fall risk. Few have succeeded. One research study, designed to introduce a structured fall-prevention program in a hospital, demonstrates the value of interdisciplinary teamwork[20] in addressing a difficult problem. The team members were identified (two physicians, two nurses, a physical therapist, an occupational therapist, and a quality manager). The group met initially to discuss the goals of the program and determine the preventive measures that would be used. They then met for 2 hours at the beginning of the study and then for short monthly meetings for the duration of the study. These members then, in turn, informed their staff about the meeting's information. The team members oriented all new hospital staff members in a 1-hour training session. No new members were introduced to the team and no members left during the project. Each team member had a well-defined role, and the procedure for identifying subjects at risk for falls was clear. Subjects identified for fall risk and their family members were immediately educated about the project. Each subject was discussed at the next team meeting. Caregivers were encouraged to attend therapy sessions. Therapeutic home visits by team members were undertaken as indicated. If deemed advisable, an ophthalmologist and an optician were added to the team for some subjects. Not surprisingly, the fall-prevention program resulted in a significant reduction in fall incidence and the relative risk of falling, regardless of the individual's level of mobility at admission. This is an excellent example of how an interdisciplinary team that functions well as a team can improve health care.

Summary

The purpose of the interdisciplinary gerontological team is to provide excellent health care. This care is improved by interdisciplinary communication of the data, analysis of the data to highlight major problems, empowerment of the team to fix any problems, and rapid adaptation of these fixes by all team members. As noted in the Geriatric Interdisciplinary Team Training Program materials, funded by the John A. Hartford

Foundation (p. 1),[11] "good teams don't just happen." Good interdisciplinary teams need to have organizational support, committed members, shared leadership, communication, and more. Evaluation and training can improve the performance of interdisciplinary teams and ultimately improve outcomes for our challenging older clients with complex health problems.

REVIEW QUESTIONS

1. Discuss the relevance of interdisciplinary/interprofessional teamwork in gerontological care settings.
2. Discuss the different types of teams and the significance of each type.
3. Identify the most common goals of health-care teams.
4. Identify and discuss the stages of team development.
5. Identify five components of behavior necessary for effective health-care teams.
6. How do "good" teams develop and maintain efficient and effective teaming?
7. Why is team communication important, and how does it relate to effective and efficient teaming?
8. When and why would the leadership role in the health-care team change?
9. Discuss conflict as it relates to teams.
10. Identify the characteristics of effective teams outlined for GITT.
11. Explain the fundamental OTR-COTA responsibilities in practice.

REFERENCES

1. American Geriatrics Society. (2012a). *Evidence supporting the effectiveness of interdisciplinary teams.* Accessed October 24, 2015. http://www.americangeriatrics.org/about_us/partnership_for_health_in_aging/interdisciplinary_team_training_statement/evidence_supporting_the_effectiveness_of_idts/.
2. American Geriatrics Society. (2012b). *Multidisciplinary competencies in care of older adult at the completion of entry-level health professional degree.* Accessed October 24, 2015. http://www.americangeriatrics.org/about_us/partnership_for_health_in_aging/multidisciplinary_competencies/.
3. Bodenheimer, T., & Yoshio Laing, B. (2007). The teamlet model of primary care. *Annals of Family Medicine, 5*(5), 457–461.
4. Bokhour, B. (2006). Communication in interdisciplinary team meetings: What are we talking about? *Journal of Interprofessional Care, 20,* 349–363.
5. Cole, M. S., Walter, F., & Bruch, H. (2008). Affective mechanisms linking dysfunctional behavior to performance in work teams: a moderated mediation study. *Journal of Applied Psychology, 93,* 945–958.
6. Drinka, T. J. K., & Clark, P. G. (2000). *Healthcare teamwork: Interdisciplinary practice and teaching.* Westport, CT: Auburn House.
7. Farrell, M. P., Schmitt, M. H., & Heinemann, G. D. (2001). Informal roles and stages of interdisciplinary team development. *Journal of Interprofessional Care, 15,* 281–295.
8. Goldsmith, J., Wittenberg-Lyles, E., Rodriguez, D., & Sanchez-Reilly, S. (2010). Interdisciplinary geriatric and palliative care team initiatives: Collaboration practices and barriers. *Qualitative Health Research, 20,* 93–104.
9. Grice, T. A., Gallois, C., Jones, F., Paulsen, N., & Callan, V. J. (2006). "We do it, but they don't": Multiple categorizations and work team communication. *Journal of Applied Communication Research, 34,* 331–348.
10. Hayward, K., Kochniuk, L., Powell, L., & Peterson T. (2005). Changes in students' perceptions of interdisciplinary practice reaching the older adult through mobile service delivery. *Journal of Allied Health, 34,* 192–198.
11. Hyer, K., Flaherty, E., Fairchild, S., Bottrell M., Mezey M., & Fulmer T. (2003). *Geriatric Interdisciplinary Team Training program (GITT): Curriculum guide.* New York, NY: GITT Resource Center, New York University.
12. Institute of Medicine. (2003). *Health professions education: A bridge to quality.* Washington, DC: National Academies Press.
13. Kane, R. A. (2002). Avoiding the dark side of geriatric teamwork. In M. D. Mezey, C. K. Cassell, M. M. Bottrell, et al. (Eds.), *Ethical patient care, a casebook for geriatric care teams* (pp. 187–207). Baltimore, MD: Johns Hopkins Press.
14. Lach, H. W. (2007). Team work: Interdisciplinary geriatric care. In A. D. Linton & H. Lach (Eds.), *Matteson & McConnell's gerontological nursing: Concepts and practice* (3rd ed., pp. 759–776). St. Louis, MO: Saunders/Elsevier.
15. Leipzig, R. M., Hyer, K., Ek, K., Wallenstein S., Vezina M. L., Fairchild S., et al. (2002). Attitudes toward working on interdisciplinary healthcare teams: A comparison by discipline. *Journal of the American Geriatrics Society, 50,* 1141–1148.
16. Mukamel, D. B., Temkin-Greener, H., Delavan, R., Peterson, D. R., Gross, D., Kunitz, S., et al. (2006). Team performance and risk-adjusted health outcomes in the Program of All-Inclusive Care for the Elderly (PACE). *The Gerontologist, 46*(2), 227–237.
17. Neill, M., Hayward, K. S., & Peterson, T. (2007). Students' perceptions of the interprofessional team in practice through application of servant leadership principles. *Journal of Interprofessional Care, 21,* 425–432.
18. O'Cathain, A., Murphy, E., & Nicholl, J. (2008). Multidisciplinary, interdisciplinary, or dysfunctional? Team working in mixed-methods research. *Qualitative Health Research, 18,* 1574–1585.
19. Ponte, P. R., Gross, A. H., Miliman-Richard, Y. J., et al. (2011). Interdisciplinary teamwork and collaboration. In C. E. Kasper (Ed.), *Annual review of nursing research* (pp. 159–191). New York, NY: Springer.
20. von Renteln-Kruse, W., & Krause, T. (2007). Incidence of in-hospital falls in geriatric patients before and after the introduction of an interdisciplinary team-based fall-intervention program. *Journal of the American Geriatrics Society, 55,* 2068–2074.
21. Rubenstein, L. Z. (2004). Comprehensive geriatric assessment: From miracle to reality. *Journal of Gerontology, 50A,* 473–477.
22. Tuckman, B. W. (1965). Developmental sequence in small groups. *Psychological Bulletin, 63*(6), 394–399.
23. Wittenberg-Lyles, E. M., Parker Oliver, D., Demiris, G., & Regehr, K. (2009). Exploring interpersonal communication in hospice interdisciplinary meetings. *Journal of Gerontological Nursing, 35,* 38–45.
24. Youngwerth, J., & Twaddle, M. (2011). Cultures of interdisciplinary teams: How to foster good dynamics. *Journal of Palliative Medicine, 14*(5), 650–654.

CHAPTER 28

Occupational Therapists as Change Agents

Kathleen Brodrick, MSOT, Althea Barry, Bsc OT

CHAPTER OUTLINE

OBJECTIVES

- Understand the nature of context and sociocultural influences in communities of aging adults
- Appreciate the challenges of daily living within marginalized populations of aging adults
- Gain an understanding of intergenerational roles and ways that occupational therapists may support related positive relationships
- Recognize the importance of relevant, meaningful, and participatory program planning with aging adults
- Understand fundamental steps in innovative program planning
- Identify qualities required to serve as an effective occupational therapy change agent in communities of aging adults

The format of this chapter differs from the others in this book in an effort to illustrate the role of occupational therapy (OT) in working with aging population groups at the community level in settings outside the traditional scope of the profession. Practical examples are used to enable students and professionals in the field to utilize what is relevant to their situations as they grapple with their roles in working with marginalized groups. A case example within a marginalized community provides an understanding of the complexity of the situations and principles in action that arise. Throughout the chapter we use examples of our OT practice in an organization called Grandmothers Against Poverty and AIDS (GAPA) to illustrate theory in practice/action.

Emerging Role of Occupational Therapy: Expansion on Practice in Traditional Settings

Occupational therapy is a long-practicing and long-serving profession with its main focus on "promoting health and well-being of people through engagement in occupation."[14,16] As such, the scope of occupational therapy is broad. Occupational therapy is concerned with people and their well-being; engagement in occupations is central to achieving this concept of well-being. There is an increasing move toward OT being practiced outside of institutions, and more and more occupational therapists are working in the places where people live. This gives the potential for the occupational therapist to utilize the person's daily environment as part of the therapeutic process. For many OT practitioners in marginalized countries, the practice of OT has found its place in environments where people's daily lives have been challenged by circumstances that threaten their well-being.[5] OT personnel in developed countries may also encounter areas in which populations are striving to survive despite economic deprivation; this chapter applies to both scenarios, where conditions of systematic marginalization are omnipresent.

Environments may be characterized by poverty, famine, violence or war, and/or epidemics such as HIV/AIDS.[1,12] In such environments the contextual stress might result in occupational deprivation of clients or groups.[14] The term *occupation deprivation* was introduced by Wilcock[15] to describe how the environment can limit the choices or opportunities afforded to people, thereby limiting their range of occupations. In such environments therapists find themselves faced by the daunting challenge of helping people to cope with the meaning and direction in their lives, their interaction with the rest of the world, and finding new ways of facing everyday challenges.

Another way in which OT is expanding beyond traditional practice is in realizing its scope in working with groups and communities and populations and not simply with individuals. This is emerging as the knowledge base of the profession is being extended to address population issues.[3] Intervening at a group or population level has become necessary due to the challenges of the limited number of occupational therapists available and the financial cost of treatment that hinders many individuals in low socioeconomic conditions from accessing OT treatment.

Occupational therapy as a profession has progressed extensively in terms of rethinking the unique contribution our profession can make. We have begun exploring concepts of occupation as a tool for promoting healthy lifestyles.[14,15] To be successful in assisting clients in these new environments, occupational therapists must become courageous in negotiating new methods for intervention/service delivery if they are to succeed in making a difference in their clients' lives. The emerging role of the occupational therapist is that of a "developer" as well as a clinician.[14]

Desirable Characteristics of an Occupational Therapist Working in Communities with Older Persons

An occupational therapist is essentially a human being who brings to his or her professionalism a unique sense of his or her character and view of the world. As with all human beings, we have characteristics we are naturally strong in and others that require some development. In this chapter we have highlighted our opinion of the characteristics that will enable an occupational therapist to practice in a community setting. It is also our opinion that where occupational therapists have a strong desire to engage in community development, they will also be driven to develop the attributes that will enhance their professional effectiveness.

Throughout the chapter, examples are used to highlight the desirable attributes of an occupational therapist working at the community level. These are not in any order of importance. Desirable attributes that occupational therapists should strive to develop are as follows. Occupational therapists should be:

- True to self
- Trustworthy and consistent
- Honest and transparent in interactions with people
- Self-aware, with the ability to set boundaries
- Courageous to challenge traditional ways of doing things
- Politically aware
- Knowledgeable about their professional limitations and able to work with other health-care professionals
- Practical, able to engage in or understand craft and other activities meaningful to people
- Empathetic and enjoy working with people, and believe in each person's potential to heal themselves
- Ready to learn and listen to other's perspectives; know when to hold their own thoughts and when to share
- Appreciative of the learning process; continuously reformulating plans as change occurs, evaluating and reflecting
- Reflective learners constantly challenging assumptions and personal worldviews
- Good at interviewing people
- Able to sum up situations quickly
- Able to promote/present projects to attract resources
- Able to anticipate necessary change to group or organizational needs
- Ethical; nonjudgmental; able to balance issues of justice, beneficence, and truthfulness; committed and reliable
- Able to creatively envision necessary change and advocate for its implementation
- Social entrepreneurs exhibiting resourcefulness, good interpersonal skills, and ability to seek opportunities
- Able to manipulate the environment to create a therapeutic setting in which healing and learning can take place, thus creating opportunities
- Flexible, knowing when to "go with the flow" and when to allow situations run their course

Developing a Project in a Marginalized Community

The next section of this chapter outlines steps taken to form a project in a marginalized community. The steps emerged from the formation of GAPA; the first author on this chapter, Kathleen Brodrick, was the founder of the organization and the second author, Althea Barry, was employed by the organization. Both are occupational therapists practicing in Cape Town, South Africa.

Figure 28-1 outlines the steps taken in the formation of GAPA; of note here is that at all stages, personal growth has an influence on and is influenced by the process. It is our opinion that the work a therapist puts into his or her own growth is vital to working in a community setting.

Step 1: Doing Personal Groundwork Before and During Community Work

First and foremost, when planning to work in communities situated in countries or cultures other than one's own, it is imperative that a therapist engage in a process of unpacking

Steps in GAPA's formation

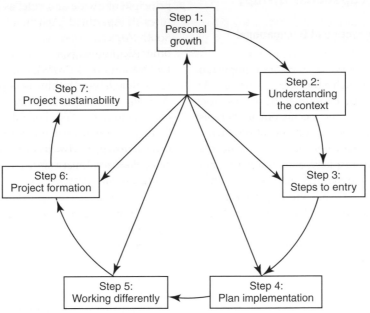

FIGURE 28-1   Diagram of the steps taken in developing projects within marginalized communities.

his or her worldview. This involves describing your assumptions about the community, how you view development, and what your goal is for your time spent in the community. What do you perceive should be changed, and how do you think the community perceives what should be changed?

The following questions may be useful in trying to unpack worldview:

- How does change begin?
- Why should change occur?
- Which aspects do not need to be changed?
- How is the process of change facilitated?

- Is it the role of the occupational therapist to be suggesting the change that should occur, listening for the change that is occurring, or merely supporting the change where necessary? The therapist has the duty of constantly reflecting on his or her role in the community to determine when input is needed or not.

It may be useful to listen to the stories of other therapists working in marginalized communities, to find out why they are working in these communities. In our experience, understanding why you want to work in a community setting gives a therapist the "edge" to make intervention successful (Box 28-1).

BOX 28-1   Roots of Passion for Occupational Therapy Practice in the Community

After graduation both authors took up placements in traditional settings, one in an old-age home and the other in a long-term psychiatric unit. Over time, through assessment and treatment of residents in the institutions, they became aware of a wider need for their services. Communities where most of their clients' families lived had no access to the services of occupational therapists. Taking up positions as community occupational therapists within the welfare sector opened up opportunities to learn about an environment that was totally different from the one in which they lived.

As one author relates:

I joined the GAPA team in 2008. My experience until then had been in mental health, a position I stretched as much as possible to work in the community. I remember one experience so vividly. An older Xhosa man had presented with his first admission to the mental health hospital. He was paranoid to

the point of not wanting to return to work. One of my first steps was to reconnect him with his family, whom he hadn't seen since admission. There we were, sitting in his little shack with his wife and their toddler, sun shining in through the holes in the roof, and this family started interacting with each other, drawing closer the bonds through playing out their roles with respect for each other. The moment just gave me goosebumps. This sensation I have experienced a few times; it happens when absolutely the right thing has happened. It's a moment when a turning point occurs in someone's life, when you look into their eyes and you know some form of hope has been ignited. The journey of gradually reintegrating into work was greatly facilitated by the subtle shift that occurred for this man on that day. This experience also brought home to me the realization that the ideal place to practice occupational therapy is in the day-to-day context in which a person lives. And so my passion for community development was cemented.

(From Barry, A. (2012). http://www.gapa.org.za/news/page/2/. Accessed October 10, 2015)

Step 2: Understanding the Context of and the Need for Occupational Therapy Intervention

Political Awareness of the Practice of Occupational Therapy

An understanding of a country's political history is important to understand the context in which a therapist is working. An occupational therapist needs to be aware of the assumptions a community may attribute to the occupational therapist given his or her cultural, economic, and educational background. Political awareness requires both an intellectual knowledge of the political atmosphere of a community and an intuitive awareness of the dynamics that exist. Furthermore, one needs to be aware of what the therapist's power position is as given by the community because of his or her background and training.

In understanding the therapist's own political position, the following questions may aid reflection:

- What is the history of my culture's interaction with this community?
- Does my educational background give me a different standing within this community?

In discovering the political atmosphere, the following are useful steps of inquiry:

- What is the history of the people who live in the community?
- Which cultural groups form part of the community, and what are their histories?
- How and why was the community formed?
- How does the community relate to the surrounding communities and population at large?
- Are there structures within the community in which people are able to voice their opinions?
- What main areas of the community can be "mapped" by taking a walk through the community?
- What are the formal and informal gathering points within the community?
- How are vulnerable groups within the community participating?

It is important to understand the power dynamic that will exist when a therapist enters a community setting. She or he may or may not be automatically given power due to his or her educational background, cultural background, socioeconomic standing, or age. These power dynamics are important to be aware of because they may influence the relationship between communities and the occupational therapist. In developing further insight regarding the therapist's own political position, the following additional question may aid reflection:

- What differences exist between my culture and that of this community?

The Context of the Authors' Practice (Grandmothers Against Poverty and AIDS) (GAPA): South Africa

South Africa is a country with a population of approximately 50.59 million people.[11] It is a country in which democracy was realized for the first time in 1994 when all citizens, regardless of race, were free to vote as equal citizens. Before the advent of democracy, the country was governed through the principle of divide and rule, as practiced through the structures of Apartheid. Apartheid meant that white and black South Africans were separated from interaction with each other. Economic gaps in the population were created by job reservation laws in which black South Africans were limited to manual labor. Within this oppressive society, black South Africans were denied many human rights, such as freedom of choice and movement. Forced separation of the population of South Africa divided along the grounds of a person's skin color created a wedge between white and black South Africans. The right of association, regardless of race, was denied to all people living in South Africa.

Khayelitsha

The authors of this chapter work in the township Khayelitsha with grandmothers who are victims of the Apartheid era with low self-esteem and limited views of their own potential for taking control of their own lives. They are now facing enormous challenges, such as caring for orphaned grandchildren and their own declining health in an environment of HIV/AIDS and poverty.

Khayelitsha is a township outside of the city of Cape Town, South Africa. The area is home to 1 million people. Poverty is rife and there is a high prevalence of HIV/AIDS. The greatest number of deaths is due to AIDS complications in the 20- to 40-year-old population group, which leaves the care of the sick, the dying, and orphans to the older women in the community.

Discovering the Need for Occupational Therapy Intervention within Khayelitsha

The first problem that confronts an occupational therapist when beginning to work in a new environment is community entry. In South Africa the results of a political system of Apartheid, with its forced segregation, violent interactions, and injustice, have led to feelings of rage and suspicion against "white" (Caucasian) people. In other countries in Africa the issue of colonization might become a factor that any Caucasian occupational therapist needs to keep in mind. Box 28-2 presents Brodrick's narrative of how the need for the organization emerged from external research.

Step 3: Steps to Entry

One of the ways in which an occupational therapist can find out where to begin working with a community is through formal research, as described earlier. Other mechanisms exist, such as promoting professional potential through the following means:

- Placement through university service learning
- Networking with organizations working within communities
- Doing an assessment of the organization's agenda
- Working through formal institutions such as hospitals
- Networking with existing projects
- Allowing individual treatment to snowball through extended family and community

BOX 28-2   Translating Evidence into Practice

In 2001 in Cape Town, knowledge about HIV/AIDS was minimal among the general population, and the stigma was high around families that were thought to harbor an affected member. Many myths surrounded the causes and sequelae of the dreaded disease rapidly took hold in South Africa. Research undertaken by Ferreira et al.[2] from the Institute of Ageing in Africa confirmed that grandmother-headed households, subjects of the research project, by their own accounting, suffered from a lack of knowledge about the disease. Households became poorer due to costs incurred in caring for the sick and job losses of bread-winners. Older women had to care for the dying and take care of the needs of orphaned children. The affected families withdrew from community life, fearing the consequences if their neighbors found out that someone was sick within their family. It was against this background that an occupational therapist was tasked to find a way to provide feedback to the community regarding the results of the research project and to design an intervention that would assist the grandmothers to cope with their lives without the support of their affected and dying children.

The key to entry is to search and listen for opportunities through interacting with people in various contexts. As an opportunity arises, a therapist needs to be ready to seize the opportunity and tap into his or her resourcefulness.

The Story of Grandmothers Against Poverty and AIDS (GAPA)

Occupational therapists are known to be innovative in their thinking, and among their strengths is the ability to analyze situations and facilitate an intervention plan to assist the community members to help themselves. This is part of creating an atmosphere of learning, in which the therapist and community engage in a process of trial and error. Box 28-3

BOX 28-3   Assessing Community Group Needs

After studying the research document outlining the plight of grandmothers who had HIV/AIDS in their families, the occupational therapist noted what the grandmothers had said in the interviews, and it became clear that their knowledge about the AIDS epidemic was sketchy and that myths about it abounded. The grandmothers also said that if they were given more money to cope with the needs of the sick they might be able to care for them better. Many thought that they might be able to start up small businesses if they were given money to do so. At the first meeting of the grandmothers with the occupational therapist, she asked the grandmothers what topics they would like to learn about in the course of the workshop series. Their collective answer was that anything would be fine. The occupational therapist realized that they had such little knowledge about the topic that they didn't know what there was to learn.

describes how the therapist engaged in this initial planning process with the community of grandmothers.

The therapist may face various challenges in forming an intervention plan. Many of these challenges arise given the experiences of the community, such as poverty and illness.

In cases of extreme hardship, the people who are in the throes of suffering the hardship may have given up all hope of ever recovering. The occupational therapist, with his or her belief that people have the capacity to heal themselves, might be, in cases such as these, the only person who is able to look beyond the difficulties and visualize a brighter future.

The occupational therapist needs to be courageous, and at the beginning of an intervention might have to take the initiative and plan a course of action without consultation or collaboration with the community. This lack of engagement of the community members in their own treatment plans goes against all of the fundamental norms of successful OT interventions. A good idea, if the occupational therapist feels uncomfortable in making all of the decisions for clients, is to seek support from another professional. This person might be a more senior occupational therapist or he or she might be a practitioner from any of the professions allied to medicine or public health who has had experience in interfacing with the clients.

Step 4: Plan Implementation

Planning of community interventions is often the most difficult process in the whole treatment plan. At this stage the occupational therapist often is working "blind" and has to rely on his or her outsider's experience and knowledge of the situation, which could be a new environment completely unlike any previous places of work. Making contact and getting people in the community to participate in the planned intervention are the first hurdles that will have to be crossed.

In the case of the planned intervention in Khayelitsha, the occupational therapist understood that there was stigma associated with HIV/AIDS from the research report, TV reports, and media articles. This meant she had to take specific steps to get around the stigma but still attract grandmothers to the workshops that she had planned (Box 28-4).

Accessing Resources within the Community

The ongoing process of planning intervention should be matched with accessing appropriate resources needed within the community. When working in underresourced communities,

BOX 28-4   Addressing Sensitive Topics

Workshops that were advertised as being about HIV/AIDS would have been boycotted because at the time, anyone having anything to do with "the dreaded unknown disease" would have been stigmatized by other people who saw that they were going to such workshops. The occupational therapist put up notices in the local language in hospitals and clinics and sent invitations to senior citizens' clubs inviting all grandmothers who were the current heads of their households to attend. The topic was advertised as "learning to live life more effectively."

where the resources are scarce and the needs are great, resources that are accessed should be used in the most effective and efficient way.[10] At all times the therapist is required to consider what is ethically appropriate; it is advised that a therapist be aware of and reflect on the ethical code of practice outlined by his or her affiliated university and/or professional body. The ultimate focus should be on facilitating resourcefulness of the community rather than simply transferring resources.[4] For example, the resources needed might be a meeting place, educators, and refreshments. It is imperative that the resources are culturally acceptable, easily accessible, and familiar to the community; these considerations relate to the ethical consideration of beneficence, or acting in the best interests of the clients.[10,16] In order that communities are not threatened, for example, this can be achieved through accessing resources in the preferred language of the community. To access the acceptable resources, the knowledge and networks of the community should be tapped into, thereby working collaboratively to do a needs assessment.[10] Sometimes the target community group is not aware of the resources and solutions available to the group. In this case the therapist will use his or her knowledge and networks to provide the best fit of resources that she or he thinks the community will find acceptable (Box 28-5).

BOX 28-5 Collaborating with Other Community Groups

In the Grandmothers Against Poverty and AIDS (GAPA) case, several community-based organizations (such as non-governmental organizations working in various areas such as food gardening, bereavement, home nursing, human rights, and HIV/AIDS education) were approached to provide support for the program that was about to take place for grandmothers who were affected by the AIDS epidemic. The therapist phoned these organizations, outlining her program, and asked whether they had anything to offer. One organization offered their premises on the grounds of a community health center, and others provided experts who were able to offer workshops in the local dialect. All organizations were happy about the choice of venue, as the venue didn't affect or disrupt their activities in the area.

The site for the GAPA workshops was therefore chosen in a community health-care facility for the following reasons: It formed a common meeting place for the target community group, and it was a public site and as such not regarded as belonging to any particular site (Khayelitsha is divided into sites, each with its own community governing body), enabling grandmothers from all sites to feel welcome without needing permission to access the venue. Occupational therapists who intend to work in community settings, especially where there is a mixture of traditional and official governing structures, have to be aware of the power dynamics on entering. This awareness can be gained by interviewing community members positioned in different areas of governance, such as traditional leaders and city officials. For example, in Khayelitsha the sites are governed by culturally appointed leaders and elected officials.

Examples of Occupational Therapy Attributes in Action
Honesty and Transparency

Forming working relationships with community stakeholders requires honesty and transparency regarding what the occupational therapist's agenda is in the community. This understanding is achieved by building trust through consistency, using formal and informal meetings/gatherings to constantly reevaluate the agenda and the roles of various parties.

It is important for the therapist to constantly evaluate and reflect on the process. This includes being aware of the assumptions and feelings of the community with regard to the means of entry used by the occupational therapist. For example, people may have a very strong set of assumptions about previous experience with research projects. They may have heard that they will be paid for information or receive goods in exchange for participation in a research project. They may have apprehensions about the organization that is your "vehicle" to community entry. If, for example, a local organization that cares for disabled children acts as the introductory body, people in the area where you begin work may think that your interest is only with disabled children and not with older people. They might also think that they will somehow be likened to disabled children if they interact with you. Be aware of when and how you clarify these assumptions and about the power dynamics at play when you are introduced with both professional and organizational power.

Professionalism

Acting in a professional manner while being engaged in these community dynamics also means being true to yourself. People in any community are sensitive to how a professional interacts with people and the attitude that the professional projects. In our experience, the community evaluates the therapist in various situations, constantly questioning if he or she is a "real" person who trusts and respects the community and is willing to remain committed versus someone with a hidden agenda.

The therapist should be aware that she or he will always remain an outsider in the community but should portray openness to constantly learning the culture of the community. Learning to greet members of the community in a culturally respectful manner goes a long way toward projecting the image that the occupational therapist is prepared to try to become part of the community.

Facilitating

As occupational therapists, we believe in the potential of each person to change his or her circumstances. We are trained to recognize this hidden potential and use the person's attributes to change his or her circumstances. It is important to hold fast to this belief because it will help to keep a therapist focused when the community members challenge him or her to assist and help them in various ways.

The "will-to-please syndrome" within a therapist may be a stumbling block when providing intervention in a community setting. Therapists who are reflective in their work will recognize that they may have fallen into the trap of wanting to please the community by "helping" in any way possible. Lorenzo, et al[6] reflect that it is not necessary for a practitioner to have all the answers to poverty and development. The ultimate result of pleasing the community is that the therapist's role becomes defined entirely by the community, and eventually the community members will think that they are dependent on the therapist for certain things, defeating the vision of sustainability and empowerment. To prevent a culture of dependency, an honest outlook is needed, and a consistent set of boundaries will go a long way toward preventing misunderstandings. When working cross culturally, the will to please might be even more difficult if the clients regard the therapist as part of an ethnic group that is wealthier or carries more authority than they do. In a situation like this, the community might unwittingly try to force the occupational therapist into acting in the manner that exhibits authority and easy access to resources.

In South Africa some older people, who had spent their entire adult lives being told what they could do and where they could live by a political system that robbed them of their freedom to take initiative, had become apathetic and had internalized the thought that they were not masters of their own destiny. The older people brought up under these conditions were very likely to adopt the attitude of "You do it for me; I can't." The danger is that an occupational therapist might fall for this kind of helplessness and unwittingly feed back into the "I'm helpless syndrome." Workshops, which normally target young people, might be a novel idea for older people. Care has to be taken in preparing workshops for older people that the workshops are not equated with "going to school," which most definitely is perceived as for children only (Box 28-6).

BOX 28-6 Facilitating Group Conflict Resolution

One day GAPA received a large donation of material; grandmothers were taught to sew with this material. Those who managed to sell their goods were met with envy and gossip from those who were less successful. The occupational therapist was left with an uncomfortable situation: Should she resolve this conflict—should she be providing more resources when none existed? It seemed that the grandmothers were requiring this of her. In a communal culture, it is viewed that each person should benefit, and it is commonly said that resources must be for "everyone or no one."[3] The therapist held on to her belief that people have the potential to help themselves.

Once the therapist realized the corner she was backing into, she held a meeting with the grandmothers. The attributes of communal problem solving were used to bring about a solution in which the grandmothers formed a management committee to address conflicts that were arising. Grandmothers with grievances could now approach the committee for communal conflict resolution.

Understanding Older People in the Community

The grandmothers or older people who are incorporated in GAPA fall outside of the strict South African definition of older person. Many developed countries define an older person as someone who is of the chronologic age of 65 years.[16] The World Health Organization (WHO) recognizes that this strict definition is not applicable to the African context, in which traditionally a person over the age of 50 years is recognized as an elder. Socially constructed factors other than chronologic age are recognized in Africa, such as a loss of roles that might accompany physical decline.[16]

In the context of the GAPA organization, it was identified by the occupational therapist that it was this strict definition of "older person" as a man of the pensionable age of 65 years or woman at the age of 60 years[9] that was creating a gap in services for grandmothers. The majority of grandmothers at GAPA are 50 years old. They are recognized as elders by their community, and although their decline in physical health would usually lead to a loss of roles, they are now reentering the roles of mother and bread-winner for their grandchildren due to the loss of their children to AIDS. However, their role as elders is not recognized by the government because they are not eligible for state grants or pensions. However, these ages are under review by government and the plan is to increase the pensionable age of men to 60 years, associated with an increase in life expectancy (p. 214).[12] Grandchildren and children brought up in townships that have access to TV, modern schooling, and Western influences also have lost the respect that older people had drummed into them in their youth. Some older people find this lack of respect bewildering and the mutual understanding between grandmothers and grandchildren to be an ever-widening gap. Other grandmothers just grumble about "the youth of today" and the challenges they face, such as teenage pregnancies, drug use, and failing education grades. In the work later done by the second author, this intergenerational gap was addressed by guiding the grandmothers through reflecting on their own childhoods and matching the "then and now."[7]

Newly qualified and young occupational therapists should guard against being viewed by the older person as someone who doesn't respect their elders and ignores cultural norms. Occupational therapists need to be mindful of what sort of behavior is accepted by the older person, and some understanding of cultural norms is required (Box 28-7). What better way of forging bond with older individuals than to ask them about their culture and their expectations? For there to be a mutual understanding, it is also a good idea for the occupational therapist to explain to the older person that she or he does things differently in his or her family, that the older person should not feel offended if the occupational therapist unknowingly exhibits a breach of good manners, and to please let the occupational therapist know if the individual feels offended.

Becoming Aware of Assumptions about Older People

Many times we hold assumptions about older people based on how the media portrays older people as or through public

Learning Appropriate Intergenerational Collaboration

As a young occupational therapist, the second I entered GAPA I was aware of the age and cultural difference between myself and the grandmothers. At times it was difficult to know how and when to address this apparent gulf between us. It became clear that this could be addressed through daily opportunities. It was a steep learning curve, but with the mutual understanding between myself and the grandmothers that I was still learning about their culture, I was fortunate to be gently and patiently "coached" by the grandmothers.

I remember a meeting in which the grandmothers were thanking me for my work. After the first speaker had said their thanks, I immediately felt that I needed to stand up and reciprocate. However, I was gently told to sit down and wait for my turn; the elders had not completed their turn to talk yet.

narratives of older people. As therapists enter a community of older people, they will need to be aware of some of their assumptions. For example, there is no truth to an anecdotal belief that to become old is to enter a phase of second childhood. Therapists should adopt the attitude that there is much to learn from the life experiences of older people; they have lived through many eras and along the way have picked up valuable life lessons.

It is rare to find an occupational therapist who is fluent in all languages and dialects spoken by clients. Often when people don't understand what one is saying, they tend to nod in agreement and leave one feeling that whatever he or she has said has been accepted. The new occupational therapist is then astonished and a little hurt when the clients don't follow what it is that the occupational therapist thinks they have agreed on after the dialogue. The older clients are left feeling confused when the OT seems annoyed that they haven't done what the occupational therapist thought was agreed. At the risk of feeling foolish, it is better that the occupational therapist ask one of the clients who speaks the occupational therapist's language fluently to confirm to the older people in their own language all that the occupational therapist thinks has been agreed. Language to be used when working with older people should be carefully considered. Generally speaking, the use of slang or jargon should be avoided because most of it may be beyond the comprehension of older people. Mother tongue, which is the language that the older person speaks at home and is most comfortable with, has to be used if the person is to understand fully the message that the occupational therapist is trying to communicate. In the case of an occupational therapist working cross culturally, interpreters are only useful to a point. When dealing with sensitive topics and when counseling an older person, it is better to refer to a like-minded professional to conduct counseling or for educational workshops to use experts in the field who speak the same language as the older person. However, the "experts"

must be cautioned to steer away from using the professional jargon of their trade, which can be just as misunderstood as someone speaking in a foreign language.

Interacting with Older People of a Different Culture
All of the norms of respectful communication with and behavior toward older people apply in whatever practice the occupational therapist finds him- or herself. In some cultures there are prescribed ways of addressing one's elders. Calling an older person by his or her first name might be a modern Western way of speaking to an older person, but it is not acceptable in developing countries. When in doubt as to how to address an older person, the occupational therapist should use the individual's surname and preface it with "Mr." or "Mrs." In Africa the indigenous people have many names, usage of which changes depending on their marital status, where they are domiciled, and whom they are speaking to. In a country, such as South Africa, where many people have adopted Western names so that their employers can address them easily, older people may expect that Caucasian people will automatically use the English name, such as Gladys or Mary, when addressing them. If a new occupational therapist, without thinking, uses the easiest name available to address the older person, the occupational therapist is regarded as being in the same category as previous employers who made no effort to be respectful toward the person. If the occupational therapist is much younger than the client, it would be a good idea to seek advice from someone familiar with respectful forms of address before embarking on a conversation.

Body language when speaking with someone also is very important. New occupational therapists going into unfamiliar territory are advised to learn to watch their own body language and try not to show feelings of disgust or uneasiness when faced with, for example, unhygienic or distressing home conditions they might encounter. They need to be aware that eating habits might be different from theirs and quite acceptable to the client population. Only once the occupational therapist has forged a strong link with clients and there is mutual respect can the occupational therapist afford to turn down something that he or she is expected to eat or drink (Box 28-8).

Bridging Cultural Norms

At one of the first workshops held in the new center, the occupational therapist asked the grandmothers to design a menu for the participants. The occupational therapist and the grandmothers went to the market to buy the ingredients. At the market the occupational therapist was nauseated to see tripe (offal) hanging on a fence and sheep heads on a table for sale. The grandmothers were thrilled that they could buy the delicacies for the meeting. On further investigation the occupational therapist discovered that although the meat was kept in non-hygienic conditions, it was in fact the most nutritious meal that most of the grandmothers would get to eat that month.

Culturally Assigned Places of Interaction: The Ritual of Eating

Sitting down and having a meal together is a very important part of forging relationships with clients. In a communal society, eating is a mainly social event with the view of sharing food and discussion.[9,13] The method of eating is also very important. Many people do not eat using the generally accepted Western way of eating with a knife and fork. A new occupational therapist organizing a meal for clients is advised to get the older clients to take over the organization of the meal and fit in with what the older client does. The occupational therapist needs to make sure that she or he is not isolated from the group by insisting on using certain utensils. The occupational therapist should make sure that he or she gets no special treatment during the meal and is not treated as the honored guest. The goal of integrating with the community's ways of interacting should be maintained (Box 28-9). If the occupational therapist is younger than others at the meal, she or her should maintain a respectful demeanor. Showing that he or she would rather be included as one of the group displays a willingness to engage clients at their own comfort level.

Step 5: Beginning Work and Thinking Differently

The best plans are those that can easily be modified to suit a sudden change. "Going with the flow" is a good attitude to adopt alongside a thoroughly professional approach to planning and execution of aims and objectives that have been set for a particular session. More time for reflection than planned for might be needed, and more time for individual responses might be needed when conducting educational sessions for older people. The therapist must be open to his or her own learning in workshop sessions and prepared to switch ownership of the teaching at certain times in the workshop. Communal communities are characterized by the principle of interdependency; the recognition of that principle enables a therapist to view the community members as a resource in development. Once a therapist embraces this principle, he or

---

| BOX 28-9 | Facilitating Intergenerational, Cross-Cultural Valuing of Group Members |

At a meal organized to celebrate the first year of operating in the new GAPA hall, the grandmothers arranged the tables so that the occupational therapist sat at a special table with some invited guests. The table was the only one with a tablecloth and knives and forks. All other tables had no cloths and only spoons. The occupational therapist asked that the arrangement be changed so that everyone ate with spoons, and the occupational therapist and guests were interspersed with the grandmothers. In this way the occupational therapist hoped to signal that the celebration was to honor and congratulate the grandmothers as much as the occupational therapist for completing a successful year.

---

she will realize that is not necessary for the therapist to have all the answers. For example, when an education workshop is being held, recipients might know more about a particular topic than the therapist. In this case key recipients might be needed as facilitators of the flow of knowledge for the flow of knowledge from one participant to the others. The therapist also needs to be aware of when it might be necessary to call in the assistance of another professional when the therapist is out of his or her practice depth and cannot assist the client.

Box 28-10 describes what happened at the first workshops planned and implemented by the occupational therapist and how the workshops resulted in the birth of the GAPA organization.

Step 6: Project Formation
Challenges of Sustainability and Role Definition

One of the challenges of working in poor communities is that occupational therapists often have to find their own resources. This often means more than acquiring goods so that activities can be conducted. The occupational therapist, by virtue of the fact that he or she is a university graduate, has access to the electronic media and also can exert pressure on authority by virtue of his or her professionalism, and can do far more to promote a cause than can an older person who has not been exposed to "modern know-how." The occupational therapist is also probably able to drive a car, which allows him or her access to a wider community than the one where the older person lives. For these reasons it falls to the community occupational therapist to locate and procure resources on behalf of the older people with whom he or she works. However, at all times the occupational therapist should be doing his or her utmost to seek out and find ways that the community members can eventually source their own materials.

During GAPA's formation the grandmothers had the expectation that the government would "give" them money if a white person asked; this belief was influenced by the political system that they had lived under for the previous 40 years when the government dictated what they could and could not have. The occupational therapist understood the rules and regulations pertaining to the formation of organizations within the community and also had a wider understanding of the new government policies than did the grandmothers. In this case it would have been easier for the occupational therapist to fulfill the requirements of constitution writing and fund-raising, but that would not have fed into her aim of empowering grandmothers to become their own agents of change. The rule then follows that whatever course the occupational therapist pursues on behalf of the community members, members of the community must agree and accompany the occupational therapist every step of the way. This incorporation of community in the development of projects is useful to add to any plan or timeline for a project.

Community Political Structures

In many communities there are levels of organization within the community. Occupational therapists entering communities

---

BOX 28-10 Respectfully Addressing Unmet Needs

The workshop series began with a local expert discussing the signs, symptoms, and causes of HIV infection and the consequences of AIDS. At the beginning the participants were very quiet and subdued. This all changed when one grandmother stood up and, amid floods of tears, related her story about the death of two of her daughters and the illness of a third. Immediately the atmosphere changed as others realized that almost all the other people in the room were suffering as much as they were. The groundswell of emotion bonded those people together and as a unit they shared their grief by singing hymns.

This workshop was repeated three times, with more and more grandmothers arriving as the word spread quietly throughout the community. The therapist could not speak the local dialect but realized that some of the grandmothers were in desperate need of counseling and further emotional support.

She sought the services of a social worker who was able to provide individual counseling services. The occupational therapist offered a psychosocial group meeting to grandmothers self-identified as having lost a family member recently or nursing a terminally ill family member. Group work began once a week for 10 women.

The occupational therapist prepared the venue and prepared the activity, which was to be patchwork.[1] Support items such as fabric, needles, thread, and scissors were all donated after the occupational therapist addressed a church group in an affluent part of town about the plight of grandmothers living in poverty in the area where she was working.

The grandmothers spoke little English, and so the occupational therapist presence was there as an organizer and "needle threader."

The grandmothers eventually took care of all emotional support issues and all methods of coping with grief among themselves. A well-bonded group was formed, and week by week their healing was obvious.

Toward the end of the workshop series the participants asked the occupational therapist what was going to happen to them once the course was over and the sponsors of the workshop withdrew. The occupational therapist asked what they wanted to happen. Their spokesperson stood up and said that the workshops had been a great success and they wanted all grandmothers to benefit in the way that they had. To do this, they said that the occupational therapist should stay with them and they would find a place to operate from. Furthermore, the occupational therapist was to ask the government for money to continue running the workshops. By this stage the occupational therapist was so inspired by the change in the grandmothers who had done the course and had seen how powerful the medium of peer support was that she agreed to return in the next year to extend the workshops and support group further. The occupational therapist asked that the grandmothers form a committee that she could work with toward drawing up a constitution and forming a registered nonprofit organization. The name of the organization was to be Grandmothers Against Poverty and AIDS (GAPA; www.gapa.org.za).

---

that are foreign to them would be wise to make finding out the pecking order within that community a priority. In some communities there are community-appointed leaders who would need to be informed of or grant permission for an activity so that it could proceed unimpeded. Sometimes there is tension between traditional leadership and modern imposed political systems. Older people in communities where traditional leaders exist are more likely to respect the old system of doing things than the modern way. In such situations, an occupational therapist could find a way to be introduced to the community leadership and prepare a presentation of his or her intended program. Similarly, if an occupational therapist intends to conduct research that involves door-to-door questions, he or she needs to let the entire community know, through the leadership, what the idea is behind the research and what will happen with the information gathered. This might be a lengthy process because deliberations often are held in the community to decide whether to allow the community members to participate in the research project or not (Box 28-11).

Step 7: Project Sustainability

An occupational therapist is but one person. However, from the moment that an occupational therapist forms a relationship with a person, she or he should be asking the question "Am I preparing this person to resume control over his or her own life?" In the case of working with groups of people who have a collective vision, the occupational therapist needs to identify potential leaders or allow potential leaders to emerge within the group to assume positions to make sure that the group works toward achieving the collective vision.

The most successful community programs are ones that an occupational therapist can eventually walk away from knowing that the people in the community will take over all aspects of the program. Furthermore, the program will continue to grow when community members have the capacity to meet new challenges that arise in their community. Communities that are richly supplied with professions allied to medicine, such as social workers, physiotherapists, dietitians, and speech therapists, can provide professional support to occupational therapists and services to the community members. However, in under resourced areas, occupational therapists will learn that they must find a way to provide services that fall outside of their normal practice or, if possible, refer to other practitioners. Occupational therapists who find themselves working alone in community settings would be well advised to make sure that they are in contact with a senior occupational therapist with whom they can have a regular supervision session in which they can psychologically unload and discuss what they have

---

Effectively Spanning Racial Differences

In the new year the occupational therapist entered a new community chosen by the committee of grandmothers and spent the first 2 months getting to know the community and allowing the community members to overcome their suspicions as to why a "white" person was in their area. After 2 months of running patchwork classes every day, a second workshop series was held. At the same time the committee of grandmothers met once a week for an update on the situation in their area of the township. Psychosocial support groups were formed using the committee members as facilitators and their homes in different suburbs of the township as venues. The occupational therapist sourced a small wooden building that was set up as the GAPA headquarters where used clothing was sold to raise funds. A third workshop series was held in a school hall that was sourced by one of the grandmothers who was particularly worried about the number of AIDS-affected families in her area. That workshop attracted 80 participants, and the occupational therapist realized that this was not ideal because each person needed follow-up and GAPA was unable to service all the participants' needs for ongoing support and education. All further workshops were put on hold while the occupational therapist investigated the legality of obtaining a piece of land that the elders in the community said that GAPA could have to build a community hall. The occupational therapist, accompanied by one of the elders, visited the local authorities to discover, much to the incomprehension of the elder, that the land had to be purchased and also rezoned. This process took a year. Further fund-raising resulted in a multipurpose hall being built, which was to be used for all future GAPA activities.

---

experienced in their workplace. Working with people who have to deal with sickness and death of loved ones, such as in a setting where HIV infection and AIDS are rife, can be a shocking and emotionally draining experience. To assist clients through traumatic periods in their lives, occupational therapists need to be empathetic and not so emotionally involved with the problem or so distressed by the situation that they lose their ability to act in a professional manner. A professional manner does not mean that the occupational therapist is forbidden from shedding tears with the bereaved people or attending funeral services with clients. Attending religious ceremonies is a personal decision that the occupational therapist has to make based on her or his own beliefs and culture. Gestures of support during bereavement are dependent on the cultural practice of the bereaved and those offering comfort. The occupational therapist is unable to ignore the occurrence of death within the community when working in the midst of poverty and sickness because death is a common occurrence where HIV/AIDS is prevalent. New occupational therapists should seek support from more experienced occupational therapists to assist them to decide on the best way for them to cope with the inevitability of death.

Generic Activities in Community Development

When working in communities there are several generic activities that an occupational therapist will have to manage. Examples include home visits, counseling, dealing with abuse, and health promotion through advertising the causes necessary to promote the well-being of the community. In addition, occupational therapists may find themselves involved in organizational development to ensure sustainability of the project.

Working in People's Homes and Communities

It is a privilege and an honor to be invited into someone's home and to meet their friends and neighbors. Occupational therapists have to become part of the community in which they work without losing any of the professional know-how to be the most effective change agents that they can be. Becoming part of the community requires political awareness. Political awareness is a sense of how communities and groups of people are structured and the subtle ways in which they interact. Much of this can be gained by observation of and involvement in community meetings. Political awareness is also about acknowledging the part that you play and the influence of your presence as you become part of the community. Maintaining your professional "edge" is achieved through constant reflection and unpacking of assumptions. Occupational therapists who work in developing communities require deepened listening (active listening) and analytical skills. Political awareness is also about knowing which battles are your own and which can be community driven, and when and where to choose your battles, but always being ready. Political awareness requires enhanced skills in mobilization of key people and constant readiness to take action when the opportunity arises. Becoming part of the community will always have one reminding point: You might be accepted but you are never fully part of the community. This awareness drives program development to constantly be paced with the community and ownership to be given to the community (Box 28-12).

Sometimes the situation might arise where the participants in a program initiated by the occupational therapist take public ownership of the achievements that the occupational therapist has worked hard to achieve. This might evoke feelings of annoyance in the occupational therapist that she or he is not receiving the prestige (kudos) the occupational therapist feels is due to him or her for having started the program. Contrary to the feeling evoked by having one's achievement discounted by the lack of any recognition for positive changes that are taking place, this is in fact a sign of success for the occupational therapist. The success of a community intervention can be measured by the extent to which participants take ownership of the process.[1,8] An occupational therapist should be prepared to let go of projects that the community takes ownership of and move on to address emerging opportunities/needs. It is important to remember to focus on the "agent" part of "agents of change" and not the "change" part. As an occupational therapist, you are not the "change"; you are the "agent," and as an agent you move from

BOX 28-12	Sensitivity in Collaborative Problem Solving

The occupational therapist at GAPA found that it was impossible to visit people individually in their homes. Apart from the language difficulties, there were far too many grandmothers affected by HIV/AIDS to visit them individually. The occupational therapist discussed the problem of too many grandmothers wanting to be visited and comforted in their homes with the committee members. After brainstorming with the grandmothers it was decided that they would each invite 10 grandmothers, whom they knew from observation and gossip in their suburbs had HIV/AIDS in their families, to their home for a meeting. Support groups were thus set up in each of the areas where the 10 grandmothers on the committee lived. Psychosocial issues were tackled by the groups. At the same time, the occupational therapist provided scraps of material to each group so that they too had a means of recruiting affected grandmothers that would not have attended any group that had HIV/AIDS as its topic of conversation. Once at a group, however, they would soon realize that all their peers were in the same predicament as they were regarding the epidemic. The occupational therapist continued to support the group leaders by holding a meeting once a week in which the group leaders could discuss any problems that they encountered with their group members.

BOX 28-13	Maximizing and Supporting Community Group Strengths

At GAPA, a core of grandmothers showed themselves to be excellent counselors. These were the grandmothers to whom other grandmothers referred visitors. Their talent was utilized by the occupational therapist whenever someone in an emotional state arrived on the doorstep. However, in a couple of cases the grandmothers referred to the occupational therapist for advice when an intervention was needed that was outside their scope of expertise. The occupational therapist was able to liaise with the state social workers on a professional level, and she was able to refer clients to psychiatric clinics and hospitals for medical treatment.

one area of change to another and maybe back again; as an agent you are invited to make changes by the community. Political awareness is about recognizing these invitations, which may come through formal and informal means. It is also useful to understand the theory of change so that an occupational therapist can recognize and be comfortable with the type of change that is occurring.

Counseling across Age and Cultural Barriers

Young occupational therapists are often regarded by older people as being of the same status as their grandchildren. Older people are also sometimes frightened by the ability of younger people to grasp all the new technologies seemingly effortlessly. Older people wouldn't unburden themselves to their grandchildren and so would find it very difficult to accept counseling from a young occupational therapist. However, a new occupational therapist understanding how she or he might superficially appear to an older person would be able to source another professional, such as a social worker or older occupational therapist, to counsel the older person. Another source that is worth accessing is the older person's spiritual guide, such as a minister of religion or wise person in the village. The occupational therapist might be invited to intervene in the situation in consultation with the person who has conducted the counseling. However, the occupational therapist might be excluded from the personal problem and should not take this as a slur on his or her professional competence. New occupational

therapists sometimes feel that they should take on all the problems that they come across, the ones they can help with and the ones for which that they can do nothing. It would be a very short time before such an occupational therapist becomes overwhelmed by all the problems and retreats from the situation, feeling that he or she is a failure. Occupational therapists should always remember that they are "agents of change." This means that they, personally, don't have to solve every problem. They need to use their expertise to facilitate the process of people finding their own solutions, and sometimes this is done by introducing the person to a more experienced health-care professional (Box 28-13).

Educational Workshops for Older People

In developing countries the educational system has in the past years been unavailable in many cases to women, and school attendance often has not been compulsory for men or women.

Lack of education or fragmented education has resulted in some older people being illiterate. In a fast-moving world characterized by complex technology, older people might hide their educational shortcomings and withdraw from the ongoing educational opportunities that might be available to them.

The drawback to any young health professional attempting to conduct an educational workshop for older people is that he or she would use the professional jargon of the discipline. Furthermore she or he is not privy to the wealth of experience by virtue of the number of years lived that older people have. The danger is that this knowledge is discounted and overlooked. Ignoring the life experience of older people is tantamount to suggesting that only the occupational therapist knows anything worth knowing about a particular subject. When workshops about health matters are to be conducted, the occupational therapist should be aware of some of the myths and preconceptions that the participants might have on the topic. Information presented in the workshop should be factual and as much as possible devoid of all technical language. Occupational therapists conducting cross-cultural workshops cannot possibly know all the cultural nuances of

BOX 28-14   Facilitating Leadership Roles

Once the building was completed, GAPA immediately began to start monthly workshop series covering all the topics of the first workshop. To do this, some grandmothers were identified as potential workshop facilitators and trained to run workshops on a particular topic. Not only did this turn out to be the best way to reach out to more grandmothers, but all new grandmothers who were brought low by their circumstances were able to look up to role models. The fact that all facilitator grandmothers had experienced loss, death, and stigmatization added weight to the idea that "there is life after AIDS." The support groups grew in number all over the township, and GAPA became known as an organization consisting of dynamic, informed, helpful grandmothers.

BOX 28-15   Supporting Community-Group Advocacy Efforts

At an awareness workshop for the new Older Person's Bill that was being rewritten in South Africa, grandmothers were introduced to the then-current legislation regarding older people in South Africa. They were also told that there were to be public hearings to which older people were invited to give their point of view to the politicians who were reviewing the bill in its draft form. The occupational therapist asked the grandmothers what they wished to share with the politicians. She then wrote out all the points made and helped choose two grandmothers who could read English and would be spokespersons for the group. The occupational therapist arranged transport and an escort for the grandmothers so that their passage to Parliament was as easy as possible. The two presentations were cited by all present as the two most outstanding contributions made at the public hearings.

the workshop recipients. It is for these reasons that, to make workshops as meaningful as possible, peer educators should be used where feasible. The occupational therapist needs to train the workshop facilitators in the technical aspects of the subject and the method of conducting workshops so that there is maximum interaction between all participants (Box 28-14).

Promoting the Community

In order for a project to continue to grow and be effective, the participants need to believe in themselves and also get others to believe in them. If older people believe that they are able to maintain their own projects and are able to convince others that they are worthy of support in their ventures, then their programs are likely to continue to exist and to grow.

Older people often begin to feel that they are living in a bewildering place that they are slowly losing track of as they continue to age. The fast pace of new developments, the rapid pace of the electronic media, and the new ways of doing business may be bewildering and frightening. It might be easier for the older person to give up trying to keep up with the fast pace and become introverted and harbor feelings of alienation. Ultimately these feelings lead to helplessness and an unhealthy retreat from society. However, it is not impossible to teach older people to use electronic media, new banking systems, and other modern inventions. Many older people enjoy a new lease on life when they are taught how to use a computer and how to write electronic letters. Many older people have been able to keep in touch with friends and family all over the world once introduced to email. Sometimes the occupational therapist has to act as an intermediary between the older person and the rest of the world. It is, however, a good idea to draw the line at actually speaking on behalf of the older person if he or she is able to speak. Preparing and role-playing situations to encourage the person to feel confident to stand up and speak on his or her own behalf are very effective, both for getting the message across and also for boosting the self-esteem of the older person (Box 28-15).

In matters of national importance, marginalized people might feel that their opinion is of no value. It is a good idea

for a new occupational therapist to find out what the country's policies are with regard to older people. If policies are available, then informing older people that they have rights under the law of the country might raise their self-esteem. Encouraging older people to exercise their civic rights contributes to making them feel like valued members of society.

Advocacy often involves promoting causes on behalf of another. An occupational therapist working in an underdeveloped community has the responsibility to show older people how to express their needs, wants, and rights. Occupational therapists might have to actually do the advocacy work because new occupational therapists probably have the ability to use and make all electronic media and modern communication methods work for any particular cause. In situations where older people have not enjoyed basic human rights or are not used to having a political voice, it is incumbent on the occupational therapist to facilitate situations where the older people can express thoughts, needs, rights, ideas, and so forth in the relevant forum (Box 28-16).

BOX 28-16   Nurturing Community-Group Public Relations

The occupational therapist at GAPA saw an opportunity to advance the story of the grandmothers' successes in overcoming the problems associated with HIV/AIDS. She arranged for a local photographic artist and a journalist to meet the grandmothers with a view to inspiring the artists to help the grandmothers advertise their successes to the world. The grandmothers and artists worked together to set up a photographic exhibition in Cape Town. The show was a success, and steps were taken to produce a book that will be available worldwide.

Abuse

Elder abuse is a known phenomenon worldwide. Abuse of older people happens in institutions and in communities. It is an issue that is difficult to deal with because in many cases the older person is afraid to speak out against the abuse, fearing worse consequences than what she or he experiences at the hands of their abuser.

As an occupational therapist becomes well known in a community, it is likely that she or he will become privy to the secrets of the community. Abuse of older persons is one such secret. In small and crowded communities, people get to know what is happening in their neighbor's homes due to the nearness of homes and the interwoven pattern of life. Reporting cases of abuse to the social workers of a community is ideal, but this is not always the correct decision to make for a particular community situation. If the social worker is an active member of the community, she or he would be the most desirable person to sort out the problem. If reporting the abuse means that strangers who make rash statements and rash decisions that are contrary to the older person's wishes come into the house, the occupational therapist needs to consider carefully what course of action to take. In most communities there is a hierarchy of authority or civic groups that could intervene in a sensitive way. These are the people to whom the occupational therapist should refer the problem. However in a case of criminal intent toward the older person, the police must be called immediately (Box 28-17).

Organizational Development of GAPA

One of the key principles of GAPA was that it should be an organization for and by grandmothers. The occupational therapist's focus was on facilitating development of the organization rather than engineering development interventions for the grandmothers. To this end, from the beginning the founding occupational therapist formed a management committee of herself and grandmothers chosen by the grandmothers participating in the initial workshops. As the

---

BOX 28-17 Supporting Effective Crisis Intervention

When one of the grandmothers stopped coming into the GAPA center and the occupational therapist asked the others what had become of her, they reported that her husband had banned her from coming to GAPA. He had beaten her and accused her of talking to others about "his business." The occupational therapist advised the grandmothers to think about what they could do, realizing that she was helpless in this situation. The grandmothers formed a delegation and went to see the local management committee, where they outlined the problem. The local committee went to the house of the abused grandmother and spoke to the husband "man to man." The grandmother never came back to GAPA, but her peers visited her in her home and took her piecework that she could do from home.

BOX 28-18 Sustaining Long-Term Organizational Development

As GAPA became well known in the community, more problems were brought to the notice of the occupational therapist by the committee and also by the community. Communication with the broader community was difficult for the occupational therapist because of language and cultural deficits, and because funding had become available, a project manager domicile in the community was employed. This moved the occupational therapist into the realm of planning, financial management, organizational development, and supervision, while the project manager dealt with running the day-to-day activities of the organization. More projects were included in the GAPA portfolio, such as a preschool bursary fund, a health club for seniors, an aftercare for primary school children who had no supervision at home in the afternoon, and an income-generation promotion aspect within the psychosocial groups. As the project incorporated more programs, it became necessary to capture the full extent of the program in a way that, at a glance, the grandmothers could conceptualize how big and how far reaching their project had become. The occupational therapist designed a pictorial model so that any grandmother could easily explain to visitors to the center the scope of GAPA.

---

organization developed, more requirements and rules were being imposed on the organization by outside agencies that were providing funding. To protect the process of development within the organization, the grandmothers were incorporated continuously in the organization's development. However, it was necessary to employ staff to assist administratively because the grandmothers were electronically illiterate. Examples of this included forming a management committee of grandmothers, maintaining grandmothers as the key facilitators for workshops, and including grandmothers as board members (Box 28-18).

GAPA Today

GAPA celebrated its 10th anniversary in October 2011. The event was hosted at GAPA's premises in Khayelitsha with the attendance of over 300 grandmothers and guests. On reflection of the journey the organization has traveled, many grandmothers voiced the importance of the organization and its influence on their occupational being, for example: "Before GAPA came into my life I was broken and tired; now I sing for joy for GAPA. GAPA has brought new hope in my life; it has wiped away my tears." The meeting of the grandmothers in various GAPA activities, facilitated by their peers, has the potential to facilitate well-being through process of collaborative problem solving and support (Figure 28-2). The GAPA model has shown us that when these processes are facilitated, maintaining their uniqueness and ownership by the community, a deep sense of collective purpose and potential can emerge.

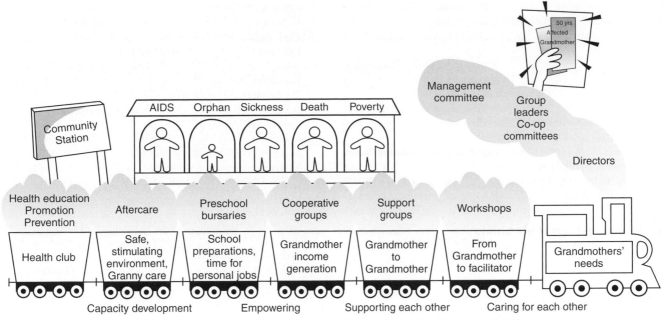

FIGURE 28-2   Model describing the activities of the Grandmothers Against Poverty and AIDS project.

Summary

Occupational therapy practice with older people is a very rewarding and exciting branch of occupational therapy. In marginalized communities, older people have had few opportunities throughout their lives to prepare for a leisurely old age. In old age they are as much concerned with struggling with daily challenges of living as they were when they were younger. In countries where there is famine and sickness that kills their adult children, they find that they never retire or give up their role in caring for children.

Mobilizing older people and facilitating their capacity to do the best that they can in meeting daily challenges is the main aim of occupational therapy in developing countries.

In this chapter we have shared some of the challenges and the successes that we have experienced in our practice of occupational therapy. The journey began with a strong belief in the basic guiding philosophy of occupational therapy—that everyone has the ability to heal themselves through activity. The journey for the occupational therapists ends when we exit the program that we initiated in the belief that the community has learned the skills to keep the program running and will adapt the program to suit the changing environment in which the community lives.

REVIEW QUESTIONS

1. Having read this chapter, do you identify with the role of OT in community development with aging population groups?
2. What are some of the ways in which occupational therapists can develop themselves as agents of change?

REFERENCES

1. Brodrick, K. (2005). Grandmothers affected by HIV/AIDS: New roles and occupations. In R. Watson & L. Swartz (Eds.), *Transformation through occupation* (pp. 233–252). London: Whurr Publishers.
2. Ferreira, M. (2004, January). HIV/AIDS and family well-being in southern Africa: towards an analysis of policies and responsiveness. In United Nations Department of Economic and Social Affairs Division for Social Policy and Development Policy Workshop.
3. Fourie, M., Galvaan, R., & Beeton, H. (2005). The impact of poverty: Potential lost. In R. Watson & L. Swartz (Eds.), *Transformation through occupation* (pp. 69–83). London: Whurr Publishers.
4. Kaplan, D., Meyer, J. B., & Brown, M. (1999). Brain drain: New data, New options. *Trade and Industry Monitor, 11,* 10–13.
5. Kronenberg, F., Pollard, N., Ramugondo, E. (2011). Introduction: Courage to dance politics. In F. Kronenberg, N. Pollard, & D. Sakellariou (Eds), *Occupational therapies without borders* (Vol. 2, pp.1–17). Edinburgh: Churchill Livingstone Elsevier.
6. Lorenzo, T., Van Niekerk, L., & Mdlokolo, P. (2007). Economic empowerment and black disabled entrepreneurs: negotiating partnerships in Cape Town, South Africa. *Disability and rehabilitation, 29*(5), 429-436.
7. Ramugondo, E., & Barry, A. (2011). Enabling play in the context of rapid change. In F. Kronenberg, N. Pollard, & D. Sakellariou (Eds.), *Occupational therapies without borders* (Vol. 2, pp. 179–185). Edinburgh: Churchill Livingstone Elsevier.
8. Rappaport, J. (1977). *Community psychology: Values, research, and action.* Harcourt School Publishers.
9. Schneider, H., Hlophe, H., & van Rensburg, D. (2008). Community health workers and the response to HIV/AIDS in South Africa: Tensions and prospects. *Health Policy and Planning, 23*(3), 179–187.
10. Swartz, L. (2005). Rethinking professional ethics. In R. Watson & L. Swartz (Eds.), *Transformation through occupation* (pp. 289–299). London: Whurr Publishers.

11. Statistics South Africa. (2011). 2011 Census Products. Accessed October 23, 2015. http://www.statsa.gov.za/.

12. The Economist. (2015). *Pocket world in figures*. London: Profile Books, Ltd.

13. Van Graan, A., Van der Walt, E., & Watson, M. (2007). Community-based care of children with HIV in Potchefstroom, South Africa. *African Journal of AIDS Research*, 6(3), 305–313.

14. Watson, R. (2005). New horizons in occupational therapy. In R. Watson & L. Swartz (Eds.), *Transformation through occupation* (pp. 3–16). London: Whurr Publishers.

15. Wilcock, A. A. (1998). *An occupational perspective of health*. Thorofare, NJ: SLACK.

16. World Federation of Occupational Therapists (WFOT). (2012). *What is occupational therapy?* Definition of an older person. www.wfot.org/AboutUs/AboutOccupationalTherapy/Whatis OccupationalTherapy.aspx.15 World Health Organization/. http://www.who.int/healthinfo/survey/ageingdefnolder/en/. Accessed 19.08.15.

RECOMMENDED READING

Brodrick, K. (2002). Correlation between scores on two screening tools for dementia in Xhosa women. *South African Journal of Occupational Therapy, 32*, 8–13.

Brodrick, K., & Drenth, N. (2009). Palliative care for older persons. In Hospice Palliative Care Association of South Africa (Ed.), *Legal aspects of palliative care*. Pinelands, South Africa: Hospice Palliative Care Association of South Africa.

Brodrick, K., & Mafuya, M. (2005). Effectiveness of the non-profit organisation, "Grandmothers Against Poverty and AIDS"—a study. *The Southern African Journal of HIV Medicine,* (19), 37–41.

Dockalova, B. (July, 2011). The Madrid Plan and you. You can be that change! *Ageways,*(77), 8–10.

Ferreira, M., & Brodrick, K. (2001). *Towards supporting older women as carers to children and grandchildren affected by AIDS: A pilot intervention project. Unpublished document Institute of Ageing in Africa,* Observatory, South Africa: Faculty of Health Sciences, University of Cape Town.

Kaplan, A. (1999). *The development of capacity, development dossier.* Geneva: Switzerland: UN Non-Governmental Liaison Service.

Wilcock, A. A. (1998). *An occupational perspective of health.* Thorofare, NJ: SLACK.

Wilcock, A. A. (2006). *An occupational perspective of health* (2nd ed.). Thorofare, NJ: SLACK, Inc.

CHAPTER 29

Community-Based Models of Practice to Address Late-Life Inequities: Examples from the UK

Nick Pollard, PhD, MSc(OT), DipCOT, Dikaios Sakellariou, PhD, MSc(OT), Linda Pollard, Clarice Harrison

CHAPTER OUTLINE

OBJECTIVES

- Identify contested understandings of aging and challenge the dominance of perspectives that have been constructed as "truths"
- Explore the relevance of Fraser's conceptualization of *recognition* and *distribution* to gerontological occupational therapy and occupational justice
- Examine socioeconomic and health-related disparities as influenced by cultural constructions of later life
- Provide examples of community-based models of gerontological occupational therapy practice to address these disparities

Equally Shared Benefits?

Distribution refers to how resources such as services and access to them, education, and wealth are shared in a population. Inequitable distribution of these resources results in social injustice.[27] Although it was initially perceived predominantly in economic terms, there has been considerable discussion of distribution focusing on the interconnections between cultural constructions such as race, gender, and age and injustices resulting from maldistribution of resources, and raising the issue of disparity of participation in daily life as a product of this interplay. In Britain, the Marmot report[41] and commentaries on the legacy of neoliberalism in health and well-being, such as Scott-Samuel et al.,[74] suggest greater inequalities. Other studies in the United States report that although inequalities certainly exist, over the long term, the picture may be very complex and require close attention to a wide range of social, cultural, health, and economic measures.[38]

On the whole, disability- and limitation-free life expectancy seems to be increasing in the United States, with improvements in mobility being reported over the years.[28] Disability-free life expectancy has been found to be positively correlated with income levels, so that the higher the income level of the population, the longer individuals are expected to remain independent and in good health.[29] An epidemiological study showed American adults (50 to 74 years of age) as being less healthy than their European peers,[4] a fact that can be partly explained by the well-documented health disparities that exist in the United States.[21] The same study showed that richer Americans were healthier than poorer ones, and that white Americans were richer than black and Hispanic Americans. Furthermore, older Americans with lower incomes who are black or of mixed race are more likely than white Americans to delay access to care due to cost, thus leading to diagnosis at a later stage and compromised chances for full treatment of the presenting conditions.[2] Prevalence of major chronic conditions, such as diabetes, high blood pressure, stroke, and rheumatoid arthritis, is higher among Americans of lower income and black Americans[2] but many social factors outside the clinical picture, such as changes in food production or increases in sedentary occupation, may influence this picture.[38]

Who Will Be There to Care?

This presents society with several issues, one of the most urgent being that of provision of services, or, as Super[82] from the National Health Policy Forum asked, *who will be there to care*? And who will pay for this care? Care in this context refers both to procedures carried out by health professionals and also practices concerned with looking after one's daily life needs.

In societies that traditionally demonstrate a communal organization of life in which family and/or community are foregrounded over the individual, such as Greek and Japanese societies, the solution to the latter aspect of care has traditionally been found within the family.[81] One or more members of the family assumed the role of the caregiver for older adult members of the family, in the anticipation that when their turn comes, they will also be cared for. Moving into a more individualistic model of organization of public and private life means that when their turn comes, they will need to find other solutions, because it is likely that family members will no longer be able to afford to take on the role of the caregiver.

This has been the case in many Western societies, including the U.S. society, in which the economic organization of the society means that care of older people has in many cases become a paid job. With fewer people being born, however, there are fewer people who can financially support the health and social care required by people who need continuous care. And there are also fewer people willing to enter what is a seriously underpaid and underrecognized industry of paid carers.

Access to appropriate care has already become a luxury. In Britain, there are cases where people living with the same conditions receive substantially different packages of care, or different health-care equipment to cover their needs, depending on which Health Trust is responsible for the area in which they reside. Furthermore, the increased needs for care by the expanding population of older people might mean that those who cannot afford individualized care might enter a system geared toward the maintenance of physical functions by covering basic needs, rather than toward the enablement of meaningful lives. These issues have been exacerbated by neoliberal health-care policies dating back to the 1980s, which first ignored the evidence of health inequalities, and then attempted to address them through health measures without sufficient attention to the wider socioeconomic context.[41] As a result, health inequalities between rich and poor, different geographical areas, and cultural groups have not lessened, but increased.[33] It is possible, although not clear, that health may be a determinant of social mobility rather than determined as a consequence, and deprivation of mobility may exert a more significant influence on health given that levels of poor health are rising in deprived areas.[9] These are aspects of a perspective on aging that require a long-term view in which the conditions of older adults are seen as outcomes of a trajectory through life, a narrative influenced by life chances, social changes, and environmental and economic factors.[18,25] Such a picture is at odds with a tendency to consider older age as something that is somehow disconnected from history, whether personal, communal, or even as a process through which a life of meaning occurs.

The Construction of Older Age as a Personal and Social Problem

In an autoethnographical account of caring for a parent with Alzheimer's disease, a neurodegenerative disease that causes dementia, Janelle Taylor[83] critically discusses notions of recognition and caring. Friends would regularly ask her if her mother recognized her, in effect equating recognition with care, with the loss of one making the expression of the other impossible.

According to Fraser,[27] recognition refers to a "...reciprocal relation between subjects in which each sees the other as its equal and also as separate from it." The very construction of aging as an undesirable process that needs to be reversed or at least halted presents a series of problems as to how older people are recognized within Western societies. The type of questions present in Taylor's account of caring for a parent with Alzheimer's disease underlines an important issue: If recognition refers to an active process of recognizing someone for who that person is, without resorting to stereotypes, then how does society recognize older people? How are people living with dementia, or people living with other degenerative or chronic diseases, recognized as persons and not as the stereotypical "sick, old body"? The answers to these questions have very tangible effects. The way people are recognized has direct implications on the kind of care they will receive, the range of treatments available to them, and, ultimately, in the value ascribed to their life.

Aging is commonly referred to as a problem, something that needs to be solved, an issue somebody needs to do something about. Who is to do what, though? The advent of what is called antiaging medicine, for example, indicates that it is the process of aging per se that is perceived as being problematic and is at the focus of professionals' efforts to tackle the *problem* of aging.[24]

The issue of aging unfolds in at least two dimensions, the personal and the social, which cannot really be separated, for the way that people are enabled to live their lives depends on the social, economic, and political environment in which they live. And in turn, these environments are being constructed by people and not by abstract ideas. Let us shift the focus to the particular case of occupational therapists and their engagements with older people. In their therapeutic goals, occupational therapists often use phrases such as *independence, engagement in occupation*, or *social skills*. These are assumed to refer to facts, whereas they actually represent social constructions. Western societies' emphasis on independence over dependence or interdependence is skewing therapeutic intervention toward individualized treatments aiming at the restoration of function or re-education. Underlying these efforts is a deep belief in the value of human occupation and its significance in people's lives. Occupation is a human right and refers to a process of doing, being, becoming, and belonging.[92] In occupational therapy, occupation is often identified with purposeful, goal-oriented, and meaningful activity. However, the assumption that occupation is a human right and is based on terms that are very similar to elements signifying life quality[56] tends to produce an uncritical regard in the profession. Occupational therapists have developed their profession in the shadow of medical practice[26] rather than an investigation of the cultural practices that "meaningful occupation" or "purposeful activity" might suggest. Ikiugu and Pollard[35] suggest that "meaningfulness" may emerge from a plethora of connections arising from the "raw material" of individual lives. These may be the experience of having survived disease, conflict, or deprivation; of having had specific working experiences; or of living in particular communities of relationships or of contact with family members. All of these elements and more build up to a sense of identity through a relationship with the wider world. The things people do, whether as individuals or part of a group, reflect some expression of this whole sense of being—unless, of course, they are accorded an identity, such as a diagnosed condition of older age, which obscures their own self-presentation. Thus, instead of seeing a person who is a grandmother who lost a husband, brought her children up in Britain through the period of wartime rationing, and worked throughout her life, we see a person who is one of 20 people on a dementia ward.

When Peter Townsend wrote his classic study of aging in a community, *The Family Life of Old People*,[84] in the mid-1950s, he remarked on the considerable increase in life expectancy that had occurred over the previous 50 years. A female child born in 1900 could expect to live 48 years; one born in 1951 had a life expectancy of 71 years. One of the themes that emerged from his interviews with 203 Bethnal Green people aged over 60 years was that of families offering each generation a sense of continuity, expressed through the changing relationship between parents and their children as they passed through various life stages. However, older people in the 1950s had smaller families than did their Victorian predecessors (e.g., author Nick Pollard's grandfather, born in 1896, was one of 18 siblings; Pollard's father, born in 1931, was one of two), and the consequence was that they would have fewer people to look after them. The extensive and rich family lives depicted in Townsend's study, in which all of the generations of siblings and cousins would gather at Christmas and have two sittings at dinners squeezed into Grandma's home (as they sometimes did during the 1960s in the Pollard family) were on the wane. In his 1963 postscript, Townsend reflected that he had not paid sufficient attention to the tensions arising in the way family relationships changed, although his study had documented them—for example, tensions over the care of older relatives.

Townsend's conclusions[85] marked an important, but largely unheeded, warning about the future balance of generations in Western society. The old are growing older and more numerous in proportion to the younger generations. In Britain today there are now more people over age 65 years, the age of retirement, than those under age 16 years, the school-leaving age. Life expectancy in many parts of the country exceeds 80 years, and the average is around 78 years. There are concerns about the viability of pension plans, particularly in the large UK public sector, where, until recently, it was possible for people to consider ceasing work in their mid-50s, if they are to support people for a quarter of a century past their maturation. An increasing number of people will be able to draw on their pensions for almost as many years as they were paying into them, and some perhaps will depend on them for longer. For much of this time they will be leading more active and healthier lives than their parents or grandparents had in similar years.

This issue is very significant, for one determinant of health, as was mentioned earlier, may be a cluster of factors around equal access to wealth and resources.[56] Townsend's study[84] explored the connection between wealth and health, drawing an implication that depreciated incomes affected many occupational dimensions of old people's lives. One problem linked to this was that of social isolation, which occurred particularly when people had few surviving relatives, had not married, or had no children of their own. In present-day Britain there has been a significant change since the 1950s of people choosing to live single lives, divorcing more frequently, and losing contact with relatives, and a growing trend in some social classes for increased internal migration connected with work opportunities. A review by Peters et al.[55] suggests that these contributors to social isolation may be among the factors increasing risk of dementia and stroke in older age groups. Although the recent policy agenda of Western governments has shifted toward healthier aging and enhanced life quality in older adults, Phillips[56] suggests that it may be difficult to effectively identify all of the contributing factors and their complex interactions. Certainly social equality and the neutralization of income differences are significant contributions to quality of life, and it is possible that body mass index may be important in relation to a range of diseases affecting cognitive and physical function. Consequently, access to the means of a good diet and facilities for exercise or physical activity may be significant, but this suggests that preventative work needs to take place in earlier life stages.

Community and Social Cohesion

One of the other factors explored by Phillips's overview[56] is that of social cohesion. Townsend's criticism[85] of his original study was that he might have emphasized some positive elements of community life in favor of more difficult issues; subsequent social theorists such as Putnam[62] maintained that the threshold of change was the period between Townsend's first and second editions of his study, the point at which most households obtained a television, reoriented their living rooms toward it in place of the hearth,[34] and turned their backs on the world around their homes. Like his 1950s predecessors hearkening back to a sense of an earlier, more vibrant, and less commercially tainted culture, Putnam's picture of communal sharing may be romantic and is not necessarily supported by evidence.[56]

These debates are important for the background to engagement with those people currently about to become older adults or who have recently attained this status. Members of this group were born in the post–World War II baby boom, which lasted from 1946 until 1964, an era of transition in social mores and material conditions in many Western countries. As Hoggart[34] recorded, along with the postwar emergence of the phenomena of adolescence, fueled by an affluence that afforded the purchase of rock-and-roll records, there was a sense that the expectations of subsequent generations would differ from their parents as a result of their rebellious individualism and desire to shock their elders with precocious smoking and chewing gum. This generation has lived through the growth of the record album, the cassette tape, and the compact disc, and perhaps now listens to its rock-and-roll memories on MP3 players.

Reminiscence is actually a favorite activity of every generation at a certain age. By late adulthood so much change has occurred that many fear their grandchildren will not believe the differences,[88] and it is also true that their grandchildren find the world their grandparents lived in hard to imagine.[8] Occupational narratives are often stories of technological adaptation—one of Blythe's interviewees,[8] for example, tells of working in a business that moved from making bicycles to crystal radio sets and finally televisions. Older people can look forward to a plethora of disability aids that were unavailable for their grandparents, and they can also recount social histories in which each era is marked by changes in household appliances. The investment in these and the dependence on them for domestic security is held to be one of the factors in social division, particularly the television and its associated entertainment systems, and the computer and its games.

Television, DVDs, and Internet streaming have not only taken people off the streets and out of the cinemas, but have replaced much of the social life in which people formerly engaged.[12] Older people have the television on for company.[31] Without television, people find it hard to relate to each other; they must rediscover conversation. The home computer is increasingly seen as a factor in improving life quality and has offered a number of silver surfers the means to make new friends and explore a new virtual world and communities within it. However, many people are not able to use the computer, cannot afford one, do not want to use one, and/or can no longer upgrade to a machine with sufficient capabilities to access the Internet.[67]

Many notions of community are perhaps inherently romantic. Williams[93] remarked that the word *community* did not have negative connotations, but that was before the neoliberal conservatism of the 1980s and 1990s passed care responsibilities to the community without allocating the resources to meet these demands. This social policy agenda is being revisited in contemporary austerity measures in the aftermath of the global financial crisis of 2008–2009. Oral narratives frequently contain an element in which people look back benignly on the past as a golden age during which, despite poverty and hardship, there were less troubles than now. Despite these pictures, there are many others that describe extreme difficulty and struggle,[35] which people have had to learn to overcome. These psychobiographical narratives, as we will later explore in this chapter, illustrate what has been called *ontological security*,[39] a sense of personal capabilities and achievements derived from experience, the groundwork for which is in the navigation of early childhood. Chodorow,[15] for example, offers a model of female contiguity in which the relation between mother and daughter stretches back continuously to prehistory, the matrilineal anchor of family life whose obverse is in Townsend's depiction[84] of the separation and reconciliation of father and son through the production of grandchildren. This theme of males navigating and reconciling their roles through the generations is

illustrated in Updike's Rabbit novels,[86,87] for example. For Rabbit, however, the community in which he lives, in which he has survived his inadequacies, has disappeared. By the final book of the quartet he has a retirement apartment in Florida and has a social life consisting of other people from the same community of retired exiles. Psychobiography[39] describes the process by which people come to understand themselves in relation to others, as both individuated and a part of a society.

However, Rabbit's story depicts considerable malaise in the generation it represents. One aspect of this, evident also in Britain, is a growing separation between the generations, evidenced by the phenomenon, for those who are able to afford it, of retirement migration.[65] Rabbit, like his UK counterparts across the southern coast of the Iberian peninsula, has visited Florida on holiday and settles into a retirement apartment in a community that is socially and geographically separate from other social groups. This parallel existence of the generations is also something that was beginning to be hinted at in Townsend's study half a century before. These changes can be observed in the community in which we live. Communities need neutral spaces in which people can meet informally, such as cafés, pubs, and even religious centers.[14,52] In Britain, the pub has been a major social institution. For Nick, as a young person in Sheffield in 1976, going to the local pubs was about participating in a lively culture in which people of all ages mixed. There were student pubs, full of other young people, but those that local people frequented could be very busy, and conversation passed easily irrespective of age. This is still part of Sheffield's social life, but the pubs are fewer and less people visit them. Many pubs have become branded and themed; much of the interior and many of the drinks and products available in them are oriented to the age of the clientele who are intended to be the market. However, as Chatfield and Hexel argue,[14] younger generations tend to meet in new and virtual environments, developing new social spaces that are replacing these physical community-based neutral spaces, for example, through online gaming.

These social developments act as barriers and exclusions in addition to issues that arise through ill health and disability. This environmental underpinning of parallelization may encourage and facilitate the perception that the older person is less interested in the new and more concerned with retaining memories of the past, as indicated in Erikson's later stages of life.[23] There may be barriers to being interested in the present imposed by the ways in which the present isolates itself from access by previous generations. But the development of older age is more complex than this succinct vision or the narrow spectrum of a marketing category.

Most people plan for a long retirement, but sometimes illness, disability, or events such as the break-up of the children's families disrupt these intentions. Grandparents have to care for children, or perhaps are still caring for their parents while themselves accumulating the symptoms of aging. Savings are used up, health is compromised, and visions have to be adjusted and downsized to more limited possibilities.

Communities within Communities

There are many conditions through which this can arise. Dementia is one of the major conditions of old age, and certainly part of the popular perception of older adults in the eyes of the younger people Blythe interviewed for his study,[8] affecting 1% of people at age 65 years and increasing in incidence with the age of individuals.[32] People often speak of their fear that in their old age they will not know what is going on around them, or of a combination of disability and loneliness.[8] However, old age is characterized by a gradually increasing accumulation of conditions. Studies have shown that community occupational therapy interventions are typically targeted at enabling personal care, domestic activities, locomotor skills, and mobility and independence issues that arise with the aging process.[78] However, reviews have also identified difficulties in establishing evidence in the efficacy of occupational therapy in relation to the older person. This appears to be due to the number, quality, and heterogeneity of the studies available. Although Steultjens et al.[78] identified a number of areas where occupational therapy could be perceived as effective in the care of older people living in the community, there were areas where more research was needed. The consequence of this continual lack of enough evidence of efficacy is that unless cost benefits can be demonstrated, as in Graff et al.'s work[32] with dementia, it is less likely that provision will be made to meet the problems that people experience.

Research evidence is not the only determinant of the visibility of a health issue or carers' needs. The People Relying on People (PROP) group, based in Doncaster, was formed of people who were experiencing early-onset dementia and their carers. They decided, because they had had so much difficulty getting their issues recognized, that they would set up a support group and raise the profile of the experience of dementia by presenting at conferences, making a DVD of poignant comedy sketches, and going out together as a group wearing their PROP T-shirts, provoking others to ask what they signified.[13,37]

The PROP group functioned as a community within the community. At the day center they were eventually provided, the program for each day was operated as if it was a continuous social occasion. Support workers organized some activities, but members of the group often wanted to do things they had always done, such as gardening and baking. These were often activities they could not do at home because their relatives were afraid of the risks. Everyone in the group (which was composed of people with mild to moderate dementia) was able to participate in "socializing," irrespective of their stage of the illness. It didn't matter, for example, if an individual had the same conversation several times with different people. There were plenty of things to do. A member might suddenly walk up the garden and start creating a new flower bed, and someone else might quietly ask this person what he or she was doing and whether he or she needed help. Occasionally differences were expressed. On one occasion the service users voted the treasurer and chairperson off the PROP committee because they felt carers were dominating the group—which was there for people with dementia.

Dementia, then, can be regarded as a clinical problem, a disease entity with probable causes that are identifiable as age-related changes occurring within the human body, but many of the aspects through which dementia is experienced cannot be visibly seen in these physical changes. Instead they are incrementally realized as barriers to occupation are met and have to be negotiated. The experience of the PROP group members was developed from their own shared narratives of social exclusion and lack of opportunities.

The current vogue in social policy for healthy aging policy is to some extent an antiaging agenda. Within this type of policy development, many of the conditions associated with old age, such as dementia, osteoporosis, and chronic heart disease, are regarded as the "symptoms" of aging.[46] The race to develop antiaging medicines and treatments is partly fueled by the realization that those who are successful will gain considerable financial gains, and partly by fears about the socioeconomic cost of aging. Mykytyn[46] also suggests that many of the practitioners involved are motivated by the possibility that these forms of medicine may reduce painful and disabling experiences for their clients. However, there are fears that such remedies would only be available to the wealthy at the expense of those who cannot afford the processes. Despite the pursuit of better treatments—even approaches that might postpone mortality—the biggest problem faced by older people remains, just as Townsend[84] found nearly 60 years ago, the limitations imposed by poverty. It is one thing to note that the relationship between well-being and reduction in poverty is very marked at lower income levels,[19] but reviewing this experience of positive or negative well-being in occupational terms allows the meaning of restricted doing to emerge. At low levels of income—Diener et al.'s figure[19] is $20,000 or below—there are increasing limitations on what a person is able to do. If people do not have adequate income to feed themselves and heat their homes in winter, they may have to prioritize food. The purchase of food can be a significant problem if public transportation is unavailable. Individuals may be reluctant to go out until they really need to buy a significant quantity of supplies, and consequently take risks with food that is so old that it may become contaminated; lack of transportation may also limit access to health treatment and facilities.[47] It is often difficult to purchase foodstuffs cost effectively if only cooking for one, especially if, due to inactivity and poor health, appetite is reduced. A person may be able to retain a small amount of savings but need to keep this in reserve in case an appliance such as a freezer or refrigerator breaks down and needs replacement. In addition to the accumulation of conditions and bereavements are many accompanying environmental factors that could precipitate events into a crisis. The choice between heating and eating may mean that one room is kept warm while the rest of the house is left cold, grows damp, becomes neglected, and eventually threatens to require serious repair work.[3]

Awareness of this, but the hope that things will last an individual until the end of his or her life, may be just one additional source of anxiety. The ability to cope is precious and may be a source of continued hope, but it can also be experienced as fragile in the face of mounting odds. A sense of creeping vulnerability can be increased in areas where there is a perception of crime and breakdown in social cohesion and trust.[36,20] Individuals may be reluctant to go out at night in case they are mugged, reluctant to talk to callers in case they are criminals who take advantage of a person's frailty to steal or extort their savings, or reluctant to leave their homes in the day in case they are burgled. Even for those who previously had the resources, the three options that Innes and Jones[36] identify as possible responses to this situation, exiting the community, remaining loyal to it, or voicing their discontent, are no longer available. The benign vision of a community of social capital that Putnam[62] pointed to is not available to those who find themselves excluded, and this vision is declining. Once excluded, access to resources, facilities, and social contact decreases,[61] and the experience of meaningfulness and life satisfaction is reduced.[20] However, research determining the consequences of chronic experiences of a range of such factors among older people is lacking.[51] Neimeyer et al.,[47] in describing the factors that contribute to the experience of grief in later life, indicate that research can only understand the contribution of complex combinations of factors through the analysis of narrative data. They warn against the pathologizing of grief, which is a natural response to the disruption of the interdependency between spouses, increasing dependency of parents on children against a paradoxical decreased dependency of children on parents, and the experience of physical and cognitive deficits. But they also suggest that people can show "resilience or even personal growth following loss."[47]

One practical intervention that is often discounted in the concerns with conditions and treatments is that of spiritual engagements.[17] Crowther et al.[17] discuss the forms that spiritual engagement may take, not only prayer and visits from local religious representatives but a whole range of active engagements in the community that occupational therapists would recognize as having a participatory occupational base. Indeed, these forms of engagement were very significant to Nick's mother as an Anglican lay reader.[58]

Through spiritual engagement people can not only experience degrees of self-efficacy as a component of well-being, but perhaps be encouraged to maintain or adopt healthier behaviors, because people with religious beliefs tend to smoke and drink less. However, Crowther et al.[17] stress the importance of client autonomy in exercising these choices concerning participation, and the need for activities to include degrees of spiritual observance through interactions with non-faith-based organizations. Such activities can be seen as a component in the development or maintenance of resources for social capital; and the spiritual element strengthens adherence, because many people will recognize the cultural and religious capital based in the authority of religious organizations and their historical but changing involvement with communities.[80] This may be more difficult for other community organizations to develop, although parallels, such as working men's or village clubs or the British Legion, may represent a more secular involvement. Few of these, however, are supported by volunteers who will reach out to the socially isolated; befriending schemes are generally developed through religious groups.[16] For more information on spirituality and aging, see chapter 17.

CASE EXAMPLE 29-1 Day-to-Day Care Work with Older People

Linda is a carer who has been working for an agency in North East Sheffield for 11 years. Her regular evening shift includes 10 people, of whom eight are over age 60 years; the age range is from 34 to 95 years, although some of her past clients were over age 100 years. On alternating weekends she visits as many as 17 people in a day and averages 40 hours a week. Her work involves helping people to get to bed in the evenings with another carer. These clients are unable to do this by themselves and need a hoist and other assistance to get into bed. On weekends, when she works from early in the morning to well into the evening, the earlier calls may involve observing people take their medication, washing, dressing, or the preparation of meals. The majority of the people she sees have had strokes, although other clients have dementia, chronic arthritis, osteoporosis, leukemia, or complications of earlier physical disabilities resulting from polio.

Many of the older clients now live alone. One client with dementia who lived alone introduced Linda to her friend, who proved to be her own reflection in the bedroom mirror, with whom she spent much of the day talking. Another is unable to see because she has cataracts in both eyes but is afraid to go to hospital for the simple operation that could treat this. Some have relatives nearby who visit, and some may be accommodated with their families or a relative. North East Sheffield is semirural, and the range of housing varies from large private homes to council properties such as flats or older people's bungalows. Linda's clients are distributed across a range of income levels.

The occupational activities available to her clients vary according to their physical ability and the assistance they can draw on from others. Many people are picked up by ambulance to attend a council-run day center 3 miles away, which offers them social activities, such as bingo with prizes, the opportunity to enjoy a pint, and occasional day trips to the coast for fish and chips and ice cream, or a local pub lunch. However, these facilities are under pressure to reduce costs: If for some reason they miss the transport due to not being ready in time, it is necessary to immediately book their place for the next visit, or they may lose their place. At the day center, clients enjoy the opportunity to catch up with each other, and often ask their paid carers how others are getting on in their own homes who they know are on the

CASE EXAMPLE 29-1   Day-to-Day Care Work with Older People—cont'd

same round. Some clients also attend church, assisted by relatives or other church members. One of the churches runs a Friday luncheon club, which also provides meals for people who are no longer able to come. Volunteers visit former luncheon club members to provide a hot meal with pudding, and sometimes homemade cakes and other goodies.

Some clients are taken out shopping by their daughters or granddaughters. One woman with dementia regularly shops on Tuesdays at the local town center; sometimes she does this independently, occasionally forgetting which day it is. Two of Linda's regular clients are older males, one using a wheelchair, whose sons take them to the pub. Some clients are able to rely on good relationships with neighbors, for example, with help around the home or with the provision of meals. With a caseload of this size there are sometimes changes in the distribution of types of personal situations, so previously Linda has had a number of clients who have no surviving relatives. One of the people she presently sees is reliant on social services for assistance with needs such as the replacement of floor covering in her home, as she has no family at all. Some people are vulnerable, and a small number have experienced break-ins or hoax callers who try to demand money for building repairs they have not done; on a couple of occasions, Linda herself has encountered people acting suspiciously around older people's homes.

Most people spend their time at home watching television; some listen to the radio. One female client likes to sit in her garden when possible, read the papers, and embroider pictures that decorate her home. Another crotchets blankets for a church orphanage charity. A woman with a stroke does all her housework and prepares her own meals from her wheelchair; another does her own washing. Most clients have routines into which they are settled, and want their carers to attend to them at regular times, not, for example, to be put to bed too early, or too late.

Part of the role of being a carer is to "cheer people up." Most of her clients maintain a positive outlook, but Linda says that "even the grumpiest people look forward to you coming round; they actually say that they don't want staff who are quiet and don't talk." Clients like to talk about things they have done, local history and experiences, and about what's going on around them. They are interested in the community around them and like to gossip. Even though some people are unable to leave their homes very often, in a village community like many of the districts of Sheffield, people know one another, and a grapevine

composed of relatives and neighbors enables them to keep informed. Although the soap operas provide some of the subject matter for conversation, perhaps somebody has a son who is a taxi driver, and is in a position to know who has been where and with whom; another may have a daughter working in a local shop and who sees many community members passing through. By the time people are in their later years they have often acquired a string of friends, neighbors, former lovers, and even enemies of whom they are still interested in keeping track. Discretion is an essential part of Linda's role. One client has a mirror positioned in her window to enable her to observe parts of the street she cannot otherwise see easily, and likes to chat about all the comings and goings she witnesses in the day. Recently a female client asked for her face to be painted with an England flag in preparation for watching an international match. The client was disappointed when Linda hadn't brought some face paint because she hadn't appreciated that the client was serious—and she asked for lipstick to be used instead. However, the time for each visit is set to a minimum number of minutes for each care task, and with cost pressures on the service and increasing need among the client group, there is less time for social interaction. It can be difficult to complete all the care tasks a person may require. Linda's agency only pays her for the time she spends with clients, and does not pay travel time between visits during the shift. Some workers find that they are actually earning less than the minimum wage. This can mean that Linda may find that her clients have not had their care needs met sufficiently in earlier visits, and she then has to deal with the consequences. For people unable to toilet, dress, medicate, or properly feed themselves, this can mean considerable discomfort and lack of dignity.

Clients sometimes say that they want to die. They feel that they have had good lives, but now there is nothing left for them, and they find little to engage their interest. They feel they are a burden on their families. Even an event like a family wedding does not excite them, because they do not want their relatives to see them in a frail and dependent condition. They are fed up, and there is nothing for them to do; they feel that they are too old to either take up new interests or to resume old ones. Some resent having carefully saved all their lives for their old age to find now that they have to pay for care that others who have either not saved or not been in a position to save can obtain without charge. "Spend your money now, while you are young enough to enjoy it," they tell her.

CASE EXAMPLE 29-2   Clarice

Clarice is 94 years old, and has lived most of her life in South Elmsall, a close West Yorkshire community in which many people have known each other all their lives. Clarice recently celebrated her 90th birthday with a party to which around 100 people came, including former neighbors, friends from the dance club she used to attend over a decade ago, and relatives from all over the country.

Clarice was widowed in 1971. She has a son in his 70s who is her main carer, five grandchildren including Linda,

16 great-grandchildren, and one great-great-granddaughter. Her son and several of her grandchildren live close to her. She keeps in touch with family members regularly on the phone. She has lived in a ground-floor flat in a complex of housing purposely built for older people since 1984, when she discovered that she would have to have a heart bypass operation. Since then she has had bilateral hip replacements and a knee replacement. She also has a dislocated left shoulder and so she is in a lot of pain. She uses a transcutaneous electrical

Continued

CASE EXAMPLE 29-2   Clarice—cont'd

nerve stimulation (TENS) machine to relieve this, but her health is variable. For several years Clarice has been unable to walk and uses an electric wheelchair to get around the flat; she needs a hoist to use the toilet and to get into bed. Since she moved in, her flat has required modifications to doorways to allow her to maneuver from room to room, but the hallway and kitchen are very narrow and difficult to negotiate without marking the walls or damaging appliances.

Clarice receives support from the local council in the form of carers who visit five times a day. They come in the morning to get her out of bed, at lunch to ensure she has a meal and a drink, in mid-afternoon for toileting and another drink, at tea time to prepare another meal and transfer her from her wheelchair to an armchair, and at night to put her to bed. Because Clarice's son lives 8 miles away, and most of her grandchildren live in the town or a few miles away, she receives regular visits. Her son and his wife come two or three times a week, taking her out to the local market to do her shopping twice a week and at other times collecting shopping items for her. Her son helps her to manage her bills. Occasionally, she hires an adapted taxi to visit the substantial market and shops at Doncaster. This can be highly variable in cost, as much as £80 (or $125) and as little as £20 (or $31) for a couple of hours between either leg of a return trip.

Clarice married her husband Bert during the war. Her mother had moved to a different part of the town and liked to sit out front of the house. This way she got to know all the shopkeepers and so did quite well during the period of rationing, which was how she came by the icing sugar for Clarice's wedding cake. It had to be worked down from a lump.

Clarice has worked hard all her life and has seen difficult times. During World War II, Bert was in the army. Her sister's husband served in the Royal Air Force in Canada. He got twice Bert's rate of pay, despite not being in active combat. Nonetheless, Clarice was the first to move out of her family's overcrowded home. Her brother-in-law's grandma read the froth in Clarice's beer and told her that she would "the first to get her feet under her own table." Shortly after, Bert wrote to her to say that she would be able to get a house through his family connections in Blackburn.

"My mother took me on one side and pointed out to me that with my son we were overcrowded in our house, and that I should take it. It was horrible, with gas lamps and a big black range. It backed onto the rail line and you could wave to the passengers; you could feel the trains rumbling by. We used to sing 'the railroad runs through the middle of the house.' But I went and took our lad to school. One of the mothers offered her a job in a shop and café for mill workers, where she made steak puddings, meat and potato pies, and loose meat and potatoes. Clarice is still friends with the owners now. One day there was a knock at the door, and Bert had come home from the war. It wasn't long before he had the range out and electricity in. But she never settled, and wanted to come back; they were still on the council list [for public housing] here and someone came to her mother's house with a key for her new council house. Her dad said 'Oh, she lives in Blackburn,' so they wouldn't let them have it. Bert went back to South Elmsall to see the council about it. Later that day the train slowed past the back of the house

as it came into the nearby station. Bert was leaning out of the carriage window shaking his head, saying 'no, no, no.'"

Eventually Clarice was able to return, and in the 1960s she was able to buy a new Wimpey house in South Elmsall with Bert, who, being a painter and decorator, knew all the builders. Because her son was also an electrician, they were able to do this work on the house for themselves, which, with Clarice going to work as well, made it affordable. She worked as a knitter in the Invicta clothing factory, interlock and wool. Clarice also used to sell dresses to neighbors, and used to get her own dresses at a discount or sometimes in exchange for doing this. After her husband died she couldn't concentrate at work and so was staring out of the window while the machine was running on and the stitches were going wrong. "So I left that job," she said, "and I lost £800 for being away from work ten days after being there 18 years. I had asked them for leave and they said I could take it. There were rumors about redundancy at the time and one of my friends told me not to take leave, but I couldn't concentrate. I used to take the girls in to work in my mini and have to throw pebbles up at the windows to wake them up." The mini had been bought new by her husband. "I kept going out in front of the house to look at it. He had to tell me 'it's only an ordinary car.'"

"When you're 90 you can't expect much," Clarice said. "I used to go dancing and now I can't even walk." Clarice now watches television, keeping up with soap operas, and likes to watch old films. She sometimes sits outside in the doorway if the weather is not too hot. She loves to go shopping when she can. "Sometimes I feel a bit lonely and bored," Clarice said. "Grandchildren were my life, I always had children around, with plenty of outdoor toys in my garden. Of course I'd like to dance again but I'm not going to be able to. I take pleasure from my visits, and from helping out with family ups and downs. I helped my son raise his children, used to do all their baking and practically helped to keep them. I used to like to take the children to the market or British Home Stores and buy them all clothes. I miss being able to do this now. I used to like to buy all the grandchildren things and even now when I go shopping I like to look at the kiddies' things, but I can't really afford to buy them now. What I bought was old fashioned and usually they didn't want what I'd bought, so I had to stop that."

Clarice gets depressed when nobody comes, but knows from her carers there are people who are not visited by anybody. Clarice is in contact with a number of her neighbors, some of whom regularly drop by, although many of those who were here when Clarice moved in have now died. People have moved in to replace them, and sometimes there are frictions about little things, like where the dustbins are. "I told them," Clarice said, "they've only just moved in; you have to give them a chance."

Clarice has her own pension and manages quite well financially, but is not very pleased with the recent election result, "as all these people have worked hard for a living, had to work or they hadn't got anything, these young men who have come to be prime ministers are all from nice families and they haven't got a clue what it's like to be poor. I've been a widow all them years. When I lost my husband because I had a widow's pension, it was taxed as unearned income, so I had more tax to pay than those who had husbands."

Narratives, Low-Key Activities, and Community

The picture Linda and Clarice give in Case Examples 29-1 and 29-2 is of older people who—just as Blythe[8] found in his investigations—have largely come to terms with their lives but enjoy and look forward to human contact, opportunities to exchange humor, news, memories, and advice. The pleasures they can afford, whether in terms of their own physical ability, the time in which they can be active during the day, the time they can demand from others, or their own ability to pay for them, are often small—a pub meal, a pint, fish and chips by the seaside, sitting in the garden, a mirror for observing. One of the ways in which such small human events can be worked with is through the development of the interest in human narratives that this pattern of activity suggests, and can also be easily afforded: Writing requires a pen or pencil and paper and a reasonable degree of cognitive and fine motor ability.

Disability is not the only factor that may limit the capacity for writing. Those of older generations, particularly women, may have experienced disruptions in schooling or have been encouraged to prioritize domestic activities over those associated with formal learning,[40] but "writing" can also be achieved through taping and transcription. Age Exchange is a charity that, since the early 1980s, has worked with groups of older people and community facilities such as museums and libraries to produce a range of "reminiscence arts" resources, including theater productions, exhibitions, and materials for schools.[71] The charity uses interviews with people to produce memory-based publications, which have included key and varied social history themes such as reminiscences of the 1930s,[1] the 1940s wartime work of women,[73] memories of health care before the development of the National Health Service,[69] retirement experiences,[70] the development of council housing around London between the wars,[66] and of hops-picking holidays in Kent.[72] A more recent publication about the experiences of people from cultural minority groups in Britain, targeted at the school curriculum, is subdivided into sections on themes such as "childhood, home and family" and "growing old in Britain."[71] These large-format publications are well illustrated with contemporary photographs and advertisements from magazines, and pictures from family albums contributed by the participants in each project. The results are widely used in Britain to stimulate reminiscence activities, and they also provide attractive resources that can be used in schools.

An extensive project by Stockport Arts and Health[79] associated writing with a range of other arts activities, including photography, drawing, and sound recordings, to produce a lavish collection of artworks, poems, and a CD. This was the culmination of a well-funded project generating a number of exhibitions and other events involving several agencies across the city over a number of years from the late 1990s.

Osmond[53] worked with a group of writers in Brighton who had experienced strokes, one of whom had already published two autobiographical works with a community publisher, QueenSpark.[89,90] Although participating in the group enabled members to discuss their experiences and to come to terms with the changes brought about by their disabilities, they also said that the process of writing and, for the carers, taping their stories for transcription, was helpful, particularly as "the focus was on content and not at all on form or method."[53] Participants in the Stockport Arts and Health[79] project even used William Burroughs–style cut-up methods to work their memories into poems, and the poems into collage-like pictures.

The use of cheap methods of publication distributed through informal networks and a market stall operated by the community publisher made it possible for Osmond's volunteer-led and virtually unfunded group activity[53] to have an external focus for its writing. One book was written by people who had experienced strokes,[63] and another was written by their carers.[57] Because of the difficulties such as memory loss experienced by the stroke group, Osmond had to edit the first book, but with the carers a collaborative process was used, and when cuts were made for a shorter edition of the book, Osmond was challenged to restore some of the changes made by other members. The books were distributed to National Health Service hospitals and local libraries, but also sold locally; each copy probably had several readers as the book was informally passed around in the community. Osmond reports that the group continued to meet, having formed a social bond through the writing experience, but he recognized that it would have been useful to have planned the group from the beginning with the intention that it would be facilitated in continuing after the project. QueenSpark continues as a community publisher, and over the years many of its titles have reflected the autobiographical experiences of older people, developing a rich community-based resource of texts describing local history with the intimacy of firsthand knowledge.* These texts are not about the experience of disability, but about a knowledge of the streets, trades, and ordinary everyday life past, such as that Clarice has enjoyed describing, in Case Example 29-2 that might otherwise be lost.

It is quite possible to develop elements of such projects using, as in some of the community publishing projects developed by Osmond,[53] no more than a photocopier and a supply of paper and colored cardstock, clear spaces on display boards where work can be mounted and appreciated by others, scrap materials, and volunteer time. Clarice, for example, describes her mobility problems, which limit the extent to which she can get out of the flat. The occasions she can go out often require some organization. However, she is part of a network of neighbors in the housing complex where she lives, and it might be possible to develop such a project around the existing links she already has.

Indeed, the OT profession has perhaps missed opportunities to engage with and realize the full potential of this source of occupational narratives,[60] or at least, has not written about its involvement in them. This is perhaps because, as Mattingly[43] suggests, much of the care process is

---

*References 5, 11, 48, 49, 50, 76, 77, and 94.

directed to technical aspects of clinical work rather than the story of the connection between individual experience and the conditions of older age. These projects can be developed in the lounges and luncheon clubs where people already meet, and the outcomes can replace the faded copies of Constable's *Haywain* or prints of flowers adorning the walls. Low-key approaches allow people to gain confidence, not to be frightened of blank paper or to be concerned with the ability to write or draw, but involved in the representation and sharing of something meaningful to the participants. At an individual level, people can point to their work, or press it into the hand of a relative, and say "I did that," but it is also very possible that such work can be celebrated in the wider community.[60] Indeed, one of the models for the development of these activities, and in which a good number of older people have always been engaged, originated largely through spontaneous community activities around developing writing and publishing as an alternative or counter-cultural practice,[54] and linked to this, community-based cooperative forms of pedagogy[75] in which people facilitate each other's learning. We have used these methods ourselves in developing this chapter, which has been written using interviews, with the copy checked over by the other participants.

This is important, because as McKee and Blair[45] have found in developing computer literacy with older people, projects have to be built around the needs the community expresses. People do not respond to things that are projected onto them. Computer literacy can be a significant means of reducing social isolation when relatives live far away, and email communication can sometimes be more effective in maintaining contact with younger generations.[67] Older people may use their new skills in working on family histories and memoirs, and can acquire new facilities by learning to "scavenge"[45] information and online resources. However, some people are very challenged by the cognitive demands using this kind of technology makes of them, or find themselves physically unable to sit comfortably at keyboards or follow the cursor on the screen. With the current rate of technological development, computers need frequent upgrading. A computer purchased 5 years ago may now be hopelessly slow and have software which is out of date; other appliances of the same age or even older and of roughly similar investment cost, such as washing machines or stereo equipment, can still function without difficulty. For people on a low income, the short life of computers may be a disincentive to their purchase;[67] and availability at public libraries, for example, can be quite limited. Of author Linda Pollard's older clients, only one couple currently uses a computer. Nonetheless, computers enable people to maintain networks across large distances, and in the case of writing and publishing, to use blogs and network websites as a form of dissemination. An example is TheFED, which has an online membership across the age ranges and to which local organizations such as Grass Roots Open Writers in Hastings and Pecket Learning Community in Halifax belong. These groups value their diversity and have a membership composed of minority

BOX 29-1   Web Links

Grass Roots Open Writers, (GROW): http://www.grow.btck.co.uk
Pecket Learning Community: http://www.pecket.org
SAGE Greenfingers: http://www.sagesheffield.org.uk/
TheFED—A Network of Writing and Community Publishers: http://www.thefed.btck.co.uk/

*All sites retrieved September 2, 2015.

cultural groups, people with disabilities, and survivors of mental distress, and a wide age range. Participation in them offers a social network and gateway to a range of other activities, such as theater and visual media (Box 29-1).[71,79] Participants can satisfy a wide range of interests through their adaptability to different subject matter, whether local history, personal autobiography, creative storywriting, or recipe books.[54] These activities can also involve the use of computer technologies, which themselves can similarly provide a gateway to a range of occupations.[45,67]

Another very broad-based and intergenerational activity is gardening. The SAGE Greenfingers project in Sheffield[59] has been developed around the needs of people with severe and enduring mental health problems living in the community. Although some of the clients are in their 20s and 30s, many are older, retired people, some in their 70s. The project has a group of three neighboring allotments of plots of land for gardening and a further allotment nearby in which members of the group can spend a couple of days a week throughout the year growing plants and eating communal meals in a large shed. The gardens feature raised beds for wheelchair users, an experimental tandoori oven, areas for just sitting and taking in the view of the Don valley and the city, a greenhouse, and a mixture of vegetable, fruit, and ornamental plants. Seasonal crops are turned into vegetarian Turkish cuisine. Members of the group can opt for gardening activities in small groups, in pairs, or alone, or just talk or sit in quiet areas. Gardening enables a group of people to be and do things together without talk always being necessary, but is also a vehicle for many occupational spin-off[54] activities—such as the trying of foods that people have not previously experienced, taking plants home to propagate, and cultivating gardens at home.

An accompanying project, the Primary Mental Health Care Project (PMHCP) is based around a writing group and a knitting group and serves severe and enduring mental health clients with an older age range, from the 30s into the late 80s. The PMHCP project is linked to a local general practice, and offers an informal basis through which the health of group members can be monitored and their general well-being maintained with the support of volunteers and part-time workers. The knitting group meets in a local café, and the writing group, although based in a room in the project offices, frequently makes trips into the community, for example, to attend the theater or to perform at community events. Through both of these projects, people are encouraged to develop other interests, attend adult education classes, or join other community groups. A recent project involved singing, for example. The members of both projects report that the groups are very important in enabling them to have regular contact with others, as one participant put it, "I'd have been just sat at home. I wouldn't have got up and gone looking for things to do,"[59] and something to talk about with other people. A simple activity, such as growing a plant in a pot, can be a focus of conversation in an otherwise uneventful life.

Billings and Brown[7] also advocate more flexible health promotion approaches that allow for individual expression. As noted earlier, horticultural interventions are increasingly popular and well established in work with older clients. [22,30,42] Martin, Miranda, and Bean's study[42] aimed in particular at reducing isolation and enabling couples to maintain their social roles. Many of the interventions developed for older adults have community outcomes: Participation in arts and voluntary programs, for example, is often connected with health promotion.[7] These strategies allow people to find their own level and to interact more freely, and for the development of occupational spin-offs from other activities. Although these interventions need to be sustainable,[7] the activities they offer clients need to have short-term and achievable goals that recognize the foreclosure of individual time.

Is It Possible to Develop a Community-Based Model of Gerontology?

Baron[6] suggests that encouraging spontaneous group formation may be one of the approaches to resolving the broken-down social cohesion identifiable in Britain, and this at least seemed to be a part of the ideology of the New Labour government. Groups such as TheFED (a network of writing groups) and Pecket Learning Community (a basic adult education cooperative), in which Nick Pollard has been involved, have found developing community activity to be difficult in the context of changing funding priorities as related to rising unemployment and the recent global financial crisis. These issues have detracted somewhat from the policy agendas around healthy aging and meeting the needs of an increasing older population.

However, to a certain extent, the development of spontaneous groups and networks depends on the availability of individual resources rather than the facilitation of local government or, for that matter, health workers. Baron[6] identified the "good social capitalist" as a person who is active in developing social networks, the kind of person identified by Putnam[62] as an older individual motivated altruistically toward his or her neighbors. In some areas, as Linda Pollard has noted in her work, neighbors do pull together in supporting each other with errands and tasks around their homes. However, in other areas, people do not have good social relations with each other or are isolated.

The activities and actions suggested here may address some of the needs of older people—if they can be developed with their active participation from the start, as, for example, the PROP group was able to do. However, membership of the PROP group was difficult for those who were unable to leave their disabled partners, or travel to a center a few miles from their homes. Although such groups and networks may enable some people, even quite large numbers of people, to belong to communities within the community in which people connect around areas of interest, a diverse strategy of engagement is needed to involve those who cannot access meeting places. This approach is also needed to enable people to continue to belong as they become unable to participate regularly through their active inclusion by, for example, visits from other members. Diversity is the key to finding ways in which people can develop and maintain a social interest, recognizing the different needs of individuals.

Many of the activities suggested here have been low-key, informally organized activities that enable people to develop as much or as little involvement as they need. Some of them, such as computer education, do require financial support; others, such as writing and local history or gardening groups, require much less, but they still need facilities in which they can meet. Many of the traditional neutral meeting grounds—the pubs, the church halls, the community centers and garden plots—are becoming threatened spaces in our communities, and traveling distance between them is getting greater as some of them are closed down and the land is sold for development. The future of social capital can be maintained if new generations can be encouraged to develop the networking skills possessed by the older generation, just as the older generation needs to be encouraged to develop and use the technological communication skills of their younger relatives. Occupational therapists may be among the community facilitators who can encourage the development of informal spaces and low-key occupational environments and practices to support the agency of social capital in an aging population.

Opportunities for Gerontological Occupational Therapists

The challenges presented by the aging population, especially the difficulty of responding from a reduced tax base among the working-age population to the complex needs of older people's health and social care, are more and more part of the current policy agenda. In some economies occupational therapy is anticipated to be very much in demand,[10,68] perhaps as part of a longer understood pattern of need in relation to demographics. One factor of concern, however, is the lack of preparedness some student cohorts feel with regard to working with older people[91] combined with an aging workforce in care professions. Strategies that encourage younger people toward working with older adults and support and retain them in these roles need to be established.[68]

Gerontological occupational therapy practice is already changing through the availability of telemedicine, although there has been uncertainty about the acceptability of these forms of intervention for older people.[44] With further advances, cheaper availability, and future generations who are more oriented to information technology, this may change.

In Britain, some of the main concerns with regard to older people are the effects of inequality and poverty, which operate in complex ways, affecting diet, physical health and mobility, proneness to falls, access to resources, experiences of loneliness, and mental health.[7]

The availability and the priority given to interventions appear to depend on professional training and the attitude of care managers. Some areas receive a particular focus, such as falls prevention, because this can be identified as a target to achieve. This appears to be a result of the use of somewhat one-dimensional evidence-gathering methods. Other approaches may have to compete with these straightforward goals by presenting complex data derived from qualitative measures. In either case, the opinions of older people about what they need are either not sought or would have difficulty finding their way through the study design. Inclusion of input from older individuals is paramount to providing effective interventions, regardless of type, to ensure compatibility, investment, and efficacy.

REVIEW QUESTIONS

1. Considering the description regarding historic understandings of aging, discuss the potential impact of anti-aging perspectives that influence Western society's view of the life course in later years.
2. Explain the relevance of Fraser's conceptualization of *recognition* and *distribution* to current and future gerontological OT practice.
3. Discuss the relationship of social constructions of later life and socioeconomic and health-related disparities.
4. Provide at least two existing or personally conceptualized community-based models of gerontological OT practice to address these disparities.

REFERENCES

1. Age Exchange. (1983). *Fifty years ago: Memories of the 1930s.* London, England: Author.
2. Agency for Healthcare Research and Quality. (2009). *National healthcare disparities report.* Rockville, MD: U.S. Department of Health and Human Services.
3. Akerman, P., Brown, P., Cooke, H., McConalogue, D., & Verne, J. (2008). *Fighting winter cold in the south west: Reducing health inequalities.* Bristol, England: South West Public Health Observatory.
4. Avendano, M., Glymour, M., Banks, J., & Mackenbach, J. (2009). Health disadvantage in US adults aged 50 to 74 years: A comparison of the health of rich and poor Americans with that of Europeans. *American Journal of Public Health, 99,* 540–548.
5. Barber, M. (1999). *A life behind bars.* Brighton, England: QueenSpark.
6. Baron, S. (2004). Social capital in British politics and policy making. In J. Franklin (Ed.), *Politics, trust and networks: Social capital in critical perspective. Families & Social Capital ESRC Research Group Working Paper No. 7* (pp. 5–16). London, England: Families & Social Capital ESRC Research Group.
7. Billings, J., & Brown, P. (2006). *Overview on health promotion for older people in the United Kingdom.* Canterbury, England: HealthPROelderly/University of Kent.
8. Blythe, R. (1979). *The view in winter. Reflections on old age.* London, England: Allen Lane.
9. Boyle, P. J., Norman, P., & Popham, F. (2009). Social mobility: Evidence that it can widen health inequalities. *Social Science & Medicine, 68,* 1835–1842.
10. Brachtesende, A. (2005). The turnaround is here! *OT Practice, 23*(1), 13–19.
11. Brighton Ourstory Project. (1992). *Daring hearts. Lesbian and gay lives of 50s and 60s Brighton.* Brighton, England: QueenSpark.
12. Bruni, L., & Stanca, L. (2008). Watching alone: Relational goods, television and happiness. *Journal of Economic Behaviour and Organisation, 64*(3-4), 506–528.
13. Chaston, D., Pollard, N., & Jubb, D. (2004). Young onset of dementia: A case for real empowerment. *Journal of Dementia Care, 12*(6), 24–26.
14. Chatfield, C., & Hexel, R. (2007). *Privacy and community connectedness: Designing intelligent environments for our cities.* Proceedings of the 19th Australasian conference on Computer-Human Interaction: Entertaining User Interfaces, 265-272. Accessed 10/22/15. http://dl.acm.org/citation.cfm?id=1324950.
15. Chodorow, N. (1978). *The reproduction of mothering.* Berkley, CA: University of California.
16. Coleman, J., Kirby, J., & Kirby, V. (2008). When the therapist met the evangelists: A story of the enablement of an inner-city community. In N. Pollard, D. Sakellariou, & F. Kronenberg (Eds.), *A political practice of occupational therapy* (pp. 167–170). Edinburgh, Scotland: Elsevier Science.
17. Crowther, M. R., Parker, M. W., Achenbaum, W. A., Larimore, W. L., & Koenig, H. G. (2002). Rowe and Kahn's model of successful aging revisited: Positive spirituality—the forgotten factor. *The Gerontologist, 45*(5), 613–620.
18. Dannefer, D. (2003). Cumulative advantage/disadvantage and the life course: Cross-fertilizing age and social science theory. *Journal of Gerontology: Social Sciences, 58B*(6), S327–S337.
19. Diener, E., Kahneman, D., Arora, R., Harter, J., & Tov, W. (2009). Income's differential influence on judgements of life versus well-being. In E. Diener (Ed.), *Assessing well-being: The collected works of Ed Diener* (pp. 233–245). Dordrecht, Netherlands: Springer.
20. Diener, E., & Seligman, M. E. P. (2009). Beyond money: Toward and economy of well-being. In E. Diener (Ed.), *The science of well-being: The collected works of Ed Diener* (pp. 201–265). Dordrecht, Netherlands: Springer.
21. Drexler, M. (2005). *Health disparities and the body politics.* Boston, MA: Harvard School of Public Health.
22. Elings, M. (2006). People–plant interaction: The physiological, psychological and sociological effects of plants on people. In J. Hassink & M. van Dijk (Eds.), *Farming for health* (pp. 43–55). Berlin, Germany: Springer.
23. Erikson, E. (1998). *The life cycle completed.* New York, NY: Norton.
24. Evert Mykytyn, C. (2006). Anti-aging medicine: Predictions, moral obligations, and biomedical intervention. *Anthropological Quarterly, 79*(1), 5–31.
25. Ferraro, K., & Shippee, T. (2009). Aging and cumulative inequality: How does inequality get under the skin? *The Gerontologist, 49*(3), 333–343.
26. Frank, G., & Zemke, R. (2008). Occupational therapy foundations for political engagement and social transformation. In N. Pollard, D. Sakellariou, & F. Kronenberg (Eds.), *A political practice of occupational therapy* (pp. 111–136). Edinburgh, Scotland: Elsevier.

27. Fraser, N. (2003). Social justice in the age of identity politics: Redistribution, recognition, and participation. In N. Fraser & A. Honneth (Eds.), *Redistribution or recognition? A political-philosophical exchange.* (pp. 7–109). London, England: Verso.

28. Freedman, V., Martin, L., & Schoemi, R. (2002). Recent trends in disability and functioning among older adults in the United States. *Journal of the American Medical Association, 288*(24), 3137–3146.

29. Geronimus, A., Bound, J., Waidmann, T., Colen, C., & Stefick, D. (2001). Inequality in life expectancy, functional status, and active life expectancy across selected black and white populations in the United States. *Demography, 38*(2), 227–251.

30. Gigliotti, C. M., Jarrott, S. E., & Yorgason, J. (2004). Harvesting health: Effects of three types of horticultural therapy activities for persons with dementia. *Dementia, 3,* 161–180.

31. Goot, M., van der. (2009). Older widows' television viewing: An interview study. In R. P. Konig, P. W. M. Nelissen & F. J. M. Huysmans (Eds.), *Meaningful media: communication research on the social construction of reality* (pp. 106–118). Nijmegen, Netherlands: Tandem Felix.

32. Graff, M., Adang, E. M. M., Vernooij-Dassen, M. J. M., Dekker, J., Jonsson, L., Thijssen, M. H. L., et al. (2008). Community occupational therapy for older patients with dementia and their care givers: Cost effectiveness study. *British Medical Journal, 336*(7636), 134–138. doi:10.1136/bmj.39408.481898.BE.

33. Green, A., Ross, D., & Mirzoev, T. (2007). Primary health care and England: The coming of age of Alma Ata? *Health Policy, 80*(1), 11–31.

34. Hoggart, R. (1957). *The uses of literacy.* London, England: Chatto and Windus.

35. Ikiugu, M., & Pollard, N. (2014). *Occupation and meaningful living: A guide for everyday activity choices (occupational therapy for a changing world).* London, England: Whting & Birch.

36. Innes, M., & Jones, V. (2006). *Neighbourhood security and urban change, risk, resilience and recovery.* York, England: Joseph Rowntree Foundation.

37. Jubb, D., Pollard, N., & Chaston, D. (2003). Developing services for younger people with dementia. *Nursing Times, 99*(22), 34–35.

38. Krieger, N., Kosheleva, A., Waterman, P. D., Chen, J. T., Beckfield, J., & Kiang, M. V. (2014). 50-year trends in US socioeconomic inequalities in health: US-born black and white Americans, 1959–2008. *International Journal of Epidemiology, 43*(4), 1294-1313 . doi: 10.1093/ije/dyu047.

39. Layder, D. (2004). *Emotion in social life.* London, England: Sage.

40. Mace, J. (1998). *Playing with time: Mothers and the meaning of literacy.* London, England: University College London.

41. Marmot, M., Allen, J., Goldblatt, P., Boyce, T., McNeish, D., Grady, M., et al. (2010). *Fair society, health lives.* London: The Marmot Review. Accessed 10/22/15. www.instituteofhealthequity. org/projects/fair-society-healthy-lives-the-marmot-review.

42. Martin, L., Miranda, B., & Bean, M. (2008). An exploration of spousal separation and adaptation to long-term disability: Six elderly couples engaged in a horticultural programme. *Occupational Therapy International, 15*(1), 45–55.

43. Mattingly, C. (1998). *Healing dramas and clinical plots.* Cambridge, England: Cambridge University Press.

44. McCreadie, C., & Tinker, A. (2005). The acceptability of assistive technology to older people. *Ageing and Society, 25*(1)91–110.

45. McKee, H., & Blair, K. (2007). Older adults and community based technological literacy programs: Barriers and benefits to learning. *Community Literacy Journal, 2,* 13–39.

46. Mykytyn, C. E. (2006). Anti-aging medicine: Predictions, moral obligations, and biomedical intervention. *Anthropological Quarterly, 79*(1), 5–31.

47. Neimeyer, R. A., Holland, J. M., Currier, J. M., & Mehta, T. (2008). Meaning reconstruction in later life: Toward a cognitive-constructivist approach to grief therapy. In D. Gallagher-Thompson, A. M. Steffen, & L. W. Thompson (Eds.), *Handbook of behavioural and cognitive therapies with older adults* (pp. 264–277). New York, NY: Springer.

48. Noakes, D. (1980a). *The town beehive—a young girl's lot, Brighton 1910-1934.* Brighton, England: QueenSpark.

49. Noakes, D. (1980b). *Faded rainbow, our married years.* Brighton, England: QueenSpark.

50. Noakes, G. (1977). *To be a farmer's boy.* Brighton, England: QueenSpark.

51. Oishi, S., Diener, E., & Lucas, R. E. (2009). Can people be too happy? In E. Diener (Ed.), *The science of well-being: The collected works of Ed Diener* (pp. 175–200). Dordrecht, Netherlands: Springer.

52. Oldenburg, R. (1989). *The great good place: Cafes, coffee shops, community centers, beauty parlors, general stores, bars, hangouts, and how they get you through the day.* New York, NY: Paragon House.

53. Osmond, N. (1995). Life after stroke: Special interest book writing groups. In M. Stuart & A. Thomson (Eds.), *Engaging with difference: The "other" in adult education* (pp. 173–186). Leicester, England: NIACE.

54. Parks, S., & Pollard, N. (2009). The extra-curricular of composition: A dialogue on community publishing. *Community Literacy Journal, 3*(2), 53–77.

55. Peters, R., & Beckett, N., Geneva, M., Tzekova, M., Hong Lu, F., Poulter, R., Bulpitt, C. (2009). Sociodemographic and lifestyle risk factors for incident dementia and cognitive decline in the HYVET. *Age and Ageing, 38,* 521–527.

56. Phillips, D. (2006). *Quality of life: Concept, policy and practice.* London, England: Routledge.

57. Player, I., Clark, K., Pearman, G., Castelfranc, G., & Roberts, J. (1993). *Stroke: Who cares? The stories of five carers.* Brighton, England: QueenSpark.

58. Pollard, N. (2006). Is dying an occupation? *Journal of Occupational Science, 13*(2), 149–152.

59. Pollard, N., & Cook, S. (2012). The power of low-key groupwork activities in mental health support work. *Groupwork, 22*(3), 7–32.

60. Pollard, N., & Parks, S. (2011). Community publishing: Occupational narratives and "local publics." In F. Kronenberg, N. Pollard, & D. Sakellariou (Eds.), *Occupational therapies without borders* (pp. 143–152). Edinburgh, Scotland: Elsevier.

61. Portes, A. (1998). Social capital: Its origins and applications in modern sociology. *Annual Review of Sociology, 24,* 1–24.

62. Putnam, R. D. (2000). *Bowling alone: The collapse and rise of American community.* New York, NY: Simon and Schuster.

63. QueenSpark. (1993). *Life after stroke: A book by survivors who have learned to live again.* Brighton, England: Author.

64. Rebeiro, K. (2001). Occupational spin-off. *Journal of Occupational Science, 8,* 33–34.

65. Rodriguez, V. (2001). Tourism as a recruiting post for retirement migration. *Tourism Geographies, 3*(1), 52–63.

66. Rubinstein, A., Andrews, A., & Schweitzer, P. (1991). *Just like the country: Memories of London families who settled in the new cottage estates 1919-1939.* London, England: Age Exchange.

67. Saunders, E. J. (2004). Maximising computer use among the elderly in rural senior centers. *Educational Gerontology, 30,* 573–585.

68. Schoo, A. M., Stagnitti, K. E., Mercer, C., & Dunbar, J. (2005). A conceptual model for recruitment and retention: Allied health workforce enhancement in Western Victoria, Australia. *Rural and Remote Health, 5,* 477. (Online.) Accessed 10/22/15. http://www.rrh.org.au/articles/subviewnew.asp?ArticleID=477.

69. Schweitzer, P. (1985). *Can we afford the doctor? Memories of health care.* London, England: Age Exchange.

70. Schweitzer, P. (1986). *Many happy retirements.* London, England: Age Exchange.

71. Schweitzer, P. (2004). *Mapping memories: Reminiscence with ethnic minority elders.* London, England: Age Exchange.

72. Schweitzer, P., & Hancock, D. (1991). *Our lovely hops: Memories of hop-picking in Kent.* London, England: Age Exchange.

73. Schweitzer, P., Hilton, L., & Moss, J. (1985). *What did you do in the war, Mum? Women recall their wartime work.* London, England: Age Exchange.

74. Scott-Samuel, A., Bambra, A., Collins, C., Hunter, D. J., McCartney, G., & Smith, K. (2014). The impact of Thatcherism on health and well-being in Britain. *International Journal of Health Services, 44*(1), 53–71.

75. Smart, P., Frost, G., Nugent, P., & Pollard, N. (2011). Pecket Learning Community: Where the stem of knowledge blossoms. In F. Kronenberg, N. Pollard, & D. Sakellariou (Eds.), *Occupational therapies without borders* (pp. 19–26). Edinburgh, Scotland: Elsevier.

76. Smith, E. (1992). *Little Ethel Smith, her story told by herself.* Brighton, England: QueenSpark.

77. Steer, A. (1994). *Brighton boy, a fifties childhood.* Brighton, England: QueenSpark.

78. Steultjens, E. M. J., Dekker, J., Bouter, L. M., Jellema, S., Bakker, E. B., & Van Den Ende, C. H. M. (2004). Occupational therapy for community dwelling elderly people: A systematic review. *Age and Ageing, 33,* 453–460.

79. Stockport Arts and Health. (2004). *Lost found time.* Stockport, England: Author.

80. Stone, L. (2001). "Misrecognition of the limits": Bourdieu's Religious Capital and social transformation. *Journal for Cultural and Religious Theory, 3*(1), 1-37.

81. Sundström, G., Malmberg, B., Sancho Castiello, M., del Barrio, É., Castejon, P., Tortosa, M. A., et al. (2008). Family care for elders in Europe: Policies and practices. In M. Szinovacz & A. Davey (Eds.), *Caregiving contexts: Cultural, familial, and societal implications* (pp. 235–268). New York, NY: Springer.

82. Super, N. (2002). *Who will be there to care? The growing gap between caregiver supply and demand. National Health Policy Forum Background Paper.* Washington, DC: National Health Policy Forum.

83. Taylor, J. (2008). On recognition, caring, and dementia. *Medical Anthropology Quarterly, 22,* 336–339.

84. Townsend, P. (1957). *The family life of old people.* London, England: Routledge and Kegan Paul.

85. Townsend, P. (1963). Postscript 1963: Moving towards a general theory of family structure. In P. Townsend (Ed.), *The family life of old people* (pp. 235–255). Harmondsworth, England: Pelican.

86. Updike, J. (1991a). *A Rabbit omnibus.* London, England: Penguin.

87. Updike, J. (1991b). *Rabbit at rest.* London, England: Penguin.

88. Vincent, D. (1981). *Bread, knowledge and freedom, a study of nineteenth-century working class autobiography.* London, England: Europa Publications.

89. Ward, M. (1988). *One camp chair in the living room.* Brighton, England: QueenSpark.

90. Ward, M. (1993). *Memories of Rottingdean 1920-1945.* Brighton, England: QueenSpark.

91. Whaley, M. M. (2009). A study of occupational therapy students' beliefs and attitudes regarding gerontological practice. *Topics in Geriatric Rehabilitation, 25*(3), 265–270.

92. Wilcock, A. (2006). *An occupational perspective of health.* Thorofare, NJ: Slack.

93. Williams, R. (1976). *Keywords.* London, England: Fontana.

94. Wren, T. (1998). *Flying sparks.* Brighton, England: QueenSpark.

CHAPTER 30

The Future of Gerontological Occupational Therapy

Karen Frank Barney, PhD, OTR/L, FAOTA, Margaret A. Perkinson, PhD

CHAPTER OUTLINE

OBJECTIVES

- Review demographic imperatives that signify future increased opportunities for occupational therapy interventions with aging adults
- Articulate the main points of the American Occupational Therapy Association's *Centennial Vision* and their relevance to the future of gerontological occupational therapy
- Review current thinking in regard to optimal aging, and discuss the implications for future gerontological occupational therapy practice
- Explain how preventive gerontology may transform future occupational therapy practice with older adults
- Consider the implications of changing health-care systems and community practice environments in regard to the profession's ability to address the occupational needs of the aging populations served
- Discuss how future occupational therapy practice with older adults might address concerns of occupational literacy and occupational justice
- Envision future continuing and unique practice scenarios that address the occupational needs of aging adults to

"Grow old along with me! The best is yet to be."
Robert Browning (1812-1889)
"Aging is not lost youth but a new stage of opportunity and strength."
Betty Friedan (1921-2006)

This chapter takes the opportunity to reflect upon the sections covered earlier in the book to forecast potential scenarios for the profession, based upon additional references and conceptualizations.

Defining aging and old age is an ongoing challenge, with many types of new evidence being discovered nearly daily. Emerging evidence challenges traditional ways of thinking about the aging process, the concept of retirement, the meaning of leisure and fundamental occupations in later life, the importance of ongoing physical and mental stimulation, the capabilities and potentials of older adults, and how families and communities can best forge intergenerational strategies to benefit individuals of all ages. Taking into account these challenges to traditional notions of aging, we revisit concepts of successful or productive aging and consider potential contributions of occupational therapy (OT) to achieving optimal states in later life.

Global Call for Action

The World Health Organization (WHO) *World Report on Aging and Health* calls for action to promote "Healthy Ageing" that especially focuses on "functional ability."[93] Rather than framing such action in terms of costs to society, fostering supports for functional ability is considered an investment that "will have valuable social and economic returns, both in terms of health and wellbeing of older people and in enabling their on-going participation in society."[93] What discipline is better positioned to support this initiative than occupational therapy?

WHO further emphasized, "'Ageing well' must be a global priority." As noted throughout this book, this imperative is driven by the burgeoning life expectancy of aging adults throughout the world, projected for the first time in history to result in the number of people aged 60 years and older outnumbering children younger than 5 years by 2020.[92] By 2050, adults 60 years and older are projected to total 2 billion, an increase from 841 million in 2014, with 80% dwelling in low- and middle-income countries. Currently 23 countries have the highest prevalence of older adults aged 60 years and older, comprising 23% to 36% of their overall population.[78] This increase in longevity is due to the use of a number of simple public-health-related strategies:

- Reduce tobacco use and high blood pressure, resulting in a decline in deaths from stroke and ischemic heart disease, especially in high-income countries
- Improve sanitation to counter infectious diseases
- Improve food storage to contribute to improved nutritional status
- Improve access to health care and the effectiveness of low-cost health interventions[92]

Productive Aging and the American Occupational Therapy Association's *Centennial Vision*

In anticipation of the 2017 100-year-anniversary celebration of the founding of the American Occupational Therapy Association (AOTA) and subsequent establishment of occupational therapy (OT) as a profession, the *Centennial Vision*[2] was conceptualized to serve as a roadmap for future development of the field. This visionary document identified productive aging as one of the six main practice areas within the profession. In response, OT research on productive aging has undergone recent rapid growth. In an attempt to assess the state of the field during the period immediately following the publication of the *Centennial Vision*, Susan Murphy[47] conducted a review of aging-related articles published from 2008-2009 in the *American Journal of Occupational Therapy* (*AJOT*), AOTA's flagship journal. Although the number of aging-related articles had increased slightly as compared with earlier times, she noted that the body of knowledge produced "was not easily translated into practice"[47](p. 172), and that evidence for the effectiveness of OT practice in aging was still limited. She concluded that the discipline was still in the "beginning stages of knowledge-building" in regard to productive aging. A subsequent update that reviewed the state of OT research on productive aging from 2009-2013[17] reflected a more positive picture, with an increase in both the quantity and quality of *AJOT* articles on aging. A notable contribution during this period was the *AJOT*'s Special Issue on Productive Aging, edited by Leland and Elliott,[38] which included a number of systematic reviews of research on occupation- and activity-based interventions for community-dwelling older adults in areas such as primary care, home modification and fall prevention programs, health management and maintenance, instrumental activities of daily living (IADLs), and occupational engagement and health outcomes. The year 2012 also saw the publication of *Occupational Therapy Practice Guidelines for Productive Aging for Community-Dwelling Older Adults*.[39]

The *Centennial Vision* projected that occupational therapy be viewed as "a powerful, widely recognized, science-driven, and evidence-based profession with a globally connected and diverse workforce meeting society's occupational needs" (p. 613).[2] It is our intent that this book reinforces the goals proposed by the *Centennial Vision* and contributes to the advancement of OT practice with aging adults around the world. Taken together, the chapters provide an overview of relevant topics on aging related to OT practice and research. All but two of the chapters have multiple authors, with one or more preeminent gerontologists reviewing the scientific evidence related to the chapter topic, coupled with the translation of that science into guidelines for evidence-based practice by gerontological occupational therapists noted for their work in that area of practice. The two single-authored chapters (7 and 10) were written by gerontological occupational therapists with significant expertise in both research and practice. By virtue of the intra-/interprofessional and international collaborations that developed in the writing of the chapters, the intended audience goes beyond U.S. OT personnel and occupational scientists, to also address a global audience of gerontologists in research, practice, education, and policy development who may be unfamiliar with the field.

Challenge: Healthful Aging within a Critical Occupational Literacy Framework

Although humans are living longer, they are not necessarily healthier, compared with earlier times. Persons aged 60 years and older account for 23% of the global burden of death and illness, due to aging-related diseases such as arthritis, cancer, cardiovascular disease, chronic respiratory diseases, osteoporosis, and mental and neurological disorders.[92] This long-term burden of illness and diminished well-being affects individuals, their families, health systems, and economies. Furthermore, recent estimates indicate that the number of people with dementia will rise from 44 million to 135 million by 2050.[62,92]

Accompanying the projected global increases in aging populations is the closely related need for aging adults to remain as engaged, empowered, and healthy as possible, for the mutual benefit of all generations. Regardless of differing cultures, lifestyles, and access to formal health care, this need presents an imperative and heretofore unparalleled opportunity for occupational science and occupational therapy to excel in promoting and supporting the fundamental well-being and quality of life of aging adults around the world. To that end, Townsend,[81] in presenting her 2014 Dr. Ruth Zemke Lecture in Occupational Science to an international audience of occupational scientists, challenged those in our field to question what we think we know about aging. Her lecture, which was published later in the *Journal of Occupational Science*, recommended that aging definitions be revised and expanded beyond the focus on older workers and health-care costs associated with aging-related morbidity and mortality. She stated that additional major emphasis should be upon occupational justice and the conditions within which people live, because these conditions determine the constraints under which they age. For example, she noted

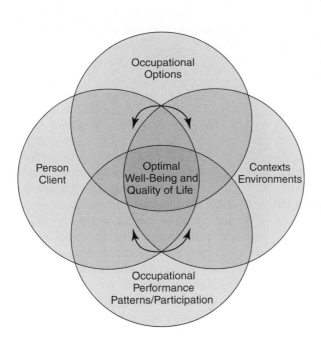

Person/Client: How are intrinsic factors uniquely expressed in this older individual/group; how may function be different now compared with the past; how can factors be optimized?

Contexts/Environment: What are the contexts/environments in which occupational options are grounded; how can we influence optimization?

Occupational Options: What are the activity participation possibilities? What does this older adult/group want/need to do; what are the current priorities and goals; how can these be optimized?

Occupational Performance/Participation: What comprises enactment of activities within the individual's/group's context; can OT optimize this process?

Outcome Goal for OT Intervention: What will enable performance of and engagement in priority activities to support overall optimal well-being and quality of life?

FIGURE 30-1   Components of well-being and quality of life applied to gerontological OT practice. (Modified from: Baum, C. M., & Christiansen, C. H. (2005). Person-environment-occupation-performance: An occupation-based framework for practice. In C. H. Christiansen, C. M. Baum, & J. Bass-Haugen (Eds.), Occupational therapy: Performance, participation, and well-being (3rd ed., pp. 242-266). Thorofare, NJ: SLACK.)

that 20% of global populations live in poverty that limits their occupational choices and options. Additionally, a hidden epidemic of malnutrition among older adults puts them at increased risk of additional morbidity and earlier mortality.[23] By introducing the concept *critical occupational literacy*, Townsend advocated new ways of thinking about occupational justice and integrating it into the everyday lives of older adults. Paraphrasing Levasseur and Carrier's definition of health literacy, we define critical occupational literacy as the ability to access, understand, evaluate, and communicate information within a framework of occupational justice, coupled with the ability to use this information to promote, maintain, and improve participation in various occupations over the life-course.[40] Townsend suggested that developing critical occupational literacy skills could help gerontological occupational therapists to challenge and expand current notions, practices, and policies of old age in order to empower individuals in later stages of life. We maintain that such challenges could empower older adults in their attempts to optimize participation in occupations and enlighten gerontological occupational therapists in their attempts to assist in this process. This chapter will consider factors that could contribute to optimal aging.

Revisiting Premises Posed in Chapter 1

The first chapter presented a model of aging-related well-being and quality of life resulting from the client's interaction with the environment, and the occupational options to which they have access and that result in occupational performance (Figure 30-1). Together with information presented in other chapters and earlier in this chapter, we now consider how the aging process and related OT practice may ideally look in the future. In the first chapter, the client's *current or existing* contextual conditions and occupational options were emphasized. In future practice, an idealized interface of the client, his/her/their environment, and occupational options resulting in occupational performance (Figure 30-2) emphasizes an occupational therapy role in lifestyle *optimization*. In this scenario, *optimal* older adult well-being and quality of life may best be supported by enhancing one or more components of the

OEWB + QoL = f (PA + EF + OA + PSP + P + OF)	
OEWB	Optimal Elder Well-Being
QoL	Quality of Life
PA	Person/Group/Population Attributes
EF	Environmental/Contextual Factors
OA	Occupations/Activities
PSP	Performance Skills and Patterns
P	Participation
OF	Optimizing Factors

FIGURE 30-2   Equation for components of optimal aging, well-being, and quality of life within the context of optimizing factors (optimal elder well-being).

model. Essentially the role of occupational therapy is, wherever possible, first to evaluate each of the separate components, also known as "the domain of occupational therapy," (p. S4)[3]. Second, via intervention that is enhanced by various optimizing factors discussed in this chapter, the profession can facilitate *optimal* function (as co-defined by the client and therapist and/or assistant) of the person/group/population attributes, together with environmental/contextual factors, occupations/activities, performance skills and patterns, and participation. This model differs from traditional OT practice in that it is conducted within a milieu of additional *optimizing factors*, which will be explicated in this chapter. The underlying aim is to promote *optimal* well-being and quality of life. Through this process the following questions should be asked:

- How can the person/client's intrinsic factors be *optimized*?
- How can OT influence *optimization* of the person/client's contexts/environments?
- What are the occupational options available to the person/client, and how can these be *optimized*?
- How can OT *optimize* the person/client's occupational performance and participation?
- By what processes will OT be able to impact the person/client's overall *optimal* well-being and quality of life?

The original model provides a diagram of existing life circumstances among different individuals, groups, or populations, regardless of socioeconomic status. This model can be used to identify target factors to address, serving as a guideline for practice; it guides decision-making for interventions. In essence, it is both a descriptive and prescriptive conceptual framework for *what is*—the current reality, and what might be. Underlying assumptions regarding the client's life circumstances within each of the model's components guide the development of the occupational assessment and intervention process. Subsequently, practice typically proceeds according to medical, legal, and/or other system policies that guide the implementation and discharge or discontinuation process. Within traditional practice settings, further interactions to address client's additional or unmet needs seldom occur.

What is missing and would provide untold opportunity for OT practice is collaborative striving for *what is optimal*—supports for function, occupational performance, and participation in meaningful occupation for the older individual, group, and/or community. Many answers to the questions may be complex, requiring the influencing of the development of health care, legal, sociopolitical, and various other systems that impact the well-being and quality of life for older adults and the generations that follow. Thus, addressing these questions may require an expanded scope and collaborative practice in a variety of new ways to support what can *optimize* well-being and quality of life for older adults. This expanded, collaborative practice approach calls OT practitioners to engage in advocacy on behalf of aging adults to address real and potential unmet enablement needs and ageism. If addressed, all generations may benefit from empowering older adults to fully function in society. Practice implications using this model are explained throughout this chapter.

The diagram initially presented in chapter 1 and replicated in Figure 30-1, which illustrates the relationships among the components of the model, has been expanded to include factors of *optimization* and will be used as a guide for our projections of optimal gerontological OT practice in the future (Figure 30-3). Utilizing many current and emerging

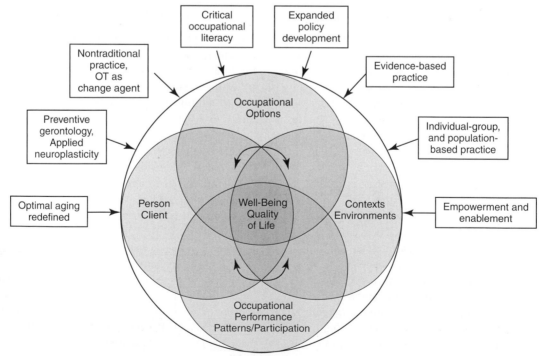

FIGURE 30-3   Model of optimal aging, well-being, and quality of life within the context of optimizing factors. (Modified from: Baum, C. M., & Christiansen, C. H. (2005). Person-environment-occupation-performance: An occupation-based framework for practice. In C. H. Christiansen, C. M. Baum, & J. Bass-Haugen (Eds.), Occupational therapy: Performance, participation, and well-being (3rd ed., pp. 242-266). Thorofare, NJ: SLACK.)

resources, the additional areas of emphasis are shown. These areas include the following:

- Redefining what is *optimal aging*, going beyond traditional perspectives of aging (the taken-for-granted views) by applying objective and potentially *new attitudes and orientation* to what is possible with aging adults
- Applying ongoing *preventive* gerontological approaches, including emerging knowledge of *neuroplasticity* to find ways to stimulate the greater cortical capacity potential of aging adults
- Exercising the extensive contextual perspectives inherent within the field to encourage OT personnel to serve as *change agents* in *nontraditional areas of practice* with aging adults
- Applying a *critical occupational literacy* perspective to influence systems of care, legal processes, businesses, organizations, communities, and other entities in order to promote occupational justice and ecological sustainability on behalf of aging adults
- In all practice contexts, thinking about and acting upon the need for *expanded policy development* to support *optimal aging*
- Using research findings to refine the development of emerging principles and routinely applying these findings via *evidence-based practice*
- Continuing to expand the scope of beyond the *individual* level to include *group- and population-based practice*
- Emphasizing the concepts of *empowerment and enablement* in all individual-, group-, and population-based interventions, regardless of the client's level of ability or frailty

Thus, this *optimal aging* model calls OT practitioners to a higher standard in addressing the full range of needs and potentials of aging individuals. If we are to address the needs and maximize the potentials of this population, we must follow additional and perhaps different avenues in addressing the *well-being and quality of life needs* of older adults.

Within the profession, it is a natural step to adopt a view of the interdependency of collective elements, based upon concepts presented earlier in this chapter and this book, together with Figure 30-3. The following discussion is based upon those assumptions regarding a collective conceptual worldview.

Age-Related Biological System Changes: The Role of Occupational Therapy in Mitigating Aging-Related Health Decline

Consider that within the human development process, at age 30 years most individuals demonstrate their peak performance potential. In subsequent years, typically, a decline in nearly all system functions occurs, unless the individual engages in consistent, systematic physical, mental, nutritional, and other practices that serve to sustain overall function and well-being.[74] Of additional importance is the individual's participation in relevant and meaningful occupations that also serve to support health and well-being.

The OT discipline has an unparalleled opportunity to influence the fundamental quality of life of individuals as they

age, in all realms of biopsychosocial function. Essentially we are the *quality of life* profession. Nearly two decades ago, Fries[20] suggested that preventive gerontology would decrease morbidity and extend life expectancy. He initiated a movement that has since focused on modifying "cumulative lifetime disability" within health-care services. Our profession has participated in this effort on many levels through national, state, and local initiatives that feature support of occupational performance at work, while driving, in managing everyday living tasks, and during leisure activities. Yet, OT personnel should be additionally vigilant for opportunities to address the need for aging-related biopsychosocial supports. For example, Park and Bischof[54] reflect upon recent developments in neuroscience, suggesting that the aging brain can increase capacity in response to prolonged stimuli, a phenomenon known as *neuroplasticity*. They found that despite aging-related neural deterioration, the brain is capable of forming new neural connections, given appropriate stimulation. Thus, cognitive training over time and "engagement in an environment that requires sustained cognitive effort may facilitate cognitive function."[54] Translating this information into practice challenges occupational therapists and assistants to not only apply current state-of-the-art approaches, but also to develop new strategies that capitalize on ever-changing and new technologies to support many aspects of potential functional decline. The development of new intervention models requires associated research to assure efficacy and effectiveness, adding to the body of evidence so critically needed in our discipline.

Age-Related Psychosocial Changes: Current Thinking on Optimal Aging and Implications for Gerontological Occupational Therapy

As reflected in several chapters in this book, our ideas about successful or optimal aging continue to evolve. Biomedically based definitions such as that proposed by Rowe and Kahn equate successful aging with "low risk of disease and disease-related disability, high mental and physical function, and active engagement with life."[66] Thus to be successful in aging, one must be physically and mentally healthy and engaged and actively pursue the steps necessary to achieve such vigor. Critics of this notion of successful aging consider the relentless emphasis on positive, active aging to be a "new form of ageism"[9,30] against frail older adults (including persons with dementia or other cognitive or mental health problems) for whom productive aging as so defined is an unrealistic goal. By advocating the extension of middle-age standards of health, activity, and independence unto later life, positive-aging discourses frame aging in a way that may limit occupational options or possibilities for frail older adults and promote occupational injustice.[8,67] Definitions of successful aging should acknowledge differences between the young-old and the old-old (or what Laslett[37] termed the "third age" and "fourth age") and come to terms with later-life conditions of transience and decline.[35] Those definitions should also take into account the views of older adults on this matter.[11,58,76] Our notions of successful aging should not equate all situations of late-life dependence, disability, and eventual mortality as "failures" in living well.[35] Indeed, mature spirituality, wisdom, and compassion may blossom in the midst of such "failed" conditions.

In affixing the concepts of "active" or "successful" aging to situations of frailty, criteria such as behavioral and emotional "plasticity,"[24] and coping, resilience, and engagement in select activities could replace attainment of high levels of physical and cognitive function and performance.[10] Berg[7] has suggested that the meaning of social engagement changes for the old-old, shifting from participation in large social networks to focus on select, emotionally close relationships. Older adults may be less actively involved in pursuing goals and more oriented to enjoying everyday occupations.[15] It is critically important for occupational therapists and assistants to be sensitive to the diversity of ways in which one can successfully and productively age, regardless of physical and cognitive function. Concepts of successful aging shape therapeutic goals and define the criteria appropriate for evaluating outcomes. One should conduct careful evaluations and maintain a client-centered approach to jointly define attainable, meaningful occupations that represent productivity and success to that particular older client. Assist clients in identifying and prioritizing their tasks in terms of meaning and value. Working as a team with your client (and possibly relevant family members), strategize how to drop and/or minimize effort on tasks deemed less important and *optimize* effort and attention on occupations of greatest significance.[5] This may require compensatory strategies to address one or more of the components illustrated in Figure 30-1 as discussed below and presented in Figure 30-3.

Context and Environment: The Role of Occupational Therapy in Optimizing Environmental Effects

Cultural Contexts

The cultural contexts in which our individual, group, or community-level clients function are resource-rich commodities of current and potential supports and occupational options for aging adults. Wherever applicable, OT personnel working with older clients should learn about and actively engage in collaborating with these resources to facilitate developing and sustaining *optimal* practice. The need for cultural education is particularly important if the client group being served is from a different culture or ethnic group from that of the OT providers. However, even if OT personnel are from the same cultural roots as the client, but are from different geographical areas and/or generations as compared with the client group, they must educate themselves on the cultural norms, historical and current practices, and expectations of the individual, group, or population they intend to serve. By taking time to self-educate via credible sources who may be members of that group, OT personnel will position themselves to most effectively intervene. Examples from Brodrick and Barry in chapter 28 highlight the role that occupational therapists and assistants can effectively play as

change agents, in any setting, demonstrating the importance of congruent perspectives between clients and therapists in understanding each other; in determining needs, problems, and priorities; in making decisions regarding intervention planning and enactment; and in achieving optimal outcomes. These outcomes will be optimal if they demonstrate a goodness of cultural fit of the intervention with the client served.

Social Environments

One's social environment affords a range of potential supports for aging individuals, from no family or significant others to large families or other accommodating groups committed to providing whatever sustaining supports are needed. Additionally, depending upon the locale, state, or country, economic, legal, and health-care supports for older members of society vary. Optimal community bases are described by Parker Palmer:[52]

> Abundance is a communal act, the joint creation of an incredibly complex ecology in which each part functions on behalf of the whole and, in return, is sustained by the whole. Community doesn't just create abundance—community *is* abundance. If we could learn that equation from the world of nature, the human world might be transformed.

His statement underscores the importance of interdependence in communities that function well and are intergenerationally and beneficially mutually reliant. How may OT personnel capitalize on this concept to foster this type of outcome? To promote holism for the greater good and facilitate compensation for services rendered, this type of outcome likely requires many layers of proactive intervention with older clients and their support systems, and with policy development for legal and health-care systems at many levels.

Physical Environments

Regardless of the location of their practice, OT practitioners should be mindful of the physical environments within which collaborative support is provided to clients, whether aging individuals, groups, or communities. In developed countries, physical environments likely represent different challenges and opportunities as compared with developing countries. In either case, occupational therapists and assistants need to be proactive in advocating for and supporting the development of physically supportive environments for all ages. Thus, therapists and assistants may need to work with governmental or nongovernmental organizations (NGOS) to promote inclusive and functionally supportive physical environments, utilizing their understanding of how accommodating spaces support function, performance, and participation in needed and meaningful occupations.

Occupational therapy personnel have unique perspectives that combine intrinsic, extrinsic, occupational performance, and options factors that can make an important contribution to big-picture thinking. This type of long-range conceptual investment may bear fruitful economic and quality-of-life outcomes that benefit the greater populace. Scharlach[70] identified aging-supportive needs in community planning, system coordination among agencies, program development, co-location of services, and the development of consumer associations. Additionally, Greenfield et al.[25] found that planning is needed to bring services in close proximity to neighborhoods, especially naturally occurring retirement communities (NORCs). Evidence regarding these needs is increasing over time, with the evolving development of instruments that objectively measure the residential environmental needs and preferences of aging adults.[13] One may postulate that supporting *optimal* aging with supportive environments is an ongoing fundamental societal need for all ages—OT perspectives need to be heard, as they are instrumental in developing supportive intergenerational communities.

Universal Design (UD) concepts, originally proposed by Ronald Mace,[42] provide a conceptual framework for OT personnel to promote such intergenerationally friendly physical environments in any location. Mace defined UD as "the design of products and environments to be usable by all people, to the greatest extent possible, without the need for adaptation or specialized design."[42] The UD approach is viewed as an inclusive strategy that supports the occupational performance of individuals of any age, regardless of level of ability or disability. UD principles and explanatory constructs promote universal access and usability for all, and need to be included in the repertoire of OT practitioners' perspectives and skills. Extensive resources on this design approach, including additional resources related to design concepts that support aging, may be found on the R. L. Mace Universal Design Institute website.[64,65]

Box 30-1 presents categories of physical environments that could be made more "age-friendly" with the application of OT-informed design or modification in one's work with planning agencies, local businesses, and community organizations. OT personnel can apply their holistic wisdom, including an understanding of aging-related changes and what physically supports *optimal* occupational performance, to influence community design in so that it maximizes *optimal* participation for aging adults and others with whom they interact.

When working with aging clients, many resources are available for recommending adaptations to home environments to support *optimal* functioning in basic activities of daily living (ADLs) and IADLs. In proceeding with recommendations, occupational therapists need to ensure that interventions focus not only on what is feasible, but also what is most meaningful for the aging adult and is likely to support their *optimal* well-being and quality of life.

Changing the design landscape toward *optimal* functional approaches may require OT personnel to join with city planners, architects, and interior designers as members of their interprofessional team. Aligning with these disciplines will allow access to influencing plans that are not only universally accessible, but especially aging-friendly. Box 30-2 notes examples of design gaps observed in categories identified in Box 30-1.

OT personnel have an incredible opportunity to impact the well-being and overall quality of life of not only older adults but all generations by collaborating with urban planners, architects, and designers. The knowledge and skills foundation that the profession "brings to the table" can potentially revolutionize how built environments are conceptualized from the beginning. Imagine the effects on *optimal* occupational performance, well-being, and quality of life! The authors of this chapter have been privileged to work collaboratively with these disciplines via consulting on the development of health-care service environments, continuum-of-care retirement communities, adult day-care settings, and personal living environments. Case Example 30-1 is based on the experiences of the first author.

BOX 30-1   Opportunities for Occupational Therapy Influence in Designing Places and Spaces

- Community development
  - Housing and neighborhoods
  - Transportation modes and hubs (e.g., mass-transit centers, railway stations, airports)
  - Shopping venues: grocery and other
  - Restaurants
  - Libraries
  - Health clubs, gyms, and other exercise facilities
  - Public restrooms
  - Historic and new buildings of any type
  - Institutional health-care environments: urgent, emergency, acute, long-term, and hospice care
  - Organizations providing services to aging adults
  - Other mobility-related amenities:
    - Roads, highways, intersections
  - Streets, sidewalks, curb cuts, traffic lights
  - Signage:, locations, wording, design
  - Parks—national, state, county/province, city, neighborhood
  - Recreational venues—theaters, theme parks, water parks, intergenerational playgrounds, museums
- Homes
  - Initial designs and furnishing
  - Retrofitting existing homes, including apartments, condominiums, and other dwellings
- Houses of worship
  - Transportation and parking space locations
  - Paths for ingress and egress
  - Accommodations for aging-related vision, hearing, and mobility limitations

BOX 30-2   Potential Gaps in Customary Designs of Places and Spaces

- Community Development
  - *Cities, housing, and neighborhoods:* There exists a lack of an overall plan for keeping walking or driving distances such that they support fitness and optimal access to grocery stores, health-care services, and other fundamental supports.
- Homes
  - *Apartments, condominiums, single or communal family:* Entrances and internal environments, even in newly constructed or spaces adapted in historic buildings, are often unsupportive of aging-related needs.
  - *Transportation modes and hubs:* Locations may not be central or easily accessible for many age groups, especially aging adults.
  - *Shopping venues:*
    - Long distances between shops without intermittent seating, including shopping malls, may discourage older shoppers from participating.
    - Access, aisle space, lighting, and items placed too high with no readily available assistance discourage optimal use.

- *Recreation Settings:* parks, museums, theaters, other venues
  - Exterior: Signage, limited or no lighting, parking availability and distance to entrance, heavy doors may discourage access
  - Interior: Low lighting, hall widths, flooring, required ambulation distances without opportunities for intermittent seating may discourage participation.
- *Potential universal unmet aging-related needs:*
  - Lighting, flooring, color choices, contrast (or lack thereof) in any environment may pose challenges to aging adults with age-related vision, mobility, or cognitive changes (e.g., dementia).
  - Signage should be explicit, using universal symbols whenever possible (e.g., for restrooms) because these tend to be "user-friendly" for all ages and cultural groups.
  - Traffic lights frequently allow limited time for crossing streets.
  - While driving, venues with signage indicating the need for quick decision making for turns may be challenging not only for aging adults, but also anyone who is unfamiliar with the territory/route.

CASE EXAMPLE 30-1   Edison Condominiums Evolvement

In 1998 the first author and her husband learned of an innovative opportunity—a plan to transform an historic landmark building in downtown St. Louis, the oldest warehouse west of the Mississippi River in the United States, into a multi-use site, including a hotel, restaurants, and condominiums. For the couple in their late 50s at the time, and who had considered condominium living for years, the meaning of this opportunity was transitioning from a single-family home in the suburbs to living in downtown St. Louis. Regarding supports for aging in place over time, this site potentially offered enormous advantages and amenities:

- Hugely reduced maintenance of exterior and interior physical spaces, with support provided by hotel staff and condominium association infrastructures
- "Just right" numbers of extra bedrooms for visits from out-of-town friends or the adult children and grandchildren; residents benefit from hotel discounts
- Resident neighbors as a unique "community" representing diverse ages, cultures, religions, occupations, and backgrounds
- Fitness room, swimming pool, and restaurants shared with the hotel
- Room service availability
- Secure parking in the building
- Patio on top of the building with gas grills for condominium residents
- Mass transit (bus, metro transit, and rail) directly across the street from the site
- Grocery stores, restaurants, library, houses of worship, parks, theaters, major sports venues, concerts, museums, courts, major parades, and other attractions within walking distance

The conversion of the building for future condominium residents meant that they were offered standard designs but could make changes to those plans. With the agreement of her husband, the author informed the developer that he should include their unit within the 20% required by law for accessible design, and she then proceeded to ensure that the new interior spaces would support their aging-related needs. Thus, all doorways were constructed wider, pocket doors were included in the guest and master bathrooms, and higher toilet seats and vanities (except for the "powder room") and grab bars were installed in all bathrooms. Furthermore, choices of lighting, carpeting, tiled flooring, wall colors, contrasting door frames, cabinetry with pull out drawers and so forth were made with aging-related needs in mind. In the original plan provided by the developer, there was no linen closet, spaces were tighter, and a large tub was included in the master bathroom. Instead, the author and her husband insisted on wider, more inclusive spaces, no large tub (one is included in the guest bathroom), and instead a large shower with no threshold, grab bars, a handheld shower head, and bath seat.

The author also advocated for accessibility and "aging-friendly" design throughout the building, resulting in modifications to the original plan in several areas. The most obvious accommodations are an elevator to the enclosed rooftop pool, and a lift into the pool for swimmers with mobility limitations.

The couple has lived in this environment for 14 years, and is thankful for the fundamental supports it provides. Most amenities are within easy reach and designed for maximum efficiency. Furthermore, the residential environment evolved with great diversity of ages, racial/ethnic groups, professions, vocations, and lifestyles and has flourished, with frequent planned and spontaneous social gatherings. Both younger individuals with disabilities and older residents with dementia, mobility limitations, dialysis dependency, post-stroke, and cardiac conditions, as well as students, athletes and other able-bodied individuals thrive together.

Glimpses into the Future

Impact of Cutting-Edge Developments in Gerotechnology on Future Occupational Therapy Practice

The rapid pace of technological development is transforming all sectors of modern life, including the experience of later life. As noted in chapter 21, occupational therapists and assistants will encounter opportunities to incorporate a wide array of technological aids in their practice with older adults. As compared with the current cohort of older adults and their family caregivers, upcoming cohorts tend to be more comfortable with technology and receptive to technological innovations in older adult care,[48] so OT personnel can expect to find a growing receptivity to new technological aids. Given the proliferation of smartphones and other technologies, even in low-income countries and rural areas, the potential for technological advances in older adult care is global in scale. Rather than summarize current offerings in technology, which previous chapters have reviewed, we briefly examine recent prototypic developments that offer promise for the future.

Ambient intelligence is a term for electronic environments that are sensitive to individual inhabitants.[1,16] An intelligent computing system recognizes and is personalized to the needs of residents, and can anticipate those needs and respond accordingly.[46,95] A well-calibrated system constantly evolves through a series of feedback loops, learning from interactions with the users, and continuously adjusts the balance between the capacity/competence of the user and the challenges or press of the environment to achieve homeostasis.[41]

Monitoring is an important component of ambient intelligence. Embedded in the physical environment, wearable, or in the form of an app, monitoring devices can track measures of physical functioning (e.g., blood pressure, heart rate, temperature, glucose and oxygen levels), biochemical processes (e.g., wound healing), amount of physical activity, harmful positioning or lifting, incidence of falls, sleep patterns, adherence to medical regimens, and changes in the home environment such as temperature or lighting.[1,53,55,59] Among its many benefits, the monitoring system can contribute to clients' safety, identify early symptoms, and enable independent living and aging in place. Pre-impact fall detectors based on accelerometers, such as the smart cane SmartFall,[36,94] represent promising ways to unobtrusively monitor for safety and sound alerts as needed. Another system designed to prevent falls among persons with Parkinson's disease (PD) monitors for "freezing of gait," a PD gait symptom strongly related to falls, and provides a rhythmic auditory signal to stimulate continued walking at signs of a halt due to "freezing"[4] (Figure 30-4 A-B).

Telerehabilitation for stroke or joint replacements can approximate in-person therapy through the use of long-distance position sensing, movement analysis, and estimation of joint angles. Engaging in rehabilitation in one's natural environment rather than in a clinic results in better functional outcomes, higher client satisfaction, lower costs, and shorter duration of treatment.[12,18] Unobtrusive monitoring of rehabilitation clients' daily physical activity provides information on the quality and amount of ambulation and exercise, which may differ from that documented in the clinic.[63]

Persons with cognitive impairment also can benefit from intelligent technology.[80] Embedded sensors combined with global positioning system (GPS) devices can provide assisted navigation and prevent wandering, both indoors and out.[21,87] (Figure 30-5). A cognitive orthotics tool, such as SenseCam,[29] records images of the day with a wearable camera and collates them with log entries to serve as a retrospective memory aid. Avatar virtual coaches and autoreminders can provide instructions to guide a person with dementia through a given task, such as hand washing.[44,51,59,60,73]

Despite seemingly boundless potential, intelligent technology has its critics. Telecare may medicalize home environments and depersonalize care.[45] Ambient intelligence may lull its users into a false sense of security and possibly reduce abilities as a result of disuse and overdependence on technological supports.[41] It is a challenge to integrate complex technological systems into health and social service systems, existing organizations, the work habits of practitioners, and the family systems and lives of older clients. Occupational therapists and assistants can facilitate this process by assisting in the selection of appropriate devices, helping to personalize them for the older client's use, instructing the older adult and his or her family members on proper use and maintenance of equipment, and helping to motivate and integrate technology into daily life routines and health-related occupations.[79] Quality-of-life technologies,[71] (e.g., person- and/or context-aware technological systems that maintain or enhance all aspects of functioning (e.g., physical, cognitive, social, or emotional) by enhancing occupational performance, entertaining or stimulating clients, offering preventive supports, facilitating information seeking and sharing, and providing venues that encourage social connectedness) all fall within the OT domain. Smart technologies generate much information relevant to the client's personal capacities and occupational performance that occupational therapists and assistants can use to inform client-centered practice. Learning how to access and interpret that information should be part of all OT curriculae.

Health-Care Environments

Health-care systems change over time throughout the world. Unlike many countries in Europe, until recently, efforts in the United States to develop national health insurance were unsuccessful, resulting in a system of voluntary health insurance that covered approximately 60% of Americans in 2008.[72] Due to high health-care costs and morbidity and mortality data revealing poorer outcomes than those in other developed countries, the current U.S. health-care system is undergoing rapid changes.[72] Since 2010, accountable care organizations

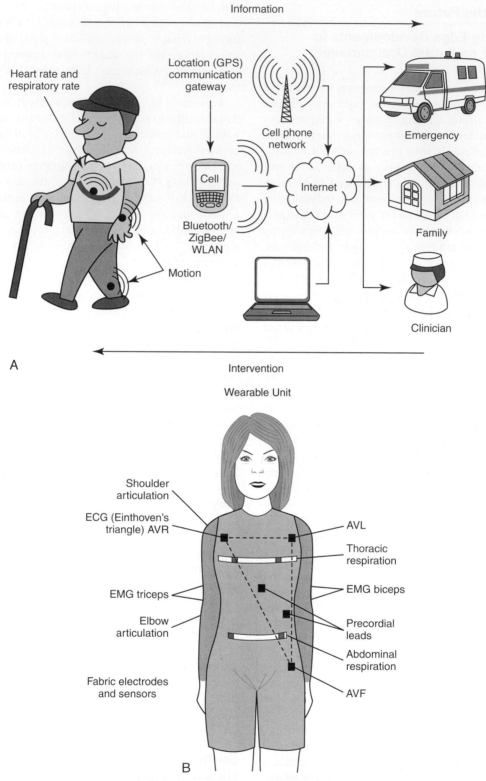

Information →

Heart rate and
respiratory rate

Location (GPS)
communication
gateway

Cell phone
network

Emergency

Cell

Bluetooth/
ZigBee/
WLAN

Internet

Family

Motion

Clinician

A

← Intervention

Wearable Unit

Shoulder
articulation

ECG (Einthoven's
triangle) AVR

AVL

Thoracic
respiration

EMG triceps

EMG biceps

Elbow
articulation

Precordial
leads

Abdominal
respiration

Fabric electrodes
and sensors

AVF

B

FIGURE 30-4 A-B   Wearable health technology.

have been forming to provide more client-centered, instead of provider-directed, care to improve outcomes and reduce health-care costs.[19] These changes have the potential to maximally humanize the delivery of services to all ages, and aging adults stand to benefit greatly.

The perennial state-of-the-art practice in which OT personnel are socialized into the profession focuses on client-centered care. Therefore the profession is well positioned, and the time is right, to work within all healthcare systems to ensure that the best interests of the recipient of services

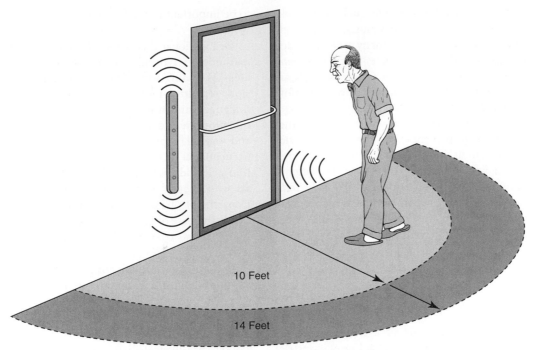

FIGURE 30-5   Electronic system prevents wandering.

are at the center of decision making. The OT voice regarding the individual client; the client's contexts and environments, including a variety of resources; and the client's individual and collective preferences for participation should be heard. Throughout the continuum of care, the profession can be at "center stage" in advocating for holistic client approaches to service delivery. Consider the intrinsic factors of aging-related changes explicated in preceding chapters along with immediate and emerging information on environmental contributors to support personal preferences for occupational performance and participation. Related to these needs, OT personnel are well positioned to collaborate in designing services in health promotion and interventions that mitigate risk for potential aging-related diseases; promote self-management of overall health, falls, and injury prevention; support intergenerational needs; assist in cost containment; and promote health-related quality of life.

Occupational Justice and Occupational Options

Although life expectancy and living standards vary throughout the world, the aim of promoting health and occupational balance for all is a purpose around which OT practitioners can rally. This effort may require "reinventing" the meaning of aging, *optimal* aging, and the occupational potential of an individual of any age, offering the potential for more freedom of choices (e.g., occupational options). Clearly, varying cultural and racial/ethnic group interpretations and values, changing demographics, and differing economic

conditions should be taken into consideration as occupationally empowering strategies are developed with individuals, families, and communities.

Townsend[81] introduced *occupational literacy* as a construct underscoring the need for reexamination of what we know about aging and how we practice with aging adults. She stressed that we need to be critical of and move beyond how aging is sociopolitically defined via data on older workers, morbidity, and related health costs. She also acknowledged the "problematizing" of aging via government reports that underscore its negative aspects.

Furthermore, she underscored the need to connect aging with the real, everyday world of occupations, to organize a more just and ecologically sustainable world. As occupational therapy personnel, we should be inspired to organize our services with older adults to maximize participation and reduce occupational deprivation, oppression, and marginalization, and thereby increase opportunities for participation in whatever roles are of interest and relevant to the individual, group, or community.[81]

Furthermore, Townsend[81] promoted linking occupation with justice and ecological sustainability. Therefore, occupational scientists and OT personnel are challenged to examine sociopolitical practices to determine strategies that will ensure the viability of aging and intergenerational populations.

Finally, Townsend[81] introduced the proactive construct of *societal enabling* versus *caregiving* as an empowering, broader perspective to apply to those populations of older adults who no longer are able to live independently. The primary aim, maintaining these care-enabled and empowered individuals in the community for as long as possible, such as for individuals with an Alzheimer's disease diagnosis, is positively supported via the collective efforts of many. She suggested that *caregiving* implies a dependent state, whereas *societal enabling* implies supportive measures at whatever levels are needed to ensure individualized occupational participation. Thus, occupational therapists can empower clients to a greater degree by inspiring them, their family members, or other supports (e.g., health-care personnel, or any related service providers) to participate in their *optimal* occupations, rather than doing for them, which *caregiving* may imply. The emphasis is on the *individual doing*, rather than *doing for the individual*. Consequences of applying this approach may expand the client's occupational options. With the client as the primary focus, rather than the routine that a caregiver/provider has established, more individualized choices that support the client's well-being and quality of life are likely to be available.

Older Workers

Growing recognition of the needs of aging workers has evolved over the past half century. The discipline of industrial gerontology was established to focus on the special needs of aging workers, especially employment and retirement needs and concerns of middle-aged and older workers.[88] Meier and Kerr[43] conducted one of the earliest cumulative accounts of older worker attributes and needs via a literature review. They found that the capabilities of these workers exceeded the physical demands of most jobs, and with appropriate placement older workers demonstrated effectiveness and greater stability, and fewer accidents and less time off from work, than their younger counterparts. Furthermore, they identified 20 studies that demonstrated that general information, judgment, and vocabulary are sustained and may increase after 60 years of age. They also determined that, overall, older workers report greater satisfaction with their work than do younger workers. Finally, gerontologists generally accept that "crystalized" intelligence, that is, knowledge or experience accumulated over time (including vocabulary), actually remains stable or improves with age (even beyond age 60 years). On the other hand, "fluid" intelligence, or abilities not based on experience or education, tends to decline with age.

Despite these positive attributes, older workers typically face negative stereotypical feedback from all age groups, and may themselves have succumbed to those beliefs.[88] When employers also hold these stereotypes, the resulting effects are great. Warr and Clapperton[88] determined that employers in industrial settings continued to encourage older workers to take early retirement buyouts. Furthermore, they continued to be reluctant to train or retrain current employees or hire or train individuals over the age of 40 years. In recent years, middle-aged and older workers were significantly affected by layoffs, downsizings, and plant closings, yet younger individuals were hired into new positions in the same companies. Clearly, continuing education, retraining, and long-range planning and coping strategies will continue

to be important in the future to maintain effectiveness in the workforce.

Occupational therapists who have worked with business and industry typically are known as specialists in numerous areas, including work-site analysis, adaptation, and/or revision; repetitive motion injury prevention; management of design, administrative, and worker changes; disability determination; residual capacity evaluations; stress reduction; and overall coping needs of workers.[26,69,90] Additionally, occupational therapists working with manufacturing workers routinely address multiple aging-related changes in individuals who engage in physically demanding work.[69] The U.S. Department of Labor Bureau of Labor Statistics reported a steady increase of older workers, especially full-time workers, in individuals over the age of 65 years, since 1970.[83] The age groups of 65 to 75 years and over 75 years demonstrated the largest increases in the labor force, with a declining number of younger full-time workers, approximately -7% in the age group of 16 to 24 years. In the United States this trend is expected to continue; aging-worker-related trends in other developed countries may be different. Nevertheless, aging workers are likely to have continuing need for support in numerous areas, and their talents are needed in the workplace. Carstensen[14] argues, "In my mind, the most pressing reason that people should work longer is that they can!" (p. 171).

Building upon many areas of expertise, with holistic understanding of the importance of considering *optimal* occupational options, continuation in the same or different work, or retirement from the workforce, OT personnel have much to offer both aging workers and their employers. With the global increased numbers of aging individuals, this area of OT practice has the potential to greatly expand.

Aging with a Disability

Within the last century, advances in medical sciences and improvements in overall quality of life in developed countries have resulted in increased life expectancy for persons with either congenital or other disabling conditions that occurred early in life. In the United States over 12 million individuals with early-onset disabilities are living to middle age and beyond;[32] however, these individuals have not experienced aging in the usual way, especially those with physical conditions such as cerebral palsy and spinal cord injury who experience much earlier changes in their 40s or 50s, similar to post–polio syndrome. Nearly 33% of individuals with Down syndrome experience Alzheimer's disease by their 50s.[32]

Individuals with disabilities present since childhood are generally psychosocially different and have greater disability than those who experience disability onset in adulthood. Additionally, poor overall health diminishes their social participation.[86] However, in middle age, despite childhood onset of disabilities, some of these individuals participate in social activities to a greater extent than individuals with adult disability onset. In both groups, social participation is primarily affected by poor overall health.[86] Large studies of persons with disabilities are rare, due to the associated high cost. Therefore, researchers in the United States, such as Verbrugge and Yang,[86] have relied upon National Health Interview Survey Disability Supplement data, compiled by the U.S. Centers for Disease Control and Prevention, to study disability-related phenomena.

The following study of disability[6] that focused on biopsychosocial factors contributing to health-related quality of life was conducted with a specific population, community dwelling individuals with spinal cord injury (SCI). Due to the sample size (n = 165) and focus (SCI), limitations are apparent, yet findings serve as an example of the impact of acquired disability upon health-related quality of life.[6] This Internet survey utilized the Medical Outcomes Study Short Form Version 2 to measure health-related quality of life within this population. The age range was 18 to 72 years, with mean age of participants at 41.3 years, mean time since injury of 15 years, with 10% who were at least 55 years of age and post-SCI as long as 30 years, reflective of long-term living with disability. Study participants' mean scores on six of the eight scales (Physical Functioning, Role Physical, General Health, Social Functioning, Role Emotional, and Mental Health) were below the 25th percentile of the norm-based scores. This finding reflects highly limited overall quality of life, when compared with able-bodied populations.[6] What are the implications of these findings for practice—for *optimizing* occupational options and occupational performance with persons aging with a disability?

Historically OT personnel have routinely encountered persons with disabilities in the medical settings in which they serve. The customary orientation has involved working with the individual toward ameliorating the effects of the disabling condition, to promote effective occupational performance and discharge to life in the community. When the time spent with these individuals is situated strictly within the health-care system (e.g. acute care, rehabilitation clinic, medical office or department), OT practitioners may have a limited view of the everyday lives of persons with disabilities. Given this situation, it seems imperative that OT personnel become routinely involved at the communitylevel to address the disability- and aging-related needs of these clients, to support lifestyles that support *optimal* health, maximize abilities, address fundamental quality-of-life needs, and support participation in their *optimal* occupational options.

Incarceration and Aging

Globally, approximately 1 in 700 persons is incarcerated (Figure 30-6). The United States historically represents the highest prison population rate, greater than five times the overall world rate, resulting in approximately 1 in 100 citizens residing in prisons.[56,78] These high rates may be explained by punitive sentencing practices,[33] the prison as a highly profitable industrialized complex, and racism.[77] Furthermore, rates of recidivism in the United States are extremely high, thus supporting the continuation of high rates of incarceration.[57]

Around the world, conditions in prisons vary. Developed countries typically apply standards regarding the nutritional value of food and health care; however, these standards may be minimal compared to what the population on "the outside" experiences, according to the International Center for Prison Studies.[31] In the *Report on International Prison Conditions*, the U.S. Department of State conveyed the following finding: "A majority of the world's prison systems do not function at the level of the United Nations' Standard Minimum Rules for the Treatment of Prisoners. In some countries, relevant international obligations and standards are deliberately disregarded." The report additionally shared the following categories of U.S. government human rights and humanitarian concerns regarding incarcerated individuals:

1. *Unsafe prison conditions*: overcrowding, poor sanitation, inadequate access to food or potable drinking water, and poor medical care, including inadequate services for people with disabilities
2. *Mistreatment of prisoners* by prison staff or other authorities
3. *Inadequate legal protections* leading to prisoners' incarceration, and failure to respect the right to legal redress while in prison

The anticipated proportion of incarcerated individuals aged 50 years and older, especially those 65 years and older, is expected to rapidly increase over the next several years, particularly in the United States. Whereas approximately 3% of the prison population was age 65 years and older in 2011, this rate is expected to triple by 2019. As a result, those 50 years and older are anticipated to constitute nearly 30% of the prison population.[33] While these incarcerated individuals are segregated from society, their bodies are experiencing the same typical aging-related changes as are characteristic of those "on the outside" in mainstream society. However, nearly all aspects of typical societal supports for occupational options and participation are highly constrained during their detention. In the United States, generally prison environments limit participation in most occupations, fostering a level of occupational deprivation not experienced in mainstream society.

The OT profession has an opportunity to affect the lives of these aging incarcerated individuals in at least four categories: jail and prison design, fostering a healthy culture for those incarcerated and staff, basic programming within the jail or prison, and pre- and postrelease services (Box 30-3). Because most incarcerated individuals return to society upon release (97% in the United States[56]), they will reside as our neighbors. Thus, how would society prefer that they be reintegrated into our communities? If jails and prisons are designed to support maintenance and/or enhancement of occupational performance, persons reentering society will be less likely to experience huge occupational performance gaps compared with those in mainstream society. Those released at older ages and who have been incarcerated for many years are more vulnerable than older adults who have lived continuously in the community, due to the occupational deprivation experienced during their incarceration term.

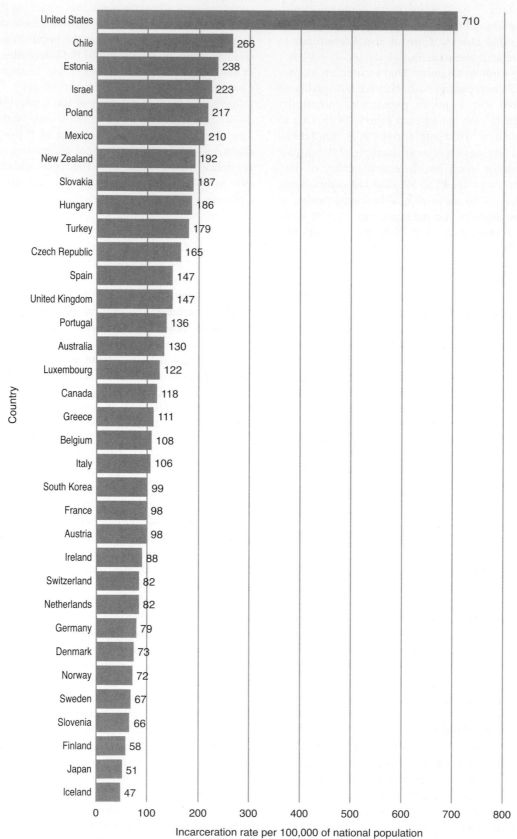

FIGURE 30-6   Global Incarceration Rates in Selected Nations. (From Organization for Economic Cooperation & Development (OECD) Factbook 2011-2012.)

BOX 30-3   Potential Occupational Therapy Roles with Incarceration Systems to Foster Optimal Function

1. <u>Modifying jail and prison design</u> that minimally supports maintenance and/or improvement of prisoner ADLs and those IADLs that are relevant to the setting, as well as psychological well-being
2. <u>Reinforcing jail and prison culture</u> that ensures safety and simultaneously supports respect and optimal health for all
3. <u>Supporting fundamental quality of life on "the inside"</u>
   a. Advocate for and develop programs that optimize the available occupational options that are available for all, including aging incarcerated persons.
   b. Educate jail and prison staff and younger incarcerated individuals on environmental and person-centered interventions that can be applied to support those who are increasingly frail and dependent upon those assisting them in the prison environment.

   c. Advocate for usual and customary health promotion and medical care as experienced on "the outside."
4. <u>Supplementing jail and prison planning efforts with those who reenter society</u>
   a. Collaborate with jail and prison staff in their work to habilitate or rehabilitate older incarcerated individuals prior to release.
   b. Assist jail, prison, and external probation, parole, and other related re-entry staff in developing transitional supports for older prisoners, especially those who have served long prison terms, and who may no longer have family, friends, or others who will assist them upon their release.

OT personnel can play a critical role in addressing these concerns; 20% of the OT profession in Japan serves this population (personal communication, Tomoko Kondo, June 20, 2014).

Mandates and Challenges in Gerontological Practice and Research

Occupational Disparities and Occupational Justice

The 2011 United Nations Report on Human Rights of Older Persons called global attention to the plight of older adults, noting that their economic and social disadvantages and status as victims of discrimination qualified them as a marginalized group, vulnerable to abuse and exploitation. The relatively low priority of older adults globally in regard to health policies, programs, and resource allocation has placed them at increased risk for disease and disability. With similar concerns for human rights, the World Federation of Occupational Therapists (WFOT) International Advisory Group on Human Rights issued recent challenges to occupational therapists with its agenda titled, "Driving Societal Change: OT, Health, and Human Rights."[28]

Attention to issues of human rights has led OT personnel to nontraditional areas of practice with vulnerable populations and the subgroups of older adults within them. Townsend and Marval[82] identified six vulnerable populations faced with continued social and economic inequities and likely to experience occupational deprivation and injustice. They singled out older adults as one of the six groups, noting their "occupational injustice persists in limited social inclusion due to restrictive and over-protective housing, lack of age-friendly transportation and technology, insufficient income assistance, and 'keep busy' activities in residential care... *Intervention should address more than just the remediation of skills and abilities*" (p. 220). The other vulnerable groups identified by Townsend and Marval, some of which have been identified earlier in this chapter, included persons with disabilities; refugees, immigrants, and survivors of disasters and war; persons in poverty; prison populations; and "persons who 'differ' from the social 'norm' of class, gender, race, religion, or sexual orientation," all of which include significant numbers of older adults.[82]

In addition to providing client-centered rehabilitation to members of such vulnerable groups, OT practice is expanding globally to include community-based interventions that promote population health.[27] Such expansion parallels a growing interest in and sense of responsibility for issues of social and occupational justice.[22,50,61,89] The increased attention to the sociopolitical nature of occupation has led to a more socially and politically engaged discipline, as OT personnel acknowledge the fact that barriers to participation in occupations can arise from social and political environments as surely as they can from individual physical or cognitive impairments.[68]

By highlighting the links between economic disparities and social marginality and increased risk of chronic disease and disability, occupational justice has emerged as an OT practice area that is highly relevant to gerontological concerns. The Framework of Occupational Justice[75] identifies four types of restricted occupational participation, all pertinent to older adults: occupational deprivation (denial of resources and opportunities to allow access to occupations), occupational alienation (having to participate in occupations that are personally meaningless and void of recognition or reward), occupational marginalization (lack of power to exercise occupational choice), and occupational imbalance (being occupied too much or too little to experience empowerment and meaning). Kronenberg, Algado, and Pollard[34] introduced another concept that sensitizes us to the nature of occupational injustice experienced by many older adults, occupational apartheid, which refers to "the segregation of groups of people through the restriction or denial of access to meaningful participation in occupations of daily life on the basis of ... age ... or other characteristics."

Building upon Carstensen's[14] perspectives regarding the likelihood that aging individuals will experience extra decades of life, OT personnel are challenged to envision how best to support healthy aging. What if individuals in their 50s and 60s are actually in mid-career, and are employed full or part time for decades longer? What if these expectations become normative, especially with the declining number of young adults in the workforce? Do we thus need to revise our thinking regarding appropriate interventions, expanding our view from those that are medical to a more holistic approach that embraces innovations in health promotion in the community and throughout the continuum of care?

Generation of Gerontological Occupational Therapy Evidence

As always, we must particularly strive for increasing research evidence that demonstrates the nature, effectiveness, and efficacy of OT interventions. Initiatives to accomplish this effort have been taken primarily over the past 25 years, yet so much more is needed. This must occur for our work with aging adults to be taken seriously, thereby increasing our visibility as a profession that is a fundamental support for developing health-promoting innovations with aging adults.

New OT personnel may link with experienced practitioners who are skilled researchers, or OT faculty who serve and/or study gerontological OT areas in their practice settings. OT personnel without ready access to experienced researchers can forge intra- and interprofessional research collaborations with partners who have strong research backgrounds to achieve the necessary level of credence regarding the need for evidence generation supporting their gerontological OT practice. These individuals may work at a distance, if necessary, especially if technological supports (e.g., access to the Internet) are available. Whether new to gerontological OT or experienced in practice or research with aging adults, all participants need to continually align their work with relevant qualitative and quantitative research questions, depending upon the nature of the need or problem to be studied regarding the client group or population served. The practitioner's area of gerontological practice may determine the type of inquiry best suited to address the research question and subsequent development of levels of evidence in a systematic way. Furthermore, in developing research questions and related studies, the profession should capitalize upon the insights of master practitioners who may best be able to inform the process by utilizing their holistic intuitive insights that are unique as compared with those of other disciplines.

Projected Employment Opportunities

In the United States, OT employment projections are very strong, with percent increase in employment for OT assistants and aides predicted to be 41%, compared with 11%

for most professions, from 2012 to 2022. For the same period, a 29% increase in demand for occupational therapists is predicted. Both of these rates are reported as much faster than average.[84] Although the sources of the demand are not specified, one must consider population aging as one of the driving forces, with the associated needs for health-care services.

The National Career Services in the United Kingdom lists occupational therapy as one of the growth professions that are most likely to address the needs of the increasing numbers of older adult citizens.[49] In addition to the United States and the United Kingdom, Japan, Germany, and Australia have the largest number of programs approved by the World Federation of Occupational Therapists (WFOT); and 34 countries are identified where OT is recognized as a shortage profession.[91] Further findings in this global OT human resource project include the following:

- Average percentage of occupational therapists working in government/public-funded posts: 63%
- Average percentage of occupational therapists working in nongovernment/public-funded posts: 33%

Reported by WFOT member organizations, the most frequently cited OT specialties experiencing labor shortages (numbers identified in parentheses) follow: mental health (23), dementia (13), older people (11), and stroke rehabilitation (10).[91]

The global demographic projections for aging and the need for OT services considered together represent outstanding prospects for the profession well into the future. Will we have the vision and tenacity to address these intergenerational societal needs, within health care system settings, within our urban and rural communities, together with influencing policy development and enactment, for the benefit of society? Opportunities abound for developing innovative interventions, creating new service-delivery models, and expanding the field to support healthy aging; we need to draw upon our holistic perspectives in pursuing this unparalleled opportunity to affect the overall *optimal* well-being and quality of life for all.

Summary

In this book we have worked to reinforce basic gerontological concepts and theoretical and disciplinary orientations, along with historical and global contexts that explain why the current epoch may well be considered revolutionary in respect to old age, and why this aging-related revolution is especially relevant to the field of occupational therapy. We further explicated many facets related to healthy aging, in an effort to inform and inspire readers to apply the information on how personal intrinsic and extrinsic factors affect the nature of occupational options and occupational performance. In chapter 1 we introduced conceptual models that relate to *typical* aging, well-being, and quality of life and presented an integrated model adapted from occupational science and OT theoretical frameworks that provided the conceptual framework for this book. The chapters that followed presented current knowledge on aging-related changes and contexts and guidelines for applying this knowledge to enhance one's practice. In this final chapter, we introduced yet another adapted version of the models, with an emphasis on *optimal* aging, to additionally reinforce and inspire the application of new insights toward the development of health-promoting interventions, structures, and policies throughout continua of care, in communities, and in governmental agencies.

Future trends in gerontological OT include a growing focus on occupational justice and ecological sustainability within a framework of occupational literacy. Client-centered, collaborative approaches that also address *optimal* enablement of those who may be marginalized in society by any of many different factors may require proactive advocacy toward policy development. Awareness of elder abuse and neglect; poverty; malnutrition; inaccessible and unsafe neighborhoods; and aging, race/ethnicity, and religious discriminatory conditions are a few examples of reasons for OT personnel to mobilize on behalf of the aging clients we serve. New, nontraditional areas of practice, including work with disaster victims, immigrants, aging workers, older veterans, and incarcerated persons, are additional professional ventures to explore for those who thrive on innovations in service delivery. One of the first author's mantras through the years has been, "Look for gaps in care; an opportunity for OT lies there." Hence, models that smoothly transition individuals from one service aspect to another may best be enacted by OT personnel who embody a "total person" (or program/system/community/population) needs and strengths perspective.

Incorporating and developing new technologies into practice will ensure proactive approaches with aging clients who can benefit from a wide range of cognitive, environmental, and lifestyle supports that these innovations offer. Occupational therapists and assistants must be ever vigilant for opportunities to invent and apply their unique professional perspective, individually or collectively, to maximize supports for healthy aging.

Finally, regardless of the area of practice one chooses in gerontological OT, one may be assured of contributing in important ways to the well-being and quality of life of aging individuals, and others: Dedication to serving aging adults serves all generations.

REVIEW QUESTIONS

1. T/F The AOTA *Centennial Vision* identified productive aging as one of the six main practice areas of OT.
2. How do you define successful/optimal aging? Discuss how your understanding of this concept would affect your future work with older adults.
3. Define *ambient intelligence*. Discuss two examples of ways ambient intelligence can contribute to the quality of life of older adults.
4. Compare and contrast the concepts of *caregiving* and *societal enabling/empowerment*, and discuss their implications for OT practice with older adults.
5. Describe how an occupational therapist might contribute to the quality of life of an older worker.
6. T/F The number of older prisoners in the United States has declined over time.
7. Discuss the types of restricted occupational participation as defined by *The Framework of Occupational Justice* and their relevance for gerontological OT.

REFERENCES

1. Acampora, G., Cook, D. J., Rashidi, P., & Vasilakos, A. V. (2013). A survey on ambient intelligence in health care. *Proceedings of the IEEE Institute of Electrical and Electronics Engineers, 101*(12), 2470–2494. doi: 10.1109/JPROC.2013.2262913.
2. American Occupational Therapy Association. (2007). AOTA's centennial vision and executive summary. *American Journal of Occupational Therapy, 61,* 613–614.
3. American Occupational Therapy Association. (2014). Occupational therapy practice framework: Domain and process (3rd ed.). *American Journal of Occupational Therapy, 68*(Suppl. 1), S1–S48. http://dx.doi.org/10.5014/ajot.2014.682006.
4. Bächlin, M., Plotnik, M., Roggen, D., Maidan, I., Hausdorff, J. M., Giladi N., et al. (2010). Wearable assistant for Parkinson's disease patients with the freezing of gait symptom. *IEEE Transactions on Information Technology in Biomedicine, 14*(2), 436–446. doi: 10.1109/TITB.2009.2036165.
5. Baltes, M. M., & Carstensen, L. L. (1996). The process of successful ageing. *Ageing and Society, 16,* 397–422.
6. Barney, K. F. (2009). *Internet research: Epidemiological study of the health related quality of life, environmental factors and orientation to life of persons with spinal cord injuries.* Saarbrucken, Germany: Verlag Dr. Muller.
7. Berg, A. I. (2008). *Life satisfaction in late life: Markers and predictors of level and change among 80+ year olds.* Gothenburg, Sweden: University of Gothenburg.
8. Biggs, S. (2004). New ageism: Age imperialism, personal experience and ageing policy. In S. O. Daatland & S. Biggs (Eds.), *Ageing and diversity.* Bristol, England: The Policy Press.
9. Boudiny, K. (2013). "Active ageing": From empty rhetoric to effective policy tool. *Ageing and Society, 33*(6), 1077–1098. doi: 10.1017/S0144686X1200030X.
10. Boudiny, K., & Mortelmans, D. (2011). A critical perspective: towards a broader understanding of "active ageing." *Electronic Journal of Applied Psychology, 7*(1), 8–14. doi: http://dx.doi.org/10.7790/ejap.v7i1.232.
11. Bowling, A., & Dieppe, P. (2005). What is successful ageing and who should define it? *British Medical Journal, 331*(7531), 1548–1551.
12. Brienza, D. M., & McCue, M. (2013). Introduction to telerehabilitation. In S. Kumar & E. R. Cohn (Eds.), *Telerehabilitation* (pp. 1–11). London: Springer-Verlag.
13. Carlsson, G., Schilling, O., Slaug, B., Fänge, A., Stahl, A., Nygren, C., et al. (2009). Towards a screening tool for housing accessibility problems: A reduced version of the housing enabler. *Journal of Applied Gerontology, 28,* 59–80.
14. Carstensen, L. L. (2009). *A long bright future: An action plan for a lifetime of happiness, health, and financial security.* New York, NY: Broadway Books.
15. Clarke, A., & Warren, L. (2007). Hopes, fears and expectations about the future: What do older people's stories tell us about active ageing? *Ageing & Society, 27*(4), 465–488.

16. Cook, D. J., Augusto, J. C., & Jakkula, V. R. (2009). Review: Ambient intelligence: technologies, applications, and opportunities. *Pervasive and Mobile Computing, 5*(4), 277–298.

17. D'Amico, M. (2014). Update on productive aging research in the American Journal of Occupational Therapy, 2013, and overview of research published 2009-2013. *American Journal of Occupational Therapy, 68*(6), 247–260.

18. Epelde, G., Carrasco, E., Rajasekharan, S., Jiménez, J. M., Vivanco, K., Gómez-Fraga, I., et al. (2014). Universal remote delivery of rehabilitation: Validation with seniors' joint rehabilitation therapy. *Cybernetics and Systems: An International Journal, 45,* 109–122.

19. Epstein, A. M., Jha, A. K., Orav, E. J., Liebman, D. L., Audet, A. M., Zezza, M. A., et al. (2014). Analysis of early accountable care organizations defines patient, structural, cost, and quality-of-care characteristics. *Health Affairs, 33*(1), 95–102.

20. Fries, J. F. (1997). Editorial: Can preventive gerontology be on the way? *American Journal of Public Health, 87*(10), 1591–1592.

21. Fudickar, S., & Schnor, B. (2009). Kopal: A mobile orientation system for dementia patients. *Intelligent Interactive Assistance and Mobile Multimedia Computing, 53,* 109–118.

22. Galheigo, S. M. (2011). What needs to be done? Occupational therapy responsibilities and challenges regarding human rights. *Australian Occupational Therapy Journal, 58,* 60–66. doi: 10.1111/j.1440-1630.2011.00922.x.

23. Gerontological Society of America. (2014). *A hidden epidemic of malnutrition. What's hot aging policy: Preventing and treating malnutrition to improve health and reduce costs.* Washington, DC: GSA.

24. Glatt, S. J., Chayavichitsilp, P., Depp, C., Schork, N. J., & Jeste, D. V. (2007). Successful aging: From phenotype to genotype. *Biological Psychiatry, 62,* 282–293.

25. Greenfield, E., Scharlach, A., Lehning, A., & Davitt, J. (2012). A conceptual framework for examining the promise of the NORC Program and Village models to promote aging in place. *Journal of Aging Studies, 26.* doi: 10.1016/j.jaging.2012.01.003.

26. Gupta, J., & Sabata, D. (2010, April 23). Maximizing occupational performance of older workers. *OT Practice* (pp. 1–7). Bethesda, MD: AOTA Press.

27. Hocking, C., Jones, M., & Reed, K. (2015). Occupational science informing occupational therapy interventions. In I. Söderback (Ed.), *International handbook of occupational therapy interventions* (pp. 127–134). New York: Springer.

28. Hocking, C., Townsend, E., Galheigo, S., Erlandsson, L-K, & de Mesquita Chagas, N. (2014). Driving societal change: occupational therapy, health and human rights. WFOT International Advisory Group: Human Rights. In: *16th International Congress of the World Federation of Occupational Therapists,* Yokohama, Japan.

29. Hodges, S., Williams, L., Berry, E., Izadi, S., Srinivasan, J., Butler, A., et al. (2006). Sensecam: A retrospective memory aid. *Ubicomp,* 177–193.

30. Holstein, M. B., & Minkler, M. (2003). Self, society and the "new gerontology." *The Gerontologist, 43*(6), 787–796.

31. Institute for Criminal Policy Research. (2014). WHO guide on prisons and health *on international prison conditions.* Accessed October 24, 2015. http://www.euro.who.int/en/health-topics/health-determinants/prisons-and-health/publications/2014/prisons-and-health

32. Kemp, B., & Mosqueda, L. A. (Eds.). (2004). *Aging with a disability: What the clinician needs to know.* Baltimore, MD: Johns Hopkins University Press.

33. Kim, K., & Peterson, B. (2014) *Aging behind bars: Trends and implications of graying prisoners in the federal prison system.* Urban Institute. Accessed October 24, 2015. http://www.urban.org/UploadedPDF/413222-Aging-Behind-Bars.pdf.

34. Kronenberg, F., Simo Algado, S., & Pollard, N. (2005). (Eds.). *Occupational therapy without borders—learning from the spirit of survivors.* Oxford, England: Elsevier Science.

35. Lamb, S. (2014). Permanent personhood or meaningful decline? Toward a critical anthropology of successful aging. *Journal of Aging Studies, 29,* 41–52.

36. Lanz, M., Nahapetianz, A., Vahdatpourz, A., Kaiserx, L. A. W., & Sarrafzadeh, M. (2009). SmartFall: An automatic fall detection system based on subsequence matching for the SmartCane. In: *International conference on body area networks.* Los Angeles, CA.

37. Laslett, P. (1991). *A fresh map of life: The emergence of the third age.* Cambridge, MA: Harvard University Press.

38. Leland, N. E., & Elliott, S. J. (Eds.). (2012). Special issue on productive aging: evidence and opportunities for occupational therapy practitioners. *American Journal of Occupational Therapy, 66*(3), 263–265.

39. Leland, N. E., Elliott, S. J., & Johnson, K. J. (2012). *Occupational therapy practice guidelines for productive aging for community-dwelling older adults.* Bethesda, MD: American Occupational Therapy Association, Inc.

40. Levasseur, M., & Carrier, A. (2012). Integrating health literacy into occupational therapy: findings from a scoping review. *Scandinavian Journal of Occupational Therapy, 19*(4), 305–314.

41. Lindenberger, U., Lövdén, M., Schellenbach, M., Li, S.-C., & Krüger, A. (2008). Psychological principles of successful aging technologies: a mini-review. *Gerontology, 54,* 59–68. doi:10.1159/000116114.

42. Mace, R. (1985). Universal design, barrier free environments for everyone. *Designers West, 33*(1), 147–152.

43. Meier, E. L., & Kerr, E. A. (1976). Capabilities of middle-aged and older workers: A survey of the literature. *Industrial Gerontology, 3*(3), 147–156.

44. Mihailidis, A., Carmichael, B., & Boger, J. (2004). The use of computer vision in an intelligent environment to support aging-in-place, safety, and independence in the home. *Information Technology in Biomedicine, IEEE Transactions, 8*(3), 238–247.

45. Milligan, C., Roberts, C., & Mort, M. (2011). Telecare and older people: Who cares where? *Social Science & Medicine, 72,* 347–354.

46. Morris, M. E., Adair, B., Miller, K., Ozanne, E., Hansen, R., Pearce, A. J., et al. (2013). Smart-home technologies to assist older people to live well at home. *Aging Science, 1,* 101. doi:10.4172/jasc.1000101.

47. Murphy, S. L. (2010). Centennial vision: Geriatric research. *American Journal of Occupational Therapy, 64*(1), 172–181.

48. National Alliance for Caregiving. (2011). *e-connected family caregiver: Bringing caregiving into the 21st century.* Bethesda, MD: National Alliance for Caregiving.

49. National Career Services. (2015). https://www.gov.uk/government/uploads/system/uploads/attachment_data/file/391911/15.01.05._UKCES_Career_Brochure_V13_reduced.pdf Accessed October 24, 2015.

50. Nilsson, I., & Townsend, E. (2010). Occupational justice—bridging theory and practice. *Scandinavian Journal of Occupational Therapy, 17*(1), 57–63. doi: 10.3109/11038120903287182.

51. Ortiz, A., Carretero, M. P., Oyarzun, D., et al. (2007). Elderly users in ambient intelligence: Does an avatar improve the interaction?

In: *Proceedings of the 9th Conference on User Interfaces for All, Universal Access in Ambient Intelligence Environments, LNCS 4397* (pp. 99–114). New York, NY: Springer.

52. Palmer, P. (2000). *Let your life speak: Listening for the voice of vocation.* San Francisco, CA: Jossey-Bass.

53. Paradiso, R., Loriga, G., & Taccini, N. (2004). Wearable system for vital signs monitoring. *Studies in Health Technology and Informatics, 108,* 253–259.

54. Park, D. C., & Bischof, G. N. (2013). The aging mind: Neuroplasticity in response to cognitive training. *Dialogues in Clinical Neuroscience, 15*(1), 109–119.

55. Patel, S., Park, H., Bonato, P., Chan, L., & Rodgers, M. (2012). A review of wearable sensors and systems with application in rehabilitation. *Journal of NeuroEngineering and Rehabilitation, 9,* 21–38. doi: 10.1186/1743-0003-9-21.

56. Pew Center on the States. (2008). *One in 100: Behind bars in America 2008.* Washington, DC: Pew Charitable Trust.

57. Pew Center on the States. (2011). *State of recidivism: The revolving door of America's prisons.* Washington, DC: Pew Charitable Trust.

58. Phelan, E. A., Anderson, L. A., La Croix, A. Z., & Larson, E. B. (2004). Older adults' views of "successful aging"—how do they compare with researchers" definitions? *Journal of the American Geriatric Society, 52*(2), 211–216.

59. Pogue, D. (2014). *Wearable tech and smarter smartphones.* AARP Bulletin, 55(10), 23. Accessed 10/24/15. http://aarp.org/bulletin.

60. Pollack, M. E., Brown, L., Colbry, D., McCarthy, C. E., Orosz, C., Peintner, B., et al. (2003). Autominder: An intelligent cognitive orthotic system for people with memory impairment. *Robotics and Autonomous Systems, 44*(3–4), 273–282.

61. Pollard, N., Sakellariou, D., & Kronenberg, F. (2008). (Eds.). *Political practice in occupational therapy.* Edinburgh, Scotland: Elsevier Science.

62. Population Reference Bureau. *Dementia cases expected to triple by 2050 as world population ages.* (2013). Accessed October 24, 2015. http://www.prb.org/Publications/Articles/2012/global-dementia.aspx.

63. Prajapati, S. K., Gage, W. H., Brooks, D., Black, S. E., & McIlroy, W. E. (2011). A novel approach to ambulatory monitoring: investigation into the quantity and control of everyday walking in patients with subacute stroke. *Neurorehabilitation and Neural Repair, 25,* 6–14. doi: 10.1177/1545968310374189.

64. R. L. Mace Universal Design Institute. (2015a). *History of universal design.* http://udinstitute.org/history.php.

65. R. L. Mace Universal Design Institute. (2015b). *Principles of universal design.* Accessed October 24, 2015. http://udinstitute.org/principles.php.

66. Rowe, J. W., & Kahn, R. L. (1998). *Successful aging.* New York, NY: Pantheon Books.

67. Rudman, D. (2006). Positive aging and its implications for occupational possibilities in later life. *Canadian Journal of Occupational Therapy, 73*(3), 188–192.

68. Rudman, D. (2014). Embracing and enacting an occupational imagination: Occupational science as transformative. *Journal of Occupational Science, 21*(4), 373–388.

69. Sanders, M., Eich, A., Porte, A., & Haversat, M. (2014, May 12). Older workers in manufacturing. *OT Practice* (pp. 7–13).

70. Scharlach, A. (2012). Creating aging-friendly communities in the United States. *Ageing International, 37,* 25–38. doi: 10.1007/s12126-011-9140-1.

71. Schulz, R., Wahl, H-W., Matthews, J. T., De Vito Dabbs, A., Beach, S. R., & Czaja, S. J. (2014). Advancing the aging and technology agenda in gerontology. *The Gerontologist, 55*(5), 724–734.

72. Shi, L., & Singh, D. A. (2015). *Delivering health care in America: A system approach* (6th ed.). Burlington, MA: Jones and Bartlett Publishers.

73. Siewiorek, D., Smailagic, A., & Dey, A. (2012). *Architecture and applications of virtual coaches.* Pittsburgh, PA: Quality of Life Technology Engineering Research Center, Carnegie Mellon University.

74. Spirduso, W., Francis, K., & MacRae, P. (2005). *Physical dimensions of aging* (2nd ed.). Champaign, IL: Human Kinetics.

75. Stadnyk, R., Townsend, E. A., & Wilcock, A. (2010). Occupational justice. In C. Christiansen & E. A. Townsend (Eds.), *Introduction to occupation: The art and science of living* (2nd ed., pp. 329–358). Englewood Cliffs, NJ: Prentice Hall.

76. Strawbridge, W. J., Wallhagen, M. I., & Cohen, R. D. (2002). Successful aging and well-being. Self-rated compared with Rowe and Kahn. *Gerontologist, 42,* 727–733.

77. Sudbury, J. (Ed.). (2013). *Global lockdown: Race, gender and the prison-industrial complex.* New York, NY: Routledge.

78. The Economist. (2014). *Pocket world in figures: 2015 edition.* London: Profile Books, Ltd.

79. Tomita, M. R., & Nochajski, S. M. (2015). Using smart home technology and health-promoting exercise. In I. Söderback (Ed.), *International handbook of occupational therapy interventions* (2nd ed., pp. 747–756). New York, NY: Springer.

80. Topo, P. (2009). Technology studies to meet the needs of people with dementia and their caregivers: A literature review. *Journal of Applied Gerontology, 28,* 5–37.

81. Townsend, E. (2015). Critical occupational literacy: Thinking about occupational justice, ecological sustainability, and aging in everyday life. *Journal of Occupational Science, 22*(4), 389–402. doi: 10.1080/14427591.2015.1071691.

82. Townsend, E., & Marval, R. (2013). Can professionals actually enable occupational justice? *Cadernos de Terapia Ocupacional da UFSCar [São Carlos], 21*(2), 215–228. doi: 10.4322/cto.2013.025.

83. U.S. Department of Labor: Bureau of Labor Statistics. (2015a). http://www.bls.gov/spotlight/2008/olderworkers/. Accessed 10.05.15.

84. U.S. Department of Labor: Bureau of Labor Statistics. (2015b). *Occupational outlook for occupational therapy assistants and aides.* Accessed October 24, 2015. http://www.bls.gov/ooh/healthcare/occupational-therapy-assistants-and-aides.htm.

85. U.S. Department of State, Bureau of Democracy, Human Rights and Labor. (2012). *Report on international prison conditions.* Accessed October 24, 2015. www.state.gov/documents/organization/210160.pdf.

86. Verbrugge, L. M., & Yang, L. (2002). Aging with disability and disability with aging. *Journal of Disability Policy Studies, 12*(4), 253–267. doi: 10.1177/104420730201200405.

87. Wan, J., Byrne, C., O'Hare, G. M., & O'Grady, M. J. (2011). Orange alerts: Lessons from an outdoor case study. Pervasive Computing Technologies for Healthcare (PervasiveHealth), In: *5th International Conference,* Dublin, Ireland. (pp. 446–451) Accessed 10/24/15. http://ieeexplore.ieee.org/xpl/articleDetails.jsp?arnumber=6038846&filter=AND(p_Publication_Number:6030000).

88. Warr, P., & Clapperton, G. (2010). *The joy of work? Jobs, happiness, and you.* New York, NY: Routledge.

89. Wilcock, A. A., & Townsend, E. (2000). Occupational terminology interactive dialogue. *Journal of Occupational Science, 7*(2), 84–86.

90. Williams, M., Sabata, D., & Zolna, J. (2008). Accommodating aging workers who have a disability. In A. Mihailidis, J. Boger, H. Kautz, & L. Normie (Eds.), *Assistive technology and research series (21), technology and aging—selected papers from the 2007 International Conference on Technology and Aging.* Fairfax, VA: ISO Press.

91. World Federation of Occupational Therapists. (2014). *Human resources project.* http://www.wfot.org/ResourceCentre.aspx.

92. World Health Organization. (2014). *"Ageing well" must be a global priority.* http://www.who.int/mediacentre/news/releases/2014/lancet-ageing-series/en/.

93. World Health Organization. (2015). *World report on ageing and health.* http://apps.who.int/iris/bitstream/10665/186463/1/9789240694811_eng.pdf. Accessed 10.06.15.

94. Wu, G., & Xue, S. (2008). Portable preimpact fall detector with inertial sensors. *IEEE Transactions on Neural Systems and Rehabilitation Engineering, 16*(2), 178–183. doi: 10.1109/TNSRE.2007.916282.

95. Zelkha, E., Epstein, B., Birrell, S., & Dodsworth, C. (1998, June). *From devices to "ambient intelligence."* Digital Living Room Conference. Accessed October 24, 2015. http://epstein.org/ambient-intelligence/.

Abandonment: When older adults abandon use of an assistive device, sometimes because they haven't been properly trained in its use, sometimes when it hasn't been properly fitted or adjusted to meet their needs, and often when the prescribing professional doesn't provide adequate support and encouragement. Abandonment threatens cost-effectiveness, treatment efficacy, and quality of life.

ACE (angiotensin-converting enzyme) inhibitors: Agents used to treat hypertension and heart failure. Examples include captopril, enalapril, and lisinopril.

Activities of daily living (ADLs): Basic activities related to self-care, including bathing, dressing, eating, feeding, and grooming.

Activity/activities: Human behaviors that are goal directed.

Activity theory: Proposed by Neugarten, it suggests that normal aging is typified by continuing engagement in meaningful occupations and relationships.

Adaptation: The process of adaptation is any trait that changes to better suit the organism for its environment.

Adaptive equipment: A wide range of devices that are used to assist in the performance of activities of daily living, including long-handled devices and durable medical equipment.

Adherence: The extent to which a person takes medications as prescribed; replaces older term *compliance*.

Adult learning: A process in which adults engage to improve their skill and knowledge.

Agent of change: An individual (collectively would be referred to as agents) who utilizes opportunities to bring about social change.

Aging in Manitoba Study (AIM): The largest and longest-running study on aging in Canada.

Aging in place: A term referring to the ability to live in one's own preferred home and community safely and independently as one ages; a model of long-term care that has slowly replaced the institutional model, which was prevalent prior to the mid-1990s. The notion now is that it is generally best to continually add an array of needed services in the home as the person ages and needs them, in order to forestall or prevent the need for generally more expensive institutional care. Assistive technology is a major area of growth that further supports the aging-in-place model.

Agnosia: The inability to recognize familiar objects by sight (visual agnosia), touch (tactile agnosia), sound (auditory agnosia), smell (olfactory agnosia), and/or taste (gustatory agnosia).

American Geriatrics Society: Health-care professionals dedicated to caring for older adults.

Analgesic: Medication to treat pain.

Anomia: Word-finding difficulty; a common form of expressive aphasia in mild Alzheimer's disease.

Anterograde amnesia: Loss of the ability to create new memories; skills and habits seem to be spared, but all short-term memory tends to be lost. It typically occurs occur during the early stages of Alzheimer's disease.

Anticholinergic effects: Group of symptoms caused by blockade or antagonism of receptors of the cholinergic system; include peripheral symptoms of dry eyes, dry mouth, constipation, and difficulty urinating and central symptoms of confusion and decreased memory. (See also Table 13-6 for a list of medications with anticholinergic effects.)

Antipyretic: Medication that reduces fever.

Aphasia: The loss of language ability; referred to as *dysphasia* if mild. Expressive aphasia is the loss of the ability to convey oral or written information to others. Receptive aphasia is the loss of ability to understand the meaning of oral and written language.

Apraxia: Characterized by loss of the ability to execute or carry out skilled movements and gestures, despite having the desire and the physical ability to perform them; referred to as *dyspraxia* if mild.

Assessment: Specific tool or instrument that is used to measure client function.

Assistive technology: Electronic and computer technologies that assist people with disabilities to be independent in their activities of daily living.

Augmentative and alternative communication (AAC): All forms of communication other than oral speech, ranging from aided (through the use of a device) to unaided communication (gestures and facial expressions). Aided AAC can be in the form of low- or high-technology devices, with low-tech devices typically not requiring electronic components and high-tech devices utilizing electronic components. Numerous types of AAC devices are available and can allow users to express simple words to long phrases and paragraphs.

Basho-fu weaving: In Okinawa, Japan, a kind of fabric woven with threads taken from Basho (banana) plants. Spinning of the threads and weaving are done manually and require a great deal of time and patience.

Beers Criteria: Explicit prescribing criteria developed in the United States; lists drugs that are potentially inappropriate for use in older adults or with certain disease states.

Biodemographic perspectives: Present ideas as to how demographic data, such as population, gender, and education, affect individuals.

Biological progression: Changes that occur to living beings from molecular, cellular, or systems changes.

Biomedical perspective: Predominantly a Western belief that disease is the result of abnormalities in structure and function of body organs and systems.

Biopsychosocial model: A theoretical position about aging asserting that to best understand the normal aging process and the acute and chronic diseases that become more prevalent with age, we must consider the joint and interacting influences of biological, psychological, and social phenomena. The biological aspect includes an understanding of various organ systems and the process of senescence in these systems. The psychological aspect considers information processing (e.g. sensation, perception, cognition, problem solving, wisdom, etc.), emotions, motivation, personality, and so forth. The social aspect includes cultural practices and beliefs, economic systems, educational and religious institutions, and so forth. Historical influences and secular change are also part of this model.

Biopsychosocial theory: Theory that includes the body, mind, and social or societal aspects of people. Believed to help occupational therapists working in community settings.

Body mass index (BMI):   Measure of body fat that is the ratio of weight to height. Obesity is defined as a BMI of 30 or greater.

Bones: The endoskeleton of vertebrates; organs that move, protect and support the body, and have functions involving mechanical, synthetic, and metabolic purposes.

Canadian Model of Occupational Performance and Engagement (CMOP-E):   A model that illustrates the relationship between person, occupation, and environment. Spirituality is the fourth dimension, placed in the center of the model to highlight its fundamental importance.

Causal relationship: The relationship between an event and the effect of that event.

Christian scripture: Writings from the New Testament, based on the teaching of Jesus Christ.

Chronic health conditions: Continuing or recurring illnesses or conditions, such as chronic obstructive pulmonary disease (COPD), muscle weakness, and so forth.

Chronological age: Actual age measured from date of birth.

Client: The recipient of occupational therapy services. Clients may be individual patients or groups of persons in the community, organizations, or populations.

Client-centered evaluation: An evaluation in which the client is considered an essential part of the evaluation process so that the evaluation will determine what the occupational clinician/practitioner will do in partnership with the client and what occupational goals are appropriate.

Client factors: Client factors, including body functions (such as neuromusculoskeletal, sensory-perceptual, visual, mental, cognitive, and pain factors) and body structures (such as cardiovascular, digestive, nervous, integumentary, and genitourinary systems, and structures related to movement), values, beliefs, and spirituality, that affect activities of daily living, instrumental activities of daily living, sleep, and socialization.

Cognitive: The process of acquiring, storing, sharing, and using information.

Community: A group of people who share a common vision and goal.

Competence–environmental press framework: A framework for understanding the transactions and outcomes between personal competencies and the "press" or demands of the environmental, which range from high to low.

Computerized assessments: Assessment tools that require the use of a computer/computer program for administration or scoring.

Continuity theory: Based on the idea that the relationship between life satisfaction and activity is an expression of enduring personality traits.

Critical perspective: A questioning or analytic stance toward any given information, to identify both positive and negative aspects and detrimental effects of power differentials. May refer to

adopting a specific viewpoint, such as feminist, Marxian, and so forth.

Cultural congruence: Extent to which an assessment is consistent with a client's cultural health beliefs.

Degenerative spinal stenosis: An acquired condition with an insidious onset that is commonly diagnosed in the elderly population.

Dementia: Chronic or persistent disorder of the mental processes caused by brain disease or injury and marked by memory disorders, personality changes, and impaired reasoning.

Developmental process: Development is viewed from several current theories, including, but not limited to, maturational, personality, behaviorist, cognitive, and psychobiological.

Dietary Supplement Health and Education Act of 1994 (DSHEA):   Directs regulation of dietary supplements, including herbal products, in the United States.

Diminishing abilities: Evidence of increasing frailty that affects individuals' ability to function as they were able to in the past.

Disengagement theory: Belief that older people withdraw from society and increasingly focus on personal meanings. It is no longer held as a valid universal theory.

Diuretics: Medications that work in the kidneys to promote excretion of salts and water and thus increase the volume of urine produced; commonly referred to as "water pills."

Ego development theory: Developed by psychologist Erik Erickson (1902–1994), proposes that development occurs as the result of crisis. His ideas about old age were refuted after his death by his wife and partner, Joan Erikson.

Electronic aids to daily living (EADLs):   Devices that enable individuals with disabilities a means to control electronic and electronically enabled devices in their environment. EADL units can range from simple units that control one device to more involved units that can control everything in an individual's environment. There are a variety of control strategies available (e.g., infrared, ultrasound, Z wave, radiofrequency) to operate the devices and numerous access methods (e.g., direct selection of buttons, voice command, scanning of an array of commands).

Environment: The aggregate of surroundings things, conditions, or influences that affect "what people do and how they do it" (Kielhofner, 2008, p. 97). It is made up of objects, spaces, occupational forms, and social groups, all of which are influenced by culture, the economy, and the political context.

Environmental docility hypothesis: Based on the idea that the environment plays a greater role in the lives of older adults as their competencies diminish.

Evaluation: The systematic collection and interpretation of data about occupational performance. Evaluation data are necessary to plan occupational therapy interventions.

Evolutionary determination: Characteristics arising from a species' genetic endowment rather than the environment, such as the age at which humans reach puberty or the maximum age a human can reach.

Executive function (EF):   A variety of higher-order cognitive processes, including initiation, planning, hypothesis generation, cognitive flexibility, decision making, regulation, judgment, feedback utilization, and self-perception.

Explanatory theory (also descriptive theory): Attempts to explain a phenomenon in terms of established theories in a field.

Factor analysis: A statistical method used as a data reduction technique or as a way to identify underlying components or factors.

Food and Drug Administration (FDA): An agency within the U.S. Department of Health and Human Services responsible for assuring the safety and effectiveness of drugs, vaccines and other biological products, medical devices, dietary supplements, and the U.S. food supply, among other areas of responsibility.

Fracture: A break in bone or cartilage that can occur anywhere in the body where these tissues reside. Hip fractures are the most common in the geriatric population.

Functional mobility: The ability to ambulate, effectively utilize wheelchairs if needed, and engage in bed transfer and mobility.

Generational differences: Identification of values that differ between groups of people (cohorts) born in different decades.

Gerontechnology: An interdisciplinary field of study and practice that evaluates the multidimensional intersections of various technological tools with the lives and well-being of older adults.

Gerontological Society of America: Promotes multi- and interdisciplinary research in gerontology, disseminates research knowledge, and supports education and training in higher education.

Gerontology: The study of the social, psychological, and biological aspects of aging.

Goal-achievement strategies: Suggest that people select goals in relation to their resources; include selection, optimization, and compensation.

Goodness of fit: The match between the needs of client and the assessment tool, including but not limited to sensitivity, standardization on a similar population, suitability for the client's cultural background, and constructive validity of the test items.

Greco-Roman: Of, or having, both Greek and Roman characteristics.

Guideline: Work consisting of a set of statements, directions, or principles presenting current or future rules or policy. Guidelines may be developed by government agencies at any level, institutions, organizations such as professional societies or governing boards, or expert panels. The term *guideline* typically relates to the general conduct and administration of health-care activities rather than to specific decisions for a particular clinical condition.

Hebrew: Ancient scriptures in the Hebrew Bible.

Holistic: Entirety; relating to or concerned with wholes or with complete systems rather than with the analysis, treatment of, or dissection into parts. Holistic medicine attempts to treat both the mind and the body. Holistic ecology views humans and the environment as a single system.

Home health agency: A public or private organization that provides skilled services (e.g., nursing and rehabilitation) and paraprofessional services (e.g. home health aide care) in the patient's home. Home health agencies are Medicare certified if they meet certain requirements, which include at a minimum skilled nursing care and one additional therapeutic service.

Home modifications: Adaptations made to the physical characteristics of the home environment that promote an individual's function and safety in daily activities.

H₂-receptor antagonists (H₂-RAs): Drugs that reduce acid production in the stomach; they treat or prevent heartburn, reflux disease, and gastric and duodenal ulcers; many are available without a prescription. Examples include famotidine and ranitidine.

Human resources: Clinician/practitioner skills, training, and time needed for completion of the assessment.

Informant data: Information that an occupational therapist may obtain from the client, caregivers, other health professionals working with the client, and past medical history from reading the client's medical chart.

Inhibition: A subcomponent of executive function referring to an ability to suppress irrelevant information in favor of important goal-related information.

Instrumental activities of daily living (IADLs): More complex activities than self-care, including financial management, meal preparation, and shopping; activities that allow an individual to live independently in the home and community.

Intelligent assistive technologies (IATs): Technologies that sense user needs and respond accordingly and thus are adaptable to changing situations in the user's environment. Most often used with individuals to compensate for physical or cognitive deficits.

International Classification of Functioning, Disability and Health (ICF): Publication of the World Health organization that explains the relationship between participation in the activities of everyday life and having a health condition.

Interval level: Constant difference between observed values in a measure.

Intervention: The process and skilled actions taken by occupational therapy practitioners in collaboration with the client to facilitate engagement in occupation related to health and participation. The intervention process includes planning, implementation, and review.

Invalid: An assessment tool that does not provide information about what is actually trying to be measured is invalid.

Islam: Religion practiced by Muslims, set forth in the Koran, who maintain a belief in one God.

Joint: Place of articulation where two or more bones make contact; constructed to allow movement and provide mechanical support; classified based on structure and function.

Lawton's (and Nahemow's 1973) Ecological Model: Proposes three function of the environment: maintenance, stimulation and support, older adults' adaptation based on their competencies, and the physical and social demands of the environment (environmental press).

Length of administration: Amount of time needed to administer the assessment protocol.

Levels of data: Measurement of data that differentiates between nominal, ordinal, interval, and ratio. (See also *nominal level, ordinal level, interval level,* and *ratio level*).

Life course perspective: Considers elements that compose the overall structure and timing of events in life, over the entire lifespan.

Life satisfaction: The way persons perceive how life has been and how they feel about where it is going in the future.

Longitudinal data: Information derived from a study conducted over time, such as days, months, years, or decades. Longitudinal studies may be experimental, in which the researcher actively manipulates the data, or retrospective, in which the event of interest has already occurred.

Lumbar spondylolisthesis: A forward movement of the body of a lumbar vertebrae on the vertebra, or sacrum, below it.

M-health/e-health (mobile health/electronic health): A rapidly expanding market of apps and programs that help to monitor health conditions and behaviors, provide wellness coaching, and offer other supports for consumer compliance with physician or other health provider recommendations. e-Health involves an even broader array of services, such as electronic health records, telehomecare, and remote patient monitoring.

Marginalized groups: Groups of people who have experienced a history of deprivation, alienation, and isolation, because of assumptions and actions imposed by another group of people.

Meaningful activities: Those activities or occupations that are personally important to the individual.

Medicaid: A joint federally funded and state-funded health insurance program for individuals of all ages who fall within certain income limits. Medicaid programs vary from state to state.

Medicare: A federal health insurance program for individuals 65 years or older, younger individuals with disabilities, and individuals with end-stage renal disease.

Medicare Part A: Referred to as hospital insurance. This type of Medicare insurance covers inpatient hospital stays, care in skilled nursing facilities, hospice care, and home health care.

Medicare Part B: Referred to as medical insurance. This type of Medicare insurance covers physician appointments, outpatient care (including physical therapy, occupational therapy, and speech-language pathology), and medical supplies. Outpatient therapy can be provided in the home and community.

Medication-related problem: An event or circumstance involving drug therapy that actually or potentially interferes with the optimum outcome of therapy. Eight categories of medication-related problems have been defined in the pharmacy literature.

Mini-Mental State Examination (MMSE): A brief screening tool for identifying cognitive impairment and measuring overall cognitive functioning, such as orientation, attention, memory, and language.

Model of Human Occupation (MOHO): Presents the idea that occupations change and develop over the lifespan, with possible diminished roles, but certain specific activities are preferred by older adults.

Nominal level: Observations that are similar with regard to a characteristic or attribute are assigned to the same category and defined by type or kind (e.g., gender, ethnicity).

Nonsteroidal anti-inflammatory drugs (NSAIDs): Used to decrease inflammation and pain in acute or chronic musculoskeletal conditions. They are considered high-risk medications in older adults because of bleeding and gastrointestinal risks, and also cardiac risks. Examples include ibuprofen, naproxen, meloxicam, and oxaprozin.

Normative values: Scores on standardized measures indicative of being within the normal range for a specific skill or characteristic in relation to a specific population group.

Occupation: All that people need, want, or are obliged to do; what it means to them; and its ever-present potential as an agent of change. It encapsulates doing, being, belonging, and becoming (Wilcock, 2006). Daily activities that reflect cultural values, provide structure to living, and provide meaning for individuals; these activities meet human needs for self-care, enjoyment, and participation in society (AOTA, 2008). "Goal-directed pursuits that typically extend over time, have meaning to their performance, and involve multiple tasks" (Christiansen, Baum, & Bass-Haugen, 2005, p. 548); "all the things that people want, need, or have to do, whether of a physical, mental, social, sexual, political, spiritual, or any other nature, including sleep and rest activities" (Wilcock & Townsend, 2009, p. 193); "activities of everyday life named, organized, and given meaning by individuals and a culture" (Law, Polatajko, Baptiste, & Townsend, 1997, p. 32).

Occupational deprivation: Being unable to access culturally important occupations because of external barriers, with observable health consequences, such as being made unnecessary when the major employer in town moves away, with little hope of finding a new job, or girls not having access to education beyond primary school because of societal attitudes about women's role and value.

Occupational models: Theories developed by occupational therapists and scientists to explain and predict people's engagement in occupation and its outcomes (concrete, symbolic, and satisfaction).

Occupational performance: The term occupational therapists use for function; the point where the person, the environment, and the person's occupations intersect to support the tasks, activities, and roles that define the person as an individual.

Occupational profile: A profile that describes the client's occupational history, pattern of daily living, interests, values, and needs.

Occupational repertoire: Number and types of activities and occupations employed by an individual: these may decrease with age as some occupations are eliminated, such as employment and leisure.

Occupational scientists: Scholars who study meaningful aspects of people's activities and roles,

Occupational therapists: Practitioners of occupational therapy.

Old: Includes youngest-old through oldest-old; criteria established by gerontologists to characterize abilities, or lack of them, as well as by chronological age (e.g., old-old may be age 85 and older).

Older person Both cultural and legislative definitions exist per community. In a cultural setting, an older person would be recognized as an elder, a person who garners culturally endowed respect given his or her age and years of experience. Legislatively, an older person would be defined in accordance to the legislative documents of that country, usually to define a group of people who would qualify for certain services.

Oral hypoglycemic agents: Refers to medications used for treating diabetes that work by increasing insulin secretion and thereby have the potential to cause excessively low blood glucose levels (e.g., glyburide, glipizide, glimepiride). In contrast, other diabetes medications work in a manner that limits their ability to cause hypoglycemia.

Ordinal level: A number that indicates an order in relation to other numbers based on some characteristic (e.g., first, second, third, and so on).

Organization for Economic Co-operation and Development (OECD): Helps governments foster prosperity and fight poverty through economic growth and financial stability; helps ensure the desired environmental implications of economic and social development.

Osteoarthritis (OA): A nonsystemic musculoskeletal condition that includes the progressive deterioration of articular cartilage, an overgrowth of periarticular bone (commonly referred to as subchondral sclerosis), and the formation of osteophytes at the margins of the joint.

Osteoporosis: A disease of bone in which the bone mineral density (BMD) is reduced, bone microarchitecture is disrupted, and the amount and variety of proteins in bone is altered, resulting in an increased risk for bone fractures.

Outcomes: What occupational therapy actually achieves for the client. Outcomes are the changes desired by the client and can focus on any area of the client's occupational performance.

Over the counter (OTC): Medications that can be obtained without a prescription.

Ownership of a project: A sense, experienced by individuals and often collectively, of agency and of freedom of choice, and the belief that that person's /group's actions and opinions matter to that project's community.

Person-Environment-Occupation-Performance (PEOP): Model, developed by Baum and Christiansen (2005), that proposes an explanation of participation in occupation; includes cultural values, social and economic systems, the built environment, technology, and social supports. Not specific to aging issues.

Personal care: Refers to assistance with dressing, feeding, washing, and toileting, and the provision of advice, encouragement, and emotional and psychological support, due to changes in abilities to perform these tasks independently.

Personality: The particular combination of emotional, attitudinal, and behavioral response patterns of an individual.

Pharmacogenomics: The study of genetic variations that lead to variable drug response.

Physical frailty: Associated with weakness, slowing, decreased energy, lower activity, and, when severe, unintended weight loss.

Place integration: The fit between a person and his or her environment, such that the person can meet environmental demands and has the resources and opportunities to sustain habitual patterns of thinking and doing.

Polypharmacy: Use of multiple medications; in research, this commonly is defined as use of five or more medications.

Positive aging: Term that suggests older adults who maintain activity will enjoy good health and remain productive.

Postmodern perspectives: Influences research and theory development by acknowledging research subjects' opinions and acceptance of greater diversity.

Practice guideline: Describes a set of directions or principles to assist the health-care practitioner with patient care decisions about appropriate diagnostic, therapeutic, or other clinical procedures for specific clinical circumstances. Practice guidelines may be developed by government agencies at any level, institutions, organizations such as professional societies or governing boards, or expert panels.

Pragmatism: An American movement in philosophy founded by C. S. Peirce and William James and marked by the doctrines that the meaning of conceptions is to be sought in their practical bearings, that the function of thought is to guide action, and that truth is preeminently to be tested by the practical consequences of belief.

Proactivity: Acting in advance to deal with an expected difficulty.

Problem solving: A core feature of the clinical reasoning process of health professionals to solve complex health conditions. Approaches to problem solving can range from broad thinking and action processes to highly structured and manualized approaches.

Productivity: The quality, state, or fact of being able to generate, create, enhance, or bring forth goods and services. Older adults who work for pay, volunteer, provide care, and engage in other social activities are regarded as "productive."

Professional reasoning: The process used by occupational therapists and practitioners to plan, direct, perform, and reflect on client care and the occupational therapy process of evaluation and intervention.

Proton pump inhibitor (PPI): Drug class that inhibits acid production in the stomach; includes esomeprazole, lansoprazole, omeprazole, and rabeprazole; used to treat or prevent heartburn, gastric or duodenal ulcers, reflux disease, and esophagitis.

Psychoneuroimmunology: Explanatory model purporting that emotions can trigger immune system illnesses, such as cardiovascular disease, frailty, and functional decline.

Psychosocial: Term that describes how one's psychological development interacts with the individual's social environment.

Public domain: A in terms of assessment, an assessment tool that does not have applicable intellectual property rights and therefore can be obtained at no cost to the user.

Public policy perspective: Considers governmental policies at all levels that affect the support or lack of support for aging individuals.

Ratio level: Observations or data that have a true zero value.

Resilience: An individual's tendency to cope with stress and adversity. This coping may result in the individual "bouncing back" to a previous state.

Re-evaluation: The process of critical analysis of client response to intervention. This analysis provides the basis for changes to the intervention plan, which are undertaken in collaboration with the client.

Referral: The practice of directing the initial request for service for a client.

Reliability: The extent to which a measurement instrument yields consistent results when repeated multiple times. (See also *validity*.)

Responsiveness: A measure of how well an assessment captures change in a client.

Rheumatoid arthritis (RA): A systemic autoimmune disease process that exhibits both articular and periarticular impairments that include joint pain and stiffness and ultimately interfere with the performance of functional activities.

Screening: Obtaining and reviewing data relevant to a potential client to determine the need for assessment and intervention. Screening is usually a relatively brief procedure in comparison with assessment, which is typically more comprehensive.

Screening Tool of Older Person's Prescriptions (STOPP): Explicit prescribing criteria developed in Europe in 2008.

Screening Tool to Alert doctors to Right Treatments (START): Explicit prescribing criteria developed in Europe in 2008.

Selection: Decision to focus on some aspects of daily life and discard or diminish other goals or activities that become more difficult to achieve.

Selective optimization with compensation: A three-pronged process of achieving one's goals by choosing goals that are generally within one's capabilities, recruiting available resources (personal and environmental), and using additional strategies to compensate for any deficits.

Sensitivity: How likely an assessment is to identify cases, that is, clients with a condition of interest.

Sensorimotor: Of, related to, or combining the functions of sensory and motor activities.

Serum creatinine: Substance derived from muscle tissue and excreted in the urine; used clinically in mathematical equations to estimate renal function.

Skeletal muscles: Are spindle-shaped, consist of a central portion called the muscle belly, and have attaching sites with tendons that connect to bone to produce strength and movements. The origin is the stationary attachment, whereas the insertion is the more movable attachment.

Skilled nursing: Daily care provided or supervised by registered nurses who perform direct care; manage, observe, and evaluate a patient's care; and teach the patient and his or her family members or caregivers.

Sleep apnea: A common disorder in which there is one or more pauses in breathing or shallow breaths while sleeping. Breathing pauses can last from a few seconds to minutes.

Social change: A change that occurs when a community or group of people shift in their understanding and actions toward situations. This is usually interpreted as a positive change for the improvement of the situation or people.

Social functioning: Term that indicates individuals' ability to interact in the normal or usual way in social settings.

Socioeconomic factors: Societal and financial elements and policies that affect individuals living within a culture or society.

Socioemotional selectivity theory: Developed by Laura Carstensen and colleagues, this life-span developmental theory examines the influence of time perception on social goals and behavior. While similar goals operate throughout the life course, the importance of specific goals fluctuates depending on place in the life cycle and perception of time constraints. When time is perceived as open-ended, information- and novelty-seeking goals take priority, prompting expansion of social networks and encounters. When time is perceived as limited, emotional goals take the fore, and people become increasingly selective of social partners, narrowing focus to emotionally meaningful activities and interactions with a smaller circle of significant others.

Specificity: Extent to which a test goes too far and identifies people as having a condition when they really do not.

Spinal stenosis: Osteoarthritis of the intervertebral discs and facet joints along with hypertrophy of the ligamentum flavum, which can begin most commonly between the disc and the vertebral bodies or at the level of the facet joint. It is a cycle of degeneration that can ultimately cause pain due to mechanical compression on the nerve roots and a compromised neural blood supply.

Spirituality: Belief in an immaterial or incorporeal nature; influences an individual's thinking, emotions, and physical well-being.

Structural issues: Refers to societal norms that are supported by law or policy, such as a mandatory retirement age, or age of entitlement to a pension.

Successful aging: Term proposed by Butler and others to categorize older adults who maintain good health, optimum functionality, productivity, resilience, and adaptation to changing circumstances. Recent research has redefined the term.

Suitability for setting: Suitability of the assessment with regard to the client population in a given practice environment.

Sustainability: In a community development context, refers to a situation in which a project has the following characteristics: the involved community has a sense of ownership of the project; the project will continue to achieve its goals despite vulnerabilities to changes in financial support and change in management/staff.

Symbolic capital: The resources available to an individual on the basis of honor, prestige, or recognition within the society.

Systematic review: A summary of the clinical literature; a critical assessment and evaluation of all research studies that address a particular clinical issue. The researchers use an organized method of locating, assembling, and evaluating a body of literature on a particular topic using a set of specific criteria. A systematic review typically includes a description of the findings of the collection of research studies. The systematic review may also include a quantitative pooling of data, called a meta-analysis.

Taoist: A Chinese mystical philosophy traditionally founded by Lao-tzu in the sixth century BCE that teaches conformity to the Tao by unassertive action and simplicity.

Task shifting: A subcomponent of executive function referring to an ability to switch between two or more tasks.

Telehealth: Delivery of clinical and nonclinical preventive, health promotion, and curative health-related services through electronic means. Can range from POTS ("plain old telephone systems") to more involved technology such as videoconferencing and devices to remotely monitor blood pressure, weight, and other vitals.

Telemedicine: Remote delivery of curative health-related clinical services through electronic means; use of telecommunication equipment and information technology to provide clinical care to individuals at distant sites. Can range from electronic transmission of medical records for remote review by practitioners, to devices that allow remote monitoring of chronic health conditions such as diabetes, to use of videoconferencing technologies that provide remote care in regions where access to health services is difficult or limited.

Theoretical proposals: Ideas advanced as an explanation of observed phenomena or to predict what will happen.

Theories of aging: Scholars' ideas of the aging process and the changes it brings.

Theory development: The process of formulating an explanation of how observed factors or events relate to one another.

Theory of goal-achievement strategies: The proposition that older adults use a combination of three strategies to achieve their goals—selection of goals they have the resources to achieve, optimization of their resources, and compensation for deficits.

Therapeutic alliance: Refers to the positive relationship purposely constructed between a health care professional and a client (or patient) to effect beneficial change in the client.

Time-sharing: A subcomponent of executive function referring to an ability to do two things at once

Transactional process of aging in place: Interaction between individuals as role competencies change or diminish due to age.

Unreliable: An assessment tool that gives a different result with repeated administration to the same client is considered unreliable.

Updating: A subcomponent of executive functioning referring to an ability to replace the contents of consciousness with the most recent relevant information.

Usual aging: Normal aging, experienced by the majority of older adults.

Validity: The extent to which an assessment reflects the concept or quantity that it is intended to measure.

Vocational choice: Ability to choose occupations and activities.

Well-being: Feelings of satisfaction with one's life at the present time.

World Health Organization (WHO): Public health section of the United Nations. Monitors disease outbreaks and assesses the performance of health systems around the globe, among other functions.

INDEX

A

Abandonment, 281
ABCX Family Crisis Model, 378, 378f
Abuse
  elder. *See* Elder abuse
  reimbursement, 24
Accountable care organizations (ACOs), 393
ACOs. *See* Accountable care organizations
  (ACOs)
"Active aging," 43, 44, 302. *See also* "Successful
  aging"
  behaviors related to, 44–45
  international uptake of, 46
  personal characteristics related to, 44–45
Activities of daily living (ADL)
  assessments of, 116, 116b
  assistive devices and, 353–354, 358–359
  avocational, 356
  basic or personal, 115–116, 115b, 354
  cars, getting into and out of, 356–357
  cleaning, 355–356
  control of, 360–361
  cooking, 354–355, 355b
  driving, 356–357, 357f
  electronic aids to, 361–363, 361b
  housing and, 353–354, 360–361
  instrumental, 115–116, 115b, 354–356
  Katz Index of, 205
  laundry, 355–356
  meal preparation, 354–355, 355b
  mobility. *See* Mobility
  vocational, 356
Activity strategy training (AST), 108–109
Activity theory, 2, 43–44
Acute rehabilitation hospital, 408
Acute/subacute care, 398, 406
  abbreviations/acronyms used in, 398, 399–400t
  acute rehabilitation hospital, 408
  aftercare options, 406, 407t
  deconditioning, 406
  definition(s) of, 398
  evaluation form, 404f
  evaluation process, 403–405
  fall-prevention team, 437
  hip fractures, 402b
  home health care, 408
  hospital departments, 401t
  hospital sequelae, 406
  intensive care units, 401f
  interdisciplinary teams for, 405–406, 437
  long-term acute care hospital, 406–408, 407b
  role of therapy in, 402–403
  skilled nursing facilities, 408
  SOAP evaluation, 403–405, 405b
  stroke, 401–402b
  telemetry equipment, 401f
  trajectory of, 400–402
ADAMS. *See* Aging, Demographics, and Memory
  Study (ADAMS)
Adaptations. *See* Environmental modifications
  and adaptations
ADL. *See* Activities of daily living (ADL)

Administration on Aging health promotion and
  wellness programs, 309
Adrenal glands, 135
Aged workforce, 480
  vocational activities, 356
AgeLine, 57–58
  search strategies, 59–60
Agency for Healthcare Research and Quality
  (AHRQ), 58–59
Aging, Demographics, and Memory Study
  (ADAMS), 34
Agoraphobia, 273
AHRQ. *See* Agency for Healthcare Research and
  Quality (AHRQ)
Alternative communication, 360
Alzheimer's disease, 34
  end-stage, 252
  informed consent in, 17
  mild, 250
  moderate, 250–251, 251b
  pre-dementia stage of, 249–250
  probable, 248–249
  severe, 251, 251b
  stages of, 249–252
  in the U.S., 34t
  vision and, 337
Ambient intelligence, 477
American Stroke Foundation (ASF), 241b, 242f
Amsler grid, 153, 153f
Andersen's Behavioral Model of Health Services
  Utilization,
  387–388, 388f
Anemia from iron-deficiency, 171
Anticholinergic drugs, 224–225, 225t
Antisocial personality disorder, 278–280t
Anxiety disorders, 270–274. *See also specific disorder(s)*
  diagnosis of, 271–272t
  medications for, 273–274
  performance deficits in, 274
  psychological treatment of, 274
AoA health promotion and wellness programs, 309
Arthritis, 34, 335–336
  interventions for, 136–137
  joint protection education, 110–111, 137f.
    See also Joint protection education
  osteoarthritis. *See* Osteoarthritis
  rheumatoid. *See* Rheumatoid arthritis
  subacute disease, 110
Arthritis Self-Management Program (ASMP), 137
ASF. *See* American Stroke Foundation (ASF)
ASMP. *See* Arthritis Self-Management Program
  (ASMP)
Aspiration pneumonia, 202–203
Aspirin, 223–224
Assessment, 74–85
  activities of daily living, 116, 116b
  cognitive impairment, 261–262, 262b
  CQI. *See* Continuous quality improvement (CQI)
  driver fitness/performance, 337–342
  executive function, 237
  feeding disorders, 176
  interdisciplinary teams, 436–437

Assessment *(Continued)*
  levels of data, 75
  low vision, 150–155
  measurement and, 75
  oral health, 204–206, 205t, 206t
  reading speed, 154
  scotoma, 153–154
  tools. *See* Assessment tools
Assessment tools
  applying, 81, 81–83b
  client considerations, 79–80
  evaluation of, 75–77
  in the public domain, 78–79
  reliability of, 76
  responsiveness of, 77
  selection of, 77, 78–79, 78b
  sensitivity of, 76–77
  specificity of, 76–77
  validity of, 76
Assistive devices/technology, 350–372
  Abeldata listing of, 351t
  activities of daily living and, 353–354, 358–359
  for cognitive impairments, 477
  communication, 357–358, 360
  computer technology, 363, 364f. *See* Computers
  cost of, 354
  definitions, 352
  environmental, 361–363, 361b
  for food preparation, 178–184, 179f
  future trends, 477
  high-tech devices, 358–367
  home automation, 361–363, 361b
  issues concerning, 352–353
  low-tech devices, 353–358, 355b, 358b
  for low vision, 156, 158b
  mobile devices, 360, 367–368
  mobility, 356–357, 359–360
  for oral health, 206, 206f, 207, 208b, 208f
  for osteoarthritis, 108, 109f, 207, 207f
  paying for, 354
  telehealth, 361
  telemedicine, 361
  wearable health technology, 477, 478f
  Websites, 359b
Assistive technologies, 77
AST. *See* Activity strategy training (AST)
Atherosclerosis, 127f
Augmentative communication, 357–358, 358b
Automobiles
  driving, 356–357. *See also* Driver fitness/
    performance
  getting into and out of, 356–357
Autonomy, 14
  informed consent and, 19
Avocational activities, 356
Avoidant personality disorder, 278–280t

B

"Baby boom" generation, 32
Back pain, 106
  interventions for, 113–114
  lower, 106